RATIONAL

HYDROTHERAPY

RATIONAL

HYDROTHERAPY

A MANUAL OF

The physiological and Therapeutic Effects of Hydriatic Procedures, and the Technique of Their Application in the Treatment of Disease

BY J. H. KELLOGG, M.D.

GYAN

Published by

Gyan Publishing House
5, Ansari Road
Daryaganj, New Delhi-110002
Phone: 011-47034999, 9811692060
E-mail: books@gyanbooks.com

Distribution Network
gyanbooks.com
India, USA, Canada, UK, Australia

ISBN: 978-93-6208-083-7 (PB)
First Published, 1918

2nd Impression 2024

Printed at: Gyan Press, Delhi.

RATIONAL HYDROTHERAPY
Author: J. H. KELLOGG

RATIONAL

HYDROTHERAPY

A MANUAL OF

The Physiological and Therapeutic Effects of Hydriatic Procedures, and the Technique of Their Application in the Treatment of Disease

---

By J. H. KELLOGG, M. D.

Member of the British Gynecological Society; the International Periodica Congress of Gynecology and Obstetrics; the British and American Associations for the Advancement of Science; the Société d' Hygiène of France; the American Society of Microscopists; the American Medical Association; Superintendent of the Battle Creek (Mich.) Sanitarium; Author of the "Art of Massage;" etc., etc.

WITH TWO HUNDRED NINETY-THREE ILLUSTRATIONS EIGHTEEN IN COLORS

PHILADELPHIA
THE F. A. DAVIS COMPANY, PUBLISHERS
1901

TO HIS FRIEND,

Dr. Wilhelm W. Winternitz,

Professor of nervous diseases in the Royal and Imperial University of Vienna, and founder of the first hydriatic clinic,

the author respectfully dedicates this volume.

PREFACE.

WHEN the famous Sydenham wrote his treatise on fevers, he apologized for departing so far from the current practice of his day as to recommend the employment of hydriatic measures as being preferable to bleeding in the treatment of febrile disorders. This innovation was made with much fear and trembling on the part of the famous old physician, who expressed his expectation that his advocacy of water as a febrifuge would render him so unpopular with the members of his profession as to destroy his practice and reputation.

Thanks to the progress made in the development of rational medicine within the last century, and especially within the last twenty-five years, it is no longer necessary to offer an apology to scientific medical men for the recommendation of a remedy which, though the simplest of all elements, has come to be recognized as one of the most powerful means of influencing the varied functions of the animal body, having, by careful clinical observation and patient laboratory research, been thoroughly rescued from the limbo of blind empiricism and placed upon a scientific and rational basis.

For years excellent scientific treatises on hydrotherapy have existed in the French and German languages, but for nearly half a century not a single systematic English work on the hydriatic treatment of disease has appeared with the exception of the translation of the article by Winternitz in Ziemssen's "System of Therapeutics" and a recent excellent work by Baruch.

The author's purpose in the preparation of this work has been to present, in a more systematic and comprehensive way than has heretofore been undertaken, the "rational" hydrotherapy which has been built up within the last century chiefly through the efforts of Currie, Fleury, and Winternitz, whose great labors have been supplemented by others too numerous for other mention than that made in the various footnotes and references which will be found in the body of this work. It has also been a part of the author's purpose to record some of the fruits of his own experience within the last twenty-five years, during which time, as superintendent of a large medical establishment, he has had opportunity to make a careful study of hydriatic principles and methods.

The general order of the book is as follows: First, a short historical sketch and a brief résumé of the physical, anatomical, and physiological facts which are especially related to the subject; second, a study of the physiological effects of thermic applications; third, a description of the technique of all useful hydriatic procedures; and, fourth, a section on hydriatic prescription making, in which is presented a brief summary of the indications presented by the diseases most commonly encountered in practice and of the hydric measures required to meet the same. The author hopes to publish later another volume in which the rational hydriatic treatment of individual diseases will be more fully discussed.

The number of procedures described in the work is about two hundred. Many more might have been mentioned, but the writer's design has been to describe only typical hydriatic processes, each possessed of a definite and characteristic therapeutic value. Of those procedures which are the outgrowth of his own experience, the author has mentioned only such as have acquired a recognized value by extended use. Of these, the most worthy of mention are the electric-light bath, the percussion douche, cold mitten friction, cold towel rub, a number of forms of hot and cold compresses and packs, and the simultaneous hot and cold douche.

If the number of procedures presented seems large, it should be remembered that they comprise three complete sets of hydriatic applications, viz.: the bath (full bath, shallow bath, sitz, foot, and other baths), the douche (jet, spray, fan, and other forms of douche in general and local application), and the wet cloth (wet sheet pack, rubbing wet sheet, wet girdle, and various other local and general applications of moistened cloths), besides a variety of procedures which a strict classification would place under the head of thermotherapy, phototherapy, and massotherapy.

Some eighteen years ago (1883) the author equipped a laboratory and began the systematic study of the physiological effects of water. Many hundreds of experimental observations have been made by the aid of the calorimeter, the plethysmograph, the ergograph, and various other instruments adapted to the purpose. The results of some of these observations are reported in this work for the purpose of presenting to the reader tangible evidence of the rational basis of this important branch of therapeutics. An earnest effort has been made to present in this work a comprehensive view of scientific hydrotherapy in its varied physiological and therapeutic aspects.

The writer has used for the foundation of this work a series of lectures which he delivered before a class of medical students in the summer of 1890. Similar courses have been given almost yearly since, to classes of increasing number, and there has been a growing demand for a text-book embodying the essentials of the subject-matter presented, and adapted for use by the medical students and nurses, as well as practitioners who desire to obtain a knowledge of the foundation facts and principles of rational hydrotherapy. The first section of the manuscript was prepared for the press in 1897, but urgent professional duties prevented the completion of the work until an opportunity was afforded by a vacation trip to Mexico in the winter of 1899-1900.

Modern scientific research has placed upon a sure foundation the great truth—dimly recognized by the earliest physicians, but wholly lost sight of during the Dark Ages—that healing power is not possessed by physicians nor by remedies, but that the curative process is simply a manifestation of the forces which dwell within the body and which are normally manifested in creating and maintaining the organism: in other words, that the body heals itself. Water, applied externally or internally, and at such temperatures as may be required, is an agent which more fully than almost any other co-operates with the healing powers of the body in resisting the onset and development of pathogenic processes. There is no other remedy by which the movements of the blood and the blood supply, both general and local, and in fact every form of vital activity, may be so readily controlled as by hydriatic applications.

While water is recognized as without doubt one of the most valuable of all natural agencies, the writer has never permitted himself to be classed with those enthusiasts who place their trust in it as an exclusive measure. It is best employed in connection with the use of electricity, massage, and medical gymnastics. Rational diet is as essential in the treatment of the majority of cases of acute and chronic disease as is water. In the treatment of chronic disorders the regulation of exercise, dress, and of other habits of life is also a matter of paramount importance; also the disuse of tea, coffee, tobacco, and alcoholic beverages, which are often found to sustain a very direct causative relation to the patient's maladies and are without doubt responsible for many failures in which the fault has been unjustly charged to the inefficiency of water as a therapeutic agent.

In the preparation of the physiological part of this work the writer has found of special service the splendid work of Landois and Sterling, the excellent "*Traité de Physiologie,*" by Morat and Doyon, and the "*Traité de Physiologie Comparée des Animaux,*" by Colin. In addition, the works of Winternitz, Bell, Currie, Fleury, Beni-Barde, Bottey, and numerous other French and German authors, besides a great mass of periodical literature, and many hundreds of monographs which have been accumulated during the last thirty years have been studied and consulted.

A most earnest effort has been made to exclude from this work every procedure and every method for which a thoroughly scientific and physiological foundation could not be presented. The author dares not, however, entertain the hope that his work will be found altogether faultless, and solicits the candid criticism of those who may do him the honor to peruse these pages, trusting that he may have the privilege of correcting in future editions such errors as may have escaped attention in this, and to record such new facts as future experience and research may develop.

In conclusion, I must not omit to express my obligations and gratitude to my colleagues of the faculty of the Battle Creek Sanitarium, and of the American Medical Missionary College, particularly Drs. David Paulson, Chas. E. Stewart, George Thomason, and Elmer Otis, for invaluable assistance in abstracting the stenographic notes of my lectures to medical classes, and for supervising and personally conducting experimental work, and to Dr. Eshelman for assistance in preparing an exhaustive index. I have also profited by the experience of my friends and colleagues for many years, Drs. Lindsay, Riley, Kress, Rand, and others, and owe much to the patient and painstaking work of a large number of my students in the experimental laboratory. I am also under obligations to my friend, Alois Strasser, M.D., assistant Professor in the Medical Department of the Royal and Imperial University of Vienna, for painstaking revision of the proof sheets and for numerous valuable suggestions. Most of all I am indebted to my friend of many years, Dr. W. W. Winternitz, Professor of Nervous Diseases in the Medical Department of the Royal and Imperial University of Vienna, to whose laborious investigations and acute observations the world is indebted more than to any other living man for the scientific data upon which modern rational hydrotherapy is based, and to whom I am proud to have permission to dedicate this volume.

J. H. KELLOGG.

BATTLE CREEK, AUGUST 1, 1901.

PREFACE TO THE SECOND EDITION.

THE author is glad to improve the opportunity afforded by the publication of a new edition of this work to correct a number of minor errors and to make a number of brief, but important, additions to the text in nearly every section of the work. He also desires to thank the profession of the United States and other English-speaking countries for the kind welcome which they have accorded the work, the cordiality of which has far exceeded his most sanguine hopes.

The interest in therapeutic agents of a non-medicinal character, including heat, light, electricity, exercise, massage, and other physical means, as well as water, is rapidly gaining ground; and, if one may judge by the frequency with which articles and treatises on these subjects are now appearing from the medical press, it may be said that an era of physiological medicine has begun. If this be true, the beginning of the twentieth century will mark the most important epoch in the history of medicine; not that drugs and allied agents must be altogether discarded, but rather that those physiological and physical measures, which during so many ages have been neglected and even despised, shall be given their proper place in practical therapeutics. Having once gained a footing, these powerful agencies, directed by modern positive and precise methods of diagnosis, will easily hold in the future the chief place in the battle against disease.

In conclusion, the author desires to thank numerous friends and reviewers for criticisms and suggestions, many of which he has put to good use in preparing this new edition for the press.

J. H. K.

JUNE 1, 1902.

CONTENTS.

PART ONE.

PART TWO.

PART THREE.

PART FOUR.

LIST OF ILLUSTRATIONS.

* This instrument is in use in the leading gymnasiums of the United States and in the Military School at West Point, and affords the only accurate means of estimating the strength of all the principal groups of muscles of the body.

RATIONAL HYDROTHERAPY.

Part One.

HISTORICAL.

WATER is without doubt the most ancient of all remedial agents for disease. This fact is evidenced by the frequent reference to its use in the earliest medical literature, as well as by the habits and customs of the most ancient peoples as brought to light more fully within recent years by the study of the old Assyrian and Egyptian records. The reason for this is clearly to be found in the fact that water is a means not only usually found ready at hand, but one which adapts itself to almost every imaginable pathological condition in a remarkable manner, thus approaching more nearly to a panacea than any other known remedy. No other agent is capable of producing so great a variety of physiological effects, no other is so universally present, and hence none is so readily adaptable for meeting the various exigencies and indications arising from accident and disease.

Hydrotherapy among the Egyptians, Chinese, and Other Ancient Nations.

The ancient Egyptians, Hebrews, Greeks, Persians, and Hindus all employed water in the treatment of disease, as do the representatives of these peoples at the present time.

According to a Chinese record dating back several centuries before Christ, a physician prescribed for a woman of that country one hundred affusions of ice-water, each followed by wrapping in a linen sheet,— a treatment in principle resembling the wet-sheet pack.

The *Tokio Medical Journal* (1881) states that the cold bath has been in use in Japan for nearly eight hundred years, especially among the native country physicians, and that nearly three hundred years ago a small treatise on the medical uses of the cold bath was published by Dr. Nakagami, in which it was especially recommended for acute mania, hysteria, asthma, and convulsions in children.

Among the Spartans of ancient Greece cold bathing was made obligatory by law. The bath in various forms is also frequently referred to in Grecian mythology.

Hippocrates on the Use of Water.

Hippocrates evidently had an excellent understanding of the physiological properties of water, both hot and cold, which he employed in the treatment of fevers, ulcers, hemorrhages, and a variety of maladies both medical and surgical, giving many directions for its use which the experience of two thousand years has not improved upon. For instance, he directed that cold baths should be of short duration, and should be preceded and followed by friction; and he evidently understood the phenomena of reaction, since he records the observation that after a cold bath the body quickly recuperates its heat and remains warm, while a hot bath produces the opposite effect.

Under the Romans the bath attained a very high degree of development. Emperors vied with one another in erecting magnificent public baths, capable of accommodating thousands of persons daily. In studying the interesting ruins of some of these structures at Rome and Pompeii, the author was astonished to find the perfection attained in every detail of the equipment of these ancient bathing establishments. Hot or cold water baths, hot-air and vapor baths, might be enjoyed at will.

Asclepiades employed water in nearly every form,—hot and cold baths, douches, compresses, etc. One of his disciples, Antonius Musa, attained great fame by curing the Emperor Augustus of a chronic catarrh by means of the cold bath, as a reward for which his statue was ordered to be erected in the temple of Esculapius ; but a lack of discrimination in the use of this powerful agent led to his downfall. Being called upon to treat the emperor's nephew, Marcellus, a popular favorite, he adopted the measures which had resulted so admirably in the cure of the athletic old soldier, but they proved too powerful for the effeminate youth, and he was prostrated to such a degree that he died soon after at Naples, where he had gone to receive treatment at the hot baths of Baiæ. This enthusiastic apostle of hydrotherapy succeeded later in redeeming his reputation by the cure of the poet Horace.

Pastor Kneipp, the Bavarian water-cure empiric, a few years ago had a similar experience. Being called upon to visit the pope, who was suffering from chronic rheumatism, he was received with great honors ; but the first cold bath given the aged prelate, entirely unaccustomed to such heroic treatment, occasioned such an exacerbation of his sufferings that the poor priest was peremptorily dismissed in disgrace. Had the patient been a sturdy young German peasant instead of a feeble Italian gentleman, the prescription might have succeeded better. A similar lack of discrimination, whether by a charlatan or a legally qualified practitioner, is always attended by disastrous results. The untoward effects thus produced should not, however, be attributed to scientific hydrotherapy, but must be charged to the stupid audacity of quackery, or to the lack of information or experience of the otherwise competent physician.

The Medical Use of the Bath by the Romans and Arabs.

According to Pliny, the bath was almost the exclusive method of treatment employed in Rome during five centuries. Celsus and other prominent Roman physicians highly extolled the bath in their works, Celsus later making it one of the three essentials of what he called a perfect therapeutic system, termed "apotheraphia," the other two being exercise and friction.

During the middle ages the Arabic physicians, the most learned men of their time, were enthusiastic advocates of the bath, especially in fevers, and their directions for the treatment of smallpox and measles could scarcely be improved upon at the present time. Rhazes recommended drinking ice-water to the extent of two or three pints within half an hour, as a means of reducing the temperature in fevers. Avicenna recommended cold water for the relief of constipation.

M. Barra, of Lyons, published in 1675 an interesting little volume entitled, "L'Usage de la Glace, de la Neige, et du Froid" (The Use of Ice, of Snow, and of Cold). In this work the author anticipated many of the therapeutic uses of cold which have, by scientific experiments within the last half century, been placed upon a sound therapeutic basis. He calls attention to the fact that the Hebrews made use of melted snow for drink, and cooled water by exposing it to the action of the wind, afterward keeping it in vessels covered with straw. He pronounced cold water to be the best of all remedies for continuous fever, and especially recommended it for "erysipelas, pestilential fevers, contagious boils, frost bite, dysentery, pleurisy, the plague, inflammation of the throat, and tightness of the stomach."

Lanzani, an Italian physician, wrote an elaborate thesis on the internal use of water for the treatment of fevers, in the early part of the last century. Fra Bernardino, about the same time, acquired the name of "the cold-water doctor" by the use of iced water in the treatment of indigestion, nervous disorders, hemorrhages, etc. He required his patients to drink from three to six glasses of ice-water daily. He avoided sweating, and aimed to stimulate the bowels and kidneys.

The Popular Use of Water 150 Years Ago.

We quote below a few interesting extracts from a small work entitled, "Primitive Physick," by John Wesley, M. A., the founder of the Methodist Church, published in 1747, which afford ample evidence of the existence at that period among the common people of a very considerable amount of knowledge respecting the use of water in a variety of ailments, as well as for the preservation of health, since the remedies recommended in Wesley's work were all such as he found in successful use among the people.

For ague or intermittent fever, "go into the cold bath just before the cold fit" (this method is still in use in Germany and France); or, "drink a quart of cold water just before the cold fit, and then go to bed and sweat."

For a tertian ague, it is recommended to "use light and sparing diet on the day between," "or use the cold bath (unless you are of advanced age or extremely weak [a wise precaution, showing no little experience]). But when you use this, on any account whatever, it is proper to go in cool; to immerge at once, but not head foremost; to stay in only two or three minutes (or less at first); never to bathe on a full stomach; to bathe twice or thrice a week at least, until you have bathed nine or ten times; to sweat immediately after it (going to bed), in palsies, rickets, etc."

"Before the cold fit begins, go to bed, and continue a large sweat by [drinking] lemonade for six or eight hours. This usually cures in three or four times. If it does not, use the cold bath between the fits." The writer found this method in use among the laity of the western part of the United States more than a quarter of a century ago, and with success in cases in which quinine and other antiperiodics had failed to effect a cure.

For apoplexy, "to prevent, use the cold bath, and drink only water."

For asthma, "take a pint of cold water every morning, washing the head therein immediately after, and using the cold bath once a fortnight." "For present relief, vomit with a quart or more of warm water. The more you drink of it the better."

For dry or convulsive asthma, "use the cold bath thrice a week."

"*To prevent swelling from a bruise*, immediately apply a cloth five or six times doubled, dipped in cold water, and new dip when it grows warm."

"*To cure a swelling from a bruise*, foment it half an hour, morning and evening, with cloths dipped in water as hot as you can bear."

For a burn or a scald, "immediately plunge the part into cold water. Keep it in an hour; or if not well before, perhaps four or five hours."

"*To prevent the rickets, tenderness, and weakness* [in children], dip them in cold water every morning, at least until they are eight or nine months old."

For whooping-cough, "use the cold bath daily."

For cholera morbus, "drink two to three quarts of cold water, if strong, or of warm water, if weak."

For a cold, "drink a pint of cold water lying down in bed."

For colic, "drink a pint of cold water, or a quart of warm water, or [apply] hot water in a bladder, or steep the legs in hot water, a quarter of an hour."

For hysteric colic, "use the cold bath. Using the cold bath two and twenty times a month has entirely cured hysteric colic fits and convulsive motions."

For chronic headache, "keep your feet in warm water a quarter of an hour before you go to bed, for two or three weeks."

For headache from heat, "apply to the forehead cloths dipped in cold water, for an hour."

For one seemingly killed by lightning or suffocation, "plunge him immediately into cold water."

For mania, "apply to the head, cloths dipped in cold water, or pour cold water on the head out of a teakettle, or let the patient eat nothing but apples for a month."

For rheumatism, "use the cold bath, with rubbing and sweating."

For rickets, "wash the child every morning in cold water."

For sciatica, "use cold bathing and sweat, together with flesh-brush twice a day; or drink half a pint of cold water daily in the morning and at four in the afternoon."

For stone, to prevent its occurrence, "drink a pint of warm water daily just before dinner."

For swelling of the joints, "pour on the part daily a stream of warm water, or a stream of cold water one day and warm water the next."

"It is also useful to use the hot bath a few days before you use the cold."

Wesley recommended cool bathing for the cure of nearly all the affections of childhood, all chronic diseases, and many surgical cases.

Although Wesley was not a physician, but simply described in his work such successful remedies as he found in common use, one can not but note the sagacity and wisdom displayed in many of these recommendations, which in many instances could scarcely be improved upon at the present day, and certainly evince extended and accurate observation of the effects of hydriatic applications.

Cullen's Use of Water in Fevers.

Cullen made some very practical observations respecting the therapeutic uses of water. In his treatise on fever he commended water as a sedative when used in such a manner as to "moderate the violence of reaction," and as a tonic when used for "supporting and increasing the action of the heart and arteries." The action of cold he described as follows:—

1. Diminished temperature and pallor of the skin.

2. Weakened action of the heart and arteries, observing that in cold countries the pulse is uniformly slow.

3. Weakness and inactivity, effects observable in the inhabitants of cold countries.

4. Prolonged and very cold applications "are capable of entirely extinguishing the vital powers," cold combined with moisture chilling the body much faster than dry cold.

5. Cold applications prepare the body for applications of heat, "producing accumulation of sensibility to the stimulus of heat."

Cullen used water according to Dr. Darwin's rule — "to warm the patient in the cold fit, and to cool him in the hot one."

Hydrotherapy in Europe.

It is very interesting to observe how few of our modern methods of employing water are really new. The moist compress was well known to the ancient Greeks under the name of "epithem." According to Sir John Floyer, who wrote in the latter part of the seventeenth century, the wet-sheet pack was employed in his time by sportsmen who wished to diminish the weight of their jockies. The method is thus described: —

"Dip the rider's shirt in cold water; and after it is put on very wet, lay the person in warm blankets to sweat him violently, and he will after lose a considerable weight, a pound or two."

The same method was used in the treatment of various maladies, particularly rickets in children. The child, being prepared for bed with a gown and nightcap, was quickly immersed in cold water, then put to bed closely wrapped in warm blankets, and left in this condition all night, sweating profusely, a portion of the clothing being removed toward morning so that the body might be gradually cooled. That it was the custom to employ this method with great perseverance is evidenced by the following suggestion made by the learned author: "If one year's dipping proves not successful, it is repeated the next year, which generally answers expectation."

Floyer also mentions that in Staffordshire and other parts of England it was a custom with the people "to go into the water in their shirts, and when they come out, they dress themselves in their wet linen, which they wear all day, and much commend that for closing the pores and keeping themselves cool; and that they do not commonly receive any injury or catch any cold thereby, I am fully convinced from the experiments I have seen made of it."

The leading features of the so-called "Kneippism" are

simply a revival of these rude practices of ignorant English peasants a century and a half ago.

Sir John Sinclair, in his "Code of Health and Longevity," gives an account of an English nobleman, born in the year 1700, who for a great part of his life was accustomed, immediately on arising in the morning, to wrap himself in a sheet just dipped in cold water — a wet-sheet pack.

In the fifteenth century, Savonarola, an Italian physician, made a systematic use of the cold bath, and Barizzi employed the cold vaginal douche in uterine affections. Cold affusions and general douches were employed by Baccio in Italy, while leading Spanish and German physicians recommended cold applications for insomnia.

Septala, in the seventeenth century, employed the cold douche for the relief of headache and sunstroke.

Herman, a Belgic physician, resorted to the use of cold water at the same period for the relief of constipation, migraine, paralysis, and mania, — maladies in the treatment of which cold water still holds its own against all other single remedies.

Hydrotherapy in England.

Sir John Floyer, in 1697, published a history of cold bathing, in which he directed that the patient should be made to sweat before taking the cold bath, by wrapping him in a wet sheet with blankets, precisely the same method employed more than a century later by Priessnitz, and now known as the wet-sheet pack. Floyer also erected a water-cure establishment at Litchfield, England, in the latter part of the seventeenth century. Two rooms were provided, one of which was used for hot baths and dry packs to produce sweating, while cold baths were administered in the adjoining room.

John Hancock published a work entitled "Febrifugum Magnum," in 1723, in which he demonstrated the value of water-drinking as a means of treatment in scarlet fever, smallpox, and measles. He cured ague by having the patient drink large quantities of cold water while wrapped in blankets, thus inducing profuse sweating.

Sir John Chardin, a celebrated English traveler of the last century, had bilious remittent fever when in Persia. His companion, a French surgeon, thinking his case hopeless, a native physician was called in, who made the patient fast five days, and drink large quantities of water previously cooled with snow, causing him to lie meanwhile upon a mat wet with water, and keeping the skin constantly wet with water. Water was also poured at intervals over the patient while two men supported him. In two days the fever disappeared.

This Persian physician evidently had a knowledge of the value of water-drinking, of the evaporating bath, and of affusion as a means of combating fever,—invaluable measures, of which Western physicians are scarcely yet making any considerable practical use.

The native physicians of Mohammedan countries still generally follow Galen, and so make use of water in many maladies in a very effective and practical way.

The Work of Currie and Jackson.

Two English physicians, Currie and Jackson, in the latter part of the last century, made a most intelligent and scientific study of the use of water in fevers, and with results which for a time commanded much attention from the profession in England. Currie discovered many important principles relating to hydrotherapy, some of which have not always been kept in mind by his successors in the use of water. For example, he says that the indications for the use of water in fevers, especially intermittent, are as follows:—

1. To diminish cold in cold stages.
2. To diminish heat in heat stages.
3. To diminish spasm of blood-vessels.
4. To support the powers of life till the diseased associations die away from the ceasing of their causes.
5. To unload the bowels.

He also advised cold water drinking in large quantities, immersion instead of effusion in warm countries, where the water is seldom at a lower temperature than 70° F., and suggested that after immersion the patient should be exposed to the air, so that the body might be cooled by evaporation. He recommended as a principle of the utmost importance for regulating the use of water, that it might be safely used "when there is no sense of chilliness present, when the heat of the surface is steadily above what is natural, and when there is no general or profuse perspiration." He observed that a cold pour could be used more safely than cold sponging, for the reason that it is "an energetic remedy," and "the system often accommodates itself to a cold which is general and stimulating, but shrinks from a cold which is slow and successive."

He also warned against fatigue occasioned by too much bathing, and recommended that after the bath the patient should be dried "hastily with towels," and recommended that when too severe effects had been obtained, causing too great depression, the extremities should be rubbed, and "a bladder of hot water applied to the stomach."

Currie also noted the evil effects of reaction in fever, and taught that short cold applications should not be made in cases of high fever, on account of their tendency to increase the fever. He also taught that great mischief might result from the use of hot applications immediately after cold in such cases. He made use of the "wet blanket," or pack, in fevers, and observed that it relieved delirium. He also applied cold to the feet in hemorrhage of the lungs, and in a case of pulmonary hemorrhage suddenly plunged the patient up to the hips in cold water, a method previously successfully used by Dr. Darwin for relief of hemorrhage from the kidneys.

Even before the time of Currie, Crawford, in 1781, had recognized as one of the physiological effects of cold, its influence upon oxidation, observing that cold "increases the difference in color between arterial and venous blood, while heat lessens this difference in color."

For some reason not easily understood, the work of Currie and Jackson, the ablest of the early pioneers of a truly scientific method of inestimable value in febrile disorders, was lost sight of, and it was not until the attention of the whole civilized world was attracted by the fame of an uneducated and blundering, but still successful, cold-water empiric, that the profession began to give this agent the serious attention that was its due; for the modern popularity of water as a remedy must without doubt be largely credited to the enterprise and ingenuity of a Silesian peasant, Vincent Priessnitz, born in the little village of Græfenburg, in Austrian Silesia, in 1790.

Hydrotherapy in America.

At a very early period, Dr. Benjamin Rush, of Philadelphia, used cold water with success in the treatment of rheumatism, gout, small-pox, measles, and many other maladies, including yellow fever. Currie declares that he found cold water "a most agreeable and powerful remedy . . . applied by means of napkins to the head, and to be injected into the bowels by means of the clyster, also washing the face and hands, and sometimes the feet, with cold water." In 1794 Rush introduced the use of broken ice in a bladder applied to the head in fevers, and claimed great advantage from the employment of this remedy.

Drs. Bard and Hosack, of the New York Hospital, began the use of cold water in fevers about the year 1795, three or four years before Currie's book on the medical uses of water appeared in America.

In 1799, Peter Edes, of Augusta, Me., published an interesting little work on the use of water, summarizing Currie's volume, and adding observations of his own.

Another American writer ingeniously suggested, in 1808, the employment of moistened clay as a cooling application for inflamed and congested parts. He used cold in the early stages of fever, but forbade its use in the latter stages.

Among the earliest scientific observations respecting the effects of the bath as regards both the physiological and the therapeutic effects of water, must be noted the careful experiments conducted by Henry Wilson Lockette, of Virginia. These experiments were published by him in the year 1801 in "An Inaugural Dissertation on the Warm Bath, presented to the Trustees of the Medical Faculty of the University of Pennsylvania for the Degree of Doctor of Medicine." In this treatise, a copy of which the author is so fortunate as to have in his library, Dr. Lockette details with great perspicacity the effects upon the pulse and general functions, of baths of different duration at varying temperatures. Among the observations that he made, were the following:—

1. That a foot bath at 110° F. increased the pulse from 76 to 92 beats a minute, the redness of the legs and the enlargement of the veins of the feet and legs and the slight but temporary pain in the head showing clearly the exciting effect of this treatment.

2. That a full bath at 107° F. raised the pulse from 72 to 114 beats, producing congestion of the veins, drowsiness, and profuse perspiration. The excitation continued for more than a quarter of an hour after the bath.

3. That a bath at 96° F. diminished the pulse from 79 to 64 beats in ten minutes, whereas an elevation of temperature to 100° raised the pulse to 80 beats, and a greater increase of temperature (to 105°) increased the pulse in fifteen minutes more to 92 beats. "The patient sweat freely and yawned after dressing, and was much debilitated, complaining of weakness in the legs,"— a very good description of the depressing effects of the hot bath.

4. That a bath at 90° F. lowered the pulse, in five minutes, from 80 to 64 beats. An elevation of temperature to 100° raised the pulse in ten minutes to 73 beats; and raising the temperature to 105° in twenty minutes more raised the pulse to 118 beats, with difficulty of breathing and profuse perspiration.

He noticed, among other effects, that a bath in which the temperature was gradually raised to 110° raised the pulse from 83 to 153 beats, producing intolerable pain in the head, partial delirium, confusion of thought, inability to speak, dimness of sight, vesical tenesmus, and "sensations which are commonly present in a violent state of fever." On leaving the bath, the experimenter nearly fainted, and sweat profusely for some time.

A bath at 95° F. for an hour lowered the pulse from 78 to 75 beats. Fifteen minutes after the bath the pulse-rate was 68. The experimenter says, "I experienced a considerable degree of lassitude, with an inclination to sleep,"—an excellent description of the effects of the neutral bath.

A bath at 92° lowered the pulse, in five minutes, from 84 to 77 beats. At the end of thirty minutes the pulse-rate was 76.

As the result of his investigations, Dr. Lockette concluded:—

1. That a temperature below 98° F. does not increase the frequency of the pulse, and may slightly lower it, and does not produce sweating.

2. That a temperature of 98° to 105° F. "accelerates the pulse and induces free perspiration, but produces no distressing symptoms."

3. That a temperature of 105° F. "is a powerful stimulant, and should never be advised or practiced in inflammatory diseases or states of fever or violently morbid action."

Dr. Lockette made similar experiments with the steam bath, which led him to conclude it to be a more convenient method of securing perspiration than the water bath. His brochure is concluded by a chapter relating to the medical uses of the warm bath, and among the most interesting observations upon the medical uses of water are found recommendations respecting its use for the relief of sick or nervous headache, which he remarks had previously been "very little attended to by physicians." He recommends the warm foot bath, fomentations to the head, and the daily cold bath, which measures, he affirms, on the authority of Dr. Dwight, have effected a cure in many cases.

During the middle decades of the present century hydropathy flourished to a considerable extent in America, and half a century ago we were much nearer the front in this line of progress than at the present time. Many institutions devoted to the carrying out of these measures were established in different parts of the United States, and scientific hydrotherapy was ably advocated by Dr. John Bell, of Philadelphia, whose work on "Baths" has, up to the present time, remained the most complete and able treatise on the subject in the English language, though it has long been out of print, and seems to be quite unknown to the profession of to-day.

The Hydropathy of Priessnitz.

When seventeen years of age, Priessnitz met with an accident whereby he received numerous bruises and other injuries, including the fracture of two of his ribs. Local physicians gave him no hope of recovery; but having been accustomed to use water in the treatment of the domestic animals for which he cared, it occurred to him to try the same remedy for himself. He covered the affected parts with cloths kept wet with cold water, and also drank freely of water, with the result that he was in a short time completely cured. This incident made so profound an impression upon the mind of Priessnitz that, although an unlearned peasant, he determined to make a thorough investigation of the merits of water as a remedial agent, used both internally and externally. He seems even to have undertaken some experiments on animals, one of which was for the purpose of determining the relative effects of hot and cold foods. Two pigs were fed, one upon cold, the other upon hot, foods; and when the animals were killed, he made a careful examination of the intestines, and asserted that in the case of the animal fed upon cold foods the intestines were well contracted, pale, and of firm resisting structure, while in the case of the animal fed upon hot food, the intestines were red, relaxed, and so easily torn that they could not be used for making sausages.

The basis of the system of Priessnitz was perspiration, followed by cold applications. His methods were exceedingly crude and were administered with comparatively little discrimination, the natural result of his total lack of medical knowledge. However, his native tact and sagacity soon led him to recognize a difference in the ability of his patients to react to cold applications, and he accordingly made it a practice to observe in each case the effects of the first application, the readiness with which the patient yielded to the means adopted to induce perspiration, and the promptness with which reaction took place on the application of cold water.

Priessnitz discovered little, perhaps, but he succeeded in calling general attention to the efficacy of various simple methods of applying water as a remedial agent which had previously been little appreciated. And he accomplished more than this. He aided to recovery a vast number of chronic invalids whose maladies were practically incurable by the measures in common use by the medical profession of that time; and though at first denounced and opposed by scientific physicians because of his empiricism, the more sagacious among them, after a time, became convinced of the genuineness of the cures effected, and many visited him for the purpose of studying his system, such as it was.

Priessnitz found nearly all the methods of employing water which entered into his system, in use among the peasantry of his country, by whom they were commonly employed at least as early as 1737, and probably even before that time. Priessnitz, however, was one of the first to organize the use of these various measures into a system, for which he deserves much credit. Crude and empirical though his system was, his success was sufficient to compel attention, and he commanded an extensive following.

The attention thus attracted led to a careful study of the physiological effects of water in its various modes of application, for the purpose of finding a scientific foundation for its therapeutic use. Among the first to undertake this study was Fleury, who published in 1852 the first extended scientific treatise upon hydrotherapy, under the title, "Traité Pratique et Raisonné d'Hydrothérapie."

Scientific Hydrotherapy. Liebermeister, Brand, and Ziemssen in Germany, and above all, Winternitz, of Vienna, revising, and his pupils greatly extending the work of Fleury and other pioneers, have within the last half century built up a scientific hydrotherapy which is based upon definite and accurate data. Before Fleury, the use of water was for the most part empirical; at the present time, however, thanks to the labors of the eminent investigators whose names have been mentioned, supplemented by those of Jürgensen, Rosbach, Bouchard, Delmas, Robin, Beni-Barde, Strasser, D'Arsonval, and others, it may be fairly stated that there is no therapeutic agent whose use rests upon a more thoroughly rational and scientific basis than water. It has thus been rescued from the hands of empirics and charlatans, and is now recognized by eminent medical men as one of the most potent of all remedial agents.

Hartshorne, of Philadelphia, published in 1847 a suggestive and thoughtful treatise on the use of water. In 1850, Bell, of the same city, published the best and most comprehensive work on the subject which had appeared in English before the translation and publication of the masterly treatise by Winternitz as a part of Ziemssen's therapeutics in 1883.

The work of Winternitz in establishing hydrotherapy upon a sound scientific basis so greatly exceeds that of all other investigators in modern times that we have given, at the close of this work, a complete list of the contributions to hydrotherapeutics made by this eminent pioneer in this line of medical research, which Dr. Winternitz, at the author's request, has kindly furnished him.

THE PHYSICS OF WATER, AIR, HEAT, AND LIGHT IN RELATION TO HYDROTHERAPY.

1 HOFFMAN, whose authority commands universal respect, declared water to be more nearly a panacea for all human ills than any other known agent. This fact, which has never been disproved, is largely due to the peculiar physical properties of this very versatile element. Water owes its value as a therapeutic agent chiefly to three most remarkable properties: (1) Its great power for absorbing and communicating heat; (2) its solvent properties, water being the one universal solvent; (3) the facility with which its physical state may be changed from a liquid to a solid or a gaseous form. These properties give to it the most perfect adaptability to the various modes of application which are required in hydrotherapy. It will be worth while to consider briefly each of these several properties, as follows:—

2 **The Specific Heat of Water.** Water absorbs more heat for a given weight than any other body, and is hence taken as the standard of "specific heat." A pound of water contains five times as much heat as an equal weight of glass; about ten times as much as the same weight of iron, zinc, copper, or brass; and thirty times as much as the same quantity of mercury, gold, or lead. The specific heat of the human body is nine tenths that of water.

3 The readiness with which water absorbs and communicates heat and the great amount of heat which it is capable of communicating or storing, exactly adapts it for use in making thermic applications of either heat or cold to the human body. There is no other substance which is at all capable of replacing it for these purposes.

4 Because of the large amount of water entering into the composition of the human body, its specific heat is near that of water, viz., .9°. A pound of water at 10° will raise the tem-

perature of one pound of iron or copper from zero to nearly 10°. A quantity of water equaling the body in weight, losing 1° of temperature through contact with the body in a full bath, will raise the temperature of the body a little more than 1°, taking no account of any change in heat production or heat elimination.

In the solidifying and freezing of water a large amount of heat is rendered latent, as shown by the fact that a pound of ice in melting absorbs, without any elevation of temperature, heat enough to raise one pound of water 142° in temperature, the temperature of the water from the melting ice remaining at 32° or slightly above it until all the ice is melted. 5

Water, in passing from the liquid to the gaseous state, likewise absorbs a considerable amount of heat. The amount depends somewhat upon the pressure, but may be reckoned at about 950 heat units, or the amount required to raise 950 pounds of water 1° in temperature. The total amount of heat required to raise a pound of water from the ordinary temperature to that of steam is about 1,130 heat units. This heat reappears when the steam is condensed at the ordinary temperature. 6

In hydrotherapy, water is most commonly used in its liquid state, but it is also employed in the form of ice, and in the form of steam, though as steam, water is never applied directly to the body. When steam is utilized, as in the Russian or vapor bath, the body is not actually exposed to steam, but to the fog or mist formed by the condensation of the steam through contact with the atmosphere. In a vapor or Russian bath the patient is not heated by the steam, but by the hot air and the suspended particles of warm water which come in contact with the body. As the steam enters the air of the apartment from the steam-pipe or other source, it is at once condensed into a mist, giving up to the air the ten or eleven hundred heat units which it contains, and thus heating the air. A pound of steam is capable of raising from 7 the ordinary temperature to 130° eighty-seven pounds of air, or 1,100 cubic feet of air, the amount contained in an apartment 10 x 10 x 11 feet in size. One pound of steam applied to the body would be capable of raising the temperature of a man weighing 150 pounds nearly 8°, or ten pounds of flesh to a temperature of over 212°. It is for this reason that steam can not be brought in contact with the tissues without destroying them.

8 A pound of ice, on the other hand, is capable of removing from the tissues of the body with which it is brought in contact 142 heat units while melting. It will not, however, lower the temperature of the tissues below 32°, unless its own temperature should happen to be considerably below the freezing point, which might be the case in very cold weather. It is apparent that in the use of ice great care must be exercised in order to avoid damaging the tissues by prolonged contact.

9 The temperatures employed in hydrotherapy are practically within the limits of 32° and 140° F. Applications are occasionally employed at a lower temperature, and very hot water may sometimes be applied, at a temperature as high as 160°, as a means of stopping hemorrhages; but great care must be used. Live steam has recently been suggested as a means of checking hemorrhage, and may possibly prove to be of service in this capacity. Vapor and hot air may be tolerated at higher temperature.

10 Water is a fairly good conductor of heat. Its conductivity is much greater than that of air, but far inferior to that of the metals. Copper conducts heat one hundred times better than water. As a conductor of electricity, copper is immensely better than water. It is for this reason that water at any given temperature, hot or cold, makes a much more intense impression upon the skin than does air at the same temperature. On the other hand, metals of all sorts feel colder or hotter than does water of the same temperatures.

Ordinary water is a good conductor of electricity, a fact which enables it to render valuable service in most percutaneous applications of electricity and in such combined procedures as the hydrofaradic, the hydrogalvanic, and similar baths. 11

The Solvent Properties of Water.

As before remarked, water is the one universal solvent. In the body it is the medium by which the foods rendered soluble by digestion are conveyed to the tissues to be assimilated, and thus rendered insoluble, while the effete matters rendered soluble by disassimilation are dissolved and conveyed back into the blood current, to be acted upon or eliminated by the liver, the kidneys, the skin, and the other excretory organs. 12

It is interesting to note that sugar and peptone, the two chief constituents of digested food, are among the most soluble of substances. Carbonic acid gas, a product of the oxidation of carbohydrates and hydrocarbons, is also highly soluble in the saline medium which constitutes the serum of the blood. Urea, a product of proteid oxidation, has a high degree of solubility in water. Uric acid, oxalic acid, and other abnormal products are, on the other hand, less easily soluble than the normal waste products, and hence, as has been shown by Haig, readily accumulate in the body, especially in those portions in which the circulation is least active. 13

Thus the value of water as a detergent agent, not only for the surface of the body but for its interior as well, is apparent. This is, indeed, one of the most important therapeutic uses of water. It may be applied by means of water drinking, the enema, or the coloclyster (this term seems to the author preferable to the French *enteroclyster*), gastric lavage, and by subdermic injection of the normal saline solution. 14

Water in the liquid form readily lends itself to application to the body in numerous ways, both active and stable, by the different forms of immersion, compresses, douches of 15 various sorts, etc. The ease with which its temperature may be varied enables us to secure by its means every degree of thermic effect desirable, while its weight renders possible various mechanical or pressure effects which are also highly valuable, as will appear later in this work.

16 **The Atmosphere.** The relation of air to the thermic effects employed in hydrotherapy is perhaps less direct and important than that of water, yet it is by no means insignificant. Air as well as water is capable of absorbing heat. Although its specific heat is scarcely more than one fifth that of water, the ease and rapidity with which it circulates about the body, its continuous contact with the skin, the variability of its temperature, and especially the fact that it is concerned in the evaporation of moisture from the skin, whereby an enormous amount of heat is constantly removed from the body, render its relations as a thermic agent important.

17 The influence of the air upon the body depends not only upon its temperature but also upon the amount of water which it contains. A cubic foot of air at 32° is capable of absorbing slightly more than two grains of water. A cubic foot of air at 96° is capable of absorbing eight times as much, while air at 72° absorbs four times as much, or eight grains. It is thus apparent that air which has had its temperature raised without the addition of moisture is capable of promoting evaporation from the skin to a high degree. This fact must be taken into consideration in the management of patients at the different seasons of the year. In the summertime the air is often completely saturated with moisture, while in the winter-time saturation of the heated air indoors rarely if ever occurs, except by the aid of artificial means. The more completely saturated the air is, the less rapidly does evaporation take place. Patients are much more likely to complain of chilliness after baths in the winter than in the summer, for the reason that the extreme dryness of the air gives rise to rapid evaporation of the small amount of mois-

ture left on the skin after leaving the bath-room, giving rise to chilliness, and occasionally resulting in a cold. On this account, patients must in the winter-time be dried with special thoroughness before leaving the bath-room, and must afterward be particularly careful about exposing themselves.

The rapid rate at which heat is removed from the body 18
by evaporation when dry warm air is brought in contact with it may be easily shown by a simple illustration: Suppose an apartment (20 x 13 x 10) contains 2,600 cubic feet of air at 96°, the temperature out of doors being 32°. The indoor air is capable of absorbing nearly fifteen grains of water, in addition to that which it already contains, for each cubic foot, or more than five and one-half pounds of water. The absorption of less than one half of this (two pounds) through evaporation from the surface of the patient's body will abstract from the body something like 2,000 heat units, and would be capable of reducing the temperature of the body more than 13°, provided no heat was in the meantime produced. The same air, if saturated with water, would absorb little water, and would take very little heat from the body. The relation of different conditions of the atmosphere to the rate of evaporation from the skin is a question which should perhaps receive more consideration in connection with hydrotherapy than has generally been accorded it.

It is also important to note that the respiratory processes 19
of both the lungs and the skin are diminished by an exceedingly dry atmosphere. Interchange of gases in the lungs is also interfered with by an atmosphere saturated with moisture.

Atmospheric pressure is likewise a matter well worthy of 20
attention in connection with hydrotherapy. In institutions located at an altitude of several thousand feet above the level of the sea, this is of special importance, on account of the tendency to pulmonary congestion due to the rarity of the atmosphere. Under such circumstances extreme care must be

taken to avoid the application of the cold douche and similar measures in such a way as to provoke disturbance of respiration; in other words, cold applications must be made to the chest only with the greatest care, and after applications have been made to other portions of the body, so that the effect may be generalized.

21 Cold air produces a less intense sensation of cold than does cold water, for the reason that its ability to absorb heat is only one fifth as great, and its conductivity of heat is enormously less. The thermic effect produced upon the skin by an object brought in contact with it is due both to the specific heat of the object and to its conductivity. Iron, copper, and other metals are such excellent conductors of heat that they may feel colder than water at ordinary room temperature even though their specific heat is many times less.

22 **Heat.** Most of the effects of hydrotherapy are obtained by means of methodical thermic applications to the skin. In other words, the specific effects of hydrotherapy are not chiefly due to water *per se*, but to the impressions of heat or cold made by this agent when brought in contact with the skin. So far as these same effects may be produced by other means, precisely the same results may be obtained.

23 Heat and cold are relative terms, what is termed a cold application being simply one that is of a temperature a definite number of degrees lower than the so-called warm or hot application. The impression made upon the skin, as elsewhere remarked, depends not only upon the temperature of the application, but upon the relation existing between the temperature of the application and the temperature of the skin.

24 The science and art of hydrotherapy include not only applications of water in its various forms, but thermic applications made by means of hot or cold air, vapor, and various heated objects, also heat and light.

Various sources of heat may be utilized in making thermic applications to the human body for therapeutic purposes. While water is generally the most convenient agent, there are conditions to which it is not adapted, and in which other means may be more advantageously employed. Heated air, the vapor of water, or rather the fog resulting from the condensation of steam in air at a temperature near that of the body, the sun's rays, and lastly the electric ray may all be utilized. The use of hot air in the form of the Turkish bath dates from remote antiquity, and the hot-air bath and the vapor bath have been used by many primitive people. The electric ray is, however, one of the most interesting sources of thermic energy; and while only recently introduced to practical therapeutics, it is certain to prove itself of the greatest practical utility. Both forms of the electric lamp, the incandescent and the arc, may be utilized as sources of heat. 25

The sun's rays, which the electric ray closely resembles in its action as a thermic agent, have been utilized in the treatment of the sick from the most ancient times. The amount of heat received hourly upon each square foot of the earth's surface is about equivalent to that produced by the burning of a sufficient amount of coal to produce one fourth of a horse-power of mechanical energy. The physical and therapeutic properties of sunlight and of the electric ray will be considered at greater length elsewhere in this work (**597**). 26

This means has the advantage over others in that the rays of radiant energy received from a luminous source penetrate the skin and the tissues to a great depth, in fact, reaching without doubt, the very innermost portions of the body. 27

When electricity meets with resistance, as in passing over a poor conductor, it is converted into heat. The same principle holds in relation to light. When light passes through a perfectly transparent medium, no heat phenomena are manifested. Very little heat accumulates in pure white glass when the sun's rays fall upon it; but if the same glass be colored or painted black, it is very quickly heated. 28

29 As the luminous rays are intercepted by opaque particles in the tissues, they are converted into heat. Thus heat is generated in the depths of the tissues, the very place where this form of vital stimulus is required, instead of being applied only to the skin, as when hot water, air, or other media are employed. This fact renders the electric-light bath or the sun bath superior to all other heating procedures.

Thermometer Scales and Heat Units.

30 The centigrade scale divides the temperature range from freezing to boiling into one hundred degrees, making the freezing point zero, whereas the freezing point is 32 in the Fahrenheit scale, and the boiling point 212. The Fahrenheit scale thus divides the range of temperature between freezing and boiling into 180 degrees. It is apparent that 100 degrees ot the centigrade scale is exactly equal to 180 degrees of the Fahrenheit scale, and that one degree Fahrenheit equals $\frac{100}{180}$, or 5–9ths, degree centigrade; while one degree centigrade equals $\frac{180}{100}$, or 9–5ths, degree Fahrenheit.

31 To find the number of degrees Fahrenheit which a given number of degrees centigrade will equal, we have only to multiply the given number by 9–5ths, or what is the same thing, but a shorter method, we may multiply by two, and subtract one tenth.

32 Example: Suppose the difference in temperature between two objects is 40° C.; what will be the difference expressed in Fahrenheit degrees?

Answer: $$40 \times \frac{9}{5} = \frac{\overset{8}{\not{40}} \times 9}{\not{5}} = 72; \text{ or,}$$

$$40 \times 2 = 80 - 8 \; (80 \div 10 = 8) = 72.$$

33 To ascertain the number of degrees centigrade which will equal a given number of degrees Fahrenheit, we have only to multiply the number of degrees centigrade by 5–9ths, or what is the same thing, divide by two and add one ninth.

Example: Suppose the difference in temperature between 34
two objects is 72° F.; how may the same difference be expressed in centigrade degrees?

Answer: $$72 \times \frac{5}{9} = \frac{\overset{8}{\cancel{72}} \times 5}{\cancel{9}} = 40; \text{ or,}$$

$$72 \div 2 = 36 + 4\ (36 \div 9 = 4) = 40.$$

But in converting Fahrenheit or centigrade temperatures 35
into equivalent expressions, we must generally take account of the fact that the zero point is not the same in both. So before beginning the calculation of converting a given fixed temperature, as shown by a Fahrenheit thermometer, into an equivalent expression in the centigrade system, we must first subtract 32; and in converting centigrade to Fahrenheit, we must add 32 at the end of the calculation.

For example: If we wish to convert 104° F. into an equivalent expression centigrade, we first subtract 32, then proceed as above (**33**). If we wish to convert 40° C. into an equivalent expression Fahrenheit, we proceed as in **31**, then add 32.

In the modern French system there are the greater and 36
the lesser calorie. The greater calorie simply represents the amount of heat required to raise the temperature of one kilogram of water one degree centigrade in temperature. The lesser calorie represents the amount of heat necessary to raise one gram one degree centigrade in temperature. In other words, the lesser calorie is the one thousandth part of the greater calorie. In the English system, which is not much in use at present, but is convenient in popularizing the principles of hydrotherapeutics, a heat unit represents the amount of heat required to raise the temperature of one pound of water one degree Fahrenheit in temperature.

To convert kilogram centigrade calories into gram centi- 37
grade calories it is only necessary to multiply by one thousand by moving the decimal point three places to the right.

38 To convert kilogram centigrade calories into pound Fahrenheit units, it must be remembered that the kilogram equals 2.2 pounds, and the centigrade degree 1.8 Fahrenheit degrees; hence the converting factor will be $\frac{22}{10} \times \frac{18}{10} = \frac{99}{25}$, or, approximately, 4; that is, we may for practical purposes simply multiply by four, to convert greater calories into an equivalent expression in pound Fahrenheit heat units. To be absolutely exact, we must subtract one per cent.

Example: We wish to convert 425 kilogram calories into pound Fahrenheit heat units.

$425 \times 4 = 1700 - 17$ (1 per cent. of 1700) $= 1683$.

39 To convert pound Fahrenheit heat units into greater calories we may multiply by $\frac{25}{99}$, or, what is practically the same thing, divide by four, and add one per cent.

Example: We wish to convert 400 pound Fahrenheit heat units into an equivalent number of greater calories.

$400 \times \frac{25}{99} = 101.01$; or,

$400 \div 4 = 100$; $100 + 1$ (one per cent. of 100) $= 101$.

40 **Medical Thermometry.** The expert hydrotherapist will give minute attention to the temperature of the patient, and of the air of the sick-room, as well as that of the water employed in remedial applications. The thermometer must be in constant requisition. It is not prudent to trust to the sensations, as these are too fickle and deceptive to serve as a reliable guide.

41 The temperature of the room must be maintained at about 65° F. In fevers a temperature of 60° is best. The sick-room is generally too warm, a fact which greatly increases the depression of the patient, and often excites a rise of temperature.

42 The temperature of the bath may be accommodated somewhat to the patient's sensations and predilections, but the exact temperature must be known, notwithstanding, and should be recorded. In an emergency, if a thermometer is not at hand, the temperature may be approximately determined by the following method: —

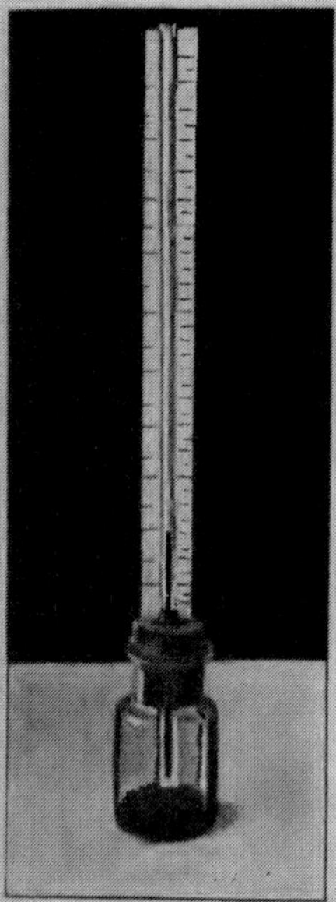

Fig. 1. AN EMERGENCY THERMOMETER (p. 50).

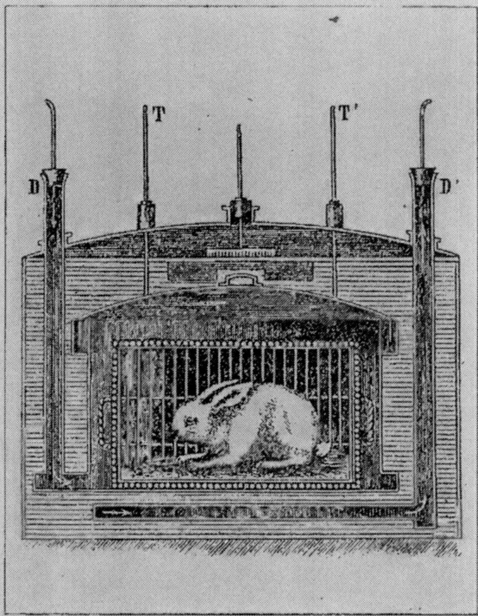

Fig. 2. WATER CALORIMETER (p. 52). (Dulong)

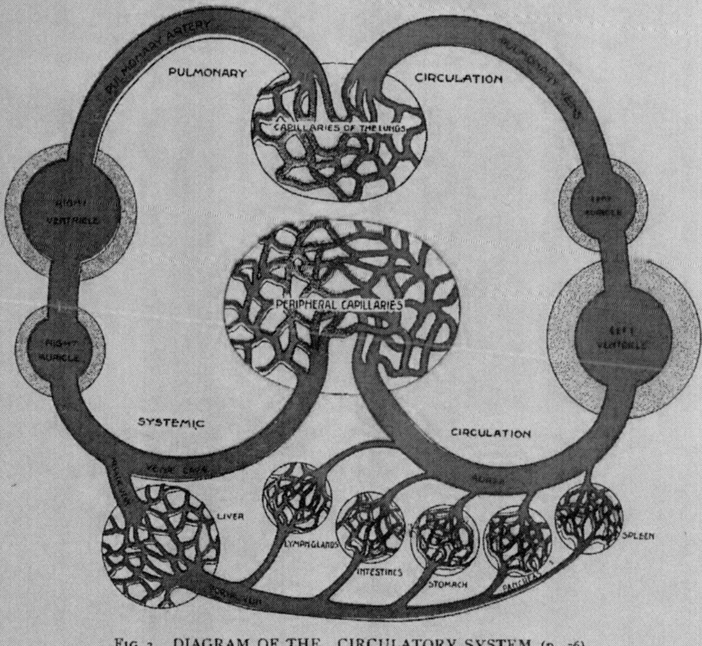

Fig. 3. DIAGRAM OF THE CIRCULATORY SYSTEM (p. 56).

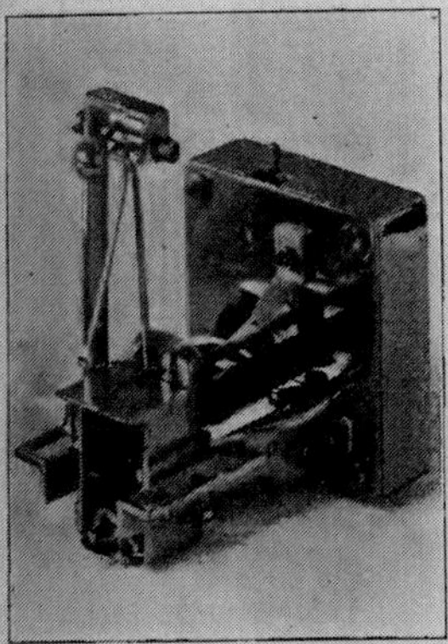

FIG. 4. SPHYGMOGRAPH (p. 60). (Dudgeon)

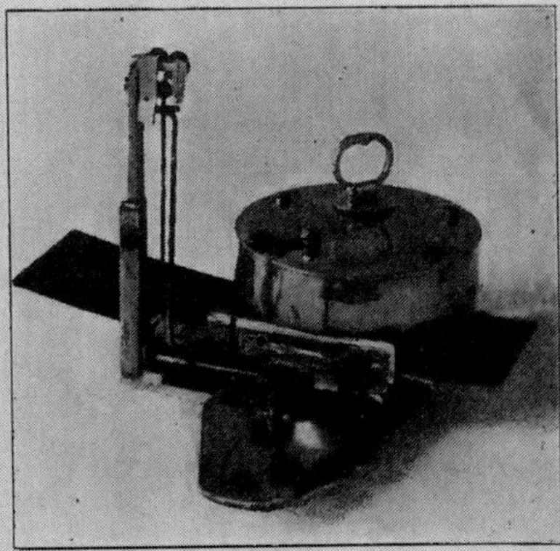

FIG. 5. SPHYGMOGRAPH (p. 60). (Granville)

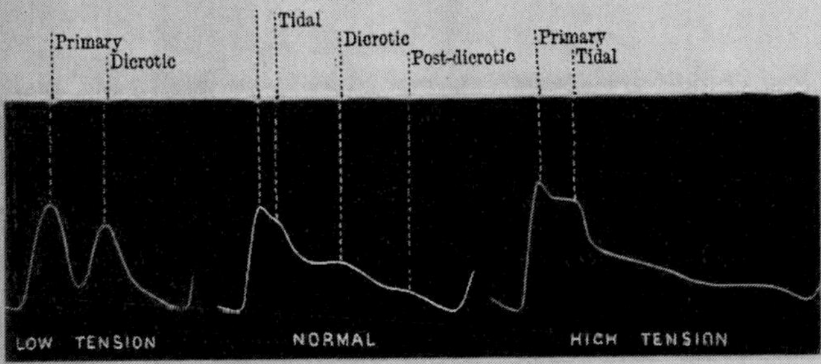

FIG. 6. DIAGRAMS OF THE PULSE (p. 60). (Waller)

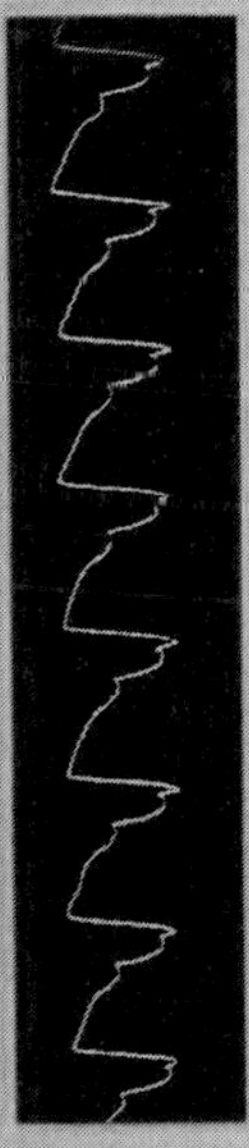

FIG. 9. SPHYGMOGRAPHIC TRACING OF PULSE OF MAN AGED SEVENTY-FOUR YEARS (p. 61).

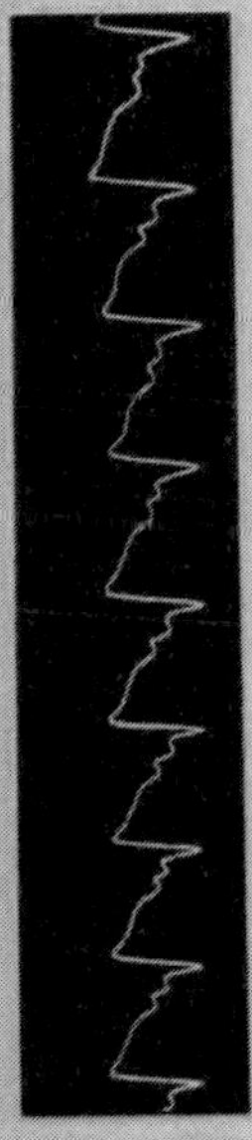

FIG. 8. SPHYGMOGRAPHIC TRACING OF NORMAL PULSE.

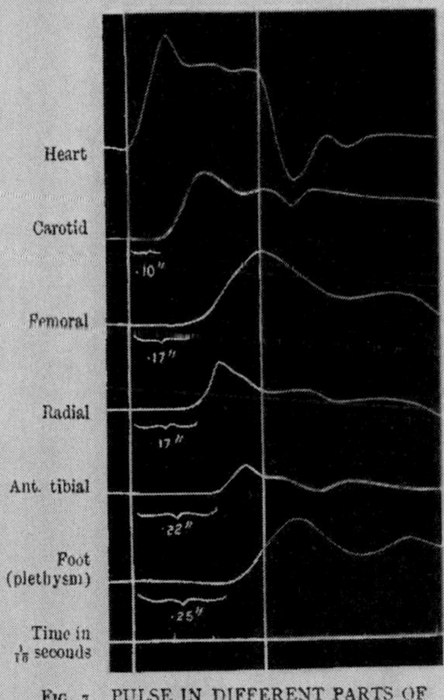

FIG. 7. PULSE IN DIFFERENT PARTS OF THE ARTERIAL SYSTEM (p. 60).

Mode of Determining and Regulating the Temperature of Water without a Thermometer.

The hand gives unreliable information respecting the temperature of water, but a more accurate judgment may be formed by plunging the whole arm to the elbow into the water, as the arm is usually protected by the clothing, and hence its temperature is more equable. When the temperature of the water is so high as to produce redness of the skin, it may be said to be hot. When there is simply a comfortable sensation of heat, it is warm. A slightly lower temperature is tepid. When the temperature is low enough to produce a goose-flesh appearance, it is cool; and a lower temperature is cold; while a temperature which within a few seconds produces pain or numbness of the parts immersed, is very cold. Water the temperature of which is so high that the hand can be held in it but a fraction of a second, perhaps, is very hot. 43

A method somewhat more accurate than the preceding, and which, with modifications, is applicable to all climates and altitudes, is as follows: The boiling-point of water at sea-level, as is well known, is 212°. In all countries the temperature of the water found in deep wells and springs is practically the same as the average of the air for the whole year. In temperate climates this is about 53°. Knowing the temperature of the well or spring water and that of boiling water, it is only necessary to combine measured quantities of water from these two sources in the necessary proportions to the amount desired. While this method is not exactly accurate, it answers for practical purposes. The following table gives the quantities to be mixed for different temperatures: — 44

Temp. 53° F.				Temp. 212° F.							
2	qts.	added	to	1	qt.	equals	3	qts.	at	106° F.	45
2½	"	"	"	1	"	"	3½	"	"	98° "	
3	"	"	"	1	"	"	4	"	"	93° "	
4	"	"	"	1	"	"	5	"	"	85° "	
5	"	"	"	1	"	"	6	"	"	80° "	
6	"	"	"	1	"	"	7	"	"	76° "	
8	"	"	"	1	"	"	9	"	"	71° "	

46 When larger quantities are needed, it is only necessary to multiply each of the combining quantities by the same number. For instance, if a gallon and a half of water is needed for a foot bath at 106°, pour into a pail or bath-tub four quarts of fresh well water and then add two quarts of boiling water. If four gallons of water are wanted for a sitz bath at 93° (a very common temperature), pour into the bath-tub three gallons of fresh well or spring water, and add one gallon of boiling water. Thus any required quantity may be obtained at the temperatures given. The cold water should be placed in the vessel first, and there should be no delay in adding the hot water, as it would rapidly lose its heat, and thus make a larger quantity necessary. The exact measurement is not necessary; it is only that the proper proportion should be maintained, the same measure being used for both hot and cold water, with both of which it is filled an indicated number of times.

47 In elevated regions, the boiling point is of course lowered, but this, being fixed, may always be known after it has once been ascertained. The temperature of deep well water or of spring water also varies little. This temperature may be ascertained, and borne in mind for use when necessary.

With ice-water and boiling water it is possible to determine the temperature of water obtained from a well, lake, or any other natural source. It is only necessary to make a mixture of ice-water and boiling water which shall have the same temperature as is noted by the hand, and to observe the percentage of each employed. For example, suppose that the proportions required are ten parts of ice-water (0° C.) to two of boiling water (100° C.). The result would be obtained thus: $10 + 2 = 12$; $200 \div 12 = 16.6°$ C., or 62° F.

48 **An Emergency Thermometer.** In Fig. 1 will be seen a simple thermometer which may be successfully used in regulating the temperature of baths, and if necessary, in determining whether or not the patient's temperature is above normal, and approximately to what degree. The instrument

consists simply of a small, thin-walled bottle, the mouth of which is closed with a cork, through which passes a tube having an opening of about one sixteenth of an inch. The tube should be about ten inches in length. In the bottom of the bottle should be placed about half an inch of a colored solution. Some aniline color dissolved in water or alcohol answers the purpose well. The tube should be passed through the cork to such a distance that when the cork is inserted in the mouth of the bottle, by pressing the cork in a little the fluid will be made to rise in the tube, and by a little management the liquid may be made to stand in the tube just at the top of the cork. Grasping the bottle in the hand, the air in the tube will be warmed and, expanding, will force the liquid farther up the tube. It is only necessary to place a foot rule behind the tube, letting the lower end rest upon the cork, and we have a very delicate thermometer with a scale which will answer a very practical purpose in the absence of a better instrument. The normal point is determined by applying the instrument to the axilla of a healthy person.

In the use of the clinical thermometer the temperature of 49
the patient should be taken in the rectum, if possible, unless enemas are being administered for cooling or nutritive purposes. If the temperature is taken in the mouth or the axilla, great care must be used to see that the lips are kept tightly closed or the arm in contact with the body.

Currie noted the fact that temperature observations made 50
by placing the thermometer in the mouth are sometimes rendered inaccurate when cold applications are administered, by the chattering of the teeth and consequent separation of the lips, admitting air.

Calorimetry. In the technical study of hydrotherapy it is 51
absolutely necessary to take into consideration not only the indications of the thermometer, or the temperature of the body as a mass, but it is of even greater importance to know what are the capabilities and the conditions of the body as a generator of heat. Information of this sort is

not afforded by the thermometer alone. The data required must be obtained by means of the calorimeter. This instrument determines the number of heat units which escape from the body in a given time, and thus, as the temperature of the body remains practically uniform, the amount of heat actually produced in the body is known (Fig. 2).

In the absence of a calorimeter, it is still possible to form a very close approximate estimate of the rate of heat loss from the surface of the body. The chief means by which the body loses its heat is by radiation, in common with all other bodies, and by the contact of its surface with atmospheric air. There is a slight loss by conduction, but for practical purposes this may be ignored. A considerable loss also occurs through the evaporation of the sensible and the insensible perspiration from the skin. A dry skin gives off heat very slowly, being a poor conductor; an oily skin radiates heat fifty per cent. more rapidly than a dry or unoiled skin. This fact the author believes he was the first to point out, although it seems as if the fact ought to have been suggested long ago by the custom of the natives of tropical Africa, who smear themselves with oil when exposed to the hot sun, and take special care to cover the head well with melted fat.

The loss of heat by evaporation ordinarily amounts to about 100 heat units per hour. By means of formulæ given elsewhere (733) it is made clear that the rate of heat loss both by radiation and by air contact may be determined by mathematical calculation based upon the laws of heat dissipation.

A consideration of the heat loss sustained by the body as determined in this manner quickly discloses the important influence of clothing, as it shows that the amount of heat actually produced and eliminated by the skin each twenty-four hours corresponds to the heat loss which would occur with the body unprotected in an atmosphere at a temperature of 78° F.,—a temperature which the primitive tribes of men readily endure without other clothing than the smallest amount necessary to satisfy the demands of savage modesty.

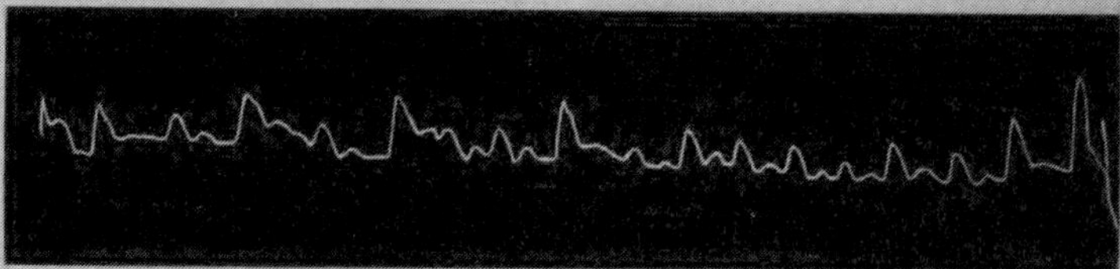

FIG. 10. PULSE OF AORTIC REGURGITATION (p. 61).

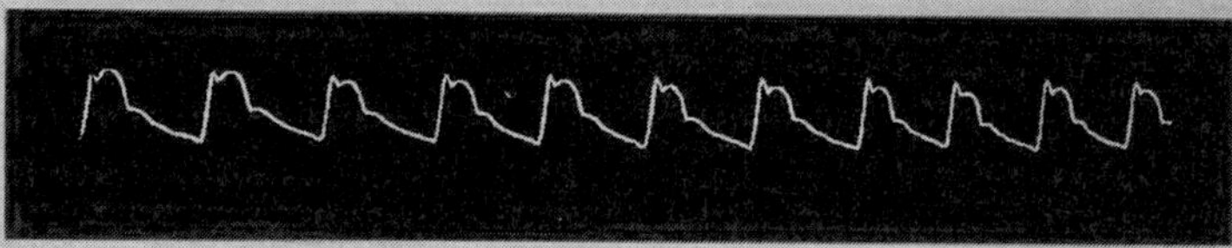

FIG. 11. SPHYGMOGRAPHIC TRACING OF A HARD (High-tension) PULSE.

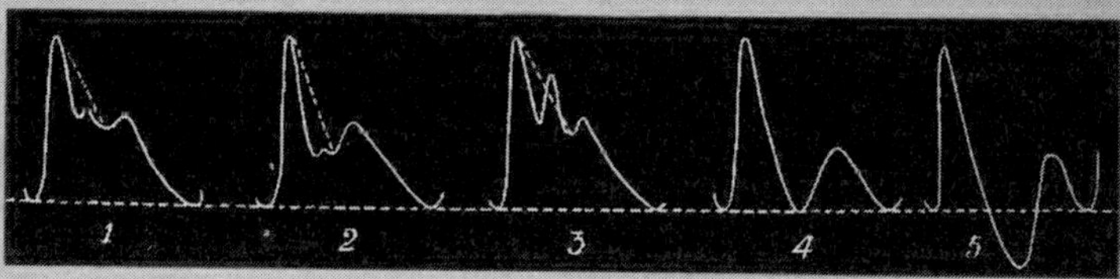

FIG. 12. DIAGRAMS OF PULSE. 1, Normal; 2, Low Tension and Soft Pulse; 3, High Tension and Hard Pulse; 4, Soft Pulse fully Dicrotic; 5, Very Soft Pulse and Hyperdicrotic. (Landois & Stering).

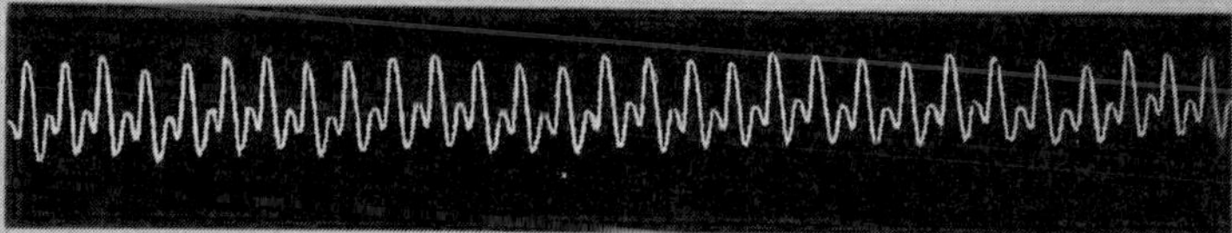

FIG. 13. DICROTIC PULSE (p. 61). (Author's Collection)

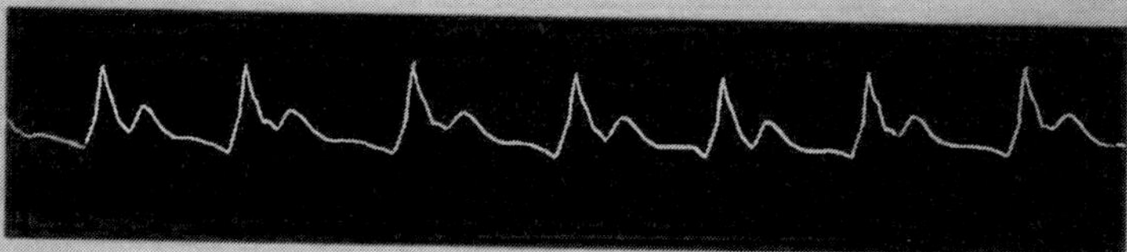

FIG. 14. SPHYGMOGRAPHIC TRACING OF A SOFT (Low-tension) PULSE.

ANATOMY AND PHYSIOLOGY IN RELATION TO HYDROTHERAPY.

THERE is no remedial agent the scientific use of which 52
demands so thoroughgoing and practical a knowledge of physiology as does hydrotherapy. Used empirically, water is certainly less likely to lead to disastrous results than some medicinal agents, the consequences of their unscientific use being only too forcibly illustrated in the terrible damage resulting from the use of patent medicines. Nevertheless, water as a remedial agent is, like powerful drugs, a two-edged sword, and its unscientific use has not infrequently produced most untoward results. Indeed, it may well be believed that the very general prejudice prevailing, among physicians as well as the laity, against the employment of water in treating disease, is largely due to the injurious effects which have followed its bungling and unsuccessful use by so-called water-cure doctors, and well-meaning, but unfortunately not well-informed, enthusiasts, who, having themselves experienced good results from the use of this simple and versatile therapeutic agent, have unwisely undertaken to cure all their sick friends by means of the same prescription through which they were themselves benefited.

Physiology the Basis of Hydrotherapy.

It is only by an exact knowledge of the 53
human body, its normal functions, and the modifications of tissue and function resulting from disease, that water can be therapeutically employed with the unrivaled results which this agent is capable of rendering. Not all cases, of course, are curable, but even in those that are incurable, it is marvelous to note the wonderful degree to which pain and various other symptoms may be mitigated by accurately adapted hydriatic prescriptions.

54 To use water intelligently, one must be a thorough physiologist, and must have an especially good understanding of the anatomy and physiology of the skin and the nervous system. Thus, for the convenience of the student, and that he may have freshly in mind those anatomical and physiological facts that are most essential to an understanding of the general principles of hydrotherapy, this chapter is devoted to a brief summary of the anatomy and physiology of the circulation, the skin, and the nervous system, so far as they are particularly concerned in the physiologic and therapeutic effects of hydriatic procedures.

THE CIRCULATION.

55 We have neither the space nor the purpose to review the whole subject of the anatomy and physiology of the circulation, but desire to recall simply the leading facts and to emphasize a few points which have a special relation to hydrotherapy.

56 The organs of the circulation are the heart, the blood-vessels (arteries, capillaries, and veins), the lymphatics (glands and ducts), and perhaps the spleen also may be included.

57 The heart is a muscular organ, having in its walls nerve ganglia which give origin to motor impulses whereby its activity is initiated and maintained. The heart's action is regulated by nerves from the cerebrospinal system: (1) The accelerator nerve, consisting of non-medullated fibers; (2) the inhibitory nerve (vagus), consisting of fine, medullated fibers.

58 The arteries, especially the smaller ones, and the smaller veins, though to a less extent, are also muscular structures capable of contracting, and, like the heart, controlled by automatic ganglia, the distal ganglia of the sympathetic system, which, like those of the heart, are capable of emitting motor impulses which cause contraction of the involuntary muscular fibers, and thus lessen the caliber of the artery. In addition, the arteries are, like the heart, controlled by two sets of nerves: (1) The vasoconstrictors, corresponding to the accel-

erator nerve of the heart, consisting of fine non-medullated fibers which pass out from the spinal cord with the anterior thoracic nerves; (2) the so-called vasodilators, which are simply inhibitory nerves, capable of retarding or counteracting the action of the vasoconstrictors, or of the muscles contracting under their influence. The vasodilators, like the inhibitory nerve of the heart, consist of fine, medullated fibers.

The capillaries are narrow tubes, the walls of which are 59
composed of nucleated cells, which, like the muscles of the heart and the small arteries, are capable of contracting, the seat of contraction being apparently in the nuclei of the cell.

It thus appears that the blood-vessels, arteries, veins, and 60
capillaries simply constitute an enormously extended and branching heart, just as the neuraxons and the nerve trunks are simply extensions of the brain and spinal cord.

The lymphatics consist of small vessels which exist in the 61
cellular spaces outside of the blood-vessels, and form a network extending throughout the entire body. The lymphatic channels connect at definite points with the lymphatic glands, which act as filters, by means of which foreign particles, germs, and other infectious elements are removed from the lymph. The walls of the lymphatics also are contractile.

The spleen is closely associated with the portal circula- 62
tion, and is also a contractile organ. It does not contract synchronously with the heart, but makes a cycle about once a minute. Its circulation is independent of blood pressure.[1]

Circulatory Systems.

There are four so-called systems of circula- 63
tion: —

1. The *systemic circulation*, consisting of the arteries, capillaries, and veins, by which the blood is propelled from the left side of the heart to the periphery, and is brought back to the right side of the heart.

2. The *pulmonary circulation*, by which the impure blood 64
sent out from the right side of the heart passes through the lungs, and is returned to the left side of the heart, to be again distributed throughout the body.

65 3. The *lymphatic circulation*, by which the lymph that escapes from the blood-vessels through the capillary walls is gathered up from the connective tissue spaces and returned to the circulation through the lymph channels and the thoracic ducts which empty into the subclavian veins.

66 4. The *portal circulation*, which consists of veins only, the venous blood from the stomach, spleen, pancreas, intestine, and liver being gathered up in one large vein and conducted to the liver, where it is filtered before being introduced into the general circulation through the hepatic vein. The accompanying diagram shows clearly the relation between the systemic, pulmonary, and portal circulations (Fig. 3).

67 The amount of blood contained in the body is about eight or nine pounds, and of this about one fifth is found in the pulmonary circulation, and four fifths in the systemic circulation. The capacity of the veins is at least twice that of the arteries. The sectional area of the capillaries is about five hundred times greater than that of the aorta, but their capacity is very small because of their short length, which is only about one twenty-fifth of an inch. The contents of the lymphatic vessels is about three or four times the quantity of the blood; that is, the lymph constitutes about one third the body weight.

The Mechanism of the Circulation.

68 Landois and others have shown that the force of the heart-beat is sufficient to account for the circulation of the blood through the entire circulatory system. The chief cause of the movement of the blood is evidently the difference in the blood pressure existing in the aorta at the heart and that in the vena cava at its junction with the right auricle. The pressure in the aorta is equivalent to about six inches of mercury, while that in the vena cava is never more than half an inch, and during inspiration, is negative. The heart is compelled to do something more, however, than simply to move the blood around the circuit of the blood-vessels. It must maintain a certain pressure, or tension, within the vessels, this be-

ing one of the means by which the various processes of secretion and other forms of metabolism are maintained and regulated.

Blood pressure results chiefly from the force of the heart- 69
beat, and the peripheral resistance at the distal end of the vascular loop in the small arteries, venules, and capillaries, through the narrowing of these parts by the contraction of their muscular walls under the influence of nerve impulses excited by various conditions and agents. In the light of present knowledge it is not, however, possible to regard the heart as the only source of energy in the circulation of the blood. For more than a score of years physiological facts have been coming to light which point with much certainty to the muscular coats of the smaller vessels, the arterioles, possibly the venules, and very probably also the capillaries, as a source of propulsive energy in maintaining the movement of the blood. Schiff showed long ago that there is a rhythmical contraction of the muscles in the arteries in mammals as well as in amphibians, the latter fact having long been recognized. Stricker observed the contraction of the capillaries, and Severini considered the contractility of the capillaries, at least of their nuclei, as of great importance in "influencing the blood stream." Roy and Graham Brown have also shown that the capillaries are contractile.[3] The writer has so long been thoroughly convinced of this fact, that in 1879, in describing the forces of the circulation in a popular work on Physiology and Hygiene, he remarked: "The contraction of the heart, which gives the blood a propulsive impulse, is followed up by the contraction of the arteries. The small arteries are supposed to be specially active in assisting the circulation. Some observers claim that the small arteries, or arterioles, keep up a constant peristaltic action, by means of which the blood is urged forward."

It may be said in short that, in addition to the heart 70
proper, the body is provided with what might be termed a *peripheral heart*, which serves several important purposes: (1) The regulation of the local nutritive and secretory proc-

esses; (2) to a certain extent the control of the heart's action by maintaining just the right degree of tension or intravascular pressure through the narrowing of the arterial outlet; (3) an active rhythmical contraction which acts like a combined suction- and force-pump at the periphery of the circulatory system, relieving the heart of a part of its burden, while at the same time aiding in maintaining the proper standard of blood pressure.

71 This action of the small vessels is of course not confined to the exterior of the body, but is doubtless present in the blood-vessels in all parts of the body, especially in the muscles. That an action of this sort is also maintained in the skin is altogether probable, as it has been observed in the ear of the rabbit. The capillaries of the skin are for the most part arranged in simple loops, which would favor a propulsive action of this sort. It is true, the arterioles of the skin have little muscular tissue in their walls; however, this lack is to a large degree compensated for by the peculiar arrangement of the yellow elastic tissue which surrounds the vessels and by the obliquely placed involuntary muscle fibers, both of which favor contraction of the vessels if they do not aid in the automatic or rhythmical action above referred to.

72 The rich vascular area of the muscles, which is capable of holding one half of all the blood in the body, may be normally more active than the skin in aiding the systemic circulation; but the remarkable readiness with which the skin responds to vascular stimuli, both those which excite the vasodilators and those which bring the vasoconstrictors into activity, shows very clearly that there is in the skin an enormous body of muscular structure connected with the circulatory system which is under the control of the nerve centers.

73 Another force which is by no means insignificant as an aid to the circulation is the inspiratory activity of the lungs acting upon the heart and the large vessels in the thorax. The negative pressure induced in the chest cavity during respiration

accelerates the movement of the blood through the heart to a marked degree. This influence is especially helpful to the portal circulation, and to the venous circulation of the brain.

The rhythmical contractility of the spleen, already referred 74
to, constitutes it a sort of heart for the portal circulation. When the spleen is contracted, the liver is slightly enlarged, showing an increase of tension in the portal circulation which must accelerate the movement in this portion of the venous system, hedged in as it is at each end by a capillary network.

The pumping action of the spleen is doubtless service- 75
able as a means of regulating the blood flow through the liver and in maintaining the necessary pressure to secure the highest degree of functional activity of this large and important gland.

The Blood Current.

When the blood leaves the heart, its move- 76
ment is at the rate of several feet per second, while in the capillaries the rate of movement is reduced to one inch in two minutes. The rapidity of movement of the blood in the vessels is constantly changing with the changes in the relative conditions of the heart and the contractile walls of the small vessels. The following table from Waller represents the several modifications which may occur, and the conditions which give rise to them. The table is so nearly self-explanatory that it is only necessary to add that in some conditions the blood pressure and the blood flow may be neither increased nor diminished, but normal.[3]

Case.	Heart.	Arterioles.	Blood Pressure.*	Blood Flow.*
1	Force constant.....	Resistance increased...	+	—
2	Force constant.....	Resistance diminished..	—	+
3	Force increased....	Resistance constant....	+	+
4	Force diminished...	Resistance constant....	—	—
5	Force increased....	Resistance diminished..	+ —	+ +
6	Force diminished...	Resistance increased...	— +	— —
7	Force increased....	Resistance increased...	+ +	+ —
8	Force diminished...	Resistance diminished..	— —	— +

* The plus sign (+) indicates increase; the negative sign (—), decrease.

77 **The Pulse.** A very good knowledge of the pulse may be obtained by its study with the finger, in the usual way, but the record afforded by the sphygmograph makes clear many peculiarities in the pulse which are difficult to understand without this graphic representation to the eye, and adds greatly to the knowledge obtained by examination with the finger.

78 The accompanying cuts (Figs. 4 and 5) show both Dudgeon's and Mortimer Granville's sphygmographs. The latter is more convenient for clinical purposes. It is, I think, very little known in this country. Figs. 6 and 7 will aid in understanding both the graphic record of the pulse and the pulse itself. The tracing is obtained by means of an arrangement which enables the upward movement of the artery to operate upon the short arm of a lever, the long arm of which rests upon a strip of smoked paper. The paper is moved along by clock-work while the instrument is in use, making a record such as is shown in Fig. 8. The curved lines between the dotted lines X and Y represent one heart-beat.

The meaning of the several parts of this curve is as follows:—

79 The first portion of the curve represents the upward stroke produced by the lever, due to the expansion of the artery under the impulse of a wave of blood sent from the heart. This is called the *primary*, or *percussion, wave*. The maximum of expansion is maintained for only a brief period, the length of which depends upon the condition of the arterial walls. At the end there is sometimes a slight rise.

80 This interruption of the decline or elevation of the curve is known as the *tidal wave*. This is followed by a slight depression, which is again followed by a slight rise, the so-called *dicrotic wave*. The depression between the dicrotic and the tidal waves often amounts to a very sharp notch, which is sometimes very deep, and is known as the *aortic notch*.

81 After the dicrotic wave there is usually one, sometimes several, small waves, which are commonly due to oscillations

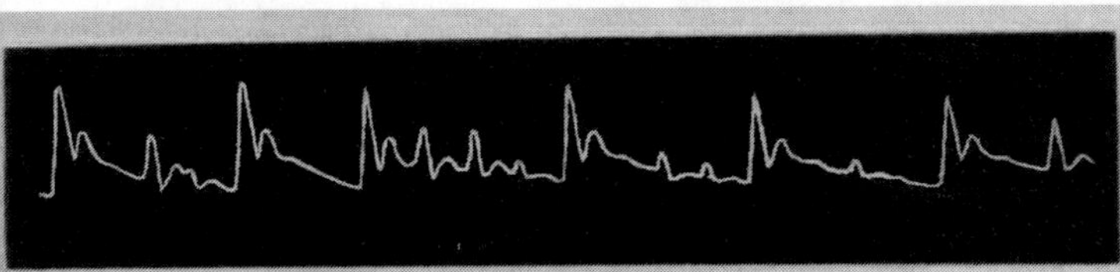

FIG. 15 (*a*). IRREGULAR PULSE (p. 62).

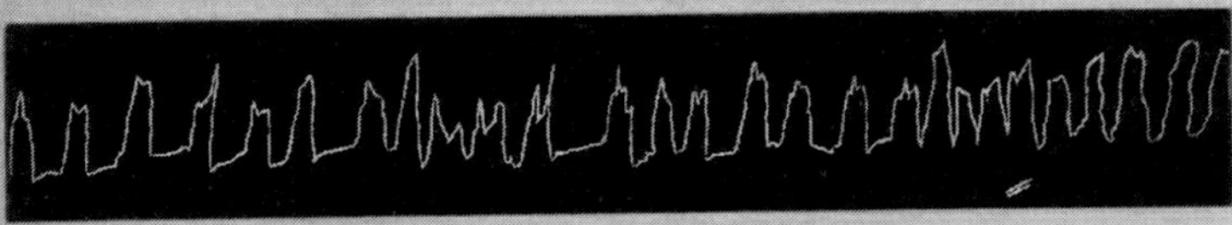

FIG. 15 (*b*). IRREGULAR PULSE OF TOBACCO USER. (WALLER)

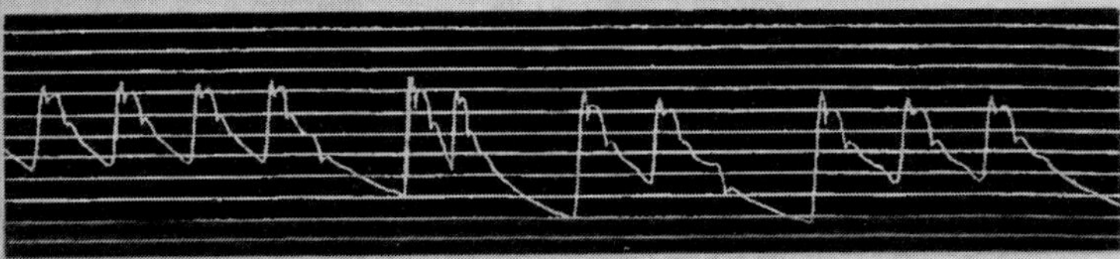

FIG. 16. INTERMITTENT PULSE (p. 62).

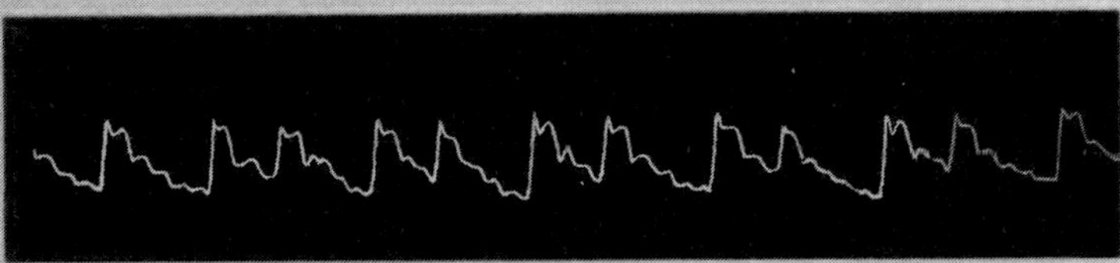

FIG. 17. INTERMITTENT PULSE.

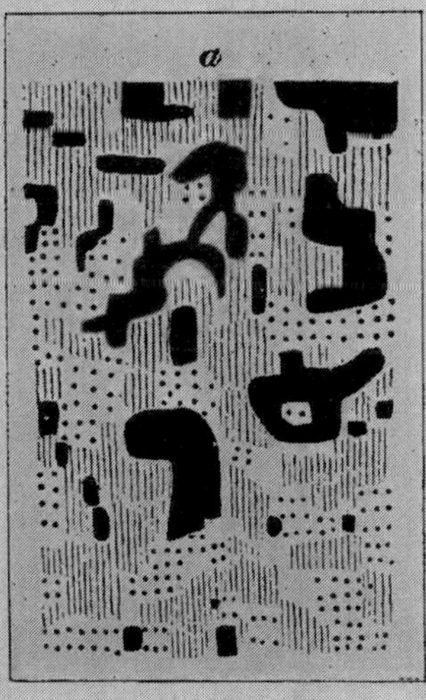

FIG. 19 (*a*). HOT SPOTS (p. 69).

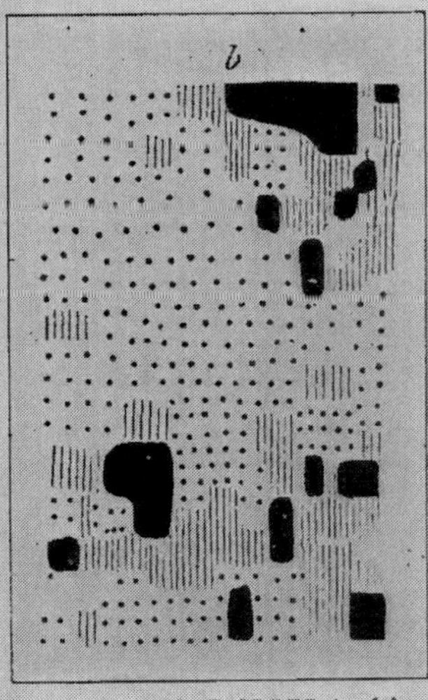

FIG. 19 (*b*). COLD SPOTS (p. 69).

of the instrument. The three points of importance to be observed in the curve are the primary, the tidal, and the dicrotic waves.

The *primary wave* marks the expansion of the artery 82
under the impulse of the wave of blood from the heart. It measures in a general way the force and amplitude of the cardiac impulse; the *tidal wave*, extending from the apex to the "aortic notch," represents the sustained propulsion of the blood resulting from the energy stored up in stretching the arteries. As the stretched arteries contract, the pressure or tension is more or less maintained, according to the degree of elasticity in the vessel walls. With a rigid, atheromatous artery, the pressure quickly falls.

The rigid arteries of old age produce a marked but short 83
tidal wave, followed by a very marked fall (Fig. 9). In aortic regurgitation, the fall is equally marked (water-hammer pulse) because of the sudden emptying of the artery into the ventricle (Fig. 10). In the high-tension pulse (Fig. 11), there is a slower and more gradual decline after the tidal wave, which is very well marked (Fig. 12). To the finger, the pulse of old age and of regurgitation feels "empty" between the beats. The pulse of high tension feels "full."

The *dicrotic wave* is little marked in high tension, but in 84
low tension is so marked that the low-tension pulse of *high fever* is often termed the *dicrotic pulse.* In such a case the dicrotic wave is so much exaggerated that it may be easily felt under the finger (Fig. 13).

In the low-tension pulse the tidal wave, if present, will 85
fall below a line drawn from the apex to the bottom of the aortic notch (Fig. 14). In the high-tension pulse the tidal wave is marked, and rises above the line described. The high-tension pulse is *hard* to the touch ; the low-tension is *soft.*

A *frequent* pulse is one in which the number of beats per 86
minute is abnormally great. In fever the pulse-rate increases ten beats (approximately) for every degree Fahrenheit rise of temperature.

87 A *quick*, or *short*, pulse is one in which the beat itself seems very sharp and quick beneath the finger. These terms are unnecessary, as the quick pulse is always a *soft*, or low-tension, pulse.

88 A *long*, or *slow*, pulse is the opposite of the quick pulse. These terms are not needed, as the long pulse is always a *hard*, or high-tension, pulse.

89 In the *irregular* pulse, the beats do not occur with rhythmical succession, but the intervals are irregular (Fig. 15).

90 An *intermittent* pulse is one in which a pulse-wave is now and then lacking, a heart-beat being omitted. Sometimes a pulse seems to be intermittent when there is no actual omission of beats, but the occurrence at regular or irregular intervals of a beat too feeble to be recognized by the finger. The sphygmograph shows the presence of pulse-beats not otherwise recognizable (Figs. 16 and 17).

The accompanying cuts of sphygmographic tracings are chiefly copied from the author's collection of many hundreds of tracings, representing a great variety of conditions, normal and pathological.

THE SKIN AND ITS FUNCTIONS.

91 Since in by far the greater share of the medical uses of water the skin is involved, it will be profitable to devote a few paragraphs to a cursory review of the anatomy and physiology of this remarkable organ.

92 Anatomically, the skin is a structure about one eighth of an inch in thickness, consisting of a framework of white and yellow elastic fibers, in which are suspended a countless number of glands, blood-vessels, and nerves. The whole is covered with cells joined by a cement-like substance (Fig. 18).

93 The deeper layers of the skin contain, in certain portions of the body, especially on the extensor surfaces, and connected with the hair follicles, an abundance of smooth muscular fibers, which are capable of contracting the skin.

The area of the skin covering the whole body is about 19.6 square feet. 94

The Sweat. The sweat-glands are, in man, present almost everywhere in the skin, but are largest and most numerous in the skin covering the palm of the hand, the sole of the foot, the forehead, and the axilla. There are very few sweat-glands in the skin covering the back. 95

Each sweat-gland receives an artery and a number of nerve filaments, and has a duct through which its product is discharged upon the surface. 96

The perspiratory ducts present an aggregate surface of nearly eleven thousand square feet. 97

The amount of perspiration produced daily is about two pints, or one sixty-fourth the weight of the body, this being double the amount of water thrown off by the lungs. The usual rate of sweat secretion is one ounce or an ounce and a half per hour. 98

Three degrees of activity of the sweat-glands are recognizable; viz.: (1) Ordinary, so-called insensible perspiration, in which the quantity is so small in amount that the water and volatile constituents of the sweat are evaporated as rapidly as formed; (2) sensible perspiration, in which the activity is so great as to produce slight moisture of the skin; (3) profuse perspiration, in which the quantity of secretion produced is so abundant that it appears in drops or minute streams coursing over the surface, and may amount to two or three pounds an hour. 99

The function of perspiration presents some interesting variations in different animals. A horse sweats, as does man, over the whole surface of the body. The same is true of the ox, but to a less extent. In the cat and the hedgehog, sweating is confined to the soles of the feet. Apes sweat in the palms of their hands. In the pig it is the skin covering the snout which sweats. The goat, rabbit, rat, and mouse do not sweat. 100

101 **Conditions that Control the Secretion of Sweat.**

The secretion of sweat is increased by the following agents and conditions: —

1. Increased temperature of the surrounding medium, as by the contact of hot air, hot water, or other heated substances with the skin. Water at 122° F., or above, *arrests the action of the sweat-glands.*

2. A diluted condition of the blood, such as results from the copious drinking of water, especially warm water.

3. Increased action of the heart, with rise of blood pressure.

4. Increased temperature of the blood. The sweat centers are excited by a rise of temperature amounting to .7° F.

5. Exercise, which increases the activity of the skin not only by increasing the activity of the heart, but by raising the temperature of the blood, and thereby stimulating the sweat centers. The temperature may be raised by violent exercise to 104° F.

6. Percussion and friction.

7. Certain drugs.

8. Stimulation of the secretory nerves by electricity or other means.

Physiological experimentation has shown that there are special sweat centers and nerves. The sweat nerves of the hind leg of a cat lie in the sciatic nerve. Stimulation of this nerve has caused sweating in the sole of the foot of a cat forty-five minutes after death. Mustard held in one side of the mouth will cause perspiration of the skin of the face of the same side. The centers of the sweat nerves for the palms lie in that portion of the cord that gives origin to the brachial plexus. Stimulation of the cervical sympathetic of one side causes sweating of the face and arm of the corresponding side.

The small blood-vessels are usually dilated in conjunction with sweating through excitement of the vasodilator nerves;

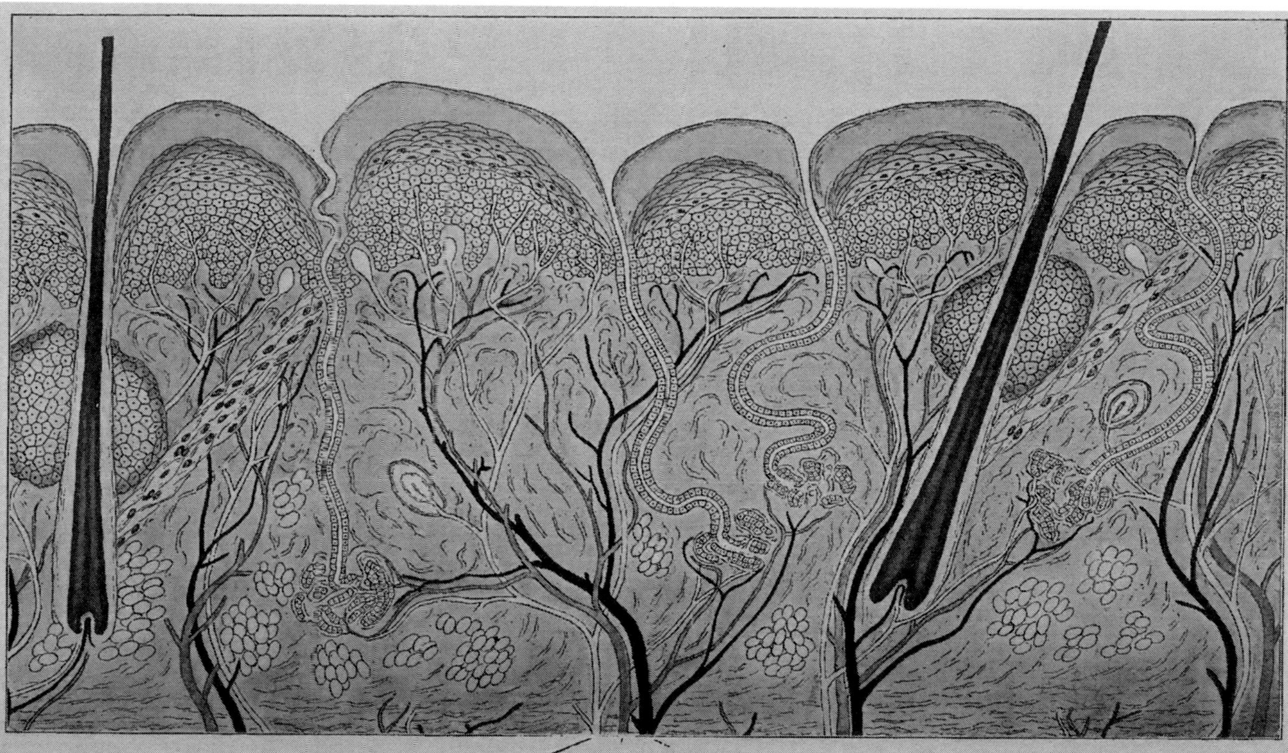

FIG. 18. VERTICAL SECTION OF THE SKIN (p. 62).

but sweating may occur with a pale skin,— the result of fear, pain, collapse, shock, or the death-agony.

Stimulation of a motor nerve causes sweating of the skin over the muscles supplied by the nerve, and of the same area of the opposite side of the body, and independently of any change in the circulation.

9. Mental excitement, as in hysteria and neurasthenia, often gives rise to sweating, especially of the head, palms, and soles, and sometimes of only one side of the face.

10. Profuse perspiration occurs as a symptom in certain diseases, as intermittent malarial fever, phthisis, and acute rheumatism.

11. The appearance of sensible perspiration is encouraged by a moist, warm atmosphere, in consequence of the lessened rapidity of evaporation.

Perspiration is decreased by — 102

1. Cold.

2. A profuse watery discharge from the kidneys or bowels. The skin and the kidneys seem to act reciprocally. When the secretion of one organ is increased, that of the other is decreased. In warm weather the volume of urine is usually diminished ; in cold weather, increased. The opposite is true of the cutaneous secretion.

3. Certain drugs, as atropia.

4. Certain forms of disease, as in some cases of paralysis, in diabetes, cancer, and many cases of chronic dyspepsia.

Perspiration is one of the most important means by 103 which the danger of excessive accumulation of heat within the body is averted. When the skin fails to perform this important function, as it not infrequently does in fever, the body temperature often rises to a most dangerous degree.

Toxins of the Sweat.

Not only uric acid and urea, but more subtle 104 and potent poisons are found in the sweat, as shown by the investigations of Bouchard. Perhaps most important of these is a peculiar substance which manifests its properties by inducing a fall of temperature.

5

The retention of this poison in the body may cause death, as has been proved by varnishing the skin of animals.

105 In diabetes the sweat frequently contains grape-sugar. Sweat from bad-smelling feet contains leucin, tyrosin, and ammonia. The sweat of rheumatism may contain albumin, and that of puerperal fever, lactic acid. Bloody sweat sometimes occurs in yellow fever, and bile pigments are found in the sweat in cases of jaundice.

106 Chromogenic microbes may give rise to red, blue, and yellow coloring matters in the perspiration. Mercuric chloride and other toxic substances have been found in the sweat after their internal administration. Pathogenic microbes have been found in the perspiration after a hot bath in infectious maladies.

The Sebaceous Glands.

107 Fat-making glands are found in connection with both the coarse and the fine hairs of the skin. They are absent only from the palms of the hands and the soles of the feet, and are largest in the skin of the nose and the labia. The purpose of these glands is to oil the hair and skin. The layer of oil covering the skin protects it to some degree. Anointing the skin with oil hinders conduction. It is a method adopted by swimmers and mountaineers for protection.

108 A minute band of involuntary muscular fibers is connected with each hair, one end being attached near the bottom of the hair pouch, the other to the skin in such a way as to form an acute angle with the hair. The sebaceous gland connected with each hair lies in the angle between this muscle and the hair. By contraction of the muscle, the hair is slightly straightened and lifted up, gently elevating the skin near the hair and compressing the gland, thus emptying it of its secretion. This action of the involuntary muscles may be excited by both heat (**536**) and cold (**328**). Heat not only causes contraction of the muscle, but softens the contents of the sac, and thus aids in their expulsion.

Absorption by the Skin. The skin absorbs substances in watery solution with difficulty, on account of the oil lying upon and in the epidermis and in the ducts. Solutions administered in a fine spray, and substances dissolved in oil and rubbed in, are more readily absorbed. Absorption takes place readily after the oil of the skin has been removed by ether, chloroform, or alcohol. By means of a galvanic current, absorption of watery solutions of iodide of potash, strychnia, and other drugs may be effected. This process is technically known as *cataphoresis*. 109

Cutaneous Respiration. Respiration by the skin in man varies in different individuals, from one half to one per cent. of the total amount of oxygen taken in by the body being received in this way. A somewhat less proportion of CO_2 is eliminated through this channel. In frogs and some other closely related animals the skin eliminates from two thirds to three fourths of the total amount of CO_2 excreted, thus becoming a more important respiratory organ than the lungs. Dipping a frog in oil and thus suspending cutaneous respiration will kill it more quickly than ligature of the trachea. Some creatures, as the earthworm, breathe wholly by the skin. 110

Respiration by the skin occurs through the thin walls of the perspiratory tubules, which present a surface of 11,000 square feet. Cutaneous respiration is most increased (1) by rise of internal temperature, (2) by increased cutaneous circulation, (3) by circumstances that hinder lung respiration, as asphyxia or dyspnea, and (4) during digestion. The amount eliminated at 94° F. is double that at 92° F.[4] 111

Nervous Functions of the Skin. The skin is without doubt one of the most important and interesting of all the sense organs, being provided with a greater variety of nerves than any other portion of the body. The nerves which supply the skin are the following:— 112

1. The nerves concerned in the tactile sense; viz., those which recognize *pressure* and *locality*.

2. The two sets of nerves concerned in the *temperature sense*, which terminate in the skin in the so-called *hot* spots and *cold* spots.

3. Nerves which recognize *pain*.

4. *Vasoconstrictor* nerves.

5. *Vasodilator* nerves.

6. *Sympathetic* nerves.

In all, at least seven distinct sets of nerves, which are connected with corresponding nerve centers.

113 In making thermic applications to the skin, the effects upon each one of these several sets of nerves must be taken into consideration. It is evident that those areas of the skin which possess the richest nerve supply must be most profoundly affected by hydriatic applications, and most capable of producing reflex effects through their connection with the internal viscera by means of their centers of origin.

114 **The Tactile Sense.** The acuteness of the pressure sense in different parts of the body is in the following order, beginning with the most sensitive: The forehead, lips, cheeks, and temples, the back of the fingers and forearm, the anterior surface of the leg and thigh, the back of the feet, the toes, the soles of the feet, and the posterior surface of the leg and thigh. The extreme delicacy of the pressure sense is shown by the fact that vibrations may be felt when exceeding the rate of 1,500 per second. This fact emphasizes the importance of giving careful attention to the exact regulation of pressure as well as temperature in hydrotherapeutic applications, a matter which has generally received less consideration than is necessary for accurate and reliable results.

115 The nerves of touch are connected with the motor centers controlling the muscles of the corresponding part. Rumpf has shown that increased sensibility of one part, whether produced by an application of heat or otherwise, is accompanied by a lessening of sensibility in the corresponding region of the opposite side.

The Temperature Sense. This is one of the most interesting of the functions of the skin, and the one most directly involved in hydrotherapy, as many of its most profound effects are the result of the influence of thermic applications upon the temperature nerves, and through them, upon the cerebrospinal and sympathetic systems. 116

The temperature sense is not uniformly distributed throughout the skin, but is confined to certain spots, of which there are two kinds,—*hot spots* and *cold spots*. These are arranged in curved lines or chains, starting from the hair roots, near which temperature spots are always to be found (Fig. 19). 117

Menthol excites the cold spots, and so produces a sensation of cold. CO_2 excites the warm spots, and thus gives rise to a sensation of heat. 118

These hot and cold spots are not sensitive to impressions of pain or pressure. 119

A "sleeping" limb recognizes heat only, and not cold. 120

The acuteness of the thermal sense differs in different portions of the body, and in the following order, the most sensitive being named first: Tip of finger, eyelids, cheeks, lips, neck, arm, back of hand, palm, thigh, leg, back. The back of the foot, the breast, and the palm of the hand have the same degree of acuteness. 121

The more acute areas recognize a difference in temperature of less than .1° F. Regions situated in the median line, as the nose, are least sensitive. 122

The temperature is estimated higher when a large surface is exposed. Water at 85° feels warmer if the whole hand is immersed than water at 90° in which the finger alone is dipped; but sudden immersion of the whole body in cold water produces a less unpleasant effect than when the body is introduced gradually. 123

Cold bodies feel heavier than warm ones. The pressure of a stream of water, as in a horizontal jet douche, feels greater when cold than when warm. 124

125 *The skin is more sensitive to cold than to heat*, impressions of cold being felt at once, while the sensation of heat develops gradually.

126 Thermic sensations are felt as warm or cold according as the temperature of the object or medium brought in contact with the skin is greater or less than that of the skin itself; hence *the temperature of the skin is the zero of the temperature sense.* Objects of a higher temperature than that of the skin are felt as warm or hot; those of a temperature below that of the skin, cool or cold.

127 Thermic impressions are most intense when the difference between the temperature of the application and that of the skin is greatest.

128 Objects that are *good conductors of heat feel warmer or cooler than poor conductors* at the same temperature. It is doubtless for this reason that hot or cold water makes a very much stronger impression than air of the same temperature.

129 *The temperature sense is most delicate at temperatures near or a little below that of the blood* (80° to 90° F.). It is less delicate at temperatures below 80° and above the temperature of the body. *Impressions of pain only are made by a temperature of 130° or above.*

130 *Rapid variations of extremes of temperature produce more marked effects than gradual changes.* The strongest impressions are made by alternations of very hot and very cold applications.

131 *The sensibility of the temperature sense improves with practice and with diminution of the blood supply.* Venous congestion of the skin diminishes the temperature sense.

132 *Fatigue of the temperature sense develops quickly;* hence marked tolerance within quite wide limits is quickly established.

133 The nerves of the temperature sense are associated with the heat-generating and heat-regulating centers of the brain and spinal cord.

Vasomotor and Secretory Nerves.

The blood-vessels are supplied with both constricting and dilating nerves, which arise from different centers, located at various levels in the spinal cord. It is through impressions made upon these nerves either singly or in succession that some of the most important effects in hydrotherapy are produced. The relation of the principal vasomotor centers to the principal surface areas and to the viscera of the chest and abdomen, is briefly stated elsewhere (**153-166**). 134

Each one of the several million sweat-glands and sebaceous glands of the skin is supplied with secretory nerves which are connected with the great sympathetic centers and with centers in the spinal cord. 135

GENERAL VIEW OF THE NERVOUS SYSTEM AS RELATED TO HYDROTHERAPY.

The skin, as has been aptly remarked, is a harp of a thousand strings, upon which one who is a master of the necessary means may play in such a manner as to produce almost any desired physiological or therapeutic effect. The skin is the keyboard, and the nerves and nerve centers are the internal mechanism. An understanding of the relation of the skin to the nerves and nerve centers is as essential to the physician who desires to employ hydrotherapy intelligently as is a knowledge of the rules of musical harmony and technique to the pianist. 136

It is necessary to understand not only the relation of the nerve endings in the skin with the nerve centers in the brain and spinal cord, but also through them the relation of the skin with the internal viscera supplied with nerves from the same or associated centers, and hence in special reflex relation. 137

Applications to the skin are sometimes made for the purpose of influencing the nervous system as a whole, but not infrequently it is desirable that the application should be limited in its effect to some single internal region. 138

139 There is no other class of therapeutic agents that requires so profound a knowledge of physiology, especially the physiology of the nervous system, and such constant employment of this knowledge, as do the various procedures included under the general term "hydrotherapy." We have space here only to call attention briefly to such physiological and anatomical data as are essential to a proper comprehension of the facts rehearsed in the chapters devoted to the physiological and therapeutic effects of water.

140 While every nerve center in the body is more or less profoundly affected by general applications to the skin, there are four sets of centers that are especially involved, as follows:—

1. The *sensory centers*, located in the brain.

2. The *heat centers*, located in the brain and spinal cord.

3. The *vasomotor centers*, located in the spinal cord.

4. The *secretory centers*, located in the spinal cord and the sympathetic system.

141 As most of the nerves connected with these ganglia are closely connected with the spinal nerves, it is of importance to bear in mind a few facts respecting the relation of the several *spinal centers* to the spine itself or to the vertebræ. These relations may be briefly stated as follows:—

1. The eight *cervical* ganglia correspond to the seven cervical vertebræ.

2. The twelve *dorsal* ganglia correspond in general to the several dorsal vertebræ, ending, however, with the eleventh.

3. The five *lumbar* ganglia are located at the level of the twelfth dorsal vertebra.

4. The ganglia of the five *sacral* and the *coccygeal* nerves are found at the level of the first and second lumbar vertebræ. No ganglia are found below this point because of the formation of the *cauda equina*.

In making applications to the spine, intended to influence the centers directly, it is essential to keep in mind the above facts respecting the location of the spinal ganglia.

The Superficial Reflexes.

As hydrotherapeutic applications are capable of exciting each and all the classes of reflexes that may be set up by stimulation of the cutaneous nerves, it is useful to bear in mind the location of the several reflex areas, and their relation to the spinal centers. 142

The *scapular reflex area* (the skin between the shoulder-blades), in relation with the first to the fourth dorsal ganglion. 143

The *epigastric reflex area* (the skin overlying the lower lateral portion of the chest), in relation with the fifth to the seventh dorsal ganglion. 144

The *abdominal reflex area* (the skin lying along the borders of the recti muscles), in relation with the eighth to the twelfth dorsal center. 145

The *gluteal reflex area* for lower portion of the nates in relation with the fourth and fifth lumbar. 146

The *cremasteric reflex area* (inner and upper portion of the thigh), in relation with the fourth and fifth lumbar ganglia. 147

The *plantar reflex area* (the soles of the feet), in relation with the five sacral and the coccygeal ganglia. 148

In the application of the douche with strong pressure, the location of the several reflex areas as described above may with advantage be kept in mind, especially in cases of organic disease of the spine.

The Vasomotor Centers.

The *controlling vasomotor centers*, both constricting and dilating, are located in the medulla. Subordinate vasomotor centers are located in the spinal cord. The vasoconstricting centers are found chiefly in the cervical and thoracic regions; the vasodilator centers are scattered throughout the cord. 149

Strong stimuli act on the vasoconstricting nerves; moderate, on the vasodilator fibers. 150

The veins and the lymph-vessels are also supplied with vasomotor nerves; and though at the present time nothing more is known of these nerves than that they exist, it is reasonable to suppose that they obey the same general laws as those connected with the small arteries. 151

152 The vasodilators differ from the vasoconstrictors in that they are made up of medullated fibers, and that they pass directly to the visceral ganglia of the blood-vessels without passing through the prevertebral ganglia. Their relation to the blood-vessels is the same as that of the vagus to the heart.

153 The blood-vessels of the head are controlled by vasomotor nerves from a center in the medulla, which pass to the head through the cervical sympathetic.

154 The lungs receive vasomotor nerves from the second to the seventh dorsal ganglion.

155 The intestines and abdominal viscera receive their vasomotor fibers through the three splanchnics. The great splanchnic is the largest vasomotor nerve in the body. Paralysis of the splanchnics causes death from accumulation of blood in the portal circulation, being equivalent to a hemorrhage, or ligature of the portal vein.

156 The principal vasoconstrictor and vasodilator nerves of the kidney leave the spinal cord with the last three dorsal nerves.

157 The liver receives its vasomotor fibers from the splanchnics and the vagus.

158 The spleen receives vasoconstrictor and vasodilator fibers from the splanchnics.

159 The pelvic organs in both sexes receive vasoconstrictor fibers from the lumbar nerves and vasodilators from the sacral nerves.

160 The arms receive their vasoconstrictor nerves from the middle dorsal region, through the first thoracic ganglion of the sympathetic.

161 The vasomotor nerves of the lower extremities pass through the lumbar and sacral plexuses to the sympathetic, thence to the lower limbs.

162 The skin of the trunk receives vasomotor fibers through the dorsal and lumbar spinal nerves.

163 The muscles receive their vasodilators through the trunks of the motor nerves.

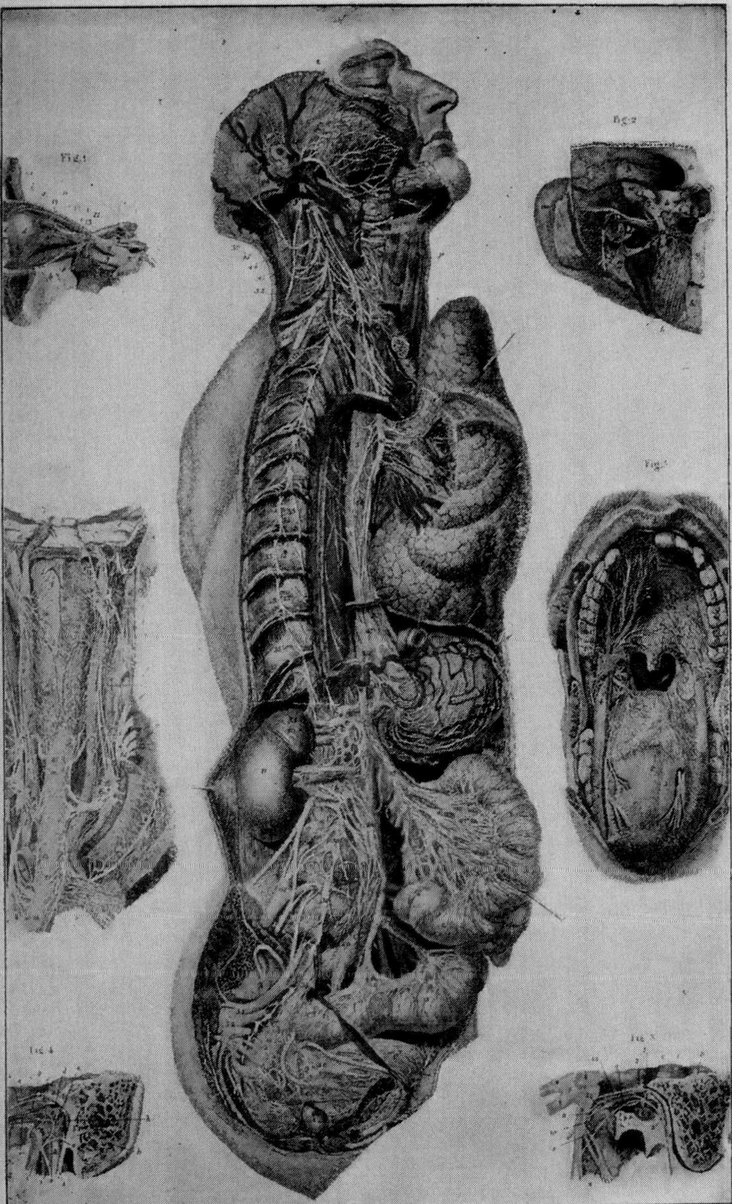

Fig. 20. SYMPATHETIC NERVOUS SYSTEM (p. 75).

The larger proportion of vasomotor nerves leave the spinal 164
cord between the fifth cervical and the first dorsal vertebra.

The richest vasomotor areas are found in the skin cover- 165
ing the palms, fingers, soles, toes, and ears.

The Visceral Motor Nerves.

The nerves that excite the peristaltic move- 166
ments of the esophagus, stomach, and intestines (excito-motor) leave the spinal cord in the upper part of the cervical region, reaching the intestines through the pneumogastric.

The Sympathetic Nervous System.

The sympathetic nervous system (Fig. 20) con- 167
sists of three distinct sets of ganglia; namely:—

1. The *lateral*, or *vertebral*, *ganglia*, consisting of a series of ganglia arranged along on either side of the anterior surface of the vertebral column, distributed as follows: three cervical, twelve dorsal, four lumbar, five sacral, one coccygeal. These two chains of ganglia form an ellipse, the ends being joined at both top and bottom in a single ganglion.

2. The *prevertebral ganglia*, or *gangliated plexuses*, con-
sisting of the *cardiac*, *solar*, and *hypogastric plexuses*, or the 168
thoracic, *abdominal*, and *pelvic* prevertebral ganglia, and the umbilical ganglia.

3. Still farther removed from the vertebral chain of gan- 169
glia are the *visceral*, *terminal*, or *automatic* ganglia, which are found in the several viscera,—the liver, kidneys, spleen, pancreas, intestines, and blood-vessels. In the intestines there are two sets of these ganglia,—one between the two muscular layers, *Auerbach's* plexus, controlling the intestinal muscles; and another lying beneath the mucous membrane, *Meissner's* plexus. The latter controls both the intestinal glands and the involuntary muscular fibers of the villi.

The Splanchnics.

The vertebral ganglia are connected with the 170
three sets of prevertebral ganglia by *visceral* or *splanchnic* nerves, which may be properly termed the *thoracic*, the *abdominal*, and the *pelvic splanchnics*. The splanchnics are in the chest known as the

three *cardiac nerves;* in the abdomen, as the *great, lesser,* and *least splanchnics.*

171 A rich supply of sympathetic nerve branches connects the prevertebral ganglia with the automatic ganglia, following the blood-vessels in their minutest ramifications.

172 **Functions of the Sympathetic.** Every ganglion is a brain, and stores up energy to be afterward used in some way in exciting or controlling some form of vital activity in the subordinate structures associated with it.

173 The prevertebral ganglia, or gangliated plexuses, act, perhaps, as reorganizing centers, receiving impulses from all parts of the body and sending them out again to the same and other parts, thus maintaining a constant universal reaction to all sorts of physical impressions received from without.

174 The distal, automatic, or visceral ganglia preside over the minute details of vital work, each controlling its own little sphere of activity.

175 The sympathetic nervous system presides over the processes of secretion and excretion, all gland action, and also the circulation. This fact alone gives to the sympathetic practical control over all the processes of nutrition and organic change, as well as of voluntary activity. Through the grasp of the sympathetic upon the cerebral circulation, mental activity, even consciousness, is under its control.

176 The automatic ganglia of the heart, the intestines, the blood- and lymph-vessels, the Fallopian tubes, and the uterus are capable of independent activity, and may perform their functions when cut off from all connection with other nerve centers, although they are, under ordinary conditions, influenced in the direction of either inhibition or excitation by nerves received from the central nervous system.

177 It is through the influence upon the great sympathetic of thermic and percutient applications to the skin that the most remarkable effects of hydrotherapy are obtained. Through the powerful impressions that may be made upon this portion of the nervous system by external and internal applications of

water, every nutritive process, indeed every vital process taking place within the body, may be modified, being augmented or retarded as circumstances may require.[8]

ANIMAL HEAT.

Since hydrotherapy consists, for the most part, in procedures which have for their object the making of thermic impressions upon the skin, it is evident that a correct knowledge of the phenomena and mechanism of heat production and regulation in the human body is essential to a proper appreciation of the methods and principles of hydrotherapy. Recent advances have been made toward the solution of the numerous difficult problems involved in the subject of heat production and regulation, which render this study especially important, interesting, and profitable from a practical point of view. 178

Sources of Animal Heat. The heat of the body is wholly derived from foods, which, as has been shown by careful calorimetric studies, produce, when completely oxidized within the body, practically the same amount of heat and energy that would be generated by their combustion outside the body. The actual caloric value is about twenty per cent. less than the estimated amount. 179

A study of the heat-producing properties of the various elements of food shows that an ounce of dried albumin produces in the body sufficient heat to raise nearly 680 pounds of water one degree in temperature; an ounce of fat produces eighty per cent. more heat, or sufficient to raise 1,200 pounds of water one degree; and an ounce of starch produces a little more than four fifths as much as an ounce of albumin, or sufficient to raise 550 pounds of water one degree F. 180

The combustion, or oxidation, of food is not direct in the body, as in a furnace, but occurs as a process of disassimilation, under the influence of special ferments which operate under the control of nerves and nerve centers. Oxygen is assimilated, CO_2 is excreted. Heat is the result of the tearing 181 down of molecules, and the reappearance in the form of molecular vibration of the energy that was previously employed in holding the molecules together in the organized state. These changes take place in all the tissues, and even, as recently shown, in the blood to some extent.[4]

182 The total amount of heat produced in the body each twenty-four hours is 2,500,000 gram centigrade calories, or sufficient to raise 10,000 pounds of water one degree F. in temperature, or to raise from the temperature of freezing to the normal body temperature, the body of a man weighing 170 pounds. This amount of heat would be obtained by the complete oxidation within the body of eighteen ounces of starch or a little less than half that quantity of fat. The generation of this large amount of heat within the body is necessary in order to maintain its temperature.

Cold-Blooded and Warm-Blooded Animals.

183 Cold-blooded animals take the temperature of the medium in which they exist, or maintain but a slight difference between the body temperature and the surrounding medium, the temperature rising and falling with that of the water or the air. The frog, in water of 68° F. or less, maintains a temperature of from two or three degrees to a few tenths of a degree above the water. In warmer water its temperature is a little below that of the water.

184 The temperature of mollusks and fish may fall to 33° F., or scarcely a degree above the freezing-point, in ice-water.

185 Most mammals have a normal temperature near that of human beings; namely, 98.6°. There are a few exceptions. The mouse has a normal temperature of 100°; birds, from 107° to 111°.

186 A warm-blooded animal maintains its normal temperature independently of the temperature of the surrounding medium within the limits of its usual conditions of life; and even when exposed to extreme or unusual temperatures, its organism struggles against any marked change of temperature until its powers of heat regulation or production are exhausted.

A young child approaches somewhat the condition of a cold-blooded animal in its susceptibility to the influence of external temperatures. This fact should be kept in mind in the employment of hydriatic processes with infants and young children. The ability to react to cold, and to adjust the body temperature to that of the environment, increases with age during the early years of life. 187

The Normal Temperature in Man.

Different observers report varying figures, but the normal temperature of man is generally considered to be approximately 98.6° F. in the axilla, the normal limits of variation being 97.2° and 99.5°. The temperature of the mouth is about .5° higher than that of the axilla, and that of the rectum and the vagina a degree higher than that of the mouth. 188

The temperature of the surface varies considerably; that of the various internal organs varies less, yet to a marked extent. 189

Surface Temperatures.

With the temperature of the room about 68°, Kunkel found the temperature of various parts of the body surface to be as follows:— 190

	Centigrade.	*Fahrenheit.*
Forehead	34.1–34.4°	93.38–93.92°
Cheek	34.4°	93.92°
Tip of ear	28.8°	83.64°
Back of hand	32.5–33.2°	90.5 –91.76°
Hollow of hand (closed)	34.8–35.1°	94.64–96.18°
Hollow of hand (open)	34.4–34.8°	93.92–94.64°
Forearm	34.3°	93.74°
Sternum	34.4°	93.92°
Pectoral region	34.7°	94.46°
Right iliac fossa	34.4°	93.92°
Upper part of thigh	34.2°	93.56°
Calf	33.6°	92.48°

The temperature of the skin is higher over muscle than over bone; over an artery than over a tendon; over an active organ than over an organ at rest. The skin of the forehead has a higher temperature than that of the occiput.

191 **Internal Temperatures.** Davy and others give the following as the temperatures found in various internal parts:—

Brain	104° F.
Left ventricle	107° F.
Right ventricle	106° F.
Liver	106.5° F.
Rectum	100° F.

192 The average temperature of the blood is about 102° F. The average temperature of the venous blood is nearly two degrees lower than that of the arterial blood. The temperature of the blood in the carotid artery is from one to four degrees higher than that in the jugular vein; in the crural artery it is from one and a half to two degrees above that of the crural vein. The coolest blood in the body is that coming from the nose and the ears. The external temperature is ten or twelve degrees below the internal (Senator).

193 The temperature varies with age; that of the infant or child is normally about one degree higher than that of the adult. After the age of thirty, the temperature gradually falls to about one degree below the average standard, while in very advanced age it rises one degree.

HEAT PRODUCTION.

194 Heat production in the body is the result of vital work. Every organ and cell participates in the work of generating animal heat. The higher the degree of activity, the greater the rate of heat production. Those organs that are most active functionally produce the greatest amount of heat.

195 In the hepatic vein during digestion the temperature is 3° or 4° F. higher than in the portal vein. The blood leaving a muscle when in a state of rest is ordinarily about .4° F. higher than that supplied to it. When the muscle is active, the difference is three times as great, or about 1.3° F.

196 The body of the average man produces each minute sufficient heat to raise seven pounds of water 1° F. in temperature. In the horse and the dog, the rate of heat

production per pound of body weight is about the same. In a child weighing fifteen pounds, the heat production is twice as great; in the guinea-pig, five times as great. In the mouse the rate of heat production is twelve times greater, and in the sparrow, twenty-four times greater, than in man. The rate of heat production in an animal appears to increase with the extension of its superficial surface.

Heat production is more active in strong and robust than 197
in weak persons. It is more active in young persons or young animals than in adult persons or full-grown animals, because of the larger proportion of radiating surface and the consequent necessity for greater heat production to retain a normal temperature.

Conditions that Increase Heat Production, and the Tendency to Temperature Rise.

There are various conditions that profoundly 198
affect the process of heat production, each of which must be recognized and remembered in dealing with febrile cases. These conditions may be enumerated as follows:—

1. *Glandular Activity.*—Freshly secreted saliva is found 199
to have a temperature of 2.7° F. above that of the blood in the carotid artery. The blood of the renal vein is warmer than that of the renal artery. Blood in the hepatic vein during digestion may have a temperature three or four degrees higher than that of the portal vein, though at other times the difference is but one degree, or even less.

2. *Muscular Activity.*—The temperature of an oarsman 200
was found to be 104° after rowing one and one-fourth miles (Experiment 1). Heat production is increased by exercise, according to Helmholtz, from 7.5 to 18.1 heat units per minute. Strong shivering also increases heat production.

3. *Mental Activity.*—Mental activity has less effect on 201
temperature than muscular or glandular activity, but an increase of one half a degree has been observed as the result of vigorous mental effort.

4. *Digestive Activity.*—Langlois proved that heat pro- 202
duction is increased thirty-five or forty per cent. during digestion. The body temperature often rises half a degree.

The contents of the stomach may have a somewhat lower temperature during digestion, owing to the fact that heat is rendered latent by the changes taking place in the food, and the low temperature at which a considerable proportion of the food is usually eaten.

203 5. *Brief Applications of Cold Water* (Exp. 2).

204 6. *A Low External Temperature.*—A temperature of 40° F. and below causes increased heat production when the body is so exposed as to cause shivering or a goose-flesh appearance. If these symptoms, which are due to muscular action, do not appear, heat production is not increased, and may even be diminished. Prolonged cold applications lessen heat production in fever.

205 7. *A High External Temperature.*—This causes, for a time at least, increased heat production through the increased tissue activity induced. The rate of heat production begins to rise slowly at 60° F., although temperatures between 60° and 70° F. may be regarded as practically neutral in their effects. Voit fixed the exact neutral point in men at 58° F. Page found the neutral point in dogs to be 77° F. With an external temperature of 104° F. the rate of heat production was three and one-half times the normal.

The influence of external temperature upon heat production is a matter of great practical importance in dealing with many classes of morbid conditions, and especially fevers.

Conditions that Decrease Heat Production.

The following conditions decrease heat production:—

206 1. *Fasting.*—Abstinence from food has a decided influence upon the temperature. At first the temperature falls one or two degrees, then marked emaciation is developed, and shortly before death the temperature declines rapidly. Fasting and badly nourished patients have little heat-making power, and bear cold applications badly.

207 2. *Sleep.*—The temperature falls half a degree or more during sleep. It is for this reason that the temperature is

usually higher at night than in the morning. The morning temperature is higher in a person who works at night and sleeps during the day. In hibernation the heat production is diminished to such an extent that the absorption of oxygen is less than one fortieth as much as during normal activity, and the elimination of CO_2 only one seventy-fifth the normal amount. According to Helmholtz, the amount of heat production is only one third that during rest when awake, or 2.4 heat units per minute as compared with 7.5.

3. Short applications of heat lessen heat production 208
while increasing heat elimination, and thereby cause a decline in the body temperature.

HEAT REGULATION.

Modern researches upon this subject apparently demon- 209
strate that the heat-producing and heat-regulating mechanism of the body consists of three elements,—*thermogenic centers*, *thermogenic nerves*, and *thermogenic tissues*.

Of the thermogenic centers there are three classes:—

1. *The automatic centers*, located in the spinal cord, which 210
have immediate charge of the thermogenic tissues, and under the control of which the process of heat production is carried on.

2. Accelerator centers, located in the brain, which in- 211
crease heat production by stimulating the automatic centers.

3. Inhibitory centers, also located in the brain, which 212
restrain the action of the automatic centers.

The automatic centers appear to be entirely uninfluenced 213
by the various forms of stimuli which influence the body temperature, while the regulating centers in the brain are extremely sensitive to such stimuli.

The Mechanism of Heat Regulation.

The inhibitory thermogenic centers of the 214
brain appear to rule in a remarkable manner a group of important functions which are utilized in heat dissipation when it is necessary to combat a tendency to temperature rise. These are—

1. Diminished production of heat through inhibition of the automatic thermogenic centers.

2. Increased activity of the heart.

3. Dilatation of the surface vessels.

4. Increase of cutaneous secretion.

5. Increased rate of breathing.

215 Heat applied to the skin acts reflexly through the nerves, and a blood temperature above normal acts directly upon the nerve cells. These two causes excite the inhibitory centers. Cold applied to the skin, and a lower temperature of the blood, in like manner excite the accelerator centers. These centers in turn diminish or increase the activity of the automatic centers of the cord, as may be required to maintain the particular temperature which the system itself seems to establish as the standard for a given set of conditions or circumstances. In sleep, for example, the temperature is lower than during waking hours, and in fever the standard for the body temperature is set higher than normal.

216 The blood is a circulating medium which is used not only to convey nutrient material from the stomach to the tissues, and excrementitious matter from the tissues to the excretory glands, but for the purpose of equalizing the temperature, conveying the surplus heat of the interior of the body to the surface, where it may be dissipated by conduction, radiation, and evaporation. Nearly nine tenths of the daily heat loss occurs from the skin. By the increased rate of heart beat, the complete exchange of blood between the center and the periphery takes place more frequently, and the blood is thus more rapidly cooled.

217 By active dilatation of the surface vessels a larger surface is exposed to the cooling influences that act upon the skin. The surface over which the blood is spread is not fully represented by the seventeen square feet of skin surface, but rather by the eleven thousand square feet of surface over which the capillaries are spread in the walls of the perspiratory tubules, —six times the surface presented by the lungs.

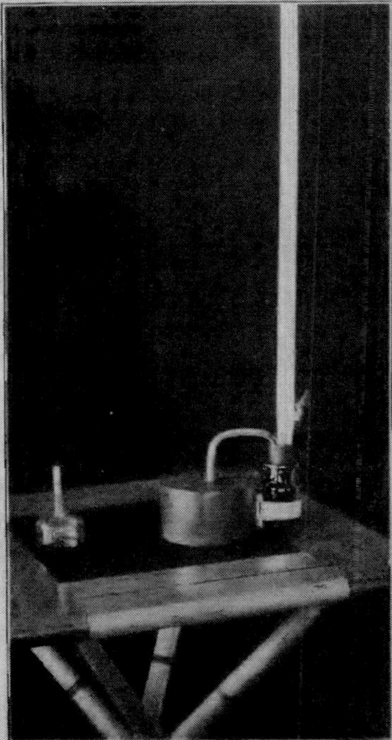

Fig. 21. FEVER CALORIMETER (p. 88). (Kellogg)

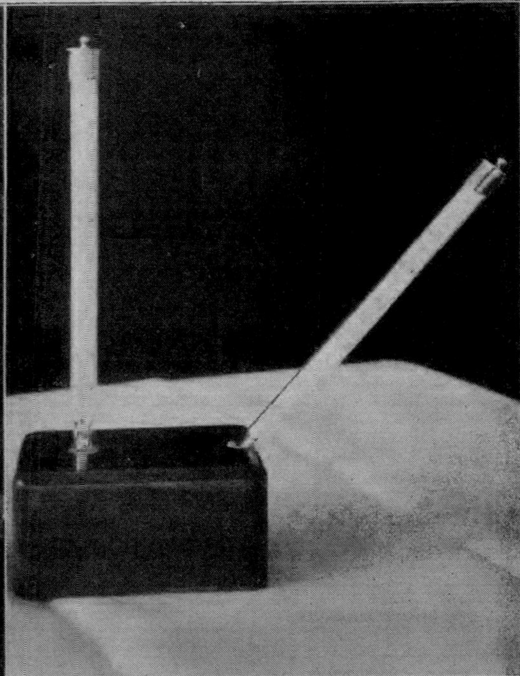

Fig. 22. FEVER CALORIMETER (p. 89). (Winternitz)

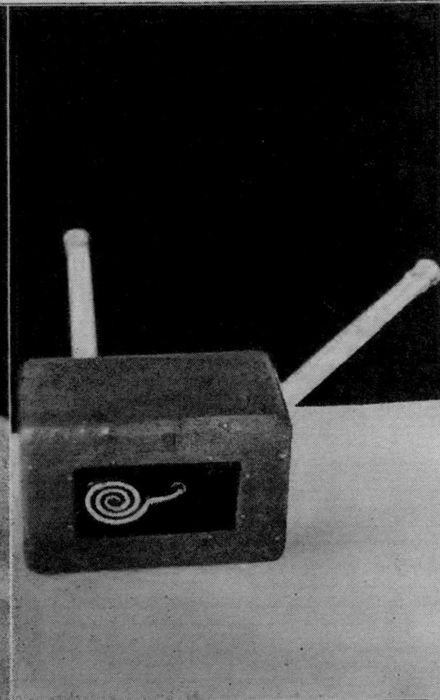

Fig. 23. FEVER CALORIMETER (p. 89). (Winternitz)

One seventh of the total heat loss by the skin is due to evaporation. Evaporation of the increased amount of water brought to the surface by profuse sweating enormously increases the heat loss. Each ounce of water evaporated from the skin absorbs heat sufficient to raise the temperature of about seventy pounds of water one degree Fahrenheit. By various means the amount of perspiration may be increased to two or three pounds an hour. 218

The increase of respiratory activity increases heat loss, not only by the increased amount of the air that is warmed, but by the evaporation of water from the two thousand square feet of surface presented by the pulmonary mucous membrane. 219

In like manner the thermogenic centers control a number of mechanisms by which heat production is increased and heat loss lessened. When cold is applied to the surface, or when the temperature of the blood is lowered, the accelerator thermogenic center is excited, and as the result — 220

1. The automatic thermogenic centers of the spinal cord are excited to increased heat production.

2. The heart's action is slowed.

3. The surface vessels contract.

4. Perspiration is checked.

5. The erector pili and other involuntary muscles of the skin contract, lessening the conductivity of the skin.

6. The respiratory movements are slowed.

The automatic thermogenic centers of the spine are excited by the accelerator center of the brain, and stimulate the thermogenic tissues to increased activity, thus increasing heat production; the decreased activity of the heart lessens the rate at which the blood is sent to the surface; the contracted vessels of the skin diminish the area of blood exposed to cooling influences, thereby lessening evaporation and heat loss; the contraction of the erector pili, by increasing the firmness of the skin, decreases its conductivity; the diminished respiratory movement lessens the amount of air heated by the 221 lungs, through which more than ten per cent. of the total loss of heat occurs. Thus, by the combined action of these various mechanisms, loss of heat is diminished while its production is increased.

222 **Heat Production and Heat Dissipation Associated.** It is interesting to note that the functions of heat production and heat dissipation are reciprocal. If heat dissipation is suddenly increased by a reflex influence acting upon the heat-regulating center, heat production is also at once increased, and measures are set in operation to conserve the body heat; while, on the other hand, if heat production is unduly increased, heat dissipation is immediately increased. Every agent that tends to increase heat dissipation, at the same time reflexly excites heat production; and whatever diminishes heat dissipation, likewise, by reflex action, diminishes heat production. This action of the thermogenic centers, whereby heat production is increased or diminished, occurs independently of any effect upon the circulation.

223 A simple illustration will make clear the necessity for this apparently paradoxical relation of heat production and heat elimination. A healthy man, whose temperature, heat production, and heat elimination are normal, is made to perspire so freely that water is evaporated from the surface of his skin at the rate of one and a half pounds an hour. The amount of heat absorbed by the water in evaporation would be about 1,500 pound Fahrenheit heat units. At the normal rate of heat production — seven heat units per minute — there should have been produced within one hour 420 units of heat. Subtracting this from 1,500, we have a net loss of 1,080 heat units, provided there were no increase of heat production. Suppose the patient's weight to be 160 pounds, his temperature would be lowered 6.75°. Upon examination of the patient's temperature, however, we find it to be normal. It is evident, then, that he has produced within the hour 6.75 heat units for each pound of his body weight, in addition to the usual amount, thus preventing the fall of temperature.

The special thermogenic tissues are found in the muscles, in which heat production is constantly taking place through the connection of these tissues with the automatic centers of the spine by means of the thermogenic nerves. Heat is constantly produced in the muscles even when at rest. When the muscle is active, four fifths of the energy consumed appears as heat, and only the remaining fifth as muscular energy. The muscles are the chief seat of heat production. They store up glycogen for heat and work. 224

Water-Bath Calorimeter.

In the clinical study of the phenomena of animal heat there has long been need for a calorimeter which could be used at the bedside. Several years ago (1890), while engaged in instructing a class of medical students in hydrotherapy, the author employed a common bath-tub for this purpose.* 225

The method is a very simple one. Water is placed in a common full bath-tub, in a room of nearly constant temperature, in quantity sufficient to immerse the patient, all but the head. The water should be carefully weighed, and its temperature accurately determined. This may be fixed at a convenient point. It must be some degrees below the body temperature, and should not be too far removed from the room temperature. The temperature of the room should be about 70° to 80° F., and as constant as possible. 226

After placing the water in the tub, it should be thoroughly stirred for fifteen minutes with a wooden paddle having a thermometer attached. Careful note should be taken of the temperature of the water every five minutes. By this means the rate of the cooling may be ascertained. It is evident that the body of a person placed in the bath will give off heat to the water, and the rate of cooling be thus diminished. By a simple calculation the rate of heat elimination by the body may be readily estimated in both normal and pathological conditions. This is a very practical and accurate method (Exp. 3, 4, 5).

---

*Since writing the above, the author has learned that Liebermeister employed the same simple calorimeter thirty years ago.

227 **The Author's Fever Calorimeter.** The author has recently (1899) devised a convenient instrument for determining quickly and approximately the rate of heat elimination in a patient under examination as compared with a normal individual. The instrument may be briefly described as follows: —

It consists of two parts (Fig. 21, *a* and *b*); first, a glass cylinder one inch in length, and of such diameter as to give its bottom an area of three square inches, making its cubic capacity three cubic inches. This cylinder is protected by a solid wooden case an inch in thickness, which may be readily removed. It is connected with a small bottle filled with colored liquid, through the cork of which is passed a piece of barometer tubing 75 cm. in length, which serves as an indicator. A scale placed behind the barometer tubing marks the height to which the column of colored liquid rises.

This instrument is extremely sensitive. When applied to the surface of the body, the column of liquid rises with great rapidity, to a greater or less height according to the temperature of the surface.

In the use of this calorimeter, the temperature of the surface is taken at the same time by a surface thermometer. The time for reaching the maximum is noted. This determines the time required to raise a given quantity of air — three cubic inches — a determined number of degrees in temperature (the difference between the room temperature and the surface temperature) by the heat thrown off from a definite area of the skin — three square inches. By means of the data thus obtained and the use of the formula given elsewhere (page 316) for determining the skin area of a body of given weight, a numerical basis is found for comparison of the amount of heat loss by a person who is in a febrile state as compared with that by a healthy person. In one patient examined with this instrument, heat elimination was found to be nearly double the normal, although the temperature was 102° F.

The Fever Calorimeter of Winternitz.

This instrument (Fig. 22) consists of two thermometers placed in a chamber with thick wooden walls, about four inches square on the inside. The chamber is open on one side, and one of the thermometers rests upon the skin when the instrument is in position with the open side next the skin. The other thermometer determines the temperature of the air in the chamber. With this instrument Winternitz has made a series of most interesting observations respecting the influence of friction and other measures upon heat elimination. This instrument, of which the writer learned on a recent visit to Vienna and Kaltenleutgeben (summer of 1899), is of great use, and renders invaluable service in the prosecution of physiological researches respecting heat elimination (Fig. 23). 228

D'Arsonval's Calorimeter.

D' Arsonval, of Paris, has devised a convenient and portable calorimeter (Fig. 24), which, while less exact than the water-bath calorimeter, is so convenient and portable that it should be briefly described, as it is an appliance which the writer has found of service in the scientific study of hydrotherapy. A cylindrical chamber made of pasteboard or binder's pressboard receives the subject. The chamber is about two and one-half feet in diameter, and about six feet in height. An opening of proper size is made in the top, and in this opening a small anemometer is placed. 229

The patient to be tested stands up while the cylindrical chamber is lifted over his head (Exp.6,7). Through a few openings in the bottom of the cylinder a current of air is allowed to pass in and through it. Coming in contact with the patient, the air is warmed and made to pass upward; and in passing out through the anemometer, its mechanism is set in operation, and a record is made upon the dial which indicates the rate at which the air current travels in passing through the instrument. It is also easy to estimate the volume of the air that has passed through the cylinder in a given time. The greater the amount of heat elimination, the more rapid will be the movement of the anemometer, and in a given time the greater the amount of heat eliminated.

This instrument is a convenient and interesting one, but we have found it much less accurate and more cumbersome than the fever calorimeter previously described, and it is certainly considerably less exact than the bath-tub calorimeter.

230 **Fever.** Fever is due to the disturbance of the heat-regulating centers. Such disturbances may result from three classes of causes; viz., (1) toxic substances, (2) nervous impressions, (3) changes in the temperature of the blood. Fever is no longer, as formerly, regarded in the light of an unmitigated evil, and to be combated irrespective of other symptoms, as it has been clearly shown that a rise of temperature is, at least in some cases, curative in its tendency. It is the result of a curative effort on the part of the body. It is not the fever, but the cause of the fever, that we must combat. An infected frog dies without rise of temperature.

The temperature has been known to rise as much as 15° above the normal in pathological conditions, and even a higher temperature has been noted just before death. Recovery rarely occurs when the temperature exceeds 107° F.

231 In fever, the functions of the heat-regulating centers are so greatly disturbed that influences which, under ordinary conditions, would not affect the body temperature, may occasion a rise of temperature of several degrees. In other words, there is, in fever, a disablement of the heat-regulating centers of such a character that the generation and elimination of heat are not properly controlled, and there is a marked loss of resistance to the causes of thermic disturbance in both directions.

232 **Influence of a Warm Atmosphere upon Heat Production.** A warm atmosphere in febrile conditions tends far more than in health to cause rise of temperature, both by decreasing heat elimination and by increasing heat production. Under normal conditions an atmospheric temperature continuously above 60° F., as elsewhere remarked, tends to

increase heat production, and at a temperature of 104° F. heat production is increased to more than three times the normal amount. In health this increase of heat production is of course very largely balanced by increased heat elimination; but in fever this balance is not maintained. The skin in fever is commonly dry under conditions which in health would induce profuse perspiration. Hence heat elimination is greatly diminished. Fortunately, heat production is increased much less in fever than in the normal state, when an equal rise of body temperature is induced by exposure to hot air or by exercise. If heat production were increased in fever to anything like the degree that the elevation of temperature might lead us to expect, the temperature would rise much higher than it does, because of the disproportionately small increase of heat elimination.

From the foregoing, the importance of proper regulation of the temperature of the air surrounding the patient in fever cases is apparent. A cold atmosphere, that is, air at a temperature below 60° F., increases heat production in fever, but to a less degree than in health. The neutral temperature for air is from 58° to 68°, while for water it is from 92° to 95°.

Exercise, either muscular or mental, even so slight as sit- 233
ting up in bed or conversing with a visitor, will affect the temperature by increasing heat production, sometimes to a very unusual degree, and may even cause relapse when a patient is just convalescing from a fever.

Although the body is at rest in bed, there is usually in 234
fever great activity in the thermogenic tissues. The predominating feature in fever is increased heat production.

Relation of Heat Production to Temperature.

For each degree centigrade (1.8° F.) elevation 235
of body temperature there is ordinarily an increase of heat production of six per cent., according to Liebermeister, or 3.3 per cent. for each degree Fahrenheit. The following table represents the percentage increase for each degree Fahrenheit within the ordinary range of fever temperatures:—

Temperature.	*Percentage Increase of Heat Production above Normal.*
98.6° F.	0
100° F.	4.6
101° F.	8.0
102° F.	11.3
103° F.	14.7
104° F.	18.0
105° F.	21.3
106° F.	24.7
107° F.	28.0

236 **Modifications of the Thermic Functions Which Cause Change of Body Temperature.** Heat dissipation is generally increased in fever, but in less proportion than heat production. When the skin is red and moist, heat elimination is more than three times the normal. The body temperature represents not the amount of either heat production or heat elimination, but the balance that is at the moment maintained between these two functions.[7]

The following table shows the various relative conditions that may result in increase or decrease of the body temperature :—

237 CONDITIONS UNDER WHICH RISE OF BODY TEMPERATURE MAY OCCUR.

1. Increased heat production with increased heat elimination. (Heat production increased more than heat elimination.)
2. Increased heat production with normal heat elimination.
3. Increased heat production with decreased heat elimination.
4. Normal heat production with diminished heat elimination.
5. Diminished heat production with diminished heat elimination. (Heat elimination diminished more than heat production.)

CONDITIONS UNDER WHICH DEPRESSION OF BODY TEMPERATURE MAY OCCUR.

1. Diminished heat production with diminished heat elimination. (Heat production diminished more than heat elimination.)
2. Diminished heat production with normal heat elimination.
3. Diminished heat production with increased heat elimination.
4. Normal heat production with increased heat elimination.
5. Increased heat production with increased heat elimination. (Heat elimination increased more than heat production.)

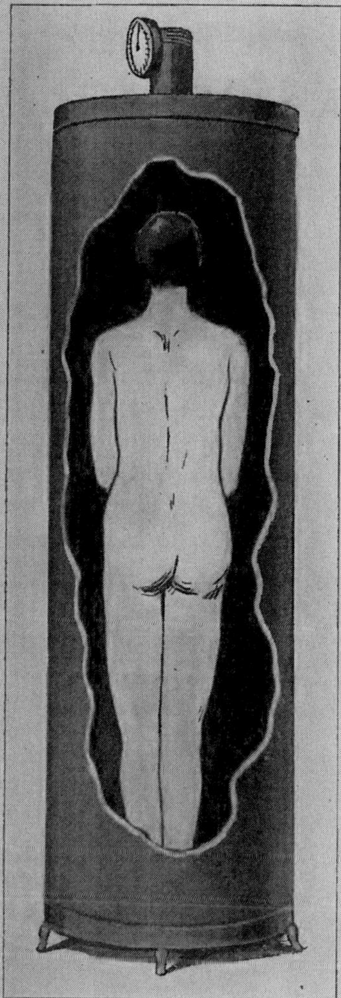

FIG. 24. CALORIMETER OF D'ARSONVAL (p. 89)

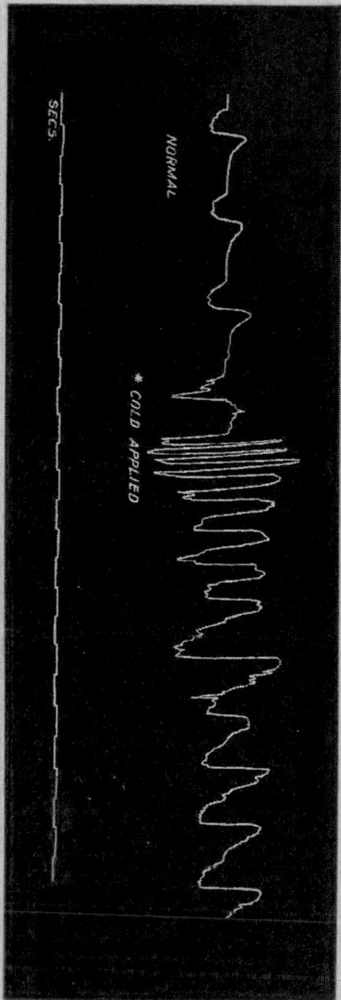

FIG. 26. PNEOGRAPHIC TRACING (p. 110).

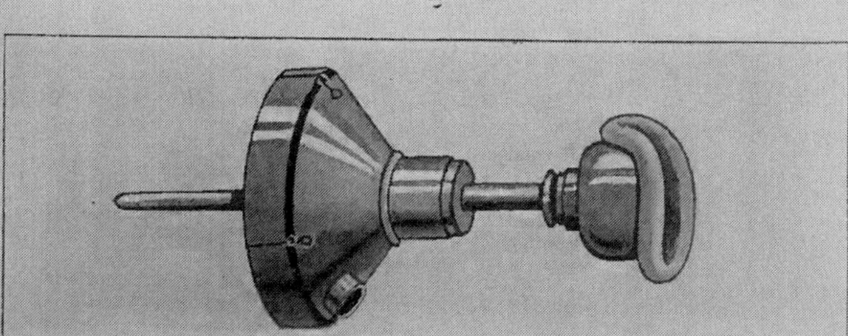

FIG. 25. PNEOGRAPH (p. 110). (Kellogg)

Control of Heat Functions.

The temperature may be reduced in fever either by diminishing heat production or increasing heat elimination, or by both means combined; and therapeutic applications may be made in such a manner as to influence either of these processes, or both of them. 238

It may not be out of place just here to mention the leading physiological means by which fever may be controlled; viz., rest, fasting, water drinking, regulation of air temperature, hydrotherapy.

A careful study of the influence of cutaneous irritation, 239
thermic applications, and changes in the condition of the blood-vessels of the skin has been made by Pospischil. The following are some of the interesting results obtained:—

Short, cold shower baths increased heat elimination to the 240
amount of from twenty-five to sixty-six per cent., according as the patient rested or exercised after the application; cold, wet rubbing caused increased heat elimination to the extent of eighty per cent.; mechanical irritation or friction produced a still greater heat loss,—ninety-five per cent.; agents producing a "goose flesh" appearance of the skin were found to diminish heat elimination more than forty-four per cent.; weak chemical irritants produced increased heat elimination to the extent of forty per cent., five times more than strong chemical irritants.

Both heat production and heat dissipation may be influ- 241
enced by various antipyretic drugs, but the effect thus produced is purely toxic in character, and involves not simply the heat-producing or heat-regulating centers, but other nerve centers as well, and thus lessens the resistance of the body and the activity of the reparative processes by which the remedial forces of the system seek to effect a cure. It is encouraging to note that the pernicious effects of fever-controlling drugs of all kinds are being recognized by physicians at the present time, and that reliance is being placed on those physiological antipyretic measures whereby the end

sought may be safely and far more efficiently attained than by the use of drugs. It is safe to predict that when these rational means of combating fevers of all types are more thoroughly understood and more generally used, the mortality from this class of diseases will be reduced to less than one third the present rate.

The experimental researches of Maragliano have shown that quinine, antipyrine, thallin, and salicylic acid cause reduction in temperature by inducing a most pronounced dilatation of the cutaneous vessels. Alcohol operates in the same way. All of these drugs depress the heart as well as the vessels, and seriously interfere with the healing process, and therefore their use is irrational and unphysiological.

Incidentally it may be mentioned that in dealing with fever by any method, it is always important to give attention to the cause of the condition, which may be simple exposure to excessive heat, sunstroke, violent exercise, exhaustion (fatigue fever), a cold (retained excretions), toxemia from the use of decomposing food or the decomposition of food by long retention in the alimentary canal, uric acid, toxins produced in infectious disease, local inflammation, gastritis, peritonitis, infected surgical wounds, nervous impressions, etc.

Heat Production after Death. The temperature may rise four or five degrees after death from tetanus or hydrophobia, oxidation and heat production continuing until all the oxygen remaining in the tissues has been consumed.

THE PHYSIOLOGICAL EFFECTS OF EXTERNAL AND INTERNAL APPLICATIONS OF WATER.

AS elsewhere remarked, Currie was the first to observe 242
and study the physiological and therapeutic uses of water in a thoroughly scientific way, he having the advantage over his predecessors in possessing a thermometer, the invention of John Hunter, whereby the temperature of the animal body might be accurately ascertained.

Soon after (1801), Henry Wilson Lockette, of Virginia, 243
published a report of important observations and experiments.

Next, Fleury, in France, conducted an extensive series of 244
researches as to the effects of water upon internal and external temperatures, making a special study of its tonic effects. His labors placed the use of the cold douche upon a scientific basis. Indeed, the efforts of Louis Fleury in this direction were so extensive and thorough that although Scoutetten, a military physician who was sent by the French government to study the work of Priessnitz, and who introduced the science of hydrotherapy into France, remarked in 1843, "Hydrotherapy is not a new medical system, but it may be made such," Raige Delorme wrote less than ten years later, "Thanks to L. Fleury, hydrotherapeutic medical practice must take its place in rational therapeutics."

Dr. John Bell, of Philadelphia, published in 1850 his re- 245
markable work on "Baths."

Schüller published in 1874 the results of a remarkable 246
series of experiments made upon trephined rabbits, in which he demonstrated the effects upon the internal circulation of thermic and mechanical applications to the surface.

Vinaj, in 1892, reported experiments upon a man whose 247
brain had been exposed by an accident, which confirmed the observations of Schüller on trephined rabbits, respecting the influence upon the brain and circulation of thermic applica-

tions to the skin in various parts and under various temperatures. These experiments of Schüller and Vinaj laid the foundation for our exact knowledge of the effects of cutaneous thermic and mechanical applications upon the circulation of the viscera.

248 The physiological effects of water are due to those qualities which enable it to be used—

1. As a nutrient, entering into the composition of every structure, and serving a useful purpose in nearly every function, especially as a vehicle for conveying food material to the tissues and removing wastes.

2. As a means of abstracting heat from the body by contact and by evaporation.

3. As a means of communicating heat to the body.

4. As a means of producing certain mechanical or percutient effects.

249 Similar effects may be obtained by other agents which are capable of impressing the system in like manner, as, for example, hot and cold air, hot vapor, the electric light, sunlight, and friction or percussion of the skin administered either by the hands of an attendant or mechanically. These means, because of the kindred effects produced by them, are universally employed in connection with water in hydrotherapy, and hence will be considered in connection with measures which are more strictly hydriatic in character.

The General Effects of Thermic Irritation upon the Circulation.

250 A very large proportion of the applications of water made to the surface of the body depend for their efficiency upon the fact that the skin is reflexly connected with the interior of the body, each portion of the skin periphery being associated, through the nerve centers which supply it with nerve filaments, with some special visceral periphery or vascular area.

251 In the study of the reflex effects of water upon the internal structures, it should be noted that whatever effect is produced upon a vascular area of the skin, is likewise produced

in the internal vascular area associated with it. The intensity of the effect produced in the internal area, is, however, generally less intense than that produced upon the surface, although this is by no means always the case.

It must be remembered, however, that in addition to the 252
reflex effect produced, there is also produced a mechanical effect, which is commonly the reverse of the reflex effect. The real effect is the sum of these two effects, and depends upon the relative intensity of the two actions. The effects of external applications of water may thus be simply divided into two classes,— reflex and mechanical.

Any sort of irritation of the cutaneous nerves which gives 253
rise to contraction of the blood-vessels of the surface, whether cold, heat, friction, percussion, pinching, or mechanical irritation, likewise causes contraction of the small blood-vessels of the interior of the body, stimulating the accelerator nerves of both the blood-vessels (vasoconstrictors) and the heart.

The duration of the reflex effect depends upon the inten- 254
sity of the stimulant and of the irritant, and also upon the area involved. When the cutaneous vessels of a large portion of the surface of the body are excited to contraction by cold, heat, friction, or otherwise, the contraction of the interior vessels is exceedingly brief. It may, indeed, be of so short duration as to escape notice. The reason for this is the development of the mechanical effect (**252**).

If the surface area to which the application is made is 255
small, the reflex effect may be confined to the internal area in sympathetic relation therewith (**349**), and will be greater and more prolonged for the reason that the reflex influence being concentrated upon the circumscribed area, the mechanical effect is distributed over the rest of the body, so it does not overshadow and wipe out, so to speak, the reflex effect on the smaller area involved.

The mechanical effect is necessarily the reverse of the 256
reflex; for when the blood-vessels of the skin are made to contract as the result of the application of an irritant of any

sort, there is an inrush of blood to the interior of the body causing mechanical distension of the internal parts. This effect follows more or less quickly the primary, universal constriction of the small vessels according to the intensity of the irritation and the extent of the application. A knowledge of these facts, to which we are chiefly indebted to Schüller and Vinaj, affords us a rational basis for the explanation of nearly all the phenomena resulting from hydriatic procedures.[3]

THE PHYSIOLOGICAL EFFECTS OF COLD.

257 **Is Cold a Sedative or an Excitant?** Cold is a vital depressant. Under all circumstances and in all modes of application this is its primary and intrinsic effect. The discussion of the question whether cold is primarily a stimulant or a depressant began soon after the first publications of Currie, and waxed especially warm half a century ago. The controversy doubtless grew out of the fact that those who maintained cold to be a stimulant, failed to observe that its so-called tonic, or stimulant, effects were reflex and secondary results.

258 A low temperature, in whatever way produced, checks cell or protoplasmic activity. This may readily be seen by a microscopic study of the pond ameba, the white blood-corpuscle, or the heart of the embryo of a chick, the movements of which are at once suspended when the temperature is lowered, but begin again with the application of heat by means of the warming stage.

259 **Hibernation.** The life processes of warm-blooded animals are slowed when the body temperature falls a few degrees below the normal standard of temperature for the individual class or species of animals under investigation. This accounts for the phenomena of hibernation. In a bear in the state of hibernation the temperature has been found as low as 35° F., the pulse eight per minute, and the respiratory chest movements entirely suspended, showing almost complete cessation of vital activity. In this state, little waste of

tissue takes place, so that the animal may pass several weeks without eating or drinking.

In fishes, whose temperature is generally only a degree or 260
two above the water in which they live, the temperature may be reduced so low that actual freezing takes place, when there seems to be complete suspension of vital activity, but not actual death, the animal living in this condition for weeks and even months.*

The depressing influence of cold upon vital activity is 261
utilized in the preservation of food, the germs which give rise to putrefactive processes being unable to multiply and produce their peculiar ferments and toxins at a temperature of 32° F. It is through this depressing influence also that diphtheria, phlegmon, and other localized maladies, even cancer, may often be beneficially controlled by applications of ice to the affected parts. The activity of the perspiratory glands is at once checked by the application of cold to the skin, and so also is the secretion of gastric juice by the peptic glands when cold water is swallowed, as witnessed by Beaumont in his observations upon the stomach of Alexis St. Martin.

Hydriatric Measures Consist Chiefly of Thermic Applications.

In the study of the physiological effects of 262
water at different temperatures upon the various structures and organs of the body, the fact must be kept in mind that as employed in hydrotherapy, water is chiefly useful as a means of communicating heat to the body or abstracting heat from it. In its internal use, the thermic effects of water are supplemented by effects arising from its solvent and nutrient properties. In its external use, certain mechanical effects are added to its thermic effects in some forms of application, particularly the several varieties of the douche.

Heat and cold, as before remarked, are relative terms, 263
objects being recognized as cold when they have a temperature less than the zero of the temperature sense,—that is, the temperature of the skin,—and the reverse. For convenience,

however, in the study of the physiological effects of water, as well as in directing its therapeutic application, it is necessary to make use of terms more accurately indicative of the approximate temperature of the application. Those which have been most commonly applied are the following: *Very cold, cold, cool, tepid, warm, hot, very hot.*

264 The terms "temperate," "nauseating," "excessively hot," and "excessively cold" are used, especially by French hydrotherapeutists, but the utility of these terms is so restricted that we have eliminated them.

265 **Classification of Temperatures.** As the classification proposed is necessarily artificial and arbitrary, it is not easy to fix the exact limits of temperature to which each term should be applied, and this fact has given rise to considerable discussion and to a diversity of views. The following table is used by the author, and is found to be very convenient in practice: —

Very cold	32° to 55° F.
Cold	55° to 65° F.
Cool	65° to 80° F.
Tepid	80° to 92° F.
Warm (neutral, 92°–95°)	92° to 98° F.
Hot	98° to 104° F.
Very hot	104° and above.

266 The effects of applications at these various temperatures differ according to the part of the body to which the application is made, and the extent of surface involved.

267 Whether or not the final effect of a cold application is sedative or excitant, depends much on the mode of application and the temperature employed, but most of all on the length of the application and the state of the patient.

268 **Primary and Secondary Effects of Cold.** When a cold application is made to the body in any form, whether internally or externally, the first effect is a lessening of the activities of the living structures with which the cold medium comes in immediate contact. If the application is

continued for a long time, this vital depression continues likewise, and is maintained for a time after withdrawal of the application. The longer the application, the longer the depression that follows. Sooner or later, however, the parts return to their normal condition; and if the depression has not been so great and so prolonged as vitally to damage the parts, in the return to normal activity the pendulum swings, so to speak, beyond the normal line, so that for a time a higher degree of vital activity is maintained than before the application. This increased physiological activity is termed *reaction;* or as the writer will undertake to show later (435), *tonic reaction.*

When the cold application is a short one, the reaction **269** follows quickly, and is as much more intense as the application made is energetic; that is, *low in temperature* and with considerable pressure, as in the form of the douche.

The application may be so managed that the primary effect **270** or action — in other words the sedation — may be diminished; or the secondary effect — the reaction or state of excitation — may be diminished; or both may be lessened.

Cold applications may be made by means of ice, cold **271** water, cold air, or by the evaporation of water or other volatile liquids from the surface of the body, which may be either spontaneous or increased by a current of air. All these means are employed in hydrotherapy. The same principles apply, however, whatever the mode of application.

In discussing the physiological effects of cold applications, **272** Currie very well says ("Medical Reports," page 68) that it is "not the cold that stimulates, but the sensations which the cold produces." This may at first seem like a distinction without a difference, yet it seems to the writer that Currie was right. The intrinsic effect of cold is depressant, while that of heat is stimulant. Nevertheless, a recognition of the thermic impressions made upon the temperature nerves of the skin, through reflex influence provokes vital activities which serve to antagonize the depressing influence of the cold, which may in a given case so far overbalance these effects that the effects which are actually apparent are those of excitation instead of sedation.

273 All discussion respecting the mode of "action" of cold must cease with the recognition of the fact that it really has no vital action whatever, serving only as a physical agent to lower the temperature of those parts with which it comes in contact. Its so-called physiological action is wholly due to the action of the body itself,—first, in recognizing the presence of an agent that interferes with its functions, and is capable of injuring the integrity of its tissues; and secondly, in rallying its forces to repel the invader, or to avert the danger arising from its presence. While cold is primarily a depressing agent, its first contact with the skin gives rise to irritant phenomena through the protective reflex activities above referred to.

Effects of Peripheral Irritation.

274 A series of interesting experiments upon animals reported by Wertheimer, in 1893, showed that the general effects of excitation of the sensory nerves of the skin by cold are in accord with the general law relating to the reflex influence of peripheral irritants of all sorts,—chemical, electrical, etc.; namely, short and intense applications cause a brief preliminary contraction of the vessels of the internal viscera, which is quickly followed by dilatation of the same; while a prolonged, more moderate application of cold to the surface results in a renewed and prolonged contraction of the small vessels in the internal regions of the body.

275 This contraction is one of the several methods by which the body defends itself against injury from the loss of heat through the application of cold. By the slowing of the rate at which the blood passes through the internal organs, these organs are deprived of less heat than if the circulation were continued at the usual rate. The vessels of the skin being contracted at the same time, it is apparent that by this wise provision of nature the body is most efficiently protected against injury from cold.

Naumann, operating upon frogs, detached all portions of 276
one of the hind legs with the exception of the sciatic nerve, and then applied cold and irritating substances to the skin of the separated leg, and noted with the microscope the effects upon the mesenteric circulation. He observed that gentle irritation of the skin of the leg produced contraction of the vessels and quickened heart action, while strong irritation produced dilatation and slowed heart action from excitation of the vagus, the inhibitory nerve of the heart, and of the vasodilators, the inhibitory nerves of the vessels. These effects are general in the body.[10]

Schüller * found that the application of cold water to a 277
nerve trunk caused contraction of the vessels of the brain; while warm water caused dilatation of the cerebral vessels, his observations agreeing in this regard with those of Naumann.

General applications to the skin by means of compresses 278
and full baths were found to produce opposite effects. A warm bath produced *dilatation* of the surface vessels, but *contraction* of the vessels of the brain; while a cold bath produced contraction of the vessels of the skin, with dilatation of the cerebral vessels.

These observations show clearly that two classes of effects 279
are produced in applications of water to the surface; viz., (1) *reflex*; (2) *mechanical*, or *derivative*.

Doubtless both of these effects are always produced. 280
When the application is general, the mechanical effect is dominant; when the area involved is limited, the reflex effect is most prominent. In general applications the primary reflex effect is quickly effaced by the succeeding mechanical effect due to the in-rush of blood from the periphery. This diversion of blood from the surface vessels to the interior of the body is termed *retrostasis*. Marked retrostasis is produced only when the cold application is made simultaneously to a very large cutaneous area.

**Archiv für Klinische Medicin*, Vol. 14, 1874, Leipsic, page 566.

281 The effects of general warm (99°–100° F.) and cold (52°) applications were observed to be transient, lasting not more than ten minutes, usually less, whether the application was continuous or interrupted. Secondary effects of an opposite character then appeared; viz., contraction of the cerebral vessels after cold and relaxation after a warm bath.

282 Dilatation of the vessels of the viscera after a short, intense general cold application follows so quickly that this may be recognized as practically its primary effect. The subject is further discussed in paragraphs 669–672, and 1256–1292.

THE EFFECTS OF COLD UPON THE SKIN.

The surface phenomena observed to follow an application of cold water to the skin are as follows: —

1. Contraction of the Small Blood-Vessels.

283 A short application of cold or very cold water (from 32° to 65°) produces pallor and coldness of the skin, due to the contraction of the small vessels (Exp. 8).[11]

284 When the application of cold is long continued, the surface becomes blue, because the muscles of the small veins, being weaker, soon become exhausted and relaxed, while those of the arterioles are still active. The capillaries being contracted, the pressure in the veins is lessened, the flow of blood is slowed, and the venules are thus distended with blood the hemoglobin of which has been reduced; and the skin consequently shows a blue or purplish color. This is the *primary* effect of cold, or rather of the vital *action* or resistance against it developed during its application.

285 When the application is withdrawn, if it has not been too greatly prolonged, the pallor or blueness quickly gives place to redness, the result of active dilatation of the small arteries of the skin. This is the *secondary* effect of cold, or so-called *reaction*, one of the most interesting and important phenomena connected with the application of water (**429**).

Percussion, or slapping, and friction have much the same effect on the small vessels as cold water, causing first excitation of the vasoconstrictors, and later the reverse (Exp. 9). 286

2. Decrease or Suspension of Perspiration.

The almost instant suspension of the glandular action of the skin as the result of the action of cold is even more remarkable than the excitation of these glands by the application of heat (Exp. 10). It is evidently a purely reflex phenomenon, as suspension of sweating takes place before the application of cold has continued long enough to occasion a lowering of the general temperature of the blood, the cessation of the action of the perspiratory glands thus taking place while the sweat centers are still experiencing the stimulating effect of a blood temperature sufficiently high to provoke intense action of the glands. 287

It is noteworthy that suspension of the action of the sweat-glands of the entire skin surface may be brought about by a cold application to a very small area, as the feet, the shoulders, and in some cases the hands or other equally limited surfaces,— evidently a reflex effect.

This sudden checking of perspiration as the result of cold applications is injurious or dangerous only when the body is in a state of fatigue, or when the perspiratory activity is the result of an effort on the part of the system to antagonize a febrile movement, as in the sweating stage of malarial fever, in sweating sickness, etc. 288

With the occurrence of reaction, the action of the sweat-glands is resumed, and may be greatly increased. 289

3. Decreased Heat Elimination and Increased Heat Production.

Cold applications, by causing contraction of the small vessels, lessen the amount of blood circulating through the skin, and thus diminish heat elimination, during the application. At the same time, the reflex effect upon the centers controlling heat production stimulates the development of animal heat in the body. 290

291 When reaction occurs, however, the result is an accelerated circulation of blood through the skin, whereby an increased quantity of blood is exposed to the cooling influences that act upon the surface of the body, so increasing heat elimination.

292 If the application of cold is long continued, the temperature of the muscles lying beneath the skin, as well as that of the skin itself, is lowered, thus checking the heat-producing processes that are active in the muscles, where about one half of the heat of the body is produced.

4. Diminished Tactile Sensibility.

293 Applications of a temperature below 92° to 98° lessen the acuteness of the tactile sense (Exp. 11). Even a very brief application of ice or very cold water will abolish tactile sensibility, and the same effect is obtained by a prolonged application of cold water. This fact is taken advantage of by dentists, who freeze the gum by the application of ether or rhigolene spray, as a means of obviating the pain of teeth extraction. Other operations are also thus rendered painless.

294 Applications below 32° F. do not excite the temperature sense, but give rise to pain. Even moderately cold applications are to most patients at first painful and shocking.

295 The impression made by a cold bath is more painful if the cold water is gradually brought into contact with the body than if the application is brought to bear upon the whole surface at once, as in the plunge bath. By sudden immersion the sensation is generalized, whereas in gradual applications it is concentrated upon the limited surface that is at each instant coming in contact with the water.

296 A fine spray feels cooler than a douche at the same temperature, for the reason that the douche stuns the skin by its mechanical effect, and thus lessens its sensibility. Immersion in cold water, for the same reason, gives rise to greater shock or pain than the douche, though at the same time it is less excitant, because of the lack of percussion effect.

297 A curious fact not infrequently noted is that more distress is experienced from the application of water at a temperature

of 55° to 65° F. than at 45° to 55°. This effect is perhaps due to the more prompt reaction at the lower temperature, as well as to the lessened sensibility.

THE EFFECTS OF COLD UPON THE CIRCULATION.

Cold slows the circulation and diminishes the frequency of 298
the heart beat. The shock occasioned by a sudden application of cold water increases momentarily the activity of the heart, but the pulse-rate quickly returns to normal, and is soon perceptibly slowed, the effect depending upon the intensity and the duration of the application. This effect is the result of the reflex influence of the stimulation of the skin upon the nervous mechanism of the heart, and is due to the fact that the accelerator nerves of the heart are first excited, and later the pneumogastric, whereby the heart's movements are slowed. It should be remembered also that in the reaction following a short cold application the increased activity of the small vessels aids the heart, while by the continuous contraction *during* a cold application the labor of the heart is greatly increased.

It thus appears that *very short applications of cold pro-* 299
duce increased activity of the heart, while prolonged applications slow its action (Exp. 12, 13, 14, 15) (Roehrig).

A short, very cold (40° to 55° F.) *application produces* 300
a very brief contraction of the visceral vessels, which is followed by dilatation lasting for a few minutes (3 to 10), which later gives rise to contraction. Through all these vascular changes, however, there is a constant elevation of blood pressure.

A prolonged cool or cold application (60° to 80° F.) *with-* 301
out percussion produces vasoconstriction in the parts which are in reflex relation to the area operated upon.

Local cold applications produce varied effects, some of 302
which may be regarded as reflex, others as due to the direct influence of cold upon the sympathetic ganglia in the vessel

walls. Some of the most important of the effects of local cold applications are the following:—

303 Plethysmographic experiments made by Franck showed that a piece of ice held in one hand causes shrinking of the other within two or three seconds, with a return to the normal at the end of a minute (Exp. 16).[12]

304 Snow rubbed on the inside of the arm at the bend of the elbow, or ice applied to the subclavian region diminishes the height of the pulse tracing (Winternitz), showing a contraction of the distal portion of the radial artery.

305 *A compensatory effect is sometimes observed.* Winternitz has noted that placing the elbow in water at 50° F. for 30 minutes gives rise to an elevation of temperature in the axilla, showing an increase in the internal temperature coincident with a lowering of the external.

306 Waller observed that the application of ice over the cubital nerve at the elbow produces a rise of temperature of 7° F. in the fourth and fifth digits, while the temperature of the other fingers falls an equal number of degrees. The muscles of the hypothenar region are at the same time paralyzed. The phenomena developed by this interesting experiment are closely akin to those observed to follow the division of the sympathetic nerve of the ear of a white rabbit, which occasions reddening of the ear of the side operated upon, while the opposite ear becomes pale.

307 *Cold applications made across the trunk of an artery cause contraction in its distal portions.* An ice-bag applied to the axilla lessens the circulation in the arm (Exp. 18). An ice cravat, or an ice-cold compress applied about the throat, lessens the cerebral circulation, through its influence upon the carotid and the vertebral arteries. The vertebral arteries alone may be influenced by an ice-bag applied to the back of the neck. An ice-bag over the femoral artery in like manner lessens the circulation in the leg. The circulation in the hand or the foot may be controlled by the application of an ice-bag to the bend of the arm or of the knee. (Exp. 18, 19).

An ice-bag applied over the heart continuously for several hours diminishes its activity and lessens rate of blood movement through the body. 308

A short, cold application over the heart acts as a tonic to the heart, increasing its force and raising arterial tension. 309

A short general cold application is a powerful heart tonic, increasing greatly the force and efficiency of the heart in appropriate cases. Direct application of cold, as by cold water dripped upon the exposed part or a cold fluid passed through it, slows and weakens it. 310

A prolonged cold application slows the heart's action, increasing arterial tension (Exp. 20). 311

Winternitz noted that *cold applications to a limited surface of the skin increased the pulse-rate for three minutes*, after which it gradually diminished in frequency. 312

The influence of cold upon the mucous membrane is essentially the same as that upon the skin, except that the mucous membrane is somewhat less sensitive to thermic impressions, having a smaller number of sensory nerve fibers. The mucous membrane is, however, richly supplied with vasomotor and sympathetic fibers, through which decided reflex effects may be produced. 313

A quantity of cold water taken into the stomach produces more marked effects than water applied to an equal area of the skin. The general temperature may be lowered by this means, and the heart's action may be slowed. Cold water drinking may lessen the pulse-rate ten to fifteen beats per minute (Exp. 21). Cold water drinking produces the same effects upon the visceral vessels and the blood pressure as do cold applications to the skin, though in less degree. The quantity of water is also an important factor. 314

Even more marked effects may be readily produced by the cool enema, which, together with water drinking, is one of the most efficient means of combating fever. The writer has often seen the general temperature fall one or two degrees in a fever case as the result of an enema administered at 80°. 315

The effect is, of course, less marked in health, which is also true of other applications of cold water (Exp. 22).

316 In this depressing effect of cold water when taken into the stomach, we have the explanation of the results that sometimes occur from drinking cold water when the body is in a state of fatigue. The power of reaction being diminished, chill and internal congestion are produced, often resulting in great injury. Cold water drinking is not contraindicated by active perspiration, but rather by fatigue, and this is true whether the skin is in a state of excessive activity or not.

THE EFFECTS OF COLD UPON RESPIRATION.

317 The observations reported by Halle, Fleury, Richter, Johnson, and others seem to indicate no regularity in the effects of cold upon the respiratory movements. One reports no appreciable effect; another, quickening of the respiratory activity, with slowing of the heart; another, sometimes quickening, sometimes slowing, of respiration. This confusion seems to be the result of failure to note the difference in the effect produced by different modes of application.

318 **Respiratory Movement.** When the cold application takes the form of the douche, the effect is to produce at first short, gasping respiratory movements, this effect being more pronounced the lower the temperature, the more abrupt the application, and the stronger the pressure employed. If, however, the patient is immersed in a cold full bath, respiratory movements after the first instant are slowed to a marked degree, and are decidedly fuller and deeper; that is, the amount of tidal air is increased.

319 The effect of the cold douche or spray in increasing the rate of the respiratory movements is especially pronounced when it is applied to the chest or upper part of the body. Thus employed, an unpleasant sensation of constriction in the chest is also produced, the very opposite of the effect following an application of warm water. These effects are clearly indicated in the tracings made by means of the author's pneograph (Figs. 25, 26) (Exp. 23).

This property of cold water must be borne in mind in the treatment of asthmatics, in whom a cold douche to the chest will generally produce a paroxysm of asthmatic breathing, and sometimes a most distressing sense of suffocation. The pulmonary vessels being made to contract suddenly by the powerful excitation of the vasoconstrictor centers of the cord, the area of blood presented for gaseous interchange in the pulmonary mucous membrane is very greatly diminished, while at the same time the demand for oxygen and for the elimination of CO_2 is increased, thus producing the painful sensation experienced in suffocation. 320

This sensation of suffocation ordinarily disappears at once when reaction occurs, and the quickened respiratory movements are succeeded by slower and fuller movements, accompanied by increased absorption of oxygen. 321

CO_2 Elimination. An examination of the expired air shows that an increased amount of oxygen is absorbed and an increased amount of CO_2 is exhaled under the influence of cold applications. 322

Crawford showed more than a century ago (1781) that cold increases the difference in color between arterial and venous blood, the result of increased oxidation. 323

The oxidation of organic waste substances which takes place in the lungs is doubtless also increased, as is the oxidation of sugar in the blood of the general circulation. 324

Liebig observed more than half a century ago that cold air, cold water, and exercise, habitually employed, are the most powerful of all means of stimulating tissue activity. 325

THE EFFECTS OF COLD UPON THE MUSCLES.

The Muscular Sense. Muscular Irritability. Prolonged applications of water at a low temperature decrease muscular irritability and muscular energy. This is shown in the stiffness and clumsiness of the fingers as the result of exposure to a low temperature. 326

A short, cold bath, as a douche or a spray, lasting for a few seconds, augments muscular energy and tone to a very 327 remarkable degree. The exaggerated tonicity thus induced is the cause of shivering. The cold bath, if short (1 to 2 secs.) and given with much pressure (25 to 35 lbs.), is a powerful restorative in fatigue resulting from severe muscular effort, but it must be immediately preceded by a short hot bath, and must be followed by rubbing and warm wrapping. The restorative effects of the cold bath are well shown in Exp. 24.[13]

328 **The Involuntary Muscles.** It is a curious and interesting fact that while cold lessens the irritability of the voluntary muscles, it excites the activity of the smooth muscular fibers of the skin, thus giving rise to the appearance known as goose-flesh. It also causes contraction of the smooth muscles of the small blood-vessels; and when applied to a large area of the skin or over special regions, as the feet or lower abdomen, may excite the involuntary muscles of the bowels and bladder, causing evacuation of these cavities.

329 Shivering is due to an involuntary action of the voluntary muscles, set up automatically as a means of combating the influence of cold by increasing heat production.

330 The application of cold water to the feet, as by means of the spray or stepping into a cold bath, may produce a goose-flesh appearance over the entire surface of the body, with shivering. The application of a cold spray or douche to one side of the body will produce a goose-flesh appearance on the opposite side, together with the usual phenomena attending the application of cold to the entire surface of the body, thus demonstrating that the powerful reflexes set up by cold applications are universal in extent within the body.

THE EFFECTS OF COLD UPON THE NERVOUS SYSTEM.

331 Nearly all the phenomena arising from applications of cold water are illustrations of the effect of cold upon the nervous system, whereby special effects are produced in various organs, as described under their respective heads. In this

section attention will be called especially to those effects of cold that are chiefly confined to the nervous system itself.

The Neuron. Recent discoveries in the minute anatomy of 332
the nervous system throw much light upon the method by which the nervous functions are influenced by cold as well as by other agents. The discovery of the fact that each nerve cell, or neuron, is an independent entity, connected with other nerve cells by contact only, and not by actual continuity of structure, and the further discovery that in its activities the nerve cell actually executes movements and undergoes distinct changes in form, retracting or protracting its dendrites and the delicate filaments constituting the end-tuft of its neuraxon, has afforded a rational explanation for much that was before mere surmise or conjecture.

The neuron is by these discoveries found to be subject to 333
precisely the same laws that govern protoplasmic structures elsewhere than in the human nervous system. A careful study of the influence of heat and cold upon the ameba and the white blood-corpuscle shows that the influence of heat is to cause increased activity of the cell, with extension of protoplasmic processes, or arms, while cold diminishes its activity, causing retraction of its processes. We may thus justly conclude that when cold applications are made in such a manner as to influence the nervous system directly, similar effects are produced.

It is held, for example, that insensibility is due to
retraction of the dendrites, or protoplasmic processes, of 334
the neurons, thus cutting off connection with the rest of the nervous system by breaking contact at the points at which connection is necessary for the maintenance of the state of consciousness. The same principle applies to all other nervous functions. Increased nervous activity of any particular sort means simply increased movement of the neurons, active protraction of their dendrites, and an increased number of contacts with other neurons by means of the neuraxons with their collateral branches, end-tufts, and innumerable gemmules, or contact globules.

335 With these facts in mind, it is not difficult to understand that cold applications to a nerve trunk may greatly diminish or even entirely abolish its functions, paralyzing the parts to which it is distributed, as Waller showed by an application of ice to the cubital nerve at the elbow.

336 **Nervous and Mental Activity.** Helmholtz showed that the application of cold to a nerve may diminish the rate of transmission of nervous impulses over it to one sixth the normal rate (Exp. 25). After such an application of cold to a nerve trunk and its withdrawal, the nerve quickly recovers, unless the application has been very intense and prolonged, and the part to which it is distributed becomes the seat of pain, sometimes very intense in character, showing that nervous sensibility is heightened in the reaction that follows the benumbing effect of a cold application.

337 If the application of cold is more intense in character and less prolonged, the sedative effect may be so slight as to be unnoticed, and the effect observed be that of excitation, which, however, as previously shown, is simply the rebound, or reaction, that naturally follows vital depression, owing to awakened resistance.

338 In like manner a short, cold application to the head results in increased cerebral activity, the reaction effect completely overshadowing the brief depression first produced. A prolonged application of intense cold to the head results, however, in a decided lessening of cerebral activity, and may give rise not only to stupidity and drowsiness, but to absolute unconsciousness, a fact which has for centuries been made use of in prisons, cold water being poured upon the head as a means of subduing refractory prisoners.

339 Schüller showed (1874) by experiments upon trephined rabbits the following interesting facts in relation to the effects of thermic applications upon the brain: —

340 1. Water at neutral temperature (92°–95° F.) applied directly to the brain produced no effect.

2. Ice applied to the brain coverings caused contraction of both veins and arteries, the contraction continuing for a short time after the withdrawal of the ice. 341

3. Ice applied to the scalp caused contraction of the cerebral vessels when carried to the point of producing general chilliness and shivering. 342

4. A cold compress applied to the spine or abdomen, or a cold full bath caused instant dilatation of the cerebral vessels, lasting from 3 to 10 minutes, then giving place to contraction. 343

5. Hot compresses or a hot full bath caused contraction of the cerebral vessels, later followed by dilatation. 344

6. Cold and warm applications applied to a nerve trunk produced an effect exactly opposite to that produced by the same applications made to the skin; that is, a cold application to a nerve trunk caused contraction of the cerebral vessels, while a warm application caused dilatation. Unquestionably the same effects, which are evidently reflex in character, occur when the sensory nerves of the skin are influenced by thermic applications, but they are overwhelmed and quickly wiped out by the mechanical dilatation of the cerebral vessels, resulting from the elevation of blood pressure and the displacement of a large quantity of blood toward the center of the body through the contraction and partial emptying of the vessels of the skin. 345

7. A heating compress or moist trunk pack of three hours' duration caused, first, dilatation, then contraction, of the cerebral vessels, and bulging of the membranes from accumulation of lymph. 346

8. Pinching the skin produced the same effects as hot applications.

These interesting experiments, which have since been confirmed by observations made upon a man whose brain had been exposed by accident, laid the foundation for a scientific therapy of the brain, which has received far less attention than 347 it deserves at the hands of medical men. These experiments show most clearly how cerebral congestion may be successfully combated by properly managed applications, and explains the relief afforded in insomnia by the moist girdle and the tonic effects of the cold douche.

348 Attention may be especially called to the effect of the moist abdominal bandage upon the blood and lymph circulation of the brain. There is normally maintained a constant balance between the blood supply of the brain and the amount of lymph present in the ventricles. The more blood in the brain, the less lymph in the ventricles and the nerves, an arrangement necessary for the protection of the delicate cerebral vessels, from the fact that the brain is inclosed in an inelastic case. The moist bandage so influences the lymph and blood circulation of the brain that the quantity of blood is notably diminished, while the quantity of lymph is greatly increased, as shown by the bulging of the membranes, thus supplying just the condition needed for normal sleep.

REFLEX EFFECTS OF COLD APPLICATIONS.

349 Edwards showed that immersion of one hand in cold water causes a lowering of temperature in the other hand. The experiments of Winternitz, and later those of Franck, showed by means of the plethysmograph that cold applied to one hand causes contraction of the vessels in the other hand.

The interesting facts already presented in relation to the influence of cold applied to the skin, both locally and upon distant parts (**339**) are examples of reflex effects. These effects include not only dilatation and constriction of the blood-vessels, but also contraction of the smooth muscles found in the bowels, bladder, and other hollow organs of the body. The muscular walls of the minute air-tubes of the lungs, the so-called ligaments which support the viscera, the secreting structures,—the liver, kidneys, digestive glands, and other allied organs,—are also influenced reflexly by applications of cold to the external areas in relation with them.

Special Effects of Applications to Muscular Reflex Areas.

In accordance with the facts just mentioned, it becomes apparent that to produce reflex effects in the muscles we have but to make cold applications to those areas the stimulation of which is capable of developing muscular contraction. These areas, as elsewhere pointed out, are:— 350

The *intra-scapular* (space between the shoulder-blades).

The *epigastric* (the sides of the chest at about the level of the fourth rib).

The *abdominal* (the borders of the recti muscles).

The *cremasteric* (the inner and upper surface of the thigh).

The *plantar* (the sole of the foot).

By gentle irritation of the skin of these several areas, the greater portion of the several muscular groups may be brought into activity. This is particularly true of the plantar surface. 351

Short, very cold applications, at high pressure, made upon these surfaces may be very serviceable in all cases in which it is desirable to stimulate the nutrition of the muscles, as in general muscular weakness, paresis or paralysis, progressive muscular atrophy, and other maladies in which there is wasting of the muscular structures. Although muscular action may not be induced, the nutritive processes in the muscles are influenced favorably by applications made to these reflex areas. Most important of all is the plantar surface.

An application of a jet of either cold or very hot water to the abdomen causes instant and vigorous contraction of the abdominal muscle, and is likewise a most valuable means of exciting intestinal peristalsis. 352

Special Skin Areas in Reflex Relation with the Internal Viscera.

Cold applications to the face and neck, short and intense, cause dilatation of the cerebral vessels. 353

A prolonged contraction of the cerebral vessels is produced if the application is greatly lengthened, and vertigo and even unconsciousness may result. This is true, however, only of very vigorous applications, as the long cold "head pour." 354

355 Short applications of intense cold to the neck and chest produce an acceleration of the pulse and of the respiratory movements, followed by a slowing of the heart and the respiration.

356 Prolonged immersion of the hands in cold water causes contraction of the vessels of the brain and of the mucous membrane of the nose. This measure is thus useful in combating cerebral hyperemia.

357 A prolonged cool foot bath causes contraction of the vessels of the uterus, and may thus be useful in combating uterine hemorrhage.

358 Very cold applications to the breasts, abdomen, hands, and feet cause contraction of the involuntary muscles of the bladder, bowels, and uterus. It is more than probable that the muscular structures of the liver, spleen, and other viscera are likewise influenced by such applications, as well as by applications made to the overlying areas of skin.

359 A short, very cold douche to the feet, with strong pressure (25 to 35 lbs.), dilates the vessels of the uterus, and is hence useful in amenorrhea.

360 A prolonged cold application to the upper dorsal region relieves congestion of the nasal mucous membrane, and is thus useful in nosebleed. The popular practice of applying cold metal to the spine to check nosebleed shows the relation of this surface to the nasal mucous membrane.

361 A prolonged cold application over the upper dorsal and lower cervical region causes contraction of the pulmonary vessels, and is useful in pulmonary congestion and hemorrhage.

362 A prolonged cold application to the occiput and neck shows the action of the heart.

363 Application of the ice-compress or ice-bag to the lumbar region produces dilatation of the vessels of the uterus and lower extremities, if prolonged, and is useful in amenorrhea.

364 A cold lumbar douche at moderate pressure, and continued from 15 to 45 seconds, produces contraction of the vessels of the uterus.

A very cold and very short douche (2 to 4 secs.), with strong pressure (25 to 30 lbs.), to the lumbar region, produces dilatation of the uterine vessels. This measure is accordingly useful in amenorrhea. 365

Prolonged cold applications to the breasts and the inner surface of the thighs produces contraction of both the vessels and the muscles of the uterus. 366

Winternitz has shown that cold applications to the thighs also influence the pulmonary circulation, combating congestion. 367

A short, cold douche applied to the lower portion of the sternum stimulates the kidneys, increasing the flow of urine. 368

A short, cold douche, with strong pressure, over the liver, stomach, spleen, or bowels, produces dilatation of the blood-vessels, with increased activity in these organs. 369

Contraction of the small vessels may be produced in the liver, spleen, stomach, bowels, and other internal viscera by prolonged cold applications of moderate intensity (60° to 75° F.) to the skin overlying these organs. This measure is of great service in the treatment of pathological conditions involving congestion of these organs. 370

Cold applications to a reflex area often give rise to a sense of constriction in the parts reflexly connected. When a cold douche is applied to the feet, a strong sensation of constriction is felt in the lower abdomen; while cold applied to the chest occasions a sensation of constriction in the thorax. 371

Summary of Methods for Reflexly Influencing the Internal Viscera.

The vessels of the important viscera may be caused either to dilate or contract by cold applications to the skin, according as the application is short and intense (1 to 4 secs., temp. 40° to 60° F., pressure 25 to 35 lbs.) (dilatation), or long and moderate (contraction), by the following methods: — 372

The *brain*, by applications to the head, neck, face, hands, and feet. 373

374 The *nasal mucous membrane*, by applications to the neck, face, upper dorsal spine, hands, and feet.

375 The *stomach*, by applications to the lower dorsal spine and the epigastrium.

376 The *kidneys*, by applications to the lumbar region, the lower portion of the sternum, and the feet.

377 The *bowels*, by applications to the feet and the abdomen.

378 The *bladder*, by applications to the feet and the lower abdomen.

379 The *liver*, by applications to the lower right chest.

380 The *spleen*, by applications to the lower left chest.

381 The *lungs*, by applications to the chest and the thighs (Winternitz), and to the upper dorsal region.

382 The *uterus*, by applications to the lumbar region, the abdomen, the breasts, the inner surfaces of the thighs, the feet, and to the cervix uteri, through the vagina. Applications made to the cervix uteri are usually very hot rather than cold.

THE EFFECTS OF COLD UPON THE BLOOD.

383 In 1893, Professor Winternitz, of Vienna, called attention to the remarkable influence of cold applications in increasing the number of blood-corpuscles, both red and white, and also the amount of hemoglobin, it being noted, however, that the white blood-corpuscles were increased in much greater proportion than the red corpuscles. In one case reported by Winternitz, the increase of blood-corpuscles by a hot bath followed by cold was 1,860,000 per c.mm. The number of white corpuscles was sometimes increased three hundred per cent. In a case observed by the writer, the increase was more than half a million.[14 15 16]

384 This remarkable phenomenon is due, according to Winternitz, not to the sudden creation of new blood-corpuscles, but to the contraction of the vessels of the viscera, caused by the application of cold to the surface, whereby great numbers of corpuscles, which have been collected in the vessels of the liver, kidneys, spleen, and other internal viscera, are driven

into the circulation. That this explanation is not entirely complete, however, is shown by the fact that local applications of cold water are followed by an increase in the number of corpuscles and of the hemoglobin at the seat of the application, though no such increase is observed elsewhere (Exp. 26).

According to Henocque, both hot and cold applications increase the rate at which the oxyhemoglobin of the blood is reduced. A freezing temperature reduces the rate one-half. 385

Crawford, of England, showed in 1781, in a paper published in the "Transactions of the London Philosophical Society," that cold baths increase the contrast of color between the arterial and the venous blood, the natural result of increased tissue activity and oxidation. 386

D'Arsonval and others have shown by the estimation of the gases contained in the blood at different points of the body simultaneously, that the interstitial combustions are increased by cold applications. These observations have been confirmed by others, who have shown that the gaseous exchanges are decidedly increased by cold applications, so that a greater amount of oxygen is passed through the body in a given amount of time. 387

Strasser (*Deutch. Med.-Zeit.*, June 15, 1896) has shown that general cold applications increase the alkalinity of the blood, the diminution in acid phosphate amounting sometimes to fifty per cent. 388

THE EFFECTS OF COLD UPON ABSORPTION.

By introducing belladonna into the rectum and observing the length of time that elapsed before dilatation of the pupil and other characteristic physiological effects appeared, Fleury showed that absorption from the alimentary canal is very greatly accelerated by the cold douche. His experiments and those of others show clearly that cold applications to the surface stimulate absorption by the gastric and intestinal mucous membrane, and consequently that such applications must favor nutrition by promoting alimentation. 389

THE EFFECTS OF COLD UPON SECRETION AND TISSUE CHANGE.

390 A short, very cold douche, administered with strong pressure (25 to 35 lbs.), over the stomach and liver, has the effect to increase the secretory activity of these organs by dilating their vessels, thus bringing a larger quantity of blood in contact with the secreting cells, and also by directly exciting cell activity.

391 The cold douche and the ice-bag or compress over the region of the stomach, increases the amount of hydrochloric acid formed by the stomach, and is thus exceedingly useful in hypopepsia (Exp. 27).

392 Experiments made upon the rabbit and the dog show that intense general applications of cold give rise to increased production of sugar, the sugar appearing in excessive quantity in the blood, and if the application is of sufficient intensity, in the urine also. Similar effects of very cold applications have been observed in man.

393 As it is generally conceded that the glycogenic function of the liver may be taken as an indicator of its activities in other directions, it is evident that cold applications may be made in such a manner as to produce greatly increased activity of the hepatic functions.

394 It is evident that all applications of water which increase the activity of the liver in the destruction and elimination of tissue poisons and pathological toxins, must be capable of rendering valuable service in the treatment of diseases in which there is an excessive production of these elements, as in typhoid fever, malarial fever, the malarial cachexia, "biliousness," many forms of dyspepsia accompanied by chronic toxemia and resulting neurasthenia, and in chronic liver disorders,—congestion, sclerosis, hypertrophy,—and other morbid states which so often accompany chronic indigestion.

395 The most pronounced effects upon the liver and stomach are to be obtained by the use of the alternate circle or horizontal douche and the percussion douche.

General cold applications, especially the cold douche, increase the production of HCl, and hence improve the quality of the gastric juice. The alternate circle douche is perhaps the most efficient of all means for promoting peptic secretion. 396

Thermic applications to the skin unquestionably produce the most profound effect upon the thermotaxic centers, but this influence is to a considerable degree masked by the fact that there is little disturbance in the body temperature. By the aid of the author's bath calorimeter, it is easy to observe that these thermic applications influence heat production and dissipation to a most profound degree (Exp. 28). 397

In an observation elsewhere described (Exp. 29), made by the author with his bath calorimeter in 1890, and many times repeated since with the same results, it was found that the patient lost, during the bath, 103,354 heat units within fifteen minutes. This represented four per cent., or one twenty-fifth of the total amount of heat produced in twenty-four hours. As the patient's temperature remained the same at the close of the bath as at the beginning, it is evident that the increase in heat distribution was compensated for by an equal increase in heat production, which must of course involve the destruction of tissue, at least the oxidation of carbohydrate material in the form of glycogen. 398

Dr. Strasser, assistant to Professor Winternitz, of Vienna, in a paper contributed to a volume published in commemoration of the fortieth anniversary of Professor Winternitz's graduation in medicine (Vienna, 1897), gave an account of a classical and exceedingly interesting study of the effects of cold water upon tissue change.[17] Strasser found, for example, that a cold bath increases the amount of urea, uric acid, ammonia, earthy phosphates, the xanthine bases or extractives, and the total nitrogen, which proves conclusively that short so-called tonic applications have the effect of stimulating to a high degree the processes of tissue change in the body. A very interesting and notable fact observed was that while 399 before the bath the quantity of imperfectly oxidized extractives constituted about 8.7 per cent. of the total amount excreted, under the influence of the bath the amount of imperfectly oxidized extractives produced was but 1.5 per cent.

It is also worthy of note that the increased amount of phosphates eliminated was almost altogether in the form of earthy phosphates, which, as Strasser states, is derived from the food, thus affording an evidence of the improved absorption due to the application of cold water to the surface. These facts account for the wonderful effects observed in the application of the cold bath in rickets, the increased absorption of earthy phosphates contributing in these cases to the development of healthy bone structures.

THE EFFECTS OF COLD UPON EXCRETION.

400 Short cold applications to the skin, being followed by dilatation of the surface vessels, favor perspiration; while prolonged cold applications have the opposite effect.

401 As a rule, an increase in the quantity of fluid eliminated through the skin is accompanied by a decrease in the quantity of urine. This is not universally the case, however; and it should also be remembered that the quantity of urine is not the true measure of renal activity, but rather the quantity of poisons removed from the system.

402 Applications of ice-water to the skin of a dog cause temporarily a decided decrease in the size of the kidneys, due to contraction of their vessels and tissues. The reaction following a cold application gives rise to dilatation of the vessels, relaxation of the tissues, and increased functional activity.[18]

The effects upon the kidneys of cold applications to the skin are so profound that they must sometimes be interdicted in cases of renal disease. In experiments upon animals, prolonged and very cold applications have caused the appearance of albumin in the urine.

Short general cold applications increase the elimination of CO_2 and the absorption of oxygen, a fact which agrees with the influence of cold upon heat production; while prolonged cold applications lessen heat production and CO_2 elimination.

Cold applications which give rise to increased heat produc- 403
tion and a corresponding increase of CO_2 do not give rise to an increase in urea unless they affect the body temperature. The production of urea seems to be regulated, to a degree at least, by the body temperature. An increase in the body temperature is accompanied by an increase of urea, as in fever; while with a depression of the body temperature, urea production and elimination are decreased.

Cold applications to the lower third of the sternum (the 404
renal douche) excite renal activity. Cold immersion and other baths also increase the amount of urine and the total solids. In cases of fever treated by the cold bath the toxicity of the urine may be increased sixfold, thus proving the great influence of cold in increasing renal efficiency.

THE EFFECTS OF COLD APPLICATIONS UPON TEMPERATURE.

Currie showed ("Medical Reports," London, 1797) 405
by thermometric observations that applications of cold water to the surface are capable of lowering not only the surface temperature, but also the internal temperature of the body. This was the beginning of scientific hydrotherapy.

In an experiment related by Currie, a healthy man was 406
put into a bath at 40° F., his temperature at the time being 97.5°. His temperature, according to the observer's statement, quickly fell to 83.1°, but rose at the end of fifteen minutes to 91.9°; at which point it remained for nineteen minutes, when it again rapidly descended, reaching in three minutes 84.9°. The subject was then removed from the cold bath, where he had been for thirty-seven minutes, and placed in a full bath at 96°. As he continued to shiver vigorously, the temperature of the bath was raised to 109°. At the end of twenty-eight minutes the body temperature was found to be normal. These observations may have been inaccurate.

407 J. Lefevre has shown that the rate of heat loss when the body is exposed to cold air or cold water does not decrease as the temperature is lowered, but increases out of proportion to the temperature lowering.

408 Fleury observed a lowering of seven degrees in temperature in a man by immersion in a bath at 50° F. for 25 minutes.[19]

409 Jurgensen observed a reduction of 6.5° in temperature as the result of a cold bath.

410 The majority of observers have not noted so great lowering of temperature from local applications as those named above. Draper obtained a fall of 1.5° from an hour's immersion in a bath of 73.5° to 75°.

411 The effect of the cold bath in lowering the temperature of the body is increased as the temperature of the bath is lowered and its duration prolonged. The effects of cold applications upon the body temperature are much more pronounced in fever than under normal conditions.

412 The surface often continues cold for some time after it has become reddened by reaction,—an evidence that cooling of the blood is still going on.

413 Fleury was the first to note that the body temperature sometimes does not begin to fall until some minutes after the subject has been removed from the bath.

414 The reduction of temperature in the cold bath is greatly increased by friction of the surface, as by this means the surface circulation is maintained, so that a larger amount of blood is brought under the influence of the cooling medium. The experiments of Winternitz showed that the rate of heat elimination from the skin in the cold bath may be increased 30 per cent. by vigorous friction of the surface (Exp. 30). Pospischil showed an increase of more than 44 per cent.

415 It must be remembered, however, that by very vigorous friction, heat production may be increased to such a degree that the antithermic effect of the bath may be undesirably diminished.

The necessity for the prolonged application of cold grows 416
out of the fact that when a cold application is made, the forces of the body instantly rally to resist its influence, heat production being increased and heat elimination diminished. The system thus endeavors to maintain the normal temperature. If the application is withdrawn before this effort is, in a measure, at least, suppressed or exhausted, the normal temperature will be quickly recovered, and may be even exceeded. This, with the other phenomena of reaction, will be discussed elsewhere.[20]

Prolonged Cold and Suppressed Reaction.

When a cold application is considerably 417
prolonged, the tendency to reaction is, to a large extent, suppressed, as a result of the exhaustion of the nerve centers involved, the lessening of the sensibility of the sensory nerves concerned in the reflex movement upon which reaction depends, as well as by the exhaustion of the powers of calorification. Thus the system gradually loses its power to resist the depressing effects of cold, and its antithermic effects are developed.

If the application is continued for a very long time, the thermal and other vital activities of the body are depressed to such a degree that two or three hours may elapse before the normal temperature is restored.

Edwards, an English investigator, has shown that repeated 418
chilling of an animal increases the length of time required for return of the normal internal temperature; hence the value of repeated cold baths in typhoid fever.

The Effects of Local Cold Applications upon the Body Temperature.

Applications of water at a temperature below 419
that of the body always lower the temperature of the part to which the application is made.

Circumscribed local applications of cold 420
water, such as immersion of the hand or foot, reduce the temperature of the part, but have no appreciable effect upon the general temperature, unless a considerable amount of surface is involved, as in the employment of large cold compresses to the trunk, except in case of

internal applications or applications to special regions, as the head.

421 Brown-Sequard showed that immersion of the hand in cold water gives rise to lowering of the temperature of the other hand.

These local applications of cold were, however, found to be without influence upon the general temperature.

422 Winternitz showed that the application of snow to the forearm produces, first, a lowering of temperature in the hand to the extent of 2° and then an elevation of 1.3° F. (Exp. 31).

423 Ice held in the mouth causes a lowering of the temperature of the cheek of the corresponding side. Copious drinking of ice-water likewise produces a fall in the temperature of the skin of the epigastrium (Exp. 32). This lowering of temperature is so marked that it may be used as a method of locating the stomach by the aid of the surface thermometer. This fact was first shown by an experiment made under the writer's supervision, by one of his students, in 1898.

424 The application of cold water to the soles of the feet, especially if in the form of a spray, lowers the temperature.

425 An ice-cap applied to the head is an efficient means of lowering the general temperature, through exercising a depressing effect upon the thermogenic centers.

426 The application of an ice-bag over the heart lowers the general temperature, slowing the circulation, and cooling the blood (Exp. 33).

427 Copious cold water drinking and the large cold water enema, although local applications, have a very decided effect in lowering the general temperature, especially in febrile conditions (Exp. 34).

THE EFFECTS OF COLD UPON THE THERMO-ELECTRICAL CURRENTS OF THE TISSUES.

Gautrelet has made the interesting suggestion that the 428
difference of temperature created between the exterior and the interior of the body by cold applications to the surface must directly augment the intensity of the organic thermo-electrical currents which are constantly playing within the body, thereby modifying, in an important way, various nutritive processes, and perhaps especially those concerned in the storing and discharge of nervous energy. This is a subject which deserves further investigation.

THE PHENOMENA AND RATIONALE OF REACTION.

Reaction, using the term as it is employed in hydro- 429
therapy, is one of the most complex and interesting of physiological phenomena. The term is perhaps somewhat misleading, as it suggests the idea of a single process, whereas there is a series of complicated actions and reactions. The most important of these are two, which may be distinguished as the *circulatory action and reaction* and the *thermic action and reaction*. Ordinarily we speak only of the circulatory reaction, as this is the one most commonly sought. Generally, however, they occur together. These reflex activities come into play in most of the process of hydrotherapy, but especially in those employed for general effects.

Suppression of Reaction.

Applications designed exclusively for local 430
effects are usually managed in such a way as to suppress reaction, either partially or wholly; as, for example, when it is desired to restrain local inflammatory processes,—pain, congestive headache, or hemorrhages, — reaction is suppressed as much as possible by continuous applications of cold of the necessary degree of intensity.

On the other hand, in the employment of the cold or cool 431
shampoo to the scalp for baldness, the cold douche to stimulate perspiration, or the heating compress to a rheumatic

joint, reaction is encouraged by means of friction, strong percussion, or high pressure, or by protection from evaporation.

432 In some general applications, also, reaction is suppressed as much as possible, as in the employment of the tepid bath for the reduction of temperature, or the neutral bath for insomnia; whereas, in other applications it is encouraged, as in the cold full bath with friction, for reduction of the temperature, and the short, cold spray or douche administered for tonic effects.

433 **Definition of Reaction.** Reaction consists of a series of vital processes which follow the making of either hot or cold applications to the skin or the mucous membrane. The reflex vital activities induced by cold applications are much more pronounced than those produced by heat, and differ in character; nevertheless, the vital reactions produced by applications of heat are clearly defined and constant in character, and may be most advantageously utilized in hydrotherapy. In view of these facts, it is indeed remarkable that the reaction of heat has been almost absolutely ignored by writers upon hydrotherapy. Even Hippocrates observed that a cold bath warms the body by reaction, while a warm bath cools it.

434 The reaction following the application of heat or cold to the skin is much more pronounced than that resulting from similar applications to the mucous membrane through the stomach and the colon.

435 **The Reaction of Cold.** We have here to consider only the reaction following short cold applications, the reaction of heat being left for consideration elsewhere (577). The phenomena resulting from a very cold application to the skin, with strong pressure and of short or moderate duration (3 to 30 secs.) may be divided into three classes:—

1. The immediate effects that accompany the application, which may be called the primary effect, or *action*.

2. The secondary effects, which constitute the phenomena of *reaction*.

3. The remote effects, that is, the final result of the application or series of applications in modifying normal or pathological nutritive processes. These later effects, being too varied and numerous to be presented in tabulated form, will be referred to elsewhere under the head of "Tonic Effects."

The most clearly defined of the phenomena included in these primary and secondary effects may be summarized as follows: — 436

ACTION.	REACTION.
1. Contraction of the small blood-vessels of the skin, with dilatation of internal vessels after a very brief contraction.	1. Dilatation of the small blood-vessels of the surface, with contraction of internal vessels.
2. Pallor of the skin.	2. Redness of the skin.
3. Goose-flesh appearance and roughness of the skin.	3. Skin soft, smooth, and supple.
4. Sensation of chilliness.	4. Sensation of warmth.
5. Trembling, shivering, chattering of the teeth, in some cases decidedly painful and distressing sensations of "constriction," etc.	5. A sensation of comfort and well-being.
6. First quickening, then slowing of the pulse, with increase of tension.	6. Slowing of the pulse, with increased tension.
7. First checked, then quick, deep, gasping respiration.	7. Respiration free, slower, and deeper.
8. Cooling of the skin.	8. Heating of the skin.
9. In most cases slight rise of internal temperature.	9. Fall of internal temperature.
10. Perspiration checked.	10. Increase of perspiration.

The initial symptoms following an application of cold water are evidence of a protective effort on the part of the system to prevent undue loss of heat by contracting the blood and lymph channels of the skin, thus decreasing its conductivity, and by increasing heat production through the muscular action of shivering. 437

If the application is very cold, at high pressure, and of short duration, the phenomena of reaction begin immediately when the application ceases. 438

439 If the patient has exercised actively just before the bath, or if vigorous friction of the skin or a hot bath has been administered, and not infrequently in healthy persons without the preparation referred to, the phenomena of reaction begin even before the termination of the application, as shown by reddening of the skin, and by the disappearance of goose-flesh and other unpleasant symptoms.

440 **Second Reaction.** If, after reaction has set in, a renewed application of cold is made, a second reaction will occur in most cases, but the vital movement will be much less prompt and pronounced; and if the subject is feeble or fatigued, a second reaction may not occur. In some very vigorous subjects, even a third or a fourth reaction may be secured by as many successive cold applications, but each time with diminished vigor; and sooner or later a point will be reached at which no reaction will occur, or only after a very long delay.

441 If, instead of administering a short, cold douche, the patient is placed in the cold bath, essentially the same thing occurs. After the first contact with cold water, the tendency to reaction appears, amounting in some cases to actual reddening of the skin, especially if the patient is rubbed. The continued contact of the water with the surface, however, prevents the complete development of reaction, and sooner or later a second chill occurs, reaction from which may be entirely suppressed.

442 **Incomplete Reaction.** The symptoms experienced by a person when prompt reaction does not occur are exceedingly unpleasant. The most prominent are prolonged chilliness, a disposition to nausea or faintness, giddiness, weakness, and great depression. The surface remains pale and cold, and the internal temperature also may be below normal, as the chill indicates the beginning of a decline of temperature below the normal level. These symptoms show that the energies of the body, by which it is naturally able to combat the disturbance created by the

application of cold to the surface, are unable to respond to the demand made upon them under existing conditions.

Conditions that Favor Reaction. The phenomena of reaction will seldom fail if the cold application is made in a proper manner. There are various controllable conditions and measures by means of which the energies of the body may be aided in developing prompt and vigorous reaction. By the employment of these in connection with the proper adaptation of the modes of applying cold to different cases, it is possible to modify at will the degree of intensity of the reaction effects obtained in any given case. **443**

These conditions and measures may be classified thus:— **444**

1. Those applicable *before the bath.*

2. Those that influence the condition of the patient *during the bath.*

3. Those that may be employed *after the bath.*

These several conditions and applications may be enumerated as follows:—

1. *Measures and Conditions which Favor Reaction, to be* **445**
Employed before the Bath: —

(1) Warm clothing.

(2) Exposure to the air of a warm room.

(3) A hot bath of some sort.

(4) Drinking hot water or some other hot beverage.

(5) The hot enema.

(6) Exercise more or less vigorous in character, according to the strength of the patient. but never carried to the degree of even incipient fatigue.

(7) Friction of the skin until warm and well reddened (Exp. 35).

(8) A warm, dry, or slightly moist skin.

(9) A state of general health and vigor.

2. *Conditions Pertaining to the Bath Itself or Acting in* **446**
Conjunction with It:—

(1) A very low temperature; the lower the temperature the more prompt the reaction.

(2) Short, sudden applications.

(3) Pressure or percussion effects, as in some form of the douche or spray (Exp. 36).

(4) Friction in the full bath, the half bath, the massage-douche, or the rubbing wet sheet (Exp. 37).

(5) Alternating and revulsive spray or douche, the difference in temperature employed being as great as possible.

447 3. *Measures that Encourage Reaction after a Bath:*—

(1) Heat in the form of hot, dry air, warm clothing, or hot-water drinking. It is even possible to induce reaction in frozen parts by rubbing with snow or ice in a warm room. The lumberman in the north woods warms his feet by taking off his shoes and stockings, and rubbing his bare feet with snow, immediately dressing them again. A high external temperature favors reaction, both by lessening heat elimination and by increasing heat production.

(2) Exercise as vigorous as the strength of the patient will allow (Exp. 38).

(3) Friction of the surface with the hand, rough towel, or flesh-brush, practised by the subject or the attendant, or both.

448 **Conditions that Discourage Reaction.** Omitting many of the specific conditions of disease that hinder reaction and contraindicate cold applications to the skin, the following may be enumerated as among the most important conditions which prevent or delay reaction, and must therefore be taken into consideration in the employment of general cold applications:—

449 1. *Old Age.* It is well to bear in mind the adage formulated by an eminent French writer, "A man is as old as his arteries." Subjects in whom arterio-sclerosis has begun, react with difficulty, and thus require special care. Very cold baths must be avoided altogether, unless the area involved is very small.

450 2. *Infancy.* Very young children react badly.

451 3. *Exhaustion,* either of a temporary nature from excessive exercise or loss of sleep, or extreme nervous exhaustion,

owing to the weak condition of the nerve centers upon which prompt reaction depends.

4. *Obesity*, owing to relative anemia of the skin. 452

5. *Rheumatic diathesis*, owing to the weakening influence 453 of uric-acid poisoning and resulting inability of the body to adjust itself readily to change of temperature.

6. *Unhealthy or inactive skin.* 454

7. *Profuse perspiration*, but only when accompanied by 455 great fatigue.

8. *Extreme nervous irritability.* 456

9. *Very low temperature of the skin.* 457

10. *An immediately preceding or impending chill.* 458

11. *Extreme aversion to cold applications.* 459

Thermic Reaction.

As the previous observations relate chiefly 460 to that portion of the phenomena of reaction designated as circulatory reaction, it may be profitable to consider briefly by itself the interesting series of vital activities which constitute what is known as thermic reaction.

Thermic reaction to cold may be defined as the effort 461 of the body to replace the heat which has been lost by exposure to cold, and to restore the equilibrium of the body temperature.

All general cold applications of whatever sort, whether 462 made to the skin or to the mucous membrane, lower both the temperature of the surface to which they are applied, and the internal or general temperature of the body. This has been abundantly proved by Fleury, Liebermeister, Bottey, and others. In a considerable proportion of the cases, however, the ultimate lowering of the internal temperature is preceded by a slight rise, which begins almost simultaneously with the cold application, and continues for 10 or 12 minutes afterward.

After the initial rise and subsequent lowering of the tem- 463 perature, there is a gradual return to the normal temperature.

This vital movement is very well shown in the following diagram, which is modified from that given by Bottey :—

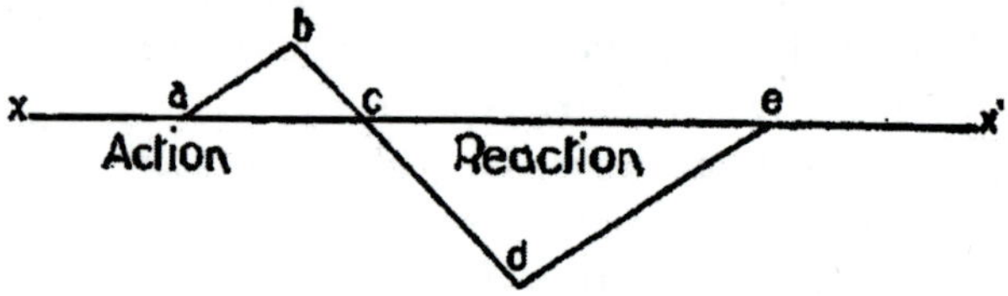

Diagram indicating the vital movement following a general cold application.

In this diagram, which represents the effect obtained from a short, very cold jet douche or spray applied to the skin with high pressure, the line *xx'* represents the normal temperature, 98.6° F.; the line *ab* represents the brief elevation of internal temperature which follows the receding of the blood from the surface the first instant after a cold application; the line *bcd* represents the fall in internal temperature which immediately succeeds the rise; and the line *de* represents the *reaction* by which the normal temperature is restored. The line *abcd* may be said to represent the *action* which precedes reaction.

464 **Modifications of Thermic Reaction.** Vigorous exercise or a hot bath taken just before a cold bath increases the initial rise of temperature, which is doubtless due to the fact that muscular activity increases heat production to so marked a degree that the cold application finds the thermogenic processes in full play, and hence more able to produce a strong thermic reaction.

465 Warm or tepid baths (80° to 92°) do not produce the initial rise of temperature. The following diagram represents the thermic action and reaction accompanying and following a tepid bath.

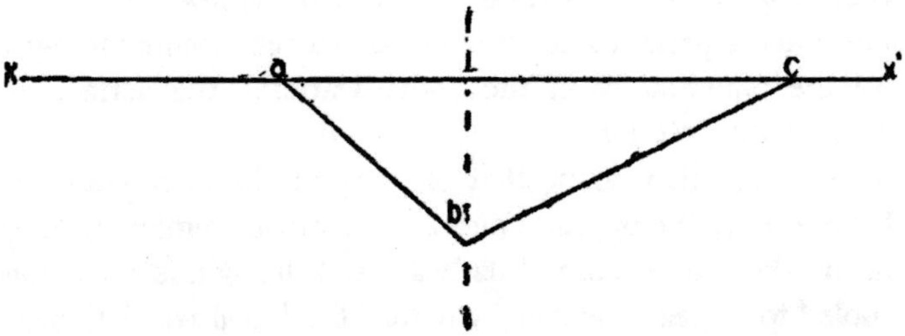

Diagram representing the vital movement following a warm or tepid bath.

In this diagram, *xx'* represents the normal temperature, 98.6° F. The line *ab* represents the action whereby the body is cooled; the line *bc*, the reaction. The perpendicular dotted line is the point of division between the two classes of phenomena.

A tepid or neutral bath causes lowering of the body tem- **466**
perature purely in a physical and mechanical way, independently of any reflex action. The surface blood-vessels do not contract, and hence the blood is rapidly cooled as it comes in contact with the water at a temperature a few degrees below the body temperature, and by the circulation of the blood current the internal temperature is lowered.

Not infrequently the rise of body temperature produced by **467**
the thermic reaction after a cold bath does not cease at the normal point, but rises slightly above it. Several oscillations of this sort may occur before the normal point is permanently gained.

The cause of the initial rise of temperature produced by a **468**
short, intensely cold application to the skin is evidently the slowing of the blood current. The blood is heated in the internal viscera, and cooled at the surface of the body. A complete circuit of the blood through the heart is effected by every twenty-seven or thirty heart-beats, or in a little less than half a minute. It is evident that the more rapidly the blood is passed through the skin, the more heat will be given

up to the skin and the air, and hence the greater will be the cooling of the whole mass of blood, and the lower will be the internal temperature, the rapid blood current tending to equalize the temperature of the body, warming the surface and cooling the interior.

469 It is equally evident that slowing of the circulation must have exactly the opposite effect: the blood, remaining longer in the skin, loses more of its heat, and the skin is accordingly cooled to a greater extent; whereas the blood which traverses the viscera, in which the thermogenic processes are most active, will remove a smaller amount of heat, thus occasioning a rise of temperature in the interior of the body, and so in a double manner increasing the difference between the external and the internal temperature. General intense cold applications to the surface cause contraction of the small arteries in every part of the body, in the viscera as well as in the skin (M. Wertheimer). The contraction of the vessels of the viscera is much briefer in duration than in the skin, but is long enough to check the movement of the blood current, thus momentarily encouraging the fall of temperature in the skin and the rise of temperature in the internal parts, as just explained.

470 Simultaneously with the development of the internal rise of temperature, there occurs an increase of heat production as the result of reflex action through the sympathetic nervous system, accompanied, as shown by Liebermeister, with increased production of CO_2, as shown by Winternitz.

471 **Counterbalancing Reaction.** Curiously enough, the influences which give rise to an increase of internal heat are antagonized by a reflex action effected through the sympathetic, or vasomotor, system, which tends to cool the body either by inhibiting the automatic thermogenic centers of the cord, or through the intervention of a special refrigerating center.

472 The initial rise of temperature in the interior of the body is very brief in duration, for the reason that by the circulatory

reaction which dilates the surface vessels, heat elimination is greatly increased, both through the enlargement of the area of blood exposed to the cooling influences acting upon the skin, and through the increased rapidity of the blood current, whereby the skin is rapidly warmed and the interior cooled. When the minimum temperature is reached, which may be from a few tenths of a degree to three or four degrees below the normal, a rise in temperature takes place, and continues until the normal point is reached, or even surpassed.

The thermic phenomena following an intense application 473
of cold to the surface may be briefly epitomized as follows:—

1. Cooling of the skin by conduction and evaporation. 474

2. Cooling of the skin and of the viscera by reflex refrig- 475
erating influences due to the action of the sympathetic nerves.

3. Elevation of the internal temperature in consequence 476
of the slowing of the blood current following contraction of the small blood-vessels throughout the body.

4. General increase of temperature internally and exter- 477
nally through reflex stimulation of the thermogenic centers.

Thermic Reaction a Useful Indicator.

The thermic reaction is a useful indicator both 478
of the extent to which the bodily functions may be modified by hot or cold applications to the surface, and of individual susceptibility. The author has found the following a useful means of testing the reactive power of an individual:—

A vessel of sufficient size to receive the arm immersed to 479
the elbow is provided with water at a temperature of 50° F. The patient immerses the bared hand and arm to the elbow for one-half minute. Note is taken of the surface temperature of the arm before immersion and every five minutes after removal, until the original temperature is restored (Exp. 39).

The appearance or non-appearance of goose-flesh and the 480
length of the continuance of this phenomenon are noted, and also the appearance and duration, or non-appearance, of reaction, as indicated by increased surface temperature and redness.

This test is a valuable means of determining the condition of the nervous system as regards the tone of the spinal and sympathetic centers, and also gives important information concerning the general vital resistance of the patient, or his power to resist disease.

A more convenient and practical, though somewhat less accurate, method of applying this test is the following: Dip the corner of a towel in ice-water, hold the saturated towel against the bared forearm of the patient for one minute, covering a surface of at least ten or twelve square inches. Do not rub the surface, simply maintain contact of the cold wet towel with the skin. On withdrawing the towel, dry the surface by light pressure with the dry end of the towel, cover to prevent slow cooling by evaporation, and note the length of time required for the occurrence of reaction, as shown by the return of redness and natural heat. General chilliness produced by this application indicates an extreme irritability of the vasomotor nerves and nerve centers and undue activity of the reflexes. A mottled blueness shows great cardiac weakness and a dangerous threatening of collapse. This fact renders this method valuable as a means of ascertaining a patient's ability to take an anesthetic without undue risk of heart failure. Good reaction ought to occur with distinct reddening of the surface, within 1 or 2 minutes after the application of ice-water.

481 **Thermic Reaction and Metabolism.** It is through thermic reaction that the cold bath produces its marvelous, renovating and alterative effects. The tissue activity set up in the thermogenic tissues of the muscles as the result of exposure of the skin to a cold medium for a short time, is participated in by every cell and tissue in the whole body. Tissue building is accelerated to keep pace with the increased rate of oxidation; and thus more food is required, more blood is in circulation, more oxygen is absorbed, more CO_2 and urea are eliminated, and all the vital functions are quickened, thus causing the stream of life to flow at a more rapid rate. This is tonic thermic reaction.

THE PHYSIOLOGICAL EFFECTS OF HEAT.

Heat may be applied to the body for therapeutic purposes 482
in a variety of ways, as by means of hot water, steam, hot air, or by radiation from an incandescent body. Illustrations of these several modes of application are to be found in the full bath, the fomentation, the Russian or vapor bath, the vapor douche, the hot air or Turkish bath, and the electric-light bath.

The effects produced in the application of heat to the 483
body depend upon (1) the mode of application, (2) the temperature, (3) the duration, and (4) the condition of the subject.

Water is recognized as hot when above the temperature of 484
the surface of the body, or between 98° and 104° F., and is termed very hot when above 104°. At a temperature of 120° a full bath becomes unendurable, although small areas, as in the hand or foot bath, or in the application of a fomentation, may be gradually trained to endure a temperature ten or fifteen degrees higher.

The mucous membrane readily endures a temperature ten 485
or fifteen degrees higher than can be tolerated by the skin.

A full bath of 120° can not be prolonged beyond 2 or 486
3 minutes without danger to life, and for some persons it would be hazardous for even a few seconds.

In the vapor or Russian bath, a temperature of from 112° 487
to 120° F. is not uncomfortable, and 130° to 145° can be tolerated for a short time.

The ordinary temperature of the Turkish bath is from 488
140° to 180° F., but it is often raised to 220° or even 250° without ill effects. Temperatures much higher than this have been endured for a short time in dry air by specially trained persons.

In the employment of the electric-light or radiant-heat 489
bath, the body is subjected to the influence of radiant heat.

A thermometer exposed upon the surface of the body in a bath of this kind has been seen by the writer to register a temperature of 116.6°, although that of the air about the patient, as measured by a thermometer protected from the direct rays of the incandescent lights, was but 95° F..

490 The body expands under the influence of heat, in this respect behaving like most other bodies. The rate of expansion is very nearly the same as that of water. The body of a man weighing 132 pounds expands 21 c.c. for every degree centigrade, or .6 cubic inches for every degree Fahrenheit, elevation in temperature, or three cubic inches for every 5° F., an amount inappreciable under ordinary conditions.

491 White fibrous tissue expands under the influence of heat, while yellow elastic tissue, like rubber, contracts. The ligaments of joints are composed of white fibrous tissue, hence they are relaxed by hot applications.

492 **Heat a Vital Stimulant.** Heat is without doubt one of the most powerful of all vital excitants. The heat of the sun is the direct source of all animal and vegetable life. Heat stimulates protoplasmic activity, as shown by many laboratory experiments. A clinical illustration of the same fact is found in the remarkable pigmentation of the skin produced by the prolonged use of fomentations or poultices.

In the following pages we shall consider the effects of heat as applied to the body by means of water in its ordinary or liquid state, except when otherwise stated.

THE EFFECTS OF HEAT UPON THE SKIN.

493 The effects of heat applied to the skin differ somewhat according to the intensity and the mode of application, but they may, in general, be stated to be as follows:—

494 **1. Dilatation of the Capillary Vessels.** The effect of moderate heat, that is, water applied at a temperature of from 100° to 104° F., is to produce a reddening of the surface, more or less intense according to the thickness or natural com-

plexion of the skin and the temperament of the subject. This reddening of the skin is due to the influence of heat upon the vasomotor nerves, which is to paralyze the vasoconstrictors and stimulate the vasodilators; while cold produces the opposite effect (Exp. 40).

Currie observed * that water at moderate heat (99° to 495
101° F.) relaxed the surface vessels, while very hot applications (104° and above) gave rise to vascular contraction in the skin.

The application of a higher temperature (110° to 130° 496
F.) produces, at first, pallor of the skin, due to stimulation of the vasoconstrictors. At the same time the surface is roughened, presenting a goose-flesh appearance, due to contraction of the involuntary muscle fibers connected with the hair bulbs. Slight shivering may also be produced, as from an application of cold, which proves that the phenomenon of shivering is not due exclusively to the influence of cold, but is, to some extent at least, connected with the excitation of the vasoconstrictor nerves from whatever cause.

The pallor and other phenomena due to excitation of the 497
vasoconstrictors from very hot applications are of but short duration. The pallor soon gives place to a dusky redness and the other appearances which accompany a hot application of more moderate degree. If the application is increased gradually in temperature from moderate heat, as from 100° to 104° F., a final temperature of 130° or even higher may be reached without excitation of the vasoconstrictors, the surface remaining reddened.

Some time after the end of a hot application, if continued 498
from 15 to 30 minutes, vasoconstrictor phenomena occur.

The effects of heat upon the circulation of the mucous 499
membrane are the same as upon the skin, except that a somewhat higher temperature is required to produce parallel results.

The stimulating effect of a high temperature upon the 500
vasoconstrictors renders very hot water useful as a means of

* "Medical Reports," 4th ed., pp. 99-101.

checking hemorrhage, and in capillary oozing from surgical wounds. It must be remembered, however, that when applied for such purposes, the water should be at a temperature of from 120° to 160° F., or hot enough to cause pain; and some allowance must be made for lowering of temperature during the application.

501 A blast of highly heated air has been successfully used as a means of checking hemorrhage in cases of metrorrhagia, also a jet of steam. The author makes use of a metallic instrument, really a hollow uterine sound, through which a stream of hot water is passed at a temperature of 170° F. The small vessels are thereby sealed up, and the hemorrhage is thus checked.

502 It is useful also to remember that hot applications to the skin produce not merely dilatation of the arteries, but especially the small veins, and a like dilatation of the lymph channels.

503 **2. Increase of Cutaneous Secretion and Respiration.** A general hot bath or even the application of heat to a comparatively small area of the surface produces a general increase of activity of the glands of the skin, both perspiratory and sebaceous. Perspiration may be induced either to the degree of producing slight moisture of the skin or profuse sweating, according to the length or intensity of the application made. The ordinary rate at which moisture is thrown off by the skin is from one to one and one-half ounces per hour; but by application of heat in the form of a very hot bath at a temperature of from 110° to 115° the rate of perspiration may be increased to more than an ounce a minute, or from fifty to sixty times the ordinary amount. The most pronounced effects possible may be secured by the electric-light bath and the sun bath.

504 These facts strongly emphasize the importance of administering water internally in connection with applications of heat. Loss of fluid from the blood has a depressing effect upon the heart similar to that produced by bleeding, though somewhat less marked; hence the vital necessity for making good the amount removed, by drinking water during as well as before and after the bath, if prolonged, or, if necessary, by means of rectal injections.

Prolonged and repeated perspiration induced by artificial 505
means weakens the skin, and thus lessens its power to react and to resist cold impressions unless counteracted by frequent cold applications.

It is interesting to note in this connection that while the 506
absorption of oxygen and the elimination of CO_2 by the lungs is diminished as the result of hot applications to the surface, the opposite effect is produced upon the skin. Ordinarily the skin performs about one per cent. of the total amount of respiratory work done by the body, but under the influence of heat this proportion is often doubled. This fact is evidently due to the dilatation of the blood-vessels of the skin, and to the moistening of the horny layer, whereby the interchange of gases between the skin and the air is facilitated.

3. Increased Loss of Heat by the Skin.

A brief application of heat to the surface 507
increases the loss of bodily heat by the skin in several ways: —

(1) By dilating the surface vessels, thus 508
increasing the area of the blood exposed to the cooling influences operating upon the surface of the body.

(2) By increasing the rate of the blood current in the skin through the stimulation of the vasodilators and the heart.

(3) By increasing the amount of evaporation from the surface through increased activity of the sweat-glands and increased osmosis, and by heating of the skin.

(4) By increasing the conductivity of the skin, thereby increasing loss of heat by radiation.

4. Decrease of Tactile Sensibility.

The tactile sensibility of the skin is greatest 509
from 95° to 98°, or the normal temperature of the surface, very hot applications (113° and upwards) having the effect to lessen sensibility (Exp. 41). This fact explains the special value of the alternating douche, or the so-called Scotch douche, which

renders such marked service in the treatment of sciatica and other forms of neuralgia. At a temperature of 130° and above, the tactile sensibility seems to be abolished, though the sensibility to pain still remains. It is a curious fact that the sensation produced by the application of intense heat is practically the same as that from intense cold.

5. Preparation of the Skin for the Application of Cold.

510 The thermic impression made by an application of any sort depends primarily upon the difference between the temperature of the skin and that of the application. By beginning the application at about the temperature of the skin, and gradually increasing it, a very high temperature may be borne without pain, as the zero of the temperature sense is thus gradually raised. This raising of the temperature of the skin has a special value in hydrotherapy as a preparation for the application of cold, the skin being thereby not only rendered more susceptible to the influence of cold, but likewise prepared to react after a cold application by reason of the increased nervous and vascular activity, and the large amount of heat stored up. For these reasons, the hot bath, contrary to what might naturally appear to be the case, prepares the skin for cold applications, — a fact which is of great importance in therapeutic applications of water.

511 When the skin is cold, or in cases of fatigue, in rheumatism with painful joints, in neuralgia, in anemic and feeble persons, and in many other conditions elsewhere indicated (1028), this preliminary heating of the skin is of the greatest importance.

THE EFFECTS OF HEAT UPON THE CIRCULATION.

512 In studying the influence of heat upon the circulation, we must consider not only the heart, as the center of this system, but especially the three great vascular areas, — the muscles, the portal system, and the skin, particularly the latter. Each of the parts named may be regarded as a great reservoir, capable of retaining a large share of all the blood

in the body. The portal area is excited and filled by digestive activity; the muscles, by vigorous exercise; and the skin, by percussion, friction, reaction from cold and heat, especially the latter.

It is impossible for each of these vascular areas to be excited to full activity or completely filled with blood at the same time. When one of these areas is in a state of congestion, the others must be in a condition of more or less marked anemia. This explains the pallor often occasioned by excessively violent exercise, and the pallor and giddiness which sometimes follow almost immediately upon the taking of food in certain forms of indigestion, also the faintness which not infrequently overcomes a person subjected suddenly to a high degree of heat in a vapor bath while sitting in an upright position. A bath at 102° F. produces venous congestion of the brain for the first three or four minutes, then cerebral anemia, which continues for some time after the bath, notwithstanding marked acceleration of the pulse. The same effect upon the cerebral circulation, though less pronounced, may be obtained by a foot or leg bath at from 104° to 108° F.[22] 513

Increased Activity of the Heart.

The effect of a general application of heat is to produce at once a notable increase in the force with temporary slowing of the heart's action (Exp. 42). This diminishes, however, as soon as free perspiration begins, owing to the lessening of the arterial tension by the dilatation of the cutaneous vessels, and the tolerance established through fatigue of the temperature sense. The final effect of a hot application is to lower arterial tension while quickening the pulse.[23] 514

The first effect of a very hot application to the skin, as already remarked (496), is to stimulate the vasoconstrictors, which results in contraction of the small blood-vessels of the surface; and this, together with the reflex stimulus received by the heart from the periphery, accounts for the sudden increase in the force and frequency of the pulse. This effect 515 is greatly increased if the water is applied in the form of a spray or a jet douche, owing to the mechanical effect thus added.

516 The first effect of a hot application to the surface is to produce a very transient contraction of the internal blood-vessels simultaneously with the surface contraction. This instantly gives way to a marked dilatation, which is in turn replaced by contraction as soon as the surface vessels are well relaxed.

517 This temporary excitation of the heart in connection with stimulation of the vasoconstrictors of the skin is liable to give rise to intense congestion of the internal viscera, especially the brain, hence the danger of administering this form of bath to plethoric persons, those who have suffered from apoplexy, or who have symptoms of incipient arterio-sclerosis. This condition of internal congestion is often indicated by a sensation of throbbing and fulness in the head, and the visible beating and pulsation of the vessels of the throat and temples, with flushing of the cheeks.

518 The reason for this increase of cardiac and vascular activity as the result of the application of heat is apparent when we consider the relation of the heart action to the condition of the surface vessels as regards heat elimination. One of the most important functions of the skin is the cooling of the blood. Now it is evident that if the temperature of the skin is raised, these cooling processes will occur at a slower rate; and thus, to secure an equal amount of cooling, the blood must be passed through the surface vessels more rapidly. Hence the nervous reflexes which regulate heat elimination are so arranged that an increase in the temperature of the skin or the media to which it is exposed, results in a quickening of the cardiac activity as well as an increase in the size of the blood-vessels of the skin, whereby a larger area of blood is exposed upon the surface of the body.

519 The very opposite of this occurs, of course, in connection with cold applications (**283**). Very hot applications also

induce, at first, a protective contraction of the surface vessels (**497**). This compensatory arrangement is continually brought into activity in the practice of hydrotherapy.

Various physiologists have noted that when a limited portion of the body is warmed, a reduction of temperature takes place in contiguous parts. This effect is purely a mechanical one. The overfilling of the blood-vessels of one portion of the area supplied by a single arterial trunk naturally results in robbing another portion of the same area, the vessels of which are not distended. **520**

THE EFFECTS OF HEAT UPON THE RESPIRATION.

General applications of heat increase the rate and facility of the respiratory movements. This is true, however, only of moist heat, so called, as dry heat, or rather the inhalation of dry hot air, produces the opposite effect, through its exciting influence upon the small air-tubes. Excessive dryness of the air also hinders the gaseous exchanges in the lungs, while moderate dryness promotes them. The increase of the chest movements in moist hot air does not indicate an increase of oxidation in the body, but is probably due to a lessened rate of CO_2 elimination. **521**

Nothing so quickly relieves an asthmatic patient as a hot full bath or a vapor or electric-light bath; but an examination of the products of respiration shows a decided decrease in the amount of CO_2, the natural result of diminution in vital combustions from the influence of heat upon the thermogenic centers. **522**

It should be noted, also, that while the respiratory movements are made with greater ease and frequency under the influence of heat, the depth of movement is considerably decreased; that is, the amount of tidal air is lessened. (Exp. 43). **523**

The effect observed *after* a hot bath is a temporarily diminished rate and depth of respiration. **524**

Such general applications of heat as raise the temperature of the blood excite the heat-controlling centers, and bring into **525** play the processes of heat dissipation, which include an increase of lung activity, as well as of skin perspiration and respiration. This fact explains the rapid respiration in high fever.

526 The influence of the hot bath upon respiration is in some respects quite similar to the effects of cold. With quite high temperatures (110° to 112° F.) a sense of constriction is felt when the body is immersed to the head in the full bath; the abdominal walls are contracted. The effect is most marked if the application is made by the aid of a douche with considerable pressure.

THE EFFECTS OF HEAT UPON THE MUSCLES.

527 Prolonged applications of heat, that is temperatures above 100°, diminish muscular excitability and capacity for muscular work to a notable extent. Maggiori and Vinaj have demonstrated this very clearly by an extended series of experiments. In one instance the muscular capacity, as shown by the results obtained by means of Mosso's ergograph, was diminished 8.043 kilogrammeters. It is this weakening of the muscles which gives rise to the very sensible enervating effects of a long hot bath. The writer has noted results in accord with those of these investigators (Fig. 27, A and B).

528 A vigorous young man experienced such great weakness after a hot full bath (Exp. 44) that he felt hardly able to walk. It is indeed surprising that the available energy of the body should by this means be so greatly reduced within so short a time. It can not be supposed that the actual store of force-producing material in the muscles or nerve centers is exhausted by the bath; hence we must conclude that the results observed are due simply to lessened muscular excitability.

529 **Lessened Irritability of the Voluntary Muscles.** Muscular irritability lessens very rapidly under the influence of a water bath at a temperature of 120° F. and above, and even at somewhat lower temperatures it is decidedly lessened. This phenomenon may be observed very readily in cold-blooded animals, in which a temperature of

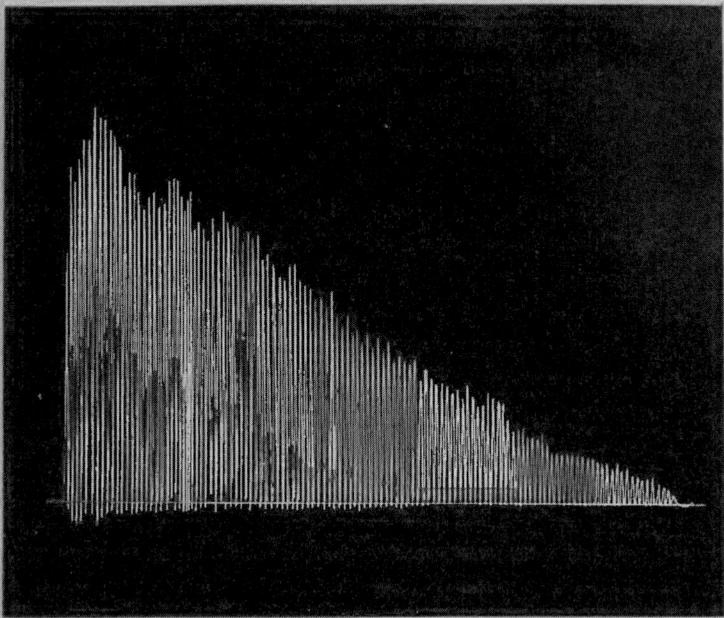

Fig. 27 *(a)*. Normal Fatigue Curve of Man Aged Twenty-four Years. Total work, 8.088 kgm.

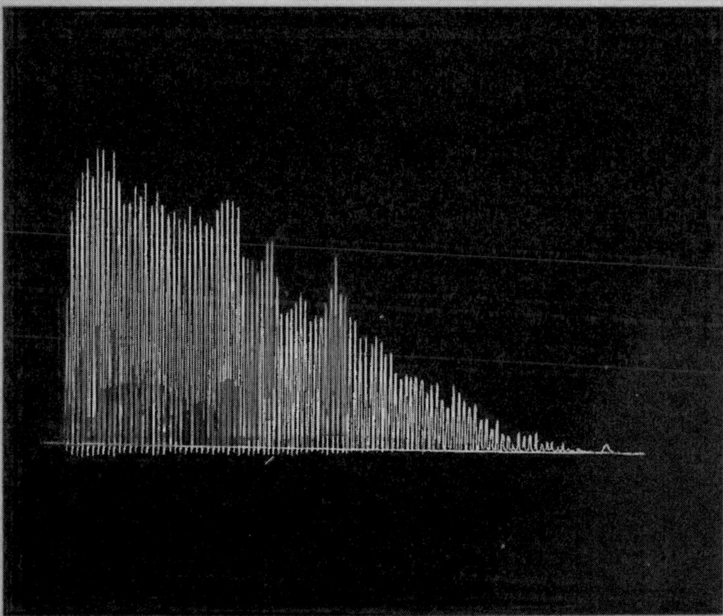

Fig. 27 *(b)*. Fatigue Curve of the Same Subject after a Hot Bath. Total work, 5,152 kgm.

a few degrees above that of the medium in which the animal lives, produces almost complete paralysis, and a few degrees higher at once gives rise to absolute muscular inactivity, through heat-stiffening of the muscles. Very prolonged hot applications at temperatures not much above the normal body temperature similarly give rise to muscular weakness in man.[24]

Notwithstanding these facts, experience shows that *very* 530
short hot applications are the best of all means for recovering a person exhausted by prolonged or violent exercise. This measure has often been employed for the relief of exhausted soldiers. An eminent English army surgeon made use of the hot enema for this purpose more than a century ago. The nerve centers of a person in a state of extreme exhaustion do not readily respond to the stimulation of cold; in other words, a person in that condition will not react to cold, hence the necessity for an application of heat. The restorative effects of an application of heat in such cases is perhaps due in part to the elimination of the fatigue poisons which is thereby encouraged, as well as to reflex stimulation of the nerve centers. The good results are rendered much more decided and lasting if the hot application is succeeded by a short cold application, such as a broken cold horizontal jet to the spine for 3 or 4 seconds, or a rubbing wet sheet, or a cold friction bath.

It is worth while to note in this connection that the 531
exhausting effects of a hot bath may be readily neutralized by an application of cold water in the form of a douche or a shower bath, since the sensation is not due to an absolute loss of strength or energy in either the muscles or the nerve centers, but is a purely nervous phenomenon, expressing the peculiar effect upon the nerve centers of impressions of heat communicated through the peripheral nerves. The restorative effect of a cold bath administered after a hot bath, the author has demonstrated frequently by clinical experience as well as by laboratory experiment (Exp. 45).

532 A young man of twenty years, when subjected to a careful dynamometric test, was found to have a total strength of 8,550 pounds, as shown by *a* on the accompanying chart. After a hot bath at a temperature of from 110° to 118° F. for ten minutes, the total strength was found to be 6,840 pounds. The details of this test are shown in the tracing marked *b* on the accompanying chart. After a cold shower bath for one minute, followed by vigorous rubbing, the same dynamometric test was again tried, with a total strength result of 8,195 pounds, as shown by the tracing *c* on the accompanying graphic.

533 To secure the maximum of restorative results, the hot bath should not be continued more than five minutes, and should be followed by a cold shower or spray douche from 5 to 20 seconds, ending in a very cold broken douche to the spine for 2 seconds.

534 Excessive muscular irritability, as in a person suffering from cramps, fidgets, or irregular muscular twitchings, is quieted by a prolonged neutral full bath (92° to 95° F.).

535 The effect of very hot applications in lessening muscular irritability is often utilized therapeutically in the treatment of deformities resulting from muscular contraction, for the relief of vaginismus, and in cases of contraction of the anal muscle.

536 **Increased Irritability of Involuntary Muscles.** Very hot applications increase the irritability of the smooth, or non-striated, muscles. This is shown by the fact that very hot applications to the skin cause contraction of the muscular walls of the small blood-vessels and the minute muscles connected with the hair bulbs, giving rise to goose-flesh and pallor. This physiological property of heat is utilized in the application of hot water to the uterus by vaginal injection for the relief not only of hemorrhage but of chronic catarrh and congestion of this organ, and in the condition known as subinvolution.

537 Hot rectal irrigation is one of the best means of combating chronic congestion and enlargement of the prostate.

A large hot enema or coloclyster will not infrequently relieve constipation when other means are ineffectual, by stimulating the involuntary muscular fibers of the intestines. **538**

THE EFFECTS OF HEAT UPON THE NERVOUS SYSTEM.

Heat may excite or exhaust the nervous system according to the mode of application. An application may be at first excitant, then depressant. The effect of a neutral bath (92° to 95° F.) is to diminish nervous irritability, thus producing a true sedative effect. This result is obtained through the protective influence of a neutral medium. The body immersed in water near its own temperature is almost entirely shut away from a variety of perturbing influences which continually play upon the nerve centers through the sensory impulses transmitted from the periphery. As a result, opportunity is afforded for the accumulation of nervous energy in the cerebro-spinal centers. To obtain a sedative effect, the bath must be considerably prolonged (from 30 minutes to an hour and a half). **539**

Baths of a high temperature (100° F. and upwards) produce, first, very exciting effects, manifested by nervousness, headache, etc.; later, symptoms of exhaustion appear. **540**

Heat Stimulates Protoplasmic Activity.

This is the fundamental fact upon which the physiological phenomenon developed by its application is based. Heat is indeed one of the most powerful of all physiological stimuli. Both the excitant and the exhaustive effects of hot applications are explainable by this single fact. The excitant effects are due to the direct influence of heat upon the nerve filaments and other tissues; while the exhausting effects are due to the fact that while the protoplasmic or vital activities of the body are excited by certain forms of hot applications, thus giving rise to an accumulation of tissue wastes or excrementitious elements, the oxidation of these wastes is diminished by the effort of the body to prevent excessive accumulation of heat through inhibition of the auto- **541** matic thermogenic centers. The result is an accumulation within the body of tissue poisons, which produce phenomena similar to those resulting from prolonged or violent exercise, — the so-called "fatigue poisons," which have been shown to possess properties almost identical with those of curari.

542 In harmony with this idea is the interesting fact recently ascertained that sunstroke is really a toxemia resulting either from the excessive accumulation of poisons within the body, or the development of special poisons under the influence of heat. May it not be possible that the well-recognized debilitating influence of excessive heat is, in part at least, due to the same cause?

543 **Reflex Effects Produced by Hot Applications.** Special reflex effects are obtainable by hot applications to certain areas of the skin, which sustain a known reflex relation to the internal viscera. These effects are obtained through impressions made on the ganglia of the great sympathetic and the vasomotor and other ganglia of the cord. To obtain effects of this sort, heat may be applied either alone or in conjunction with cold water in the alternating douche. The reflex effects thus obtained are either those of vasodilatation or vasoconstriction, according to the degree of heat employed. Warm or hot water stimulates the vasodilators, while very hot water (115° to 130° F.) produces vasoconstriction.

544 Winternitz, Brown-Sequard, Tholozan, Rosbach, and others have experimentally worked out the topography of this reflex action with reference to all the more important internal viscera, pointing out the exact area of the surface which must be operated upon in order to obtain the effects desired. Among the most important of these associated areas are the following:—

545 1. The face and the back of the neck, which are in relation with the brain.

546 2. The upper portion of the spine, the chest, and the shoulders, which are intimately associated reflexly with the lungs through the pneumogastric.

3. The hands and feet, which are associated with the brain, the mucous membrane of the nose, and the organs of the chest. 547

4. The middle dorsal region, with the stomach. 548

5. The breasts, with the uterus. 549

6. The skin covering the lumbar region, with the kidneys. 550

7. The lower lumbar region, with the uterus and the lower extremities. 551

8. The internal surface of the thighs, with the uterus. 552

9. The plantar region, with the uterus. 553

10. The feet, with the kidneys. 554

11. The skin covering the lower third of the sternum, with the kidneys. 555

12. The skin surface over the liver, spleen, stomach, bowels, and bladder, with the corresponding organs. 556

Very hot applications made over these surfaces stimulate simultaneously the vasoconstrictors of the area to which the application is made, and those of the internal region which is in reflex relation with it, as just designated. The explanation of these interesting relations will be found in a study of the anatomical relations of the vasomotor centers of the spine and other special ganglia with the areas innervated by them. 557

The reflex effects of these localized applications at a high temperature are of great service in hydrotherapy; for example, cerebral congestion may be relieved by the hot foot bath, which, as Mosso proved by experiments on a man a portion of whose skull had been removed, is capable of producing even cerebral anemia. The temperature should be from 105° to 110° F. A hot full bath at 102° F. is often most effective in relieving cerebral hyperemia. Bathing the face with very hot water is a most effective means of checking nosebleed. Hot sponging of the head and neck often gives complete relief in insomnia from cerebral congestion. 558

Splenic and hepatic congestion, the usual accompaniment of malarial disease, is relieved by very hot fomentations 559 applied over these organs. Uterine hemorrhage may often be checked by a short, very hot foot bath (105° to 115° F.), although the warm foot bath (92° to 100° F.) causes dilatation of the uterine vessels. Relief from congestive headache is obtained by very hot sponging of the back of the neck.

560 In employing heat to the spine for the relief of pulmonary hemorrhage, the best effects are obtained by making the application to the skin overlying the first dorsal vertebra, as the vasomotor center controlling the vessels of the lungs is situated at this level of the spinal cord.

THE EFFECTS OF HEAT UPON THE BLOOD.

561 Winternitz and many other observers have pointed out the interesting fact that under the influence of hot baths the blood count is considerably diminished, through detention of blood cells in the viscera, as shown by Breitenstein.

562 There is also observed a diminution in the percentage of hemoglobin present in proportion to the decrease of red blood-corpuscles. Winternitz has also pointed out the remarkable fact that, while there is a marked increase in the number of leucocytes in the circumscribed part subjected to the influence of heat, there is a decided decrease in the number of red cells, while Henocque has observed an increase in the rate of reduction of oxyhemoglobin.[25] These effects in part at least explain the mottled appearance of the skin induced by hot applications.

563 Strasser showed (*Deutsche med.-Zeit.*, 1896) that general hot applications diminish the alkalinity of the blood by increasing the amount of acid phosphate, often to the extent of double the normal quantity.

THE EFFECTS OF HEAT UPON NUTRITION.

564 The stimulating effects of heat upon cell life may be easily studied under the microscope by the application of heat to the ameba, or the white blood-corpuscle. Nothing could be more interesting than to note the readiness with which

these cells respond to the very slightest increase of temperature. When heat is applied to the surface of the body, not only the skin, but the entire body is to some degree excited thereby, both through the transmission of heat by the conductivity of the tissues to the internal parts, and its transportation by the blood current from the skin to the viscera. The result is an increase of the activity of the cell life of the body so far as is possible without increased absorption of oxygen. Oxidation is diminished, as is indicated by the diminished absorption of oxygen and exhalation of CO_2. But the increase of cell activity is nevertheless shown by the greater amount of nitrogen eliminated, largely in the form of uric acid.

The diminution of oxidation may occur to such a degree 565
as to produce an increase of sugar in the blood, and may even give rise to its appearance in the urine. It is for this reason that hot baths must be used with great discretion in diabetes and in all other maladies characterized by deficient oxidation.

That heat stimulates vital activity is clearly shown by its 566
influence upon the skin. A patient who has worn the moist abdominal bandage for some time, or has been subjected to the daily application of fomentations to some portion of the body for a few weeks, will present a mottled appearance of the skin of the part to which the application has been made, — a very striking illustration of the stimulating effects of heat upon the pigment cells. The heat from the direct rays of the sun produces a similar effect, giving rise to freckles, and deepening the color of the complexion often to a remarkable degree. The same effects are likewise produced by the electric light, and even by the newly discovered X-ray. The stimulating effect of the electric light upon the growth of plants and the ripening of fruits affords further evidence that heat and light act powerfully in stimulating vital activity.

Elevation of the body temperature above normal increases 567
the oxidation of nitrogen. This is shown by the increase of urea and other proteid wastes, and accounts for the rapid wasting of the muscles during febrile disease under the influence of high temperature.

THE EFFECTS OF HEAT UPON THE STOMACH, LIVER, AND OTHER DIGESTIVE ORGANS.

568 It has been experimentally proved that the amount of hydrochloric acid secreted by the peptic glands may be very perceptibly increased by means of fomentations placed over the stomach for an hour or two after eating. A hot water bag may be more conveniently employed for this purpose.

569 The hot douche over the stomach and spine opposite diminish the secretion of HCl in hyperpepsia. General hot baths produce the same effect (Simon), perhaps from excessive loss of sodium chloride in the perspiration.

570 Hot applications made over the region of the liver by means of hot compresses or fomentations also unquestionably increase the flow of bile, and doubtless stimulate all the other activities of the liver.

571 Applications of heat over the abdomen may also increase the activity of the digestive processes in the intestines and the functional activity of the pancreas and the spleen.

THE EFFECTS OF HEAT UPON BODY TEMPERATURE AND HEAT PRODUCTION.

572 The immediate effect of a general application of heat to the body is to occasion a rise of temperature; in fact, immersion of the body in a bath at the body temperature will in the course of an hour cause a rise of temperature of 1.8° F., while water at 104° F. may occasion a rise of three or four degrees within fifteen minutes (Exp. 46, 47).

573 An interesting observation first made by Hippocrates, and verified by all students of hydrotherapy, is that a short application of heat to the body is followed by a lowering of the temperature, with increased susceptibility to the influence of cold. Modern calorimetric studies have shown that the effect of short applications of heat to the body is to diminish heat production, while at the same time heat elimination is encour-

aged, as shown by increased perspiration, relaxation of the surface vessels, and increased activity of the heart. This is the *atonic reaction* of heat.

Prolonged applications of heat always give rise to increase of temperature, both by diminishing heat elimination and by increasing heat production. Heat stimulates vital activity; indeed, there is perhaps no other agent capable of exerting so remarkable an influence upon vital processes. By a prolonged bath at a few degrees above the normal temperature, heat production and heat accumulation may be so increased as to become dangerous to life in a few minutes. 574

Even warm air increases heat production to a most remarkable degree. An external temperature a few degrees above the body temperature may increase heat production more than 300 per cent. This fact is illustrated by the prevalence of heat-stroke, or thermic fever, during a period of hot weather, especially in damp climates. Whatever causes a rise of the body temperature increases heat production, at least in all physiological conditions, although there may be exceptions in some conditions of disease. So also whatever increases heat elimination tends to increase heat production. 575

A rise of 20° F. in external temperature occasions an elevation of 1° F. in body temperature, and a further elevation of 1° takes place for each additional rise of 20° F. 576

It is not necessary in order to obtain the effects of heat that the application made should be above the temperature of the body. A bath at the exact temperature of the body will cause a general rise of temperature (Exp. 48.) 577

REACTION FOLLOWING AN APPLICATION OF HEAT.

For most purposes it is doubtless true that the reaction effects resulting from cold are to be preferred to those from hot applications: nevertheless, the peculiar effects obtainable from heat will sometimes be found better suited to the case in hand than those arising from cold. Indeed, not infrequently the dread of cold water on the part of the patient 578 is so intense as to make its use inadmissible without a course of gradual training. In these cases, the effects obtainable from heat are particularly serviceable, and its employment may prevent the development of a positive idiosyncracy against cold.

579 The general reaction effects produced by intense, short, general applications of heat are as follows: —

ACTION.	REACTION.
1. Brief contraction, then dilatation of the surface blood-vessels, especially of the small veins.	1. Vasoconstriction.
2. Slight pallor if previously red, followed by dusky redness.	2. Pallor.
3. Sometimes goose-flesh appearance and slight shivering.	3. Skin smooth, soft, and moist.
4. Slowed, then quickened high-tension pulse.	4. Pulse frequent, tension low.
5. Respiration at first checked, then frequent, CO_2 diminished.	5. Respiration frequent, free, superficial.
6. Perspiration at first checked, then increased.	6. Perspiration lessened.
7. Heating of the skin.	7. Gradual cooling of the skin.
8. Rise of internal temperature from diminished heat elimination.	8. Depression of internal temperature from increased heat elimination and decreased heat production.
9. General nervous excitation; at moderate temperature, sense of comfort and relief.	9. Diminished nervous and mental irritability, drowsiness, and depression.
10. Increased muscular irritability.	10. Muscular weakness and indisposition to muscular effort.

From the above it will be readily apparent that the general and usual reaction effects of heat are of an atonic or depressant character.

580 **The Neutral Bath.** A bath which is absolutely neutral is practically impossible, for the reason that a bath exactly at the temperature of the skin checks the elimination of heat, and hence occasions a rise of the

body temperature, while a bath a few degrees below the temperature of the body excites the temperature sense, and thus gives rise to increased heat production and other reflex effects.

The vital perturbations set up by the warm bath, how- 581
ever, are so slight as to be scarcely perceptible, and the characteristic effect of the bath is its calmative or quieting effect. This result is not obtained by any depressing action, but by the protection afforded by the medium of water so employed as to be absolutely unirritating, without percussion, and of such a temperature as to shield the body from the continued excitation resulting from the contact of the skin with the clothing, constantly changing temperature, force of movement, and various other disturbing influences.

As the result of this protection, the nerve centers, being completely at rest, are afforded an opportunity to accumulate a store of energy, so that the warm, or so-called neutral, bath is, after all, not really neutral in its physiological effects, but is recuperative and energizing through promotion of the nutritive processes, and the accumulation of force-producing material in the nerve cells. The irritability of the cutaneous nerves is perhaps lessened by the imbibition of water.

THE EFFECTS OF ALTERNATE HOT AND COLD APPLICATIONS TO THE SKIN.

The Scotch Douche.

In this form of application the skin is first 582
heated considerably above its normal temperature, then the temperature is lowered by the use of cold water. In alternate applications the heating and cooling are several times repeated. The reaction which takes place as the result of the Scotch or the alternating douche may be made chiefly circulatory in character, or both circulatory and thermic. This form of application is therefore a most efficient means of stimulating nutritive changes, obtaining derivative effects, etc., and that without creating thermic disturbances of any kind in the body.

583 Pflüger found that a short hot bath following a cold bath increased the reduction of temperature.[26]

584 Vinaj based upon this observation the recommendation to follow the cold bath employed for reducing temperature in fever with a hot bath, continued for two or three minutes. For further considerations respecting alternate applications, see paragraphs **677, 681.**

GENERAL VITAL REACTIONS RESULTING FROM HYDRIC PROCEDURES.

585 As previously intimated, the circulatory and thermic reactions which occur from cold applications to the surface are only two of a considerable number of distinct reactions resulting from the cutaneous excitation occasioned by an intense application of cold. A consideration of the effects of this form of stimulation in the light of modern physiological research, leads at once to the conclusion that the reactions produced involve not only the nerve centers, blood-vessels, and involuntary muscles, but every cell and tissue in the body.

586 A careful study of the effects of local application leads to the conclusion that there are many subtle and not easily observed reactions to which many of the effects of hydrotherapy may be properly attributable. Doubtless every viscus, even every gland and probably every individual cell has its own mode of reacting to the powerful stimulus of thermic impressions made upon the skin.

587 The profound effects produced upon the nervous system by the application of water to the skin enables us through this agent to influence every bodily function, for, as one has well said, "The nervous system dominates all the phenomena of organic life directly or indirectly; all depends upon it. Nothing transpires in the body of the animal without its intervention. The cells are the artisans in the organic workshop, but the nerves are the overseers."

588 Whatever agent affects the heat-producing processes of the body, affects, likewise, in a most pronounced degree, all the vital processes. As Lubansky has well said: "To touch

calorification is, in a certain sense, to touch the springs of existence; and disturbance of the heat-making functions of the body produces a corresponding disturbance in the most important functions of the system. It is to create the necessity for repair, and to impress directly and profoundly the general nervous system."

SUMMARY OF ORGANIC CHANGES PRODUCED BY HEAT AND COLD.

1. Elevation of body temperature is accompanied by 589
increase of metabolism.

2. A fall of temperature is accompanied by decreased metabolic change.

3. Short cold applications cause rise of temperature and increase of metabolism.

4. Prolonged cold applications cause fall of temperature and diminished metabolism.

5. Short hot applications cause fall of temperature with diminished metabolism.

6. Prolonged hot applications cause rise of temperature and increased metabolism, especially increased oxidation of albumin.

7. No disturbance of metabolism occurs as the result of baths at neutral temperatures, or while the body temperature remains normal.

8. Strasser showed increased alkalinity of the blood after cold baths, and diminution after hot baths.

9. Jardet has shown that the acidity of the urine is decreased by warm baths, and may even become alkaline.

In febrile conditions, when heat production is increased, antipyretic applications do not lessen the heat production unless applied in such a way as to cool the muscles and produce a diminution in the general body temperature.

The primary effect of cold applications is to increase CO_2 production. In the reaction period there is elevation of temperature, which, if sufficiently pronounced, is accompanied by an increased oxidation of albumin.

THE PHYSIOLOGICAL EFFECTS OF FRICTION OR MECHANICAL IRRITATION OF THE SKIN.

590 MECHANICAL irritation of the skin produces effects so closely allied to those of hydric applications, and in the practical employment of hydriatic measures is so constantly and so intimately associated with the use of water, that it is proper to devote a few paragraphs to the consideration of the physiological effects of this powerful means of vasomotor excitation, which may be properly classed as mechanical rather than chemical or thermic stimuli.

The forms of mechanical stimulation especially utilized in hydrotherapy are *friction* and *percussion*.

591 **Friction.** This procedure consists in rubbing the surface of the body with the bare hand, or with the hand reinforced by a mitt, glove, or towel, either dry or moistened with water at any desired temperature. Percussion may be applied by the hand, usually in connection with friction, but this mechanical effect is usually obtained in connection with water in the different forms of the douche.

Physiological Effects. The effects of friction and percussion are essentially the same, the magnitude and the intensity of the effect depending upon the force employed and the duration of the application. The effects of percussion as connected with the douche will be described elsewhere (**1015**). The physiological effects of friction have been carefully studied by Naumann (1867), Röhrig (1873), Winternitz, and other eminent investigators. Three grades or degrees of friction are recognized; namely, "light," "energetic," and "very vigorous." Briefly summarized, their effects may be described as follows : —

592 1. *Light Friction.*— Light centripetal friction applied to the surface accelerates the circulation, causing rise of blood

pressure, increases the force and frequency of the pulse, and lessens the frequency of respiration.

Very light friction continued for some time gives rise to contraction of the small blood-vessels, which may persist for several hours. There is also a slight rise of temperature, due to a small increase of heat production and a slight diminution of heat elimination.

2. *Energetic friction* causes first very marked contraction 593
of the blood-vessels, which is quickly followed by dilatation of the vessels, arteries, veins, capillaries, and lymphatics, with great acceleration of the blood current.

The increase of heat elimination reduces the temperature several tenths of a degree.

3. *Very vigorous friction*, or violent irritation of the 594
skin, produces almost instant and very marked dilatation of the cutaneous vessels, the preliminary period of contraction being so brief as be practically imperceptible.

The heart's action is slowed, as is also the respiration.

Heat elimination is increased nearly fifty per cent (Winternitz, Pospischil), and the temperature may fall as much as 1° or 2° F. (Mantegazza).

Examination of the products of respiration show marked increase of CO_2 (Pflüger), which would indicate increased heat production, notwithstanding the lowered temperature, showing that the increase of heat elimination is much greater in proportion than that of heat production.

There is, also, according to Pflüger, a marked increase in the production of urea, showing that there is a general increase of catabolism, since both nitrogenous and carbonaceous wastes are augmented.

Very violent friction or irritation produces marked weakness of the heart, dyspnea, and in rabbits, albumin in the urine (Walkenstein), in which again we see an effect identical with that which follows an excessively severe cold application.

All the functions of the skin are stimulated by friction. Under its application a dry skin becomes moist and oily, through the increased activity of the perspiratory and sebaceous glands. It is also a common observation that friction promotes the development of hair upon the parts to which it is applied. Weyrich and Winternitz have shown that by the application of friction to the skin, the amount of moisture thrown off may be increased more than fifty per cent. Under the influence of friction the temperature of the skin is raised to a very marked degree, through dilatation of the surface vessels, which brings an increased amount of blood to the surface. This is, of course, the cause of the increased heat dissipation under the influence of friction. This fact explains the interesting observation of Winternitz, that friction of the patient in the cold bath very greatly increases its temperature-lowering power. In experiments made by the writer, a rise of surface temperature amounting to 2° F. has been observed as a result of friction of the skin of a healthy person (Exp. 49). This would represent an increase of heat elimination of at least eight per cent. In a person with a cold skin the increase may be sixty or even seventy-five per cent.

The mechanical effects of friction vary with its direction. When the friction is applied in the direction of the blood current in the veins (centripetal friction), the movement of blood toward the heart is accelerated, and thus the activities of the part are increased. The circulation of lymph is also encouraged, there is an increase in the rapidity of the vital exchanges, and a promotion of all the metabolic processes.

On the other hand, friction made in the direction opposite to that in which the blood moves in the veins (centrifugal friction) slows the circulation, diminishes metabolic activity, and thus produces a sedative effect.

The foregoing facts demonstrate most clearly the potency of mechanical irritation as a means of vasomotor stimulation, and through this powerful influence upon one of the most vital functions of organic life, its importance as a rational therapeutic procedure. The practical application of the principles thus set forth will be dwelt upon elsewhere (**1209**).

Dermographism. The phenomenon to which the term "dermographism" is applied is closely allied to urticaria. Pressure made upon the skin, as in drawing a line with the tip of the finger or the end of a lead-pencil, ordinarily produces but a very slight effect, merely a temporary pallor, quickly followed by a barely perceptible redness of the skin. In certain persons, however, a simple stroke with the finger tip produces a raised white or rose-colored area corresponding to the surface touched. 595

Dermographism indicates a disordered state of the vasomotor nerves or nerve centers. These structures are affected by some poisonous substance, received from without or produced in the alimentary canal, and in such a manner that the vessels have lost their tone, or are unable to maintain their normal equilibrium. Demographism also affords information respecting the condition of the nervous system in general. It indicates that there exists in the body of the patient some toxic agent against which the nervous system has ceased to be able to defend itself.

This curious symptom is most often present in certain forms of neurasthenia, especially gastric neurasthenia, in hysteria, diabetes, rheumatism, stomach dilatation, and gastro-intestinal fermentations.*

This test is one of the means whereby the physician may judge of the susceptibility of his patient to hydric applications. The test should be applied to each patient received for treatment as a means of determining his power of reaction to mechanical stimulation. Persistent spasm of the vessels, as shown by pallor remaining for some minutes, indicates an abnormal irritability of the vasomotor nerves or of the visceral ganglia of the small vessels. A quickly appearing and prolonged redness indicates that the vessels lose their tone with abnormal readiness. All these facts should be noted and considered in the hydriatic treatment of invalids.

---

* "Étude sur le Demographisme," T. Barthélemy, Paris.

THE PHYSIOLOGICAL EFFECTS OF LIGHT.

596 THE therapeutic use of light is so closely associated with hydriatry that it seems proper to make here a brief statement of the physiological effects of this powerful agent, which, though in use from ancient times, has never been scientifically studied until within recent years. Limited space will, however, permit nothing more than an exceedingly brief summary of the important fundamental facts bearing upon this subject.

Considered from the standpoint of physics, light is not a force, but a mode of motion,—a movement of the ether particles resulting from the energy set free by the sun or some other incandescent body. For a minute study of the physical properties of light, and for purposes of spectrum analysis, and in the study of the physiology of vision, light is considered as being composed of three primary colors,—red, green, and violet; but in a study of the question from a therapeutic basis, another classification of the nature of the sun's rays is more practical and useful. Thus, the sun's rays may be divided into three classes; viz., *heat* rays, *luminous* rays, and *actinic*, or *chemical*, rays. The whole gamut of light rays, if considered analogous to the musical scale for the purpose of comparison, is found to extend through about four octaves, of which the luminous rays occupy as much space as would be represented by the interval of the sixth in music. Two of the four octaves are found below the luminous rays, and another octave above. The heat rays occupy the lower two octaves, and include also the red and ultrared, while the chemical rays include the violet, the ultraviolet, and the upper octave of non-luminous rays.

Of these three classes of rays, the heat rays and the chemical rays are those of special interest in therapeutics. The heat rays while in the form of radiant energy passing through space do not manifest heat, but when they come in contact with objects which offer resistance to their passage,—in other words, objects opaque to heat rays,—they are transformed into heat, and the temperature of the opaque object is raised. So likewise the actinic, or chemical, rays manifest their special properties only when they come in contact with substances in which they are capable of setting up molecular changes, the radiant energy being then transformed into chemical energy.

It has long been known that the three sets of rays may be separated by the employment of glass of different colors. Red glass, for example, gives passage to rays which are almost wholly thermal in character, while blue or violet glass allows only the chemical, or actinic, rays to pass through it. Yellow and green glass, on the other hand, while transparent to the luminous rays, permit also the passage through of a few of the thermal and actinic rays.

The art of photography illustrates the action of the chemical ray upon various chemical substances. Its action may also be observed in the coloration of flowers and leaves and other phenomena in the animal and vegetable world. One of the most interesting illustrations of the action of the actinic ray upon animals is to be observed in the curious phenomenon known as "sunburn." That this is not really a burn, but erythema due to the noxious action of the actinic rays, is shown, first, by the fact that the swelling, redness, and pain do not appear until several hours after exposure to the sun's rays; and secondly, by the fact that exposure of the skin to light from which the actinic rays have been separated, but which present the heat rays in all their original intensity, prevents entirely the ordinary effects of the intense rays of the sun upon nude surfaces unaccustomed to such exposure. The term "solar erythema" is preferable to the expression "sunburn."

Within the last few years numerous experiments have 597
been made by Arloing, d'Arsonval, Geisler, and others, for

the purpose of determining the influence of different classes of rays — luminous, thermal, and actinic — upon microbic life. Investigations have shown that the chemical rays — violet and ultraviolet — are unfavorable to the growth of bacteria, at least such pathogenic bacteria as the bacillus anthracis, the bacillus pyocyaneus, and the typhoid bacillus. Graber showed that the earthworm, which habitually hides itself away from the light, behaves toward a red light as toward absolute darkness, while the violet and ultraviolet have the same effect upon it as ordinary light. Experiments made by Paul Bert, Du Bois, and others have given similar results.

The influence of light in producing pigmentation of the skin in human beings is a matter of common observation. Solar erythema, or so-called sunburn, is always followed by a deepened color of the skin; after this pigmentation has taken place, the surface involved is less subject to sunburn, and may be wholly protected so long as this deepened color is retained. This process in the skin may accordingly be looked upon as a protective action for the purpose of preserving the deeper and more important structures of the body from injury through the noxious influence of the chemical rays. Negroes and other dark-skinned races are not subject to solar erythema, their skins having by long residence in a hot climate, and through the action of heredity, acquired a natural protection against the chemical ray. We are doubtless unaware how much our ordinary life depends upon the action of the thermal and actinic rays of the sun, especially the latter. The fact that an excessive action of the chemical rays gives rise to an acute inflammatory process in the superficial layers of the skin, is sufficient evidence of its powerful influence upon animal life. In conditions of disease persons have been found so sensitive that exposure to even the diffused light of day was sufficient to give rise to a marked erythema of the face.

598 A most remarkable and interesting fact, first pointed out by Picton in 1832, and more recently studied by Black and Barlow

in England, Lindholm of Norway, and Finsen of Copenhagen, is the noxious influence of the actinic ray in smallpox. It has been found that if the chemical rays are excluded by hanging thick red curtains before the windows of the sick-room during the suppurative stage of the eruption and the consequent secondary fever, ulceration may be almost uniformly averted. Finsen has within the last half dozen years undertaken an extensive series of observations for the purpose of studying more accurately the physiological effect of the actinic ray, making numerous experiments upon flies, worms, embryos, and other forms of animal life. These experiments have demonstrated very clearly that the chemical ray is an excitant of the nervous system; and that under ordinary circumstances it may be considered as one of the most important promoters of animal life and energy. The importance of the thermic influences derived from heat rays need not be emphasized, as this has long been well known and appreciated; but the fact that the actinic ray is a direct stimulant of the functions of animal and vegetable life, and thus a means of supporting vital energy in all its forms, is a discovery of the highest importance, and one which will doubtless prove of great utility in the future. To the chemical rays rather than to the thermic rays must in all probability be attributed the greater part of the wonderful results which have long been recognized as following the proper employment of the sun bath, or so-called insolation.

Upon the discovery of the electric light and practical 599
methods of producing it, numerous experiments were undertaken for the purpose of ascertaining whether this excellent artificial substitute for sunlight possessed the property of stimulating the vital processes of plant life in a manner analogous to the action of sunlight. An interesting paper by Wm. Siemens, published in March, 1880, contained a detailed account of experiments made for the purpose of determining the influence of the electric light upon vegetation, with the following conclusions:—

1. That the electric light is efficacious in producing chlorophyl in the leaves of plants and in promoting growth.

2. That an electric center of light equal to 1,400 candles, placed at a distance of two meters from growing plants, appeared to be equal in effect to average daylight at this season of the year (March), but that more economical effects may be attained by more powerful light centers.

3. That the carbonic acid and nitrogenous compounds generated in diminutive quantities in the electric arc, produce no sensible deleterious effects upon plants enclosed in the same space.

4. That plants do not appear to require a period of rest during the twenty-four hours of the day, but make increased and vigorous progress if subjected during the daytime to sunlight, and during the night to electric light.

5. That the radiation of heat from powerful electric arcs can be made available to counteract the effect of night frosts, and is likely to promote the setting and ripening of fruit in the open air.

6. That while under the influence of the electric light, plants can sustain increased stove heat without collapsing,—a circumstance favorable to forcing by electric light, and showing the influence of light as a vital stimulant.

Similar experiments have been made by others, the pioneer in this line of investigation being Hervé-Mangon (Compt. Rend. 53, 243). These experiments showed that the electric light is capable of causing the development of chlorophyl and inducing heliotropism, or the phenomenon of turning or bending toward the light.

Prillieux (Compt. Rend. 69, 410) showed that the electric light is capable of promoting assimilation in plants, or decomposition of carbon dioxide and water.

Siemens found that plants exposed to ordinary daylight and six hours of electric light in addition "far surpassed the others in darkness of green and vigorous appearance generally." Strawberries and other fruits were fully equal to those raised under ordinary conditions, and grapes were of stronger flavor than usual. Melons were remarkably large and aromatic, and bananas were pronounced by expert judges to be "unsurpassed in flavor."

Many of these experiments have been repeated in this country with similar results. The most important experiments were those conducted at the Cornell University Agricultural Station in 1889–90. The results obtained showed clearly—

1. That the electric light may be used under such conditions as to make it fairly comparable to sunlight in its power to promote protoplasmic activity.

2. That the electric light acts as a tonic to plants, so that they are able to endure adverse conditions which otherwise would cause them to collapse.

3. That the electric light is a true vital stimulus, since the effect of its use at night, upon plants, is essentially the same as that of the longer day of the Arctics upon plants growing in that region.

De Fontaine, in an article in *Semaine Médicale*, 1888, entitled "Coup de Soleil Électrique," gives an interesting account of the results of exposure to a powerful electric light, undertaken for experimental purposes by a physician, M. Maklakow, surgeon to a large factory near Moscow, in which the electric arc is employed in soldering metals. The first symptoms felt were tingling of the skin; a few moments later, pronounced coryza and lachrymation, the eyes being swollen so that they could not be opened. There was marked photophobia, and a sensation of burning heat upon the right side of the face and neck. After a short sleep, the experimenter awoke with all his symptoms aggravated. By evening of the same day the face had become brick-red in appearance, was very much swollen; there was marked chemosis of the conjunctiva, and all parts which had been exposed to the light were greatly inflamed, the investigator suffering much during the entire night. An interesting fact noted was that while the whole conjunctiva covering the ball of the eye was intensely inflamed, the mucous lining of the lids was not at all affected, evidently because not directly exposed to the light rays. The following day the erythema increased, becoming edematous, hot, dry, and painful to the touch. The night of the second day the symptoms began to abate considerably, and toward night of the following day the epidermis began to separate, and a few days later desquamation of the skin took place in large scales, as after scarlet fever. The pigmentation of the skin remained for some time after the acute symptoms had disappeared. The amount of heat to which the individual was subjected in this experiment was not sufficient to occasion any inconvenience, and the painful symptoms did not appear until some hours after the exposure.

This experiment proves very clearly not only that the noxious effects of light are due to the chemical rays, but that the electric light is capable of producing results identical with those produced by the sun's rays.

600 According to Dolbear, the earth receives in the form of sunlight about one-fourth horse-power for each square foot of its surface, or about one forty-thousandth of the amount of energy thrown off by the sun from each square foot of its surface. The ordinary electric arc light presents an intense radiating surface having an area a little less than one tenth of an inch square. The temperature of this radiating surface is more than 6,000° F. If this area could be increased so as to present a square foot of surface, the amount of energy would be practically the same as that emitted from an equal area of the surface of the sun. It thus appears that the electric arc light is an exceedingly efficient source of light, and that it may be used as a substitute for sunlight, over which it enjoys the advantage of being more easily controlled and manipulated, and always available.

The influence of sunlight upon the vital processes has been recognized from the most ancient times. The old Greeks and Romans employed the sun bath, or insolation, very frequently in the treatment of chronic maladies of all sorts. The natives of the South Sea Islands and other primitive peoples still utilize this powerful agent in the treatment of the sick. The natives of the *terre caliente* of Mexico have long practiced exposure to the sunlight on the sea-beach, partially covered with sand, as a means of treatment for syphilis, the patients thus treated being made to drink large quantities of infusions of leaves of various sorts while exposed to the sun. The natives of Haiti are said by M. Delow to employ similar practices.

All physicians place the highest value upon exposure to the sun by an out-of-door life as a means of stimulating the nutritive processes of the body in many chronic disorders, as anemia, chlorosis, tuberculosis, in convalescence from fevers, and other similar conditions. The value of the sun bath as a therapeutic measure will be readily appreciated by noting the facts respecting its remarkable physiological influence, which must be very largely attributed to the actinic ray, although a share of it must be attributed to the calorific effect of the sun's rays. But though its value has been so long and so generally recognized, the various practical difficulties in the way of utilizing the sun's rays for therapeutic purposes, and the great uncertainty of sunshine in the larger part of this and other civilized countries, have been so great obstacles that little use has thus far been made of this powerful agent, even in institutions largely devoted to the use of physiological measures.

The author has made more or less use of the sun bath 601
during the twenty-five years in which he has been engaged in institutional medical work, but the difficulties encountered, long ago led him to the study of the electric light as a substitute for sunlight. The most definite and practical experiments along this line were begun by him about ten years ago. In a paper read before the American Electrotherapeutic Association at its meeting in New York City, in September, 1894, he presented a description of a new method of apply-

ing heat to the body, in which the incandescent electric light was utilized as the source of heat. This paper gave the details of many experiments which had been conducted for the purpose of determining the physiological effects of this bath, and also a comparison of the effects obtained by this bath with those obtained by the Turkish and Russian baths. The general conclusions resulting from his investigations were as follows: —

1. The electric-light bath stimulates the elimination of CO_2 in a very marked degree. In an electric-light bath lasting 30 minutes, the percentage of CO_2 elimination during the last ten minutes was 5.13 as compared with 3.60, the average of CO_2 elimination before the bath. In a Russian bath the percentage of elimination was 3.96. In a Turkish bath of 30 minutes' duration, the percentage of CO_2 elimination was 4.01, while the elimination of urea was diminished.

2. The elimination of nitrogenous wastes represented by urea, and also the elimination of total solids, was greatest in the Russian bath, and least in the electric-light bath.

3. The amount of perspiration produced by the electric-light bath was fully double that induced by the Turkish bath in the same length of time. The time required for the first appearance of perspiration was, in the electric-light bath, about one half the time of that in the Turkish and Russian baths. The reason for this is apparent when one recalls the fact observed by Bouchard, that perspiration begins when the temperature of the blood has risen .7° F. above the normal. In the study of the physiological effects of the electric-light bath in 1891, when the author made his first experiments upon this subject, he found the internal temperature was raised by the bath 1.6° F. in five and one-half minutes, the surface temperature rising, in the same time, 2.3° F.

602 From these facts it is evident that the electric-light bath raises the temperature of the blood more quickly than any other form of bath. The reason for this is apparent when it is remembered that the skin and other structures of the body

readily permit the transmission of the radiant energy of the electric light, which, entering the body as light, becomes, by the resistance which it meets, transformed into heat. Thus heat is developed in the deeper tissues instead of being slowly carried in by conduction from the surface. The skin is, like glass, a poor conductor, but at the same time allows the passage of radiant energy in the form of light. This fact explains the readiness with which perspiration is induced by the electric-light bath.

Prior to the author's experiments upon this subject, there had been no scientific study of the physiological effects of the incandescent electric-light bath upon human beings. He had constructed, as early as 1891, various experimental forms of baths, which he has gradually perfected. Some of these admit the whole body in a sitting posture, others lying down. Some are adapted to the application of heat to a circumscribed portion of the body, as the trunk, the feet, or the spine. The photo-reproductions show the principal forms of the bath in use at the present time. These baths are now employed in various places in this country and in foreign lands. Fig. 133-138 (p. 707, 708).

The electric-light bath has been received into special 603
favor in Germany. Professor Winternitz, the greatest living authority on hydrotherapy, speaks as follows respecting it in his recently published treatise, "Physiologische Grundlagen der Hydrotherapie:"—

"The electric-light bath is a method of recent origin, and equal to the sun bath. It was at first employed empirically. [Only the arc light was thus employed, and in the most inefficient and unscientific manner.] Dr. Kellogg (Battle Creek, Mich., U. S. A.) has constructed one for the entire body as well as for the separate parts thereof, various-shaped cabinets which are supplied with mirrors internally and a great number of electric lights.

"It has been undoubtedly demonstrated that radiant heat penetrates the tissues much better than conducted heat, and it is quite probable that cellular activity is powerfully modified by these rays of heat (either qualitatively or quantitatively). The effects of the vapor bath can be brought about in the cabinet, and the differences thus far determined are the following:—

"The giving off of the CO_2 is more abundant than in the vapor bath, and what is especially noteworthy is that the perspiration appears very soon and at a very low temperature, and is very profuse. We notice the earlier appearance at 95° F. (Kellogg averaging 85° F.), while in the vapor bath a much higher temperature is generally required to produce the same effect. The time at which perspiration in the electric-light bath appeared averaged three and one-half minutes, while in the vapor bath almost five minutes was required. Finally, the quantity of perspiration in the electric-light bath is considerably larger. That the rays of heat here play the most important part, and that it is not on account of the temperature of the air in the cabinet, is further shown, for instance, by the fact that the external surfaces of the thighs, which were directly opposed to the light, perspired much more rapidly and profusely than the inner surfaces, which received only reflected rays. Within ten to thirty minutes, the temperature reached 104° F., pulse 160, respiration 42, with symptoms of fever-like condition. We have, thus far, employed the electric-light bath like the vapor bath in only a few disorders, such as chlorosis, chronic rheumatism, and gout, and have obtained satisfactory results. More extensive experience is wanted. Kellogg reports very favorable results in the treatment of chlorosis, gout, and a number of cases in which there is need of increased metabolism. Lehmann reports regarding psoriasis.

"As we now possess a thermic method in the electric-light bath by means of which we are able to measure the exact dose, and knowing the powerful influence on cell life and the entire organism, we believe this method of thermic application should receive an important place. It enables us to influence a number of maladies much more rapidly, better, and more intensely than we have heretofore been able to do."

The skin, as well as the air, is to a large extent trans- 604
parent to light, and the same is true of all the living tissues. This is evidenced by the phenomenon of trans-illumination. By a speculum placed in the vagina or rectum, and a suitably arranged electric light of 16 or 32 candle-power placed over the abdomen, one may see the interior of the pelvis illuminated and glowing with a bright red light, the red color being due to reflection from the red corpuscles of the blood. Even the bones when in a living state are translucent to light. This is clearly shown by placing the hand between an electric light and the eyes, with the fingers in close contact. The hand being placed near enough to the light, the whole of each finger will be seen to be illuminated by the light, and not simply the soft part. Light penetrates the body in the same manner as it penetrates any other transparent or translucent medium.

That the actinic ray penetrates the body to a considerable depth is readily shown by the following experiment:—

The hand is placed over a piece of sensitive film, such as is used by photographers, the opaque object being placed between the hand and the paper, and exposure made in such a manner that the light which reaches the sensitive tissue must pass through the hand. The fact that the chemical rays are transmitted is shown by their action upon the sensitive paper beneath the hand, and the complete absence of their action upon the surface protected by the opaque object placed between the hand and the paper.

In case of the water bath, the Turkish bath, the vapor and hot-air baths, heat reaches the interior of the body by conduction, passing through successive layers of living tissue, which, while affording great resistance to the conduction of heat, readily allow the passage of the luminous rays from the incandescent film.

The electric-light bath does not depend for its effect upon the heat of the air surrounding the patient, but upon the radiant energy which passes in straight lines from the incandescent filament into the patient's body without heating the air, the air about the patient being of the ordinary temperature; just as a person standing before a log fire out of doors on a frosty night may expose one side of his body to intense heat, while the other is chilled by the zero atmosphere which surrounds him.

The incandescent-light bath enjoys a great advantage over other methods of applying heat in that it produces strong tonic effects at the same time that it encourages powerful elimination.

605 The electric arc-light bath has been used more or less both in this country and in France, but its physiological effects have not thus far been accurately ascertained. The author is at the present time engaged in a series of studies of this subject, the results of which, it is hoped, will place the use of this form of bath upon a sound scientific basis. The apparatus employed is described elsewhere in this work (**1251**).

The technique of the incandescent electric-light bath and of the electric arc-light bath will be found in the section devoted to the technique of hydric applications.

Part Two.

THE GENERAL PRINCIPLES OF HYDRIATICS

BEFORE entering upon the consideration of hydrotherapeutics proper, it will be profitable to review briefly the physiological effects of hydric applications.

SUMMARY OF THE PHYSIOLOGICAL EFFECTS OF COLD APPLICATIONS.

General Effects. 1. Cold is ***primarily*** depressant or sedative in 606
its effects, lowering the temperature and lessening vital activity (**257, 261, 267, 268**).

2. A *secondary* excitant effect follows a short cold application, as the result of the reaction of the body against the depressing influence of cold; hence the practical result of a short cold application is exciting (**269, 273**).

3. Short cold applications cause contraction of the small vessels both of the skin and of the internal organs, quickly followed, however, by active dilatation, the internal dilatation occurring almost instantaneously, the external later.

4. A prolonged moderately cold application to the skin (65° to 80°) causes prolonged contraction of the vessels of the internal part in reflex relation therewith (**274**).

Effects upon the Skin. 1. General cold applications first diminish, then increase, the perspiration (**287, 289**).

2. Cold applications cause first pallor from spasm of the smaller arteries, veins, and capillaries of the skin, later (with reaction) flushing from active dilatation of the vessels.

3. Cold causes contraction of both the muscular and the connective tissues of the skin.

4. Prolonged very cold applications to the skin lessen its sensibility and diminish reflex effects (**293–296**).

5. The mucous membrane, though less sensitive, reacts to cold in essentially the same manner as does the skin (**313**), both local and general effects resulting.

Effects upon the Circulation.

1. General cold applications first quicken, then slow the heart-beat, increase tension, and cause active dilatation of the small vessels (**298**).

2. Cold applied to one hand causes contraction of the vessels of the other hand. Similar relations exist between other symmetrically related organs (**303, 421**).

3. Cold applied over an arterial trunk causes contraction of its distal branches (**307**).

4. A continuous cold application over the heart depresses its action, and lowers arterial tension.

5. Short cold applications over the heart at first increase its activity and force, then lessen the pulse-rate and raise the arterial tension (**309**).

6. Short cold applications to a limited area of any portion of the body temporarily increase the pulse-rate (**312**).

7. A compensatory effect sometimes appears in increased heat production. A thermometer placed in the axilla shows increase of temperature when the elbow is held in water at 50° F. for some time (**305**).

Effects upon Respiration.

1. A general cold douche causes quick, gasping respiration.

2. A non-percutient cold application causes deepened and slowed respiratory movements (**318, 319**).

3. Oxidation of the tissues is increased by cold applications, and the amount of CO_2 in the expired air is correspondingly increased (**322**).

4. An atmospheric temperature of 40° F., or below, causes increase of heat production and CO_2 elimination when the body is so exposed as to cause shivering.

Effects upon the Muscles.

1. Prolonged cold applications decrease muscular irritability and energy (**327**).

2. A short cold application, general or local, increases the excitability and capacity of striated muscles.

3. Cold applications excite the smooth muscular fibers, as those of the skin, blood-vessels, bladder, bowels, etc. (328).

4. Cold applications to a relatively small area, as the skin of the back or the feet, may cause general pallor, goose-flesh appearance, and shivering (330).

Effects upon the Nervous System.

1. Cold applied to a nerve trunk paralyzes the parts supplied by it (335).

2. Cold diminishes the rate of transmission of nerve impulses (336).

3. Prolonged very cold applications to the head diminish mental activity, and may produce unconsciousness, while short applications are in a high degree excitant to the brain (338).

Reflex Effect of Cold Applications.

1. Short, very cold applications, with high pressure, to a reflex area, cause vasodilatation in the related viscera (372).

2. Prolonged non-percutient cold applications produce internal vasoconstriction (372).

3. Short applications to the face and neck stimulate the circulation and activity of the brain (373).

4. A short, very cold douche to the chest first excites, then slows, the pulse (355).

5. Prolonged immersion of the hands in cold water causes contraction of the vessels of the brain and of the nasal mucous membrane (356).

6. Short, very cold applications to the hands cause contraction of the uterine muscles (358).

7. A short, very cold douche to the feet, with strong pressure, dilates the vessels of the uterus (359).

8. Immersion of the legs in cold water causes contraction of the vessels of the lungs and the kidneys.

9. Short cold applications to the mammæ give rise to vigorous contraction of the muscles of the uterus. This simple measure is much utilized for this purpose in obstetrics.

10. Short, very cold applications to the abdomen, the hands, and the feet cause contraction of the muscles of the bladder, bowels, and uterus (**358**).

11. Prolonged applications of cold to the upper dorsal region cause contraction of the vessels of the nasal mucous membrane and of the lungs (**360**).

12. An ice-bag to the dorsal region causes contraction of the vessels of the stomach.

13. A cold lumbar douche at moderate pressure (duration from 15 to 45 sec.) causes contraction of the uterine vessels (**364**).

14. A very short, cold douche to the lumbar region (duration from 2 to 4 sec.), with strong pressure, causes dilatation of the uterine vessels (**365**).

15. A short cold douche to the thighs causes dilatation of the vessels of the uterus (**366**).

16. A short cold douche to the lower portion of the sternum causes increased activity of the kidneys (**368**).

17. Short cold applications, with strong pressure, over the stomach, liver, spleen, and bowels, cause first contraction, then active dilatation, of the vessels of these organs (**369**).

18. Prolonged cold applications over an internal organ, without pressure, produce contraction of its blood-vessels (**370**).

The Blood.

1. The reaction following cold applications increases the number of corpuscles in circulation.

2. Cold applications increase the amount of oxygen absorbed by the blood, and the rate of oxidation, the result of which is increased reduction of oxyhemoglobin (**385-387**).

Effects upon Absorption, Secretion, and Nutrition.

1. General cold applications increase absorption from the alimentary canal (**388**).

2. Short general and more prolonged local cold applications increase the activity of the glands of the stomach, liver, kidneys, and other secreting viscera (**390**).

3. Short general cold applications to the skin cause a quickening of all the vital functions, hastening the blood and lymph currents, stimulating assimilation and disintegration, and augmenting vital resistance.

Effects upon Animal Heat and Temperature.

1. General cold applications diminish the temperature of the skin and the general temperature.

2. A cold spray to the soles of the feet produces slight lowering of the general temperature (**425**).

3. Cold applications to the head lower the temperature by depressing the thermogenic centers.

4. Cold applications to the surface increase the thermo-electrical phenomena (**428**).

5. Short cold applications stimulate heat production (**416**).

6. Prolonged cold applications at first increase, then decrease, heat production (**411–418**).

7. General shivering under an application of cold is an evidence of lowered internal temperature and the beginning of increased heat production.

8. Circulatory reaction is produced by the reflex influence of cold applications upon the vasomotor centers and perhaps also by direct action upon the visceral sympathetic ganglia of the blood-vessels.

9. Cold applications produce thermic reaction by lowering the temperature of the skin and of the blood.

SUMMARY OF THE EFFECTS OF HOT APPLICATIONS.

Water is said to be warm at a temperature of 92° to 98° **607**
F., hot at 98° to 104° F., and very hot at 104° F. or above.

General Effects.

1. Heat is *primarily* an excitant. It is, indeed, one of the most powerful of all vital stimulants. It increases vital activity, elevates the temperature, and excites the brain and nerve centers (**492, 564, 566**).

2. The secondary effect of heat is depressant through atonic reaction. The temperature is lowered through reflex action, which produces lessened heat production and increased heat elimination, with generally diminished tissue activity. Long-continued applications of heat increase heat production.

3. Short hot applications to the surface cause passive dilatation of the small vessels (venules) of the skin, with strong revulsive effects upon the internal parts (**516**).

4. Prolonged hot applications may give rise to mixed effects of excitation and exhaustion, either of which may predominate.

Effects upon the Skin. 1. Contraction of the yellow elastic tissue, relaxation of the white fibrous tissue.

2. Goose-flesh appearance from contraction of the smooth muscle fibers (**496**).

3. Reddening of the skin, or, if suddenly applied at a temperature of from 110° to 130° F., brief pallor, from strong stimulation of the vasoconstrictors, followed by reddening of the skin due to dilatation of the small veins.

4. Contraction of the vessels of the skin with pallor after the heat is withdrawn, when the application has been prolonged (**498**).

5. Increased perspiratory and respiratory activity (**503**).

6. Increase of tactile sensibility at 98°, decrease at 113°, extinction at 130°.

7. Increased heat elimination from the skin (*a*) through dilatation of the surface vessels, (*b*) increase of the flow of blood through the skin, (*c*) increased evaporation of moisture from the surface, and (*d*) increased conductivity of the skin (**508**).

8. Heat prepares the skin for cold applications (**510**).

Effects upon the Circulation. 1. A general application of heat first slows, then quickens the pulse. Pulse rate and tension diminish when free perspiration begins (**514**).

2. Very hot applications (115° F. and upwards) cause slight contraction of the small vessels of the skin, soon followed by relaxation. Warm and hot applications cause dila-

tation of the surface vessels, especially of the small veins.

3. Hot applications raise blood pressure when accompanied by friction, percussion, or other mechanical effects.

Effects upon Respiration. 1. A general application of moist heat (air or vapor) increases the rate and ease of respiration.

2. Hot dry applications (hot air) hinder respiration (**521**).

3. After the withdrawal of a very hot application there is for a time diminished rate and depth of respiration (**524**).

4. An external temperature above 60° to 70° F. increases CO_2 elimination, while a temperature below 40° F. also decidedly increases CO_2 elimination.

Effects upon the Muscles. 1. Short hot applications (98° to 104° F.) increase the excitability and energy of striated, or voluntary, muscles (**529**).

2. Prolonged hot applications (106° to 120° F.) lessen the energy and excitability of the voluntary muscles (**529**).

3. Very hot applications increase the excitability of the non-striated, or involuntary, muscles, as shown by the goose-flesh appearance of the skin following a very hot application, and the contraction of the small vessels of the skin (**527**).

4. Neutral temperatures (92° to 96° F.) have no influence upon the excitability of the striated muscles. The sedative effect produced depends upon the influence on the cutaneous nerves.

Effects upon the Nervous System. 1. Very hot baths produce various nervous disturbances, as sleeplessness, nervousness, headache, and other symptoms of nervous excitation and exhaustion (**540**).

2. Extreme heat, as in sunstroke, may give rise to the development of special poisons, which act upon the nerve centers of the brain and cord, producing grave and even fatal collapse. Hence the danger of a very hot bath if prolonged.

3. A short hot application powerfully excites the nerves and nerve centers.

4. The excitant effects of heat are followed by depressant effects or atonic reaction (**579**).

Effects upon the Blood. Heat, unless followed by cold, decreases the red and increases the white cells.

Effects upon General Nutrition. At very high temperatures heat is a powerful vital stimulant or excitant. It increases CO_2 production and the oxidation of nitrogen.

Effects upon the Stomach, Liver, and Other Abdominal Organs. 1. Prolonged applications of heat over the region of the stomach after eating, either fomentations or dry heat, increase the amount of hydrochloric acid secreted by that organ.

2. Short hot applications, especially the short hot douche, diminish the secretion of HCl, at least in cases of hyperpepsia (**569**).

3. Prolonged applications of heat over the region of the liver and other viscera increase their activity.

4. Short hot applications, especially the short very hot hepatic douche, relieve visceral congestion.

5. Large fomentations over internal parts lessen their blood supply and functional activity.

Effects of Hot Applications upon Heat Production and Body Temperature. 1. General applications of heat cause immediate rise of temperature. This is true even when the temperature of the bath is no higher than that of the body itself (**572**).

2. An external temperature above 60° to 70° F. occasions increase of heat production. An atmospheric temperature of 104° F. increases heat production three hundred and fifty per cent. in dogs.

3. An application of heat is followed by a fall of temperature, the result of atonic reaction (**578**).

COMPARATIVE SUMMARY OF THE CHIEF EFFECTS OF COLD AND HEAT.

COLD.	HEAT.
General.	*General.*
Primary, depressant.	*Primary*, excitant.
Short, excitant by tonic reaction.	*Short*, depressant by atonic reaction.
Prolonged, depressant.	*Prolonged*, mixed, excitant, and depressant.
Special.	*Special.*
Skin: Action, diminished activity.	*Skin:* Action, increased activity.
Reaction, increased activity.	Reaction, diminished activity.
Diminished sensibility.	Diminished sensibility.

COLD.	HEAT.
Heart: First quickened, then slowed. Increased force.	*Heart:* First slowed, then quickened. Decreased force.
Vessels: Action, contraction. *Reaction*, dilatation. Increased tone and activity. Local anemia, collateral hyperemia. *With reaction*, local hyperemia, collateral anemia. *Short*, reflex dilatation of visceral vessels.	*Vessels: Action*, contraction, then dilatation. *Reaction*, contraction. Lowered tone—paralysis. Local hyperemia, collateral anemia. *With reaction*, local anemia, collateral hyperemia. *Short*, reflex fluxion and derivative effects.
Nerves: Benumbs and paralyzes. *Excites* by tonic reaction.	*Nerves:* Excites. *Depresses* by atonic reaction.
Muscles: Short, increased excitability and capacity. *Prolonged*, lessened excitability and capacity.	*Muscles: Short*, lessening fatigue effects. *Prolonged*, diminished capacity and excitability.
Lungs: Slows and deepens respiration. Increased amount of respired air. Increased CO_2. Increased respiratory quotient.	*Lungs:* Quickens and facilitates respiration. Diminished am't of respired air. Decreased CO_2. Diminished respiratory quotient.
Stomach: Increased HCl and motor activity.	*Stomach:* Decreased HCl and motor activity.
Kidneys: Congests and excites.	*Kidneys:* renders anemic and lessens activity.
Animal Heat: Short, increased heat production. *Prolonged*, diminished heat production.	*Animal Heat: Short*, diminished heat production. *Prolonged*, increased heat production.
Blood: Increased blood count, especially leucocytes.	*Blood:* Decrease in number of red cells, increase in number of leucocytes.
Metabolism: Increased CO_2. Increased urea, and improved oxidation.	*Metabolism:* Decreased CO_2. Increased urea and general proteid waste.

TONIC REACTION.	ATONIC REACTION.
1. Vasodilatation.	1. Vasoconstriction.
2. Skin red.	2. Skin pale.
3. Pulse slowed.	3. Pulse rate increased.
4. Arterial tension increased.	4. Arterial tension diminished.
5. Skin action increased.	5. Skin action decreased.
6. Temperature lowered.	6. Temperature lowered.
7. Feeling of invigoration.	7. Languor.
8. Muscular capacity increased.	8. Muscular capacity decreased.
9. Amount of respired air increased.	9. Amount of respired air decreased.
10. Heat production increased.	10. Heat production decreased.

THE THERAPEUTIC EFFECTS OF HYDRIATIC APPLICATIONS.

608 THE classification of hydrotherapeutic procedures has given rise to much discussion among writers and practitioners, growing out of the fact that thermic applications are capable of producing a great variety of effects, which are not infrequently so intermingled that it is not easy, in all cases, to decide which is the dominant effect.

It has also been observed that an application of water made in a definite manner and of a definite temperature may, at one time and under one set of circumstances, produce an effect radically different from that produced by an identical application at another time and under different circumstances; for example, an application which in one patient might prove to be exciting or tonic, in another would produce decidedly sedative or depressing effects, and the reverse.

This characteristic, however, is not peculiar to water; it applies to all classes of therapeutic agents. No two persons are exactly alike, and the state of the system in every individual is constantly varying from hour to hour and from day to day, the condition at each moment differing from that of every other moment, past or future. Particular individuals also present special peculiarities or idiosyncrasies of constitution, which must be taken into account in the employment of thermic applications as well as in the use of other therapeutic measures. Nevertheless, amid this apparent confusion, there is a sufficient amount of stability and unity to permit a basis for a simple and comprehensive classification of the effects which may be expected from definite and exact hydric applications under clearly and accurately defined conditions.

609 From a careful study of the physiological effects of water, it is evident that, in general, two classes of effects are produced. These are *excitation* and *depression*. This naturally

leads to a simple grouping of therapeutic applications of water into two general classes: (1) *Excitant;* (2) *Sedative.*

These two groups of effects may be almost indefinitely subdivided, but the leading and essential subdivisions the author believes will be found included in the following table, which is offered as an attempt at a scientific classification of the therapeutic effects which may be obtained from hydriatic procedures:— 610

CLASSIFICATION OF HYDRIATIC EFFECTS.

I. Excitant.

II. Sedative.

I. EXCITANT EFFECTS.

A. Primary effects.

B. Secondary effects.

A. Primary Excitant Effects.

1. General.
2. Local.

a. Hemostatic { Direct. / Indirect or Reflex.

b. Cardiac.

c. Uterine.

d. Vesical.

e. Peristaltic.

B. Secondary Excitant Effects.

1. General.

a. Restorative.

b. Tonic.

c. Calorific.

2. Local.

a. Sudorific { (*a*) Spoliative or Reducing. / (*b*) Eliminative.

b. Expectorant.

c. Diuretic.

d. Cholagogic.

e. Peptogenic.

f. Emmenagogic.

g. Revulsive.

h. Derivative.

i. Resolutive.

j. Alterative.

k. Calorific.

II. SEDATIVE EFFECTS.
1. Circulatory.
 a. Antiphlogistic.
  (*a*) Vascular.
  (*b*) Cardiac.
 b. Hemostatic.
2. Nervous.
 a. Hypnotic.
 b. Calmative.
 c. Analgesic.
 d. Anesthetic.
 e. Antispasmodic.
3. Thermic.
 a. Antithermic.
 b. Antipyretic.
4. Secretory.

GENERAL PRINCIPLES.

611 The following brief statement of the general principles which determine the effects of hot, cold, and neutral applications, may be found of service:—

612 **Respecting Hot Applications.**

1. *The primary effect* (*action*) *of an application of heat is excitant.*

2. *The secondary effect* (*reaction*) *of an application of heat is depressant, sedative, atonic.*

3. *The actual effect of an application of heat depends upon many factors, as the condition of the patient, the intensity and length of the application, the form of the application, etc.* In general, it may be said that—

(*a*) *The effect of a very short application at very high temperature is strongly excitant,* the depressant effects being practically imperceptible.

(*b*) *The effect of a less intense and slightly prolonged application of heat is moderately excitant* during the application; after the application, *decidedly depressant* effects appear, resulting from a lessening of thermic and other tissue activities through atonic reaction.

(*c*) *The effect of a prolonged application of heat at a high temperature is both excitant and exhausting or depress-*

ant, the excitation resulting from the elevation of the temperature of the body, the depression being due to the exhaustion of nervous energy. Practically, *cold contracts* while *heat dilates* the vessels *at the moment of application.*

Respecting Cold Applications.

1. *Cold is intrinsically sedative, but practically the primary effect* (*action*) *of a cold application is excitant.* 613

2. *The secondary effect* (*reaction*) *is invigorating, restorative, tonic.*

3. *The actual effect of an application of cold depends upon the method of making the application, the temperature, the susceptibility and condition of the patient, and many other factors.* In general, it may be said that —

(a) A short application of intense cold is excitant, and, if repeated daily, *tonic.*

(b) A more prolonged application at a moderately low temperature is less excitant and less tonic.

(c) A prolonged cold application is first excitant, then sedative, the depressant effects resulting from the exhaustion of the nerve centers from prolonged excitation and the lowering of the temperature of the body.

Respecting Neutral and Intermediate Applications.

1. *A neutral bath* (92° to 95° F.) produces no reaction, circulatory or thermic, but *suppresses reflex activity* by lessening the sensibility of the cutaneous nerves; consequently the effect is calmative. A neutral bath is also restorative by checking or abolishing the loss of energy and encouraging cutaneous and renal activity. 614

2. Baths at *intermediate temperatures* produce *mixed effects*, the *dominant effects being* those of the class most nearly approached, cold, neutral, or hot.

The characteristic effects of baths, either hot or cold, may be intensified by the mechanical effects of percussion,— as by means of the douche in various forms,— by friction with the hand, towel, sheet, or by other suitable means.

The effects of baths may also be intensified by various

means which favor or delay reaction, applied *before*, *during*, *or after* the bath, such as *exercise*, *artificial heat*, etc. (443)

I. EXCITANT (Action) EFFECTS.

615 The excitant effects of thermic applications are chiefly reflex in character. They may be divided into two classes: (A) *Primary;* (B) *Secondary*.

A. PRIMARY EXCITANT EFFECTS.

616 Primary excitant effects are those which are the immediate results of the motor impulses sent out by the nerve centers under the stimulus of the impression produced upon the skin or mucous membrane by the application made. All thermic applications, whether at a temperature above or below that of the body, which produce decided sensations or impressions are excitant in character; but only those applications are classed as excitant which are managed in such a way that the excitant effects are the sole or dominant effects; hence as will readily be seen by a study of the foregoing statement of principles, applications for excitant effects must necessarily be short (from 2 or 3 secs. to 1 or 2 min.). As a rule, the shorter the application, the more purely excitant will be the effect, provided the temperature is very hot or very cold.

Excitant effects may be produced by either hot or cold applications. *Very cold* applications are much more excitant than cold or cool applications. Likewise *very hot* applications are more highly excitant than applications which are simply hot or warm. The greater the difference between the temperature of the application and that of the skin surface to which it is applied, the more highly exciting will the effect be, whether hot or cold applications are employed.

Applications producing excitant effects may be subdivided into *general* and *local* applications.

617 *1. General Primary Excitant Effects.*— General applications are usually employed for general excitant effects, the most important of which are the very hot douche—shower, spray,

or jet — temperature 110°–130° F., continued from 15 seconds to 4 minutes; very hot affusion 110°–115° F., from 30 seconds to 5 minutes; hot-blanket pack, 105°–112° F.; hot-water drinking; general alternate hot and cold sponging; full bath, 105°–110° F., 5 to 10 minutes; hot enema, hot sitz bath. Hot applications to the head and spine, and very hot applications over the heart are powerfully excitant.

The effect of alternate hot and cold applications is continually to renew the exciting effect of the heat; the cold application should be long enough to remove the heat absorbed by the skin from the hot application, but not long enough to produce lowering of the general temperature, as announced by chill, shivering, or any other indication of thermic reaction. As a rule, in alternate applications the applications should be made of equal length, — about fifteen seconds each, — but the time during which the heat is applied may often be increased with advantage (638).

Alternate hot and cold applications are the exciting applications *par excellence*, for the following reasons:—

(*a*) For primary excitant effects it is desirable to arouse the nerve centers without exhausting them by decided reaction effects, and to suppress atonic thermic reaction by making the hot application very short, and following it by a short cold application.

(*b*) If a cold application is prolonged, the effect is to abstract heat from the skin and from the blood, and thus either directly lower the vigor of the patient or provoke an undesirable thermic reaction whereby the weakened resources of the body will be still further exhausted.

(*c*) By a short application of heat, immediately followed by an application of cold of equal length, the heat impression is made of only sufficient intensity and length to produce the desired nervous impression, any further effect being prevented by the neutralizing influence of the succeeding cold application, which restores the normal temperature of the skin, and thus prepares it for the new excitant impression to be produced by the succeeding hot application. This renders possible an almost indefinite extension of the effect.

Although the strongest excitant effects may be obtained by the alternate douche, very powerful excitant effects may be made by alternate hot and cold sponging, compresses, affusions, etc.

The sun bath is a most valuable and practical exciting measure. It owes its properties to the three sets of rays of which it is composed, viz., heat, luminous, and actinic or chemical rays. The heat and luminous rays are directly stimulating to the cells of the tissues, causing a development and accumulation of heat, while the actinic rays (597) act upon the nervous system in a most powerful manner.

The electric-light bath possesses the same properties as the sunlight; hence the importance of utilizing this simple measure especially in countries blessed with little sunlight and at seasons of the year when sunlight is uncertain. By the use of colored lamps or screens the patient may be exposed to the action of the red or heat rays only, or to the chemic or violet rays, or to the full-light rays. The actinic rays may be used when stimulation of the nervous system is especially desired, independently of any calorific effect. When the heating effect alone is desired, the red rays should be employed.

In the employment of such non-percutient applications as the compress and the fomentation, or hot and cold friction, greater extremes of temperature may be employed than with the douche. As a rule, the temperature should be as extreme as can be borne without actual pain, except, of course, with extremely nervous patients, who may easily be over-excited by a too strong stimulation of the sensory nerves.

When to Employ Excitant Measures.

The general excitant effects of heat or of alternate applications of heat and cold are indicated in cases of extreme exhaustion, collapse, surgical shock, collapse under anesthesia, drowning, suffocation, and syncope from hemorrhage, fright, or any similar cause.

The excitant effect of cold may be occasionally used with advantage in cases of collapse or asphyxia. The reaction must be quick and general; hence the colder the water and the greater the force with which it is applied, the better will be the effect produced. Cold friction may be used instead of the douche when more convenient.

As a rule, the excitant effect of heat is to be preferred to that of cold in conditions of collapse or pain. Depressant effects from heat may be prevented by making the application short and by a very short cold application following.

Contra-indications. In the employment of the hot full bath and the hot douche, great care must be taken to avoid cerebral excitement. To accomplish this, apply a cold compress or an ice-cap to the head when hot applications are being made to any large area of the skin. Care must also be taken to avoid overexcitement of the heart. General very hot applications are contraindicated in cases of weak heart, arteriosclerosis, advanced age, and infancy (below seven years), also in cases of previous injury from sun-stroke or heat-stroke.

2. *Local Primary Excitant Effects.*—The primary exci- 618
tant effects of thermic applications may be usefully employed for numerous local therapeutic effects, the most important of which are the following:—

Hemostatic Effects. The hemostatic effects of thermic applications 619
may be obtained either directly through application to the bleeding vessels, or indirectly through reflex action.

To obtain direct hemostatic effects, either very hot (140° to 160°) or very cold (32° to 40°) applications must be employed.

Of hot applications, the hot douche (**1024**) and the hot compress (**1289**) are the most valuable. A jet of hot steam has been used with success (**1422**).

Of cold applications, ice, ice compresses, and the ether or rhigolene spray are the most convenient methods of checking hemorrhage by the direct application of cold to the bleeding part, or across the trunk of a main artery supplying a bleeding part, as the ice-collar or cravat for nosebleed.

This method of checking hemorrhage is, of course, not adapted to cases of bleeding from large vessels, and applies rather to cases of capillary oozing than to those in which the hemorrhage occurs from arteries or veins which have been cut or otherwise ruptured.

Other methods which are found efficient are the following: The hot nasal douche and sponging the face with very hot water for nosebleed; the hot vaginal douche for menorrhagia, hot uterine irrigation in metrorrhagia and post-partum hemorrhage; the hot bladder irrigation in vesical hemorrhage.

Indirect Hemostatic Effects.

Cold applications to the upper spine constitute a most excellent measure for checking nosebleed. Placing the hands in ice-water, and the application of ice to the base of the cranium, and especially to the cervical and the upper dorsal portion of the spine, are also very effective means of checking nosebleed when other measures have proved futile. Placing the feet in cold water constricts the blood-vessels of the nasal mucous membrane, and may be advantageously combined with the other measures mentioned.

For pulmonary hemorrhage there is no better remedy than cold compresses over the chest and very hot fomentations between the shoulders. Care should be taken to cover both the lower cervical and the upper dorsal region. The vasomotor nerves which supply the lungs find exit from the spine in this region, and hence applications made at this point are especially effective. The application of ice to the nostrils also contracts the pulmonary vessels (Brown-Séquard).

In cases of hemorrhage from the stomach, lumps of ice may be swallowed, and large ice compresses should be placed over the epigastrium.

In apoplexy, the ice-cap **(1314)** and ice-cold compresses to the head, face, and neck are most appropriate and valuable measures.

In hemorrhage from the uterus, short, very hot fomentations (**1328**) or the hot douche (**1024**) may be applied to the thighs and spine, and an ice-bag (**1314**) placed over the lower abdomen, while a hot vaginal douche is administered.

Among the most useful measures of this sort are a very short hot douche to the lumbar region, the inner surfaces of the thighs, and the soles of the feet, to combat uterine hemorrhage. Prolonged cold applications (55°–70°) to the same surfaces produce like effects. These applications may be made either with or without a simultaneous use of the hot uterine or vaginal douche, according to the severity of the case. It should be stated, however, that cold applications can not be used in cases of menorrhagia, without the utmost care and discretion, at the beginning of a catamenial period, on account of the danger of producing hematoma or hematosalpinx, through the sudden checking of the outflow of blood. On this account, less violent measures should be employed during the first twenty-four or thirty-six hours, the application of cold water being reserved to a later period. The hot vaginal douche, and even the astringent douche, may be employed with greater safety during the first day in menorrhagia. The danger of producing hematoma is, in the author's opinion, very small after the first day.

A case which came under the author's observation in practice some twenty years ago illustrates very well the value of cold applications of this sort: A girl about fifteen years of age had suffered for nearly a year with most extreme menorrhagia, until she had become exsanguinated to a very remarkable extent, and was frequently in a state bordering on collapse. The attending physician had employed every sort of medicinal and many non-medicinal means for checking the hemorrhage, but without avail. Packing the uterus had not been tried, but tamponment of the vagina with alum and other astringents had been thoroughly employed, yet without material results. The patient was placed at once in a sitz bath of about 50° F. for fifteen minutes, the feet being placed in cold water at the same time, with the result that the hemorrhage ceased at once, and by continued and repeated application of the cool sitz bath for a few weeks, the difficulty was relieved.

The great value of this principle as a means of controlling hemorrhage was recently illustrated in a case of menorrhagia in which the author was consulted by a medical colleague. The patient had been flowing continuously for a month, the hemorrhage following a curettement. The usual remedies had been employed most assiduously, but without result, tamponment of the uterine cavity having failed to control the hemorrhage even temporarily. The application of a cold pelvic pack controlled the difficulty at once, and completely for twenty-four hours, when a slight return of the flow occurred; another application of the same simple measure, however, resulted in permanent relief.

This measure will not control a hemorrhage due to vegetations, a uterine fibroid, or malignant disease, though even in cases of this sort it will often be found of value ; but for menorrhagia or metrorrhagia due to uterine or ovarian congestion, it is a most valuable resource. In cases of hemorrhage accompanied by severe neuralgic pain or by acute pelvic inflammation of any kind, very hot rather than very cold applications should be made to the inside of the thighs and the lumbar region. The application should be brief, and the temperature sufficiently high to be somewhat painful. It is most satisfactorily made by sponging the parts with water at a temperature of 140° F., or by the application, for 1 or 2 minutes, of cloths wrung from water of the same temperature. This measure acts in the same way as the hot nasal douche, or bathing the face with hot water, in relieving nosebleed.

620 **Hydriatic Heart Tonics.** There is no more powerful means of exciting increased activity of the heart than hydriatic applications. Short, very hot fomentations over the heart, the application of large, very hot or very cold compresses over the entire chest and trunk or to other large areas, hot and cold applications to the spine,

hot water drinking, and the hot enema are all efficient means of stimulating a flagging heart to increased action. The measures named are especially serviceable in cases of collapse under chloroform.

Prolonged cold quickens, then slows and energizes the heart. Prolonged heat slows, then quickens and weakens it.

Hot applications over the heart should be avoided where there is any considerable degree of cardiac dilatation, as in cases of this kind the indication is for withdrawal of the blood from the heart, through dilatation of the surface vessels by means of revulsive applications to the general surface, as the effervescing bath, cold friction, and carefully graduated passive exercises, rather than for excitation of the heart muscle.

A very short application of cold to almost any part of the body, but especially to the face and chest, stimulates the heart. The common practice of sprinkling cold water upon the face of a fainting person affords an excellent illustration of the primary exciting influence of cold in rousing the flagging energies of the heart to increased activity. The most excellent effects may be obtained from the application of cold over the heart in cases of cardiac insufficiency.

Cold applications excite the vasomotor constrictors, or accelerator nerves of the blood-vessels, as is clearly shown in the ordinary phenomena of reaction to cold, in which there is first a spasmodic and continuous contraction of the small vessels, later an active dilatation, accompanied by a vigorous rhythmical action of the vasoconstrictor muscles, whereby the movement of the blood is accelerated. The heart participates in this action. Its accelerator nerves, like those of the vessels, are derived from the sympathetic. Whatever affects the activity of the peripheral heart,— the small vessels,— affects in like manner the central heart.

Cold applications, through their influence upon the nerve centers which control the heart and vessels, cause an increased outflow of energy to the muscular structures of these organs, whereby they are brought into more effective activity. The heart contracts with greater force, and more completely empties itself. The small vessels contract more vigorously, while at the same time dilating more fully, thus acting more efficiently in their capacity as a peripheral pump; and so the movement of the blood is hastened by increased activity at both ends of the vascular loop.

The most powerful effect upon both the heart and the vessels results from an application of cold to the whole cutaneous surface. Marked effects may also be produced by applications to the mucous surface, as by hot or cold water drinking and the hot or cold enema. For effects purely cardiac, the application should be confined to the precordia, the cutaneous surface overlying the heart, which is in special reflex relation with it. Cold applications made to this surface powerfully excite the accelerators of the heart, whereby the force of its contractions is greatly increased. The pneumogastric is also acted upon in such a manner that while the force of the heart-beat is increased, its frequency is diminished, thus giving greater efficiency to its action, by allowing more time for rest and repair of its tissues between beats. A continuous feeble action of the heart soon wears it out by depriving it of rest and interfering with its nutrition, while a slower action enables it to maintain its vigor and freshness. Cold applications to strengthen the heart action may consist of the following measures: —

1. The ice-bag or ice compress over the heart. The application must not be continuous, as the cutaneous nerves will soon become insensitive, whereupon the stimulating reflex effects will cease, and effects the very opposite of those desired will be produced. Thus the cold applications must be withdrawn frequently, and long enough to allow the nerves of the skin to regain their sensibility. An ice-cold application may be made for half an hour three times a day, or in cases requiring more vigorous treatment, once in two or three hours. Friction should afterward be applied to the cooled surface to maintain the circulation and normal sensibility.

2. The cold compress, consisting of a folded towel or half a dozen thicknesses of cheese-cloth, of sufficient size to cover half the front of the chest, and wet in water at the ordinary living-room temperature (60° to 70° F.). The compress should cover the cardiac area, extending over a portion of the chest wall contiguous. In cases of cardiac weakness, accompanied by pulmonary congestion, the compress may with great advantage cover the entire front of the chest. This moderately cold application maintains a constant stimulation of the cardiac centers, thus sustaining the heart tone and activity, as indicated by a slowed and strengthened pulse, and shown in a graphic manner by the sphygmograph. The increased cardiac force may be easily measured by the sphygmodynamometer. I have seen as the result of the cold cardiac compress, an increase of tension from 12 to 20 in a normal subject, and from a tension too low to be measured to 8 in a patient suffering from great cardiac weakness. The longer upstroke shows also that the arteries are better filled, as the result of a strong ventricular contraction.

To obtain from hydric applications the best results in energizing the heart, it is necessary in almost all cases to apply at the same time such measures as will lessen the peripheral resistance, and increase the movement of the blood in the vessels by stimulating the contractile activity of the peripheral heart (the small vessels). This is best accomplished by cold applications to the skin of such a character as to produce pronounced circulatory reaction. Cold friction, the rubbing shallow, the cold douche, the Scotch douche, the rubbing wet sheet, and the wet-sheet pack are all excellent means for this purpose. In cases of extreme cardiac weakness with degeneration of the heart muscle, or valvular disease, cold friction is the best of all measures, for the reason that complete general reaction is produced, but without sudden displacement of blood to the interior. In some cases the ice-bag protected by a single thickness of flannel may be applied over the heart continuously for several hours with advantage.

This measure is equally superior in cases in which cardiac weakness sometimes complicates apoplexy, hemorrhage, and visceral congestions.

The very short hot bath, the short hot-blanket pack, the hot and cold immersion bath, and moderate dry friction are all efficient means of stimulating the action of both the central heart and the peripheral heart. Cold applications to the gastric and rectal mucous membranes stimulate the heart and the pulmonary circulation.

In cases of nephritis with uremic poisoning and cardiac failure, I have seen most striking results from the cold trunk pack. In one case the patient was unconscious, pulse 160, and almost imperceptible at the wrist. The hot-blanket pack had been administered to relieve the renal congestion. Being consulted with reference to the cardiac weakness, I suggested the application about the trunk, excluding the arms, of a half-sheet wrung as dry as possible from very cold water. The result was magical. The pulse became strong, was reduced in frequency from 160 to 100, and the patient's entire condition rapidly improved. Such an application may be safely made even in cases of renal and other visceral congestions when preceded by a general hot application. With this preparation the cold application does not produce the usual intense internal congestion while the cutaneous reaction is being established, but the reaction of heat is simply converted into the reaction characteristic of cold, in which the cardiac and vasoconstrictor centers are powerfully energized and the circulatory functions accelerated and regulated.

When cardiac weakness demands therapeutic interference, there are three things to be done: (1) Increase the power of the heart; (2) Decrease the amount of work it has to do; and (3) Remove the cause or causes of the morbid conditions of the heart and vessels. In other words, we must, if possible, simultaneously lessen the work of the heart while we increase its ability to work, and remove the causes of the increase of work and the decrease of cardiac power. By means of appropriate hydric applications, all these indications may be simultaneously and most efficiently met. The heart is energized, the small vessels dilate widely and contract more vigorously, behaving in this respect in the same manner as does the heart. At the same time the increased movement of blood secures better oxidation and elimination of the poisons which depress the heart and cause contraction of the small vessels, and thus increase the work of the heart while lessening its ability to work.

It will be in place to devote a few lines just here to the consideration of the remedies most commonly used in cases of cardiac weakness or failure; viz., alcohol and digitalis. While alcohol lessens the power of the heart, as shown by the experiments of Hare and other observers, it at the same time weakens the constrictors of the vessels, and so dilates the small vessels and lessens the blood pressure. In other words, alcohol, while lessening the power of the heart, at the same time lessens the amount of work it has to do. If the work is lessened more than the cardiac power is weakened, there may be a temporary gain to the patient in a given case.

Digitalis produces an effect the opposite of that of alcohol, causing the heart to contract with greater vigor, and also lessening the caliber of the small vessels, thus increasing peripheral resistance in the blood circuit. In other words, digitalis increases the vigor of the heart, and at the same time increases its work. If in a given case the heart's power is increased more than its work is increased, then there may be a temporary gain, but this advantage is not always secured

It is most profitable to note the difference between the effects of water and those of alcohol and digitalis. Alcohol diminishes the work, but also the working power. Digitalis increases the working power, but at the same time increases the work. *Cold increases the working power, while diminishing the work.* Moreover, alcohol and digitalis, both being toxic substances, add to the toxemia which is often a cause of cardiac inefficiency, while, on the contrary, hydric applications aid in the removal of the disturbing poisons. No condition requiring the use of a heart tonic or stimulant can be named in which a hydriatic application of some sort will not answer the indication far more efficiently than any drug known to the pharmacopeia.

621 **Uterine Excitation—Emmenagogic Effects.** Cold applications over the abdominal surface, especially over the lower abdomen, short and sudden cold applications to the mammary glands, the hot vaginal douche, and also alternate hot and cold applications applied to the breasts and lower abdomen, are efficient in stimulating uterine contractions in cases of delayed labor.

In cases of amenorrhea, the short cold douche to the lumbar region is a measure of very great efficiency. It operates by stimulating the circulation of the ovaries and the uterus, and, by improving the nutrition of the parts, restores the suspended function.

622 **Vesical Excitation.** A cold douche to the feet and over the bladder is a powerful means of exciting vesical contractions, and, used judicially, is applicable in many cases of motor insufficiency of the bladder. This remedy should, of course, be withheld in cases of retention of urine from obstruction.

623 **Intestinal Excitation.** The hot enema, the cold enema, the graduated enema, cold and alternating douches, and other applications over the loins and the entire abdomen, especially about the umbilicus, are measures which are highly efficient in exciting intestinal activity through the impressions made upon the sympathetic centers and splanchnic nerves.

The hot and cold rectal douche (**1410**) is an excellent means of arousing nervous activity in semiparalyzed conditions of the rectum, often so prolific a cause of constipation in cases where the bowels have become inactive through neglect to attend regularly to their daily evacuation.

There is no means by which gastric motility can be so efficiently excited as by cold applications made to the epigastrium or the dorsal spine. Sipping half a glass of cold water or the application of an ice-bag to the epigastrium for half an hour before eating powerfully stimulates gastric motility in atonic states.

B. SECONDARY EXCITANT (Reaction) EFFECTS.

Secondary excitant effects are altogether derived from cold applications, as the reaction effects of hot applications are atonic or sedative. Heat may, in many cases, be advantageously used in connection with cold, in the production of excitant effects by reaction, as in the alternate douche (**1044**) and other alternate applications. The use of heat is not merely to renew or intensify the effect of the cold application by a preparation of the tissues which are to receive it, an important service, but to produce its own specific excitation, in accordance with principles elsewhere explained (**482**). 624

Secondary excitant effects may be either (*a*) general or (*b*) local, according to the form of the application.

1. *General Secondary Excitant Effects.*— The general excitant effects of cold water occupy an important place in the hydriatic armamentarium. Indeed, there is no therapeutic measure known to modern medical science which is capable of producing more powerful general excitation of the entire system than a scientific application of cold water. A short application of very cold water is excitant, in whatever manner it is applied. When, to the influence of a low temperature, is added the percussion effect obtained by the douche with considerable pressure, the excitation resulting is of a most intense character, and is capable of arousing to action every nerve fiber and every cell, and awakening every form of activity in the entire body. 625

In the practical therapeutic employment of water, two important general excitant effects, quite similar, but differing in use, are especially recognized. These two classes of effects may be distinguished as (*a*) *Restorative*, and (*b*) *Tonic*.

626 **Restorative Effects.** A single short application of cold water in the form of a douche, affusion, rubbing wet sheet, immersion, or any other measure in which cold water is brought in contact with the general surface of the body, is always restorative and invigorating in its influence. A man who has been exhausted by laborious effort in a highly heated atmosphere, finds his muscular strength wonderfully re-enforced by an affusion of cold water, cold immersion, a cold shower bath, and especially by a cold douche.

The application of cold water to the face and head has a wonderfully refreshing effect. The brightened expression, the increased vigor, and the relief which follows a simple bathing of the head, face, and neck with cold water when exhausted, are the result of the reflex stimulation of the nerve centers of the brain and spinal cord and the tonic reaction which follows such an application. When the whole surface of the body instead of a small area is acted upon, the effect is proportionally greater.

During the heated term, thousands of lives have been saved in our great cities by the timely opening of free shower baths in crowded tenement-house districts, whereby the depressing and exhausting effects of a superheated atmosphere have been successfully antagonized and antidoted by the restorative influence of the cold bath.

In this connection it is important to mention the necessity of exercising care in the use of the general cold bath in cases of extreme exhaustion from violent exercise, and when, either with or without exhaustion, a sensation of chilliness exists. A general cold application should never be made when the surface is cold, blue, or covered with cold perspiration, nor when the body is in a state of extreme fatigue from violent exertion of any sort, nor when the patient is chilly.

When the surface is hot and dry, a cold bath may be administered without risk, and usually the presence of perspiration, even though it may be quite profuse, is not a contraindication to cold applications, provided, however, that the patient is not at the same time suffering from an infectious fever; but the application must be short, and must be followed by sufficient exercise or friction to secure proper reaction. Care must be taken, however, to see that the exercise be not such as to produce too violent a reaction, especially in cases in which the skin is hot and perspiring.

In cases of extreme exhaustion in which it is not prudent to administer a general cold bath, cold applications may be made to the head, face, neck, and spine, with advantage. The hands and feet may also be bathed in cold water, care being taken to keep the remainder of the body covered if there is cold perspiration. General cold friction may be applied safely in nearly all cases.

A short hot bath (2 to 4 min., 104° to 110°) followed by cold friction is one of the most efficient means of combating a state of collapse, such as often occurs in fever.

Tonic Effects. Tonic measures are such as increase vital 627
activity in a healthful direction. The most powerful tonics are the most powerful excitants, it being understood that by excitants is meant exclusively physiological means, such as thermic influence, light, and electricity. It must be remembered, also, that an excitant may be employed in such a manner as to exhaust the nerve centers, and thus produce effects the very opposite of those desired.

The tonic effect of cold water is its most constant and regular effect, this tonic influence being exerted whenever water is applied at a temperature below that of the body.

Trousseau defined a tonic as an agent having for its object to give tone to the tissues, to restore the functions of nutrition and assimilation, and to increase vital resistance. A more modern definition of a tonic would be an agent which, when systematically employed, aids in the restoration of normal tissue activities, both constructive and destructive, thereby promoting a renewal of the body and a recuperation of its forces, and an increase of vital resistance.

The tonic effects of water are, of all the remarkable therapeutic properties of this versatile agent, the most important and the most extensively used. They are obtained by the repetition of excitant measures, and are due to the reaction which, under ordinary conditions, always follows a short cold application.

Water, by its accessibility, its convenience in use, and its high specific heat, more readily lends itself to the assistance of the physician in producing restorative and permanent tonic effects than any other agent.

628 **Cold Water vs. Medicinal Tonics.** The numerous medicinal tonics, so called, are universally toxic in character. Whatever tonic effects they may seem to produce are due to the fact that the system is aroused to resist their influence and to expel them from the body; and while a certain amount of benefit is perhaps derived from the use of such agents, there is always a possibility of serious damage; and doubtless in all cases a considerable amount of harm is done through the toxic influence of the drug, which falls with especial weight upon those organs which are most concerned in its elimination,— the liver and the kidneys.

A medicinal stimulant is a mortgage placed upon the vital capital of the body, which must be paid sooner or later. It is a draft upon the constitution. A stimulant is simply a means by which the nerve centers are made to give up a little more of the energy which they have stored up; and unless the stimulus is of such a character that the storing power as well as the expending power of the nerve centers is increased, there must be a loss from its employment.

A toxic agent like strychnia may provoke the expenditure of nervous energy, but it does not replenish energy; while it does lessen the activity of the kidneys in eliminating tissue poisons and the efficiency of the liver in the destruction of toxins and leucomains, thus encouraging the development and maintenance of a condition which is, in itself, an indication for the necessity of employing tonic measures; in other words, a medicinal tonic or stimulant aggravates the very condition it is intended to cure.

Nervous Energy.

The establishment in modern times of labo- 629
ratories for psychological and neurological research has been the means of throwing much light upon the nature of mental and nervous activity. Nervous energy no longer means, as formerly, an intangible, mysterious something, but, as has now been clearly demonstrated, is immediately and definitely connected with material elements found in the interior of the nerve cell. For example, a nerve cell, when in a state of rest, shows a large number of grayish granules, which have been shown to be intimately connected with the storage of energy; so that when the granules are abundant, the cell is like a fully charged battery, ready to discharge under the influence of the right sort of stimulus the maximum of energy which it is capable of exhibiting. On the other hand, when the cell is fatigued, as after prolonged, energetic work, the granules are found to be very few and small, and the cells shrunken and pale.

With these facts in mind, it is easy to understand why such disappointing results have followed the use of strychnia and a very large number of medicinal agents, so-called nerve tonics, since it is evidently impossible that these drugs should in any way increase the store of energy in the cell; and the most that can be expected of them is the excitement of the cell to activity when it has become exhausted to such a degree that a sense of fatigue supervenes as a warning that the store of nervous energy is reduced to a point where any further demand upon it is dangerous, and that rest is imperatively demanded.

The only way that the energy granules of a cell can be augmented is by the assimilation of food from the blood, and the development of energy-containing particles. Cold water surpasses all other agents in its power to promote the normal energy-storing processes. Cold applications also facilitate to a very remarkable degree the discharge of nervous energy when a sufficient store exists, though sometimes it may not be available because its useful application is hindered by the influence of retained excretions or nerve-benumbing toxins generated within the tissues or absorbed from the alimentary canal. This effect of water is readily apparent in the influence of the cold bath upon muscular energy, to which attention is called elsewhere (**327**), and also in the sensation of well-being, buoyancy, and readiness for exertion which results from the application of cold water.

The tonic effects of cold water are unquestionably to a large degree due to the influence of cold impressions acting through the nerves of the skin upon the sympathetic nerve centers. The great sympathetic nerve controls the blood-vessels, glands, heart, the functions of secretion and excretion, and, in fact, all the vital functions of the body. The awakening of the sympathetic to renewed activity, or a balancing of its action, is what is specially needed by the great majority of chronic invalids. The functions of the brain and spinal cord, and through them all forms of nervous activity, are to a remarkable extent influenced by the sympathetic. The sensation of well-being which accompanies the reaction following a general cold application is largely due to the increased activity of the cerebral circulation, brought about through the stimulation of the sympathetic. By its power to influence the sympathetic, hydrotherapy is capable of controlling, restraining, reorganizing, balancing, all the processes of organic life, and through them modifying the functions of animal life to a marvelous degree.

630 **Cold Water a Physiological Tonic.** Cold water is a physiological tonic, and has the advantage over medicinal tonics of all sorts, in that it awakens nervous activity without the imposition of any extra burden upon any vital organ, and without hampering the activity of any function. The cold bath employed in such a manner as to produce tonic effects accomplishes its results by increasing vital resistance to the causes of pathological processes, by making the wheels of life run more smoothly, by lifting the whole vital economy to a higher level. The impression made upon that harp of a million strings, the skin, with its vast network of sensory, motor, sympathetic, vasomotor, and thermic nerves, arouses every nerve center, every sympathetic ganglion, every sensory and motor filament in the entire body to heightened life and activity. Every blood-vessel throbs and every cell quivers with a new life; the whole body thrills with quickened impulses, the whole being is translated into a new state of existence.

A person who has never experienced the glow of exhilaration, the invigoration and buoyancy of body and mind, which accompany the state of reaction from a short, general cold application, can not well appreciate the value or significance of the cold bath as a physiological stimulant. It is not too much to say that it is of all measures known to man, the most valuable as a means of arousing to activity the flagging energies of the body, and lifting the enervated invalid out of the morasses and quagmires of chronic disease.

Tonic Effects of the Cold Bath Due to Repetition.

The reaction produced by tonic applications 631
fills the skin with blood; and if it is daily repeated, the blood is finally fixed in the skin, thus permanently increasing its vascular activity, and relieving internal congestion.

The hidebound animal suffers from visceral congestion because of the deficient amount of blood in the skin and the excessive massing of blood in the internal organs.

In the employment of the cold bath as a tonic, there are a few principles which it is important to keep constantly in mind. Especially must it be remembered that the cold bath is, like other tonic agents, a two-edged sword,—it is capable of acting in opposite ways. The cold bath may be used in such a manner as still further to weaken and debilitate the patient who is already nervously exhausted. Indeed, it is so easy to produce such a result that it is not improper to say that no physician should ever undertake the use of the cold bath as a tonic without an exact knowledge of the principles and methods of hydrotherapy and the most precise and complete information respecting the condition of the patient to whom the application is to be made.

All applications of water of a temperature low enough to provoke vital resistance are tonic; hence tonic effects are produced by all temperatures below 90° F.

It should be remembered that those forms of hydric application which are tonic when of short duration, become sedative when sufficiently prolonged. The sedative effect is accompanied and indicated by the lowering of the rectal temperature a few tenths of a degree. The length of time required to render a cold application sedative in character depends, of course, upon the condition and the susceptibility of the patient.

Although all baths at a temperature below 90° may be employed for tonic effects, the most certain and pronounced results are obtained from the douche in every form, which adds mechanical impact to the thermic effects of cold.

The tonic effects of non-percutient baths may be increased by vigorous friction during the bath.

632 The most durable tonic effects are obtained by the frequent use of very cold and very short baths. Short tonic baths may, in many cases, be employed twice daily with advantage.

Of the several forms of douche, the *rain douche*, or shower bath, is the most strongly refrigerant, since it impresses at each instant the largest portion of the surface. The next most vigorous purely hydriatic measure is the horizontal jet. The massage douche combines with the mechanical and thermic effects of the douche, the powerful influence of massage upon circulatory reaction and metabolism.

The horizontal jet, the spinal douche, the circle douche, the pail douche or affusion, the wet-sheet rub, the towel rub, cold friction, the wet-hand rub, the plunge or swimming bath, the sitz bath, the full or immersion bath, the Scotch douche, the alternate douche, the percussion douche, and various modifications of these baths may be employed in such a way as to produce tonic effects varying in degree according to the method of application, the temperature, the length of the bath, and the conditions under which the application is made.

As tonic effects are obtained almost altogether from the use of cold water, great care must be taken to observe the general directions and precautions given elsewhere with reference to the use of the cold bath (767).

Indications for Tonic Applications.

Tonic measures are applicable in nearly all 633
forms of disease. Although tonic baths can not always be employed at the outset of a course of treatment, it should be the constant aim to prepare the patient for them; and after the beginning with tonic measures, there should be a progressive training in the direction of more and more vigorous applications.

Tonic measures are especially indicated in cases of anemia, all forms of nervous exhaustion, or neurasthenia, hysteria, in the numerous varieties of dyspepsia in which enteroptosis and consequent irritation of the sympathetic nerve gives rise to general nervous irritability and exhaustion, in chronic inebriety, in many cases of insomnia, in obesity, in exophthalmic goiter, in convalescence from fevers, and most other chronic morbid conditions.

Tonic applications are also indicated in cases of irritable weakness, such as delirium tremens; in the extreme nervousness and agitation which often accompanies fevers of grave type, as typhoid and typhus; in chlorosis; in many reflex neuralgias growing out of irritation of the abdominal sympathetic; in insomnia; and in cases under treatment for the cure of the alcohol, chloral, opium, or other drug habit.

In depressed conditions of the nervous system, such as hypochondria, nervous dyspepsia, many cases of melancholia, and general nervous exhaustion, without excessive excitability, very exciting applications may be employed, such as the different forms of the douche,—jet, percussion, spray, and rain,—in which the excitant effects of cold are supplemented by percussion effects. The rubbing shallow bath, cold friction, the wet-sheet rub, the cold-towel rub (wrung as dry as possible), the salt glow, and the shallow bath are also valuable. In very weak persons, simple dry friction may be employed for a few days at the beginning of the treatment, or a short hot bath may be administered just before the cold water applications are made.

There is no class of cases in which the tonic effects of cold water are of greater importance than in the treatment of acute infectious febrile disorders. Tonic hydriatic applications build up the bodily resistance as no other measures can do.

634 **Suggestions and Precautions Respecting Cold Applications.** A few words may be useful in relation to the adaptation of tonic measures to the various classes of invalids that require tonic treatment.

Extremely feeble persons are in the greatest need of tonic treatment, and yet have the least tolerance for cold water; hence in the beginning the very gentlest measures must be employed, such as the cold wet-hand rub, cold friction, the salt glow, alternate hot and cold applications to the spine, and similar means.

In many cases it is necessary at first to confine the application to small areas, passing from one part of the body to another in rapid succession, as first a hand, then an arm, a foot, a leg, the chest, the upper portion of the back, the lower portion of the back, etc., carefully drying, rubbing, and covering each part before proceeding to the next. It is best to make the application symmetrical; that is, if the right hand and arm are first treated, the next parts to be treated should be the left hand and arm. This brings into action adjacent and related nerve centers practically simultaneously, and so secures the maximum effect.

In feeble patients a very unpleasant and discouraging 635
sense of fatigue is often experienced after tonic applications, especially at the beginning of a course of treatment. This arises from a deficiency in vital capital to support the loss of heat and the expenditure of nervous energy required by the reaction. The irritable condition of the nervous system occasions a very quick reaction, whereby heat dissipation, through the increased surface circulation, begins before the production of heat has proceeded far enough to repair the loss occasioned by the contact of cold water, and thus an unpleasant nervous perturbation continues, sometimes accompanied by chilliness and various nervous symptoms which only too clearly indicate the fact that the patient's vital resources are at a very low level. In such cases the greatest care is demanded to avoid producing so great a degree of exhaustion as to discourage the patient and blight his prospects for recovery. It must never be forgotten that cold water is a most powerful therapeutic agent, and potent for mischief as well as for good, and that an application which, if wisely managed, may produce powerful tonic effects, may, from lack of care or judgment, become equally depressing and highly injurious.

It must be remembered, also, in making tonic applications of water, and especially in the use of the cold douche, that the skin is abundantly supplied with sympathetic nerves; that these nerves are connected with the great ganglionic system, including the abdominal brain, which controls every vital process in the body, and that there is an intimate association between the sympathetic nervous system and the pneumogastric nerve, which exercises so profound an influence upon the functions of the lungs and heart.

The coughing, oppression, and distress experienced in the region of the chest as the result of a very cold application to this part of the body, are indicative of the profound influence thus exerted upon the respiratory center. This fact must be kept in mind in the treatment of persons of a nervous temperament, especially those subject to asthmatic attacks, or suffering from dyspnea or cardiac weakness.

636 **The Cold Douche to the Chest to be Avoided.** Mechanical stimulation of the pneumogastric stimulates the inspiratory movements. This fact explains the effect of the douche with strong pressure when applied to the upper part of the chest; hence the necessity for avoiding strong percutient applications in cases in which there is an irritable and congested condition of the pulmonary structures, or a hypersensitive state of the pulmonary area of the pneumogastric.

Applications of the cold douche over the stomach, loins, and abdomen should be avoided in cases of hyperpepsia, ulceration of the stomach, hemorrhage from the bowels, or any form of uterine hemorrhage, as menorrhagia or metrorrhagia.

Very anemic persons, such as convalescents from fevers and other wasting diseases, or those who have suffered severe hemorrhage, and especially those who are greatly emaciated as well as weak, must be treated with careful regard for the precautions suggested.

Extremely nervous or neurasthenic patients invariably rebel at the application of very cold water. Such persons must be humored at the start until their confidence is secured. The author has found it a very good plan to prescribe at first for such a patient a hot bath, as the electric-light, vapor, or warm electro-hydric bath, which is likely to please the patient, especially as the immediate effect is usually quieting and comforting. But the application is made short (3 to 10 min.), and immediately followed by a cold application, from 65° to 70° F., very short (4 or 6 secs.), or if at a more moderate temperature, as from 75° to 80°, for 10 to 20 seconds.

637 **The Cold Bath in Anemia.** For very feeble and anemic patients the Scotch douche generally secures the best effects, as in such cases the heat-producing powers are weak. This is especially true with patients who are very susceptible and excitable. The bath should be

graduated by extending the length of the concluding cold application each time until it is well borne for ten to thirty seconds.

If the patient is so sensitive that the douche can not be tolerated, employ the wet-sheet rub, fomentations to the spine followed by affusion with water at 80° F., the electric-light bath, followed by affusion at the same temperature, or the hot-air or vapor bath, also followed by the tepid affusion or some similar measure. The patient must, however, be progressively trained to employ water at lower and lower temperatures until short applications of very cold water can be borne (55° to 60° from 1 to 3 secs.).

It is sometimes a good plan to have the patient, while taking the cold jet or spray douche, stand in a foot bath with the water so hot that he can scarcely stand still in it. His attention is thus diverted to his feet, and the impression of heat is so generalized that a brief general cold application is tolerated without complaint.

Or, the patient may be prepared for the cold application by a very hot spray or shower (110°–120°) lasting from one to three minutes, and of gradually increasing temperature. The hot shower may be instantly succeeded by the cold douche to the spine, or to the spine and lower extremities, or the temperature may be gradually lowered to 70° or 60°. Care must be taken to avoid the abdomen, the chest, and particularly the region of the heart in nervous cases, especially those in which hysteria is a well-marked symptom, and in cardiac disease and asthma. The author finds an arrangement of the electric-light bath in combination with the shower and douche very excellent in these cases.

In anemia, and especially anemia of the brain, whether 638
accompanying general anemia or an independent condition, there is an excessive accumulation of lymph in the ventricles and between the dura and the brain substance. As a result of this stagnation of the lymph, the nutrition of the brain is seriously interfered with, waste matters accumulate, the

nerve cells are unable to store energy, and chronic mental and nervous exhaustion is the result. Tonic applications of water afford the most efficient of all means of correcting this condition. As long ago shown by Schüller, cold applications to the surface cause a sudden filling of the blood-vessels of the brain, whereby a vigorous movement of the lymph current is produced; and when the applications are so managed as to create strong respiratory movements, as in applications to the chest, rapid fluctuations are induced in the volume of the brain, which are attended by a simultaneous agitation of the lymph, which can not be experienced without a salutary effect in cases of this sort.

The observations of Virchow, however, should be borne in mind in dealing with these cases. He showed that chronic anemia is liable to be accompanied by degeneration of the heart and blood-vessels, so that care must be taken to avoid violent measures whereby such strong reflex impressions may be made upon the weakened structures as to paralyze the heart or produce irreparable injury to the vessels. Cold friction, the sitz or shallow bath, and the tonic pack, with the water at a moderate temperature (70° to 80°), are the measures most suitable for these cases.

639 **The Tonic Bath in Cerebral Congestion.** In most cases of chronic congestion of the brain, the difficulty is really due to a paralysis of the vasoconstrictors, though possibly in some cases the difficulty may be due to irritation of the vasodilators. In any case, the normal balance of action between these two sets of nerves is disturbed. It is evident that the most effective measures for securing permanent relief must be those whereby the caliber of the cerebral vessels may be lessened. By means of general warm baths, a large quantity of blood may be drawn to the surface, and the cerebral vessels contracted. But this effect is purely mechanical. Better effects are obtained by cold applications to the lower extremities (the broken douche, rubbing wet sheet, cold

friction), whereby the cerebral vessels may be brought reflexly into a state of vigorous contraction. This effect is, of course, transient, but the nutritive changes set up, and especially the stimulation of the flow of lymph in the ventricles and lymph channels of the brain, when repeated by daily applications of measures of the sort suggested, produce most happy results. These partial tonic applications must be accompanied by short and very moderate general applications. In cases where considerable irritability exists in connection with the cerebral congestion, the cold douche should not be employed, but warm and neutral baths, the shallow bath, wet-sheet rub, rubbing sitz, or tonic wet-sheet pack must be used.

In passive cerebral congestion, and especially in the congestion of the brain which frequently accompanies anemic conditions, these mild tonic measures are of the very greatest value, and will produce most happy results when carefully managed.

The Tonic Bath in Hypochondria and Rheumatism.

In hypochondria, tonic measures are of the highest importance, and are generally well tolerated. It is necessary, however, to precede the cold application by a short hot bath carried to the extent of perspiration, so as to secure the elimination of the poisons to which the depression is due. 640

Rheumatics can comfortably and safely receive cold applications only after a heating bath of some sort. The cold application must be very moderate in degree, and the painful joints must be avoided. These observations apply also to cases of painful gout, and to cases of neuralgia in which large nerve trunks or extensive areas are involved, as in sciatica, spinal irritation, and myalgia involving many groups of muscles.

In persons suffering from cardiac disease with deficient compensation, in arteriosclerosis, in apepsia, in hypopepsia, in acute mania, in advanced cases of consumption, especially those in which pulmonary hemorrhage is a marked symptom, in diabetes with emaciation, in both acute and chronic Bright's disease, in locomotor ataxia, in persons who have an idiosyncrasy against cold, in conditions of fatigue from extreme exhaustion, as violent muscular exertion, or exhaustion from loss of sleep, or excessive expenditure of nervous energy in other ways,—in all these conditions very cold baths must be avoided, as also in the case of very young (children under seven years of age) and very aged persons. These remarks respecting the contraindications for the cold bath must be understood, however, as applying only to the very cold douche, the cold immersion, and like vigorous procedures. Cold applications are useful and necessary in all these cases, and may be safely made by means of cold friction, the cold rubbing sheet, the graduated Scotch douche, and other mild tonic measures.

It should be here noted that age must be judged not entirely by the number of years lived, but by the evidences of senile decay. One person may be older at fifty than another at seventy. An elderly person who has been in the habit of taking a cold bath daily may be able to tolerate the cold douche without injury, while another person of the same age, who has not been accustomed to cold bathing, might be greatly harmed unless gradually trained to it. The presence of arteriosclerosis is always an evidence of senility.

Calorific Effects. All tonic and restorative procedures are accompanied by general thermic or calorific effects. It is necessary, however, in some cases, to secure strong calorific effects independently of other effects, or at least to emphasize thermic reaction and the resulting calorification. The short cold immersion bath (20 secs. to 2 min.), the cold douche with little pressure, cold affusion, and especially the wet-sheet pack prolonged to beginning perspiration, are most efficient calorific measures

641 2. *Local Secondary (Reaction) Excitant Effects*—Applications of water at suitable temperatures may be made in such a manner as to affect the function of any organ or set

of organs in the body. The chief local effects, however, to which it is here desirable to call attention, are the following: Sudorific, expectorant, cholagogic, peptogenic, emmenagogic, hemostatic, revulsive, derivative, resolutive, alterative, and calorific. We will briefly consider each of these local excitant effects, which, as previously intimated, are for the most part to be obtained by applications of cold water, either by itself or in connection with heat.

Sudorific Effects.

Sudorific effects, or stimulation of the perspir- 642
atory function, are obtained by various means which are capable of raising the body temperature. Bouchard has shown that an elevation of the temperature of the blood .7° F. is sufficient to induce general sensible perspiration by stimulation of the sweat centers.

Local perspiration may be induced by circumscribed hot applications or by retention of the natural heat of the part by warm or impervious coverings.

The measures which may be most conveniently employed for the production of active perspiration are, the electric-light bath, the Turkish bath, the Russian bath, the hot-air bath, the vapor bath, the hot full bath, the wet-sheet pack, the dry pack, the hot douche, the vapor douche, the hot blanket pack, the hot sitz bath, hot water drinking, the hot enema, hot fomentations to the spine, and the sun bath. Any one of these measures may be found the most convenient and serviceable in individual cases, and under special conditions.

The electric-light bath is without doubt the most efficient and satisfactory of all modes of inducing perspiration, as it produces such powerful stimulation of the perspiratory glands and other structures of the skin as to cause the perspiration to appear in a remarkably short space of time, thus avoiding the necessity of subjecting the body to the exhausting effect of prolonged exposure to heat. Profuse perspiration generally appears in the electric-light bath in from three to five minutes, and often when the temperature of the air surrounding the patient is not above 85° F. Winternitz has noted a case in which sweating began at a still lower temperature. The dry pack not infrequently fails to produce perspiration within less than an hour and a half or two hours.

643 **Importance of Attention to the Skin in Chronic Diseases.** When the extent of secreting surface presented by the skin is taken into consideration (the area of the perspiratory ducts being more than eleven thousand square feet), it appears evident that this organ is the most extensive of all the eliminating structures of the body. The skin throws off each hour from an ounce to an ounce and a half of insensible perspiration in the form of invisible vapor. Practically, the whole skin takes part in the function of perspiration, acting essentially in the same manner as does the mucous membrane lining the lungs, which the skin still further resembles in its ability to eliminate carbonic acid gas. In profuse perspiration, the sudoriparous glands are brought into vigorous activity, sometimes pouring out their secretion at the rate of from thirty to sixty ounces per hour, or from twenty to forty times the normal amount.

The secretion produced by the sweat-glands closely resembles urine in its character, containing urea and various other toxic matters, and particularly, as has been shown by Bouchard, a ptomain or toxin capable of causing a fall of the body temperature when injected into the veins of an animal. Formic acid, butyric acid, and various other acid substances and poisonous matters are also eliminated in the perspiration.

The healthful activity of the skin is one of the conditions most essential to physical well-being. The state of inactivity and disease of this organ found present in nearly all chronic maladies is not only a consequence but a cause of a large number of serious morbid conditions of the body; and it is in a great majority of cases quite impossible to effect a cure until the skin has, by patient and persevering treatment and training, been brought into a healthy state.

The dry, sallow, dingy skin so often observed in the chronic dyspeptic—indeed, in most forms of chronic disease—is not only a symptom of the disordered bodily state, but a cause of the perpetuation of this condition. This appearance of the skin is due to the accumulation of effete matters in it, and to its impaired nutrition, which state exists not only in the skin, but in the entire body. Hence the correctness of the observations of the empirical but not infrequently very sagacious practitioners of the cold-water cure in the early part of the present century, which led them to rely so largely upon the state of the skin as a perfect index to the patient's general vital condition, and as a test of his progress toward recovery.

As previously stated, it is practically impossible to effect a permanent cure in a large number of chronic disorders without first restoring the skin to a normal state. Diseased conditions of the skin are common among the civilized races because of the disease-producing influence of clothing and the neglect of the daily bath.

Sweating baths are of the highest value as a means of ridding the skin of its accumulated impurities, opening up the obstructed lymph channels and spaces, thereby encouraging the circulation of the nutritive fluids and the development of normal nerve and gland structures, unloading obstructed sebaceous follicles of their hardened contents, as well as arousing to activity the nerve ganglia and the secreting cells of the internal organs, through the reflex movements set up by the cutaneous sensory impressions made.

A diseased state of the skin is always connected with a 644
congested or otherwise disordered condition of important internal viscera, and the restoration of the skin to activity is the most important means of relief from visceral congestion and other functional disturbances.

Neglect of Heating Procedures by Hydrotherapeutists.

The value of heating measures as therapeutic means has not generally been sufficiently appreciated by those who have undertaken to employ water in a scientific manner. Indeed, many hydrotherapeutists, as Fleury and his followers, have held that scientific hydrotherapy is confined to the use of cold water exclusively. On the other hand, there are a large number of those employing baths, in this country at least, who make excessive use of hot applications, particularly the Turkish bath, the Russian bath, hot mineral baths, mud baths, etc. A vast deal of harm has unquestionably been done by the depressing effects of frequently repeated and prolonged hot baths without the association therewith of the cold douche or some other means of producing tonic effects whereby the excessive sedative and spoliative effects of the hot applications may be antidoted or antagonized. This very serious fault exists almost universally in the methods employed at mineral bath establishments and other popular bathing resorts, especially those connected with natural sources of hot water.

The author was pleased, however, in visiting various European bathing establishments some years ago, to note an exception to the general rule, in the practice prevalent at Leukerbad, Switzerland. At this quaint old resort, the patient sometimes spends six or eight hours "soaking" in a great tank filled with alkaline waters derived from artesian wells at a temperature of about 100° F., but on leaving the bath the massage douche is employed, and produces decidedly tonic effects. The massage douche consists of the application of a jet douche chiefly to the spine and the posterior parts of the body and over the region of the liver, the water being applied with high pressure while the attendant vigorously rubs and kneads the tissues with the hand covered with a hair mitten. In taking the massage douche, at the end of an hour's seance in the tank, I found it necessary to lay fast hold of a strong iron bar arranged for the purpose, and to keep my feet firmly braced, to avoid being thrown down and carried away by the force of the large stream of cold water directed upon me by the attendant. By a powerfully tonic application of this sort, the debilitating effect of the warm bath is prevented; but it is certain that equally good effects might be produced by less tedious means and milder measures.

The cold bath in some form should be universally employed after sweating baths, except when contraindicated, as in Bright's disease, rheumatism, neuralgia, and cases in which the sedative effect of heat is desirable.

Alterative or Spoliative Effects. Sweating baths may be employed advantageously for the purpose of reducing the weight, or to remove serous deposits in the tissues, as in anasarca, or in the abdominal or pleural cavities, and also as a hygienic or prophylactic measure for the purpose of atoning, to some degree, for the neglect of active muscular exercise. It is perhaps most valuable as a hydriatic means in the rational treatment of obesity. It must be remembered, however, that the sweating produced by heat is by no means so efficient in reducing flesh as that induced by exercise. It is by a combination of the two means that the most pronounced effects obtainable may be realized. 645

In cases of obesity there is great danger of overheating the blood in consequence of the obstacle to heat elimination presented by the thick layer of non-conducting fat. Therefore, hot applications for the reduction of flesh should never be too greatly prolonged, and the bath should always be finished off by a vigorous cold application. 646

The sudden removal from the blood of a large quantity of serum has to some degree the same effect as bleeding from a vein, weakening the heart's action by lessening the volume of the blood, and thus exposing the patient to risk from cardiac failure, a tendency to which is not infrequently present in cases of extreme obesity, either from actual fatty degeneration or from accumulation of fat about the heart or beneath the serous lining of the chest and the mediastinum.

A short general cold application following an application of heat for the purpose of producing perspiration to reduce weight in obesity has the effect to restore and increase the disposition for muscular effort, in addition to the tonic effect upon the general nervous system, thus enabling the patient to add to the spoliative effects of the hot bath the still more positive effects of prolonged muscular exercise.

647 In administering a sweating bath for the purpose of reducing flesh, it is an excellent plan to interrupt the hot application at intervals by a cold application, a cold shower bath, a cold horizontal douche, or an affusion being best employed for this purpose. The temperature should be from 50° to 60° F., and the application continued not only long enough to remove from the skin the surplus heat which has been absorbed, but from five to twenty seconds longer, so as to produce a strong reaction. The atonic reaction of the hot bath, whereby heat production and tissue activity in general are reduced, will thus be antagonized, oxidation will be encouraged, and effete matters and surplus tissue broken down and prepared for the elimination which will be effected by the succeeding application of heat. By the adoption of this plan the hot bath may be prolonged to two or three times the period otherwise admissible.

Hot Baths Must be Used Carefully in Dropsy.

648 In the application of hot baths for the relief of dropsy, great care must be exercised, especially in cases of cardiac disease. The appearance of dropsy in a case indicates that the small blood-vessels have lost their power of active contraction, and the heart is weak and dilated. The stimulating effect of strong applications of heat may cause still further dilatation of the heart, which is already so weak as to be unable completely to empty itself of its contents, while the depression resulting from the atonic reaction of heat will still further weaken the organ, and may result in so embarrassing it as to induce grave symptoms. Death from cardiac weakness has not infrequently occurred in Turkish bath establishments. The danger is even greater in the Russian bath, and the vapor bath is not wholly free from danger.

Attention should be called to the fact that in cases of edema due to anemia, especially when associated with obesity, sweating baths, even when quite prolonged, are often borne without inconvenience and with decided benefit. The same is true of cases in which edema of the legs is associated with chlorosis, provided that marked cardiac weakness from fatty degeneration or other cause is not also present.

A cold application following a hot bath in dropsy due to 649
cardiac disease is especially important as a means of increasing the tone of both the blood-vessels and the heart; but it must be remembered that a severe cold application to the surface brings, for the moment, a very great strain upon the heart during the primary contraction of the small vessels which is induced throughout the entire body; hence the application must be managed with great care, and extreme temperatures should not be employed.

A douche at 75° or 80° is better suited to these cases than lower temperatures. The application should be made first to the feet and legs, then to the arms and back, and lastly to the chest. It is well to mitigate the shock to the lungs and heart by dipping the hand or a towel in cold water and applying to the face, neck, and chest before making a general cold application. In cases of well-marked cardiac insufficiency the douche must be altogether avoided, and such milder measures as the rubbing shallow bath and cold friction employed instead.

The Hot Bath in Bright's Disease.

The hot bath is also an invaluable measure in 650
certain cases of dropsy of renal origin. It is of special value in acute dropsy due to the nephritis sometimes encountered as a complication in scarlet fever, smallpox, diphtheria, and in the puerperal or pre-puerperal state. In these cases it proves beneficial chiefly by drawing a large quantity of blood to the surface, and thus relieving the congestion of the inflamed organs. It is, of course, also of some service by the elimination of toxins through the sudoriparous glands, but the amount of urea and other toxins thus carried off, even during the most profuse perspiration, is comparatively small.

The hot-blanket pack is a most serviceable measure in cases of this sort. The author has employed this very convenient mode of inducing perspiration in numerous cases, and with most excellent results. The hot-blanket pack is admirably adapted for use in cases of acute nephritis in children. Care must be taken to keep the head moistened with cool water during the application, but it should not be cooled to such a degree as to antagonize the effect of the pack.

In the dropsy of chronic nephritis the hot bath is less serviceable, in consequence of the organic nature of the affection, which leads to the almost certain reappearance of dropsical symptoms after they may have been removed. In these cases there is also great constitutional weakness as a result of the disease, so that the system is poorly prepared to endure the depressing effect of the hot bath.

651 The hot bath also has the effect of leaving the patient in a condition of diminished resistance to colds, which is one of the most serious dangers to the chronic sufferer from Bright's disease. On this account, some eminent authorities wholly forbid the use of hot baths in this class of cases. In the author's experience, however, the hot bath has been found invaluable in these cases, in one special condition; namely, when the sufferer from chronic nephritis has suddenly become dropsical through an exacerbation of the disease, as the result of exposure to cold, or through some departure from the required diet or regimen, or other similar cause. Under these circumstances, the hot bath may be employed with advantage, and, if properly managed, without injury; but the application must be short (10 to 20 min.) and it must be administered so as to give the patient as little fatigue as possible, never so hot nor so long as to be weakening or exhausting. The heart may be protected by a cold compress (**1383**).

In most chronic cases of renal disease, the neutral bath at a temperature of 92° to 95° F., and especially the effervescing bath (**1139**), has proved more serviceable than the sweating bath, as it produces stimulation of the skin circulation without inducing depressing effects. The well-known effect of the neutral bath in exciting renal activity is also here made serviceable.

The electric-light bath is far superior to any other form of 652
sweating bath for cases of Bright's disease, for the reason that the skin may be excited to a high degree of activity by a very short application and without exposing the patient to the risk involved in the breathing of highly heated air or a hot atmosphere saturated with moisture, as in the Turkish or the Russian bath. During the last seven years the author has employed this bath in a very large number of cases, and without witnessing any untoward effects, but with advantages not afforded by other methods of applying heat. One great advantage of this bath is that the medium about the patient is not overheated. The air may be readily maintained at a temperature of 85° to 90°, so that heat elimination may go on normally, which can not be the case in any other form of hot bath.

In the hot immersion bath, heat elimination, except through the lungs, is entirely suspended. In the Russian bath, heat elimination from both the skin and the lungs is almost wholly interrupted. In the Turkish bath, heat elimination takes place by evaporation only, both the skin and the mucous membrane receiving heat by conduction from the highly heated atmosphere surrounding the body.

Another advantage of the electric-light bath is that heat is produced in the depth of the tissues as well as at the surface, through the resistance encountered by the rays of light in passing through the numerous layers of tissue which it penetrates, reaching, with some degree of intensity at least, the innermost recesses of the body.

The Sweating Bath in Dropsy.

In dropsy due to anemia, sweating baths may 653
be employed, if carefully administered, but they should be very short, owing to the extreme degree of cardiac weakness usually present in these cases, and the general vital and nervous

weakness resulting from the impoverished condition of the blood and the general interference with nutrition. Here again the electric-light bath shows itself superior to other measures for applying heat to induce perspiration, for the reasons already pointed out.

In these cases the sweating bath is particularly serviceable as a means of preparing the body for an application of cold, the combination of these two measures having been shown by Winternitz and others to be among the most effective means for the enrichment of the blood, if not by the actual production of blood-corpuscles, by bringing into the blood current a vast number of blood cells previously hidden away in the vessels of the liver, spleen, and other internal viscera, perhaps exposed to excessive destruction, as these organs have, for one of their functions, the destruction of blood cells.

The sweating bath may be advantageously employed in many cases of dropsy of the abdomen and of the chest. Not infrequently absorption takes place at such a rapid rate that within a few days there is a very marked diminution or a complete disappearance of the effused fluid, which had previously resisted with stubbornness tapping, counter-irritation, and all other ordinary means of treatment. The sweating bath is certainly not a panacea for cases of this sort, but it is a most serviceable measure.

654 It must be remembered that a cold application should always be administered after a sweating bath when employed for spoliative purposes, as well as in most other cases. Great care, however, is needed in the adaptation of the cold application at the conclusion of the bath to the serious morbid conditions which are almost invariably present in connection with dropsy, whether local or general in character. The remarks previously made with reference to cold applications after the sweating bath in cases of obesity are equally applicable to cases of dropsy. Respecting the application of cold in cardiac cases, it is only necessary to add that usually the cold-towel rub or cold friction, and, in persons sufficiently

strong and vigorous, the wet-sheet rub or the rubbing shallow bath, in all cases followed by vigorous dry friction, are measures to be preferred to the cold douche, the cold immersion, or other stronger measures of treatment.

The Cold Bath in Renal Disease.

In cases of dropsy with renal disease also, 655
cold applications must be administered with the very greatest care. If the application of cold be so intense as to produce the slightest indications of chill, it will be accompanied by congestion of all the viscera, and consequently increased activity of the renal disease. The cold douche and similar percutient applications must be entirely avoided. The cooling off after a hot bath must also be managed with great care. The best method of doing this is to wrap the patient in blankets after the hot bath, and cool the skin by cool or tepid sponging of limited portions of the surface, taking first one arm or leg, then the other, and thus proceeding to extend the cooling to various parts of the body until the whole surface has been treated. It is sometimes necessary to go over the whole surface two or three times to complete the cooling in a satisfactory manner. The covering should be at the same time gradually withdrawn. If too strongly sedative effects are produced by the bath managed in this way, a tonic effect may be secured by supplementing the bath, after the general surface has been cooled and dried, by cold friction.

To avoid the possibility of taking cold, the patient must not be allowed to dress nor to leave the treatment-room until the surface has thoroughly cooled and the pulse returned to its normal rate. The skin must be not only superficially dry, but thoroughly dried out by the evaporation of the absorbed moisture, as will be indicated by its condition of smoothness and firmness. By reason of the great liability to chilling after a warm bath, it is preferable in cases of renal disease that the patient should be confined to his room for several hours after treatment. It is better, on this account, to administer the treatment in the evening, so that the patient may retire at once. By morning the normal equilibrium will have been so completely established as to obviate the risk of taking cold.

In cold applications following a sweating bath in cases of abdominal dropsy and dropsy of the chest, special regard should be paid to the local condition present. In abdominal dropsy, cold applications should be made first and chiefly to the arms and the upper portion of the back, while in dropsy of the chest the chief part of the application should be made to the lower half of the body, the purpose of this being to prevent too strong a reaction in the congested and disabled parts by first producing reaction in the parts of the body most remote from the diseased structures.

The Sweating Bath in Icterus. The sweating bath is of great value in icterus, both as a means of relieving the intolerable itching, and of aiding the elimination of bile. The electric-light bath is especially useful for this purpose. The sweating process should, however, in these cases be employed only until profuse perspiration is induced. The neutral bath should then be administered for twenty or thirty minutes, at a temperature of from 92° to 95° F. Very hot sponging frequently relieves pruritus when other measures fail.

656 **Surgical Uses of the Sweating Bath.** Sweating baths may be advantageously used as a means of producing general muscular relaxation for the purpose of aiding in the reduction of a hernia or a dislocated limb. The relief thus afforded by a hot bath is partly due to the diminished muscular tone, which lessens the tension of the muscles controlling the joint, and in part to the peculiar influence of heat upon the white fibrous tissues, the chief constituent of the ligaments which bind together the bony structures entering into the formation of a joint. Heat expands white fibrous tissue, thus relaxing the tissues.

The general sweating bath should be employed in cases of hernia not readily reducible by skilful taxis without the bath. The hot immersion bath is perhaps the most appropriate measure for this purpose, and has often proved very effective. The patient lies in the bath with the head (not the shoulders) raised, and the knees well drawn forward. After the bath has been continued long enough to induce active perspiration, the physician employs the usual means for reducing the hernia, the patient still remaining in the bath.

In case of dislocation, the general sweating bath is not always required. It is usually sufficient to apply a large fomentation or a hot pack over the joint and the muscles controlling it, to secure the necessary relaxation of the muscles and ligaments.

Depurative or Eliminative Effects.

The value of the sweating bath as an elimina- 657
tive measure is perhaps not so great as it has been popularly believed to be, as the percentage of urea and other toxins contained in the sweat, especially when profuse perspiration is induced, is small,— indeed, very small when compared with the percentage of these tissue poisons ordinarily found in the urine. That a considerable amount of the waste elements ordinarily eliminated through the urine may be, however, under some circumstances, carried off through the skin, is evidenced by the peculiar urinous odor noticeable when profuse perspiration is induced in a patient suffering from renal insufficiency.

The author has often seen most excellent results from the application of a hot-blanket pack and other forms of the sweating bath in cases of uremic poisoning arising from sudden suppression of renal activity as a complication of the latter stages of pregnancy, and in urinary suppression occurring in surgical cases, especially after a severe abdominal operation, as a hysterectomy or a prolonged operation for the removal of diseased uterine appendages.

The sweating bath is occasionally valuable as a means of 658
averting or aborting a threatened attack of uremic convulsions. A patient under the author's care many years ago, who had for some years suffered from chronic Bright's

disease, discovered for himself that the characteristic symptoms of incipient uremic poisoning might be thoroughly controlled by a hot bath, and had, accordingly, fitted up in his own home a vapor bath, into which he entered whenever threatened with an attack of convulsions, remaining in the bath until the symptoms had entirely disappeared. He stated that he sometimes remained in the bath more than forty-eight hours continuously. Such prolonged applications are not, however, to be commended as generally useful, at least not without interruption every hour or two by the application of cold in the form of a cold trunk pack, applied by means of a single thickness of linen wrung very dry out of very cold water and well covered, so as to secure prompt reaction; by cold over the heart, or by cold friction.

Eliminative Baths in Toxemia.

659 The eliminative effects of the sweating bath may be resorted to with advantage in all forms of chronic toxemia due to the retention of tissue poisons, as gastric neurasthenia, migraine, jaundice, and chronic "biliousness." To be of the greatest service in these cases, however, the sweating bath should not be too prolonged, and should be immediately followed by short tonic applications of cold water, in the form of the cold douche (**1020**), cold wet-sheet rub (**1216**), or cold plunge (**1108**). The electric light (**1250**) is one of the most suitable means of applying heat in cases of this sort, as it induces profuse perspiration without long exposure of the body to a high temperature, and produces tonic as well as eliminative effects.

Sweating applications may be made to a limited portion of the body when desirable, as in the treatment of exudates, the enlarged and stiffened joints of chronic rheumatism, pluritic adhesions in the chest, chronic peritonitis, and in certain forms of neuralgia, as sciatica.

The most serious objection to the application of heat in many of the cases mentioned, especially in rheumatism and gout, is the danger of diminishing the general bodily resistance, leading to the contracting of colds through slight exposures, by which the good effects of the treatment may be more than lost. With care, however, this may be avoided.

In diabetes with emaciation, and when the perspiration does not contain sugar, the sweating bath must be avoided, or at least used with extreme care. In cases of skin disease accompanied by painful eruptions, furuncles, or other evidences of extreme excitation and irritation, if the sweating bath must be employed, it should be in the form of the vapor, the Russian, the hot-water, or the electric-light bath. The Turkish and dry-air baths irritate the skin, while the wet-sheet pack is too exciting.

Expectorant Effects. The mucous membrane is closely allied to the 660
skin in its structure and functions. Thus, applications which produce general perspiration of the skin at the same time encourage increased activity of the mucous membrane, through its close sympathy with the skin. This explains the great relief experienced by persons suffering from a severe cold and obstruction of the respiratory passages within a few moments after entering a Russian or vapor bath. A dry, painful cough is quickly loosened and relieved under the influence of a warm bath; but if great care is not exercised, the condition is likely to be decidedly aggravated by a fresh cold acquired through the diminished vital resistance naturally resulting from the atonic reaction of heat. Persons suffering from hay fever, so called, and other forms of asthma are often quickly relieved by the Russian bath, but the distressing symptoms are very likely to return with redoubled force as the result of some inadvertent exposure, unless the cutaneous activity is maintained, which is likely to be very exhausting if long continued. This measure is useful only as a palliative. Cold applications are required for the tonic effects absolutely essential to permanent relief from chronic asthma. Hay asthma, of course, requires change of climate and the services of a specialist, as well as general tonic baths.

Local applications of vapor in the form of steam inhalations are also of great value in the treatment of those forms of throat, ear, and nose affections in which increased secretion is desirable, the expectorant effects of these measures being very marked.

The chest pack (1373) is an invaluable means of favorably influencing the pulmonary mucous membrane. In a febrile state, or acute congestion, do not cover with oiled muslin or other impervious material; but if chronic passive congestion is present, as in bronchial catarrh, apply an impervious covering, so as to procure more decided revulsive and derivative effects.

The expectorant effects of water, particularly in the form of the sweating bath, are often of service in breaking up a hard cold, if it is taken at the beginning. If, however, several days have elapsed since the exposure, the sweating bath is not likely to effect a radical cure, but it may be the means of shortening the attack, provided, of course, that sufficient precaution is taken against exposure to chill subsequent to the bath.

Water drinking, and especially the free use of hot water internally, is of the highest value as a means of encouraging activity of the skin and mucous membranes. A copious draft of hot water should always be taken before entering a sweating bath of any kind. Cold water may be substituted, if greatly preferred, provided it is not swallowed so rapidly and in such quantity as to produce a chill.

661 **Diuretic Effects.** The cold douche applied over the lower portion of the sternum has long been recognized as a means of stimulating the kidneys to activity. A short cold douche to the loins is effective in the same way.[87]

The cold trunk pack is also a very efficient method of stimulating activity of the kidneys. When used for this purpose, the pack may be confined to the central and lower portions of the trunk, the sheet with which it is applied being wrung as dry as possible out of very cold water. The pack may be allowed to remain in place for two or three hours, or until dry. It may be renewed every hour or two in cases in which active diuresis is required.

Fomentations to the lumbar region may be advantageously employed in cases of renal insufficiency, and for the purpose of obtaining revulsive effects in cases of pain in the kidneys.

Cholagogic Effects. The cold hepatic douche is certainly one of 662 the most effective means of stimulating the liver. Both the circulation and the functional activity of the liver may be profoundly influenced by the application of cold water by means of the horizontal jet, with considerable pressure, over the lower portion of the right chest and the epigastrium. The alternating douche is a more agreeable and in most cases an equally exciting measure. Where congestion or pain is present, the hot or Scotch fan douche, without pressure, may be substituted for the cold or the alternate douche (**1044**), or if the douche can not be conveniently administered because of the feebleness of the patient, or for any other reason, the fomentation may be substituted. The effect of the fomentation will be prolonged and intensified if followed by the heating compress.

In painful affections of the liver, fomentations repeated every two or three hours, with the heating compress applied during the interim, may be commended as a most efficient means of relieving pain and restoring the organ to its normal state. The hot douche and fomentation followed by the wet girdle, are of the highest value in cases of infectious jaundice, gall-stones, and in all acute congestions and inflammations of the liver.

Peptogenic Effects The cold douche (50° to 70° F.) applied over 663 the region of the stomach by means of the horizontal jet with considerable pressure (20 to 30 lbs.), is the most efficient means of stimulating the production of an abundant quantity of gastric juice of efficient quality. This is the measure par excellence to be employed in the treatment of hypopepsia. The alternate douche may be employed to better advantage than the cold douche in many cases. The author makes use of the circle douche or the percussion douche, which produces more pronounced effects than the ordinary horizontal douche. The percussion douche should be employed if possible, especially in the cold application.

664 The ice-bag over the stomach for an hour before eating is a most powerful peptogenic procedure, and is of the highest value in cases of atonic dyspepsia or apepsia and hypopepsia. The good effect of the treatment is quickly shown in improved appetite and digestive vigor.

The application of heat over the stomach for an hour or two after eating is also a peptogenic measure of high value. The constricted gastric vessels are thus relaxed and the anemic stomach provided with an abundant blood supply.

665 In cases of hyperpepsia in which it is desirable to diminish the secretion of hydrochloric acid or lessen the production of gastric juice, as in gastrorrhea, it is necessary to employ measures of a character opposite to those used for peptogenic effects: in other words, to secure antipeptogenic effects. This may be best accomplished by means of the hot douche over the region of the stomach. The heating trunk compress and the hot and cold trunk pack (**1367**), applied just before eating and retained for an hour or two afterward, are most excellent means for relieving gastric irritability and combating painful hyperpepsia.

666 **Emmenagogic Effects.** Of all methods whereby the menstrual function may be stimulated, hydric measures are both the safest and the most effective.

Perhaps the most powerful of all excitants of the menstrual function is the cold douche to the loins (horizontal jet or spray; temperature, 50° to 70° F.; time, 2 to 10 secs.; pressure, 20 to 40 lbs.).

The prolonged hot foot bath (temperature, 100° to 104° F.), the hot sitz (temperature, 100° to 104° F.), the hot enema (temperature, 105°), the hot immersion, the tonic hip pack daily in the intermenstrual period, and the hot hip pack (temperature, 110°, 10 to 15 min.) are among the best measures for use in cases of this sort. General tonic measures are, of course, needed when the amenorrhea is due to anemia.

Revulsive and Derivative Effects.

The revulsive effects obtainable by water con- 667
stitute one of its most interesting and valuable therapeutic uses. This effect is nothing more nor less than a strong circulatory reaction localized in accordance with the indication present. The anatomical basis of this therapeutic action is the association of vascular areas in the skin with definite and well-understood visceral vascular areas. These associations have been elsewhere carefully pointed out, so that we need not here devote space to a lengthy description of them. It will only be necessary to point out the principle upon which the revulsive method rests, and the best methods of utilizing it.

As previously stated, applications of cold water to the surface of the body set up both *circulatory* and *thermic* reactions. In revulsion pure and simple, it is desirable to obtain only the circulatory reaction; hence the application should be so managed as to avoid *thermic* reaction except in those cases in which the excitement of tissue activity by the aid of the thermic reaction will not interfere with the results sought, as in cases of passive congestion without pain (673).

When this circulatory reaction is produced in an area 668
of the skin supplied by an artery, a branch of which supplies some deeper structure, as in the case of an inflamed muscle or joint, a congested nerve, or an alveolar abscess, a considerable amount of blood may be by this means diverted away from the inflamed or congested part, thus affording relief from urgent symptoms by producing a local hyperemia of the skin and a collateral anemia of the affected part. By continuous cold applications, local anemia and collateral hyperemia may be produced.

669 **Fluxion.** Fluxion, or movement of the blood, is one of the most important of all the functional modifications which may be affected by hydric applications. The permanency of chronic disease is generally due to a disordered state of the blood-vessels of the affected parts.

The most important thing that can be done therapeutically in relation to a chronically congested organ is to increase the supply of healthy blood, not necessarily by augmenting the volume of blood which the organ contains at any moment, but by quickening the rate at which the blood passes through it. This may be accomplished by increasing the energy and activity of the heart as well as the activity of the blood-vessels of the affected parts, and by concentrating the blood in the diseased organ by the use of appropriate measures.

The blood is the great healer. In the words of Holy Writ, "The blood is the life." It washes out of the tissues the waste and toxic products which they contain, and brings new vitalizing and energizing elements to take their place. The only way in which a diseased organ can be restored to permanent health is by complete renovation in its tissues, since function depends upon structure. This requires a tearing down and a rebuilding through increased movement of the blood and lymph.

670 **Revulsive Methods for Combating Superficial Anemia.** Some of the measures most useful for this purpose are, first, short cold applications followed by vigorous rubbing. The cold application must not be too long, otherwise the anemia will be increased; but the rubbing should be sufficiently prolonged and vigorous to insure thorough circulatory reaction, which is the end sought. The cold percussion douche, temperature 20° to 60°, duration 4 to 10 seconds, is most efficient. Cold affusion and other measures are efficient just in the proportion in which mechanical and thermic effects are combined. When the anemia is general, the cold bath should be preceded by the incandescent electric-light bath or some other form of hot bath, from 3 to 5 minutes, or

a sufficient time to heat the skin, as in these cases the heat-generating powers of the body are lowered, and the abstraction of heat is not well borne. The application should be intense, as a douche at high pressure, vigorous wet-sheet rubbing, or a vigorous shallow bath of short duration. The temperature may be, for the general douche, 60° to 70° F.; the shallow bath, 70° to 75°; the wet-sheet rub, 60°.

The hot and cold compress is a powerful revulsive measure; the heating compress, preceded by a fomentation or rubbing of the parts sufficiently prolonged, is also very efficient. The compress should be covered with flannel, but with no impervious covering, so that the slight cooling effect produced by evaporation may maintain vigorous skin activity, and prevent superheating and resulting vascular paralysis. Fomentations at a temperature of 104° to 106°, prolonged from 15 to 20 minutes, is another valuable means in many cases. The fomentation should not be too hot, as Max Runge has shown that prolonged application at a temperature above 104° produces paralysis of the small vessels, with turgescence from slowed movement of the blood. What is desired is not paralysis and congestion, but activity of the vessels. In anemia there is intense tonic spasm, which is ordinarily overcome by the relaxing effect of heat; but if the heat is at too high a temperature, or the application too prolonged, the vessels of the parts may be paralyzed instead of energized. Increased activity through vital stimulation of the tissues is the end sought by hydric applications, and this object may be readily attained by the varied means suggested, which individually meet the peculiarities encountered in the treatment of special cases.

Methods Adapted to Anemia of Deep-Seated Organs.

In deep anemias, general cold applications are of special service, especially when many of the large viscera are involved in the morbid state, a condition which, though generally overlooked, is, in the opinion of the author, of very frequent occurrence. Tonic spasm of the vessels set up by the irritation resulting from these anemias is usually due to a strain upon the sympathetic nerves occasioned by prolapse of the stomach, colon, viscera, and other forms of visceral displacement. Contraction of the muscular walls of the hollow viscera, such as the colon, resulting in obstinate constipation, as well as contraction of the visceral blood-vessels, is not an uncommon condition due to this cause.

671 Renal insufficiency, hepatic inactivity, and functional feebleness of all the viscera are also conditions due to this cause. Amenorrhea is another illustration often encountered of anemia due to vascular spasm. In these cases the condition of the viscera is precisely the same as that of the feet and hands of the nervous dyspeptic, which are often pale, cold, and bloodless, not because of feebleness of the heart, but because of vascular spasm.

For the relief of conditions in which there is general visceral anemia, as in enteroptosis, nephroptosis, gastroptosis, and atony of the pelvic viscera, general cold applications, such as the douche at 80° for 30 to 60 seconds, the shallow bath at 80° to 85° for 5 to 6 minutes, the tonic half-pack, cold friction, and the wet-sheet rub, are means possessed of wonderful curative power. Very low and very high temperatures must be avoided on account of excessive excitation of the skin. What is desired is moderate fluxion between the surface and the interior of the body, with general increase in the movement of the blood and moderate concentration of the blood in the internal viscera. This *retrostasis*, if excessive, may be followed by reaction, leaving the parts in a condition of greater anemia than before.

Such local anemias as occur in amenorrhea, and also in general atony of the genitals, indicated by coldness of the external parts, and infantile uterus, are combated by ice-bags and ice compresses to the spine. A very cold lumbar douche, a cold douche to the hypogastric region and the inner surfaces of the thighs, and the tonic pelvic pack may be advantageously used in most cases. In amenorrhea, the best results will be obtained from the measures named, supplemented by vaginal irrigation at 110° for 10 minutes and 80° for 1 minute. In the treatment of these visceral anemias it is not only important to concentrate the blood in the affected part, but to increase the activity of the entire circulation of the body by improvement in its general conditions, so that the whole vital tone may be elevated and the blood supply increased.

Hydriatic Measures for Relief of Deep Congestions. Visceral congestion is illustrated in gastro-duodenal catarrh, intestinal catarrh, infectious jaundice, splenic and hepatic congestion, congestion of the spinal cord, menorrhagia, subinvolution and general relaxation of the uterus and appendages, congestion of the prostate, catarrh of the bladder, catarrh of the rectum, hemorrhoids. Congestion of the sympathetic ganglia, giving rise to hyperesthesia and vascular spasm of the parts supplied by these ganglia, as indicated by tenderness of the epigastrium and the umbilical points (**168**), is a condition responsible for a great variety of morbid phenomena expressed for the most part in remote symptoms rather than by local indications. 672

For pelvic congestions, very hot fomentations or a hot douche administered to the lumbar spine and the inner surfaces of the thighs, render invaluable service. For congestion of the spine, fomentations, followed by the heating spinal compress (**1355**) covered with flannel only, is an excellent measure, especially in cases in which spinal congestion and irritation coexist.

In deep passive congestions, alternate hot and cold compresses may be applied to the related cutaneous area, followed by a heating compress covered with flannel, to be changed once in 40 minutes. By this means the dilated blood-vessels of the congested parts are made to contract and relax alternately, so that the organ is emptied of its venous blood, and the muscular walls of its vessels, being fed by fresh blood, are better prepared for vigorous and sustained contraction under the influence of the cold compress.

In the treatment of acute inflammation, whether near the surface (but not involving the skin) or affecting a deeply seated viscus, great care must be observed to avoid such procedures as may cause increased fluxion of blood toward the inflamed organ. For example, in inflammation of a muscle, a cold application over the affected part will cause local anemia of the skin and collateral hyperemia of the inflamed tissues, thus aggravating the condition, unless the application is very intense in character, as an ice-bag or an ice poultice long continued. The fomentation, on the other hand, by producing hyperemia of the skin, causes collateral anemia of the muscle, and so relieves pain. A simple compress at 60°, changed every half hour or every hour, succeeds better than very cold applications, maintaining after fluxion through reaction, while to a degree reflexly affecting the inflamed area in a favorable way through vasomotor influence.

In the case of deeply seated inflammations, prolonged applications to the associated cutaneous areas, with renewals every 20 to 40 minutes, succeed better than continuous very cold applications, as renewed contraction is produced at each renewal, thus maintaining both the vessel tonus of the affected part and an active fluxion of healing blood through its vessels.

The term revulsion is perhaps most properly applied to effects produced in an internal organ, as the abdominal viscera or the brain, by applications to a cutaneous area in reflex relation therewith. In relation to these effects it may be sufficient here to remark that the vessels of the internal area are, in general, affected in the same manner as those of the skin. A short cold application causes temporary contraction of the vessels of the skin, and likewise of the associated internal vascular area, and is quickly followed by reaction, with dilatation of the vessels of both areas.

A prolonged cool application causes continuous contraction of the vessels of both the external and the internal associated areas.

Very hot applications produce effects similar to those of cold applications. Warm applications produce little or no reflex effects.

Very hot applications to the abdominal surface afford the most efficient revulsive means of relieving visceral pain in this region of the body, whether the pain is neuralgic or inflammatory in character; but the application must be very hot (115° to 130°), and the high temperature must be maintained by frequent renewal of the application. The surface vessels become filled with blood by exhaustion of the constrictors through the accumulation of heat in the skin; but the internal associated vascular area is constantly cooled by the blood currents passing through it, so that the first, or vasoconstricting, effect is maintained.

From the above it is evident that we must depend upon very cold, cold, cool, hot, or very hot applications for producing revulsive effects. Neutral or warm applications are incapable of awakening the nervous activities which are the essential factor in this class of hydriatic effects.

Simple Revulsive Effects.

For purely revulsive effects, we seek to obtain 673
results very different from those which follow a short cold application, but we depend upon the same reflex activities and the same exciting measures for accomplishing the desired end. We are able to do this by a carefully managed combination of the atonic reaction of heat with the tonic reaction of cold, so manipulating the measures employed as to secure the strongest possible circulatory reaction while wholly suppressing thermic reaction.

As inflammation involves increased cell activity, it is evident that the suppression of thermic reaction in obtaining revulsive effects is a matter of primary importance; but, singularly enough, it is a thing which has generally been entirely overlooked, and hence the frequent failure of attempts to employ water for revulsive effects. The physician or attendant who knows how to apply, under varied circumstances, hydriatic measures so as to produce the best revulsive effects, is an adept in the employment of water for curative purposes, and is entitled to be called a hydrotherapeutist.

674 The true revulsive application invariably begins with an application of heat. The application may take the form of a douche, a fomentation, dry heat, as a hot bag, an electric-light bath, immersion, affusion, etc. Powerful revulsive effects may be obtained from the application of heat alone, provided the temperature is sufficiently high. The temperature required is from 110° to 130° F. If the surface involved is very small, even higher temperatures may be used. The effect of such an application is to dilate the surface vessels, particularly the venules, and thus to divert to the surface a considerable amount of blood.

The revulsive effect of heat is often inconvenient, however, in cases in which it is necessary to extend the application to a very large area, or to the whole surface of the body, for the reason that such extensive applications of heat give rise to excitation of the cerebral and spinal centers, which interferes with the application, and produces untoward effects.

675 Revulsive effects are also obtainable by the application of cold, but in revulsion by cold a strong thermic reaction is set up in connection with the desired circulatory reaction, which is often most undesirable and injurious. By a proper combination of heat and cold, we are able to obtain not only a more powerful circulatory reaction, and hence more powerful revulsive effects, but the thermic reaction may be either wholly suppressed, or may be permitted to any degree, more or less, as may be advantageous to the results sought.

When a hot application is made to the surface, a considerable amount of artificial heat is absorbed by the skin and underlying tissues. If the hot application be followed by a suitable cold application so adjusted and manipulated as to absorb just the amount of heat which has been absorbed by the skin,—in other words, so as to antidote and neutralize the artificial heat to which the skin has been subjected,—the skin is left at its normal temperature. Thermic reaction is set up only when the temperature of the skin is lowered below the normal point; hence, if the application of cold is barely sufficient to bring the skin to the normal temperature, no thermic reaction will take place.

How may this be accomplished? It is certainly apparent that it is practically impossible to make such use of a thermometer as to enable one to apply cold in just the measure to balance exactly the previous application of heat. But, fortunately, nature has given us a perfect indicator whereby this may be accomplished. The reaction produced by heat results in a dilatation of the surface vessels, but this dilatation involves the small veins to a much greater degree than the small arteries; in other words, heat relaxes the venules more than the arterioles, thus giving rise to a disproportionate increase of venous blood in the skin. The result is a dusky or purplish red color, as a characteristic effect of hot applications to the skin. The reaction induced by cold, on the other hand, produces an active dilatation of all the surface vessels, both arterioles and venules, thus producing a quickened circulation through the skin rather than stagnation.

This effect of cold, in increasing the circulation of the 676
blood through the skin and dilating the small arteries as well as the veins, gives rise to a crimson or bright-red color, which is easily distinguished by a practiced eye from the dusky hue resulting from a hot application.

It is evident that if an application of cold follows an application of heat upon the same surface, a change of color will appear. This change of color begins the instant the heat communicated to the skin has been absorbed by the cold application; hence the change in the color of the skin becomes a perfect guide in the employment of revulsive measures, showing just the right instant to check the cold application in order to secure a purely circulatory reaction and wholly to suppress all thermic reaction.

A little practice is required to enable one to distinguish, at a glance, the color produced by reaction to heat from that produced by reaction to cold. It is, of course, evident that the effect of the cold application must be watched with the greatest care, and must be interrupted the instant the looked-for change in color appears. The time usually required with the cold douche is ten to fifteen seconds.

In the employment of heat for revulsive effects, the result will be (within certain limits) as much more intense as the temperature is high and the application prolonged. The maximum effects are usually reached in from ten to fifteen minutes.

In the employment of cold applications for revulsive effects, the effect will be as much more intense as the temperature is low and the percussion strong.

677 **Revulsion by Means of Hot and Cold Applications.** In the production of revulsive effects by the combined use of heat and cold, the effects will be more intense the greater the difference in temperature between the hot and the cold applications; hence, for the strongest effects the hot application should be as hot as can be borne. If the area is small, the temperature may be from 115° to 130° F., though a temperature of from 110° to 120° is generally safer. The higher temperature may be readily used if the horizontal jet or spray is employed instead of the immersion bath, since the current of water may be applied with aspersions, and made in rapid succession upon different portions of the surface. In the alternate douche a temperature of from 50° to 60° for the cold application is desirable, and a still lower temperature may sometimes be employed, though ice-water and ice are seldom used except when the application is confined to very limited areas.

Revulsive effects may be produced either by percutient or non-percutient applications, or by a combination of percutient and non-percutient means; for example, revulsion to the lower extremities may be obtained by a very hot foot or leg bath followed by a cold douche, as well as by the hot and cold douche. The leg or foot bath may be of seven to ten minutes' duration, but generally an exposure of the surface to an application of heat for four or five minutes is sufficient to obtain the effects desired.

During the application of the cold spray, the color of the surface acted upon must be carefully watched, and the instant the bright red produced by the reaction of cold begins to make its appearance, the cold application should cease. By subsequent friction the circulatory reaction may be increased. Equally good effects are obtained, and somewhat more speedily, by the employment of the hot douche, especially the vapor douche, preceding the cold douche. Three or four minutes will suffice for the hot application, and from ten to fifteen seconds for the cold application.

When neither hot immersion nor the cold douche can be employed, a fomentation followed by a cold compress or cold friction may be used. The latter is an excellent measure in the case of bedridden patients. When the skin surface to be acted upon is so sensitive that percutient applications can not be tolerated, a towel wrung as dry as possible out of very cold water should be applied for twenty to thirty seconds after a fomentation.

One of the most generally useful of all the various revulsive applications which can be made is the revulsive Scotch douche, which consists of a very hot horizontal jet or spray for three or four minutes, followed by a very cold douche from five to fifteen seconds."[33]

Revulsion as an Analgesic Measure.

Revulsion is perhaps most valuable as a means 678
of relieving pain. When analgesic effects are desired, the greatest care must be taken to avoid all thermic reaction, by the methods which have been already explained. The Scotch douche has been used with great success in hundreds of cases of sciatic neuralgia, to the relief of which it seems to be especially adapted.

The Scotch douche may be used with equal success in neuralgia in other regions, though sometimes with less convenience. In cases of neuralgia accompanied by extreme sensitiveness of the skin, strong pressure must be avoided; in some cases, also, extremes of temperature give pain. In such cases the neutral douche with little pressure (3 to 5 lbs.) must be used until the surface pain is lessened, as a preparation for the Scotch douche, which should at first be employed at very moderate temperatures, and with little pressure, both temperature extremes and pressure being progressively increased as tolerance is established.

679 **Analgesic Effects of the Scotch Douche.** In spinal irritation, in intercostal neuralgia, in lumbago, in crural neuralgia, and even in cases of facial neuralgia, the Scotch douche may be relied upon as a sovereign remedy, though the application must be more or less modified to suit the varying conditions under which it may be employed. For enteralgia and gastralgia, apply the fomentation for 10 or 20 minutes.

In chronic visceral congestion, the Scotch revulsive douche may be administered to those areas of the skin which are in reflex relation with the several viscera. When it is desired to draw the blood away from the upper part of the body, it is necessary to localize the application to the lower extremities by means of the Scotch douche or by a hot leg or sitz bath, followed by a short cold application.

When it is desirable to produce revulsion in the opposite direction, the Scotch douche may be administered to the upper part of the back and the arms. Such an application is often useful is cases of pelvic congestion or hemorrhage, while at the same time efforts are being made to reduce the congestion of the affected parts by other suitable measures.

The Hot and Cold Trunk Pack. This ingenious hydriatic application, first described by Winternitz, is one of the most valuable of all revulsive measures. It is especially serviceable as a means of relieving gastric irritability associated with hyperesthesia of the great abdominal sympathetic centers. The various forms of the hot and cold compress, and their several applications, will be found fully described elsewhere.

General Revulsive Effects. General revulsive effects may be advantageously employed in such disorders as cholera, chronic rheumatism when the joints are universally affected, and in cases of heat-stroke in which the surface is pale. It is a useful measure in all forms of shock and collapse, as a means of combating internal congestion. Revulsion in these cases may be sought without care to suppress the thermic reaction; hence it is not always necessary to precede the cold application by a hot one, although as a rule this is desirable when it can be accomplished without too much delay, and the cold application may be continued long enough to obtain the excitant or tonic effect. 680

The lumberman brings the blood to his blanched and freezing feet by pulling off his boots and socks and rubbing the parts with snow. The Persians combat the collapse from cholera by vigorously rubbing the surface with cold water. In accordance with this idea, it has been the practice from time immemorial in Persian cities to place upon every street-corner vessels of water during epidemics of cholera; and if a person falls upon the street, the bystanders immediately deluge him with water, and rub the whole surface of the body with the greatest vigor.

The author has for many years made use of similar means in collapse under anesthesia, in surgical shock, and in similar cases, preferring, however, whenever possible, to make the cold application short, and to precede or alternate it with a hot application. In this manner both an excellent circulatory reaction and simultaneously a calorific effect may be obtained.

The hot immersion bath may sometimes be used with advantage as a revulsive measure for the relief of visceral congestion, as in acute nephritis, especially in the nephritis of scarlet fever. It is equally useful in cerebrospinal meningitis. The hot-blanket pack may be successfully used in the same conditions. Care must, however, be taken to guard the head by a large towel saturated with cold water; and if the heart is feeble, or seems unduly excited, it should be protected by an ice-bag placed over it during the bath, or by a cold chest compress.

681 When the suppression of thermic reaction is not necessary, as when purely revulsive effects are not required, the *alternate douche* may be employed instead of the Scotch douche. In this douche, as elsewhere explained, the applications of heat and cold are of equal length. The extremes of temperature are as great as can be borne, provided the exciting effects of such an application are not contraindicated; the alternations should be eight or ten in number. The application may be renewed several times a day, or as frequently as required.

In place of the alternate douche, the alternate foot bath, alternate affusion, alternate compresses, and various other forms of applying heat and cold in alternation may be used, the measure being adapted to the case in hand.

The alternate douche differs from the Scotch douche in that it is primarily exciting rather than calmative or sedative in its effects. It is one of the most exciting of all hydriatic applications. Nevertheless, it often relieves pain by its powerful revulsive effects.

682 **Derivative Effects.** So-called derivative effects do not differ essentially from revulsive effects, except that they are generally somewhat less intense in character, and the term is applied to the relief afforded a congested organ by diverting the blood into a distant part, as in relief of cerebral congestion by a hot foot bath. All the measures suggested for producing revulsive effects are equally useful for inducing derivative effects. Ordinarily, however, it is not necessary to avoid thermic reaction in producing derivative effects. Any measure whereby the blood can be drawn

into a part distant from the congested part to be relieved may be utilized for this purpose. The most generally useful procedures are the following: The hot leg bath; hot sitz; short cold sitz; rubbing sitz; leg pack; half pack; hot, cold, or alternate douche to legs or arms, as may be indicated; cold friction; rubbing shallow pelvic pack; heating abdominal compress. General derivative effects may often be advantageously procured by the wet-sheet pack, the rubbing wet sheet, and general cold friction. Derivative measures are of the greatest possible service in the treatment of insomnia, pulmonary congestion or hemorrhage, apoplexy, acute mania, and cerebral congestion.

By a reversal of the method, cerebral anemia may be 683
combated as successfully as the opposite state. For example, a short cold douche to the feet powerfully stimulates the circulation of the brain, and the short cold douche to the lumbar region and feet is an excellent means of combating amenorrhea.

In this connection may be properly mentioned an important application of the principle of derivation which may be utilized by one skilled in hydriatry to most excellent advantage in the use of the cold douche and many other general cold applications.

It will be recalled that the contraction of the surface vessels set up by the application of cold water is accompanied by a similar but more brief contraction of that particular vascular area which is in reflex nervous relation with the area operated upon. An application made to the entire surface of the body causes a momentary contraction of the peripheral vessels throughout the entire body, raising the blood pressure and forcing the surplus blood into the large venous channels, especially those of the portal circulation and the associated viscera,—the spleen, the liver, the stomach, the pancreas, and the intestines. Reaction and dilatation quickly follow if the cold application is a short one,—more quickly, in fact, in internal parts than at the surface, for the reason that the internal tissues are surrounded by heated organs, and are not exposed to the continued influence of cold through evaporation, and because of the inrush of blood from the surface to the interior of the body.

When the application is made to a circumscribed portion of the surface, the reaction which follows, both external and internal, is likewise circumscribed, and particularly as regards the viscus or viscera associated with the area operated upon, which may be the stomach, the liver, the kidneys, the brain, the uterus, or some other internal part. The circulatory activity of the skin following such an application, indicated by redness and heat, is an outward indication of the quickened activity in the internal parts under the influence of the application.

684 While this vascular and cellular activity is sometimes desirable, it must often be suppressed as much as possible. When, in such cases, general cold applications must be made, any part that is likely to be damaged by the congestion following the first contact of cold water with the skin, may be protected by the application to the cutaneous area associated reflexly with the part, of water at a lower temperature than that to be used in the general application, or in case the douche is used, both lower temperature and higher pressure may be employed. The effect is to cause so vigorous a primary contraction of the visceral vessels that the part will be protected against the mechanical distension arising from the sudden inrush of blood from the surface when the general application is made. The brain should be always thus protected before either a cold or a hot bath, by bathing the face, neck, and scalp with cold water, and applying a cold wet towel. The liver, when congested, may be protected by a short hepatic douche before the general douche. Congested pelvic viscera should be protected by the douche to the lumbar region and the thighs. In pulmonary congestion, the douche should be first applied to the arms, and then generalized. The brain and lungs may also be protected by a preliminary Scotch douche to the legs. The

hydriatist must have in mind all these interesting and important principles of protection and adaptation, and the facilities for applying them at command, if he would avoid many most unnecessary and unfortunate failures in the use of general cold applications.

Resolvent Effects. The alternate douche is extremely useful as a means of stimulating the absorption of exudates in joints or muscles and about tendons. The *resolvent* effects obtainable by means of it are highly valuable. Similar effects, though less vigorous, may be obtained by non-percutient applications, such as the fomentation followed by the heating compress, or by alternate hot and cold compresses, the alternate pail douche etc. In the employment of alternate hot and cold compresses or other applications for resolvent effects, the length of the hot and the cold applications should usually be approximately equal, about fifteen seconds each. 685

When the part under treatment is painful, the hot application should be somewhat prolonged, the times of duration being as follows: Heat, 60 seconds, cold, 15 seconds; or heat, 2 minutes, cold, 15 seconds. By this means strongly resolvent effects may be obtained, while at the same time pain is mitigated if not wholly relieved.

Alterative Effects. The multiple reflex activities set up in the body through the agency of therapeutic applications of water to the surface, may give rise to effects to which the term "alterative" has been applied; and these are quite unequaled by any other known therapeutic agent. An alterative effect may be roughly defined as an agitation, a change, a disturbance. The beneficial effects of such an application are perhaps not easily explained, but there may be something more than a rhetorical figure in the suggestion of Fonssagrives, that such an application lifts the patient out of an abnormal state by untying a bundle of pathological habits, thus giving nature, relieved of embarrassing obstacles, an opportunity to organize her resources and to 686 set in operation favorable vital processes or recuperative actions.

The alterative effects of water are obtained by the cold douche, the alternating douche, the wet-sheet pack, the full or immersion bath, sweating procedures, and in fact nearly all general applications, both hot and cold. The most effective, however, are cold applications, and especially those accompanied by strong percussion, as the horizontal douche or spray. The percussion douche and the massage douche are perhaps the most powerful of all means for producing general alterative effects.

Local alterative effects are likewise produced by circumscribed applications, such as the various forms of special douches which have been elsewhere described,— the hepatic douche, the splenic douche, etc.

The general alterative effects of water are the most efficient of all means of treating refractory cases of malarial infection, a variety of chronic neuroses, neuralgias, headaches, and neurasthenias. In fact, the alterative effects of cold water may be regarded as among the most important and fundamental means by which this agent proves serviceable in the treatment of the majority of chronic affections.

687 **Calorific Effects.** Local heating or calorific effects may be obtained by various hydric procedures, one of the most efficient being the short cold douche with strong pressure. The colder the water and the higher the pressure, the greater the calorific effect produced. If the application be greatly prolonged, the ability of the tissues to react may be exhausted, and then the effect becomes sedative instead of exciting. The aim in an application of this sort is to produce as decided thermic reaction as possible (**460**). Short cold applications produce local calorific effects.

The heating compress is an excellent measure for this purpose. The compress must be wrung very dry, out of very cold water, and should be well covered first with flannel and then with mackintosh or some other impervious material.

The heating compress managed thus not only stimulates heat production, but diminishes the local elimination of heat, and is thus very appropriately named.

Cold friction of a part, either with the hand or with the friction mitt, is an efficient means of stimulating local heat production.

Immersion of a part in cold water for a short time (15 secs. to 3 min.) is a successful calorific measure if accompanied by constant and vigorous friction.

Prolonged hot applications, as the hot bag or the fomentation, are important means not only of accumulating heat, but of stimulating local heat production. The local hot air, vapor, or electric-light bath are also invaluable means of local calorification. The special apparatus required for this purpose are described elsewhere in this work (**1250**).

In the use of the local electric-light bath for purely calorific effects, lamps with red globes or covered with red screens may be used instead of the ordinary clear-glass globe so as to exclude the chemical rays; but this is scarcely necessary, as the actinic effects of the incandescent ray is very feeble. (It may perhaps be questioned whether hot applications are not direct or primary rather than secondary excitants of thermic action. This is a matter for further study.)

Applications capable of producing local calorific effects are 688
indicated in all cases in which it is desired to quicken the functional activities of a part. Heat production is so intimately associated with all other forms of vital activity that it may be considered as a good measure of vital action in general. A subnormal temperature means vital depression, whether general or local. By increasing the calorification of a part, we at the same time increase its activities in all directions,—glandular, nervous, catalytic, etc. Calorific measures are thus applicable in all cases in which there is need of increased local activity of any kind. They are very generally useful, and form the basis of many of the most important of the various therapeutic uses of hydric procedures.

Calorific measures, both general and local, are of great service in preparing the body for cold applications. For this purpose, heat is generally preferable; but we may also employ friction with water at a temperature lower than that of the proposed application.

C. SEDATIVE EFFECTS.

689 A sedative is an agent which moderates the abnormally increased action of an organ or set of organs. There are three general classes of sedative effects which are therapeutically indicated: —

1. *Sedative of the circulatory system.*
   - *a.* Antiphlogistic
     - (*a*) Vascular.
     - (*b*) Cardiac.
   - *b.* Hemostatic.
2. *Sedative of the nervous system.*
   - *a.* Hypnotic.
   - *b.* Calmative.
   - *c.* Antispasmodic.
   - *d.* Analgesic.
   - *e.* Anesthetic.
3. *Sedative of metabolic activity.*
   - *a.* Antithermic or Antipyretic.
   - *c.* Antifebrile.

Sedative applications and effects may be either general or local. Antiphlogistic and hemostatic remedies are usually employed for local effects. The same is true of anesthetic and analgesic measures; while antithermic and antipyretic measures are necessarily general in character, owing to the nature of the indications to be met. There are, however, cases in which a general febrile state may be combated by local means applied to subdue the pathological processes to which the rise of temperature is due.

Sedative or depressant effects may be produced by precisely the same means as are employed for excitant and tonic effects, differently managed. Whether a particular application of water at a given temperature is to prove tonic or sedative, may also depend as much upon the temperament of the patient and the special conditions in which he may happen to be for the time being, as on the particular method of procedure itself. The only hydriatic procedure which is immediately, directly, and always sedative is the full or immersion bath, at 92° to 97° F.,—the neutral bath.

Sedative effects may be either immediate or remote. Remote sedative effects may often be produced by the application of excitant or tonic measures, whereby the irritation which exists,—the condition which an eminent clinical teacher has so well defined as "irritable weakness,"—is made to disappear under the tonic influence of cold applications systematically employed.

Sedative effects may be obtained— 690

1. By cold applications.

2. By warm applications; and in two ways by each class of measures.

Sedative effects may be obtained by *cold* applications:—

(*a*) By restoring nerve tone through the use of tonic applications systematically employed for the necessary length of time (remote effect); and—

(*b*) By the prolonged application of water at some temperature below 92° (immediate effect). Water at a temperature below 92° produces at first an excitant effect, through arousing the resistance of the body, the thermic reaction provoked extending to every cell and tissue of the body. If the application be short, as has been elsewhere shown, the excitant effect is dominant; but if the application is sufficiently prolonged, the reactive powers of the system are at last exhausted, and after many oscillatory attempts at reaction of gradually decreasing intensity, the ability to react is finally wholly exhausted, and a decidedly sedative effect is established.

Sedative effects from *warm* applications may be produced in two ways, as follows:—

(*a*) Short applications of hot water, which produce an excitant or stimulant effect, followed by an atonic or asthenic reaction, the reverse of the reaction produced by cold.

(*b*) By prolonged applications of water at a neutral temperature, from 92° to 97° F.

The leading sedative effects which are obtainable by water, and the most convenient methods for obtaining them are the following:—

691 **Sedatives of the Circulatory System.** The effect of cold, when directly applied to the skin, is to cause contraction of the small blood-vessels throughout the body, thereby diminishing the blood current. Cold applications of sufficient intensity may even absolutely arrest the blood stream in the small vessels. In order, however, that this effect may be obtained, it is necessary that reaction should be wholly suppressed, for in the state of reaction which follows an application of cold there is active dilatation of the small vessels, both venules and arterioles, giving rise to a greatly increased rate of flow of the blood current throughout the whole system.

For the suppression of tonic reaction, it is necessary—

1. That the cold application should be prolonged.

2. That percussion and friction should be avoided in the mode of application, since these mechanical stimuli encourage tonic reaction.

Cold causes at first a strong contraction of the blood-vessels, which is quickly followed by a dilatation of all the small vessels of the skin, continuing for a considerable time, as illustrated by the ruddy nose and cheeks of the woodchopper. On the other hand, the application of heat produces, after the first instant, strong dilatation of the small veins, which after withdrawal of the heat is followed by prolonged contraction. A prolonged application of cold and a short application of heat are alike in producing at first stimulation, later sedation. The fully developed effect of *cold* is *sedative*, while that of *heat* is *stimulant*. The subsequent, or reaction, effect of *cold* is *excitant*, or *tonic;* of *heat*, *depressant*, or *atonic*. This is true of all forms of functional activity, since all vital activity depends upon blood supply and blood pressure.

Sedative Applications Useful only when Well Borne.

Sedative baths are beneficial only when well borne. Weakness after the bath, secondary chill, headache, and nervousness are evidences of too low a temperature or too prolonged an application; or in case the hot bath has been employed, the indication is that the hot application was too intense or prolonged, or that the concluding cold application was not employed for a sufficient length of time to obliterate the exciting effects of the heat.

Water, properly employed, is superior to all other remedial agents as a sedative. Of the various classes of sedatives,—*hypnotics*, *heart sedatives*, and *pain sedatives* or *anodynes*,—those of a medicinal character are all powerful toxic agents. Bromide of potash, chloral, sulphonal, paraldehyde, and all the rest of the long list of hypnotics are each and all productive of most pernicious effects when employed for any considerable length of time, and often untoward effects follow immediately upon their use.

In a recent discussion of this subject in the *British Medical Journal*, most pronounced views against the use of medicinal hypnotics of any sort were recorded by leading English and American authorities. It was shown by indubitable evidence that all hypnotic drugs are poisons, and capable of doing great mischief if habitually used. The neutral bath at bedtime is worth more as a genuine and efficient hypnotic than all the medicinal agents known to pharmacy.

All the medicinal *heart sedatives* are toxic agents, which may produce highly untoward or even fatal effects. There is no drug sedative which can be used for any considerable length of time that will not produce injurious effects.

Water, on the other hand, may be made to produce prompt and highly sedative effects without leaving behind any damaging influence.

By cold applications the pulse rate may be reduced from 692
150 to 100 beats per minute, and the volume of blood in a part reduced 20 times.

693 **Nerve Sedative Effects.** Those measures which are sedative to the circulation, and which have been described as antiphlogistic, are without exception also sedative in their effect upon the nervous system, as the circulatory system is controlled by the vasomotor and sympathetic nerves. It is not easy, in fact, to distinguish definitely between circulatory and nerve sedatives, though for convenience we may specially designate by the latter name those measures which are particularly helpful in lessening the activity of the cerebrospinal system of nerves. Measures of this sort are usually classed as *hypnotic*, *calmative*, *antispasmodic*, *analgesic*, and *anesthetic*.

For hypnotic or general sedative effects there is no measure superior to the warm bath, which should be employed at a temperature of 92° to 97° F., and may be continued from thirty minutes to two hours. It should be taken at bedtime.

The wet-sheet pack is very similar in its effects. It should not be given very cold, but at a temperature of from 70° to 75° F. The sheet should be wrung very dry, and the patient should not be too warmly covered, in order that the tendency to perspire may be avoided.

The broken jet douche at 85° to 92° F. for three minutes, the ice-cap or cold compress to the head, the evaporating head-cap, revulsive compresses to the spine, are measures of the highest value. The alternate application to the spine may consist of compresses, hot and cold sponging, the alternate hot and cold pour, or the alternate hot and cold douche. Avoid percussion effects or shock from too strong impressions, the effect being to excite the nerves.

The moist girdle, or heating compress, applied over the abdomen and worn at night, and in some instances during the day, is also a measure of great value, and one which is much relied upon in Germany as a brain sedative for the relief of insomnia. The wet girdle, or Neptune's girdle, owes its hypnotic effects to the diversion of a large amount of blood into the portal veins, whereby the brain is relieved.

The wet-sheet pack is a very effective means of relieving sleeplessness due to nervousness or "fidgets." It is also a valuable remedy in acute mania, often quieting the patient when other measures fail, and obviating the need of drugs also in the delirium of typhoid fever, especially when the skin is hot and dry, but the temperature not excessively high.

The spinal pack (**1355**) is a valuable means of combating insomnia, when spinal irritation is a marked symptom.

Local Analgesic Effects. For local quieting effects the neutral rain douche, from 5 to 15 minutes, with little pressure, is a means of great value. In cases of locomotor ataxia, sclerosis of the spine, and in neurasthenia with marked exaggeration of the deep reflexes, the warm fan douche (92°) to the spine, from 3 to 15 minutes, will usually be found highly useful. The heating compress also proves highly serviceable in cases in which a circumscribed irritation exists without inflammatory action or active congestion, as in hyperesthesia of the lumbar ganglia of the abdominal sympathetic or of the solar plexus. 694

The pain of circumscribed acute inflammations and certain neuralgias accompanied by inflammatory conditions is frequently relieved in an almost marvelous manner by the prolonged cold compress, the ice pack, or the evaporating compress. As a rule, the cold application should be moderate in degree (60° to 70°), and continued for several hours if necessary. After the acute stage of the onset is passed, fomentations should be employed for 10 to 15 minutes at intervals of from 2 to 6 hours, and the cold compress should be exchanged for the cool compress (60°) every hour, well covered with flannel.

For chronic pains, revulsive applications (**678**) are the most generally useful. Derivative applications are useful in both acute and chronic painful conditions (**1341**).

Hot applications may be continued for hours, if necessary to control pain, in nearly all cases except those in which the pain is located in the head or the eyes. As a rule, however, it is wise to remove the hot application once an hour, applying in its place a tepid compress for a time, or, what is better in many cases, a towel wrung as dry as possible out of very cold water, for half a minute. In applications to the head and eyes the hot application should be interrupted by a short cold compress at least once every thirty minutes, and often better results are obtained by a change every ten minutes.

The pain of pleurisy is best relieved by very hot applications, as fomentations, a rubber bag filled with hot water, hot bricks, hot sand-bags, or similar means. The same means may be employed for the relief of pain in the stomach, as in colic, gastralgia, gastric crises, also in hepatic colic, renal colic, and other painful affections. For the relief of pain, the fomentations should be as hot as can be borne (140° to 160°).

In chronic cases and in deep-seated acute inflammations the heating compress renewed every half hour (60°) with fomentations for 15 min. every two to four hours is a better method than continuous heat.

Pain in the bowels, when not due to inflammation, generally yields to large fomentations; the hot enema, however, is highly useful in a large proportion of cases in which the pain is not of an inflammatory origin, as in the case of intestinal colic, enteralgia, and pain due to hyperesthesia of the abdominal ganglia, also in renal and hepatic colic.

Fomentations are also useful when the pain in the bowels or abdominal region is due to local inflammation of some sort, as enteritis, colitis, peritonitis, or other inflammatory affections of the abdominal or pelvic viscera, but should not in these cases be long continued. The temperature should be as hot as can be borne; but the application should not be continued more than 15 or 20 minutes, when the cool compress should be applied for an hour or two, after which the fomentations may be again renewed.

The hot enema is valuable in some cases in which the pain is due to inflammation, as in inflammation of the ovaries or tubes. This application may be repeated two or three times a day. The quantity of water introduced at once should not be more than one or two pints after the bowels have been emptied, as the application is designed for the lower pelvis. The water should be retained for five minutes, when it may be allowed to escape, and a fresh quantity introduced, this being repeated from 3 to 6 times. It is not necessary to remove the rectal tube. By detaching the tube from the fountain, and lowering the end, the water may be allowed to escape into a suitable vessel, as directed for the cold enema.

The patient should lie upon the back, to avoid filling the colon at a higher level than is necessary. In most cases hot irrigation by means of the author's rectal irrigator (page 902) is preferable to the enema.

The pain of hemorrhoids and rectal ulcer generally yields to fomentations applied over the inflamed region. A very hot sitz bath is also effective in cases of this sort. The water need not be more than two or three inches deep, but should be as hot as can be borne, the temperature being gradually raised, after the patient enters the bath, to 115° or 120° F. The pain of inflamed hemorrhoids is sometimes best relieved by an alternation of heat and cold. In cases in which there is great pain at stool, relief is often experienced by sitting over a pail or slop-jar half filled with boiling water while moving the bowels. The hot steam relaxes the muscles, and exercises a powerful analgesic effect upon the painful tissues.

A short, very hot sitz bath (112° to 120°) is a most excellent means of relieving chronic pelvic pain. The duration should be from 3 to 5 minutes, and it should be instantly followed by a dash of cold water upon the hips or rapid cold friction of the parts. This is a most excellent and serviceable analgesic measure, and may be advantageously employed in chronic ovarian and uterine pains, painful affections of the rectum, and chronic inflammation of the prostate.

The pain of sciatica and other forms of neuralgia is best relieved by either revulsive applications, which may consist of very hot fomentations continued for 15 or 20 minutes, followed by a well wrung, very cold compress for 30 to 60 seconds, or by cold friction. The Scotch douche is, however, probably the most effective of all means which can be employed for the relief of sciatica. The hot fan douche should be applied with moderate force at a temperature of 120° to 130° F., or as hot as can be borne, over the lower part of the back and along the track of the affected nerve. The hot application should continue for 4 or 5 minutes, being immediately followed by a very cold jet (50° to 60°), broken when the skin is sensitive, or the fan douche, continued from 6 to 10 seconds.

The prolonged leg pack following a fomentation (**1313**) is an analgesic measure of great potency and value in cases of sciatica and crural neuralgia.

The pain of congestion, as congestive headache, is best relieved by rubber bags filled with ice, or the ice compress. The application may be made not only to the head, but to the face and about the neck, with excellent effect. Indeed, ice-cold water is in all cases an excellent remedy for the relief of inflamed parts, as inflamed hemorrhoids, painful wounds, burns, etc. Cold irrigation with water at a somewhat higher temperature, 60° to 70° F., is almost equally effective, and often more convenient and agreeable.

For the pain of sprains and bruises administer very hot applications, followed by cold compresses or ice-bags. The fomentation may be renewed every two or three hours for 15 minutes, cold compresses being maintained in the interval.

For the relief of painful affections of the eye, either hot or cold applications may be employed, according to the case. In pain due to inflammation of the lids, very thin cold compresses are most efficacious, the compress being kept cold by evaporation, stimulated by fanning, either with an ordinary fan or the electric fan, or by dripping on ice-water. A very good plan is to have two sets of compresses, cooling them by laying upon a block of ice, so that a fresh cool compress is ready for immediate use when the one in contact with the tissues, having become slightly warm, is removed.

Painful affections of the eyeball are generally best relieved by very hot applications; but heavy fomentations, bags filled with hot water, and similar hot masses should never be applied to the eye. Instead, thin compresses should be employed, not more than five or six thicknesses of cheese-cloth, three or four inches square; these should be wrung out of very hot water and applied to the eye, covered, and changed every 1 to 2 minutes. The application should not be continued long without a brief cold application. A good plan is to apply heat for 3 to 5 minutes, then cold for 15 to 30 seconds. By these applications to the skin over and about the eye, a vigorous revulsive effect with collateral hyperemia of the skin is produced, and the pain thus relieved.

The analgesic effect of cold applications is well illustrated in the use of a continuous cold compress in the case of burns. On one occasion in which the author was involved in a serious railway wreck in a Mexican desert, he succeeded in bringing almost immediate relief to two badly scalded porters by wrapping their burned legs in wet sheets, which were kept cool by pouring water over them continuously. In ten minutes the poor fellows, who had been writhing and groaning in agony, were almost entirely at ease, and both secured a good night's rest.

For the relief of pain in conditions unaccompanied by inflammation, fomentations, the local hot douche, the revulsive douche, and other revulsive and derivative applications are generally most effective. Dry heat is sometimes more serviceable than moist heat. Occasionally, alternate applications are most efficient. The fomentation, followed by a heating compress to be worn overnight or for several hours, is also a means which can be highly commended in this class of cases.

695 **Anesthetic Effects.** It is unnecessary to do more than call attention to the well-known anesthetic effects of cold. When the temperature of the skin is lowered very much below normal, the sensibility of the numerous classes of nerve filaments which it contains, and especially of the sensory nerves, is diminished to a marked degree. Thus the application of ice for a few minutes will almost completely abolish sensibility in the part. By the employment of freezing mixtures of salt and ice or an ether or rhigolene spray, the skin and subjacent parts may be so benumbed as to render minor operations painless.

696 **Antispasmodic Effects.** For true antispasmodic effects we are obliged to rely wholly upon applications of such a temperature that the exciting effects of both heat and cold are avoided. The neutral full bath is precisely adapted to the indications presented in cases of hysteria, extreme nervous agitation, insomnia from restlessness, etc. The full or immersion bath should be employed at a temperature of 92° to 97°, duration from 15 minutes to an hour or more. This is a sovereign remedy for hysteria, and will usually avert a threatened attack if perseveringly employed.

The neutral fan douche, which is especially serviceable in cases of nervous agitation with insomnia, should be given at a temperature of 95° to 97°, duration 1 to 5 minutes.

The neutral fan douche and the hot bath should be employed only as an introductory or palliative measure, to be followed by tonic applications as rapidly as the patient can be trained to endure them.

Local antispasmodic effects may be obtained by the application of the neutral douche, warm (not hot) compresses, the neutral pour, and when the extremities are involved, by the neutral spinal douche, without pressure, or the spinal pour.

In constipation due to spastic contraction of the colon or the anus, and in gall-stones and renal colic, hot fomentations, the hot sitz, and the hot enema are measures which rarely fail to give satisfactory results.

Hemostatic Effects. The sedative influence of cold may be 697 employed as an efficient means of checking hemorrhage, as in the application of ice to a wound to check capillary oozing, plugging the nostrils with ice in epistaxis, the ice-cap in apoplexy, swallowing ice pills in hemorrhage from the stomach, the application of the ice pack to the loins in hemorrhage from the kidneys, the ice-bag or compress over the abdomen in case of hemorrhage from the bowels, and the application of ice-cold compresses to the vulva and perineum in uterine hemorrhage.

It must be remembered that in the use of cold for the purpose of controlling hemorrhage, great care must be exercised to prevent reaction, since this involves dilatation of the vessels, and defeats the object sought. Hence the applications must be absolutely continuous. If compresses are employed, a freshly cooled compress must be ready for instant application when the warm one is removed.

Very hot as well as very cold applications of water are effective means of controlling hemorrhage. A sponge or napkin saturated with water at a temperature of 140° to 160° F. is a most efficient means of checking capillary oozing. This means of controlling hemorrhage is very generally used in operations involving the peritoneal cavity, and is not infrequently of very great service in shortening the time required for the completion of an operation by facilitating the preparation of wounds for closing. The application of water at a temperature of from 125° to 130° F. to the interior of the uterus will almost instantaneously control uterine hemorrhage. The application must not be longer than 4 or 5 minutes, for, as shown by Runge, prolonged very hot applications produce paralysis of the uterine vessels, with stasis. Cold applications following hot often produce the best results.

Heat may also be applied to the uterine cavity by means of a hollow metal sound **(1416)**, through which a stream of hot water is allowed to flow. The author has made use in this way of water at a temperature of 160° with advantage. Cold may be applied in the same manner.

698 **Antiphlogistic Effects.** Under this head are included applications which have for their purpose to suppress or combat a local acute congestion or inflammation, such as a boil, a felon, an acutely inflamed joint, a pneumonia, a pleurisy, a peritonitis, an iritis, a phlebitis, an erythema, and also a circumscribed erysipelatous inflammation.

In the use of antiphlogistic measures, the various conditions involved in local congestion or hyperemia must be constantly kept in mind. The hyperemia may be due either to mechanical injuries or obstructions, or to vasomotor disturbances. The several conditions which should be especially noted and provided for in the arrangement of a hydriatic prescription, together with the appropriate measures for use in the conditions named, may be briefly mentioned as follows:—

1. Mechanical congestion of the viscera in cardiac insufficiency and certain forms of valvular incompetency.

2. Congestion of the organs connected with the portal system from hepatic sclerosis.

3. Hyperemia from the pressure of a tumor or other morbid growth, or mechanical obstruction, as in congestive headache due to overloaded bowels from enteroptosis or other cause.

4. Vasomotor spasm in some other portion of the body, proximate or remote, causing congestion by retrostasis.

5. An atonic or paretic state of the vaso constrictors of the affected part, as in solar erythema, erysipelas, and other inflammations.

6. Overstimulation of the vasodilators through visceral irritation or some other reflex influence, as in cerebral congestion due to digestive disturbance or to pelvic disorder.

Each of these conditions requires a careful adaptation of special hydriatic measures, either palliative or curative as may be possible in a given case. According to the indications in each of these several classes of cases the following among other means may be suggested:—

1. Improve the heart tone by a cold compress to the pericardium for half an hour three times a day. Energize the peripheral heart and dilate the surface vessels by the neutral bath with friction, the effervescent bath, cold friction, and the rubbing wet sheet.

2. Stimulate the circulation of the liver by the broken douche to the chest (60°), the alternate hepatic douche (100° to 60°), and the heating compress, and drain off a portion of the portal blood into the lower extremities by means of the warm leg bath, the heating leg pack, or the Scotch douche to the legs.

3. In this class of cases, hydrotherapy offers small assistance in a curative way, but great relief may often be secured through the use of very simple measures, such as increasing the tone of the congested parts by means of cool compresses, thus enabling them better to resist the disturbing cause. Constipation, if present, must be combated by special means.

4. Spasm of the vessels of the feet and legs, causing congestive headaches, may be relieved by the Scotch douche, the prolonged hot leg or foot bath, and the heating pack to the legs. Fomentations to the abdomen, followed by the heating abdominal compress, will remove the cause of the vascular spasm of the legs by relieving the irritation of the sympathetic ganglia in which the disturbing reflex influence originates.

5. Prolonged cold compresses (60° to 70°), alternate hot and cold applications, or very hot compresses or douches, are measures by which the vascular tone of the affected part may be raised, and the stagnated blood moved on to make room for an influx of pure blood with its supply of normal nutrient and healing properties.

In changing the hot and cold compresses, great care must be taken to avoid the slightest delay, as the occurrence of reaction between the applications will destroy the effect obtained by the cold application and cause a return of the pain and swelling. A freshly cooled compress should be ready to replace the warm one the instant it is removed, or the desired temperature may be attained by irrigation, the cold water being trickled in a small stream upon the affected part protected by a suitable compress of cheese-cloth or linen. Make changes with the greatest care, to avoid irritating the inflamed or congested surface.

6. Cold to the congested part by means of the frequently renewed cool compress or the evaporating compress, while at the same time soothing applications are made to the affected ganglia by the abdominal fomentation, the heating compress, or a wet girdle; the prolonged neutral bath; derivative applications to the feet and legs, such as the leg pack, the Scotch douche, and the prolonged leg or foot bath at 104° to 110°, are measures applicable in this class of cases.

In the application of cold for antiphlogistic effects, it is, as above stated, of the highest importance to avoid percussion and friction, and to make the applications continuous until the desired effect is obtained. Compresses saturated with cold water, rubber bags filled with ice or iced water, cold immersion, and the evaporating compress are the chief and most convenient methods for producing antiphlogistic effects by means of cold.

It must be always borne in mind that if a cold application becomes warmed by contact with the skin, it is because reaction has occurred, and to the extent to which there has been reaction, the antiphlogistic effect has been neutralized. Thus care should be taken to renew the cold compress as soon as it begins to approach the temperature of the skin. A large, thick, well-saturated compress may retain its efficiency for five minutes, or even a little longer; while a compress of two or three thicknesses of cotton or linen cloth will need to be renewed every minute.

In the use of the ice-bag or the ice-compress, a piece of rather thick, well-saturated woolen cloth should generally be placed next the body to avoid excessive chilling of the skin. If this precaution is omitted, great care must be exercised to prevent injury, and the application must be removed for a few minutes every half hour, so that partial reaction may be allowed to occur, thus maintaining the vitality of the part.

In cases in which there are acute inflammatory conditions involving the hands and feet, the proximal compress may be used to good advantage.

This compress has the advantage over direct applications to the part affected, in that it avoids irritation of the part. In the use of the proximal compress, cool applications should be made to the inflamed part, and cold or very cold applications applied between the part and the heart. For example, in applications to control inflammation in the hand, the arm should be wrapped in cloths wrung out of very cold water, while cool water is applied to the hand. Both applications should be made continuous by allowing a stream of water of the proper temperature to trickle upon the parts, or by frequently drenching the parts with water at the right temperature. The compress upon the hand may be kept cool by evaporation, if not too thick. No more than four to six thicknesses of cheese-cloth should be employed. These should be moistened as often as necessary, and should never be allowed to become dry. An ice poultice may be applied to the arm, or wet cloths may be laid next the skin, and the ice-bags laid over these. The ice-collar or ice-bag applied over the carotid in this manner is a most excellent method of reducing cerebral hyperemia. In cases of cerebral meningitis, the ice-collar may be used in conjunction with cold applications to the head.

In the case of organs lying within the trunk, as the kidneys, liver, and other viscera, a different principle must be employed. By the warm bath (92° to 98°), dilatation of the surface vessels with contraction of the internal vessels may be produced. This should be followed by an application of water at 60° to the affected part. If a very cold application is made, it must be removed at short intervals, particularly in the treatment of visceral inflammation, so that there may be opportunity for full reaction and complete dilatation of the surface vessels in reflex relation with the interior. When this occurs, there is doubtless a reactionary contraction of the dilated vessels of the inflamed viscus; whereas, when a very cold application is continuous, the cutaneous nerves are benumbed, the reflex stimulation ceases, and the result is passive dilatation. For best effects apply compresses at 60° and change every 10 to 40 minutes, or when warm.

Revulsive measures may be brought into service in conjunction with other means by making cold applications to the reflex cutaneous area connected with the affected part. Cold to the feet causes contraction of the vessels of the brain, with lowering of the temperature of the mouth and of the axilla. The cold running hand-bath causes contraction of the vessels of the chest; cold to the lumbar region causes contraction of the uterine vessels, as do also cold applications to the buttocks, the perineum, the vulva, the hypogastrium, the inner portion of the thighs, and the soles of the feet.

For derivative effects in relieving congestion of a hyperemic part, the vessels of a large area in some remote part of the body are dilated by suitable hydriatic procedures, and thus the blood is drawn off from the congested part. It should always, when possible, be ascertained whether anemia does not exist in some part as the result of a disturbed distribution of blood; if so, the application should be made in such a way as to influence this anemic part, restoring to it its normal blood supply. For example, congestion of the brain is commonly connected with coldness of the hands and feet through excessive contraction of the vessels of these parts. The circulation should be restored by short cold applications followed by vigorous rubbing, the Scotch douche or hot baths, the partial vapor bath, the hot-air bath or the electric-light bath, dry friction, or the hot-blanket pack, followed by vigorous friction.

Lowering the temperature of the blood helps to diminish

congestion by influencing favorably the central nervous system and the heart. General or local refrigerating measures may be used for this purpose, as the cool enema, the cooling bath, the wet-sheet pack, the half pack, the cold precordial compress.

The mesenteric circulation is a blood reservoir which may frequently be used as a means of regulating the blood supply. The almost instant relief from headache which is sometimes experienced from taking food is due to dilatation of the mesenteric vessels under the stimulation of the food. The mesenteric circulation may be stimulated by massage, especially by hacking movements, by short applications to the abdomen or trunk, and by the enema. A very short cold enema results in reaction in the portal circulation and filling of these vessels. The large enema of water (100° to 104°), retained for a few minutes, produces dilatation of the portal vessels.

By bringing these various measures to bear in concert, most powerful effects may be produced, as, for example, in a case of cerebral hyperemia, a bath of 92° for a half hour to an hour may be administered, care being taken by gentle rubbing to keep the surface vessels well dilated, so as to avoid the slightest tendency to chilliness, which produces excitation of the central nervous system. This will reduce the temperature. The same may be accomplished by the wet-sheet pack of 30 minutes' duration or continued to the end of the neutral stage. Either of these procedures should be followed by a Scotch douche to the feet and legs, the patient afterward being put to bed with the heating abdominal bandage, and an evaporating compress to the head. The whole may be preceded by an enema of a pint and a half to two pints of water at 70°. The evaporating or cool compress should be applied to the head during the neutral bath, to insure lowering of the cerebral temperature.

Application of cold should be confined to the early stages of inflammation. Passive hyperemia, which appears after the most acute stage of the inflammatory process, favors exudate and morbid changes in the structure and functions of the parts. A good supply of healthy blood is the best means of antagonizing this condition and bringing the part to a normal state. The blood is a sort of traveling physician, which, moving from part to part, repairs injuries by the same marvelous methods by which it builds up and maintains the body in health,— through normal nutritive processes. Recovery from diseased conditions is effected by means of the cell and tissue activities by which the ordinary functions of the body are maintained.

The cure for inflammation after the first stage is passed is accomplished by improving the circulation; hence continuous cold application should cease after the first stage, which in erysipelas and pneumonia never includes more than the first day or two, and in some cases but a few hours. Hot applications should be made once in two or three hours, with simply cool or tepid applications during the intervals to maintain active fluxion through the affected part. It is necessary to study each case carefully to know just when to cease the employment of antiphlogistic measures, and to introduce those calculated to induce active congestion or fluxion. After the first onset of the disease is passed, the heating compress may be applied. At first, change every hour; later, every three or four hours, increasing the intervals from day to day. Thus employed, the heating compress, by aiding the circulation in the diseased part, may aid in bringing the morbid process to a favorable termination without suppuration. The cotton poultice similarly employed still later may aid in establishing resolution. These measures are very valuable in the treatment of pleurisy, either with or without affusion, and in lobar- and broncho-pneumonia, greatly aiding the absorption of morbid products and in restoring normal conditions.

By the repetition of a cold application as soon as reaction begins, a new contraction of the small blood-vessels of the parts and of the internal associated area is produced. For this reason a frequently renewed cool or cold application may sometimes produce better effects than continuous cold in the hydriatic management of deeply seated congestions or inflammations.

In the use of cold, care must be taken to avoid producing a harmful collateral hyperemia in cases of deeply seated inflammation by prolonged cold application to the surface (672).

To obtain the atonic antiphlogistic effects of heat (642), fomentations, the cotton poultice, the hot-water bag, hot irrigation, and hot immersion are the chief measures. The neutral pour or irrigation and neutral immersion are also highly useful. Fonssagrives maintains that the relief obtained by warm or emollient applications in acute congestions and inflammations may be in part attributed to dilution of the blood by absorption of the fluid from the moist mass in contact with the skin, producing a local hydremia, whereby the blood is rendered less stimulating to the irritated tissues. This idea, expressed more than a dozen years ago, seems to be sustained by our present notions respecting the part played by toxins of bacterial origin in provoking and maintaining local congestive and inflammatory processes. The dilution and hastened removal of these poisons must certainly tend to lessen the intensity of the morbid changes set up by them, and to aid the tissues in their efforts to combat the disturbing elements present, whatever they may be.

Recent observations have developed the interesting fact that nervous irritability is notably lessened when a nerve is made to take up a quantity of water. This may be the true explanation of the relief always afforded by warm compresses, the neutral bath, and many other sedative hydriatic procedures.

It seems reasonable, also, that dilution of the blood may serve to lessen the activity of morbid processes in a congested or inflamed part, by diminishing the proportion of blood cells present and diluting the blood serum.

The employment of the hot foot bath for the relief and

prevention of congestion and inflammation in sprains of the ankle and other joints affords an excellent illustration of the antiphlogistic effect of hot applications.

Prolonged immersion (for several weeks if necessary) of a part in water at a temperature of from 95° to 97° F. is a most effective means of preventing inflammation in cases of badly contused and lacerated wounds. Dr. Frank Hamilton, of Bellevue Hospital, New York, when the author was a student in that institution twenty-five years ago, made large use of the neutral immersion bath in the treatment of injuries resulting from street railway accidents, and demonstrated the value of this method by saving a large number of badly bruised limbs which his colleagues had condemned to amputation.

This is also a most excellent method of preventing inflammation and other complications in case of severe burns. Some seventeen years ago the author, while visiting the great Hospital for Skin Diseases at Vienna, learned of a patient who had suffered from a severe burn, and who had been kept immersed in a full bath for a number of months. He ultimately made a good recovery from an injury which, without the advantage of this measure, would probably have proved fatal.

699 **General Antiphlogistic Effects.** For general antiphlogistic effects, that is, for subduing a condition commonly known as feverishness, but without actual rise of temperature, the neutral bath at 92° to 95° for 20 minutes to an hour or more has been found a sovereign remedy. The excessive action of the heart is controlled, the bounding, feverish pulse becomes soft and returns to the normal rate, the flushed face acquires its normal hue, and the patient finds complete relief.

Care should be taken to avoid friction in the bath or after it (**1130**), and the patient should also avoid exercise soon after the bath. Immediately on removal from the bath, the patient should be wrapped in a Turkish sheet and woolen blanket, and dried by allowing the moisture upon the surface to be absorbed by the sheet, without any friction whatever. He should remain quiet for some hours after the bath, in order that the tendency to reaction may be suppressed.

Tepid sponging and the evaporating compress are antiphlogistic measures of value in feverish states, whether of inflammatory or non-inflammatory origin.

Use of Cold in Pneumonia, Pleurisy, and Other Acute Disorders.

In cases of acute inflammation accompanied 700
by exudate, as in pneumonia the frequently renewed heating compress (1284, 1318) should be employed during the early stages of the disease; but after the acute inflammatory stage is passed, the cold application should be exchanged for intermittent hot applications. Fomentations and equivalent measures may be applied regularly every two or three hours, the heating compress being employed in the interval.

In the transition stage between the first and second periods of the disease, the cold applications may be interrupted every two or three hours by hot applications for 10 or 15 minutes. This method the author has found eminently successful in the treatment of pneumonia, erysipelas, acute arthritis, and similar conditions. Care must be observed, however, in making continuous cold applications at very low temperatures, not to destroy the vitality of the tissues by complete interruption of the circulation. To avoid this, the applications, if the temperature employed is below 50°, should be removed every hour or two for a short time, so as to allow partial reaction for restoration of the circulation.

After the very first onset of an acute inflammatory affection; that is, after the first twelve or twenty-four hours, hot applications may be made for 3 or 4 minutes with advantage every two or three hours. The application of heat in such cases must be short, and the temperature as high as can be borne.

Of sedative measures especially applicable to particular regions of the body, the most useful are the following:—

701 *Applications for the relief of cerebral congestion,*—cold to the back of the head and about the neck; cold compress to the scalp and face; evaporating compress to the head and face; heat to the upper spine; cold to the face and top of head; the short cold douche to the hands, arms, feet, and legs; leg or hip bath at 105° to 110° for 3 or 4 minutes, followed by a cold douche for 15 or 20 seconds; heating pack to the trunk; heating half-pack to legs and hips; heating wet-sheet pack at 70°, followed by wet rubbing sheet, cold pour to the head or back of neck, 1 or 2 minutes, at 60° to 70°.

To diminish cardiac activity and blood pressure, ice-bag over the heart continuously. The heart's action may also be lessened by cold water drinking, the water being sipped slowly.

702 *Congestion of the stomach,* as in hyperpepsia and chronic gastritis, is best relieved by the prolonged hot douche over the stomach and the spine opposite, or by the revulsive circle douche or revulsive compresses.

As a general sedative measure, applicable to almost all classes of cases and all parts of the body, there is no better procedure than the cool compress, consisting of a folded linen towel or a half dozen thicknesses of cheese-cloth saturated with water at a temperature of 60° to 70° F. This compress should be changed about once in twenty to thirty minutes when much heat is present, or once an hour when the morbid process is less active. The effect of an application of this sort is to cause a maintained contraction of the vessels of the skin surface with which it is in contact, and of the corresponding internal visceral area. When applied to the chest, it causes contraction of the pulmonary vessels; applied to the abdomen, the mesenteric vessels are contracted; applied to the lower abdomen, upper thighs, perineum, and external genital organs, the pelvic viscera are de-congested; applied to the head and neck continuously, cerebral congestion is relieved; while application to the spine contracts the vessels of the cord; application to a congested or inflamed part affords relief from pain, and controls inflammatory processes in a wonderful manner. The cool or cold compress applied over the heart is a heart sedative of inestimable value.

Ice-cold or very cold applications provoke powerful reaction effects, dilating the vessels; but cold and cool applications induce a sustained contraction.

Antithermic Effects. When a procedure is such as to abstract heat, 703
it is *antithermic*. When it not only abstracts heat but lessens heat production, it is *antipyretic*. The effects of antithermic applications are often defeated by imperfect methods. A passive cold application, as a cold immersion bath, stimulates heat production to a greater extent than heat elimination, so that the temperature after the bath may be higher than before. Many persons have for this reason been led to renounce water treatment altogether, not understanding that the lack of success was due to the faulty method rather than to failure of the hydriatic principle.

In combating fever, the principal point to be borne in mind is so to manage the antithermic measures employed as to avoid the thermic reflex; that is, the automatic increase of heat production. The method of accomplishing this was pointed out by Winternitz more than twenty years ago, but has been too little appreciated, unfortunately, by those who have undertaken to use water in fevers. The method is simple: it consists in maintaining dilatation of the cutaneous vessels and active movement of blood through the periphery by means of friction. Thus accumulation of blood in the muscles and the thermic reflex set up by cooling of the nerves in the skin, which cause increased heat production, are prevented.

Whatever measure is employed it should be long enough in duration to produce a decided effect upon the patient's temperature. A single wet-sheet pack, for example, would certainly increase heat production, and elevation of temperature (**719**). A short cold bath has the same effect.

Winternitz has shown that the wet-sheet pack, continued for 30 minutes, the sheet being renewed every 5 to 8 minutes, reduces temperature more effectively than any other procedure. For example, in a test case, during the second week the average results obtained for the half-bath were .87°; for the wet-sheet pack, 1.21°; for the half-bath, followed by the trunk compress, .73°. At the end of five hours after the half-bath the patient's temperature was .4° *above* the original temperature, while after the wet pack and the half-bath, followed by cold compresses, the temperature was still *below* the original. During the fourth week the same results were obtained. The wet-sheet pack produced a much more decided and durable reduction of temperature than the half-bath alone or the half-bath accompanied by the trunk compress.

Next to the pack, the best measure is the graduated or the Brand bath, followed by the abdominal or trunk compress changed every half hour. By means of the trunk compress the refrigerating effect of the half-bath is prolonged. It is not sufficient to abstract heat at intervals in febrile cases. We must constantly maintain heat discharge by maintaining dilatation of the surface vessels. In combating fever, care should be taken to keep the temperature down during the whole course of the disease. Every threatened exascerbation of the temperature should be met with prompt measures. When neglected, the fever acquires a sort of momentum, so to speak, which greatly increases the difficulty of controlling it. The gastric secretion ceases when the temperature is very high, and the gastric juice loses its power to act upon albuminous substances during the existence of high fever (Winternitz). When the temperature is very high, the action of the salivary glands is also suppressed; the mouth is hot, dry, and parched; the lips and tongue are covered with dried secretion, while with the lower temperature which may be maintained by proper hydriatic procedures, the mouth is moist, the stomach continues to secrete an active gastric juice, thus changing the whole aspect of the case.

The antithermic or refrigerant effects of water are among the most important and valuable therapeutic uses to which this agent can be put. It has been recognized from the earliest ages, certainly since the time of Hippocrates, that the application of water at a temperature below that of the body is a most perfect means of antagonizing the elevation of temperature which occurs in connection with fevers of all classes.

From the time the value of water as an antipyretic was brought to the notice of the profession by Currie and Jackson in the latter part of the last century, up to the present time, no one has undertaken to deny that the death-rate has been uniformly lessened to a very marked degree whenever hydriatic measures have been systematically and intelligently used for reducing febrile activity, from whatever cause. A long list of eminent physicians, both English and Continental, as well as American, have given their adherence unreservedly to the use of water as the most valuable means known for this purpose.

In the treatment of a long series of cases of typhoid fever by the cold bath in the New York Hospital, the mortality was reduced to 7.5 per cent. The rate of mortality in over thirteen hundred cases previously treated by the usual method was from twenty to thirty per cent.

The author and his colleagues of the Battle Creek Sanitarium are able to report over two hundred cases of typhoid fever treated by these methods with a mortality of less than four per cent. In one series of thirty-six successive cases, all the patients recovered, although in several instances the symptoms were very grave, owing to delay in beginning treatment. The measures chiefly relied upon were water-drinking, the enema, and the cooling pack. No medicinal antipyretics were employed.

J. C. Wilson, a few years ago, reported sixty-four cases of typhoid fever treated in the German hospital, Philadelphia, Pa., without a single death. In one hundred and eight cases of pneumonia reported by Fenwick, in which the treatment was entirely by cold applications, the mortality was only ten per cent.; while in another series of nine hundred cases in which the ordinary methods were employed, the mortality was twenty per cent.

Any of the various applications of water, used at a temperature lower than that of the body, may be utilized for combating a tendency to excessive heat production.

A few general principles should be borne in mind in the application of water for the reduction of temperature:—

1. *The greater the difference in the temperature of the body and that of the water, the more decided the effect, other things being equal.*

2. *The application, to be of permanent value, must be prolonged.* The length of the application may vary from ten or fifteen minutes to half an hour or even longer, according to the nature of the application. The average time of a cold bath for lowering the temperature, as in typhoid fever, is about twenty minutes. The time, of course, must be made to depend upon the condition of the patient, the degree of the elevation of his temperature above normal, and the temperature of the bath. The tepid (88° F.) bath may be prolonged to the extent of from one to several hours, if necessary.

3. *All forms of the bath which are accompanied by percussion effects must be avoided,* as must also friction after the patient is removed from the bath, unless there should be very pronounced shivering or other symptoms indicating the need of assistance to produce sufficient reaction to insure the viscera against injury from prolonged congestion.

4. *Friction should always be employed while the patient is in the cold bath,* as by this means the circulatory reaction is promoted, and, while the lowering of the body temperature is encouraged, shivering is prevented, and thus increased heat production is avoided. Winternitz has shown that friction in the cold bath increases the rate of heat elimination more than thirty per cent.

Antipyretic Effects.

The antipyretic effects of cold water are 704
obtained by the systematic employment of antithermic measures. There has within the last few years been a very strong reaction against the use of antipyretic drugs, and in favor of this truly physiological and rational remedy, and at the present time no respectable medical authority disputes the extreme value of water as an antipyretic measure. Modern observations have demonstrated that the danger from elevation of temperature is not so great as was formerly supposed, that in fact the rise in the body temperature accompanying febrile activity is really a part of the remedial effort put forth by the system in combating the morbid process to which the rise of temperature is due; and it has been clearly shown by Winternitz, and by many others, that the mere lowering of the body temperature by means of antipyretic drugs is not only not in any way beneficial to the patient, but, on the contrary, is decidedly detrimental, since the system is thus compelled to struggle not only with the toxins which are produced in connection with the special morbid processes present, but with the toxic drug introduced with therapeutic intent.

In visiting the fever ward of a large city hospital some years ago, the author was particularly struck by the fact that patients whose temperature was normal as the result of the administration of large doses of antipyrin, had the expression of persons in a state of collapse or extreme shock, the evident result of the combined influence of the bacterial toxins and the toxic effect of the antipyretic drug.[30]

In the reduction of temperature by means of hydriatic measures, not only is no toxic substance introduced into the body, but the cold applications, which lessen to some degree the pathological thermogenic processes which are in operation, at the same time act as a true tonic to the reparative forces of the body, and stimulate the elimination of the toxic substances to which the special symptoms characteristic of the disease are due.

Effects of Cold on the Heart in Typhoid Fever. Indeed, as the result of the antipyretic application of water, the heart's action is improved, the vital resistance of the patient is strengthened, the eliminative action of both the skin and the kidneys is encouraged, and all the graver symptoms of the disease are mitigated, often to such a degree that the disease is scarcely recognizable from the symptoms as set forth in the text-books, which frequently describe not natural diseases, but maladies aggravated by artificial and irrational therapeutics.

705 **Antipyretic Effects of Hot Applications.** From the practice and the teachings of most hydrotherapeutists, it would appear that antipyretic hydriatic means consist wholly in applications of *cold* water. It is probable that in the first attempts to combat febrile conditions by means of baths, cold water was exclusively employed; but modern laboratory researches and clinical experience have demonstrated the fact that hot water as well as water at a temperature below that of the body, may be employed in such a manner as to secure a considerable reduction of temperature in febrile states. Short, very hot applications stimulate the surface circulation, and thus aid heat elimination, while lessening heat production. By a judicious combination of very hot and cool or cold applications, the most energetic antipyretic effects may be produced.

It should be noted that in the febrile state the thermogenetic and thermotaxic mechanisms of the body are always profoundly disturbed, and in such a manner that they are influenced by causes which may have no effect whatever upon the body temperature in the non-febrile state. A rise of a few degrees in the temperature of the air of the sick-room, sitting up in bed, talking with a friend, reading, taking a slight excess of food,—these and other similar causes are sufficient to occasion a considerable rise of temperature in a febrile patient, and sometimes even to give rise to a relapse in a patient recently become convalescent.

Likewise, hydric applications which are not capable of

producing a marked lowering of temperature in a well person may have a decided effect in the febrile state.

Relation of Heat Production and Heat Elimination to Antipyretic Methods.

A general rise of the body temperature may 706
result (*a*) from increased heat production, (*b*) from diminished heat elimination, or (*c*) both increased heat production and diminished heat elimination may be present, or still other disturbances of the thermogenic or thermotaxic functions may exist (**227**).

In the majority of cases there are, in fact, both increased heat production and increased heat elimination, the rise of temperature being due to the fact that the heat production is greater than the heat elimination. In many cases, as shown by Rosenthal, Botkin, Leyden, and Winternitz, the rise of temperature is due to diminished heat elimination alone.

There is always a disturbance of the thermotaxic, or heat-regulating, function in fever. It is important in any given case to ascertain as nearly as possible the conditions present; and before making a hydriatic application of any sort, it should be determined, if possible, whether the rise of temperature in the case is chiefly due to increased heat production or to diminished heat elimination. The neglect to do this is responsible for many failures in the use of hydriatic measures in fever.

The temperature in fever may be reduced either by diminishing heat production or increasing heat elimination, or by both means combined, and by hydric applications either or both of these processes may be influenced.

Conditions are sometimes present in which there is a great increase in both heat production and heat elimination, and in which it is apparent that nature is doing all that can be done to combat the rise of temperature; therefore, interference on the part of the physician would be not only unnecessary, but possibly injurious. This is practically true in cases of fever in which there is profuse perspiration. In such a case, neither hot nor cold applications are needed for temperature control. It is only necessary that the perspiration should be gently removed every few minutes by means of a soft linen cloth. By keeping the surface free from sensible perspiration or visible moisture, evaporation will be greatly promoted, and thus a cooling effect be produced. To apply a cold wet-sheet pack, a cold bath, a cold sponge bath, or in fact any other measure than the simple means mentioned, in such a case, would be to run great risk of inflicting serious, and possibly irreparable, damage.

707 **Heat Elimination by Evaporation from the Skin.** An enormous amount of heat is absorbed by the evaporation of water from the surface, the ordinary amount being about one to one and one-half ounces per hour. Suppose this to be increased to sixteen ounces per hour, as might possibly be the case; if the perspiration were completely evaporated, the result would be the removal by evaporation alone of nearly one thousand heat units. In case of a patient weighing 160 pounds, this would be equivalent to a fall of six degrees in temperature. The normal rate of heat production is about 1.8 calories, or 7.2 pounds Fahrenheit heat units, per minute, or 432 heat units per hour. If heat production were doubled, the total for the hour would be 864 heat units. Subtracting (1000—864), we have 136. Dividing by 160, we have .85. Hence there would be an actual reduction of temperature to the amount of nearly one degree.

Of course the rate of heat production may be more than doubled, and such profuse sweating can not always be induced; but when present, it must not be interfered with. When not present, we see how much may be accomplished by applying to the skin the moisture that nature fails to supply. It has been shown that in fever there is retention of water by the tissues, and that by friction the loss of water may be increased more than fifty per cent (Weyrich). Hence the value of this measure when the skin is cool and dry.

It should be remembered that cold applications, while aiding heat elimination in some ways, in other ways diminish it, as by lessening the conducting power of the skin, by decreasing the blood supply, and by checking perspiration. It is consequently evident that to give a general cold bath in a case in which the surface is pale, cold, and dry,—in other words, when there is a decided diminution in heat elimination,—would be ill-advised, and likely to do harm. Indeed, the persistent application of such a measure in a case of that kind might induce a fatal result.

It is true that in persons possessed of considerable vitality, a very cold bath might awaken such vigorous resistance on the part of the system as to produce reaction to the surface, thus increasing the heat elimination, and so restoring the heat-eliminating power of the skin. Indeed, it is more than probable that this result might occur in quite a large proportion of cases; so that the danger from the application of cold water in a manner theoretically wrong would not always be so great as might at first seem; nevertheless, it is far better to recognize the exact condition present, and to select the most appropriate measures for meeting existing indications. The physician who depends upon the reserve forces of the body and the versatile powers of nature to avert the consequences of his blundering methods in the therapeutic uses of water, can hardly be regarded as a scientific hydriatrist.

Indications of a Condition of Increased Heat Production.

In cases presenting an abnormally high temperature, the following symptoms may be regarded as indicating that the elevation of temperature is the result of *increased* heat production:— 708

1. A flushed face, with full pulse.
2. A warm, moist skin.
3. A hot, dry skin.

Symptoms Indicating Decreased Heat Elimination.

The following symptoms accompanying an elevation of temperature may be regarded as indicating that the rise in temperature is, at the moment at least, associated with decreased heat elimination:— 709

1. Cold, dry skin.
2. Cold, moist skin.
3. Goose-flesh appearance.
4. Blueness of the skin.
5. Chilly sensations.
6. Shivering.

Both heat production and heat elimination are often increased in fever, but heat production more than heat elimination. When heat production and heat elimination are equally increased or equally diminished, no change in temperature occurs. Winternitz has shown, however, that the deviations from the normal in febrile states may be almost wholly accounted for by disturbance of heat elimination.

Increase of both heat production and heat elimination, but with excessive increase of heat production, is a condition present in sthenic fevers and inflammations. In this condition the skin may be either flushed, hot, and dry, or warm and moist. A similar condition is found when an elevation of temperature results from violent exercise.

A condition of increased heat production, associated with normal or diminished heat elimination, exists in cases of fever in which the skin is cool and dry.

In the febrile condition resulting from sunstroke (thermal fever), the rise in temperature is in part, at least, due to the diminished heat elimination. A similar rise of temperature occurs in the Turkish bath and other sweating procedures before perspiration begins. The decrease of heat elimination is due to spasm of the small vessels of the skin, a condition which is best combated by cold friction or by a short hot application, as a hot affusion, for example, followed by cold friction.

When elevation of temperature occurs without increase of heat production, there must be an accompanying diminution of heat elimination. This condition sometimes exists in connection with an ordinary cold.

Exposure to an overheated atmosphere, as during a

prolonged period of hot weather, is often productive of a vast number of cases of febrile disease, especially in infants.

When a person is in a hot bath or a dry pack, although the rate of heat production may remain normal, there will be diminished heat elimination and rise of temperature.

An elevation of temperature may occur while both heat production and heat elimination are diminished, in case the heat elimination is diminished to a greater extent than heat production. This condition is often found in fever cases in which the patient is bordering on collapse, with a cold, pale, dry, or moist skin, and when present, calls for the immediate employment of vigorous measures, before the symptoms of collapse shall have reached so serious a stage as to render recovery impossible.

Principles that Govern the Application of Hydriatic Measures for the Reduction of Temperature in Fevers.

1. A general cold application increases both 710
heat production and heat elimination. Which of these effects is dominant depends upon the duration and intensity of the bath.

2. A general cold application, if very brief, causes no perceptible loss of heat, and may occasion, by thermic reaction, a slight temporary rise of temperature.

3. A prolonged cold application lowers the temperature by increasing heat elimination, and also finally by diminishing heat production, through the general sedative effect upon the nervous system and the cooling of the thermogenic tissues in the muscles.

4. The prolonged tepid bath lowers the temperature, by increasing heat elimination without increasing heat production.

5. The appearance of chill and shivering marks the beginning of the lowering of the body temperature, and diminished elimination accompanies it as a conservative measure, while increased heat production begins.

6. Coldness and dryness of the skin, goose-flesh appearance, chilliness, blueness of the surface, are indications for

the use of measures to increase heat elimination; that is, means to encourage the cutaneous circulation.

7. A short general hot application ($\frac{1}{2}$ to 2 min.) diminishes heat production by its reflex effect upon the heat centers, and increases heat elimination by increasing the skin circulation and the production and evaporation of perspiration.

8. A long hot bath raises the temperature by heating the body and increasing heat production.

9. In general, tonic thermic reaction should be, so far as possible, suppressed in fever cases by avoiding short cold applications and measures involving mechanical effects, such as the douche.

10. Gentle friction during a cold bath increases heat elimination by stimulating the surface circulation, and controls heat production by maintaining the skin temperature and thus preventing shivering.

Laschkiewitsch showed that death after varnishing is due to excessive cooling from paralytic dilatation of the cutaneous vessels.

The notion that hydrotherapy is chiefly useful in fevers as a means of lowering the temperature is based upon a very superficial knowledge of the rationale of this marvelous therapeutic agent. Winternitz wrote nearly twenty years ago:—

"The hydriatic antipyretic method consists in an antithermal procedure, together with applications which act upon the nervous system and the circulation in a manner analogous to nerve tonics and sedatives, and in tonic-raising features which influence nutrition in a favorable manner as well as in local measures, or reducing hyperemia and congestion, whereby morbid processes may be controlled."

In view of this important fact, which is still quite too rarely recognized, it is evident that a routine practice, even in the treatment of fevers, is quite impossible. The procedure must be carefully chosen, and adapted to the needs of the individual case. In certain cases of fever, thermic reaction must be wholly suppressed, or as nearly so as possible; in others a moderate amount of thermic reaction will prove beneficial. In threatened collapse, thermic reaction must be encouraged.

Methods that May be Efficiently Employed in the Various Morbid Conditions Accompanied by a Rise in Temperature.

Of the various measures which may be em- 711
ployed for the reduction of temperature, the following may be mentioned as having been tested in actual clinical experience, not only by the author, but by numerous able clinicians. All have been found useful and efficient, some being best adapted to one particular set of circumstances, others to other conditions, but each having its particular utility; for rational hydrotherapy gives no countenance to routine methods, and recognizes no panacea:—

1. *The Cold or Tepid Affusion.*—This method, first employed by Hippocrates, and in recent times revived by Currie and Jackson, is efficient in lowering temperature. The mortality rate in scarlet and typhoid fevers is reduced by its use from thirty or forty per cent. to almost nothing. The patient simply sits in a large tub, while several pails of water at the ordinary temperature, or about 70° F., are poured over him, this procedure being repeated as often as the temperature reaches 102° F.

Currie observed that the warm affusion (87° to 97° F.) is more effective in reducing temperature than the cold, offering in proof the following excellent reasons, which are certainly highly creditable to the sagacity and medical knowledge of this pioneer of rational hydrotherapy, considering the fact that his observations were made more than a hundred years ago:—

"I find that, in many cases at least, the heat of the living body is lowered as speedily by the affusion of tepid water as by the affusion of water that is cold. If I mistake not, in some cases the heat is lowered more speedily by the tepid water."

The principal reason for the greater effect of the tepid bath in lowering the temperature, Currie finds in the fact that it is "little if at all stimulating, and does not, like the cold affusion, arouse the system to those actions by which heat is evolved and the effects of external cold are produced. If the object is to diminish the heat, this may be obtained with great certainty by the repeated use of tepid affusions."

He further makes the following very wise observation: "I have accordingly employed the tepid affusion very generally in those feverish affections where the morbid actions are weakly associated, depending rather on the stimulus of preternatural heat than upon contagion, miasmata. . . . It is also applicable to every case of fever in which the cold affusion is recommended." *

Currie also used the "cool bath" (75° to 85°), but employed it most in chronic diseases. He preferred, however, the cold bath in contagious and infectious fevers, evidently for the reason that baths of this temperature are the most effective in arousing the vital forces of the body to resist and antagonize disease.

712 2. *The Cold Immersion Bath* (1112).—This bath was first systematically employed by Brand, who by its means reduced the mortality from typhoid fever more than two thirds. The method of Brand requires that the patient be placed every three hours, day and night, in a bath at 68° F. for fifteen minutes. Brand requires the administration of the bath whenever the rectal temperature of the patient reaches 102° F. At the beginning of the bath, he directs that an affusion of water at 59° F. should be slowly poured upon the back of the patient's neck for two minutes, and that the patient should drink freely of water during the bath.

After the bath, the patient is placed in a sheet in which he is wrapped and carefully dried, but without rubbing the abdomen. The patient is only slightly covered after drying,

* "Medical Reports on the Effects of Water, Cold and Warm," by James Currie, Vol. I, pp. 64, 65.

and may continue to shiver slightly for some time after the bath, as an indication of the actual lowering of the body temperature occasioned by the bath. Twenty minutes after the bath the temperature is taken and recorded.

The amount of reduction of the temperature by the cold bath may be from half a degree to three or four degrees, seldom more than one or two degrees, and not infrequently there is a slight rise immediately after the bath. This is especially true at the beginning of a fever. Later the effect is greater.

Therapeutic Substitutes for Alcohol. The question of the use of alcohol in connection with the cold bath is one which is deserving of more than mere passing mention. Most German and some American authorities who recommend the use of cold water insist that just before putting the patient into the cold bath, at least in febrile cases, alcohol should be administered. The idea upon which this practice is based is evidently the supposition that alcohol is a stimulant, at least that it in some way sustains the heart or the vital powers. But this theory was long ago rendered thoroughly untenable by a multitude of carefully conducted experiments upon healthy subjects, showing that alcohol is always and in all doses a narcotic, and not a stimulant; that it depresses, and does not excite the heart and other vital organs; that it lessens vital resistance to disease; and that it is a toxic agent which the body must cast out, and not a food to be assimilated, nor a source of energy or aid to any vital organ or function.

The relation of alcohol to the heart and the circulation is a matter of most profound importance in the class of cases in which the cold bath is most frequently employed. In relation to this point the fact should be recalled that the heart is not the only force involved in the circulation of the blood. It is doubtless the great engine of the circulation, but it has been clearly shown by Schiff and numerous other physiologists that the movement of the blood is greatly aided by a rhythmic action of the small vessels, both arterioles and capillaries. These contractions are not simultaneous with those of the heart, hence do not interfere with its action; but as the pressure in the veins is very much below that of the arteries, these contractile movements serve most efficiently in pushing the blood along toward the veins. The heart keeps the large arteries pumped full of blood, while by means of the contractile movements of the peripheral vessels, the blood is, so to speak, milked out into the veins. We may say, in fact, that there are two hearts concerned in the systemic circulation, the work of the central organ being supplemented by the peripheral heart,—the small vessels,—working at the distal end of the vascular loop, where the resistance is greatest.

Active congestion, or hyperemia, is simply a state in which the movements of the small vessels are very vigorous, and have a wide swing, so that a large amount of blood is passed through the tissues. In passive congestion there is dilatation of the small vessels without increased activity. One condition results from increased action of the vessels through stimulation of both the vasodilators and the vasoconstrictors; the other from paralysis of the vasoconstrictors or excitation of the vasodilators, or both, resulting in dilatation of the small vessels, with stagnation of their contents. In active congestion, the aid afforded by the rhythmic movement of the small vessels is increased. In passive congestion this action is greatly diminished or entirely lost. The difference in the rate of the movement of the blood gives rise to the difference in color,—scarlet in active hyperemia or congestion, cherry red in passive congestion. In the one case a rich supply of fresh, oxygenated arterial blood is passing through the small vessels into the veins, the movement of the blood is rapid, and all the vital processes are quickened; the heart, as well as all other organs, is thus better nourished and energized. In passive congestion and all conditions of the circulation in which a cyanotic appearance is present, the usual condition in slowed circulation, the blood current is slow through cardiac weakness, or the lack of the active assistance of the peripheral heart; as a consequence, an insufficient amount of oxygen is introduced into the body, the blood is charged with CO_2 and other tissue poisons, and all the vital processes are depressed. To aid the heart and the circulation the thing needed is not simply an increased rate of activity of the heart, or an increased volume of the pulse, but an increased movement of the blood current throughout the entire system.

Pallor is due to contraction of all the vessels of the skin. 713
Local cyanosis is due to greatly slowed movement of the blood, either from passive congestion or spasm of the arterioles, resulting in excessive absorption of oxygen and accumulation of CO_2 in the blood.

In the application of any agent for the purpose of relieving conditions of this kind, the peripheral heart as well as the heart itself must be taken into consideration. In fact, the whole circulatory system must be regarded as one. The heart and the arteries are composed of essentially the same kind of tissue, and have practically the same functions. The arteries and capillaries as well as the heart are capable of contracting. Both the heart and the arteries are controlled by excitory and inhibitory nerves. These two classes of nerves controlling the heart and the vessels respectively are kindred in structure and origin, the vagus and the vasodilators being medullated and of spinal origin, while the accelerators of the heart and the vasoconstrictors of the arteries are non-medullated.

Winternitz and other authorities have frequently called attention to the value of cold as a cardiac stimulant or tonic. The tonic effect of this agent is greater than that of any medicinal agent which can be administered.

The cold compress applied over the cardiac area of the 714
chest may well replace alcohol, as a heart tonic. The thing necessary to encourage the heart's action is not mere relaxa-

tion of the peripheral vessels, but, as Winternitz has shown, increased activity of the peripheral circulation in the skin, muscles, and elsewhere. Alcohol paralyzes the vasoconstrictors, and so dilates the small vessels and lessens the resistance to the heart action; but at the same time it lessens the energy of the nerve centers which control the heart, diminishes the power of the heart muscles, and lessens that rhythmical activity of the small vessels whereby the circulation is so efficiently aided at that portion of the blood circuit most remote from the heart. A cold application to that portion of the chest overlying the heart reflexly stimulates and energizes the heart through the cardiac nerves. This reflex action is not confined to the heart muscle; the stimulation of the activity of the cardiac vessels improves the circulation through the heart structure, refreshing and energizing it in the same manner in which a voluntary muscle is energized by a cold application, as is so well shown by the ergograph (Exp. 50).

It is well to remember that the vasoconstrictor nerves are one in kind with the excitor nerves of the heart, while the vasodilators are in like manner associated with the vagus. With this in mind, it is easy to see that while alcohol paralyzes the vasoconstrictors, it at the same time weakens the nerves and the ganglia which initiate and maintain the activity of the heart. Cold, on the other hand, excites to activity these nerves and centers, and thus produces the opposite effect.

The apparent increase of strength which follows the giving of alcohol in cases of cardiac weakness is delusive. There is increased volume of the pulse for the reason that the small arteries and capillaries are dilated, thus lessening resistance and cardiac work; but this apparent improvement is very evanescent, as naturally results from the fact that while the heart is relieved momentarily by the sudden dilatation of the peripheral vessels, the accumulation of blood in the venous system through the loss of the normal activity of the peripheral heart, gradually raises the resistance again by increasing the load of blood which has to be pushed along in the venous system. This loss of the action of the peripheral heart thus in the end more than counterbalances the temporary relief secured by the paralysis of the vasoconstrictors. This accumulation and sluggish movement of blood in the venous system is shown by the purplish hue of the skin in a person under the influence of alcohol,—a wide contrast to the ruddy glow presented by the skin in which the small vessels are actively engaged in pumping the blood out of the arteries into the veins, an action in which the whole body may be made to participate by a general cold douche or other suitable application of cold water to the surface. Cold applications, general and local, may be safely affirmed to be the true physiological heart tonic.

It is evident, then, that in the use of alcohol in connec- 715
tion with the cold bath, we are not enhancing its effects, but are simply lessening its influence. If it is desired to mitigate the tonic or excitant effect of cold water upon the heart or vessels, this may be accomplished by employing water at a higher temperature, or, if it is desired simply to get the patient over the preliminary shock of the application, we may accomplish this much more efficiently by a preliminary heating of the skin, as by a fomentation to the spine, a hot-blanket pack, a hot enema, or even hot-water drinking.

3. *The Cold Friction Bath* (1150).—The utility of the cold 716
bath as originally practiced by Brand can not be questioned; but Winternitz has shown that the rate of heat elimination may be very greatly increased by rubbing the patient continuously during the bath. At the present time Brand and his followers, who are adepts in the use of the cold bath in fever, uniformly employ vigorous friction during the entire bath. Those authors who forbid friction during the bath because of the supposition that heat production may thereby be increased evidently do not recognize the fact that by the maintenance of a vigorous surface circulation the rate of heat elimination is increased out of proportion to the slight increase of heat pro-

duction, so that there is a decided gain to the patient by friction employed during the bath; and especially do these writers neglect the important fact that the greatest benefit derived from the cold bath is not the simple heat abstraction, but the general rousing of the vital powers, the increase of resistance, and the quickening of the recuperative and reparative activities of the body.

Another advantage of this method is that the patient is much more comfortable in the bath, and will tolerate the application for a longer time and at a lower temperature as well as more frequently than when it is administered without friction. As elsewhere shown, friction also averts increase of heat production by preventing shivering (**200, 1151**).

The claim made by some authorities that friction during the bath lessens the permanency of its effect in temperature reduction, is perhaps correct, to a degree, but this only necessitates the more frequent use of the bath, which the friction renders readily tolerable.

How, then, may we explain the good effects obtained by the method of Brand? The explanation is to be found, not in the subtraction of heat alone, but especially in the tonic effects of cold water, and in the sedative influence upon the nervous reflexes concerned in the febrile process and in the powerful diuretic effects of the bath.

717 4. *The Tepid or Neutral Bath* (**1130**).—A bath at 92° to 95° F. would produce little or no fall of temperature in a healthy person, but experience has shown that by the employment of the neutral bath in fever cases, a marked fall of temperature may often be induced. The reason for this is that when the patient's temperature is three or four degrees above the normal, the difference in the temperature of the body and that of the bath is much greater than under ordinary circumstances, and consequently the temperature-reducing effect of the bath is proportionately greater. Riess made a special study of this bath (**1136**).

The late Professor Dujardin-Beaumetz, the eminent French

clinician, a few years ago expressed himself in very decided terms against the cold bath as a means of reducing temperature. He remarked: "Relying exclusively upon physiological experimentation, the method of cold baths applied for antithermic effects in the treatment of febrile phenomena is an irrational practice. It subtracts heat from the patient, but increases organic disintegration." *

Laur, of Lyon, in 1874, and later other French clinicians, showed the superiority of tepid baths over cold baths as a means of reducing temperature and relieving the nervous phenomena characteristic of typhoid and other continued fevers. The temperature of the bath was 86° to 95° F., or ten or twelve degrees below the temperature of the body, continued for a half or three quarters of an hour.

A bath administered at a temperature of 88° to 92° is highly effective in reducing temperature if sufficiently prolonged, and a bath of this temperature has the decided advantage that it does not provoke thermic reaction to any considerable degree, and hence does not increase heat production, either during or after the bath. A temperature of 88° to 92° F. is often tolerated without difficulty by a feeble typhoid fever patient who could not support a more vigorous application, and is found to be most effective in lowering the body temperature. It must be remembered, however, that a temperature of 80° or 85° makes upon the hot skin of a nervous fever patient an impression very little different from that produced by water at a temperature five or even ten degrees lower in a normal person. In other words, the neutral zone is raised in febrile conditions. If the temperature is three or four degrees above normal, the neutral zone is raised to about the same extent.

5. *The Graduated Bath.*—Ziemssen first, and later Glen- 718
ard, recommended in high terms the so-called graduated bath, in which the patient is placed in an immersion bath, the

* "L' Hygiène Thérapeutique," by Dujardin-Beaumetz, Paris, 1888.

temperature of which is 3.5° to 4° below that of the body. The temperature is then steadily lowered at the rate of about one degree every three minutes, until a temperature of 86° is reached. This method has the advantage that no shock is produced, as when the patient is placed in water at 68°, by the Brand method. There is, accordingly, no marked thermic reaction. If desirable, the temperature may be lowered still more, or until the patient becomes slightly chilly, but he should not be allowed to shiver. The bath should be accompanied by gentle friction for the purpose of preventing chill and to increase heat elimination (Exp. 51).

With feeble patients who chill easily, the lowest temperature of the bath may be made 90° or 92° F. in the first application, the bath being more prolonged than when the lower temperature is employed. In such cases the temperature of the bath should be lowered one or two degrees at each application until the temperature of 70° or 75° is reached.

The graduated bath obviates the danger from syncope, which is one of the inconveniences of the cold bath. It may be employed in cases in which the cold bath is contra-indicated, as in cases of typhoid with serious renal or cardiac complications.

The results in temperature reduction obtained by the graduated bath are more permanent than those obtained from the cold bath of Brand or the cold affusion of Currie; and after several years' experience with this bath, the author considers the graduated bath one of the most efficient and satisfactory of all the methods employed for reducing temperature in fever. Unfortunately, it is much less convenient for use in the ordinary home or in private practice than in hospitals. There are, however, other means by which very similar, and perhaps equally good, effects may be secured.

719 6. *The Cooling Wet-Sheet Pack* (**1189**).—When employed for the reduction of temperature, the sheet should be wet in cold or cool water, and should be wrung out slightly, then wrapped about the patient in such a manner as to come into

immediate contact with every part of the body, being tucked in closely around each limb and about the neck. The patient should be covered very lightly if at all. In a few moments the temperature of the sheet will be raised to nearly that of the body, when it should be renewed, a fresh pail of cold water being employed each time for wetting the sheet, which should be wrung out as dry as possible, in order to remove the warm water which it contains, before dipping into the cold water for the second application. It is better to use two sheets, having the freshly prepared sheet on another couch.

The application may be renewed in this manner five or six times in succession, or even more. When the temperature of the body is very high, the sheet is so rapidly heated that it must be renewed every five to seven minutes, to make the cooling effect continuous. The applications should be renewed until the temperature has been lowered one degree or more, or until reduced to 101° or less, each successive application being longer than the preceding. There should be good circulatory reaction to maintain an active cutaneous circulation. It is often well to secure this by friction with the hand outside the sheet.

7. *The Cold Shower Pack* (**1190**).—Instead of removing 720
the sheet from the patient, the same effect may be accomplished by opening the sheet and sprinkling the body as well as the sheet with cold water. The patient should be made to turn, first upon one side and then the other, so that the back and whole body may be exposed to the cold application.

A better method still is to place the patient upon a cot covered with oilcloth, so arranged in relation to a tub placed at the foot of the cot that any surplus water may be caught as it runs away; then the water may be turned upon the patient from a watering-pot or poured over him either from a dipper or other convenient vessel. By this means the cooling effect of the sheet may be made continuous, and almost as intense as that of the cold bath.

The late Dr. Austin Flint introduced this form of cooling bath in 1874, when the author was a pupil under him in Bellevue Hospital. In a paper read by him before the Academy of Medicine at that time, he reported several obstinate and protracted cases of remittent malarial fever with very high temperature, that were rapidly cured by this measure repeated daily.

Water at any desired temperature may be used. If the patient does not well tolerate cold applications, water at a temperature of 80° or even 85° F. will be found efficient in lowering the temperature, provided the application is continued for a sufficient length of time.

When very cold water is employed, the disposition to chill may be prevented by friction with the hands applied outside the sheet.

721 8. *The Cold Compress* (**1318**).—The cold compress may be efficiently used for reducing temperature in cases in which the febrile action is not so intense as to require more vigorous measures. The compress should consist of two or three thicknesses of linen, or twice as many thicknesses of cheese-cloth. The fabric should be soft, so that it will fit the surface perfectly. It is necessary that the compress should be changed and recooled as soon as it approaches the body temperature. It should not remain long without change.

The compress should be wet in cool or cold water, and should be but slightly wrung. The more water it contains, the less frequently will a change be required. The compress must be large enough to cover more than one fourth of the skin surface, or about five square feet for a person weighing one hundred and eighty pounds. Several compresses may be used, one for the front of the trunk, another for the back, and one for each limb. Nervous patients and children often tolerate the compress better than the wet-sheet pack, and it may be changed more easily than the wet sheet. The compress may be covered with dry flannel, or, if desired, it may be left uncovered, and will thus cool by evaporation.

9. *The Cold Sponge Bath* (**1204**).—This is an exceedingly useful measure in cases of fever in which the temperature is not very high, but the skin flushed and dry, and the patient restless and uncomfortable. If a sponge is used, it should be as wet as possible, so that the surface will not be simply moistened, but thoroughly wet. The intensity of the bath is increased if a large amount of surface is exposed at one time. If the patient is very sensitive to cold, and complains much of the disagreeable sensations produced, small areas, as a single limb, may be sponged in succession, each part being covered as soon as gone over with the sponge. When a stronger effect is desired, the whole body may be sponged, and left uncovered to cool by evaporation. In general this is not an efficient or satisfactory method of combating elevation of temperature. It is useful only when the skin is hot and dry. 722

10. *The Wet-Towel Rub* (**1213**).—The cold towel bath is essentially the same as the cold sponge bath, only applied somewhat differently. A towel of ordinary size is wrung out of cool or cold water, and spread out quickly over as large an area as possible. The hands are applied with a rubbing movement, outside, not under, the towel, first one part, then another, until the whole towel is slightly warmed, when it is quickly renewed by dipping in cold water and wringing slightly, and applied to an adjacent or corresponding surface; and so on, until the entire body has been gone over, the operation being continued as long as may be necessary to procure the desired results. This method is applicable only to cases in which there is but a slight rise of temperature, or where the patient is too feeble to be subjected to more vigorous measures. Each part must be quickly dried, rubbed, and covered after the application before proceeding to the next. 723

The cold-towel rub, the towel being wrung as dry as possible, is of great service in cases in which the patient is in an adynamic state, with cold extremities, pinched features, and marked depression. Especial attention should be given to the limbs, and the application must be short and instantly followed by vigorous rubbing. Partial cold rubbings test the patient's reaction and preparation for more vigorous applications, such as the cooling pack and the graduated bath.

724 11. *Cold Wet Friction* (**1209**).—This bath, administered by means of the cold friction mitt, as elsewhere described, is a most useful measure in cases of fever in which the condition of the patient demands a cold application to lower the temperature, energize the heart, and increase vital resistance, but in which there are conditions that contraindicate the ordinary cold immersion, or Brand bath. It is a most valuable antipyretic measure, and is always indicated in fever, except in cases in which cold applications must be forbidden altogether, as when the patient is perspiring freely. It may even be employed when the skin is cold or cyanotic. It is possible to use water at a very low temperature, even ice-water, in administering this treatment. It is of the greatest possible service in the adynamic or ataxo-adynamic conditions of typhoid fever, in cases in which serious cardiac or renal complications have appeared, in intestinal hemorrhage, and in collapse from hemorrhage or perforation. It rouses the vital powers in a wonderful manner, brings to the surface the blood which is stagnating in the viscera, awakens the lethargic brain, slows and strengthens the fluttering pulse, and completely changes the aspect of an apparently desperate case, and that often in a very brief space of time, a few hours, even. The bath may be perfectly graduated. At first the mitt should be only moistened. As the circulation improves, it may at the next application be saturated, and later it may be filled.

725 12. *The Cold Evaporating Sheet* (**1200**).—A linen sheet should be wrung out of cold water and wrapped about the patient, who is left uncovered. The skin is cooled by evaporation of water from the sheet, which may be encouraged by vigorous fanning with an ordinary fan or by means of a current of air from an electric fan. By this means a degree of

refrigeration as intense as the patient is able to endure may easily be produced. It is only necessary to keep the sheet moist to continue the effect as long as may be desired. Moderate friction should be employed by the hands applied outside the sheet. Leyden has shown that the dryness of the skin and retention of water in fever is a cause of diminished heat elimination. Hence the value of this and other similar hydric measures.

13. *The Hot Evaporating Sheet* (1200).— This measure 726
is precisely the same as the preceding, except that the sheet is wrung out of hot water. The temperature of the water should be as high as can be borne, 130° to 140° F. The purpose of the hot evaporating sheet is to obtain the combined effects of heat and cold. The impression of heat which lasts for a few seconds at the beginning of the application produces an atonic thermic reaction, diminishing heat production, and preparing the way for the largest benefit to be derived from the cold impression which quickly follows as the sheet is cooled by the rapid evaporation. Evaporation may be stimulated by fanning, as in the case of the cold evaporating sheet. Repeat in five to eight minutes, or as soon as chilly sensations are felt. Apply gentle friction as the sheet is cooled.

This measure is especially valuable in cases in which the patient is very nervous, and dreads the contact with cold water. In one such case the temperature was lowered two degrees during an hour as the result of repeated applications of the hot sheet.

14. *The Hot Sponge Bath.*—The hot sponge bath is an 727
application sometimes useful in febrile conditions. The brief impression of heat produces an atonic reaction, with diminished heat production, while the evaporation taking place from the moistened surface subsequently produces cooling effects. This method is of comparatively limited value, but it nevertheless often proves useful in special conditions, as in cases in which there is cyanosis, shivering, chilliness, or a dread of cold water, and in mild febrile cases.

The hot sponge is of the greatest service in connection with cold friction or the cold-towel rub. It should be applied to each part just before the cold application, as a preparation for it. It promotes the reaction whereby the surface vessels are filled, and thus encourages the antipyretic effect desired, also reflexly acting to reduce heat production. The water employed should be as hot as can be borne, 130° to 140°. The sponge should be squeezed quite dry, and should be applied quickly, and to a small area, as an arm, a thigh, or a leg. The hot sponging should be continued, rewetting the sponge every half minute, until the surface reddens slightly. Then the cold application should be instantly applied with rubbing, allowing no interval for chilling.

728 15. *The Hot-Blanket Pack* (**1197**).—This is a very useful means for reducing temperature in certain cases in which cold applications can not be employed without serious risk, and hence are contraindicated. The hot-blanket pack acts, of course, by producing an atonic reaction, thus lessening heat production, and is in some cases especially useful as a preparation for a subsequent cold application, the heat preparing the skin for rapid heat elimination.

The hot-blanket pack is of the greatest service as a means of aiding the reduction of temperature in cases in which there is decreased heat elimination (**237**). The duration, however, should be brief—3 to 10 minutes—and as hot as can be borne.

The following instance illustrates very clearly the advantages of the hot-blanket pack in cases requiring increased heat elimination: A number of years ago the author was called in consultation in the case of a child of four years, who was suffering from malignant diphtheria. The patient was found with a temperature of 106°, comatose, the skin pale and cold. A hot-blanket pack was ordered immediately, which quickly brought the blood to the surface. In fifteen minutes the patient was revived to consciousness, and in two hours the temperature had fallen to 102°. The recovery was rapid and excellent. Numerous similar cases might be cited, in which a high temperature with diminished heat elimination accompanying typhoid fever and other febrile states has been promptly relieved by a preliminary hot application followed by cool compresses, the wet-sheet pack, and allied means.

It must be remembered, also, that heat is a sedative of great power; hence the presence of cardiac weakness, a condition very commonly accompanying the adynamic state in which the hot pack is indicated, must be most carefully considered in making an application of heat of any sort. Fortunately, short hot applications are depressing only in very slight degree, and very short applications (1 to 3 min.) are stimulating in their effects. Any depressant effect arising from the hot-blanket pack may be overcome by means of the cold precordial compress, or an ice-bag over the heart during the application.

16. *Fomentation to the Spine* (1328).—It would perhaps 729
be more proper to describe this measure as a fomentation to the back, as the application should not be confined to the spine, but should extend to the whole posterior surface of the trunk. A fomentation to the spine acts in a manner similar to the hot-blanket pack, but its effect is of course less intense. The application often produces profuse perspiration, whereby a considerable amount of heat is carried off. The hot pack is also a good preparation for a cold application, and is especially useful when the cold bath is contraindicated.

In some cases, alternate hot and cold compresses to the spine are more effective in producing perspiration than fomentations alone, and hence greatly promote heat elimination. A hot application to the spine encourages heat elimination by stimulation of the sweat centers.

17. *Fomentation to the Abdomen.*—This procedure, in 730
combination with other measures, aids in reducing temperature. When the patient complains of chilliness or is inclined to shiver, the abdominal fomentation will at once dissipate these unpleasant symptoms, and prevent the increased heat

production which would otherwise result from the muscular action induced. The fomentation aids in maintaining the surface circulation, and is an excellent means of preparing the patient for the cooling pack and the cold bath. In cases in which the cold bath produces abdominal pain or cramps, the fomentation for ten minutes just before the bath relieves this inconvenient symptom. The fomentation may be usefully employed in connection with the cold enema when this measure causes unpleasant shivering. It is useful, likewise, as a means of increasing tolerance for the cool abdominal compress, for which purpose the compress should be removed once in two hours and the fomentation applied for ten or fifteen minutes at as high a temperature as the patient can bear. Used in this manner, the fomentation materially aids the compress as a means of combating visceral congestion.

731 18. *The Hot and Cold Bath.*—In many cases, and especially in persons in whom the surface circulation is sluggish, more pronounced antipyretic effects may be produced by immediately preceding the cold bath with a hot bath at a temperature of 105° to 107° for 3 or 4 minutes, than by the use of the cold bath alone. Galen treated fever cases by rubbing with cold water after a warm bath.

Vinaj claims that the hot bath for three minutes, followed by a bath at 95°, gradually lowered to 80° during 5 to 15 minutes, is more effective in lowering the temperature than the cold bath of Brand, and produces more permanent results. The author has confirmed this in certain cases.

Pflüger found that greater refrigerant effects were produced by the hot spray for one minute, followed by a short cold spray, than by the cold spray alone. Finkler confirmed these results in experiments upon febrile rabbits.

This result is doubtless attributable to the increased heat elimination due to dilatation of the surface vessels, and to the atonic thermic reaction.

The observers mentioned noted also that a greater effect was produced by a short cold bath, if the body was sprinkled with very hot water at the moment of emerging from the bath than if the cold bath were prolonged. This may prove an excellent method. The heat impression made upon the skin induces lessened heat production, without communicating a sufficient amount of heat to the body to cause a rise of temperature.

19. *Cold Applications to the Head, Spine, Heart, and* 732
Abdomen.— The application of the cooling compress (**1318**), ice bag or cap, or the cold coil to the head or abdomen or to both regions, is a powerful means of reducing the general temperature, and was successfully employed by Spencer Wells and others in the treatment of patients suffering from a high temperature due to peritonitis. Benjamin Rush used an ox-bladder filled with broken ice in yellow fever more than one hundred years ago.

Cold applications to the head should never be neglected in fever cases, care being taken to wet the hair thoroughly, as it is an excellent non-conductor unless saturated with moisture.

A continuous application of cold to the head and abdomen produces in some cases such marked effects that no other measures are required for controlling febrile action. Care must be exercised, however, in the application of cold to the head, that too pronounced depressing effects are not produced.

Winternitz has shown that the prolonged application of an ice-bag or an ice-water coil over the heart cools the blood, and thus lowers the general temperature. This measure may be advantageously associated with others in the treatment of fever cases.

Neale advocates the use of the ice-bag to the spine as a means of lowering the temperature. The antipyretic effect of this measure is doubtless due, in part at least, to its influence upon the circulation, as it dilates the surface vessels of the extremities.

20. *The Cold-Air Bath.*— The temperature of the air 733
in the sick-room has a most decided influence upon the body

temperature in the case of a fever patient, an increase of a few degrees in the temperature being often responsible for a rise of temperature in the patient which could not otherwise be accounted for. The fever patient is somewhat in the condition of the so-called cold-blooded animal, whose temperature rises and falls with that of the surrounding medium; for the body has lost the power of regulating its temperature, as it does when in a normal condition.

It should be remembered that while atmospheric temperatures below 58° F. cause increase of heat production, air at a temperature above 60° has a like tendency. Air is practically neutral between 60° and 70°, while at 104° the heat production may be three and one-half times the normal amount. Whenever the body temperature is above normal, tissue metabolism and heat production are increased.

Breathing air of a low temperature, as well as exposing the skin to cold air, has a decided effect in lowering the temperature. This method has been adopted as a definite procedure, the patient being made to breathe artificially cooled air, brought to him through a tube. It is interesting to recall in this connection that Currie relates a case of fever treated in 1801 in which the temperature was reduced from 104° to 101° by an air bath at 65°. The patient's body was exposed uncovered to the air, being placed between an open window and a large chimney. The pulse fell in a short time from 120 to 114. He also relates the case of an Arab traveler suffering from the plague who escaped from a caravan during a violent delirium, and wandered naked in the desert for three weeks, until he finally recovered. He subsisted during this time on sorrel.

The lungs present a surface of about two thousand square feet, while the skin has a surface of only seventeen square feet. It should be noted, however, that the surface presented by the perspiratory ducts of the skin aggregates more than eleven thousand square feet. All the blood in the body is spread out just beneath the lining surface of the air-cells of the lungs every two and a half minutes, making this a very important cooling surface. But, unfortunately, the amount of air which can be introduced into the lungs is so small that the effect obtained, even when the rate of breathing is doubled and the volume of tidal air considerably increased, can not be very large. I have, however, succeeded in lowering the temperature in fever cases by means of re-enforced respiration, causing the patient to breathe deeply of cold air while the arms were raised above his head to aid the respiratory effort.

By making a patient breathe very cold air, say at 5° F., taking in 125 cubic inches at a breath, and breathing fourteen times a minute, he would take into his lungs about sixty cubic feet of air per hour. To raise this air from 5° to the temperature of the patient, supposing the patient's temperature to be 105°, would require the addition of about 120 heat units, representing an equal amount of heat abstracted from the body, or a lowering of the temperature of 1° F. in a person weighing 120 pounds. So good a result can not be obtained in practice, however, for the reason that the air inhaled at 5° F. does not reach body temperature before being exhaled, and ordinarily the temperature of the inspired air is much higher. Yet a considerable degree of cooling may be effected through the breathing of cold air, provided pains is taken to increase the volume of air inspired. It is apparent, however, that the breathing of cold air is by no means so powerful a refrigerative measure as the exposure of the surface to cold air or cold water. Its beneficial action is doubtless largely due to the stimulation of the pulmonary circulation and the tonic reflex influence upon the heart.

The human body obeys the same physical laws as do other bodies as regards cooling by contact with air or radiation of heat toward masses of lower temperature. The experiments of Peclet show that the body cools by radiation at the rate of about one heat unit for each square foot of exposed skin surface per hour for each degree of difference between the temperature of the skin and the temperature of the walls of the room in which the patient is exposed, while the rate of heat loss by contact with moving air is about one-half heat unit for each square foot of skin surface exposed to each degree of difference between the temperature of the skin and the temperature of the air in contact with the body. From these facts one may easily deduce the probable amount of cooling which will result from the administration of a cold-air bath. Suppose the temperature of the walls of the room to be about 60°, the temperature of the air 70°, the average skin temperature 95°, and the amount of skin surface exposed 10 square feet. We shall have, by application of the above rules, a loss of 350 heat units by radiation and 125 heat units by contact with the air, or 475 heat units in all. Supposing the weight of the patient to be 160 lbs., there would be a loss of 3 heat units per pound, or a lowering of the general body temperature of about 3 degrees. If the patient lies upon a hard surface, the amount of skin exposure will be greater than if the body rests upon a soft mattress. By frequently changing the position of the patient, turning first on one side and then on the other, the cooling surface may be considerably increased.

If it is desired to calculate the amount of skin surface actually active in a given case, it may be done by means of a simple formula: A man weighing 180 pounds has a skin surface of about 19.6 square feet. Applying the well-known law pertaining to the relation of the contents of a solid body to its surface, we obtain the following proportion, in which W represents the weight of the patient under consideration, and S the skin surface:—

$$180 : W :: 19.6^{\frac{3}{2}} : S^{\frac{3}{2}}$$

This may be simplified into the following formula:—

$$87\ W = 180\ S^{\frac{3}{2}};\ \text{or,}\ \frac{W}{2.07} = S^{\frac{3}{2}}$$

Or, if we divide the weight by 2.57, and square this quotient, and extract the cube root of the result, we shall have the number of square feet of skin surface in a person of given weight.

If the patient weighs 130 pounds, the skin area would be 15.5 square feet. Supposing the amount of surface exposed to be two thirds of the whole, or about ten square feet; we require to know further only the surface temperature of the patient, the temperature of the walls of the room, and of the air about the patient, to be able to determine the rate of heat loss during an air bath of one hour's duration. This rate of cooling may be sufficient to compensate for heat production of nearly double the normal rate.

Since the heat production, as shown by the experiments of Winternitz, is rarely or never increased to this extent in febrile conditions, it is evident that the continuous cold-air bath, accompanied by rubbing to prevent chilling, is a most efficient antipyretic means.

Continuous moderate rubbing greatly enhances the effect of the air bath by maintaining a vigorous surface circulation. If the skin becomes cooled, the rate of heat elimination is greatly lessened. Under ordinary conditions, the skin eliminates 66.6 per cent. more heat with a surface temperature of 95° than with one of 85°. The employment of olive-oil, cocoa butter, or vaseline as a lubricant facilitates the rubbing, and increases the rate of radiation to the extent of perhaps forty or fifty per cent.

21. *The Graduated Compress.*—The compress (1313), as 734
well as the full bath, may be graduated. The first application should be made at a temperature a few degrees below that of the body, the temperature of each succeeding application being lowered two or three degrees. In patients who are very sensitive, the first compress may be wrung out of water at 130°. Apply for 3 minutes. Such a compress, by producing an atonic thermic reaction, prepares the way for the fullest effect to be derived from the cold applications to follow.

735 22. *Water-Drinking* (**1423**).—The free drinking of cold water is an efficient means of lowering the temperature. Drinking two or three pints of water at a temperature of 40°, within ten minutes, has caused a fall of temperature of one and one half to two degrees. This method, first empirically used by John Hancocke nearly two centuries ago, has been employed by a number of observers, with interesting results, but its chief utility is as an accompaniment of other antipyretic measures. Water-drinking lowers the temperature not only by absorbing heat, but by diluting the blood, and thus promoting evaporation from the surface and exciting the kidneys to increased activity, thereby encouraging the elimination of the toxins to which the rise of temperature is due. A glass of cold water every hour is an excellent rule for fever patients when the febrile action has any considerable degree of intensity. Cantani considered water-drinking superior to all other means of reducing the temperature, and Beverly-Robinson, after an extended experience, highly recommends it, directing that the patient should swallow not less than six or seven quarts every twenty-four hours.

736 23. *The Tepid or Cold Enema* (**1405**).—The enema affords a much more convenient means of introducing cold water into the alimentary canal than does water-drinking, for the reason that the patient usually refuses to swallow the amount of water required to produce any decided effects. Two or three pints of tepid or cool water may easily be introduced into the colon, if care be taken to avoid the introduction of air and to allow the water to flow in slowly and with little pressure. The water should be retained from 5 to 10 minutes, or as long as the patient does not suffer great inconvenience. The amount introduced should not be so large as to produce uncomfortable fulness or a painful desire for evacuation, but the patient should be instructed to make forcible efforts to retain the water, and, if necessary, assistance should be rendered by pressure with a napkin (Exp. 52). A long rectal tube should be used in introducing it.

The principle of graduation may be employed with the enema as with the cold bath. Beginning with a temperature of 98°, the water introduced may be steadily cooled until it is reduced to 70° or even lower. As a rule, however, a temperature of 80° is sufficient to accomplish the desired result.

A simple illustration will show the efficiency of the enema as a means of lowering the temperature. Suppose, for example, the quantity of water introduced to be five pounds (pints), and its temperature 70°, the patient's temperature being 105°, and his weight 150 pounds. If, on the withdrawal of the water, its temperature is found to be increased to 85°, the water has absorbed 75 pound Fahrenheit heat units (5x15=75), which would be an equivalent of one-half heat unit to each pound of the body weight, or .5° of temperature fall for the whole body. In other words, if there had been, in the meantime, no increase of heat production, the temperature of the body would be lowered .5°. By repeating the enema every fifteen minutes for an hour we may remove in four applications three hundred heat units, whereby the temperature of the body would be lowered 2°; but as the effect of a cool application of this sort is to stimulate heat production to some extent, we should not always expect quite so great effects as this, but rather a reduction of one to one and one-half degrees, which would certainly be an excellent result.

If water of a higher temperature — say 80° to 85° — is employed, which is sometimes necessary to avoid shivering and other discomforts to the patient, the rate of heat abstraction would be less; but on the other hand, the increase of heat production would also be less, and the measure may be continued for a longer time, and thus the net result may be equally great. On the whole, the results of clinical experience are decidedly in favor of long applications of moderate temperature, rather than short applications at a low temperature, as a means of temperature reduction.

Halm and Stolz reduced the temperature 3.6° and the pulse twenty-five beats per minute by using the cold enema in quantity of one liter, at a temperature of 46°, repeating eight times in succession, at intervals of from 5 to 10 minutes. Jacques employed the cold enema and water drinking in fever cases in 1839 with great success.

A very convenient method of administering the enema is to supplement the ordinary tubing of the fountain syringe by a shorter piece of tubing two or three feet in length, connected to it in such a way that it may be easily disconnected. It is better to have the short piece of tubing somewhat larger than the ordinary size, so that it will not be easily obstructed. After being slowly introduced, the water should be retained for 5, 10, or 15 minutes if possible. Then, by disconnecting the short tube and without removing the rectal tube, the water may be allowed to escape into a suitable vessel, and another portion of cool or tepid water may be immediately introduced. In a fever case under the author's care a number of years ago, the cold enema was employed in this manner continuously for two or three hours, and with the result that the temperature of the patient, which was at the beginning of the treatment between 105° and 106°, and had proved refractory to every other measure, was reduced to 102°, and was thereafter readily controlled by a repetition of the same procedure.

The author has constantly made use of the enema at different temperatures in the treatment of fever patients during the last twenty years, and finds it, when properly used, one of the most efficacious of all antipyretic measures.

The larger the quantity of water introduced, the greater will be the cooling effect, for the reason that it will come in contact with a larger extent of surface. With the patient lying on his back, it is generally difficult to introduce more than one or two pints of water; but by placing him upon the left side, with the limbs drawn up, or by elevating the hips six or eight inches, a much larger amount of water may be introduced, as by this means the liquid may be made to enter the transverse colon and even the cæcum. It is thus easy to introduce two or three quarts of water. If no more than one quart of water is used, the amount of surface with which the water is brought in contact is so small that comparatively slight effects are produced.

24. *Partial Cold Applications.*—When the general febrile action is the result of a local inflammatory process, as in many pelvic inflammations, appendicitis, pneumonia, pleurisy, peritonitis, acute arthritis, phlegmon, felon, and otitis media, the temperature may be best reduced in many instances by a very cold circumscribed application made to the affected part. Cold irrigation, the cold compress, and the ice-bag are among the most suitable measures in these cases, employed either alone or in combination with fomentations or other hot applications, used either as a preliminary measure or at intervals, as special conditions may indicate. 737

In certain cases, as in compound fracture of the limbs, in which the surgical dressing for maintenance of the parts in proper position prohibits the employment of cold water to the affected part, the principle of the "proximal compress" (**1327**), so much used by Priessnitz, may be employed. In head injuries, apply the ice-collar. In injuries of the hand, employ the cold elbow bath. In injury or inflammation of the foot, apply an ice-bag to the groin or the bend of the knee. This method is based upon the well-known fact that an application of cold to the trunk of an artery causes contraction in all its branches beyond the point of application.

Conditions Giving Rise to Elevation of Temperature. As previously pointed out, elevation of temperature may occur in five different cases as regards the condition of the heat-regulating functions (**237**). 738

In the application of measures for the reduction of temperature, it must first be ascertained to which of the several classes the case in hand belongs. It may be that no hydriatic application of any sort should be made, or that hot instead of cold applications are required. It may be profitable to note briefly the special indications in each of these classes of cases: —

In cases in which there is very great increase of heat production, with heat elimination increased, but to a less extent, by noticing the skin, the condition of which gives the best indication of the state of the patient as regards heat elimination, we may find any one of the following conditions: (*a*) Perspiring skin; (*b*) warm, moist skin; (*c*) hot, dry skin. We certainly would not find a cold skin, for heat elimination is increased.

What is to be done in cases of this sort? Certainly, if the skin is hot and the patient is perspiring freely, heat elimination is taking place as rapidly as possible, and usually no hydriatic applications should be made. We should simply dry the skin by wiping frequently with a soft warm cloth. If the skin is cold, even though it may be covered with moisture, elimination is not increased, for water will not evaporate quickly from a cold skin. The application of a cold bath, a cold enema, or any other refrigerating measure would be in the highest degree detrimental in cases of this sort, for it would check the perspiration and thus further diminish heat elimination, and would probably produce a chill, with internal congestion. This is a matter of great importance, especially in the treatment of pneumonia, and other fevers accompanied by an internal inflammation, and in dealing with such disorders as sweating sickness, which has prevailed so extensively in the southern part of the United States, in the West Indies, and in many other countries. Wiping frequently with a soft linen cloth promotes the cooling process by removing the surplus water and thus increasing the amount of radiating and evaporating surface.

In cases in which the skin is warm and slightly moist, but not perspiring freely, perspiration may be promoted by hot-water drinking, by hot sponging of the spine, and by a small hot enema. The patient should otherwise be treated the same as when perspiration is profuse. If the skin is cold and moist or perspiring, hot applications should be made. The hot application may consist of a fomentation to the spine, a hot enema, a short hot-blanket pack, or an immersion bath at 102° for 3 or 4 minutes. Cold friction may be applied with great advantage immediately after the hot application in most cases.

Heat elimination may be encouraged by two general **739**
methods: (1) By the application of cooling measures; (2) by employing measures to induce perspiration. It is by no means easy to induce perspiration in cases of continued fever, the condition of the perspiratory glands being such that it is generally impossible to induce active sudation. When the patient does perspire, it is generally an indication of an improved condition, usually of a lowered temperature, except when other grave symptoms appear coincidently. On the other hand, the skin may be cooled at will, and to any extent desired; no matter how active may be the production of heat in the body, it is possible to apply to the skin cooling measures of such intensity that the heat produced within the body may be eliminated as rapidly as it is generated. The thick stove-cover becomes red-hot, but the temperature of the boiling kettle does not rise above 212°, the rate of heat elimination in the boiling kettle keeping pace with the rate at which the heat is communicated to its bottom.

Three different methods may be conveniently employed for **740**
the encouragement of heat elimination by cooling the skin. These are (1) the application of cold water; (2) the application of cold air; (3) evaporation of moisture from the skin.

Cold water may be applied by various hydriatic measures, of which methods 1 to 19 (**744**) are most appropriate and convenient for a case in which there is fever, with increase of both heat elimination and heat production.

The method of cooling the body by contact with cold air has been elsewhere described (**733**).

To cool the skin by evaporation it is only necessary to substitute ordinary water for the perspiration which nature is unable to produce. The evaporating sheet (**725**) and the sponge bath are the most efficient means of accomplishing this.

In cases in which there is an increase of heat production with normal heat elimination, there is evidently a greater need for an increase of heat elimination than in cases in which there is less active heat production, and consequently less necessity for the application of vigorous cold procedures. The first indication in cases of this sort is to stimulate activity of the peripheral circulation. This may usually be accomplished by friction of the skin; but if the temperature is high, vigorous friction will not be desirable, as mechanical irritation of this sort may stimulate heat production as well as heat elimination. Those measures most serviceable are the graduated bath, the tepid bath, the cold friction bath, and the graduated compress.

741 Friction should accompany all cold applications made in a case of this sort, as it is desirable to produce circulatory reaction, while thermic reaction should as far as possible be suppressed. The graduated bath and the tepid bath, with friction, are especially to be commended in cases of this class. The cold friction bath and cold immersion bath, cold affusion, the cooling shower pack, and other cold applications may be employed, provided a hot bath of some sort, as the hot-blanket pack for 5 minutes, hot immersion for 3 to 5 minutes, or some similar procedure is administered just before the cold application. The hot application must be short and intense (105° to 110°), and must be instantly followed by the cold application before the skin has been chilled by evaporation or contact with the air.

In cases of increased heat production with diminished heat elimination, the most important indication is to increase heat elimination. Heat production can not be so easily controlled, but heat elimination is entirely under the control of the physician, if the proper measures are employed.

At the same time that heat elimination is increased, thermic reaction must be avoided, or there will be heat increase. However, the elevation of temperature in a given case of this kind may be due as much to diminished heat elimination as to the increase of heat production. The most suitable measures to be employed for restoring the normal temperature are essentially the same as those recommended above. Care must be taken, however, in cases of this sort, to avoid too long-continued cold applications. The patient should be well covered after the bath, and must be well rubbed in the bath to insure vigorous surface circulation.

In cases in which heat production is normal, with heat elimination decreased,—a condition comparatively rare,—the skin is always cool. A hot skin generally implies increased heat elimination, although Herz, of Vienna, has shown that dryness of the skin greatly lessens heat elimination. Clamminess of the skin may be present, but this does not necessarily involve an increase of heat elimination by evaporation. The measures most serviceable in cases of this sort are, the Scotch douche, the hot-blanket pack followed by a short cold immersion bath with friction, or fomentations to the spine, followed by general cold friction.

In cases in which there is diminished heat production with 742
diminished heat elimination, but to a lesser degree, a hot bath (5 to 10 min.) followed by a short cold bath ($\frac{1}{2}$ min.) will be found a most efficient means of restoring the temperature equilibrium. The cold bath should be accompanied by vigorous rubbing, to secure thorough circulatory reaction. Rubbing should also be practiced in the bath to encourage both circulatory and thermic reaction. If the bath is continued too long, thermic reaction may be suppressed. In cases of this sort both thermic and circulatory reaction are to be encouraged. The hot enema, or fomentations to the spine, followed or accompanied by cold friction and dry friction afterward, are also valuable measures. The important thing is to increase the surface circulation. Pallor, blueness, or coldness

are always indications for the application of heat and friction to the skin. The effect of hot applications in stimulating the surface circulation, however, is transient; hence the importance of following the hot application by a very brief cold application, thereby exciting circulatory reaction, by means of which the blood is more permanently fixed in the skin and heat elimination encouraged. No harm is done if the application is carried to the extent of slight chilliness, provided the patient is afterward quickly warmed up by rubbing. Reaction must necessarily be encouraged by wrapping the patient warmly for a few moments after the cold application. Cold friction is a measure well adapted to cases of this sort, the pack following a fomentation to the spine or abdomen, the short hot full bath, or any other measure whereby the general surface of the body has been thoroughly heated.

748 In the treatment of febrile disorders it is important to take into account in each case and on each occasion, whether or not the dominant condition is increased heat production or diminished heat elimination. Winternitz has shown that variations in heat elimination may be sufficiently extensive to account for all changes in body temperature; nevertheless, it is quite certain that variations in heat production are also an important determining factor in deviations from the normal temperature mean.

In addition to the subjective and objective indications relating to the processes of heat production and elimination, there are calorimetric and other means by which more definite and exact information may be obtained. For example, by means of the formulæ given elsewhere (pp. 315, 316), we may determine the rate of heat elimination by radiation and air contact. Let us suppose, for example, in the case of a febrile patient, that the surface of the skin feels cold, and has an average temperature of 80° F., while the temperature of the walls of the room is 70° and that of the air 70°. By the formulæ the heat loss per hour for each square foot of surface will be 15 heat units. The weight of the patient is 120 pounds. By the formula already given (p. 316) we find the skin area to be 15 square feet ($180:120::87:S^1$; $S=15$). At the rate of 10,000 heat units' daily loss for a skin area of 19.6 square feet, the normal heat loss for a skin area of 15 square feet would be about 7,650 heat units. But the actual loss is only 5,400 ($15 \times 15 \times 24 = 5{,}400$), a diminution of 2,250 heat units, or 30 per cent. less than the normal rate of heat elimination. By this simple mathematical calculation it is possible in any case to determine approximately the rate of heat elimination to normal; and if the loss is found less than normal, while the rectal temperature is above normal, it will be at once evident that the febrile temperature may be readily accounted for by the retention of heat, and that the therapeutic indication is for the use of such measures as will increase heat elimination. In such a case, the Brand bath would of course be contraindicated; the measures required would be dry friction, or short hot baths followed by partial cold applications with vigorous friction. The use of the friction mitt with water at 50° to 60° would be especially indicated.

Let us suppose, on the other hand, that the patient's surface temperature is found to be high, the skin hot to the hand, and 100° by the surface thermometer. The heat loss will be at the rate of 16,200 heat units *per diem* ($45 \times 15 \times 24 = 16{,}200$), or an increase of 112 per cent. The rectal temperature being above normal, it is evident that there must be at least an equal percentage increase in heat production; and vigorous measures to diminish heat production and to increase heat elimination are required.

The use of the author's calorimeter and of the bath calorimeter first employed by Liebermeister more than thirty years ago, have been referred to elsewhere (**225**, **226**).

Hydriatic Applications to be Employed in Cases in which 744
Both Heat Production and Heat Elimination are Increased.—In the following list the aim has been to arrange the various therapeutic measures suggested in the order of their greatest efficiency, naming the most valuable first:—

1. The graduated bath (**718**).

2. The cooling wet-sheet pack (**719**).

3. The Brand, or cold friction, bath (**716**).

4. The prolonged tepid immersion bath (88° F.) (**717**).

5. The cold immersion bath (**712, 731**), followed by a short hot immersion, affusion, or sprinkling.

6. Tepid affusion (**711**).

7. Cold affusion (**711**).

8. The shower pack (**720**).

9. The cold compress (**721**)

10. The graduated compress (**734**).

11. The evaporating sheet (**725**).

12. Cold to head and neck (**732**).

13. Cold to spine (**732**).

14. Cold to abdomen (**732**).

15. Cold over heart (**732**).

16. Cold irrigation (**1294**).

17. The tepid or cold enema (**736**).

18. Cold water drinking (**735**), a measure that should be combined with all the other measures named.

19. The cold air bath (**733**).

745 *Hydriatic Measures to be Employed in Cases in which Heat Elimination is Diminished or not Increased.*—The following list comprises the most serviceable measures for increasing heat elimination when fever is present and the cold bath contraindicated:—

1. Hot bath (2 to 3 min.) followed by a cold bath with friction (1 min.) (**731**).

2. Hot-blanket pack (**728**).

3. Hot evaporating sheet (**726**).

4. Hot sponge bath (**727**).

5. Fomentation to the back (**729**).

6. Fomentation to the abdomen, followed by the cold enema (**730, 736**).

7. Fomentation to the back, followed by a cold wet-sheet pack (**719**).

8. Hot-blanket pack, followed by graduated bath (718).
9. Hot-blanket pack followed by prolonged tepid bath.
10. Hot-blanket pack followed by cold friction.
11. Dry friction.
12. Cold friction.

Suggestions and Cautions Respecting the Use of Water for Antipyretic Effects.

Cold applications alone are contraindicated in fever cases in which the skin is cold, the lips or skin blue, when goose-flesh, perspiration, general shivering, or chilliness are present, and when cold applications are particularly disagreeable to the patient. In most cases of this sort, however, the contraindication may be made to disappear by a short general hot application, by which both the skin and the nervous system are prepared to receive beneficial effects from refrigerant measures. 746

When the cold enema produces colic pains or chilliness, a fomentation over the abdomen may be employed at the same time.

The same measures may be employed after any application the refrigerant effects of which appear to be more intense than was desired.

General cold applications, especially prolonged applications, must be avoided in cases in which there is a general febrile condition due to some internal local inflammation, as in acute ovaritis or salpingitis, or other pelvic inflammations, gastritis, nephritis, etc. The inrush of blood produced by the cold application in cases of this sort increases the congestion which already exists in the affected parts, and thus adds to the intensity of the inflammatory processes. Prolonged neutral and tepid applications or local revulsive applications are to be preferred in these cases. The general temperature may be most efficiently lowered by controlling the local inflammatory processes by appropriate measures.

Currie well recognized the importance of avoiding general cold applications in cases of general fever due to some local inflammatory affection, and recommended the tepid bath in these conditions, with careful avoidance of the cold affusion or other applications likely to produce excitation or stimulation, remarking, "It appears to me probable that in the proportion of this stimulation is the difficulty of reducing the actual temperature."*

747 In the employment of the hot-blanket pack, fomentations, and the hot bath, care must be taken to avoid too *prolonged* applications. In an experiment, one of my assistants, a healthy young man, found that his temperature rose two degrees in half an hour in a hot-blanket pack. In a full bath at the temperature of the body, or a few degrees above, the temperature is found to rise at about the same rate.

In febrile conditions, the effect of a long hot bath in causing elevation of temperature will be still more pronounced. It is clearly evident that such an application, if prolonged, might become seriously dangerous in a case in which the temperature was already elevated. For example, if a patient with a temperature at 105° were kept in a hot-blanket pack or a hot bath for half an hour, the result might be an elevation of the temperature to 107° or 108°, with serious if not fatal results. The writer has known of several cases in which, under similar circumstances, the patient became delirious from the hyperpyrexia, and though quickly restored by the withdrawal of the heat and the application of cool sponging and cold compresses, was greatly excited for some time, remaining in a state of very great exhaustion for several hours.

The duration of a hot-blanket pack or hot bath of any sort for the purpose of warming the surface and exciting vascularity of the skin should be usually not more than five or ten minutes.

Hydrotherapy, to be effective as an antipyretic, must be employed with vigor and unremitting perseverance. An ordinary sponge bath two or three times a day may afford a little comfort to a patient burning up with fever, but it is of no

*"Medical Reports," 4th edition, p. 204.

value whatever as a means of lowering the temperature or of combating the causes of the disease.

The readiness with which a high temperature yields to an application will depend upon the time of day and the stage of the disease, as well as upon the thoroughness of the application. The regular typhoid fever curve shows a rise of temperature from 7 A. M. to 3 P. M. After 3 P. M. a decline occurs, with another rise having its maximum at midnight, and followed again by a decline. It is evident that a bath given when the temperature is rising may have no other effect than to lessen the rate of the elevation of temperature and to lower the maximum point reached, while a bath given while the temperature is naturally falling will have the effect to accelerate the fall, and thus seem to be more efficient and beneficial, when the actual influence of the bath may be precisely the same in the two cases. This fact must be taken into account in estimating the value of any particular mode of treatment or any particular application. 748

The effect of the treatment upon the temperature must be judged not only by the immediate effect, but by the effect upon the daily curve, which should be carefully watched. A case rightly managed ought to show a steady decline in the maximum temperature for each day, after the first week, and the physician and nurse should consider it their duty to see that the temperature of the patient does not at any time rise above the maximum for the day on which treatment was begun. This result is nearly always possible except in those rare cases in which the patient is under observation from the very beginning of the malady, when there may be a gradual rise for the first few days, in spite of all measures to the contrary, due to the development of the disease. But every case seen at so early a period ought to be brought to a favorable issue. 749

Most authorities resort to the bath whenever the temperature reaches 102°, even though this may require the application of the bath six or eight times a day. This rule 750 may be a good one for the first week, but after that time, in the author's opinion, the temperature may easily be kept at a lower point by the intelligent employment of efficacious measures, in harmony with the principles which have been pointed out, with less frequent applications.

By the end of the second week, the temperature is much more easily controlled than during the first week, and if the fever continues for three or four weeks, the heat-producing powers of the body may be so much reduced that the more vigorous applications must be employed with the greatest care, if not wholly interdicted, because of the readiness with which the patient's temperature may be made to fall. In these cases the prolonged graduated bath lowered to a temperature of 92° or 88° is sufficient to control the temperature. The cold enema, the hot evaporating sheet, and the wet-sheet pack are often to be preferred to stronger measures.

The temperature is more easily controlled in mild than in severe cases. Unnecessarily extreme or severe measures should not be employed.

When hydrotherapeutic measures are properly directed and efficiently administered, the effect upon the temperature will be not only to lower it at the time of the bath, but to cause it to fall for half an hour or more after the bath, the effect being apparent for two or three hours. When the temperature is excessively high (104°-106° and above) and when normal or nearly normal (99°-100°), it is very difficult to lower it; but febrile temperatures between 100° and 104° generally yield quite readily to the persevering application of suitable measures.

As a rule, one need not expect to see all the characteristic symptoms of typhoid or other grave fevers present when hydriatic measures are thoroughly employed from the beginning, since the course of the disease is likely to be so favorably modified that the worst symptoms will not appear. This is especially true of coma, delirium, and other adynamic and atonic symptoms.

Hemorrhages sometimes appear as the natural result of the separation of the sphacelated structures when the ulceration happens to involve vessels of considerable size, but the danger of hemorrhage is in nowise increased by hydrotherapeutic applications, neither is it a contraindication for the use of these measures, except as regards certain of the more severe general cold applications.

The influence of hydrotherapy in lessening the frequency of grave symptoms is clearly indicated by the fact that when the bath has been systematically and efficiently used in cases of extensive epidemics, the mortality has uniformly been reduced to a small fraction of the usual rate.

Hydrotherapy is entirely safe when judiciously employed, 751
and its use is free from serious objections; while the use of medicinal antipyretics is attended by many objectionable features, of which the following are but a few:—

1. In the use of antipyrin and other temperature-lowering drugs, the depression is usually followed by an elevation to a point higher than before.

2. The depression of temperature is short, and the patient's condition while under the influence of the drug is often one closely bordering on collapse. When the use of quinine as an antipyretic was advocated by Dr. Austin Flint, some twenty-five years ago, the author made trial of its use in comparison with baths, and found that though it produced a fall of temperature, the effect was very transient. Bouchard pointed out a few years later that after obtaining an antipyretic effect with quinine, the second dose, even though a large one, produced practically no effect unless a period of three days was allowed to elapse after the first.

Hydrotherapy shortens the duration of febrile disease, renders grave cases mild, and lowers its mortality from twenty per cent. to three or four per cent., or even less.

The numerous other advantages of the hydriatic method of dealing with all febrile disorders will be further discussed in other chapters of this work.

752 **Conditions in which there is Disturbance of the Heat-Regulating Functions with Depression of Temperature.**

As conditions of temperature depression are occasionally encountered in connection with the treatment of fevers, it is important to know their significance and the remedies which should be employed to combat them.

In conditions in which there is a depression of temperature while heat elimination is increased, it is evident that heat production must be, if not normal or less than normal, at least increased to a less extent than heat elimination. This is a condition which naturally results from exposure to a low temperature without proper protection. Prolonged profuse perspiration from any cause, particularly night sweats and the perspiration following the chill and fever of ague, is often a cause of subnormal temperature.

There may be a lowering of temperature with diminished heat production, and with either normal, diminished, or increased heat elimination. All these conditions are sometimes encountered in cases of starvation from obstruction of the esophagus and in cases of semi-starvation due to chronic indigestion with anorexia.

In surgical shock or severe vital collapse of any sort, we may find both heat production and heat elimination diminished.

In every case a careful inquiry should be made to determine as nearly as possible the relation of heat production and heat elimination to each other, to the normal degree of activity, and to the abnormal rise of temperature. All the symptoms and the conditions of the patient should be carefully considered, so that a correct judgment may be formed with reference to the therapeutic indications of the case, and that the appropriate remedy may be employed.

If a patient's temperature is subnormal because of excessive heat elimination, nothing more may be required than additional protection, a few blankets, hot water bottles, an elevation of the room temperature, hot drinks, the hot enema, and dry rubbing. The application of oil to the surface is a measure not to be neglected as one of the most efficient means of lessening heat elimination, so long as the body is covered.

If the temperature depression is due to colliquative sweating, hot saline sponging is indicated.

If the subnormal temperature is due to diminished heat production from the results of starvation from any cause, the remedy here again is clearly indicated,—such food must be selected as will furnish heat-supporting elements in abundant quantity and in a form easy of assimilation; nutritive enemas may be employed; and the patient should be given absolute rest, with sufficient protection, hot water bags, etc., to restore the balance between heat elimination and heat production.

Temperature depression from shock requires artificial heat, internally and externally. A large hot enema (**736**), fomentations to the spine (**729**), hot bags, hot blankets, and rubbing of the surface are especially indicated.

Contraindications for the Cold, or Brand Bath.

The cold bath is a measure capable of much mischief as well as much good. It is of the highest importance to understand its limitations and contraindications. The conditions which forbid its use or which render necessary the most extraordinary caution and circumspection in its employment, may be briefly stated as follows:— **753**

1. *Sweating.*—Under ordinary circumstances the presence of perspiration is evidence either that the febrile action is subsiding or that nature is doing all that can be done to lower the temperature and eliminate the toxin which is the disturbing element. **754**

In the disease known as sweating sickness a persistent high temperature long continued renders necessary the use of cold as a heart tonic and to promote vital resistance; it is not best, however, to resort to so severe a measure as the Brand bath. The desired effect may be secured by means of cold friction (**1209**). At first, water at the ordinary temperature (70° to 75°) should be employed, and the mitt should be moistened only, not filled with water, as in ordinary cases of fever. Care should be taken to apply the friction to small areas successively, and to secure reaction as quickly as possible, and to avoid provoking general chilliness. The application may be repeated every two or three hours, but two or three daily applications will be found sufficient in ordinary cases. If the application of cold friction to the whole surface is not well tolerated, it may be confined to the back and chest. The application to the chest stimulates the heart action in a most powerful manner, while the application to the back arouses the central nervous system, and promotes general vital resistance almost as much as an application to the general surface. The surface should be dried and rubbed before the cold mitt is applied.

755 2. *Goose-Flesh Appearance.*—This physiological evidence of chill and a lowered temperature of the blood is sometimes present when the internal temperature is several degrees above normal, as the result of the action of toxic substances in the circulation. This symptom indicates that there is a persistent contraction of the small blood-vessels of the skin which directly antagonizes heat elimination. To put a patient in such a condition into a bath at 65° F. or even at 75° is not only an irrational but a hazardous proceeding, and is as unnecessary as it is unwise. Every indication which would be met by the cold bath can be better answered by other perfectly safe and efficient means. Rubbing with the friction mitt moistened in water at a temperature of 60° to 70° is usually sufficiently exciting, but ice-water may be used when more powerfully excitant effects are required. The same precautions must be observed as when perspiration is present. It is always desirable to precede the cold friction by a fomentation or some other hot application to the spine. Cold friction produces reaction by a powerful thermic impression combined with the mechanical effect.

3. *Cyanosis.*—Here again the cold bath of Brand is decidedly contraindicated. This symptom is an indication that the movement of the blood is slowed as the result of cardiac weakness, and the heart is not prepared to sustain the shock of sudden and prolonged contact of cold water with the whole surface of the body, while the internal viscera, already profoundly congested in consequence of the cardiac inefficiency, would be endangered, especially the lungs, liver, and spleen. Administer a short hot bath, a hot enema, or a fomentation to the spine followed by cold friction, beginning with the chest, then the back, and last of all the legs. In these cases applications of cold by means of the friction mitt are of the greatest service, not only in lowering the temperature, but in stimulating cardiac action, arousing the peripheral heart to activity, exciting increased renal activity, and promoting oxidation and increased vital resistance. By its use most of the advantages of the cold bath may be secured, with none of its disadvantages. 756

4. *Pronounced Cardiac Weakness.*—The dicrotic pulse, marked weakening of the first sound of the heart, and especially the "pendulum" action of the heart, in which the two silent periods of the heart's action are equal or nearly equal, are indications of an asthenic state of the heart, in which it is wholly unprepared to meet the tremendous demands temporarily made upon it by placing the patient suddenly in a tub of cold water. By means of the cold precordial compress, hot and cold sponging of the spine, and general cold friction, the energy of the heart may be re-enforced and its work diminished by increased activity of the peripheral heart. Under this simple treatment the pulse rapidly improves, the temperature is lowered as the result of the increased movement of the blood, and the general improved appearance of the patient, his easier breathing, and the disappearance of various nervous symptoms afford evidence that he is better. 757

Areolar cyanosis following a local cold application is an indication of great cardiac weakness and impending

collapse, which may, by aid of this warning symptom, be foreseen and prevented by general cold friction and the
758 cardiac compress often repeated.

5. *Myocarditis.*— The remarks respecting cardiac weakness apply with added emphasis to conditions in which the heart is the seat of an inflammatory process, as in endocarditis, pericarditis, and especially myocarditis. The last-named complication, which is not infrequently encountered in typhoid and other continued fevers, especially requires circumspection in the use of the cold bath. The sudden inrush of blood attending a general cold bath may easily overwhelm a heart whose muscular structures are crippled by an inflammatory process, while its nerve centers are depressed by the toxins characteristic of the general maladies present. If such patients escape alive, notwithstanding the severe treatment to which they are subjected by overzealous disciples of the hydriatic method of dealing with febrile disorders, the fact must be attributed to the wonderful energizing properties of the cold bath, and the marvelous resources of nature.

759 6. *Intestinal Perforation.*—The cold bath, when employed from the beginning in typhoid fever, greatly lessens the liability to this grave complication. When begun late in the disease, however, perforation sometimes occurs in spite of the ameliorating influence of cold bathing. When the symptoms of perforation occur, the general cold bath must be suspended, as its use not only involves considerable disturbance of the patient, but powerfully excites intestinal peristalsis, thus increasing the dangers incident to the perforation. Cold friction to the chest, the cold precordial compress, and general cold friction, carefully applied, may be employed to meet pressing symptoms of heart failure or collapse, and to improve the patient's resisting powers.

760 7. *Peritonitis.*—It may be said of this complication, as of the preceding, that it rarely occurs in typhoid fever when the cold bath is systematically employed from the beginning. It is, in fact, practically unknown in such cases. When

present in connection with general fever, it is a contraindication for the general cold bath. Fomentations, revulsive applications, and the cooling compress may be applied to the abdomen, but the general cold bath is decidedly contraindicated. The prolonged tepid bath (88°)and the short hot bath followed by cold friction are suitable measures for meeting the indications to which the cold bath is applicable under other circumstances.

8. *Pleurisy and Pneumonia.*— Both of these conditions, 761
when occurring in connection with typhoid fever, smallpox, or any other continued fever, are a contraindication of the cold bath. The neutral bath, the hot bath followed by cold friction, the cooling pack carefully managed, and especially the cooling chest compress with fomentations to the chest every two or three hours, are proper hydriatic measures to be employed in connection with these complications.

9. *Tuberculosis.*— When this complication occurs in con- 762
nection with typhoid fever, as it occasionally does, or in connection with any other continued fever, the cold bath must be interdicted on account of the intense visceral congestion occasioned by it. The wet-sheet pack and cold friction with the mitt well filled with water when the temperature is high, are suitable measures for a case of this sort. The cooling chest compress should also be employed.

10. *Infancy.*— The immersion bath at low temperature is 763
contraindicated in infancy because of the small heat-making capacity of the young child and the large radiating surface as compared with the weight. The vital powers of an infant, that is, a child under seven years of age, are not sufficiently vigorous to react to the ordinary Brand bath. The tepid bath, the cooling pack, and cold friction are suitable measures for this condition.

11. *Old Age.*— The conditions in old age, while decidedly 764
different from those in infancy, also constitute a contraindication to the use of the cold bath. The presence of arteriosclerosis is always a contraindication for the cold bath, what-

ever the age of the patient. The condition of the arteries, rather than the number of years, constitutes the physical condition referred to in this connection by the term "old age." The inactive skin, the weak heart, the general sluggishness of the bodily functions, low vital resistance, the diminished heat-making capacity,—these conditions, characteristic of senility, afford sufficient grounds for forbidding the use of the Brand bath, even though the person is not advanced in years. The prolonged tepid bath, the repeated wet-sheet pack, cold friction, the rubbing wet sheet (reclining), cold water drinking, are the measures to be employed in old age. With proper management these procedures may afford as good results as those obtained from the use of the Brand bath, and without the danger involved in the use of this vigorous procedure.

765 12. *Late or Neglected Cases.*—While cold baths may be used with impunity in ordinary cases of fever in which the general resistance of the body is good, and before the vital forces have been depressed by the long continuance of the disease, this is by no means true in cases in which hydriatric treatment has been neglected during the first week or ten days of the malady; hence great care must be taken in the use of the cold bath in cases which come under observation at an advanced period of the disease. In these neglected cases the condition of the patient is generally one of great nervous exhaustion, with cardiac weakness, not infrequently beginning degenerations; the nerve centers are weakened through starvation and malnutrition and the long-continued action of the toxins characteristic of the disease; heat production is limited, while heat elimination is deficient through spasm of the surface vessels. Ataxia or adynamic symptoms are marked, and not infrequently these conditions are found associated. There is a tendency to hypostatic congestion of the lungs, and, indeed, this condition may be already present. The liver, spleen, and other viscera are intensely congested, their functions are thereby seriously impaired, and their structure

may be injured. To plunge such a patient into a bath at 65° to 70° and retain him there for 10 or 15 minutes will most certainly imperil his life. The tonic influence of cold is in the highest degree desirable, but the patient is too weak to react to so powerful an impression as is made by the contact of cold water with the entire surface of the body at the same instant. By means of partial cold rubbings applied to different portions of the body successively, the cutaneous circulation may be marvelously improved without increasing, even momentarily, internal congestion. By increasing the movement of the blood, and especially by producing a hyperemic condition of the skin, the internal congestion may be definitely relieved. The heart is reflexly energized at the same time its labor is lessened, by the increased activity of the peripheral heart accompanying the reaction resulting from the cold friction. Similar though vigorous effects may be obtained by rubbing the skin with dry, warm flannels. The prolonged neutral bath (92° to 95°) and a hot-blanket pack for 10 minutes, followed by cold friction, are the best measures for aiding heat elimination. Hot and cold sponging of the spine, or, better, the alternate hot and cold spray to the spine, produces an excellent effect upon the central nervous system. The bed-sores likely to be present in these late cases render the full bath inconvenient, but do not interfere with the application of packs, compresses, cold friction, and allied measures. The hot enema followed by cold friction is a most effective means for aiding heat elimination, through stimulation of the kidneys and arousing of the depressed energies of the patient to resist the disease.

In the management of these grave cases, in which the life of the patient depends so much upon the exact and judicious employment of effective therapeutic procedures, it is important to remember that death in these cases, when attributed to so-called heart failure, is really due to general collapse of the vital powers. The weak condition of the heart is a true index to the condition of the body as a whole. The heart continues its work until the body as a whole is ready to surrender, then fails with the rest.

It may be remembered with advantage, also, that cardiac weakness is not the only, nor always the chief, cause of the feeble circulation in adynamic conditions in fever. The blood movement depends upon several other important factors in addition to the cardiac activity: respiratory movements, rhythmical action of the small vessels, the caliber of the small vessels, the tone of the tissues, cell activity, the mass of the blood,—each and all of these factors may be modified by hydric applications over the heart and to the general cutaneous and mucous surfaces, as has been pointed out elsewhere.

A brief cold application to the skin stirs the whole bodily fabric to its deepest foundations. Every cell and fiber vibrates in response, so to speak, and quivers with a new life, a reinforced energy, which appears not only in the surface reaction which follows, but in the quickening of its own proper functions as well as improvement in the quality of the work performed. Tonic applications of water are the most effective of all known means for setting in motion and maintaining those renovating and restorative processes in which the recovery of the sick chiefly depends.

Secretory Sedative Effects Cold applications made in such a way as to lower the temperature of the secreting structures of a gland, produce an important and very marked diminuation in secretory activity while heat produces the opposite effect. The activity of the mammary glands may be by this means controlled to a remarkable extent, and salivary activity may likewise be to some degree influenced. The most striking illustration of this action is seen in the instantaneous control of profuse perspiration by cold application to the surface. The activity of an internal gland is reflexly excited by cold applications made upon the overlying skin. The opposite effect, or sedation, is produced by neutral and hot applications (92°-104°). Very hot applications may produce excitant effects allied to those resulting from cold applications.

GENERAL RULES, PRINCIPLES, AND SUGGESTIONS RELATING TO THE PRACTICAL EMPLOYMENT OF HYDROTHERAPY.

IN the employment of water as a therapeutic means, it is first of all important to keep in mind the principle that it is the patient, not his disease, who is to be treated. The fundamental idea in hydrotherapy, as with all rational measures of treatment, is that the curative force resides in the body, and that the office of the physician, aided by intelligent and trained assistants and nurses, and by the co-operation of the patient, is to supply such conditions as will aid the natural forces of the body in combating the disease. It is hence of the utmost importance that the general plan of treatment adopted for the relief of any particular case shall first of all take into account the causes by which the patient's maladies may have been induced. These will usually be found to exist in some wrong habits of life, of which the patient himself may have been wholly ignorant, at least as regards their deleterious character.

All cases of chronic disease may be roughly divided into 766
two general classes: —

1. Those in which the seat of the disease is a local irritation of mechanical or other origin, such as eye-strain, catarrh of the nose, stomach, liver, or bladder; or in which there is a local mechanical or tissue injury, as in dilatation or prolapse of the stomach, floating kidney, displacement of the pelvic organs, ulceration of the stomach, etc.

2. Those due to a diathesis, or a constitutional condition, as in diabetes, obesity, migraine, neurasthenia, chronic uric acid poisoning, Bright's disease, and the various degenerations.

In order, then, to form an intelligent idea of the proper course to be pursued in the treatment of any given case, there must be a careful scrutiny of the causes which have led up to it, and of the exact pathological conditions existing. For example, in indigestion we must ascertain with accuracy, in order to employ the proper measures, whether or not a patient is suffering from apepsia, hypopepsia, hyperpepsia, or simple dyspepsia, and whether or not there exists so-called chronic or subacute gastritis or a condition of increased or diminished sensory or motor irritability. Insomnia may be due to local irritation of some sort, to chronic toxemia, or to cerebral anemia or congestion. An anemia found present may be the result of a recent hemorrhage from a wound, of profuse menorrhagia, hemorrhoids, gastric ulcer, a surgical operation, a fever, tuberculosis, malaria.

General Directions for the Use of the Bath.

767 1. Before beginning a course of general applications of cold water, careful investigation should be made respecting the condition of the heart, the nervous system, the liver, the kidneys, and other viscera, so that all contra-indications may be at once apprehended and the proper allowance made therefor. It is also important to ascertain in each case a patient's reaction power by means of a partial cold bath of some sort, and by the dermographic test.

In very feeble patients, there may be sufficient nervous energy to react well when an application of cold is very limited in extent, but not enough to secure prompt and vigorous reaction when the application extends to the entire surface of the body; in such cases, the effects produced by the first bath should be carefully noted, and the prescription should be arranged in accordance with the indications thus obtained.

If any of the symptoms of imperfect reaction occur, those measures necessary to encourage reaction should be adopted, as elsewhere indicated (**443**). If the reaction is excessive, less strongly stimulating measures should be employed; that is, (*a*) raise the temperature a few degrees; (*b*) substitute a non-percutient form of bath for the douche, as a cold friction bath, a wet-sheet or a towel rub, a sitz, immersion, or affusion;

(*c*) have the patient exercise less long or vigorously before or after the bath; or (*d*) follow the cold application by a short cool or tepid non-percutient application, as a wet-sheet rub or affusion at 75° or 80° F., cover less warmly in bed, or otherwise modify the measures which promote reaction.

2. After short, very cold applications, watch carefully for the appearance of the bright-red color which indicates normal reaction. If this does not, under vigorous friction, appear within one minute or less, it will usually be found wise to precede the cold application by the hot rain or jet douche, hot bath, steam bath, or some other general hot application. The hot application should be continued from three to five minutes, followed by a cold application, when a good reaction will be assured, even in patients whose power in this direction is quite limited. The application of heat in this manner greatly diminishes the unpleasant impression of cold applications, while at the same time promoting to a high degree the circulatory reaction. After a very hot bath it is sometimes well to diminish the shock resulting from the contact of very cold water by an intermediate tepid or cool application.

3. *The Duration of Applications.*—The lower the tem- 768
perature of the water, the shorter should be the application.

For very cold applications, the duration should be 1 to 5 seconds. The duration of the cool douche may be 10 to 30 seconds.

Tepid, warm, and hot douches may be much more prolonged, especially when moderate pressure is employed. The duration may be from 1 or 2 minutes to 10 or 15 minutes.

Very hot applications should be of moderate length, rarely more than one minute.

When employed to reduce the temperature in fever, and for antiphlogistic effects, non-percutient, cool applications may be prolonged to 15 or 20 minutes.

The neutral bath may be continued as long as circumstances require. It may be made practically continuous for several months, if care is taken to regulate the temperature so carefully that thermic reaction is wholly suppressed. For sedative effects, from 30 minutes to 1 or 2 hours is the usual time required.

769 4. *The Temperature of Applications.*—In general, it should be the constant aim to train the patient progressively to react to water at as low a temperature as possible, the temperature of the water being steadily lowered day by day.

5. The best and most durable effects are produced by short cold applications, frequently repeated.

6. Long cold applications may be too exciting by producing a too strong reaction, or the effect may prove to be sedative or exhausting instead of tonic. This is especially true of emaciated and anemic persons, and those suffering from sclerosis. In emaciated persons the amount of fuel for heat production is diminished, and the amount of oxygen taken into the blood is also below the normal standard; hence the calorific, or heat-making, powers are deficient and easily exhausted, so that a too prolonged cold application may result in an excessive loss of heat, as indicated by delayed reaction, prolonged chill, or the frequent recurrence of chill or chilliness after the application.

7. In persons suffering from nervous exhaustion, especially, the reaction ability of the nerve centers is speedily exhausted; hence the importance of making cold applications very short in duration.

770 **The Therapeutic Significance of Reaction.** The phenomena of reaction under physiological and pathological states is a subject which must be thoroughly understood by the hydriatist. Elsewhere (**429–480, 577, 578**) the rationale of reaction under physiological conditions has been fully explained; here the subject will be considered briefly from the standpoint of practical therapeutics.

First of all, it may be remarked that a large share of the therapeutic applications of water require either the production or the suppression of reaction, or the production of atonic reaction effects. Hence it is of the utmost importance not only that every patient should be carefully studied in relation to his ability to react at the beginning of a course of hydriatic treatment, but that the reaction of the system to each different procedure employed, and to each daily application, should be carefully noted, and any necessary readjustment of the prescription made at once. Hydriatic treatment must be under the immediate supervision of a competent medically educated person, and must never be left to the inaccuracies of a bath attendant, no matter how well trained.

Conditions that Control Reaction.

The intensity of the reaction effects following 771
a given application depend upon —

1. The method of application, especially whether percutient or non-percutient (Exp. 53).

2. The temperature of the water.

3. The length of the application.

4. The condition of the patient, whether (*a*) febrile or non-febrile, (*b*) weak or strong, (*c*) fat or thin, (*d*) rested or fatigued, (*e*) warm or chilly.

5. The ability to develop animal heat.

6. The ability to repair quickly the loss of heat, and to support its loss without serious inconvenience to important vital processes.

7. The condition of the nervous system at the time of the application.

8. Whether accustomed to cold bathing.

9. The mental state of the patient, whether apprehensive and fearful, or resigned, cheerful, and in a condition of mind to co-operate with the treatment.

It is well to recall that in cases in which a patient does not react well to low temperatures, the reaction effect desired may be encouraged by strong friction or by increased pressure if the douche is employed.

Oscillatory Reaction.

Several oscillations of reaction are sometimes 772
observed following a cold bath, each recurrent reaction being weaker than the preceding. These oscillations are doubtless due to the swift rush

of blood to the skin during the first reaction, whereby it is rapidly cooled by evaporation from the moist surface which has perhaps been insufficiently dried, and also through the consumption of heat energy by its conversion into mechanical work by friction and exercise.

773 **Suppression of Reaction.** While it is usually the aim to promote reaction, there are cases in which the suppression of reaction (**432**) is of the highest importance. Sometimes reaction must be suppressed altogether,—when sedative effects are desired, as in cases of fever, inflammation, nervous irritability or insomnia, burns, wounds of various sorts, and hemorrhages. The means by which reaction may be diminished or increased have been fully described elsewhere (**443–459**).

EXERCISE IN CONNECTION WITH HYDRIATIC APPLICATIONS.

774 From the days of the earliest cold-water cures, the importance of exercise in connection with water treatment, especially applications of cold water, has been fully recognized. Priessnitz kept his patients sawing and chopping wood a considerable part of the time when they were not occupied with the multitudinous drinkings, packings, douchings, cold plunges, etc., to which they were subjected under the heroic regimen in vogue at Graefenberg. It is more than likely that a large share of the benefit obtained from treatment under the old water-cure system was the result of the muscular activity required in connection with the routine of baths to which each patient was required to submit himself. Extended trips along the steep paths of the neighboring mountains and hard work at the wood-pile were required of all patients able to endure any considerable degree of physical exertion, those who were not able to exercise being considered too weak to be subjected to cold-water applications. No doubt many persons were damaged by the excessive amount of muscular work required of them; but as a large

share of the patients who visited Priessnitz were persons of robust constitution who were suffering chiefly from the effects of high living, sedentary habits, and wine drinking, the measures employed were for the most part successful.

Exercise not only encourages circulatory reaction, but especially stimulates thermic reaction. It has been clearly demonstrated by experience that the temperature lowering which begins from five to fifteen minutes after a cold bath is continued and increased by exercise, so that the maximum diminution is fully half a degree greater with moderate exercise than without it.

Exercise before the Bath.

In persons able to take exercise, a sufficient 775
amount of physical activity to produce slight perspiration before a bath favors the tonic effect of the application, and re-enforces it to a very considerable extent. Care should be taken, however, to avoid profuse perspiration in feeble persons, for the result would be so great an expenditure of energy that both circulatory and thermic reaction might fail, producing a secondary chill and most unfavorable effects. The bath should be taken immediately after the termination of the exercise, and before there has been opportunity for cooling of the skin by evaporation, which takes place with great rapidity when the skin is exposed. If there must be even the slightest interval between the removal of the clothing and the administration of the douche, the body should be protected by wrapping in a blanket or Turkish sheet.

Exercise should not be sufficiently vigorous to induce excessive action of either the heart or the lungs, as a cold bath should never be administered when these organs are excited. The best forms of exercise are walking, Swedish gymnastics, bicycle riding, dumb-bell exercise, club swinging, self-resistive exercises,* and moderate exercise with chest-weights.

---

* For description of a system of self-resistive exercises, see paper by the author, in *Modern Medicine* for December, 1898.

Persons who are unable to take exercise may be prepared for a cold bath by massage, by vigorous friction, by manual Swedish movements, or by an application of heat.

A preparation by exercise, either active or passive, is to be preferred to a preparatory hot bath; but when necessary, the hot douche, hot immersion, vapor douche, Turkish bath, or best of all, the electric-light bath, may be employed. The electric-light bath is preferable to all other means of heating the skin, aside from exercise, for the reason that it quickly warms the skin, and does not produce a depressing effect. The douche should be applied before profuse perspiration has been induced.

Violent exercise should always be avoided, for the reason that the skin and the body become thereby so strongly overheated that the absorption of the surplus heat requires so prolonged an application of the cold douche or other cold application that the nerve centers are apt to be quite exhausted by the too strong reflex activities set up, especially in feeble persons, resulting in incomplete reaction and depression.

776 **Exercise after the Bath.** Imperfect reaction after the cold bath is in the highest degree injurious, and lack of knowledge as to how to avoid this exceedingly disagreeable and inconvenient accident is responsible for much of the prejudice existing against the employment of the cold bath as a hygienic or therapeutic measure.

Incomplete reaction not only frequently results in a secondary chill, but in successive chills or an almost continuous chill, not only for an hour or two, but often for several hours, after the bath. The hands and feet are cold, there is headache, not infrequently diarrhea, and other evidences of internal congestion, such as abdominal and ovarian pains, rheumatic pains in the joints, neuralgic pains in various parts of the body, vertigo, lassitude, and an increase of catarrhal discharge from the nose, throat, lungs, or other mucous surfaces, when there is actively present a catarrhal affection of these parts.

As a rule, exercise should always be taken after a cold bath when the patient is sufficiently strong to walk.

Reaction may be favored by covering the patient with blankets or surrounding him with hot-water bags or other means of artificial heating, or by his remaining in a warm room; but the reaction effects obtained are far less beneficial than those which result from exercise. The reason of this will appear when it is remembered that exercise favors thermic reaction, and that thermic reaction means activity, not only in the nerve-muscular thermogenetic apparatus, but in every cell and tissue of the body, and an exaltation of function.

The application of artificial heat, on the other hand, lessens thermic reaction by the atonic reaction effect which is connected with hot applications of all sorts. Thus exercise promotes the most efficient element of the reaction following cold applications when tonic and reconstructive effects are desired, viz., the thermic reaction, whereas artificial heat diminishes this most important factor.

Exercise immediately following the bath favors regular and complete circulatory and thermic reaction, thus increasing the fall of temperature, and making the bath more thoroughgoing and efficient in its effects upon the system. The fall of temperature produced by exercise following a cold bath may amount to nearly one degree Fahrenheit.

An interesting fact has been pointed out by Delmas, to which attention should be called in this connection. Increase of blood pressure, whether induced by exercise or other agents, ordinarily causes a slowing of the pulse-rate; but under the influence of cold, the increased blood pressure induced by stimulation of the heart and contraction of the peripheral vessels is accompanied by a quickened pulse.

The reason for this is obvious. When the blood pressure is raised by cold applications to the surface, nature increases the rate of the heart's action through the specific influence of cold upon the heart-regulating mechanism, so that an increased amount of blood may be carried to the surface, thus compensating, to some degree, for the diminished caliber of the surface vessels, and protecting the parts, so far as possible, from the evil effects of refrigeration. When reaction begins, and the blood pressure falls (though not below normal) with the dilatation of the surface vessels, the heart's action is slowed—the reverse of what ordinarily happens under diminished blood pressure.

The result of this slowing of the circulation is to delay reaction, which under ordinary conditions is desirable, for otherwise slight changes in the atmospheric temperature might result in excessive and exhausting perturbations of the nervous and vascular systems; as it is the purpose of therapeutic applications which promote reaction to produce systemic perturbations and metabolic and catabolic changes, it is desirable that the tendency to slowing of the heart's action, which sets in with the beginning of reaction, should be antagonized by means of exercise whereby the heart's action will be quickened and the blood promptly forced to the surface of the body.

The increased vascularity of the skin thus induced, encourages heat dissipation, and both thermic and circulatory reaction. If the exercise is moderate in degree, the heat elimination developed by it exceeds the heat production resulting from the muscular activity; but if it is too violent in character, heat production may be in excess of heat elimination, in which case there will be a rise in temperature, and the effect of the bath will be antagonized. It is thus apparent that exercise after a bath, in order to be effective and helpful, must be moderate in character.

Walking at a moderate rate for twenty to sixty minutes after a vigorous cold douche is the most generally useful form of exercise. Very vigorous exercise for a short time can not, however, be substituted for moderate exercise for a longer time, for the reason that time must be allowed for heat elimination; besides, vigorous exercise for even a short time might, by overexciting heat production, place the balance between heat production and heat elimination on the wrong side, and thus occasion a rise of temperature, and to a considerable degree destroy the good effects of the bath. It is for this reason, in the author's opinion, that better results are obtained from reaction when the process takes place regularly and slowly, as has long been known to be the case from clinical observation.

There are, of course, cases in which cold applications are indicated, but in which the patient is too feeble to take the necessary amount of exercise by walking or by other means. In such cases, vigorous massage, especially friction and percussion movements, or manual Swedish movements and deep breathing, may be employed until the return of warmth to the surface, indicating that active reaction has begun.

Occasionally cases are met in which the patient is so fee- 777
ble that he can not react spontaneously, even by the aid of massage, and it is necessary to employ artificial means to assist the reaction. The patient should be wrapped in a Turkish sheet as quickly as possible after the bath, covered with blankets, and dried by vigorous rubbing underneath the blankets. The moist sheet should be removed, the woolen blanket placed next the body should be tucked carefully around each limb and close about the neck, and hot bags placed to the feet and the sides, extra blankets being thrown over all. The patient must be carefully watched by observing the condition of the skin of the face, and noting the pulse, and the hot bags and blankets carefully withdrawn as reaction sets in, so that excessive reaction with sweating may be prevented, as this will destroy the tonic effect of the cold application.

Avoid Excessive Heat.

A rule which was insisted upon by Priessnitz, 778
and which is quite universally followed by hydrotherapeutists, is that the sun, excessive clothing, heated rooms, and especially stove heat or other artificial heat, should be sedulously avoided after a bath. By this artificial heating of the skin the heat elimination and

thermic reaction necessary for a general systemic vital perturbation, upon which the tonic and restorative effect of cold applications depends, are arrested before being fully developed by atonic thermic reaction.

Great care should be taken after a cold bath to avoid any circumstance or condition which will cause perspiration, which, when produced in any manner after a cold bath, is followed by an undesirable sedative effect, whereby vital resistance is lessened, the tonic effect desired is antagonized, and the patient is exposed to the risk of taking cold.

Many times patients imagine that they have taken cold in a bath from the application of cold water, when the untoward effects are really the result of either incomplete reaction after the bath or a reaction accompanied by perspiration.

A THOROUGH SCIENTIFIC EXAMINATION NECESSARY AS A FOUNDATION FOR A HYDRIATIC PRESCRIPTION.

779 1. A careful investigation of the urine is necessary in every case, not merely for the determination of the presence or absence of albumin, sugar, blood, urinary casts, or other morbid elements, but for the determination of the coefficient of elimination of nitrogenous wastes. Careful note must be taken of the relation of the total solids to the urea, as an indicator of the relative activity of destructive tissue processes.

2. An examination of the blood is essential for a determination of the color coefficient, the blood-count, and the relative proportion of white and red cells. It is also important, in cases of anemia, to note the relative proportion of the different varieties of white cells. There is no means by which the blood-count and the quality of the blood can be so profoundly and so quickly modified as by the resources of hydrotherapy.

3. Headache may mean cerebral congestion, cerebral anemia, or simple sympathetic nerve irritation. Fever may be the result of toxins of bacterial origin, as in typhoid fever, pneumonia, septic infection; or it may indicate the presence of an

excess of ordinary tissue poisons, or leucomains, either from diminished excretion, as from cold, or from overproduction, as in exhaustion or fatigue fever from muscular exertion. Neurasthenic symptoms of various sorts may be due either to the presence in excess of nitrogenous wastes, the so-called uric acid diathesis, or sympathetic irritation arising from enteroptosis.

4. Every case must be carefully investigated with reference to the existence of pathological changes, either functional or structural.

(1) The functional disturbances which it is especially important to note are hypopepsia, apepsia, or hyperpepsia; local congestion or irritation of the bowels, bladder, uterus, or ovaries; irritability of heart or lungs or sympathetic centers; cardiac weakness; catarrh of respiratory or digestive tracts; hyperesthesias of the skin, of the joints, or of the internal viscera. Each of these conditions requires special adaptation of the measures of treatment employed so as to avoid untoward effects which might at least discourage the patient, and not infrequently be the cause of more serious damage.

(2) Structural changes, such as those which are commonly found present in advanced cases of lithemia, in arteriosclerosis, Bright's disease, hepatic enlargement or sclerosis, must be carefully considered in arranging a hydrotherapeutic prescription. The same may be said respecting other structural changes, such as those found present in paresis or paralysis, from apoplexy or organic changes in the brain and spine; neuritis, chronic muscular spasm; epilepsy; chronic affections of the heart; varicose veins in the legs or other parts; fatty degeneration of the heart, liver, spleen, etc.

5. The general physical state of the patient must be considered: Is he fat or lean? Is he weak or strong? Has he a thin or a thick skin? Is he a person of resolution and strong will, or a weak-willed, irresolute individual? Is he of a persevering, reliable disposition? or is he unstable, vac-

illating, easily discouraged? The treatment must be carefully planned with reference to all these considerations.

780 **Physical Coefficients.** 6. It is of immense advantage to make a careful study of the patient's *physical coefficients.* By means of a graphic representation of the principal physical coefficients, more may be learned at a glance respecting the general vital capabilities and the physical peculiarities of a patient than by weeks of "cut-and-try" experience.* The chief practical deductions to be drawn from physical coefficients are the following:—

(1) A *high height-weight* coefficient indicates an excess of reserve tissue or fat, and hence ability to endure reducing or spoliative measures, if otherwise indicated.

(2) A *low height-weight* coefficient gives contrary indications as regards the prolonged use of tissue-wasting measures, though not forbidding their temporary or careful use.

(3) A *high strength-weight* coefficient may indicate either a deficiency of fat or an unusual muscular development. This coefficient must accordingly be considered in connection with the height-weight and strength-weight coefficients.

(4) A *high strength-weight* coefficient with *normal height-weight* coefficient, indicates a good foundation for thermic reaction to cold applications, a constitution not greatly impaired, nutrition well sustained.

(5) A *high strength-weight* coefficient with *high height-weight* coefficient indicates the ability to bear vigorous reducing measures and a probable constitutional predisposition to obesity, that ought to be combated by frequent sweating baths, followed by cold baths.

(6) A *high strength-weight* coefficient, with *low height-weight* coefficient, indicates that with a deficiency of reserve tissue and hence lack of ability for sustained resistance to cold applications, there is at least fairly good vitality and power to

*See paper entitled "Physical Coefficients," by the author, published in *Modern Medicine*, July, 1895.

effect a good reaction; but the cold applications must be short and not too frequent.

(7) A *low strength-weight* coefficient with a *normal height-weight* coefficient indicates diminished muscular and nervous energy and the need of great care in the use of hydrotherapeutic measures. Very short cold applications will be best borne, especially douches with high pressure. Hot baths and all spoliative measures must be avoided, except in cases of toxemia in which short sweating baths accompanied by copious water-drinking may be employed, especially the electric-light bath; but care must be taken to follow the hot application with a short cold douche at high pressure.

(8) A *low strength-weight* coefficient with a *high height-weight* coefficient indicates in general the need of spoliative measures, but small ability to bear general hot applications or sweating baths. There being good ability for sustained heat production, the patient should have frequent cold baths, with abundance of exercise. Sweating baths may be employed later, as the strength increases, and may be used at the beginning if very short, and not too frequently administered, provided the actual total strength of the patient is not much below the normal average for a person of his height, and provided also that the strength-weight coefficient is nearly normal.

(9) A *low strength-weight* coefficient with a *low height-weight* coefficient indicates a state of great debility and impairment of nutrition, little power to support either the sedative effect of hot baths or the calorification required by cold baths. Strongly tonic measures are needed, with careful avoidance of spoliative procedures; but the patient will tolerate cold badly and will be easily overstimulated. The very short hot douche will be invaluable as a preparation for the short cold douche. Neutral baths may be needed to encourage elimination without depression, also the cold hepatic and renal douches and the epigastric douche (cold in hypopepsia and hot in hyperpepsia).

(10) The *strength-height* coefficient is a good indication of the general neuro-muscular condition of the patient. A normal or *high strength-height* coefficient indicates a good store of nerve energy and good power of circulatory and thermic reaction, the muscles being the seat of the most active heat-making processes. The nerve tone and muscular development are good, and, unless otherwise contraindicated, all kinds of rational hydriatic means will be well tolerated.

(11) A *low strength-height* coefficient indicates a low state of nerve and muscular energy, little reaction power, and necessity for the use of all precautions in the arrangement of a hydriatic prescription. Tonic applications are specially needed, but any form of cold application must be preceded by a short hot application, preferably the hot douche or the electric-light bath. Strongly percutient measures must be used, or in the absence of a douche apparatus, cold friction or the wet-sheet rub may be employed. The patient should have vigorous rubbing after the bath to promote reaction, but should not be required to exercise very freely until the muscular power is considerably increased.

Other deductions may be drawn from physical coefficients, as will be obvious without further elucidation here.

781 **Adaptation to Individual Cases.** 7. The patient's physical aptitudes or temperament must also be carefully considered. Is he phlegmatic, nervous, or sanguine? Is he afraid of cold water, or has he any idiosyncrasy against it? Has he good powers of calorification; that is, has he good ability to endure cold, or does he become easily chilled by exposure to cold air or water? Has he good reaction powers? Determine this by a test (**480, 596**). Before prescribing treatment for a new patient, Priessnitz invariably made a careful examination of the skin, and was always present at the application of the first bath, noting carefully the intensity of the reaction produced and the rapidity with which it occurred. Although an empiric, he was a remarkably sagacious one, and his success was largely due to his acute powers of ob-

servation. For example, he reasoned that if chilling the feet will cause congestion and inflammation of the internal organs, there must be some important relation existing between these parts capable of use in the treatment of diseased parts. This he accomplished by studying and utilizing the principle of reaction.

8. It is impossible to make a routine prescription of hydriatic measures. These powerful agencies must be regulated with even greater nicety than medicinal agents, as the difference of a few degrees of temperature or a few seconds in the length of an application may not only negative the results expected, but produce results the very opposite in character, which, under some circumstances, might inflict irreparable injury upon the patient.

9. The patient's habits of life,—whether he has been accustomed to cold bathing and regular active exercise; what have been his habits as regards clothing, especially whether or not excessive clothing has been habitually worn; the length of time he intends to remain under treatment,—these and other kindred matters must be carefully considered.

Organotherapy and Symptomatic Treatment to be Avoided.

10. Before making a prescription in any case, 782
it is also necessary to determine which most requires immediate attention—some urgent symptom, or the fundamental morbid condition which furnishes the background for the pathological picture presented. In general, the treatment must be both palliative and curative. Patients generally need to be encouraged by the relief from distressing and annoying symptoms, even though the measures employed therefor may not be radically curative in their character; at the same time, there must be a systematic employment of those measures which, if perseveringly used, may ultimately result in abolishing the symptoms altogether. It is above all things important to avoid falling into the error of making the course of treatment merely a running fight with the ever-changing symptoms presented in most cases of chronic disease.

Of all the so-called systems of treatment which have appeared and disappeared within the last century and which have been so prolific with novel medical ideas, "organopathy" has perhaps the least to commend it to rational consideration. Dyspeptics never get well by the treatment of their stomachs only; neurasthenics never get well by the treatment of their nerves alone. Equally futile is the exclusive treatment of the skin in most forms of cutaneous disease. It is the patient himself who is sick, not some circumscribed portion of his anatomy. The organ which seems to be the chief seat of the disorder is simply that portion of the body which, being the point of least resistance, suffers greatest disturbance of structure or function, or both, and thus becomes the medium through which the morbid condition is most distinctly expressed.

Patients usually clamor for the relief of those symptoms which most urgently obtrude themselves upon their attention, and judge of their progress toward recovery by the extent to which a chronic pain, a palpitation, a gastric acidity, a chronic discharge, or some other definitely recognizable symptom, is relieved by the measures of treatment employed.

The fact that certain symptoms, and, in particular, painful symptoms, such as neuralgia, migraine, and nervous attacks, which have been aptly termed "nerve storms," sometimes become more frequent during the first few weeks of treatment, often presents a perplexing problem to the inexperienced hydriatist, and occasions him much inconvenience because of the necessity of maintaining the patient's courage, so that he may be induced to persevere in his efforts. But that some patients under a course of treatment by physiological measures which are addressed to the removal of causes, the reconstruction of disordered tissues, and the reorganization of disordered functions, must thus pass through a period in which many symptoms and various functional disturbances appear to undergo a temporary exacerbation, is a matter of common observation.

Exaggeration of Symptoms under Treatment.

In French and German hydropathic estab- 783
lishments the more experienced patients often encourage novices with the remark, "You must expect to feel worse before you feel better." After carefully studying this question in thousands of cases during a quarter of a century of experience in the use of hydriatic measures, the author feels confirmed in the view which he formulated many years ago; namely, that this exaggeration of symptoms and the occasional appearance of symptoms quite new must be attributed to the intensity of the visceral activity set up by the strong stimulation of the sympathetic nervous system produced by hydriatic applications. This being true, it is evident that the increased intensity of symptoms occurring within the first few weeks after the patient begins a course of treatment need not necessarily be regarded as an indication that he is getting worse, or that his treatment does not agree with him. It is only an indication that the treatment is producing a powerful effect upon the system, and that a reorganization of functions and forces is taking place.

Haig has observed that when a highly nitrogenous diet is exchanged for a strictly non-flesh diet in a case of chronic migraine, for example, there is likely to be, within the first few weeks, an increased frequency in the occurrence of the paroxysms. This he explains by the supposition that a change in the character of the blood results in the dissolving out of the tissues of a larger amount of uric acid, which, being brought into the circulation, irritates the nerve ends with which it comes in contact, particularly those of the sympathetic, thus giving rise to recurrence of the paroxysms.

This explanation seems rational, and the principle may aid us in explaining the exaggeration of other unpleasant symptoms which not infrequently occurs during the first few weeks of a systematic course of hydriatic treatment. Whatever the explanation may be, experience shows that if the patient can be induced to persevere, and the treatment is properly managed, the unpleasant symptoms soon disappear, and usually do not reappear, although it sometimes happens that they disappear in an oscillatory manner, being less pronounced at each reappearance until they finally pass away entirely. This is likely to be the case with such disorders as epilepsy, hysteria, periodical migraine, chronic malarial affections with intermittent paroxysms, and other maladies in which periodicity is more or less marked.

It is well to encourage patients to dwell less upon symptoms and to consider more the fundamental morbid conditions out of which they grow. Symptoms are nothing more than the leaves and fruit of the pathological tree, the roots of which are deeply seated in the intimate recesses of the tissues, and consist in disturbed nutritive processes.

If too much attention is given to the treatment of symptoms, the results may be so great exhaustion of the vital resources of the patient that he will not be able to respond to the more thoroughgoing measures which look toward the actual eradication of his real malady.

Let us suppose, for example, that a patient is suffering from spinal irritation, a pain in the region of the liver, epigastric pain or tenderness, or from general muscular pain. He finds applications of heat very comforting; indeed, the Turkish bath, the hot spray bath, fomentations, the hot bag to the spine, and similar measures afford such great comfort that the patient is likely to resort to them to such an extent as to suffer seriously from the depressing effects of heat; while, on the other hand, cold applications may temporarily aggravate some of these symptoms in spite of the greatest care that can be exercised. The patient will naturally feel very sure that hot applications do him good, and that cold applications do him harm; whereas, the former afford only temporary relief, while the latter, by increasing the general nerve tone, improving the character of the tissue processes and of visceral activity, are laying the foundation for ultimate cure. No small degree of tact, scientific knowledge, and intuitive judgment are required so to combine local and systemic measures with palliative and systematic treatment that the greatest degree of comfort to the patient shall be secured simultaneously with the most rapid progress toward recovery.

It must not be forgotten, however, that though symptoms are only the voice of nature declaring the existence of pathological conditions, yet the intensity of a symptom or of a group of symptoms is, on the whole, the best measure of the pathological state which gave rise to it; so that one can not consistently say to a patient for an indefinite period that the condition which gives rise to a certain symptom is being removed when the symptom itself is steadily becoming more pronounced. No encouragement even should be given unless there is some reliable diagnostic means or data at hand whereby the fundamental pathological condition in question may be measured, and an improvement definitely recognized.

There are also cases in which symptoms may be so urgent in character as to require, for the time at least, the principal or even exclusive attention of the physician, as in the hemorrhage of pulmonary tuberculosis, ulcer of the stomach, hemorrhoids, metrorrhagia, or menorrhagia. In many cases, also, fever, though ordinarily demanding attention only secondarily, reaches so high a point that vital damage is threatened, making this the capital feature which should attract the attention of the physician, just as a carpenter engaged in repairing the roof of a house or in replacing a shattered window or door, might leave his work to assist in putting out a fire on the premises.

Why Real Progress Must be Slow.

11. In the organization of a plan of treatment 784
in a given case, it is necessary to determine not only the course of treatment to be employed, but the length of each treatment and the number of daily applications, and the time of day when the applications should be made. The settlement of each of these questions depends upon the object to be accomplished by treatment, upon the mode of treatment employed, upon the strength and susceptibility of the patient, etc.

A general plan should be made also respecting the length of time during which the course of treatment is to be continued. If the patient can devote but a few days or a few weeks to treatment, the plan employed may be quite different from that which would be pursued if he were willing or able to devote a sufficient amount of time to render possible a more thoroughgoing renovation of his system and reorganization of his vital processes.

Patients should be made to appreciate the fact that in the employment of rational and physiological measures of treatment, the co-operation of the system is required; that whatever real progress is made is the result of a growth which takes place within the body, just as growth takes place in a tree or a flower. Recovery from a chronic disease is simply the growing out of a condition of disease into a state of health. Time is required for the development of health just as for the growth of a crop of grain. The physician tills the soil and plants the seed, to use an agricultural illustration, but nature grows the crop; and the patient must be content to wait for the harvest.

It may be said, however, for the encouragement of patients, that in not a small proportion of cases, immediate relief is experienced from those symptoms which have occasioned the greatest distress and inconvenience. There is certainly no therapeutic agent, or class of agents, which so promptly affords such real and permanent relief as may be obtained from the diversity of the resources of hydrotherapy.

If there is at first an increase in intensity of symptoms, it is usually due to the leaving off of opiates, hypnotics, medicinal tonics, and other remedies which have simply obscured the patient's condition by hiding his symptoms; in other words, by silencing the voice of nature, of which pain and a vast number of other symptoms recognized as evidence of disease, constitute the vocabulary. An opiate may cure a pain, but it does not remove the cause of it; and when it is withdrawn, the patient will of course be made to appreciate his real condition. The brief interval which elapses between the withdrawal of symptom-obscuring remedies and the amelioration of symptoms which come from the accumulation of hydriatic applications is sometimes a pretty severe ordeal for the patient to pass through; but with proper moral support and encouragement, he may be carried along until he begins to appreciate for himself that he is making real, not fancied, progress toward health, that the fetters of his morbid condition are being loosened, and that he himself is being reconstructed upon a sounder foundation — that he is growing out of disease into health.

If the patient can remain under treatment but a few days, or two or three weeks, perhaps the best that can be done for him is to teach him how to correct his wrong habits of life, how to adjust diet, exercise, work, etc., to the morbid conditions which exist in his system, how to employ such palliative means as will give him some relief, and encourage him to continue in a direction which may ultimately result in his cure. Moderately tonic measures may be added, but measures of treatment calculated to produce a high degree of perturbation, such as frequently repeated very cold applications, strongly eliminative treatment, and other powerful measures, should be used only with the very greatest care.

With patients who are undertaking a systematic course of treatment for tonic effects, applications should be made daily, in some cases twice daily, very rarely three times a day. In acute disorders, applications may be repeated hourly, or many times a day, as when antipyretic effects are sought, and in many instances continuous treatment is required, especially when local antiphlogistic effects are desired.

12. Patients should be taught that they can not usually expect to realize the best results of treatment during the first few weeks. If there is no unpleasant exacerbation of symptoms, there may be no diminution in the intensity of the chronic symptoms for some time, a fact which is often a source of great discouragement to the patient.

It is astonishing, however, how obstinate and distressing symptoms will in some cases seem to disappear all of a sudden, after many weeks in which there has been no perceptible change for the better. In many instances, a patient who has been under treatment for several months without apparent relief, will arise on a certain morning entirely free from annoying symptoms which have been incessantly present for months or even years. Sometimes this result will take place after only a few weeks of treatment. In one case, a patient who had suffered for several years with pain in the back, after a few weeks' treatment, while bending forward one day, felt, as he expressed it, a sudden "letting up" in the back, and from that moment he was entirely free from the pain which had obstinately resisted the efforts of the most eminent physicians of the United States and Europe. And this relief was permanent.

It is not easy to explain what happens in a case like this; nevertheless, in this instance something did happen which brought deliverance to the patient; and the thing which happened was without doubt the sudden culmination of the beneficial effects which had been developed during the preceding weeks of treatment. Chronic symptoms often yield to therapeutic blows persistently administered by the physician, just as does the rock to the sledge-hammer of the stone-mason. Even after long and persistent hammering upon the same spot, there may be no evidence of progress; but at the very next blow the rock may be shattered. It is true, however, that in a majority of cases gradually progressive relief from symptoms is experienced from the first.

It is very important for the permanency of the effects obtained that the patient under treatment for chronic disease should continue treatment until there has been a disappearance of all the symptoms of his malady, and not only this, but until the body has been so fortified by an increase of its vital resistance that the symptoms will not again return, provided, of course, that the patient pursue such a course of life regarding diet, exercise, and other matters of regimen, as his particular malady may require.

13. It is important for the physician, as well as for the patient, to remember that chronic disease is rarely entirely cured; in fact, we may almost say that a complete cure of a chronic malady never occurs. The symptoms may disappear, but the patient's constitution has been permanently weakened in certain directions, so that his condition is analogous to that of a steam-boiler which has been strained by overpressure. There is a weak spot somewhere, which is likely to give way, and it can not be safely used except at low pressure. A person who once succumbs to the causes of chronic disease will ever afterward be liable to another break-down of the same sort. Hence, he should sedulously guard himself against those causes which his system has lost the power to resist.

The chief benefits to be derived from a course of hydro therapeutic or other rational treatment are the result of constitutional changes which require a considerable length of time for development, and consequently the best results of treatment are not experienced for some time, often many months, after it is begun.

Not infrequently, in fact, the patient does not really appreciate the full benefit which he has received until some months after the course of treatment has been discontinued. This, however, should not lead the patient to abbreviate his course of treatment, which is almost certain to be quite too limited, but should rather encourage him to lay a broad foundation in a prolonged and thoroughgoing course, which may be expected to develop large and excellent results subsequently, when the processes of regeneration of tissue and reorganization of function have been completed by those natural curative forces within the body which it is the purpose of rational hydriatic treatment to organize and set in operation.

It sometimes happens that the prolonged use of tonic measures results in a condition of nervous weakness following a period of apparent marked improvement. In such a case, the treatment should be at once suspended or modified; but the same measures should be again employed as soon as the evidences of therapeutic overwork have passed away. Often patients feel so much improved, when such a suspension of treatment takes place, that they imagine that the treatment has been doing them harm, and that they are better off without it than with it. They should be made to understand that the improvement experienced after the suspension of treatment is but the legitimate result of the therapeutic applications made, and that it is simply a foretaste of the greater improvement and permanent benefit which they will experience later as the result of the internal vital work which it is the purpose of the treatment to organize and maintain.

It is, most of all, important to keep always before the patient the great fact that disease is only normal vital energy manifested under abnormal conditions. When a sick person recovers, it is by the operation of forces within him, the same forces by which the ordinary processes of growth and repair are carried on. Nature, not the doctor, heals. The healing agency is within the man, not outside of him. No new force or principle comes into operation in the struggle of the body under the abnormal conditions which we call disease. The disease itself is not the thing to make war upon; it is rather the causes of disease which we should combat. The chief concern of the physician, then, should be to discover and remove the causes which have made his patient ill, and to aid, by supplying favorable conditions, the remedial effort which constitutes the pathological picture we call disease.

GENERAL INDICATIONS AND CONTRAINDICATIONS.

As suggestive of the general principles of adaptation of methods to cases, the following observations may be made: —

Anemic patients require short cold treatment. Special care should be taken to see that the patient is warm when the treatment is applied. Long hot baths should not be administered, however, because of their exhausting effects. A short exposure of one or two minutes in the electric-light bath, just long enough to heat the skin thoroughly, is an excellent preparation for a cold application in the case of a pale, bloodless patient. The short hot shower and other heating measures may also be employed.

Nervous Disorders.

Feeble neurasthenics, patients who are ex- 785
hausted by loss of sleep or other causes, chronic inebriates, and cases of hysteria with emaciation and general feebleness, require such moderate measures as the Scotch douche, cold friction, the wet-sheet rub, the affusion, or the full bath at a moderate temperature. Affusion constitutes an excellent method in these conditions.

An excellent measure in many cases is a bath at 92° to 96° F. for 10 minutes, 103° for 2 to 3 minutes, followed by affusion at 80°, four to six pails.

Cases of neuralgia, myalgia, painful congestions, chronic 786
rheumatism with painful joints, require the Scotch douche or very short (2 to 3 secs.) cool douches. All douches must be avoided in cases complicated with neuritis, or tenderness. Such cases require fomentations, the heating compress, and half-baths at 85° to 78° F.

What is required is thorough circulatory reaction without thermic reaction; hence measures involving strong percussion should be employed. Cold baths should in these cases seldom be employed alone, but must be preceded by heat, the succeeding cold application being short, or just long enough to remove from the skin the surplus heat absorbed.

In the case of very sensitive and timid persons, treatment should be begun with the very short cold douche or the Scotch douche. An excellent plan of dealing with these cases is to make the patient stand in a hot foot bath while the temperature of the water is increased until the heat is almost unendurable, and the patient can hardly stand still. The heat impression made by the foot bath thus administered is so generalized that a short application of cold may then be simultaneously made without occasioning much inconvenience or complaint.

787 If cold applications cause unpleasant after-effects in very sensitive patients, the method should be modified by employing less force, using non-percutient measures, or employing a higher temperature, as for example, 70° to 80° instead of 60° to 70° F., or a lower temperature. Some authorities recommend in such cases that the bath be prolonged, instead of moderated in temperature; but the author's experience has been that the longer the application in such cases, the more intense the unpleasant after-effects. Where the douche is not well tolerated, a wet-sheet rub, cold friction, a sponge bath, the graduated Scotch douche, or a tepid immersion bath may be advantageously employed.

788 Neurasthenics and persons suffering from enteroptosis with extreme irritability of the lumbar ganglia of the abdominal sympathetic can not endure a cold douche to the abdomen. A hot douche without pressure may be employed, and cold friction with the hand or with a towel, but percutient measures must be avoided.

789 Hypochondriacs are often very sensitive, and unable to bear the cold douche. In such cases the neutral bath should be employed, the patient being gradually trained to water at a lower temperature until a short cold application can be tolerated. Cold friction, the tepid affusion, the cool wet-sheet rub, and finally the Scotch douche may be applied. The same is true of opium habitués.

In very nervous persons the irritable state of the reflex

and automatic centers is indicated by palpitation of the heart, a sense of weight in the chest, by prickling, numbness, and other peculiar sensations, wandering pains, headache, and malaise after cold treatment. In certain persons it is not infrequently difficult to avoid such effects altogether. It is advisable in some cases to precede the use of the douche in its various forms by a period of training by means of cold friction, the towel rub, the short wet-sheet pack, and the wet-sheet rub. The temperature should not be low, and the towel or sheet employed should be wrung as dry as possible, so that the effect of the cold applications may not be too prolonged. Short affusions, a very short douche applied to the spine only, or to the spine and legs, with very light pressure and of moderate temperature (60° to 80° F.), the Scotch douche, or the hot bath in some form for 3 or 4 minutes prior to the cold application, are other measures which may be recommended.

If short cold applications are not well borne, a slightly 790
higher temperature should be used, with stronger percussion. This method is preferable to that suggested by Beni-Barde and others; viz., to attempt to avoid the excitant effects of short, very cold applications by increasing the duration of the application, and thereby producing a slight sedation, or lessened excitation. While this method seems to be theoretically rational, in practice it fails; for the sensitive patient who can not tolerate a short cold application because of too great reaction, generally fails to react well to a longer application, and thus suffers greater inconvenience than from the short cold bath. The better plan is to raise the temperature and increase the pressure. This secures a good circulatory reaction, with a less intense sensory stimulation.

Cardiac Diseases.

The presence of cardiac disease, either as a 791
complication or otherwise, especially demands consideration in the adjustment of a course of treatment. In cases of cardiac hypertrophy with overcompensation, and in cases of functional irritation of the heart,

all extremes of temperature should be avoided. Neutral baths are indicated. The patient may be trained to endure a douche at 75° to 85° F.; but in administering it, care should be taken to begin at the feet, each day rising a little higher, until the upper portion of the body is reached. The chest, and especially the precordia, should always be avoided.

In cases of weak heart the general indication is for baths at 85° to 90° F. for 5 to 10 minutes, accompanied by friction, followed by the short Scotch douche at 104° for 1 or 2 minutes, a cold douche at 75° for 10 to 12 seconds, the water being allowed to fall upon the legs, back, and arms only.

792 In the treatment of cases of organic cardiac disease, it is important to observe which of the four phases of the disease the patient presents, and to this end the following queries should be answered; viz.:—

1. Is cardiac irritability present?

2. Is there incipient dilatation of the heart, as shown by loss of power in the cardiac muscle?

3. Have the small arteries lost, or are they beginning to lose, their contracting power, as indicated by edema of dependent portions of the body?

4. Are there evidences of lesions in the viscera, such as passive congestion or hypertrophy of the liver, congestion of the stomach, etc.?

In cases in which excessive compensation exists, exciting measures must of course be avoided; whereas in the opposite class of cases, in which the vessels have lost their power to contract, there is likewise a loss of ability to react; hence vigorous cold treatment can not be successfully employed except in a limited way.

Cold applications, when used, should be applied to small areas by means of the friction mitt or a towel wrung very dry from very cold water, and the application should be accompanied by vigorous friction. When made in this way, cold applications may sometimes be employed with advantage in exciting a weak heart to increased activity.

Very hot and very cold applications should be avoided in cases of cardiac disease with aortic insufficiency, in which sudden death sometimes occurs, having in a few instances been occasioned by a cold douche or exposure to excessive heat in the Russian bath. In aneurism of the aorta, in advanced arteriosclerosis, and in apoplexy, the same precautions must be observed. Very hot baths should be avoided in aortic stenosis. Non-percutient measures are best in these cases, and moderate temperatures only should be used.

In *Bright's disease* and other forms of renal disease, very 793
cold treatment must be avoided; but short very hot applications are valuable, especially in acute nephritis.

Very *fleshy persons* do not at first react so well as lean persons, but they bear prolonged treatment much better, in consequence of their large heat-making resources. Lean persons react well, but their powers of reaction are quickly exhausted; hence they are more likely to suffer from secondary chill and untoward results.

Thick-skinned persons of phlegmatic temperament readily tolerate the very cold douche and a very high pressure; that is, if no contraindicating symptom is present.

The Field of Hydrotherapy.

Cold water as a therapeutic agent is especially 794
adapted to the treatment of *acute maladies* in which fever or pain is present or in which diminished activity or overactivity of special organs is a fundamental condition.

It must be remembered that cold applications with percussion should be avoided when acute inflammation is present, as the strong reaction set up by an application of this sort will surely give rise to exaggeration of the condition. Very hot applications followed by tepid compresses are more serviceable in cases of this sort.

Hydriatic measures may always be employed with great advantage in *chronic disease*, the tonic effects of cold water being almost universally required in the treatment of these maladies.

795 Surgical cases involving *pain, fever, or danger of inflammation,* such as compound fractures and wounds of various sorts; burns, scalds, and many other kinds of accidents and injuries, afford most excellent opportunity for the therapeutic employment of water.

Those who have assigned to hydrotherapy a more limited sphere of usefulness than that here claimed for it have been led to this narrowness of view by the failure to recognize to the fullest extent the great advantages to be obtained by employing a wide range of temperatures.

Hydrotherapy is especially helpful in the treatment of *fevers* from whatever cause, there being no other means by which a febrile action may be more quickly or permanently controlled than by the scientific employment of water.

796 The modern science of *obstetrics* owes much to hydrotherapy in a variety of ways. The proper use of water during the lying-in period greatly assists in conducting both mother and child through the perils of this critical period, and in quickly restoring the patient to a normal condition. The author is hardly prepared to adopt the cold sitz bath immediately after delivery, as recommended by Pingler; but during twenty-five years of the practical use of hydrotherapy in obstetrics, he has found it of invaluable service, especially in the form of the hot vaginal douche, the hot uterine douche, the enema, the daily sitz bath as a preparatory measure, the neutral bath to relieve nervous irritability and insomnia (both before and after confinement), and cold friction as a general tonic.

797 *Organic degenerations* are of course incurable, but by the appropriate use of water their progress may often be greatly delayed, and not a few instances have occurred in which the degenerations which accompany locomotor ataxia, general paresis, etc., have been so entirely arrested as to be held in abeyance for years. Whatever develops general vital vigor and resistance must delay the development of degenerative processes, malignant as well as non-malignant.

In organic disease of the brain and spinal cord, an arrest of the disease may often be accomplished, and it is rare indeed that some benefit is not obtained in cases of this sort.

Brilliant results could scarcely be expected in cases of hyperplasia or hypertrophy, and yet even in these conditions marked improvement has not infrequently been effected, atrophied parts having been stimulated to renewed development, so that functions almost entirely lost were restored.

There is no more useful agent than hydrotherapy in 798
dropsy due to *chlorosis*, *anemia*, and other *cachexias*. When caused by disease of the heart or kidneys, hydrotherapeutic applications are still highly useful, but must be employed with the greatest circumspection.

Hemorrhages from the nose, stomach, lungs, or pelvic viscera may be successfully combated by suitable applications of water, as elsewhere explained.

In *gastric disorders*, hydrotherapy affords more assistance 799
than any other remedial agent. The cold douche in hypopepsia and apepsia, and the hot douche in hyperpepsia meet the indications of these morbid conditions in a more effective manner than any other known therapeutic agent, the cold douche increasing the production of HCl, while the hot douche diminishes the formation of this acid in cases in which it is already present in excess.

The cold douche applied to the abdomen stimulates intestinal peristalsis, and thus combats constipation.

Genito-urinary and renal disorders present many condi- 800
tions which are in the highest degree amenable to hydriatic treatment. The sitz bath, rectal irrigation, the vaginal and uterine douches, the pelvic pack, the fan or jet douche, and general tonic applications are invaluable in this class of disorders. It must be remembered, however, that general cold applications must be avoided or greatly modified when acute inflammatory conditions are present in the pelvic organs or any other of the viscera. Cold friction (1209) is about the only tonic measure permissible in these cases.

801 *Pulmonary disorders* present a large variety of conditions in which hydriatic applications are capable of rendering invaluable service. It is important to remember, however, that very cold general applications must be carefully avoided in most cases of this sort. For example, in the application of the cold douche in a case of chronic bronchitis or where there is a tendency to pulmonary hemorrhage, the application should be confined to the feet and legs. A moist pack applied to the chest is a most valuable measure, which may be supplemented by cool sponging of the upper parts of the body, followed by vigorous rubbing.

802 In *catarrhal affections* of the throat and lungs, the heating compress may be applied systematically to great advantage, but care must be taken not to cover it too warmly, thus producing the effect of a poultice, which is highly sedative and relaxing. A healthy skin is an indication of a healthy mucous membrane, and disorders of the mucous membrane may not infrequently be caused to disappear by the employment of tonic means calculated to bring the skin into a thoroughly healthy condition.

803 In *affections of the skin*, neutral baths are often of the highest service. In scaly eruptions, the curative value is enhanced by adding alkalies to the bath. The tepid douche may also be employed with advantage in many cases. Skin eruptions are usually due to general toxemia. The enema and hot-water drinking should be freely employed as a means of tissue cleansing. Cold baths must be avoided.

In *chronic eczema*, with thickening of the skin, the daily hot douche to the affected parts has proved a most effective means of restoring the diseased parts to a normal state.

In cases of skin disease in which a considerable portion of the skin structure is destroyed, as in pemphigus, the prolonged neutral immersion bath of Hebra may sometimes be employed with great advantage. In some cases of this sort patients have remained in the bath for several months.

The *diatheses* and *cachexias* especially require the alterative and tonic effects of hydrotherapy, yet the lowered vital tone existing in these morbid states requires that great care be exercised.

The three leading diatheses, which are typically repre- 804
sented by *chronic rheumatism*, *obesity*, and *diabetes*, all present as their characteristic feature, deficient oxidation. In the rheumatic diathesis there is a deficient oxidation of the proteid wastes; in diabetes, a deficient oxidation of sugar; and in obesity, deficient oxidation of fat.

The cold bath excites oxidation, and hence is especially indicated in these cases; but there being, at the same time, diminished vital resistance, lowered nerve tone, and lessened ability to react in consequence of the prolonged perversion of nutrition, through exposure to the influence of depressing toxic agents and retained excrementitious matters, tonic measures must at first be administered with great care, and the patient must be trained by carefully graduated applications to react to the contact of cool water.

Obese patients require cold baths, followed by prolonged moderate exercise, to energize the muscles and lower the body temperature. Rheumatics require hot, sweating baths, followed by very short cold baths and exercise.

Diabetics, if emaciated, require long neutral baths. Very hot and very cold applications should be avoided. If the patient is in good flesh and strong, the Scotch douche, the short cold douche (4 to 8 secs.), short cold immersion (2 to 3 secs.), and other cold applications are admissible and advantageous, especially if immediately followed by moderate exercise.

In the training of feeble patients to the use of cold water, either one of two methods of training may be adopted. In some cases it is necessary to apply first one and then the other. The first of these is —

The Method of Graduation.

If some form of douche is the mode of appli- 805
cation selected, the water should be employed at a moderate temperature, as 80° to 85° F. The application should be 10 to 20 seconds, and followed by

energetic friction. From day to day, as the patient's nerve tone increases, the temperature may be gradually lowered to 65° or even 60° F. As the temperature is lowered, the time of the application should be shortened, until at 60° it should not be more than 6 to 10 seconds, and at 55°, 3 or 4 seconds.

In obese persons who still have a moderate amount of energy, a somewhat lower temperature may sometimes be reached after long training. The same is true in reference to diabetic patients who are still in good flesh and in whom there is no marked tendency to emaciation.

In the rheumatic diathesis, and in persons who are very sensitive to cold, we may begin with the tepid douche at 85° to 90°.

In cases in which the percussion effects of the douche are badly tolerated, non-percutient measures may be at first employed, such as affusion at 80° to 85°, the wet-sheet rub at the same temperature, the immersion bath for 3 minutes at 85° to 90°, with friction, the sitting shallow at 80°, the towel rub, and cold friction.

It should ever be borne in mind that in beginning a course of treatment it is better to commence with too moderate than with too severe measures, as otherwise the patient is likely to become discouraged and lose confidence. Moderate applications two or three times a day may be made to accomplish the same results as a more severe procedure daily.

806 **Training by the Scotch Douche.** A second method of training for the cold bath is preliminary heating of the skin followed by a very short cold application. This succeeds in some cases better than the method of graduation. Reaction as a rule develops more promptly and regularly after a short cold or very cold application than after a prolonged application of higher temperature. For many patients also an application at 75° to 80° is quite as disagreeable as a colder one. It is consequently advisable in some cases to begin with the application of cold or very cold water at the

outset, but making the application so short in duration that untoward effects are obviated. The preliminary heating of the skin greatly diminishes the unpleasant sensation attending the cold application, as well as the untoward after-effects which occasionally occur. The hot application should be at a high temperature, usually 105° to 110°, and should be continued 3 to 6 minutes, or until the patient is so thoroughly heated that he experiences an intense desire for a deluge of cold water, which is an evidence that the system has been prepared to receive the cold application with benefit.

The hot douche, the hot immersion bath, the electric-light bath, the vapor and hot-air baths, are excellent means of preparing the patient for a cold application in cases requiring preparation. The electric-light bath is to be preferred to the other measures mentioned, when it is accessible. Unless the patient is quite emaciated, the bath may without injury be carried to the point of slight perspiration; and in cases of obesity and rheumatism, when the patient's general strength is good, profuse perspiration may be produced without injury, and in most cases with benefit, but must not be carried to the point of exhaustion.

The longer the hot application is continued, the longer the time required for removal of the heat communicated to the skin by the bath; hence the length of the cold application must be regulated by that of the hot one, the time of the cold application, however, being measured in seconds, while the hot application is measured in minutes. As a rule, the time of a cold or very cold application will be not more than 2 to 4 seconds after a hot application of as many minutes, and should not exceed 10 to 15 seconds, after a hot application of 6 to 10 minutes.

Cool or tepid applications, which are often required in diabetic and rheumatic cases and in chronic Bright's disease and neuralgia, may be continued 1 or 2 minutes in many cases. The required effect must be secured; viz., cooling of the skin until proper but not excessive reaction is secured.

807 The cold application should follow the hot bath immediately and before there has been the slightest opportunity for cooling of the skin. To accomplish this, the vertical rain-douche or shower apparatus may be advantageously placed in the same compartment in which the vapor or Russian bath is administered, so that the patient may receive a stream of cold water upon his body immediately, thus avoiding the preliminary chill, which, if it does not altogether spoil the effect desired, greatly lessens it.

808 The author has had constructed for this purpose an electric-light bath and douche apparatus combined, in which the electric lamps are protected from the action of the water by an inner lining of plate-glass, so that the patient may receive a cold douche at the same time that the heat-rays from the incandescent filaments are falling upon the surface of the body with full intensity. By means of this apparatus the applications of heat and cold are really simultaneous, so that there is no possibility of chilling the surface by evaporation.

809 In very sensitive persons the full jet should not be applied to the whole surface. The stream of water should be at first directed upon the feet and legs from the knees down, the amount of surface being increased at each succeeding application until the whole body is subjected to the influence of cold water under high pressure. The broken jet should be applied to the rest of the body, or cold friction may be applied before the douche. The applications should be made with great rapidity, however, and should not last more than 1 or 2 seconds at first, and later, 2 to 5 seconds.

810 In cases of rheumatism with very painful joints, care should be taken to avoid allowing the stream of cold water to fall upon those joints which are sensitive, otherwise the thermic reaction set up may increase the irritation and congestion of the joints, and consequently aggravate the pain and discourage the patient.

In anemia accompanied by menorrhagia, a condition not

uncommon, the cold douche should be preceded by a very short hot shower bath, or a fomentation to the spine, or both. Care should, however, be taken in the application of the douche to avoid the lumbar and abdominal regions.

In anemia with amenorrhea, a general cold douche may 811
be administered, but should be preceded by a hot douche to the hips, thighs, and feet; or a short hot sitz and hot foot bath; or a hot foot bath, and a warm circle douche to the hips.

Incurable Maladies. Even in disorders which are not curable, much 812
can be done for the patient by the palliation of the most distressing symptoms, as in cancer of the stomach accompanied by vomiting; uterine tumor or cancer giving rise to hemorrhage; advanced locomotor ataxia accompanied by lightning pains; and a variety of other symptoms connected with disorders which can not be wholly cured. Thus the vomiting of cancer may be checked and a very considerable degree of improvement secured; the consumptive cough may be controlled, and night sweats, fever, and other symptoms of this disease mitigated to a remarkable extent by suitable hydriatic measures; and if the patient can at the same time be so situated as to enjoy the advantages of a climatic change at an elevation of about five thousand feet, a cure can be effected in a large number of otherwise hopeless cases. By the prolonged hot douche or the revulsive douche, the lightning pains of locomotor ataxia may often be relieved with a promptness which seems truly magical; and out of the scores of cases of locomotor ataxia which have been under the author's care within the last twenty years, recovery from nearly all the symptoms present has occurred in a considerable number of cases, and great improvement in nearly all.

Thus no case of chronic disease, no matter how inveterate, unless it has reached an absolutely hopeless stage, should be abandoned as incurable without giving hydrotherapy, with the accompanying regimen of diet and exercise, active or passive, an intelligent and persevering trial.

THE UNTOWARD EFFECTS OF HYDROTHERAPY.

There is no remedy, however valuable, which is not capable of misapplication or abuse. That untoward effects sometimes result from applications of water is not an objection to its use, but is rather an argument for its scientific employment, and suggests the necessity of giving the same attention to the study of this important therapeutic agent that is given to the study of the various remedial agents enumerated in the materia medica.

813 **Headache.** Perhaps the most common of the unpleasant effects which sometimes follow remedial applications of water is headache in some form. The pain is most commonly located in the forehead, but the top of the head, the back of the head, or the whole head may be involved. This condition indicates that the application has been (*a*) too extreme in temperature — either too hot or too cold, (*b*) too long in duration, (*c*) that the reaction has been excessive, or (*d*) incomplete.

Headache more commonly follows the cold plunge, the cold douche, or a hot bath of some sort, than any other form of application. Some patients are so susceptible, indeed, that placing the feet in very hot water will induce a severe pain in the head. In others, strong reaction induced by any form of cold bath will occasion this difficulty. In some instances, the headache thus occasioned is extremely violent, and may last for several hours.

The explanations of headache under these conditions are various. Some hydriatrists contend that it is always congestive, others that it is always anemic. The author's view is that the headache following hydriatic applications is sometimes congestive, sometimes anemic, and sometimes purely reflex or sympathetic in character, due to overstimulation of the sympathetic centers.

When the headache occurs immediately or soon after a cold bath, the indication is that the bath was too cold, too prolonged, administered with too much percussion, or that reaction either failed or was too intense, any of these conditions constituting sufficient cause.

The headache which sometimes accompanies or follows a hot bath is due to neither congestion nor anemia, but rather to a swelling of the ganglion cells or of the nerve endings in the brain under the excitation of heat.

Applications which are found to produce headache should be modified at once, as definite and serious injury may result from the prolonged employment of measures which induce an unpleasant symptom of this sort.

Vertigo. Vertigo and sweating may occur either in con- 814
nection with headache or without. Vertigo is due to the same causes which have been mentioned as productive of headache. Sweating of the head indicates too strong determination of blood to this part.

The three symptoms named indicate the necessity of some modification of the measures employed; as, for example, a towel rub or the wet-sheet rub, an affusion at 80°, or a short full bath at 85° to 90° should be substituted for the horizontal jet or other percutient measures. Too strong reaction to the head may also be obviated by wetting the face, neck, and head just before the application of the bath; by the application of a cold compress about the neck and to the head; and by the hot foot bath just before, during, or after the bath.

Insomnia, Palpitation, etc. Insomnia, nervousness, wandering pains, pal- 815
pitation, fidgets, uneasiness, and indefinable but unpleasant sensations following a bath, indicate the necessity for the employment of less strongly exciting measures. The Scotch douche should be substituted for the cold douche, or perhaps the douche should be suspended, the rubbing wet sheet, the towel rub, or the neutral bath being substituted. The last-named measure is one of the best of all known remedies for insomnia. In cases in which strongly tonic results are desirable, these applications should not be made in the evening, but in the forenoon. A

disposition to insomnia may be combated by a neutral bath taken just before retiring at night.

Insomnia, or a persistent sensation of fatigue occurring after three or four weeks' tonic treatment, indicates a necessity for the substitution of dry friction, short electric-light baths, the wet-sheet rub, the neutral douche with little pressure, and similar measures in the place of the cold douche or other strongly excitant treatment, so that the central nervous system may have an opportunity to recuperate the energy which has been expended in reaction and reparative work.

816 **Neurasthenia and Hysteria.** In neurasthenia and in many cases of hysteria, in which pain is generally expressed chiefly at certain points, care should be taken to avoid exciting or tonic applications to these points. This precaution is sometimes rather difficult to carry out; nevertheless it is necessary to exercise the greatest care to avoid the so-called hysterogenous zones, and especially the abdomen in cases in which the patient complains of decided pain or tenderness in this region, as the application of cold water will sometimes precipitate an attack.

Hot and cold applications to the spine will usually give temporary relief from such an attack, if it does occur, and the neutral bath may be employed daily for a few days until the peculiar susceptibility of the nervous system is somewhat modified. In such cases, the patient must be carefully trained to endure cold applications, the first attempts being made with water at a temperature of 75° to 80° F., and the temperature systematically lowered from day to day, as the patient gains power to react.

817 When enlarged or ruptured veins are present, percutient applications to the affected areas should be carefully avoided.

Taking Cold. At the beginning of a course of hydropathic treatment, the patient not infrequently complains of an increase in susceptibility to changes of temperature. This, however, passes off in a short time, for the continued use of cold water hardens the skin and increases its resistance. Great care must be taken to dry the skin thoroughly after baths of all sorts, by removing not only all sensible moisture from the surface, but also that which has been imbibed by the skin, the subsequent evaporation of which may produce chill.

Colds, sore throats, and catarrh of the nose and throat are usually due to neglect completely to dry the skin, thus exposing the patient to secondary chill and resulting visceral congestion and acute catarrh, which very readily becomes chronic. For relief of the cold in cases of this sort, the cold applications should be preceded by a hot Scotch douche, an electric bath, or some other form of sweating bath.

Rheumatic Pains; Skin Disease.

Rheumatic pains, which not infrequently fol- 818
low hydrotherapeutic applications, are not due to taking cold, as is often feared, but to incomplete reaction, or to the setting free of uric acid, and the consequent effects of an excess of this irritating substance in the blood. Slow cooling by evaporation after incomplete drying, and the prolonged application of "dry cold" by means of rubber bags filled with ice, are often the cause of rheumatic pains.

Chronic skin disease sometimes presents a serious obstacle to the employment of hydrotherapy. If suppurating pimples or furuncles, erythemas, or acute eczemas appear, the indication is that cold baths should be suspended and that neutral baths should be employed. Zinc ointment may be advantageously applied to the affected surfaces after each bath. The application of vaseline is also wise. Furuncles following the stimulating compress are due to infection by the compress. It may be prevented by daily boiling the compress and washing the parts well with yellow soap and hot water.

Crises or Fever of Reaction.

Priessnitz and the early water-cure doctors 819
made much of so-called "crises," but the modern scientific study of hydrotherapy has shown that "crises" are the result of too violent measures,

or of strong measures employed for too great a length of time. The principal symptoms mentioned in connection with crises are fever, boils, suppurating eruptions, salivation, hemorrhoids, diarrhea, and vomiting. The application of too strong measures to the surface is likely to give rise to eruptions and irritation of various sorts, boils, etc.; while excessive water-drinking may cause intestinal disturbances.

There are no salutary effects arising from crises which can not be obtained by far better means. The practice of producing crises was based upon the supposition that all disease is due to impurities, and that these impurities may be gotten rid of by means of purulent discharges from the skin, artificially created. No one at all familiar with modern medical ideas can for a moment entertain faith in this antiquated, inconvenient, and, happily, now obsolete measure.

820 Slight symptoms of general systemic disturbance, as malaise accompanied by indigestion, headache, weakness, and other indications recognized by the water-cure doctors of the last century as the beginning of a crisis, should not be regarded as unfavorable, but, on the contrary, as affording positive evidence that the treatment is sufficiently vigorous in character to induce pronounced systemic effects. The symptoms should not be encouraged, however, but should rather be checked by some modification of the prescription, such as has been already suggested, and the patient may be encouraged that he will soon be able to realize that he is making rapid strides toward health.

821 In making hydriatic prescriptions, special care must be taken so to adjust the procedures as to produce just the amount and kind of reaction desired. In febrile diseases it is always desirable to repress thermic reaction as far as possible, and to encourage circulatory reaction. It is best also that the reaction should be developed slowly, as thus it will not be excessive. It is this feature that gives to the cooling pack its advantage over the Brand bath as an antipyretic. Applications for the relief of pain should always produce circulatory

reaction. In these cases it is best to develop the reaction as quickly as possible, so that the procedure shall not be fatiguing.

In applications for the reduction of temperature, a cer- 822
tain amount of thermic reaction can scarcely be avoided; but by employing cold applications accompanied by continuous friction, both the skin circulation and the temperature are maintained, and thus the cutaneous nerves are not cooled to a sufficient degree to set up powerful thermic reflexes, and heat production is but slightly increased. Cold douches must, of course, be avoided in cases in which there is elevation of temperature. It is not desirable, however, to altogether suppress the thermic reaction in fever, as it is important to develop strongly the resistance of the body, and this can be done only by such an application as will moderately stimulate metabolism as well as other functions. The cooling pack accomplishes this in a most satisfactory manner.

In fevers, circulatory reaction must be encouraged, so as 823
to aid heat elimination while thermic reaction is suppressed. In chronic disorders requiring tonic measures, quick thermic and circulatory reaction must be secured; and after all general procedures, complete reaction must be attained, or the results sought will not be secured.

The influence upon metabolism must be watched by noting 824
constantly the effect of the treatment upon the weight, the muscular strength as shown by the dynamometer as well as by the patient's general feeling, the appetite, and by the urine. An excess of solids, especially chlorides, signifies excessive tissue waste. Urea in excess indicates too long or too frequent hot baths, or too much exercise.

The temperature must also be noted. Excessive tempera-
ture elevation after cold baths, or an elevation of temperature 825
followed by perspiration, resembling a febrile movement, indicates excessive stimulation and thermic reaction. The procedures must be modified or treatment suspended, else an actual fever, the so-called hydropathic crisis, may result.

THE HYGIENIC OR PROPHYLACTIC EMPLOYMENT OF HYDROTHERAPY.

826 Rational medicine, as Dr. Horatio C. Wood, of Philadelphia, has so clearly pointed out, consists essentially in the application of prophylactic measures; that is, the employment of means which are capable of maintaining a normal individual in a state of health. It may be suggested as a corollary from this proposition, that by the employment of those physiological measures which are most effective in the restoration of a sick person to health, the individual may be maintained in good health.

However applicable this principle may be to other therapeutic means, experience has shown most positively that the cold bath, while one of the most powerful tonics and most efficient of restoratives, is at the same time one of the most valuable of all known prophylactic or hygienic measures. The cold bath acts powerfully upon the sympathetic nervous system,— that great regulator of nutrition. It likewise affords a gymnastic means for the vasomotor system of nerves and centers, and develops by exercise the contractile activity of the small blood-vessels. Cold water, in common parlance, hardens the skin; technically, we would say, it increases the vital resistance of the skin. If habitually employed, the cold bath protects against taking cold, not by closing the pores, but by increasing the activity of the cutaneous circulation and developing the vital resistance of the body in general, and especially the ability of the body to reheat the skin after it has been chilled by exposure or cold applications.

Through the influence of the cold bath upon the sympathetic nervous system, all the processes of nutrition and assimilation are quickened. The amount of hydrochloric acid produced by the glands of the stomach is increased, as the result of which appetite and digestion are improved; and the stomach, being provided with a better quality of gastric juice, is better prepared to protect itself against injury from intruding microbes. Modern investigations have shown that typhoid fever germs, cholera germs, and, in fact, all varieties of germs, succumb to the attack of a thoroughly healthy gastric juice; hence the daily cold bath, by maintaining a sound digestion, as well as by increasing the general vital resistance of the body, serves as a most valuable protection against infectious disorders, even those which are communicated by virulent living organisms of various sorts.

One of the most interesting effects of the cold bath is the increased number of blood-corpuscles found in the surface vessels after the establishment of the reaction which follows these cold applications. The blood is the means by which oxygen is conveyed to the tissues, and carbonic acid gas to the lungs, whence it is discharged from the body. Certain of the blood cells are also useful in destroying the germs which may find their way into the blood-vessels, and in removing dead and useless particles of various sorts.

It is thus apparent that the number of corpuscles contained in the blood is a matter of the greatest importance in relation to the degree of vital resistance, or the ability of the body to maintain itself in health under adverse circumstances or against the destructive influence of disease-producing causes.

The total surface area of the blood cells contained in the body of an average man is 3,100 square yards. It has been shown by Winternitz and others that by the application of a cold bath the number of blood cells may be increased thirty and even fifty per cent. This means an increase of 1,000 to 1,500 square yards of surface available for use in conveying oxygen to the tissues, and removing carbonic acid gas. It means also an increase of thousands of millions in the number of active protective cells scattered throughout the circulation. This effect of cold upon the blood is one of its most valuable and important uses, and easily accounts for the freshness of color, clearness of complexion, and general buoyancy and vigor which result from the habitual daily employment of the cold bath.

In the application of cold water as a hygienic means, care must be taken, however, to adapt both the temperature and the mode of application to the age, and also to some extent to the sex, as well as to the temperament and to individual susceptibilities.

827 **Cold Bathing in Infancy and Early Childhood.** Children under seven years of age do not well bear the application of very cold water; therefore, the douche in all forms should be avoided, cold friction, the rubbing shallow, or the immersion bath with rubbing being used instead, and never at a very low temperature. A temperature of 70° to 80° F. will produce sufficiently strong impressions to develop good reaction in children under seven years of age. After seven years of age, as the child advances in years, the temperature may be lowered somewhat, and more vigorous applications may be made, such as the affusion and the light douche with water at 70° to 75° F. in temperature. After fourteen or fifteen, lower temperatures may be employed.

The daily cool douche, or affusion, is an excellent means of relieving urinary incontinence in children, a difficulty indicating weakness of the inhibitory centers, which later may develop serious nervous disorders.

The daily cold bath is an important aid to general development in growing children, and increases not only muscular vigor and energy, but nerve tone. It prevents the development of neurotic conditions in young persons just entering upon manhood and womanhood, relieves so-called growing pains, and promotes vigorous and normal development.

828 **The Cold Bath for Adults.** Adults must adapt the form of the bath to their conditions of life, their special predispositions and individual susceptibilities.

Sedentary persons especially need the benefit of the cold bath. Such persons may advantageously employ, before the cold douche, a hot bath for three or four minutes.

Adults who are predisposed to rheumatism, gout, gravel, 829 migraine, Bright's disease, neurasthenia, and other maladies which for the most part are the result of the retention within the body of the products of nitrogenous wastes, will be greatly benefited by the employment of a cold bath daily, but it should be carefully administered. Very cold water must be avoided, and the cold application (68° to 80°) should be preceded by the hot bath for three or four minutes, or until sweating is produced. In feeble persons, cold friction should be employed instead of cold applications in which the whole surface is wet at once.

The Cold Bath for Women. The daily cold bath is especially useful for 830 women of civilized nations, because of the deteriorating influences of their artificial life. The harmful customs of civilization, rather than nature, have made woman "the weaker vessel." The cold bath gives nerve tone, combats nervous weakness of various sorts, is a most excellent prophylactic against hysteria, and to a very considerable degree combats the unwholesome tendency of the indoor and sedentary life to which most women are subjected.

The cold bath favors the development of the menstrual function in young girls, and if habitually employed, affords great assistance at the menopause. A woman who has made regular and persistent use of the cold bath for some years preceding the "change of life" is very little subject to the vasomotor disturbances, the flushings, sweating, etc., which render the lives of so many women miserable for months, sometimes years, at this period.

The cold bath should be avoided during menstruation. Although several authorities recommend that the cold bath be continued during the menstrual period, the author believes it to be, on the whole, safest to suspend it at that time, and to substitute the tepid bath. The cold bath taken at the beginning of the menstrual period may easily result in serious injury. In one reported case, a fatal hematocele was produced. In febrile diseases, cold bathing may be continued, but the intensity should be modified somewhat.

In cases of dysmenorrhea, menorrhagia, and relapsing inflammation, suitable hydriatic applications may be made at the menstrual period with great benefit. By the aid of proper measures of this kind, these disorders may be more profoundly and favorably influenced than by any other nonsurgical means. Hot fomentations, the revulsive sitz, the hot vaginal douche, render most valuable assistance at this period, when appropriately employed.

In pregnancy, the cold douche should be avoided in all forms. Short cold frictions at a temperature of 60° to 70° may be employed with advantage, but the cold douche about the abdomen and lumbar regions should be avoided.

During lactation, the cold bath may be employed with good effect, but cold applications about the lumbar and abdominal regions should be avoided as likely to cause a premature establishment of the catamenia. It is on this account better to confine the application chiefly to the upper part of the body. Cold friction, in strong women even the shallow bath, is safer than the douche or any measure accompanied by percussion.

831 **The Cold Bath in Old Age.** Old age involves the liability to the existence of arteriosclerosis and allied forms of degeneration, in either an incipient or an advanced stage. The skin is inactive, rigid, and comparatively bloodless, and the heat-making powers of the body are greatly diminished, so that the thermic as well as the circulatory reaction is likely to be incomplete, thus giving rise to numerous untoward and distressing symptoms. On this account, great extremes in temperature must be avoided. The neutral bath, douches at a temperature of 75° to 85° F., the wet-sheet rub at the same temperatures, and the cold friction or towel

rub, are the most appropriate measures. Cardiac weakness, emphysema, and bronchitis are conditions so likely to be present in aged persons that they must be kept constantly in mind in the treatment of the old.

The cold bath affords one of the best means for reviving a person who has been exhausted by heat, and especially by heat accompanied by profuse sweating.

The hot sponge bath taken in the morning is sometimes preferable in very hot weather to the cold bath. As the result of a short hot application, an atonic reaction is produced, which lessens heat production, and thus enables a person better to endure exposure to a high temperature.

In the winter season, the habitual employment of the cold bath trains the skin to react promptly, and thus lessens the danger of taking cold or of suffering from pulmonary congestion, as the result of chilling the surface of the body. With a change of season, however, it is sometimes necessary to modify the form of the bath.

The importance of the daily cold bath is a matter of far greater moment than is generally comprehended. In the opinion of the author, every public school should have connected with it a shower-bath, a swimming-tank, and a gymnasium, and all pupils should be required to undergo physical training not only in the gymnasium but in the swimming and shower-baths as well, under careful medical supervision. By this means the physical development of the young may be greatly encouraged, and evil moral tendencies combated, and thus the present rapid deterioration of the race may be stayed. The universal introduction of these measures would certainly result, within a generation, in the production of a much more vigorous race of men and women than we now see.

The Sweating Process.

The sweating bath is a hygienic measure of 832
the greatest value for persons of sedentary habits, constituting to some extent a compensation for lack of exercise. It is a noticeable fact that the people who inhabit very cold countries, as the

natives of Northern Russia, etc., are great devotees of the sweating bath.

The Finns, who for a considerable portion of the year are confined indoors and have little or no exercise, have been intuitively led to seek a compensation for the lack of exercise in the sweating bath, followed by a vigorous cold application. Every house in Finland has its sweat-room attached, in which hot steam is produced by pouring water upon heated stones. After remaining in the sweat-house until sweltering with heat and dripping with perspiration, the bather rushes out and rolls in the snow, thus producing a most vigorous reaction.

The sweating bath, followed by a cold application, though in no means a perfect substitute for exercise, does nevertheless to a very considerable degree relieve the system of the excrementitious wastes which accumulate within the body when a sufficient amount of exercise is not habitually taken. This it accomplishes by increasing oxidation and renewing the body by stimulating tissue changes.

Sweating softens the sebaceous matter which often accumulates in the ducts of the skin, and loosens the dry epithelium by means of which the outlets of the perspiratory ducts are often greatly obstructed, but its greatest benefit is through the stimulation of the circulation of the skin, the excitement of all its functions, and especially in the reflex influences upon the internal structures which are set in operation, and the vigorous fluxion of the blood which is created by the intense hyperemia of the cutaneous envelope produced by prolonged exposure to heat followed by cold.

The skin is capable of containing one half to two thirds of all the blood in the body. When its vessels are dilated to their fullest extent, mechanical displacement of the blood toward the surface causes a temporary anemia of the internal viscera, with contraction of their vessels. By this means, internal congestions are relieved. The cold application following the sweating bath causes an inrush of blood to the interior, distending the visceral vessels and stimulating their functions by increased blood pressure and accelerated movement of blood. By the fluxion of blood between the interior and the exterior of the body, the various vital activities of the organism are stimulated to the highest degree, all the nutritive processes are accelerated, and the most powerful alterative and tonic effects result.

Sedentary persons should take a sweating bath of some sort at least once or twice a week, care being taken, however, to follow the sweating bath by a cold bath of some kind sufficiently prolonged to remove from the skin the heat imparted to it during the sweating process, and to produce vigorous circulatory and thermic reaction. By this means the skin is strengthened and protected from the disturbing influence of atmospheric changes, appetite and digestion are improved, blood pressure and nerve tone are raised, and the wheels of life, so to speak, are made to run more smoothly and quickly. The sweating bath should always be taken at night, and just before retiring.

The Neutral Bath. The bath at 92° to 95° is of special value for business men, teachers, orators, physicians, and all engaged in professions which associate comparatively little bodily activity with an undue degree of mental and nervous strain. The temperature should be 92° to 95° F., duration 15 to 30 minutes, or even longer. This bath should be taken at bed-time, as it possesses soporific power to a wonderful degree, inducing sleep even when hypnotics fail, and by its timely use the employment of sleep-producing drugs may be avoided. The individual who finds himself unable to get to sleep on going to bed, or who awakens after two or three hours unable to continue his slumbers, will find in the neutral bath a sovereign remedy, which, by the sound sleep thus induced, and the accompanying vital recuperation, will enable him to maintain good health under conditions to which he must otherwise succumb. The loss of sound sleep soon results in complete nervous break-down, and not infrequently in mental 833 failure as well. The neutral bath at the temperature named may be taken every night for a prolonged period without injury, provided that the cold morning bath is habitually employed. When the rain douche or the horizontal jet is available, it may well take the place of the neutral bath, as good effects being obtained from the application of the douche for five to ten minutes as from a neutral full bath of three times as great duration.

834 **Precautions.** 1. When fatigued as the result of the loss of sleep or severe muscular exercise, a cold application should be preceded by a hot douche or immersion bath for 3 to 7 minutes.

2. If but slightly fatigued, a short cool or tepid douche, or cold friction may be substituted for the cold bath.

3. A very cold bath should always be short, and should never be administered when the body surface is cold or chilly. The hot bath carried to the point of gentle perspiration is an excellent preparation for a cold application.

4. The temperature of the air of the room in which a cold bath is taken should always be higher than that of the bath.

5. Avoid frequent hot baths at all seasons, and especially in winter, as they are depressing, and lessen vital resistance to cold and other disturbing influences. The best time for a hot or warm bath in cold weather is just before retiring.

HYDRIATIC INSTITUTIONS AND THEIR EQUIPMENT, AND THE GENERAL MANAGEMENT OF CASES.

IN the scientific use of water in the treatment of disease elaborate apparatus is not essential for effectiveness. 900
Indeed, it is possible to secure the most valuable of the therapeutic advantages of water by the aid of sheets, towels, blankets, a pail, a bath-tub, and a thermometer, if coupled with the consummate skill which comes from long experience. There can be no doubt, however, that the best results of hydrotherapy are most readily and quickly attained by the aid of perfected apparatus especially designed and suited for bringing to bear upon the body the thermic and mechanical impressions which may be elicited from water. It may also be added in this connection, that, while it is true that no remedy lends itself so readily to all conditions and environments as does water, and while there are few morbid conditions which may not be greatly benefited by the use of such simple appliances as are usually found at hand, it is true beyond question that a very large number of cases, especially those of a chronic nature, may be much more satisfactorily treated and far more quickly restored to health by treatment in an establishment furnished with all the appliances for the most efficient use of water. It is not always necessary for the patient to live in such an institution, though he should be sufficiently near to make daily treatment possible without too great inconvenience; but in quite a large proportion of chronic cases it is important that the patient's whole life should be controlled,—the diet, exercise, and the entire regimen regulated in harmony with rational living,—in other words, that the patient should give himself for the time being wholly to the cultivation of health, in order to secure the desired results. Hence a few words may not be out of place in regard to the

equipment requisite for an establishment devoted to the use of hydriatic measures.

901 The most necessary thing is an abundant supply of water. Soft water is preferable to hard, because of its better effects upon the skin, but mineral water offers no real advantage over the purest soft water. The slight advantages which may possibly be claimed for certain alkaline mineral waters, especially those containing carbonic acid gas and chloride of calcium, in the production of circulatory reaction at neutral temperatures, may, when desirable, be easily attained by the addition of the proper chemical substances. Soft water is much more readily absorbed than hard water or mineral waters, as has been shown by laboratory experiment. This gives it greater value when used at neutral temperatures for sedative effects.

902 A consideration of the greatest importance in relation to the water supply is the temperature, a low temperature being a very desirable quality. The summer temperature should not be higher than 55° F., and five to ten degrees lower is desirable. At a temperature above 60° it is difficult to obtain some of the most desirable hydriatric effects. It is not every case in which the powerfully tonic effects of water at 50° can be utilized, but means should be at hand for the production of the profound thermic and circulatory reaction which may be secured by water at this temperature, administered with proper pressure, in cases which may require it. In temperate climates there is no difficulty in obtaining water at a sufficiently low temperature during the cold months, but during the summer-time the temperature of water conveyed for some distance in pipes often rises to 70° or even 75°. In such cases artificial means of cooling may be employed. The accompanying cut (Fig. 28) shows a method of cooling which the author has found very satisfactory. Water at a temperature of 70°, after circulating through this apparatus, is delivered at a temperature of 50° or less. Water from deep wells and mountain streams is generally of a sufficiently low temperature for practical purposes.

In the empirical hydropathy of Priessnitz and his followers, cold water was the one thing needful; but in modern rational hydrotherapy water is employed at all temperatures possible without injury to the skin; hence some suitable means of affording an abundant supply of hot water is required. Water may be conveniently heated by means of such a water-heater as is commonly used in laundries; or when the bathing establishment is heated by steam, it is usually most convenient and economical to heat the water in a boiler through which the steam is made to circulate by means of brass or copper pipes. If an engine is used for running a pump, elevator, or other machinery, the exhaust steam may be utilized in heating the water. Another method recently invented is the heating faucet, into which a steam pipe and a cold-water pipe are connected in such a manner that by the proper adjustment of the valve the steam and water may be mixed at the moment of escape, and thus water at any temperature desired instantly obtained. Water may also be heated by passing a steam pipe directly into the tank of cold water. This method, however, has the disadvantage of being extremely noisy. The noise may be somewhat lessened by fastening a suitable head to the open end of the pipe, but can never be entirely overcome. 903

Live steam is needed for the vapor bath, the Russian bath, and especially for the vapor douche. 904

Adequate pressure is a matter of utmost importance for a complete hydriatic establishment, it being essential for the different forms of the douche,— the most powerful if not the most essential of hydriatic procedures. The pressure needed is at least thirty to fifty pounds, representing a water column seventy-five to one hundred feet in height. A higher pressure is in no way undesirable, though not often required. When city water pressure can not be utilized, water may be pumped up into a tank placed at an elevation sufficient to give the necessary pressure. Each foot of elevation gives a pressure of about .45 of a pound. The pressure required may be obtained by means of a closed steel tank and an air-pump, an arrangement shown in the accompanying cut (Fig. 29). This device is much used in France, and is very satisfactory. In the absence of a better appliance, it is possible to administer the douche, and that in quite effective fashion, by means of an ordinary green-house spray pump. But in order to secure all the advantages of this most potent and admirable therapeutic agent, a complete and well-constructed apparatus must be provided. The douche apparatus being naturally the central feature of a well-equipped scientific establishment for the employment of hydrotherapy, it should not be clumsy or incomplete. The cost of a proper outfit, including a percussion douche nozzle with air-pump and tank to operate, need not be more than $500 to $600 at the most.

905 The apartments devoted to the administration of baths should be carefully constructed for the purpose, and when possible, should comprise the following distinct compartments: An office, a waiting-room (the office and waiting-room may often be combined), a series of dressing-rooms with cooling-room adjacent, general treatment-room, a room for douches of various sorts, a room for the administration of massage, packs, and fomentations. In addition to these there must be a water-closet, and provision for the administration of enemas and vaginal and rectal douches.

Special attention should be given to the ventilation of the apartments. The amount of air required per hour in living-rooms is estimated by Parkes at 3,000 cubic feet. In bath-rooms provision should be made for at least twice this amount of air, because of the great activity of the lungs and skin of patients during hydriatic treatment, and also because of the fact that the rooms are to be occupied by diseased persons, in consequence of which the air will become contaminated more rapidly than under ordinary circumstances. The maximum number of patients likely to occupy the rooms at any one time should be estimated, and provision made for 5,000 to 6,000 cubic feet of air per hour for each person. The air should be warmed before it enters the room. It may enter

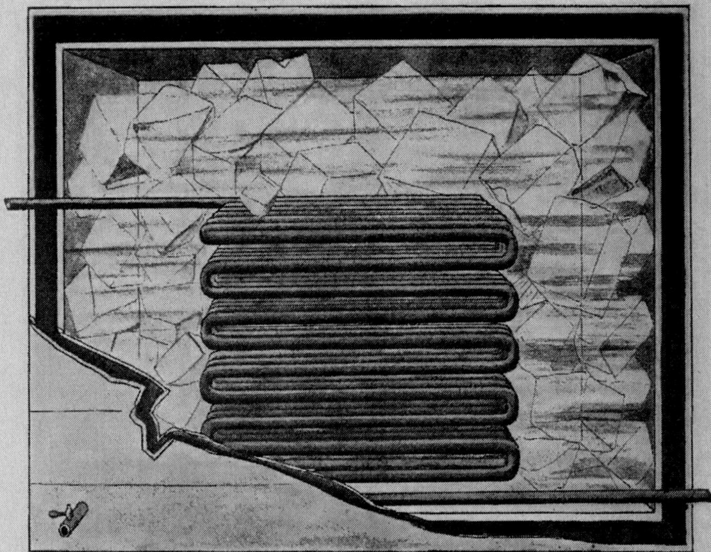

FIG. 28. WATER COOLING APPARATUS (p. 398)

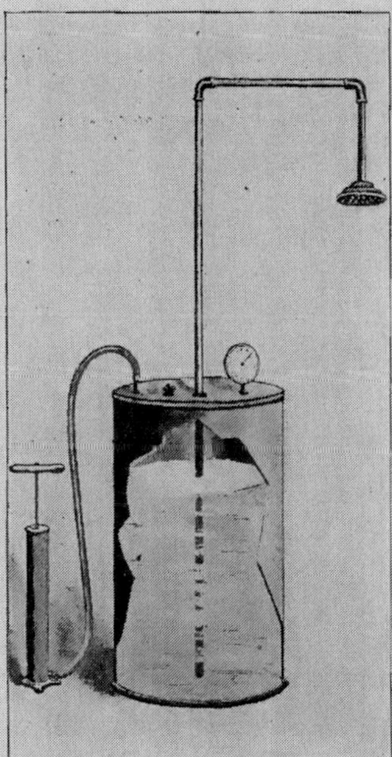

FIG. 29. COMPRESSION-TANK DOUCHE. APPARATUS (p. 400).

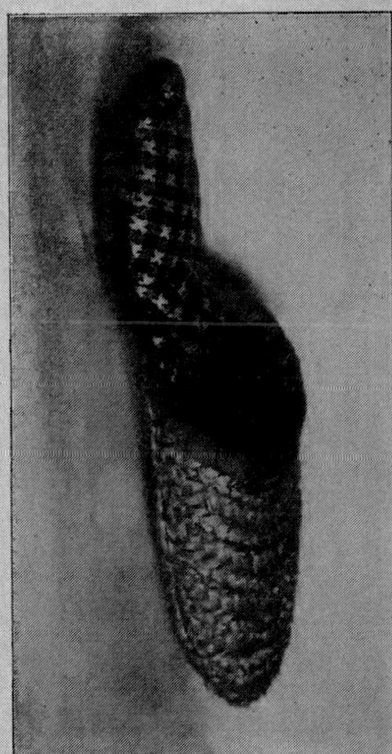

FIG. 30. BATH SLIPPER (p. 404).

at any rate desired, but should not leave the room at a rate of more than five to seven feet per second. The outlets should be numerous and located on, or at, the floor and beneath the windows, so as to prevent the cold air which falls along the outer walls from collecting at the floor, thus chilling the feet of the bathers. Ventilating shafts should be located in the inside walls, so that they will always be warm. If it is impossible to carry the shaft high enough to secure a strong draft, a suction-fan may be introduced, it being operated by steam, water, or electricity. Great care should be taken to avoid drafts, as the rapid evaporation from the skin produced by moving air readily gives rise to chill and most unpleasant effects. The temperature of the bath-rooms should not be higher than 75° to 78° F. A temperature of 65° to 70° is preferable for the waiting- and cooling-rooms; while a temperature five to ten degrees higher may be allowed for the general treatment-rooms.

The floors of the waiting- and dressing-rooms should be 906
made of hard wood, and waxed. If necessary, the floor may be covered with soft rugs, which should be taken out and shaken and sunned daily. The floors should never be covered with carpets, as these collect the dust, and often become musty, and contaminate the air. In apartments in which the floor is likely to be wet, as the douche and the general treatment-rooms, the floor, or at least a portion of it, should be covered with tile, marble, slate, or concrete. The walls should also be of impervious material, preferably marble, and no crack should be left into which the water can enter, or to become filled with decomposable material.

If gutters are employed for carrying off the water (these should be depended upon as little as possible), they should be along the outer wall, and should be deep enough so that they will not readily overflow, and should be readily accessible so that they may be cleaned daily. No pipes of any sort should pass through the gutters, and there should be sufficient fall so that they will empty themselves rapidly.

Partitions should, as far as possible, be made of waterproof material. No woodwork of any sort should come in contact with the floor.

For fully equipped bath apartments at least the following appliances will be required: —

907 Bath-tubs of proper construction for full, sitz, foot, running foot, shallow, and leg baths. An apparatus for administering douches of all sorts, including the vapor douche, is one of the most important necessities, and should be provided regardless of expense.

For good heat effects an electric-light bath and vapor or hot-air baths are needed, and for a large establishment it is well also to add the Russian bath. Electric-light apparatus should be provided for the administration of local light-baths to the spine, legs, abdomen, and other parts.

Several large dippers, and pails properly constructed for the pail douche, should be provided, and there should be an abundant supply of linen and Turkish towels, linen and Turkish sheets, large soft woolen blankets, double blankets for the wet-sheet pack, friction mitts, a shampoo slab, manila or excelsior for shampooing, fomentation cloths, cheese-cloth for compresses, hot-water bags, both square and long, hot-water bags for the throat, and properly constructed sofas and couches. Several thermometers should be hung about the bath apartments in various places, by which to regulate the temperature. The thermophore, when obtainable, may be employed instead of the hot-water bag.

It may be properly added, however, that the most elegantly equipped establishment for the administration of hydriatic procedures may be only the means for bungling and unscientific dabbling with human ailments, unless conducted under skilled medical direction and by the aid of attendants well trained in the versatile procedures of hydriatry. The hydriatrist must know not only that his apparatus and appliances are perfect and in perfect condition, but he must know exactly the condition of the patient to be treated, and must have a clearly defined rationale for each application made. Every prescription must have a sound physiological basis. Empiricism is bad anywhere, but especially so in practical hydrotherapy. A profound knowledge of physiology and pathology is essential to success.

It may be profitable to note a few of those conditions of 908
the patient aside from distinct pathological states which have an important bearing upon the effects of hydriatic procedures.

The exact condition of the patient as he comes to the bath should be noted and taken into account, as it may be necessary to modify a procedure which was designated for him the day before or even the hour before. If he is in a state of exhaustion, for example, from overexercise or loss of sleep or other cause, any very cold application will probably be inappropriate. If the patient is chilly, he must be warmed. Simply warming the feet by a hot foot bath may be the only heating measure needed; but if necessary, fomentations to the spine, a short hot immersion bath, a hot-blanket pack, or a hot rain douche just before the cold douche, may be employed as most convenient or as may seem to be indicated. If the patient is able, a few minutes' exercise, until gentle perspiration is induced, will, in ordinary cases, be found a more excellent means of preliminary heating than any form of hot bath, for the reason that exercise brings into full action the heat-making processes which the cold bath is designed to stimulate. If the patient is unaccustomed to cold water, his feelings should be respected, and the cold applications graduated in such a way as to avoid so unpleasant a shock as to distress or discourage him. If a patient is too feeble to help himself without more than ordinary assistance, the method of application must be modified to suit his case; as, for example, the shallow bath should be used rather than the rubbing wet sheet. If the patient has little power to react, his reactive ability must be stimulated by thorough heating before the bath by means of exercise, perhaps supplemented with a heating bath of some sort, as a vapor or an electric-light bath.

909 It is important to remember that patients are as likely to take cold in the treatment-rooms as elsewhere. The patient generally attributes his cold to a cold application, because during such an application he has experienced sensations of chill or shivering; but in this he is in error. If he has taken cold, it is because of the slow cooling which takes place by evaporation from an imperfectly dried skin after the bath, or because of a secondary chill occasioned by improper administration of the treatment. He can not take cold from a short, vigorous cold application followed by rubbing and a good reaction. The secondary chill (441) must be carefully avoided. Chill is not infrequently produced by evaporation from the skin while the patient, who has perhaps had a heating procedure of some sort, is waiting for the completion of his treatment. The attendant should take care to see that such dangerous pauses in the treatment do not occur. The cold treatment must follow instantly upon the completion of the heating procedure. If from some accident or emergency a few seconds' delay occurs, the patient must be warmed up again by the administration of a hot rain or needle douche for a minute before the cold douche is given. Chilling of the feet by walking upon cold floors is doubtless in some cases the cause of taking cold. This may be obviated by the use of slippers. The heelless bath slippers, such as are generally used in the bathing establishments of Italy and Germany (Fig. 30), are very convenient.

The subject of exercise in connection with baths has been considered elsewhere (774). Suffice it to say here, that, in general, moderate exercise for 15 to 30 minutes should be taken both before and after a cold bath by patients able to exercise, but after a hot bath the patient should rest.

910 The training of patients to endure cold applications is a matter of the utmost consequence, and it requires considerable intelligence on the part of the attendant as well as the physician himself to conduct the process skilfully. While as a rule the temperature should be lowered a little each day,

there will be occasionally a day when the patient's nerve tone is not quite up to par, when it may be necessary to return to the higher temperature employed two or three days previously. The day following, however, with improved nerve tone, rapid advance may be made toward the goal constantly aimed at in the average case; namely, the administration of water at a temperature properly designated as cold or very cold.

This training is especially necessary in the case of seden- 911
tary persons, such as are represented by the average business or professional man, teachers, and the wives and daughters from wealthy homes. Americans are as a class less able to bear water at a low temperature than are the English, the Germans, or the French. The reason for this is that Americans generally maintain their living rooms at a higher temperature in winter, and load themselves with a mass of unnecessary clothing at night as well as during waking hours, so that the skin is generally relaxed, and possessed of little ability to react. The necessary reactive power may, however, be acquired by careful training, and the rapidity with which the patient comes to enjoy the most vigorous cold procedures is frequently very surprising. The exhilaration which comes with the reaction following the bath is soon recognized as more than ample compensation for the slight unpleasantness occasioned during its application, and indeed it requires only short training to bring the patient to a point at which the really unpleasant symptoms at first experienced are no longer felt, or are mitigated to such a degree as to be scarcely noticeable.

It should never be forgotten, however, that very old, very 912
young, and very feeble persons are incapable of enduring the very cold procedures suitable for ordinary adults, as their heat-producing powers are much less. Very cold baths must also be avoided in rheumatism, cardiac weakness, valvular disease of the heart, organic diseases of the brain and spinal cord, and degenerations of the kidneys, liver, heart, lungs, and other internal organs.

913 Very cold or very hot baths should be avoided just before or just after meals. The sitz bath should always be taken with the stomach empty, and the moist abdominal bandage should be removed during the meal, except in cases of gastric irritation in which it may be specially indicated.

914 From Schüller's experiments * it is evident that the condition of the cerebral vessels should always be taken into consideration in the arrangement of a hydriatric prescription. Warm baths are contraindicated in cerebral anemia, for the reason that they would mechanically cause still further contraction of the cerebral vessels; while in pronounced cerebral congestion the application of very cold baths may be equally inappropriate in consequence of the intense though temporary cerebral congestion which they induce.

915 The success of hydriatic procedures depends as much upon the faithfulness and thoroughness of the attendant as upon the nature of the procedure itself. Every little detail must receive conscientious attention. No person can become qualified to administer hydriatric treatment in a satisfactory manner unless capable of following a prescription with absolute precision; and no person should be employed to administer treatment of this sort unless it is known that he can be fully relied upon to administer it in the manner indicated.

916 The attendant must never forget that nearly all procedures require a thorough cooling of the head, which demands bathing of the face and neck with cold water as well as complete saturation of the hair and wetting of the scalp. Women generally decline to have the hair wet, protecting it with a rubber cap so as to avoid the long delay necessary for drying the hair after the bath. This disadvantage may be obviated to a considerable degree by a thorough bathing of the face and neck with water colder than that of the proposed bath, and the application of a cold compress about the neck during the treatment.

* *Archiv für Klin. Med.*, 1874.

If the bath is one requiring rubbing, it must be faithfully done, but not overdone, and as a rule it must be continuous from the beginning of the bath to the end of it. Interruption of the rubbing for half a minute may be sufficient to spoil the effect of the procedure altogether. When the patient is able, he must be constantly encouraged to assist in the rubbing, as the physical exercise thus involved is relied upon as a means of assisting reaction, and is an important factor in securing the good results expected of the procedure. 917

In procedures like the wet-sheet pack and the neutral bath, care should be taken to secure the greatest possible degree of quiet about the patient. Bright sunlight should be excluded by drawing down the curtains a little. Conversation, if allowed at all, should be suppressed. The patient should be disturbed as little as possible, no attention generally being required further than the changing of the cold compress applied to the head. If the patient is inclined to sleep during the bath, he should be allowed to do so. If the purpose of the bath is to obtain sleep, its duration may be extended beyond the usual limit, so long as the patient remains quietly sleeping, care being taken that no untoward effects are provoked by the accumulation of heat or other change in the conditions essential to the proper effects of the bath. 918

Quiet should always be maintained in the bath-room. Noisy talking, whistling, singing, and a bustling manner are entirely out of place there. Patients should not be encouraged to converse while taking treatment.

Particular attention must be given to drying and rubbing the patient after the bath. This portion of the procedure is almost as important as any other, yet it is frequently neglected, even in the best-equipped and ably managed establishments. Attendants should see that the bath sheet is thoroughly dry, but it should not be heated for a tonic application, as the contact of the heated sheet with the skin is likely to produce an atonic reaction, thus antagonizing the tonic effects of the bath. 919

The warm sheet may be applied after the neutral bath without harm, and the temperature of the sheet should at least be such that it will not produce the impression of cold when brought in contact with the skin. A Turkish sheet is to be preferred to the ordinary linen or muslin sheet for drying after the bath.

Extreme care must be taken to avoid chilling by evaporation after the neutral bath, as by this means the effect of the bath may be wholly destroyed. To this end the patient must be closely covered instantly when removed from the bath, special care being taken to avoid air currents about the neck and feet. Gentle rubbing over the sheet will facilitate the absorption of water by the sheet, and the patient may thus be rapidly dried without producing an undesirable reaction, either circulatory or thermic.

920 After a cold bath the patient must be thoroughly rubbed until a good reaction has occurred. Special attention must be given to the feet and legs, as these parts, particularly the feet, are very likely to become cold soon after the bath, through defective reaction, and may remain in this condition for several hours unless the patient's ability to react is good. When the circulation of the lower extremities is disturbed in this way, the cerebral vessels are dilated, and headache is likely to result. The patient should be first rubbed thoroughly with a towel or sheet, and afterward vigorously with the bare hand, the warm fleshy hand of the attendant greatly facilitating reaction. The patient is by no means dry when the skin ceases to feel wet. So long as the skin is soft and spongy, it still contains moisture which has been absorbed by the superficial layers of the epidermis. This absorbed moisture being left to evaporate after the bath, the patient becomes chilly, and contracts a cold, which he erroneously attributes to the bath, whereas the difficulty is wholly due to the ignorance or neglect of the attendant, or perhaps to the patient's own failure to observe the precautions suggested to him by his attendant or physician.

Rubbing, though thorough, should never be so vigorous as to produce irritation of the skin or to bruise or exhaust the patient. Excessive friction depresses the heart. 921

It is necessary to exercise great care to avoid burning patients when making hot applications. This accident is liable to occur in the treatment of patients who are in a state of insensibility from any cause, as from syncope due to chloroform, the stupor of fever, or sensory paralysis. In various forms of spinal disease there is a diminished sensibility and lowered vitality due to the presence of toxins, which greatly decrease the patient's ability to resist high temperatures, so that severe burns may occur from the application of a fomentation at a temperature which would produce no unpleasant effect when applied to sound tissue. The same is true of patients under the influence of an anesthetic, and in some forms of cardiac weakness on account of the slowed movement of the blood. 922

Equal care must be taken to avoid freezing parts to which very cold applications are made continuously for a considerable length of time, especially in the use of the ice compress, the ice-bag, or the carbonic acid gas compress, especial care being necessary in the use of the last-named measure. Parts which may be completely surrounded by the cold application, as the hand, the foot, the scrotum, the ear, and parts in which the bones are thinly covered by flesh, are much more likely to suffer than are other parts of the body. In some parts, as the face, the cutaneous circulation is so active that there is very little danger of injury from this cause. It should be remembered, however, that in patients who are in a low condition, as in the ataxo-adynamic state of typhoid fever, the circulation is so sluggish that freezing occurs much more readily than in normal individuals.

Before putting the patient into a continuous bath, the 923
skin should be oiled to prevent masceration and resulting irritation. The same precaution must be taken when fomentations are applied daily to a part, as for relief of pain in

sciatica and in chronic joint disease. Oiling of the skin is also essential as a protection against taking cold for patients who are under hydriatic treatment, especially during the cold season of the year. A little refined vaseline or cacao butter should be applied daily or every other day, after drying the patient.

924 Great care must be taken to keep the towels, sheets, and blankets employed about the bath-room in a thoroughly aseptic condition by frequent laundering. Towels should be boiled daily. The rashes resulting from the continuous use of the abdominal girdle on which the empirical hydropaths dote so much, are in large part due to neglect to properly cleanse the wet bandage, which, being used day after day, accumulates fetid matter from the skin, and affords a favorable culture medium for the various forms of pus-producing microbes which are always present upon the skin. These rashes are never desirable, and may generally be prevented entirely by taking the precaution to apply vaseline to the skin and to boil the bandage daily. If the bandage is worn both night and day, it is well to employ a fresh one each night and morning.

925 The hydriatrist should always be sharply on the lookout for untoward effects from the applications which the patient is receiving at his hands, and should be ready to apply at once the necessary remedy, whether in the form of a hydriatic antidote or such an adjustment of the prescription as will obviate these untoward effects, which have been dwelt upon more fully elsewhere, but may be here again briefly enumerated, with a few words of suggestion, as follows: —

926 *Loss of Flesh.*— If the patient's weight is normal, as indicated by the height-weight coefficient (the height-weight coefficient of the average man is 37; that is, he weighs 37 kilograms (1¼ oz.) for each millimeter (one twenty-fifth of an inch) of height, as the author has elsewhere pointed out),* a loss of flesh probably indicates overtreatment or

* "A New Dynamometer for Use in Anthropometry," read before the American Association for the Advancement of Physical Culture, 1893.

advance of the disease. There are many cases, however, in which metabolism has been so sluggish, allowing an accumulation of imperfectly oxidized waste matters in the body, that the first effect of active stimulation of the nutritive processes is disproportionately to increase destructive metabolism. Under these circumstances there is necessarily a slight decrease in the weight. The rubbish must be removed and old defective structures broken down before new and more highly organized tissues can be deposited It is hence apparent that a slight loss of weight need not give rise to any apprehension; but if this loss is considerable, or continues for some time, especially if accompanied by a loss of strength or appetite, it is a matter requiring immediate attention, and there should be a readjustment of the patient's prescription.

As Bouchard has so clearly pointed out, a great number 927
of chronic invalids are suffering from a slowed or enfeebled condition of the general nutrition, where there is deficient metabolism, either constructive or destructive. There are, of course, morbid conditions in which metabolism is accelerated. Hydrotherapy affords more effective means than any other known agent for the control of these tissue changes, as has been clearly shown in the chapters devoted to the physiological effects of water; but it is of course necessary that they should be intelligently applied, so that the loss will not be so rapid as to discourage the patient or reduce his strength unduly.

A very common cause of the loss of flesh referred to is the 928
excessive employment of heating measures. When this is the case, these should be at once suspended, and short cold applications at 60° to 65°, duration 4 to 10 seconds, or as cold as the patient can bear, should be substituted. Long cold applications should be avoided. In some cases very vigorous cold procedures can not be tolerated, and only very mild tonic measures, such as cold friction, should be employed alone or alternated with neutral baths.

929 A gain in flesh is to be effected by means of neutral temperatures, as by neutral baths, the neutral pack, or the rain douche, combined with wholesome food and plenty of rest. In many such cases it is necessary to employ hydriatric measures in such a way as to produce activity of internal parts, as in hypopepsia with anorexia and emaciation. The increased movement of blood and diminished outflow of energy resulting from the application of sedative measures, with just sufficient stimulation by cold friction or wet-sheet rubbing to maintain active nutrition, are effects which may be advantageously employed in cases in which loss of flesh is to be combated. When pain or irritability exists, higher temperatures are required.

On the other hand, the failure of an overfat patient to decrease in flesh indicates the need of more vigorous procedures. Obesity may be best combated by the application of measures which will produce powerful stimulation of the nerve centers. The wet-sheet pack, vapor bath, or electric-light bath not too greatly prolonged, followed by the cold bath, cold shower bath, with affusions to the abdomen, constitute a rational treatment for persons who have been properly trained to the employment of such powerful measures.

930 *Loss of Appetite.*—The loss of appetite in hydriatric treatment is a matter requiring immediate attention, as the usual effect of the treatment is to increase the appetite at once. As a rule, short very cold applications made when the patient is fasting, powerfully stimulate the appetite. A cold bag applied over the stomach half an hour before meals is highly useful for this purpose.

931 *Loss of Strength.*—This, like loss of appetite, is a symptom which is indirectly of great significance, and one which should receive attention without delay. Tonic hydriatric procedures energize in a wonderful way both the nerve centers and the muscular system. Gradual loss of strength indicates the necessity for more highly tonic applications; or if the patient is feeble, it may be possible that the applications

are too vigorous, so that the patient's energies are overtaxed by the strong reaction induced. The employment of the author's universal dynamometer* in connection with hydriatric treatment furnishes a ready means for determining the constitutional effects of the measures employed. A study of the coefficients which may be obtained by the use of this instrument instantly furnishes a clue to the patient's vital condition, and affords a means by which any change, whether favorable or unfavorable, may be at once observed. The height-weight, strength-weight, strength-height, and respiratory-height and -weight coefficients are especially valuable. The significance of these coefficients and their use in hydriatic prescriptions has been dwelt upon elsewhere (780).

The blood-count and the percentage of hemoglobin may 932 be watched with great profit. A diminution indicates that excessive demands are being made upon the system in the stimulation of eliminative and oxidizing processes. The appearance of an excessive amount of uric acid or urates in the urine, while generally accompanied by unpleasant symptoms, such as headache, malaise, etc., is not necessarily a discouraging feature, though it is a symptom the significance of which the patient will often need to have explained. In cases in which this symptom appears there has been for a long time an accumulation or storing-up of uric acid in the tissues. The increased alkalinity of the blood resulting from tonic and alterative hydriatic procedures renders possible the solution and elimination of this toxic element, the product of the deficient oxidation of nitrogenous wastes, which accounts for the sedementary deposits referred to. This symptom should be welcomed as an indication that the treatment employed is accomplishing the results expected of it; and no matter how depressed in mind the patient is, he may be assured that he is making real progress toward recovery.

The appearance of *an excessive amount of urea or a trace* 933 *of albumin or sugar* may be an indication that the procedures

* "Physical Coefficients," Modern Medicine Pub. Co., Battle Creek, Mich.

employed are too intense. The temperature should be elevated and the pressure reduced. The possibility of the appearance of these symptoms should lead to a frequent examination of the urinary secretions. Such an examination should be made at least once a week. The author has arranged a scheme for graphically representing the several features developed by the clinical examination, together with the different coefficients which represent mathematically a number of important relations. A glance at the graphic (page 415) which may be prepared by the aid of this schedule shows instantly what is the effect of the treatment upon the general metabolism, and also reveals any untoward effects upon the kidneys.

934 An excessively active destructive metabolism may be at once suspected from the presence of an excess of chlorides, while an excess of phosphates indicates great excitation of the nervous system. In such cases the intensity of the treatment must be diminished, applications at a more neutral temperature being employed. Excessive nitrogenous waste usually results from too prolonged hot baths, leading to abnormal destruction of the proteid tissue elements. Such a waste is usually attended by a loss of nervous and muscular energy.

935 *Palpitation of the heart* indicates either that the application has been at too extreme a temperature,—too hot or too cold,—or that it has been managed in such a way as to produce an improper excitation of the heart. When this symptom is troublesome, more moderate temperatures should be employed, and with less pressure, and in making the application care should be taken to avoid the region of the heart and chest. In some instances, this unpleasant symptom may be entirely avoided by the application of a cold compress or an ice-bag over the heart during the procedure. The application of the Scotch douche to the legs at the beginning of a general cold application, by dilating the blood-vessels of the lower extremities, aids in lessening the tendency to palpitation of the heart, as does also the application of cold water

Sanitarium Laboratory of Hygiene.

ANALYSIS OF URINE. (Men.)

NORMAL CONSTITUENTS.

Amount.	Specific Gravity.	Acidity.	Urea.	Uric Acid.	Total Nitrogen.	Chlorides.	Phosphates.	Fixed Sulphates.	Conjugate Sulphates.	Total Solids.
6000.	1.075	11.00	80.0	3.25	38.0	31.0	5.60	6.00	2.50	134.0
5200.	1.067	7.00	72.0	2.70	34.0	27.0	5.00	5.00	2.10	114.0
4400.	1.059	5.00	64.0	2.20	30.0	24.0	4.50	4.50	1.70	97.0
3700.	1.052	3.90	57.0	1.80	26.0	21.0	4.00	4.00	1.30	82.0
3000.	1.045	3.10	50.0	1.40	23.0	18.0	3.50	3.60	1.00	60.0
2400.	1.039	2.40	43.0	1.10	20.0	15.0	3.00	3.20	.70	60.0
1900.	1.034	2.00	37.0	.80	17.0	13.0	2.00	2.80	.50	54.0
1500.	1.029	1.60	32.0	.60	13.0	11.0	2.30	2.40	.35	50.0
1200.	1.026	1.30	28.0	.45	13.0	9.0	2.00	2.00	.25	47.0
1000.	1.024	1.10	26.0	.30	12.0	8.0	1.70	1.50	.20	45.0
800.	1.022	.95	24.0	.23	11.2	7.7	1.40	1.30	.15	43.9
750.	1.020	.70	22.0	.20	10.0	7.0	1.20	1.30	.12	42.0
650.	1.018	.40	20.0	.18	9.0	6.5	1.00	1.10	.11	40.0
550.	1.016	.10	18.0	.16	8.0	6.0	.80	0.90	.09	37.0
450.	1.014	.0	15.0	.14	7.0	5.4	.60	.70	.07	34.0
350.	1.012	.10	12.0	.12	6.0	4.8	.40	.50	.05	30.0
250.	1.009	.40	9.0	.10	5.0	4.2	.25	.40	.04	25.0
170.	1.006	.80	6.0	.08	4.0	3.5	.15	.30	.03	20.0
100.	1.003	1.50	3.0	.05	2.5	2.0	.10	.20	.02	13.0
50.	1.001	2.00	1.0	.02	1.0	1.0	.05	.10	.01	6.0
0.	1.000	3.00	0.0	.00	0.0	0.0	.00	.00	.00	0.0

ABNORMAL SUBSTANCES.

Albumen.*	Sugar.
30.0	500.0
20.0	250.0
18.0	125.0
8.0	60.0
5.0	25.0
3.0	10.0
2.0	4.0
1.5	2.0
1.0	1.0
0.5	0.5
0.0	0.0

Bile.	Ind.	Ammonia.	Hemoglobin.	Blood Cells.	Pus.	Bacteria.	Spermatozoa.	Epithelium.	Casts.	*Crystals.	Mucus.	Toxins.
Great Quantity.	Great Quantity.	Great Quantity.	Great Quantity.	Very Numerous.	Very Numerous.	Very Numerous.	Very Numerous.	Very Numerous.	Very Numerous.	Very Numerous.	Great Quantity.	Great Quantity.
Strong Test.	Strong Test.	Strong Test.	Strong Test.	Many.	Many.	Many.	Many.	Many.	Many.	Many.	Much.	Strong Test.
Fair Test.	Fair Test.	Fair Test.	Fair Test.	Several in Each Field.	Several in Each Field.	Several in Each Field.	Several in Each Field.	Several in Each Field.	Several in Each Field.	Several in Each Field.	Small Amount.	Fair Test.
Trace.	Trace.	Trace.	Trace.	One in Several Fields.	One in Several Fields.	One in Several Fields.	One in Several Fields.	One in Several Fields.	One in Several Fields.	One in Several Fields.	Trace.	Trace.
0	0	0	0	0	0	0	0	0	0	0	0	0

The accompanying figures represent averages based upon the exact examination of many thousands of urines, normal and pathological. By the line drawn across the chart is shown the relation to normal of the specimen, the details of the examination of which are given on the preceding page. The several quantities are indicated as follows:—

Amount:—In cubic centimeters.

Specific Gravity:—By Urinometer.

Acidity:—Phosphoric acid in grams, and when below 0 Sodium oxide in grams.

Urea, Phosphates, Uric Acid, Chlorides, Total Nitrogen, Total Solids, Sulphates, Albumen, Sugar, each in grams.

Coefficients:—See last page for explanation.

The figures running across the middle of chart between double lines are the average normal quantities. The points above the central line indicate the degree of excess over the normal quantities. The points below the line indicate deficiencies.

* This refers only to number of crystals and not to kind.

(OVER.)

COEFFICIENTS.

Urea.	Uric Acid.	Relation of Uric Acid to Urea.	Total Nitrogen.	Fixed and Conjugate Sulphates.	Total Solids.	Urotoxic.
4.00	16.80	51.20	4.00	16.66	3.04	3.00
3.30	12.00	30.00	3.30	13.0	3.10	2.60
2.80	9.00	17.00	2.80	9.30	2.60	2.30
2.40	6.50	9.00	2.40	6.75	2.20	2.00
2.10	5.00	6.00	2.10	5.50	1.90	1.70
1.80	3.75	4.00	1.80	3.75	1.70	1.40
1.60	2.75	3.00	1.60	2.75	1.50	1.10
1.40	2.00	2.00	1.40	2.00	1.35	.90
1.25	1.30	1.40	1.25	1.50	1.20	.75
1.10	1.20	1.20	1.10	1.20	1.10	.60
1.00	1.00	1.00	1.00	1.00	1.00	.50
0.90	0.90	0.90	0.90	.90	0.90	.40
0.80	0.80	0.80	0.80	.80	0.80	.35
0.70	0.70	0.70	0.70	.70	0.70	.30
0.60	0.60	0.60	0.60	.60	0.60	.25
0.50	0.50	0.50	0.50	.50	0.50	.20
0.40	0.40	0.40	0.40	.40	0.40	.15
0.30	0.30	0.30	0.30	.30	0.30	.10
0.20	0.20	0.20	0.20	.20	0.20	.05
0.10	0.10	0.10	0.10	.10	0.10	.02
0.00	0.00	0.00	0.00	.00	0.00	.00

to the head and chest, especially the precordial region, previously to the general application of the douche.

936 *Dyspnea* rarely occurs except in persons suffering from emphysema, or who are subject to attacks of nervous asthma. The indication is either that the application made is too intense, or that sufficient care has not been taken to avoid the region of the chest, especially the front part of it. More moderate applications or the employment of a somewhat prolonged (10 to 15 sec.) cold douche (65° to 70°), with low pressure, before the general application, will generally suppress this symptom; or it may be relieved by a neutral compress to the chest and a Scotch douche to the legs.

937 *Malaise*, *nervousness*, and *depression* are symptoms commonly resulting from overtreatment or excessive employment of heating procedures. The last-mentioned cause is most frequent. Depression and malaise may generally be quickly overcome by vigorous general cold applications or the cold dorsal percussion douche daily. The Scotch douche to the back or the prolonged neutral affusion to the spine (93° to 96°, 10 min.) relieves nervousness and other symptoms of excitation.

Vertigo and *fainting* are symptoms likely to occur in connection with hot applications when too greatly prolonged, but are quickly relieved by cold applications, especially cold affusion to the chest and shoulders. Their recurrence indicates the necessity for a change in the prescription by lowering the temperature or by increasing the pressure of the bath.

938 *Sleeplessness* may result from excessive stimulation by intense cold procedures or by the excitement arising from heating processes. When these procedures are necessary in persons subject to sleeplessness, they should be administered in the early part of the day instead of the evening, and if necessary, the neutral bath may be employed at bed-time to counteract any excitation which may remain from the treatment in the early part of the day. If the difficulty is not thus controlled, the exciting measures may be suspended for

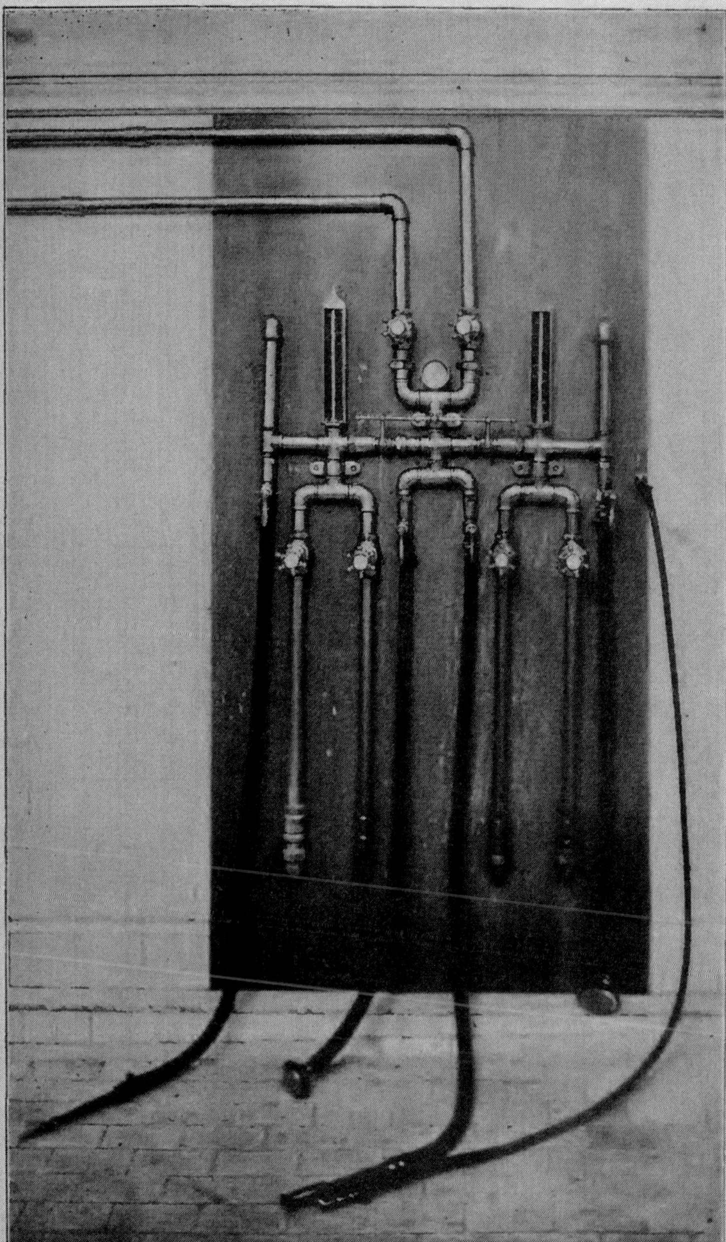

FIG. 31. GENERAL DOUCHE APPARATUS (p. 427). (Kellogg)

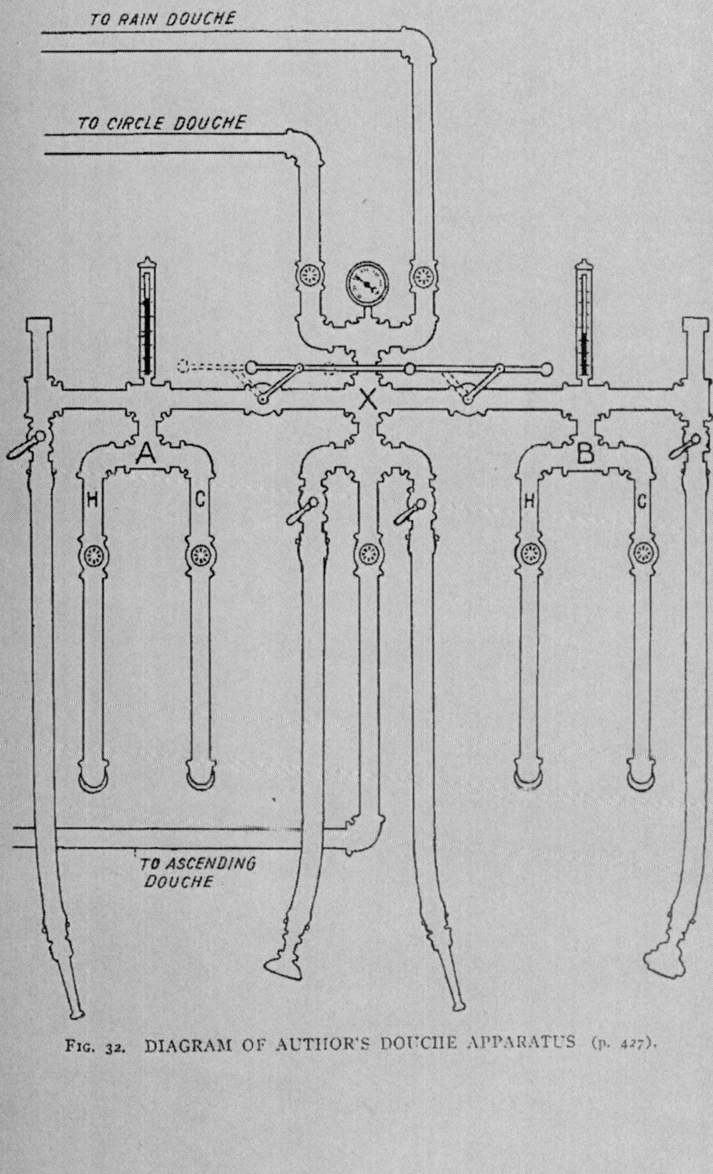

FIG. 32. DIAGRAM OF AUTHOR'S DOUCHE APPARATUS (p. 427).

a time, such quieting means as the tonic pack, the neutral immersion bath, the neutral douche, or cold friction being employed instead of the douche or the shallow bath.

Pain may be the result of excessive congestion of some 939
part induced by misapplied or mismanaged procedures, or it may be simply the awakening of some chronic neuralgic affection. The cold douche often gives rise to sciatic or intercostal pains in persons who have been subject to those difficulties. Pain is very likely to result from cold applications which have not been followed by complete and thorough reaction.

Headache is one of the most common results of misman- 940
aged or too intense hydriatic procedures. "The hydropathic headache" is a well-known phrase among the frequenters of Continental hydropathic institutions. Headache is very likely to result from excessively cold or excessively hot procedures, and may be due either to congestion from imperfect regulation of the circulation or to excessive excitation of the cerebrum.

Deficient reaction, as shown by long-continued pallor and 941
coldness of the skin, with chilliness, cold extremities, and generally headache, indicates that the duration of the application has been excessive, or that the patient was not properly prepared for the application. The last-named cause is perhaps the most frequent. The patient who is chilly or exhausted when the cold application is made, is likely to suffer in this way. Deficient reaction not infrequently occurs as the result of neglect to employ, after the bath, the proper measures to encourage reaction, the most important of which are rubbing and exercise. Exercise is by far the best means of encouraging reaction, as it sets in operation most fully the forces necessary for perfectly balancing the circulation, increasing heat production, and energizing all the vital functions.

Very short and very cold applications are most likely to be followed by complete and thorough reaction. Reaction is quite certain to fail, especially in feeble patients, when a succession of cold applications is made with an interval between, as, for example, a rubbing wet sheet followed by a prolonged cold sitz bath, or the sitz bath followed by a cold douche. A patient not possessed of very vigorous reactive powers would be almost certain to suffer the evil results of defective reaction following secondary chill, if subjected to such a formula as the above. The author has known many similar and worse combinations to be employed, and yet wonderment was expressed that the results were not such as had been expected.

942 When the patient fails to react during or after a cold application, as the wet-sheet pack, the shallow bath, the wet-sheet rubbing, or the cold douche, a hot application should be made at once, the temperature of which should be about 100° F. at the beginning, being rapidly raised until a temperature as high as the patient can endure is reached — 108° to 110°. When the patient has become so thoroughly heated that he longs for some cooling drops to fall upon him (1 to 3 min.), the cold application should be renewed; but unless he has been accustomed to the use of cold applications, the temperature should not be lower than 65° to 75°, and the duration should be brief. If a douche apparatus is not convenient, the patient may be put into a hot immersion bath at 100°, the temperature being afterward raised to 106° or 108° until he is thoroughly warmed, as indicated by flushing of the face and a full pulse. The cold affusion (70° to 80°) may then be employed while the patient sits or stands in a partially filled tub. The patient should not be allowed to leave the hands of the attendant until good reaction has been produced and the circulation has become well balanced, as shown by a full, steady pulse.

943 *Excessive reaction,* as shown by overexcitation of the heart, perspiration, and prolonged sensation of heat, fulness of the head, perhaps headache, indicates a too intense or too short application. In the employment of the Scotch douche the symptoms named are very likely to occur when the cold application is not employed for a sufficient length of time to

allay the exciting effects of the heat, and develop the tonic-sedative influence of cold. Excessive reaction calls for a reapplication of cold at moderate temperature (65° to 80°), with little pressure.

Eruptions of the skin indicate excessive cutaneous excita- 944
tion, and interdict the use of the sweating pack and similar procedures. In some instances the vapor bath or the electric-light bath must be substituted for more exciting sweating procedures, or the prolonged neutral bath, followed by cold affusion, must be employed instead of more highly tonic applications, until the irritated condition of the skin is relieved. Cold friction, the rubbing wet sheet, the hot immersion bath, and similar processes must of course be avoided in cases of this kind.

Winternitz has made the interesting discovery that hydro- 945
therapy may be employed as a sort of diagnostic "reagent" to determine, in doubtful cases, whether or not syphilitic infection exists. In persons in whom this dyscrasia is present, the characteristic eruptions occur under hydriatic treatment, especially from the stimulating effect of the sweating pack and other sweating processes and cold shower baths.

The occurrence of *spasm* of the *voluntary or involuntary* 946
muscles is a symptom that may require special attention. Cramps in the muscles of the legs sometimes occur in the prolonged cold bath administered for antifebrile effects in continued fevers. This may be obviated by rubbing the parts with cold water before the bath or by wrapping the legs with flannels wrung out of very cold water just before the patient enters the bath. Special attention should be given to rubbing the legs in the Brand bath and the shallow bath to prevent the occurrence of this unpleasant symptom in persons especially subject to muscular cramps, in whom this symptom is very likely to occur whenever cold water is entered, or even water at a temperature of 70° to 75°, thus rendering swimming dangerous. In such cases the limbs must be rubbed vigorously and continuously during cold baths of any sort, special

attention being given to the muscles in which the cramp is most likely to occur.

947 Another symptom of excitation, which not infrequently occurs when very cold baths are employed, is increase of seminal losses in cases of spermatorrhea due to irritation of the spinal genito-urinary center. In these cases cold applications, if employed at all, should be exceedingly brief,—not more than one-half minute in duration,—and not infrequently cold applications must be entirely suspended, the neutral sitz bath for half an hour to two hours being substituted.

948 At the beginning of treatment, patients sometimes complain of a slight or even decided *exacerbation of morbid symptoms* as the result of the procedures to which they are subjected. This may indicate either that the treatment is not yet accurately adjusted to the patient's conditions, or that the curative processes employed are so powerfully alterative or perturbing in their effects that there is an intensification of the effort to restore the patient to a normal condition, the symptoms from which the patient suffers being simply an indication that such a remedial process is in operation. In the latter case an increase of these symptoms need not be considered in any sense discouraging, the patient being, on the contrary, thus assured that the measures employed are aiding nature in her curative work.

949 Measures which are radically curative in character by no means always produce an amelioration of symptoms as soon as they are applied. Time must be allowed for the healing processes of nature to proceed to completion. Recovery from disease is a thing which requires time, like the growth of a plant. Good judgment and good sense are necessary for interpreting the meaning of an exacerbation of the symptoms in a case under hydriatic treatment, whether they are what might be termed accidental, or merely functional symptoms, as, for example, pain, loss of appetite or of energy, or whether they are of a destructive character, as manifested by ulceration, suppuration, sloughing, etc. In any case they

can not be regarded as in any way favorable, and demand an immediate change of the prescription or the application of measures for their suppression.

On the other hand, the recurrence of biliary obstruction 950 in the attempt to discharge a collection of gall-stones or a similar recurrence of renal colic may indicate an advance in the curative process. The same may be said with reference to various remedial processes in which there is an evident effort to eliminate some foreign substance or to purify the tissues, as an increased frequency of the recurrence of attacks of headache, an effect sometimes observed in cases of chronic migraine soon after the beginning of a course of hydriatic treatment.

The hydriatrist, of all physicians, must be thoroughly acquainted with the language of disease, with all its pathological processes, and must especially be familiar with the conditions of health as expressed in human physiology. No hydric application for therapeutic purposes is safe or likely to prove successful unless made with the full knowledge of the patient's condition at the moment, and in harmony with the physiological and therapeutic principles involved in the particular case in hand. Routine treatment is always bad enough, but in hydriatic practice it is absolutely dangerous and destructive alike to the reputation of the physician and to the comfort and possibly even the life of the patient.

The application of cold water without friction is one of 951 the best known means of testing a patient's vital state. If reaction is slow, his vitality is at a low ebb. If a mottled, cyanotic appearance remains for some time after the cold application, the indication is proof of cardiac weakness, with possibility of impending collapse. This test should be frequently applied in cases of typhoid fever or other grave febrile disorders, and may be used with much advantage as a test for determining the advisability of administering an anesthetic in a case in which there may be some question of the ability of the patient to receive it with safety.

952 **The Average Temperature of Baths.** It will be helpful to the beginner in the use of hydriatic measures to find brought together in small space a statement of the average temperatures required for efficient results with the leading forms of baths. These may be briefly stated as follows, the extremes being indicated in ordinary type, the average in bold:—

Douche: cold, 50° to 70°, **60°**; hot, 104° to 125°, **115°**; neutral, 92° to 97°, **95°**.

Affusion: cold, 55° to 65°, **60°**; cool, 70° to 80°, **75°**; hot, 104° to 122°, **113°**.

Plunge: cold, 50° to 70°, **60°**.

Immersion: cold, 50° to 70°, **60°**; cool, 70° to 80°, **75°**; hot, 100° to 106°, **102°**; very hot, 104° to 115°, **108°**; neutral, 92° to 97°, **95°**.

Brand bath: **70° F.**

Shallow: cold, 55° to 65°, **60°**; cool, 70° to 80°, **75°**.

Cold wet-sheet pack: **60° F.**

Hot-blanket pack: **130° F.**

Sponge bath: 60° to 75°, **70°**.

Wet-hand rubbing: 45° to 75°, **60°**.

Cold friction: 32° to 70°, **50°**.

Cold towel rubbing: 40° to 75°, **60°**.

Wet-sheet rubbing: **60°**.

Hot-air bath: 110° to 180°, **160°**.

Local hot-air bath: 200° to 300°, **250°**.

Turkish bath: 140° to 250°, **180°**.

Russian bath: 110° to 140°, **125°**.

Vapor bath: 110° to 140°, **130°**.

Foot bath: cold, 45° to 65°, **55°**; hot, 105° to 120°, **115°**.

Sitz bath: cold, 55° to 65°, **60°**; hot, 106° to 120°, **115°**; neutral, 92° to 97°, **95°**.

Fomentation: 120° to 160°, **140°**.

Part Three.

THE TECHNIQUE OF HYDROTHERAPY.

THE modes in which water may be applied to the human body therapeutically are almost infinite in form and variety. It is not proposed in this section to undertake to exhaust the subject, but only to describe those procedures which are capable of being employed in an exact and scientific manner, and have been shown by the test of practical experience to be really essential to enable the hydrotherapeutist to produce each and all of the various therapeutic effects which belong to scientific hydrotherapy.

Disregarding temperature, all hydrotherapeutic measures may be divided into two general classes: —

1. *Applications in which thermic effects alone are pro-* 1000
duced. This class comprises all forms of water baths in which the application itself is not accompanied by rubbings or frictions, percussions with the hand, or the mechanical effects produced by water in motion, the applications being purely passive in character. Of this class are immersions, general and partial, when not accompanied by friction; compresses, hot and cold; packs; hot air, vapor, and electric-light baths; irrigations; applications of coils or rubber bags filled with hot or cold water,—in short, all purely passive applications of heat and cold to the body, either internal or external.

2. *Applications in which thermic impressions are supple-* 1001
mented by mechanical effects, either (*a*) by giving more or less vigorous movement to the mass of water brought in contact with the skin, or (*b*) by manual manipulations, such as rubbing or friction, and percussion. In this class are included

douches of all sorts, also the so-called *percutient* measures, wet and dry friction, rubbing sheets, affusions, and immersions accompanied by friction, such as the Brand bath, the shallow bath, the rubbing sitz.

In most general hydriatic procedures mechanical effects of some sort are employed to a greater or less extent as a necessary aid to reaction. It is only in comparatively exceptional cases, in which reaction must be prevented, or is not required, as in most hot applications, that mechanical effects are absolutely excluded.

In certain cases it is desirable to secure mechanical effects alone. The thermic effects of water are then suppressed by the employment of neutral temperatures (92° to 97°), or of such purely mechanical measures as dry friction and percussion. The last-named procedures belong properly to the province of massage; but, as elsewhere remarked, the effects produced by massage and by thermic applications are so closely allied, and these procedures so constantly and intimately associated, that it is almost impossible to avoid considering both under the same head. Indeed, hydrotherapy in practice is essentially a thermo-mechanico-therapy; but we lack a convenient word to express this compound idea, and so are by the poverty of our nomenclature compelled to describe and discuss under the general heading "Hydrotherapy" some procedures into which water does not enter at all.

In the description of the various hydriatic processes, it is not possible to follow closely the above classification, although in the therapeutic application of the resources of hydrotherapy, it is of the highest importance that it should be held constantly in mind.

The discussion of the therapeutic application of individual hydriatic processes is rendered not a little difficult by the fact that almost every one of the procedures described in this work, numbering more than two hundred, is possessed of such versatility and capacity for modification that it constitutes in itself almost a complete hydriatic armamentarium. In general, it may be said that the therapeutic applications which have been indicated for individual procedures are those to which the measure in question most conveniently or aptly lends itself, and those the value of which has been proved by clinical experience. It is true that a physician possessed of a sufficient amount of knowledge, skill, and experience will be able to secure nearly all and perhaps the very best results of hydrotherapy by the aid of comparatively few and simple measures. Indeed, there are very few effects which can not be secured by such extraordinarily simple means as a sheet, a few towels, a pail, and an ample supply of hot and cold water, provided the requisite experience and skill are added. But the ability to accomplish large and efficient results with such small means can be attained only by long practice and training, while they may be much more readily reached by the employment of means more exactly adapted to the purpose required. An expert, with a pocket-knife alone, can accomplish nearly all that is produced with the varied tools of the wood-carver and the cabinet-maker, but certainly not with the same facility or rapidity. An expert may be able to do more even with a single implement than a bungler with a hundred tools. But the best results of all will be attained by the expert who has at command a full complement of instruments of precision adapted to the work in hand.

It is also a purpose of this work to present in a methodical form the varied resources of the most versatile and marvelously potent curative agent which a beneficent Creator has given to man, and not to him only, but to the whole animal kingdom.

In describing the various hydriatic procedures in the following pages, those which are similar in method of application will be grouped together, although their physiological effects may be quite different, the various therapeutic effects of water and the methods by which each may be produced having already been systematically discussed at considerable length in the preceding section of this work.

DOUCHES.

1002 A douche consists of a single or multiple column of water directed against some portion of the body. In the therapeutic employment of the douche, three factors are active: (1) *Temperature*, (2) *Pressure*, (3) *Mass*.

The range of temperatures employed in douches is from 45° to 125° F. The pressure ordinarily employed is from 10 to 60 pounds, represented by a water column of 25 to 150 feet. The mass varies greatly, according to the effect desired. For the single horizontal jet, a nozzle with an aperture of one fourth to three eighths of an inch is commonly employed. In the filiform douche, the column of water is scarcely larger than a fine hair. Both the pressure and the mass effect may be easily regulated by means of the finger placed in the water column near the mouth of the nozzle, thus breaking or dispersing the stream. More exact and certain means of regulating the pressure should be employed, however, in regular hydriatic practice.

1003 The douche apparatus should be constructed with pipe of ample size (at least one and a half inches in diameter), and should be directly connected with the sources of both hot and cold water, the connections being so arranged that the use of hot and cold water elsewhere in the bath-rooms or in the establishment shall not cause a variation of the temperature of the water delivered to the apparatus after it has once been adjusted for use. This is not always easy to accomplish, but can always be done if sufficient intelligence and experience are brought to bear upon the problem.

An accurate pressure gauge and thermometer should be connected with the apparatus, so that pressure and temperature may be accurately determined. For facility in the use of the douche, and for the most efficient work, it is highly important to have the apparatus so constructed that it may be quickly adjusted for any form of douche, and for any temperature desired, and in rapid alternation if required.

The author has devised and used for a number of years 1004
(1899) a very convenient apparatus, the general form of construction of which may be seen in the accompanying cuts (Figs. 31, 32). With this apparatus it is possible to administer the douche in every required form, at any required temperature, and to regulate to a nicety both the pressure and the temperature of the application.

As will be seen by reference to the figure, the apparatus consists of two ordinary douche apparatuses (A and B) connected by a pipe (X). Each of these is supplied with a thermometer. A pressure gauge placed between the two valves indicates the pressure for both. By means of a switch connecting the two valves so that they move together, water from either of these sets of pipes may be directed upon the patient with the same service hose. By this means the attendant has complete and instant control of both the temperature and the pressure in the administration of the douche. The temperature range is from 45° to 125°, and the pressure from one-half pound to 45 pounds. In giving the Scotch douche and the alternate douche, the temperature is carefully regulated in each of the twin apparatuses to suit the needs of the case. By adjustment of the proper valves the pressure may be regulated instantly, and the switch permits the alternations of different temperatures to be made instantaneously. An extra service hose for each side permits the simultaneous employment of water at any desired temperature.

With this apparatus for supplying water at any temperature and pressure desired, there are connected short pieces of rubber hose with variously shaped nozzles and other appliances for determining the form of the douche, as the jet, fan, rain, needle, percussion. The rain douche and the multiple circle or needle douche are each supplied by a pipe from each one of the twin apparatuses, so that in making successive applications at different temperatures, as in the use of the Scotch or alternating douche, there may be no delay on account of the time required for heating or cooling the service pipe.

A steam-pipe with service hose and a suitable nozzle supplies the means for the vapor douche when required.

With an instrument of precision of this sort, water may be applied to the body with the same accuracy as electricity is employed by the aid of a galvanometer.

This apparatus has been used by the author and his colleagues in the Battle Creek (Mich.) Sanitarium and its branches in several hundred thousand applications, and has proved to be eminently satisfactory.

In regulating the temperature of the douche it must be remembered that considerable cooling takes place in the column of water while it is passing from the apparatus to the patient. Descantes* showed that in giving a cold douche at 48° F. in a room at a temperature of 72° F., the temperature fell 1.8° in a distance of 3½ meters (11½ ft.). In giving a hot douche under the same conditions, the loss of temperature was 4½°.

1005 Douches are named according to the form or direction of the stream, the part to which they are directly applied, or the organ or set of organs which they are intended to influence.

Douches are classified according to their form, as the *horizontal jet*, *vertical jet*, *fan*, *broken jet*, *vertical rain* or *shower*, *horizontal rain* or *spray*, *filiform*, *percussion*, *circle*, *multiple circle* or *needle bath*, *Scotch*, *alternate*, *massage douche*, *irrigation*.

Localized Douches. Special applications of the douche to particular parts of the body are described under the following names: *Cephalic*, *dorsal*, *lumbar*, *thoracic*, *epigastric*, *hypogastric*, *abdominal*, *plantar*, *perineal*, *anal*.

Visceral Douches. A number of special applications of the douche are described and designated by the names of the organs or internal parts which they are specially designed to influence, as follows: *Cerebral*, *cerebro-*

* Descantes, *Revue d'Hydrologie*, Paris, 1896, p. 51.

spinal, pulmonary, cardiac, gastric, enteric, hepatic, splenic, renal, genito-urinary, articular, muscular.

In some instances the visceral douche is a compound or complex procedure involving several different successive or simultaneous applications, as in the case of the renal and the gastric douche.

The principal applications of irrigation are to the nose, eye, ear, stomach, rectum, colon (coloclyster), bladder, urethra, and vagina.

Physiological Effects.—The douche, combining as it does 1006
both thermal and percussion effects, is essentially an exciting procedure, and is capable of producing the most powerful effects which can be elicited by hydrotherapeutic procedures of any sort.

The precise effects obtained by the application of the douche depend upon (1) the temperature of the water, (2) pressure, (3) duration, (4) form of the stream as determined by the shape of the outlet, (5) whether it is general or local, and if local (6) the part to which it is applied. According to Schüller's experiments,* the temperature of the water employed in the douche, though important, is of less importance than the mechanical effect. The special adaptation of the several forms of the douche to individual morbid conditions will be indicated in connection with the description of the several forms of this procedure.

The douche, like the centripetal stroking of massage, aids 1007
the movement of blood through the heart, and accelerates the current of lymph in the lymph channels, in this action co-operating with the peripheral heart and other normal agencies by which a constant movement of blood through the vessels is maintained. As Winternitz wrote years ago (1882), "The *vis a tergo* of the blood by the *normal rhythmical contraction of the vessels so like peristaltic action*, prevents a retrograde movement." Ludwig has shown that the movement of

---

* *Arch. für Klin. Med.*, 1874.

lymph is accelerated by the increase of blood pressure in the capillaries.

The blood pressure of the part upon which the column of water plays is increased under the influence of the douche, and Ludwig has shown that increase of pressure in the capillaries accelerates the movement of the lymph and increases the flow of lymph from the blood-vessels out through the lymph spaces. The douche, like the stroking of massage, accelerates the movement of lymph in the vessels.

The effect of the douche upon cutaneous sensibility differs chiefly according to its duration. The short douche (either hot or cold) increases sensibility of all kinds; while if sufficiently prolonged, the douche, either hot or cold, may diminish all the sensory functions of the skin.

Muscular capacity is increased by the *short cold* douche, as shown by the experiments of Vinaj and Maggiori. In paresis the patient sometimes finds himself perfectly able, after a short cold douche with strong pressure over the affected parts, to control voluntary muscles which previously were almost wholly useless. The hot douche may lessen muscular capacity to one fifth the normal amount.

The reaction effects produced by the cold douche are not necessarily more *vigorous* than those following any other hydriatic application of the same temperature, but are more *immediate*.

1008 The interesting experiments of Couette on the effects of different forms of the bath upon the body temperature showed that a short cold douche (5 to 30 secs.) may cause a fall of temperature amounting to half a degree by the end of 20 minutes, after a brief rise of a few tenths of a degree. A cold douche of 3 minutes' duration causes an immediate fall of temperature amounting to nearly 1½° F. within 20 minutes after the douche. The temperature still remains below normal more than an hour after the application of the cold douche, even when vigorous measures to encourage reheating are employed.

The *warm* and the *neutral* douche have no effect upon the temperature.

The hot douche always elevates the general temperature; the longer the bath and the higher its temperature, the greater the elevation.

The form of the bath seems to have little relation to its effect upon the temperature. The controlling factors are the temperature of the bath, its duration, and the amount of exercise following it. Pressure apparently has no effect.* Pressure hastens reaction, but has little or no effect upon metabolic processes. Hence the most important element in the douche is the temperature. Pressure plays an important but secondary rôle.

The general cold douche is one of the most powerful of all tonics. It creates an appetite for food and a disposition to, and capacity for, both mental and muscular activity to a remarkable degree.

The douche encourages both thermic and circulatory reaction to a high degree — thermic reaction because of the rapid cooling of the skin, and circulatory reaction by reason of the massage effect produced by the intermittent pressure of the stream of water upon the cutaneous surface.

In the employment of *non-percutient* hydriatic measures, *temperature* and *duration* are the principal factors to be regulated; but in the employment of the douche, as the horizontal jet, for example, two other factors of importance must be taken into consideration; viz., *volume* and *pressure.* These factors may be controlled in various ways. Pressure is regulated primarily by the elevation of the source from which the water supply comes, or the pressure in the general system with which the pipes supplying the douche apparatus are connected. It may likewise be regulated by valves, by the distance of the patient from the nozzle, and by breaking and partially dispersing the stream by the finger. The volume

*Couette, "Étude Experimentale sur l'Action Thermique de l'Eau Froide en Applications Hydrotherapeutiques."

of the stream in size and form determines to a considerable degree the effect produced as regards the thermic as well as the mechanical effects. The greater the volume, the greater the effect produced, both thermically and mechanically, other things being equal.

1009 **Therapeutic Applications.**—The douche is one of the most universally useful of all hydrotherapeutic measures. In some Continental hydriatic establishments, especially in France, the writer found the douche used almost to the exclusion of every other measure. The *cold* douche is perhaps the most powerful of all known tonics. The alternating douche and the Scotch douche are excitant measures of most extraordinary power. The *warm* or *neutral* douche is decidedly sedative or calmative in its effects. The *hot* or *very hot* douche, with strong pressure, produces exciting effects similar to those of the cold douche, but being often followed by atonic reaction, is inferior to the cold for tonic effects.

Used with little pressure, the hot douche is a powerful analgesic measure, especially when employed in connection with cold, as in the Scotch or revulsive douche. The very hot or revulsive douche is indicated in such painful affections as *sciatica*, *painful rheumatic joints*, *sprains*, *neuralgic affections*, *visceral disease* accompanied by pain, as *chronic gastritis*, *hyperpepsia*, *gastric ulcer*, *congestions* of the *liver* and *spleen*, and in some cases of *pelvic congestion*, and in so-called *inflammation of the uterus* and *ovaries*.

Contraindications.—The douche is contraindicated in cases in which it is desirable to suppress reaction as much as possible, as in *acute inflammation*, and when *acute nervous irritability* or *excitability* exists. Other contraindications are referred to elsewhere (803–807, 1023).

THE HORIZONTAL JET.

1010 This is the most useful and generally employed of all forms of the douche; and in this work, when the word *douche* is used without a definite description indicating some particu-

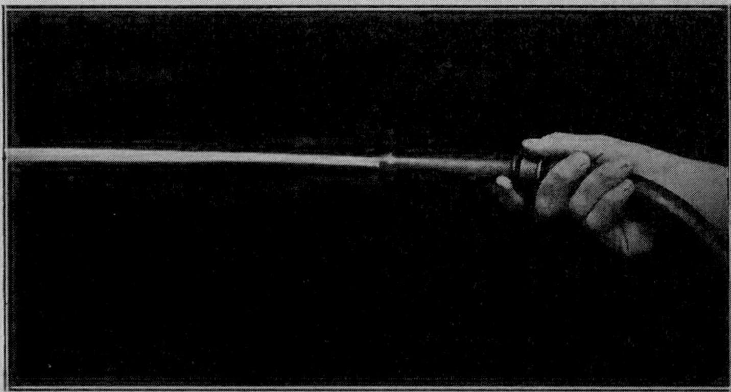

FIG. 33. DOUCHE — Horizontal Jet (p. 433).

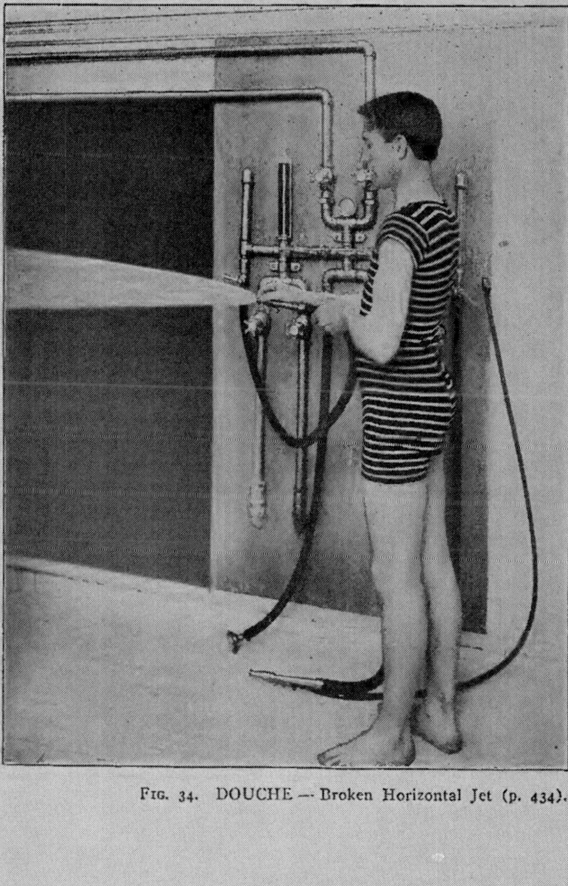

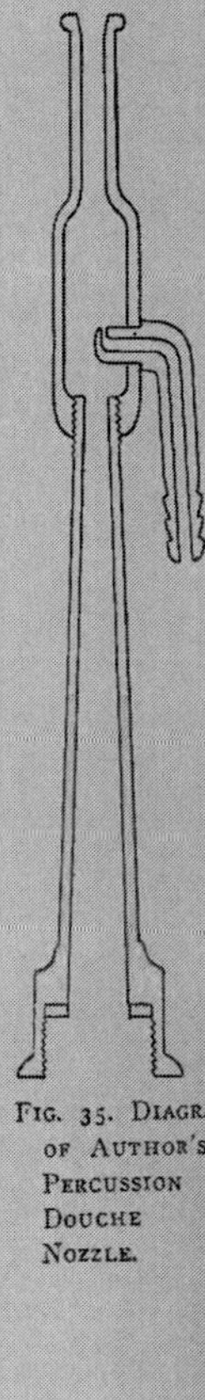

FIG. 35. DIAGRAM OF AUTHOR'S PERCUSSION DOUCHE NOZZLE.

FIG. 34. DOUCHE — Broken Horizontal Jet (p. 434).

lar form of douche, the horizontal jet is the form of procedure referred to.

The jet douche consists of a single stream, varying in diameter from a millimeter or less (the filiform douche) to an inch or even more. The usual size is about three eighths to half an inch. The horizontal jet is applied by means of a nozzle not unlike that of a garden hose, attached to a piece of rubber tubing two or three feet in length, so as to permit free movement (Fig. 33).

Method.—In administering the horizontal jet, water may be employed at any temperature applicable to therapeutic purposes. The full force of the stream may be used where indicated, or the pressure may be broken, either by adjustment of the pressure-regulating valve or by breaking the force of the stream by placing the end of the finger in the stream near the mouth of the nozzle so as to scatter the column of water to the extent desired. The last-named means of lessening the pressure is always available, and must be used in all general applications in adapting the force of the stream to the different regions of the body.

Lemarchand* employed water at a pressure of ten to fifteen atmospheres, but so great a force is certainly not required for securing the good effects of the douche, and is exceedingly liable to abuse. It is a most excellent thing, however, to have in reserve an ample force for use in any special case which may demand powerful mechanical effects.

The pressure employed may vary from 5 to 50 pounds. Still higher pressures may be employed with proper precautions. The degree of pressure should be carefully measured in each case by the pressure gauge.

To insist, however, that the douche can not be scientifically administered without the pressure gauge is an error; but if the application of the douche is left to nurses or attendants, the pressure gauge is quite essential. In the author's opinion, the employment of so vigorous a therapeutic pro-

* Lemarchand, *Annales de la Société d'Hydrologie*, 1893.

cedure as the cold douche should always be conducted under the immediate supervision of an intelligent person who has been medically trained.

The *broken jet* (Fig. 34) is used over the heart and anterior portions of the chest; to the cervical region; and to all sensitive parts, as over the stomach, liver, bowels, and uterus, in inflammation of these organs; *to inflamed or sensitive points; and over painful nerves.* The *full jet* (Fig. 33), at appropriate pressure, may be used upon the back, arms, legs, feet, and over the liver and spleen when not contraindicated.

The head must be very thoroughly cooled before the douche, and should be protected by a cold towel around the head or neck or both. The jet is usually first applied to the back for a few seconds, then the legs and arms, then over the anterior portions of the body and the liver, ending with a strong dash upon the feet. The whole body may be gone over several times in the manner suggested, each particular region being carefully respected as regards the appropriate degree of pressure, the patient turning around as directed by the attendant.

When the cold douche is employed for other than general tonic effects; in other words, when this measure is used as a means of exciting activity in some special organ, the application should first be made to the back, arms, and legs, then over the part in which it is desired to produce the most pronounced effects, as over the stomach in hypopepsia, over the lumbar region in cases of amenorrhea, etc. At the close of the application, a few aspersions should be made to the whole body, and at the last the stream should be directed upon the feet for 2 to 5 seconds.

When it is desired to protect a congested organ against the inrush of blood produced by a general cold application, the douche should first be applied for 3 to 5 seconds to the reflex area connected with the part concerned, before the general application is made. By this means the blood-vessels of the congested part are strongly contracted before the general inrush of blood occurs, and thus the part is protected. This practical fact has led to the application of the douche over the liver and stomach first after the back, and before the general application, on account of the almost universal feebleness of these organs and the need of both protecting and energizing them.

In the general application of the douche, it should be remembered that the stream should not be allowed to fall steadily upon one spot, except in case of the *localized* douche, in which a very pronounced effect is required. By constant movements of the nozzle, the stream should be directed upon different portions of the surface in succession, in dashes or aspersions. In a very short application, two or three aspersions will suffice.

When the patient has previously been prepared for the cold douche by a heating process of some sort, which is generally the case, great care must be taken that he does not become chilled by exposure to the cooling effect of evaporation. To avoid this a cold procedure should follow the hot application instantly; or if a short interval must intervene, a few seconds perhaps, the patient must be protected by a warm woolen blanket. If there is the slightest cooling off by evaporation, causing chilliness, or if an interval of a minute or two has elapsed by reason of some emergency, the skin must be thoroughly warmed up again by a hot rain or needle douche before the cold jet is applied. The condition of the patient should be such that the cold water will not be regarded with extreme aversion and dread.

The patient usually stands in taking the douche. If quite feeble, he may sit, or better, may be supported.

The duration of the douche is from 3 or 4 seconds (cold) to as many minutes (hot or neutral). For prolonged applications, other means are, with rare exceptions, better suited.

In many cases it is well to combine the different forms of the douche in an application, beginning perhaps with the warm rain douche, applying the cold fan douche over the liver, abdomen, and chest, and ending with the full jet to the spine, legs, and feet.

The temperature of the *cold* douche is from 45° to 65°; of the *cool* douche, from 65° to 80°; of the *tepid* douche, from 80° to 92°; of the *neutral* douche, from 92° to 97°; and of the *hot* douche, from 104° to 125°.

The exact temperature as well as the duration must be indicated in each individual case, unless the application is to be made by the physician himself, in which case the immediate effects produced may serve as a useful aid to the knowledge of the case obtained by previous examination. The douche must be regarded as a therapeutic agent of too great power for evil as well as good to permit of careless or routine employment; and the German and French physicians who make use of this potent hydriatic procedure have much foundation for maintaining that no one but a physician can be fully competent to apply so powerful a measure.

1011 **Physiological Effects.**—This extremely versatile hydriatic procedure, though constantly used by Priessnitz and the early empirical hydropaths, was systematized and developed by Fleury about the middle of the present century at his establishment at Belleville, France. Charcot made large use of the douche in certain forms, especially the dorsal, or spinal, douche; and to the use of this simple agent he doubtless owed, in large measure, the successes which gave him a world-wide reputation, not only as a pathologist and an original investigator, but as a medical practitioner. The cold spinal douche is sometimes known as the Charcot douche, though not devised by him. In 1883 and also in 1889 the author found the douche in great use in the hospital Salpêtrière, under the supervision of Charcot, and on visiting this great medical workshop in 1899, he found this and other hydriatic measures occupying a most prominent place in the therapeutics of neurasthenia, hysteria, and all forms of nervous maladies. The same may be said of the hospital Charité and other great centers of scientific medicine in Paris.

The douche is a compound procedure, combining both thermic and mechanical effects. When used in its most vigorous and efficient form, it is capable of producing the most profound effects, both general and local, which can be obtained by any hydriatic measure. It may be usefully employed at all temperatures, and at varying degrees of pressure. It is invaluable both as a general and as a local procedure.

The effects of cold applied in the form of the douche are those which have been described in the section of this work devoted to the physiological effects of water at various temperatures, with the addition of such special features as result from the localization of the procedure, or such modifications as may arise from the special forms in which it may be administered, the combination of thermic and mechanical effects serving to intensify the influence of both these means of impressing the nervous system. The thermic effect may be varied at will by modifying the temperature of the water, while the mechanical effect may be modified by changes in the form and size of the column of water used, or the number of streams employed simultaneously.

Wertheimer* showed that cold applications, as the cold douche to the cutaneous surface, produce vascular changes in the kidney and mesenteric vessels. That similar changes take place in the brain has been demonstrated by Schüller and others.

Carefully conducted experiments made by Storoscheff, of 1012
Moscow, showed conclusively the powerful effects of the cold douche upon metabolism. The consumption of nitrogen was found to be considerably increased; the temperature immediately after the application was lowered a few tenths of a degree and slightly elevated later; respiration during and after the application was lowered eight breaths per minute; the pulse was diminished ten to sixteen beats per minute; the tactile sense was diminished, while the muscular response

* M. Wertheimer, *Académie des Sciences*, 1893, p. 44.

to both the galvanic and the faradic currents was decidedly increased.

The author has undertaken some experiments for the purpose of ascertaining whether or not the last-named effect was the result of increased conductivity of the skin due to saturation with water, or to an actual increase in the muscular excitability. The details of this experiment are given elsewhere (Exp. 54).

1013 The exhaustive researches of Vinaj and Maggiori have shown clearly the remarkable effects of the douche upon the muscles. The cold douche shows by its modification of the fatigue curve an enormous increase of muscular irritability and capacity for work (Exp. 55).

The hot douche produces an effect in an opposite direction even more pronounced, hence its great value in relieving muscular spasm (Exp. 56). The Scotch douche may produce either increase or decrease of muscular excitability and capacity, according to the way in which it is managed.

The rise of blood pressure produced by the cold douche may be followed somewhat later by a diminution in pressure, when the blood-vessels are well dilated by a strong circulatory reaction. This is due to the fact that the influence of the douche upon the surface vessels may endure longer than its effect upon the heart. This is especially true of a very short and energetic application (45° to 55°, at 40 lbs. pressure, 3 to 5 secs.).

The most powerful effects of the douche are produced at from 45° to 60°; time, 4 to 30 seconds. A good working temperature is between 55° and 70°. *The higher the temperature, the longer must be the duration and the greater the pressure required to produce decided tonic effects.* At a low temperature a transient but powerful impression is made upon the skin and through the strong reflexes produced upon the entire organism, manifested chiefly through the thermic and circulatory reactions.

When the douche is administered at a higher temperature (80°), in some instances undesirable nervous phenomena are produced, as headache, lassitude, and imperfect reaction. In such cases it is necessary to educate the patient to the use of low temperatures by very short cold or even very cold applications. 1014

In the administration of a cold jet douche with strong pressure and an unbroken stream, it will be noted that at the exact point upon which the column of water falls the skin becomes instantly blanched, the color reappearing as soon as the stream is allowed to fall upon some other part. Each time that the water column impinges upon any point of the cutaneous surface, this phenomenon is repeated. The blood-vessels are not only made to contract by the thermic impression of cold water, but the weight of the stream of water, the force of impact, compresses the tissues, and forces the blood out of the vessels, leaving them free to dilate again as soon as the pressure is removed. Thus the tissues are alternately compressed and released; in other words, a veritable massage is produced, whereby the circulation is excited and accelerated; and the thermic effect of the douche is thus materially aided by the purely mechanical or percussion effects of the moving water as really as if friction or percussion movements had been executed with the hand. 1015

When the pressure employed is sufficient to produce a decided stinging sensation at each point of contact, a powerful reflex effect is produced by stimulation of the various sets of nerves which recognize temperature, pressure, pain, and tactile impressions. When we recall that in addition to the nerves mentioned, the douche, in common with other procedures, influences the vasoconstrictors, the vasodilators, and the sympathetic ganglia of the vessel walls, it is apparent that this procedure excels all others as a means of awakening or controlling local activity in the skin, also, through the wide-spreading reflexes set up by it, of arousing or otherwise impressing metabolic processes and all other vital activities.

The douche is unquestionably the most powerful and most versatile of all hydriatic procedures, and one which may be most readily and perfectly adapted to all conditions and indications. The only disadvantage which can be mentioned is the fact that it can not be administered without apparatus of some sort. In an emergency, some simple device may be adopted, such as allowing water to fall from a height. In the old water-cure at Graefenberg, this was the only form of douche employed. The stream of the principal douche was of the size of the arm, and fell from a height of fifteen feet. The temperature of the water employed was often that of ice-water, or 32° F. But these crude measures were by no means capable of accomplishing the results which may be obtained by the use of the scientific instrument previously described, and for which the world is chiefly indebted to the ingenuity and sagacity of that eminent French clinician and hydrotherapist, Fleury. In the absence of any more convenient apparatus, a greenhouse pump may be used, with good effect.

1016 **Therapeutic Applications.**—The powerful perturbing influence of the cold douche gives to it the very highest value as an alterative and restorative procedure. Under its influence the whole organism is aroused to the highest degree of activity; the intensity of every function is heightened; the whole body is lifted upon a higher plane of being; the vital resistance is increased; digestive activity is augmented, both by increase of motility and by the production of a greater quantity of hydrochloric acid; glandular activity of every sort is quickened; the processes of assimilation and disintegration are hastened; oxidation and elimination are increased; all the wheels of life move with a quickened vigor and regularity. The individual begins to live a more vigorous and vital life, physically, mentally, and we may even say morally.

The versatility of the douche permits its adaptation to every morbid condition. Fleury depended almost wholly upon this measure in the hydriatic treatment of invalids of all classes, as do the majority of physicians who practice hydriatry in France at the present time. While not underestimating the value of the douche, the author does not share in this extreme partiality to it. Many of the therapeutic purposes for which it is employed by Duval, Beni-Barde, Bottey, and many other leading French specialists, may be more conveniently obtained by the employment of other simple measures requiring no apparatus of any kind. It must be said, however, that the douche is the most powerful and valuable of all tonic measures. There is no drug known to man that is possessed of such marvelous renovating and permanently restorative properties.

As a tonic, the cold douche may be advantageously **1017**
employed in almost every case of chronic disease. If not appropriate at the beginning of a course of treatment, the constant aim should be to train the patient, by a series of carefully graduated measures, to a condition which will admit of the employment of the cold douche. This training may be accomplished by a variety of means. In general, it will begin with nonpercutient measures, such as wet-hand rubbing, cold friction, the cold-towel rub, the wet-sheet rub, and the half bath. When the patient's strength and ability to develop strong reaction have been increased to a sufficient degree, the douche may be employed, at first at a moderate temperature, beginning at 75°, or 80°, or even 90° in very extreme cases, and being gradually lowered from day to day as the patient's strength and resistance increase. The pressure is also gradually increased, beginning with 10 or 15 pounds and gradually increasing to 20, 25, or even 40 pounds, and finally reaching that of the percussion douche.

There is room for discussion as to which is the better method of graduating the cold douche,— whether it is better to apply it at first with higher temperature, less pressure, and longer application ; or to employ at once the lowest temperature likely to be used at all, making the application at first very brief, perhaps not more than 2 or 3 seconds, and gradually increasing the duration from day to day.

It must be admitted that both methods may be employed, and perhaps the two are equally serviceable, provided discrimination is used in their application, and care taken to apply each plan to the class of cases to which it is especially adapted. From the observations which the author has made upon this point, he is, however, of the opinion that in most cases it is better that the patient should begin with cool or cold, but very short, applications, rather than with tepid and prolonged ones, as the cold application, though short, is certain to produce vigorous reaction by the powerful stimulation of the vasomotor centers, while not infrequently a prolonged application of higher temperature results in imperfect reaction and the development of the many disagreeable symptoms which accompany this condition.

In persons suffering from *rheumatism* and *neuralgia*, however, it is evident that the very cold douche can not be employed at the beginning of a course of treatment. This is likewise true of persons suffering from *Bright's disease* of the kidneys, *gastric ulcer*, *locomotor ataxia*, *spinal sclerosis*, and most organic affections of the brain and spinal cord. In these cases it is preferable to begin a course of treatment with very mild non-percutient measures, as the tepid fan douche (90° to 80°) with little pressure (4 to 8 lbs.).

1018 It is in some cases necessary to employ at the beginning of treatment a very much lower pressure (8 to 10 lbs.) than will be readily tolerated after the patient has had the benefit of a few weeks' training. Low pressures (1 to 4 lbs.) are especially indicated in cases in which great *hyperesthesia* of the skin exists, and also in relation to special regions which are the seat of tenderness or pain, as in douches to the joints in *chronic rheumatism*, with much pain or tenderness, to the chest in *intercostal neuralgia*, to the abdomen in *chronic hyperesthesia* of the solar plexus and the *sympathetic ganglia*, and to all parts in which much irritability is present.

As nonpercutient measures of training, arranged in the order in which they may be advantageously introduced into the prescription for a feeble patient in training for the douche, the following may be enumerated: Dry rubbing, wet-hand rubbing, cold wet friction, the salt glow, the towel rub, wet-sheet rubbing, rubbing sitz, the shallow bath. Each of the above measures is capable of being graduated to a nicety, and through a wide range of intensity. **1019**

In the majority of cases, the cold douche requires a preliminary preparation of the skin by a short application of heat. When the douche is used for this purpose, a temperature of 104° to 120° may be readily employed; 125° may be tolerated for a few seconds, rapidly moving over the surface treated. **1020**

It is apparent that the douche may be advantageously combined with a variety of other hydriatic procedures, especially such as produce heating effects, as the heating or sweating pack, the electric-light bath, the vapor, Turkish, Russian, and hot-air baths, the immersion bath, the hot immersion bath, fomentations to the spine and abdomen, the hot enema, etc. It forms a fitting conclusion for any heating procedure in which its mechanical effects are not contraindicated.

No other therapeutic agent is of such value as the cold douche in the treatment of *neurasthenia* in most of its forms. In nearly all chronic cases the cold douche sooner or later becomes the sheet-anchor of treatment. In *chlorosis* and all the curable forms of *anemia*, the cold douche daily wins successes in scientific hydriatic establishments when iron and all the other usual remedies have failed.

As a general awakener and regulator of *nutrition*, the cold douche has no equal; and it is also unrivaled as a curative agent in *chronic atonic dyspepsia* or *hypopepsia*, and in most cases of *chronic toxemia* from chronic infections of the alimentary canal. It may even be employed, after careful training, and with the exercise of great care, in quite a large proportion of cases of *cardiac insufficiency* and *renal disease*,

In *chronic inebriety*, and in the treatment of the *opium* and other *drug habits*, cold water holds a high place, not simply as a means of aiding escape from the thraldom of the drug, but especially as a means of building up the patient's vital resistance, restoring the tone and equilibrium of his nervous system, and establishing a condition of perfect health and independence of narcotic or stimulant drugs of any kind, and so removing the excuse and temptation to relapse.

The cold douche may be used to relieve *insomnia* due to cerebral congestion. It acts by producing powerful derivative effects toward the lower extremities when reaction is established, and also through reflex contraction of the cerebral vessels, from stimulation of the rich network of vasomotor nerves distributed in the plantar region of the foot.

1021 In the administration of the cold douche to relieve *cerebral congestion* the following method is to be recommended: —

A thick, dry woolen sheet is wrapped about the patient, being drawn tightly about the neck so as to protect the body. Standing in a foot bath of hot water (104° to 110°), he bends forward while one to two gallons of water at 60° is poured upon the vertex of the head and the back of the neck. A towel wet with water at 50° is then wrapped about the head, and the patient stands erect while the cold broken jet or spray douche is administered to the feet from half a minute to two minutes. If an apparatus for the administration of the plantar douche is not at hand, the patient, standing with his face toward the attendant, turns half around at intervals of 15 to 20 seconds, and raises first one foot and then the other so as to receive the force of the stream upon the plantar surface of each foot for about 10 seconds. The application to the dorsum of the feet and to the ankles is then continued as before, thus repeating for 1 or 2 minutes.

1022 A short cold douche (10 to 30 sec.) or a very hot douche (110°–122°) of the same duration may be advantageously employed in cases of *hysterical anesthesia*. The douche often has the effect to transfer the anesthesia to the opposite side.

The cold douche is equally useful in *hysterical hyperesthesias*, though in such cases the application should be made to the symmetrical part of the opposite side of the body; as, for example, if the hyperesthesia is in the right leg, the douche should be applied to the left leg. It is well to apply the hot douche or fomentation to the affected limb at the same time that the cold application is being made to the sound part.

The general cold douche administered while an ice-bag is applied to the throat is a valuable measure in *hysterical aphonia*. In *hysterical paralysis* of the lower extremities the cold douche at 50° may be applied to the dorsal and lumbar spine with advantage. Strong pressure may be used, but the stream should be small. The parts should be well rubbed with flannel after the application.

Contraindications.—Care must be taken to avoid the 1023
employment of the cold douche in all cases in which an active inflammation exists, and especially in cases of inflammation of the *uterus*, *ovaries*, *kidneys*, *stomach*, *liver*, *bladder*, or *bowels*.

In many cases of so-called *chronic inflammation*, as *intestinal catarrh*, *myelitis*, *chronic gastritis*, *cystitis*, and *general neuritis*, the cold douche *must be avoided*. The cold douche is of high value, however, in cases of *passive congestion* of the *liver*, *stomach*, *spleen*, and *other viscera*.

In *acute rheumatism* the cold douche is contraindicated, and may even be dangerous; but in *chronic rheumatism*, after proper training, it may be employed with benefit for constitutional effects. Special care must be taken to avoid the use of the cold douche in cases of *arteriosclerosis*, *apoplexy*, *valvular disease* of the *heart* with *deficient compensation*, *cardiac insufficiency* from *fatty degeneration*, *renal disease*, or from any other cause when marked in degree. In *acute* or *chronic nephritis;* in *painful nervous affections*, as *sciatica*, *locomotor ataxia*, *multiple neuritis*, in *hyperpepsia*, and in *gastric ulcer;* in *varicose* conditions of the *portal* or *mesenteric veins,* such as sometimes accompany *hepatic sclerosis;* and in cases of extreme general *nervous irritability,* the cold douche must be avoided. The douche at all temperatures is contraindicated in *eruptive disorders* of the *skin,* and in *hyperesthesia* and *neuralgia* of the *skin.* Heggelin has pointed out the danger of pulmonary hemorrhage during the cold douche in persons liable to this accident, on account of the temporary rise of pressure in the left auricle, and stasis of blood in the lungs. General cold applications of all sorts must on this account be avoided in these cases, but such partial applications as cold friction and the cold-towel rub may be employed at any desired temperature.

THE HOT DOUCHE.

1024 The temperature of the water employed may vary from 100° to 130°. The duration varies from 15 or 30 seconds to 4 or 5 minutes. Very strong pressure is less essential than with the cold douche, as its effects depend almost wholly upon the thermic impression. As the hot douche is very largely used for the relief of pain, little pressure is commonly employed. When water at a very high temperature is used, as 120° to 125°, care must be taken to keep the nozzle in constant motion, so that the stream shall not fall constantly upon the same spot. By this means the accumulation of heat at any one point is prevented, and a most powerful sensory impression is made without injury to the tissues.

In the use of the very hot douche the application should be begun at a nearly neutral temperature, as 100° to 102°, the temperature being gradually but rapidly increased, reaching the highest point in from 30 to 60 seconds. Too much time must not be lost in the graduation, otherwise the maximum effect for the time specified will not be obtained. The patient's sensations are a reliable guide. The temperature should be raised as rapidly as possible without producing a decidedly painful sensation, thus causing excessive nervous excitation. In order to give the best effects in relieving deep-seated pain, the temperature must at the end be high enough to cause a slightly painful sensation.

Physiological Effects.— The general hot douche is a very 1025
exciting procedure. Its physiological effects are very similar to those of the hot immersion bath, with the addition of mechanical effects. Excitation of the vasomotor centers is produced by the impact of the water when considerable pressure is employed. The blood pressure is on this account increased instead of being lowered, as in the hot immersion bath. The immediate effects of a *very hot* douche are in many respects similar to those of a cold douche, except that they are transient, and followed by an atonic reaction. The hot douche is thus at first excitant, later relaxing, depressant, or sedative.

The very hot douche is one of the most exciting of all hydrotherapeutic measures. The nature of the application permits of the employment of a temperature higher than can be employed with the immersion or other forms of the bath in which a thermic impression is made upon the entire surface at the same instant, so that the nervous impression produced is greater.

The duration of the hot douche is usually too brief to produce any very marked effect upon metabolic processes, but it produces very prompt and decided effects upon the circulatory and nervous systems. When the temperature is sufficiently high to cause slight pain, a very brief contraction of the small vessels occurs at the beginning of the application. This effect is the more pronounced the greater the pressure employed. This contraction is almost instantly followed by dilatation of the vessels, causing a very pronounced passive congestion of the skin, which at once assumes a dusky or cherry-red hue. If the application is very short, this redness quickly disappears, but if prolonged and at a high temperature, there is paralysis of the vessels, which persists for a very considerable length of time after the conclusion of the application. This is not an active but a passive or paralytic dilatation of the vessels, and is quite different from the active dilatation produced by a cold douche.

1026 At the beginning of a very hot douche, the heart action is slowed; later, it is quickened. This preliminary slowing of the heart is due to the contraction of the surface vessels, which is greater in proportion as the pressure of the douche is increased. This quickened action results from the powerful sensory impression made upon the cutaneous nerves, and the storm of reflex impulses sent in upon the nerve centers in consequence. The heart shares in the general excitation, and by its greatly increased activity the blood pressure is temporarily raised by the rapid filling of the arteries, in spite of the passive dilatation of the small vessels. There is a rapid fall of pressure, however, soon after the conclusion of the application (Exp. 57).

Simultaneously with the passive dilatation of the surface vessels there is a mechanical contraction of the vessels of the interior of the body. The withdrawal of one third to one half of the entire blood of the body into the vessels of the skin necessarily leaves the vessels of the brain and the viscera in a depleted condition.

1027 It should be remembered, however, that when very hot applications are made to the skin, the excitant effects upon the heart and brain are such as to cause at the first a very decided cerebral congestion. This was well shown by Max Schüller in his experiments upon trephined rabbits in 1874. In his experiments the very hot immersion bath was employed. This congestive effect is doubtless due in part to the preliminary contraction of the cutaneous vessels, but that it is not wholly due to this cause is evidenced by the fact that it continues much longer than does the vasoconstriction referred to, and disappears only when the temperature of the application has been very considerably lowered. The cerebral congestion accompanying a very hot application must be due, then, to the reflex excitation of the brain and heart and the elevation of blood pressure.

A knowledge of these facts sufficiently emphasizes the necessity for protecting the head when a very hot douche or other general application is to be made by a thorough cooling of the head, face, and neck, and the application of a cold towel to the head or neck, or both.

The effect of the hot douche upon the central nervous system is at first excitant, but this state is quickly followed by a very pronounced sedation and relaxation.

Therapeutic Applications.—For simple revulsive effects 1028
by excitation of the circulation of the skin, the hot douche from 1 to 5 minutes at a temperature of 100° to 125° gives excellent results. Ordinarily, water at a temperature from 104° to 110° should be employed, the duration being 3 to 5 minutes.

The most vigorous effects of which the hot douche is capable are produced by raising the temperature until the limit of endurance is reached. Few persons can bear a temperature much above 120°, but by taking care not to allow the column of water to fall for more than an instant upon the same spot, a temperature of 124° or 125° may be reached in most cases, and 130° may sometimes be attained. Applied in this manner, the hot douche acts vigorously upon both the blood-vessels and the nerves of the structures subjected to its action, and produces most powerful revulsive and derivative effects.

The general hot douche is most frequently used as a preparation for the cold douche, as in the general Scotch douche and the alternating douche. It should be employed before the cold douche whenever the patient feels an instinctive dread of the contact of cold water, when the skin is cold or the patient inclined to shiver, and especially when the patient has had a prolonged cold application, or when a hot application has been made and the skin has afterward been cooled by evaporation, as during an accidental delay.

The general hot douche, with very slight pressure, is exceedingly useful as a means of relieving *general superficial pain*, *hyperesthesia*, *neuralgia*, and *paresthesia*. It is, in some cases, valuable in relieving the distressing irritation of *pruritis*, *urticaria*, and *jaundice*. A very hot general douche (110° to 122°, 15 to 30 secs., 30 to 40 lbs.) may also be used with advantage in a relaxed condition of the skin accompanied by general and copious perspiration occurring without excitation by heat or exercise, as frequently observed in *neurasthenics*.

1029 The hot douche applied at a very high temperature and of very short duration, may sometimes be employed with excellent advantage in cases which can not tolerate cold applications because of unpleasant after effects. For an application of this sort, a temperature of 110° to 122° is required, and the duration should not be more than 5 to 10 seconds (30 to 40 lbs.). This application is useful in depressed conditions, such as occur in *advanced cardiac* and *renal disease*. Care should be taken to avoid the precordial region in cardiac cases, and the application must not be extended much beyond the time named.

1030 Lemarchand * maintains that equally as good tonic effects may be obtained with the very hot douche (122° F.) as with the cold douche, and notes that it may be tolerated in a great number of cases in which cold water can not be employed, and without the inconvenience of the laborious process of training the patient to the use of cold water. He finds the very hot douche always well borne, and declares that it "concedes nothing to the cold douche" in its value and efficiency. For tonic effects the highest pressure available should be employed. For the best results, a pressure of 35 to 45 pounds is required.

The very hot douche is an excellent excitant measure in cases of *exhaustion* from prolonged or violent exertion. For

* Lemarchand, *Ann. Soc. d' Hydrol. Med.*, Paris, Compt. rend. 1892–93, XXXVIII, 247–275.

such a purpose the application must be greatly prolonged, and should be administered with a considerable degree of pressure (30 to 40 lbs., 1 or 2 secs.).

The general hot douche, as well as the hot-blanket pack, the hot full bath, and other general hot applications, is an *antidote* for an *excessive* application of *cold* which may have been made through inadvertence or as the result of lack of acquaintance with the exact physical condition of the patient or his individual susceptibility. This fact may be borne in mind with great profit by those who are inexperienced in the employment of hydriatic procedures.

In connection with the cold douche, the hot douche may be employed in such a manner as to relieve *pain* or *congestion*, to excite *physiological activity*, or to control a *morbid process* which may be present, according to the methods of application, which will be explained under the respective headings, "The Revulsive Douche" (**1041**) and "The Alternating Douche" (**1044**).

THE NEUTRAL DOUCHE.

Temperature, 92° to 97°; duration, 2 to 30 minutes; **1031**
pressure, from 2 to 20 pounds, according to the effect desired. The ordinary duration of the general neutral douche is from 3 to 15 minutes, pressure, 5 to 20 pounds. Care must be taken to cover the whole surface as completely as possible, so as to prevent cooling by evaporation. When used for simple quieting or sedative effects, the pressure should not be more than 5 to 10 pounds; when employed for derivative effects, that is, to dilate the surface vessels, and so contract the vessels of the brain by displacement of blood to the surface, considerable pressure may be employed; but the pressure should not be so strong in irritable cases as to produce an undesirable excitant effect.

For purely sedative effects, the rain or fan douche should be employed; for derivative effects, the stronger mechanical properties of the full jet may be utilized with advantage.

1032 **Physiological Effects.**—The mechanical effect upon the skin causes widening of the cutaneous vessels, an effect resembling ordinary circulatory reaction from other hydric applications, but without thermic effects either tonic or atonic, and without marked reflex influence, so that the central nervous system is little influenced. The congested brain is thus drained of blood, and at the same time not disturbed by a storm of sensory impressions, as in the hot or the cold douche. The physiological effects of the prolonged neutral douche are essentially the same as those of the neutral immersion bath. This procedure, like other applications of the same temperature, decidedly lessens the muscular tone and capacity. It is on this account well adapted to cases in which there is a decided tendency to muscular cramp or convulsions.

1033 The effects of the neutral douche differ from those of the neutral immersion bath chiefly in the fact that the decided mechanical effect serves to increase the efficiency of the application as a means of increasing the volume and movement of blood in the skin, thus relieving the brain and the thoracic, abdominal, and pelvic viscera. Another advantage of the neutral douche over the neutral full bath is the fact that its action is considerably more rapid than that of the full bath, so that the same results may be obtained by a shorter application. This is a decided advantage in many cases of insomnia, and especially in the treatment of cases of seminal weakness and other forms of genito-urinary irritation of spinal origin. This increased rapidity of effect is doubtless due to its power to decongest the central nervous system. A neutral douche of 5 minutes' duration is equal in effect to a full bath of 30 minutes.

The neutral douche offers an advantage over the hot and the cold douche as a derivative measure in that it is capable of producing physiological congestion of the skin without provoking a preliminary congestion of the brain and internal viscera, and without exciting thermic reaction.

1034 **Therapeutic Applications.**—The application of the neutral douche (92° to 97°) to the back, along either side of the spinal column, is one of the most effective means of quieting *reflex excitability of the spinal centers.* For this purpose, the application should be somewhat prolonged, usually from 4 to 6 minutes, or even 2 or 3 minutes longer. This effect of the neutral douche renders it of great service in the treatment of *St. Vitus's dance, locomotor ataxia*, the irritable spine of *neurasthenia*, certain genito-urinary disorders due to irritation of the genito-urinary center, as *nocturnal enuresis, seminal weakness, vesical irritation*, some cases of *vaginismus*, and *erotomania* in both sexes.

The neutral douche is very useful in general *nervous irritability* as a means of relieving *hyperesthesia* of the skin, *dermalgia*, the itching of *pruritis* or *jaundice*, and general *paresthesias* of various sorts. In all cases in which excessive nervous irritability is present to a marked extent, the application should be made with as little pressure as possible.

(See paragraphs **614** and **1130** for further remarks upon the neutral bath, one of the most useful and interesting of hydriatic measures.)

THE PERCUSSION DOUCHE.

As the special characteristic of the douche is the percu- **1035**
tient effect produced by it, it occurred to the author some years ago (1883) to undertake to improve this hydriatic measure by the development of means whereby its one special characteristic property might be intensified so as to increase the range of its capabilities, especially in cases in which only a low or at most a moderately strong pressure can be obtained from the general water supply. As the result of a dozen years' experimentation, at intervals, an apparatus was perfected which accomplishes this in an admirable manner. An air current under pressure is led into a specially constructed nozzle, near the orifice. This device is shown in the accompanying cut (Fig. 35). The effect of the combination of air

and water is to break up the single column of water into a series of short columns, which are projected upon the surface of the skin with any degree of force desired, each separate mass of water receiving from the expanding mass of air behind it an addition to its initial pressure, just as it issues from the mouth of the nozzle. By regulating the relative pressures of the air and the water, any desired form of the water column may be obtained, from a widely scattered shower, with large drops, or even the *fog douche* to a compact stream, which, falling upon the skin, creates the impression of a fusillade of water bullets, which may be compared to the stream of lead bullets from a Gatling-gun (Fig. 36).

The solid stream of the ordinary horizontal jet produces a more or less constant pressure. If means are adopted to diminish this solidarity, as in the so-called broken jet, the result is greatly to diminish the force with which the water is projected upon the surface; but in the percussion douche, the stream is broken, while at the same time its force is augmented to such an extent as to produce, if desired, a decided stinging sensation as the flying particles of water impinge upon the skin.

1036 The observations which have been made respecting the modes of application and the physiological effects of the horizontal jet in ordinary form, apply equally to the percussion douche. The special advantages which it offers are these:—

1. More powerful effects can be obtained with the ordinary form of douche at the pressure available because of the stronger percutient effects. This remark applies especially to the circulatory reaction produced. Strong percussion of the skin alone will produce strong circulatory reaction, as in slapping the skin with the hand. When the percussion douche is applied with sufficient force, a marked tingling or smarting sensation is produced, as in dry percussion, and the skin is very quickly reddened. Thus the blood supply of the skin is increased, the thermic impression is accordingly

intensified as more heat is abstracted, while the evil effects of the prolonged retrostasis resulting from a nonpercutient general cold application are almost altogether avoided. As the application progresses from one part of the body to another, a reddened, congested skin surface is left behind.

2. The stunning effects of the hydriatic fusillade, which, by means of the percussion douche is made to play upon the skin, render it possible to employ water at a lower temperature than can be employed with the ordinary form of the douche with the same water pressure, thus securing better reaction and more pronounced tonic effects.

3. The very pronounced percutient action renders it possible to obtain by this means excellent and decided effects with water at a higher temperature than is required with the ordinary jet douche,—a fact of great value in the treatment of a very large class of neurasthenics, who, not having been accustomed to cold bathing, are exceedingly rebellious to the application of very cold water.

4. The force and form of the douche can be instantly controlled to suit the will of the operator, without modifying the volume of the water column, by slight adjustment of the nozzle itself held in the hand of the operator.

Therapeutic Applications.— The percussion douche is useful and is indicated in all cases in which the full jet douche can be employed. It is the author's practice to employ it in connection with other forms of the douche in general applications, administering the percussion douche to the back and legs.

The percussion douche to the spine at a temperature of 65° F. is a most admirable tonic measure for phlegmatic neurasthenics. The percussion douche at 45° to 55° is one of the most powerful of all means whereby the central nervous system may be energized. The tissues of the back are supplied with nerves from each of the ganglia of the spinal cord, so that the entire cord is represented in this small portion of the body surface. The area of skin covering the back being small compared with the entire cutaneous surface, applications at a much lower temperature and at a much higher pressure can be made than when the entire skin surface is involved. The general retrostasis which results from the application of cold to the entire body surface and the resulting internal congestion are avoided, and reaction is assisted by the activity of the circulation in the general cutaneous surface. It is thus possible by means of the cold percussion douche to the spine not only to influence the entire spinal cord, but to bring to bear more intense applications than can be tolerated by the general surface. This fact gives to the dorsal percussion douche a high value in the treatment of all forms of disease in which it is important to energize the motor or vasomotor centers of the spinal cord. It is especially useful in *neurasthenia* and *hysteria*, in paralytic forms of *writers' cramp*, in *Raynaud's disease*, in *chronic intoxications*, and in *hypopepsia*, *enteroptosis*, and *constipation*.

The *neutral* percussion douche is valuable as an application to the hips for producing collateral hyperemia to relieve neuralgia of the pelvic viscera when hot or cold applications are too exciting.

By the use of water at a neutral temperature (92° to 96°) powerful circulatory reaction can be produced with no thermic reaction, a point of great value in the treatment of affections requiring suppression of thermic effects, such as the lightning pains of *locomotor ataxia*, *spinal neuralgia*, and the *hyperesthetic* states of the *sympathetic ganglia*, which are responsible for a host of obscure *reflex pains* and *paresthesias*.

The *hot* percussion douche is less often of service than the same procedure applied at a temperature of 55° to 70°; but it may be very useful in cases in which it is desirable to produce analgesic and derivative effects with strong circulatory reaction, as in applications to the legs in *asthma*, to the lumbar spine in *lumbago*, to the thigh in *sciatica*, over the liver in the passive *hepatic congestion* accompanying the malarial cachexias and so-called bilious dyspepsia, ascites, rheumatic joints not sensitive to pressure, loss of normal sensibility in *paraplegia*, *hemiplegia*, and *spinal sclerosis*, and to relieve the lightning pains of *locomotor ataxia*.

The hot percussion douche may also serve a most excellent purpose in the treatment of a certain class of neurasthenics who have a natural dread of contact with cold water. It is true that this dread can in most cases be overcome by a little patient training and systematic lowering of the temperature of the bath from day to day; but many patients have neither the patience nor the fortitude to endure this training process, and are likely to break down in the midst of it, and suspend their visits before the point has been reached at which tangible good results may be expected to appear. In such cases the *very hot* general percussion douche (110° to 125°) may be employed for tonic effects, and with most satisfactory results. After a few days or weeks, the graduated Scotch, and finally the cold douche may be employed.

THE SCOTCH DOUCHE.

The Scotch douche consists in the application of hot 1037
water followed by a short cold application. Any desired form of douche may be employed. The hot application must be relatively long (1 to 4 min.), and the cold application must be short (3 to 30 secs.). Employed in this way, the effect of the cold application is to greatly intensify the derivative or revulsive effect of the hot water, and to increase its duration. The application may be general; that is, applied to the whole surface, or it may localized, according to the effect desired.

The Scotch douche in many cases follows a sweating application of some sort, especially in dealing with cases of sciatica, rheumatism, gout, dropsy, and neuralgia, particularly when accompanied by general toxemia or obesity. The vapor, Turkish, Russian, or electric-light bath may be used for the preliminary heating of the skin, or a general hot rain douche may be employed. The best of all means is the electric-light bath so arranged as to permit the employment of the douche while the patient is exposed to the heat rays (**832**). Next to this in efficiency is the Russian bath and the cold rain douche in combination (**831**).

In the Scotch douche the stream may assume any form, as the jet, fan, spray, rain, or percussion douche; usually the fan or spray douche is employed.

The cold application should follow the hot instantly, with no interval whatever, as a wet surface is rapidly cooled by evaporation, so that the heating effect produced by the hot application may be in large part destroyed in an interval of exposure lasting only a few seconds.

When employed for general tonic effects,—its most common application,—the purpose of the Scotch douche is to serve as a means of training the patient to the application of the cold douche. The purpose of the hot application is in many cases to warm the skin so as to prepare it for the succeeding cold application. It is especially useful in cases of feeble persons who are not able to take a sufficient amount of exercise to accumulate the heat necessary to secure prompt and complete reaction. The warm or hot rain douche (98° to 106°) is admirably adapted for this purpose. The duration should be 1 to 3 minutes, as may be required. The patient's sensations must generally determine the duration. The temperature and duration should be such that the patient becomes thoroughly warm, and feels that the contact of the cold water will be agreeable.

Care should be taken to allow the water to fall upon the arms and legs, as well as upon the shoulders, so as to thoroughly warm the extremities. To avoid overheating the head, the hair should be thoroughly saturated with cold water, and the head protected by a thick towel saturated with water at 60°. In neurotic patients who have a decided tendency to cerebral congestion, it is in some cases necessary to place about the neck a towel wet with cold water (60°).

For the cold application the best effects are obtained by the full jet to the arms and legs, the broken or fan jet over the chest and abdomen, and the percussion douche to the back. In very sensitive patients, the spray or the fan douche may be employed instead of the horizontal jet until the patient has been trained to more vigorous measures. The temperature of the cold application must be adapted to the patient's condition. When purely tonic effects are desired, the temperature should be as low as the patient can endure,—from 65° to 50°, duration 5 to 20 seconds. In cases in which very cold applications are contraindicated (**636, 803, 1023**), higher temperatures may be employed (70° to 85°), and the duration must be extended from 20 to 60 seconds. The higher the temperature, the longer should be the duration of the cooling application. It is also important, when the temperature is elevated, to increase the pressure, in order to secure good circulatory reaction.

The Graduated Scotch Douche. Although the Scotch douche depends for its effectiveness upon the transition from heat to cold, it is not essential that this change should be abrupt; yet the more sudden the change, and the greater the extremes of temperature employed, the more pronounced will be the effects. In persons who can not endure a sudden change from heat to cold, the temperature may be gradually lowered, occupying from half a minute to a minute in the transition.

In some cases in which there is great susceptibility to thermic changes, the application should begin at a temperature near that of the body (100°). The heat of the application is gradually increased until a temperature of 110° to 120° is reached, held at this point for 2 or 3 minutes, or longer if necessary, then gradually but rapidly reduced to the minimum temperature desired.

With very sensitive patients it is better at first to make the extremes of temperature not greater than 20° to 30°; but this limit may be gradually extended from day to day until a difference of 40° or even 50° is reached.

The most pronounced effects are produced by managing in such a manner as to make the applications to the skin at extremes of temperature as great as possible. The method of gradual transition is to be employed only in cases in which this less vigorous measure is positively indicated.

The Simultaneous Scotch Douche. The simultaneous application of hot and cold water possesses, in certain cases, very decided advantages, as has been mentioned elsewhere in the discussion of the hot and cold compress (**1290, 1356**). The principles defined in the paragraphs referred to apply equally well to the simultaneous application of the douche. This mode of applying the douche, which, so far as the writer knows, he was the first to employ and call attention to, is especially applicable to cases in which ordinary cold applications are badly borne or wholly intolerable because of some individual idiosyncrasy. In certain neurasthenics, the dread and apprehension of cold water is so great that the patient will not allow an application at a sufficiently low temperature to produce any decided tonic effects, even after a hot application. This is especially true of neurasthenics in whom paresthesias of various sorts are particularly common, affecting chiefly the temperature of the nerves, and manifested by subjective chilliness or coldness of the arms and legs, of the skin between the shoulders, and of other parts. In such cases it is often possible to administer with benefit a strong percussion dorsal douche simultaneously with a rain douche at 100° to 102°. By a little training the general cold douche may, with careful management, be administered in these cases. While receiving the warm rain douche, the patient projects from the area of the falling streams, different parts of the body in succession, to receive the cold application, until the whole body has been gone over. The duration of the application upon each part should be 2 to 5 seconds, and if desirable, the intensity of the application may be increased by rapidly going over the whole surface two or even more times. By this method the entire surface of the body, with the exception of the part to which the cold application is being made, is under the influence of the warm douche. This renders impossible general chilliness with retrostasis and the resulting general vascular and nervous disturbances connected therewith, which follow general cold applications to the surface, and which in sensitive persons follow the application of cold to a small area even, as the chest, abdomen, back, or a hand or foot. At the same time the whole surface is acted upon by the cold douche, and thus each nerve center in the body is successively excited by reflex influence through the impressions made upon the skin, and so a general tonic and restorative effect may be secured.

This method may be adopted as a means of training sensitive patients to the application of cold water. It resembles in principle the combined cold shower and Russian bath (**831**), and the combined cold douche and electric-light bath (**832**).

Special forms of the simultaneous Scotch douche which may be advantageously employed are the following: —

1. *The Dorsal Cold Douche (65° to 80°) Combined with the Abdominal Hot Douche (106° to 125°).* — This measure is chiefly useful in the treatment of chronic congestive conditions of the stomach, liver, intestines, and spleen, accompanied by pain. The duration of the application should be 5 to 20 minutes. The prolonged cold application to the spine causes contraction of the visceral vessels by reflex stimulation of the vasomotor centers, while the hot application to the abdominal wall produces a collateral hyperemia, whereby the amount of blood entering the mesenteric vessels and the portal circulation is diminished, thus simultaneously bringing to bear upon the congested viscera two powerful means of relieving the morbid condition present. The analgesic effect of the hot application renders tolerable the cold dorsal douche in cases in which its use would otherwise be inadmissible. Applications of this sort should be made with the patient sitting

upon a stool. The pressure should be moderate, 5 to 15 pounds. This application may be usefully employed in cases of *chronic gastric catarrh*, *chronic intestinal catarrh*, *hyperesthesia* of the *lumbar ganglia* of the abdominal sympathetic, *hepatic congestion*, *splenic congestion*, *renal congestion*, and *enteroptosis*, especially if pain is present.

2. *The Cold Lumbar and Hot Hypogastric Douche.*—The method of application of this douche is the same as that described for the preceding, except that it is localized upon the lumbar and sacral spine and the hypogastrium. This procedure is especially useful in cases of *chronic pelvic congestion*, so-called *metritis*, *ovarian congestion*, *chronic inflammation* of the *tubes*, and atonic conditions of the pelvic viscera accompanied by *passive congestion* and *pain*. It is contraindicated in cases in which acute inflammation or suppurative processes are present.

3. *The Combined Spinal Douche and Hot Douche to the Feet.*—The cold percussion douche is applied to the spine simultaneously with the hot douche (110°–122°) to the feet and legs. The fan or spray douche may be employed for the hot douche to the feet. By this procedure, it is possible to apply a very cold (50°–60°) percussion douche to the spine, even continuing it 30 to 60 seconds, in cases of very sensitive persons who have little power to react and yet who require the powerful nerve stimulating effect of the cold spinal douche. This is one of the most effective measures which can be employed in many cases of neurasthenia. It is especially applicable to cases in which the general cold douche alone can not be tolerated. The application should end with two or three quick applications of cold water over the entire surface of the body, and the application of the cold spray to the feet and legs for two or three seconds.

4. *The Symmetrical Combined Scotch Douche.*—In certain hysterical cases, especially in *hyperesthesias* affecting one side of the body, a transference of the affection to the opposite side and a rapid mitigation of the symptoms may be effected

by the simultaneous application of the hot douche to the affected part and of the cold douche to the symmetrical part of the opposite side of the body. By the daily application of this measure, the nutrition of the affected part may be improved, and with the improvement of the general health secured by general tonic measures, the symptom may be made gradually to disappear.

Physiological Effects.— The physiological effects produced by the Scotch douche combine those of both the very hot and the cold douche, though not in their entirety. The hot application causes passive dilatation of the cutaneous vessels, with increased heart action and elevation of blood pressure, with a reflex influence in general tending to atonic reaction. The cold application slows the heart, augments the blood pressure, converts the passive dilatation of the surface vessels into an active dilatation, and by reflex influence produces a tonic reaction in which every cell and fiber of the whole body participates, provided the intensity of the cold application is such that the tonic effect produced by it more than counterbalances any atonic effects of the hot application. 1038

It thus appears that very versatile effects may be produced by the Scotch douche, according as the hot or the cold impression is dominant. Upon the exact balancing or regulation of the effects of heat and cold this bath depends for its special physiological and therapeutic properties. If so managed that the cold application is dominant, the preliminary heating being just sufficient to warm the skin and prepare it to react to the cold douche, the effects are excitant, or tonic, and correspond exactly to those of the cold douche. The brain and viscera are, however, protected to some degree by the preliminary congestion of the skin, so that the retrostatic congestion of these organs which immediately follows an ordinary cold application, is less marked and of much shorter duration,— a fact of great practical importance in dealing with cases requiring tonic cold applications, while complicated with chronic cerebral, hepatic, articular, and other internal congestions. The physiological effects of cold are dominant when the concluding cold application is continued for a sufficient length of time to cause pallor of the skin, chilliness, and the thermic reaction of cold. To produce such effects, the cold application must continue for 30 or 40 seconds, or even longer, unless very cold water is employed.

When the cold application is brief (5 to 10 secs.), producing neither shivering nor other evidence of refrigeration, no tonic thermic reaction occurs. The reaction is purely circulatory, and hence derivative or sedative rather than tonic in character. A very brief cold application (1 to 3 secs.) after a hot application of ordinary length may leave the body under the atonic or depressing influence of the hot application. Such an effect as this is rarely desirable, except when it may be necessary to counteract to a partial extent the depressing effect of a long hot application employed for analgesic or derivative effects, but in which the excitant effects of cold are undesirable, as in acute or subacute sciatica, ovarian neuralgia, enteralgia, or spinal neuralgia.

In many cases it is desirable to balance exactly the hot and cold effects; the method of accomplishing this will be explained under the heading, "Revulsive Douche."

1039 **Therapeutic Applications.**—The therapeutic uses of the Scotch douche are even more general than those of the cold douche. It may be used in all cases to which the cold douche is applicable, as the hot douche preceding the cold only intensifies the effect of the latter, when rightly managed, and can be employed in many cases in which the cold douche could not be utilized, either because the patient will not submit to the application or because his system is unable to react to cold without the preparation afforded by the preceding heating procedure.

The merits of the Scotch douche in a variety of morbid states have been energetically championed in France by Lemarchand.* The author has found the Scotch douche

*Lemarchand, *Ann. de la Soc. d' Hydrol. Med.*, Paris, 1893.

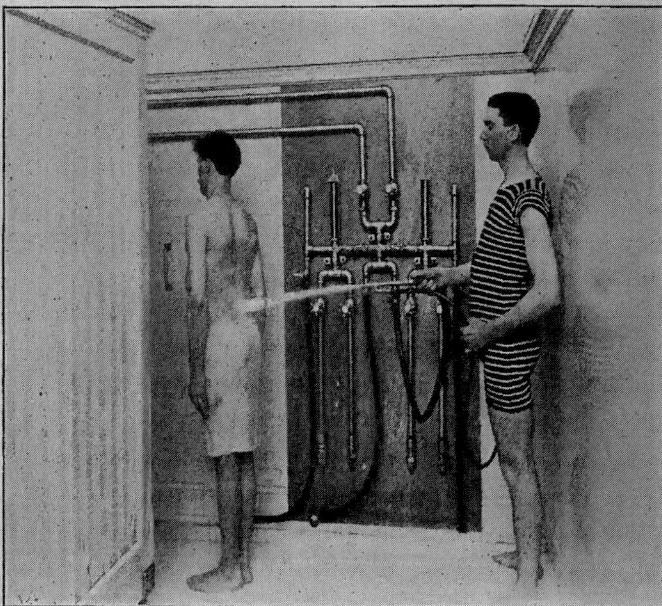

FIG. 36. PERCUSSION DOUCHE (p. 454).

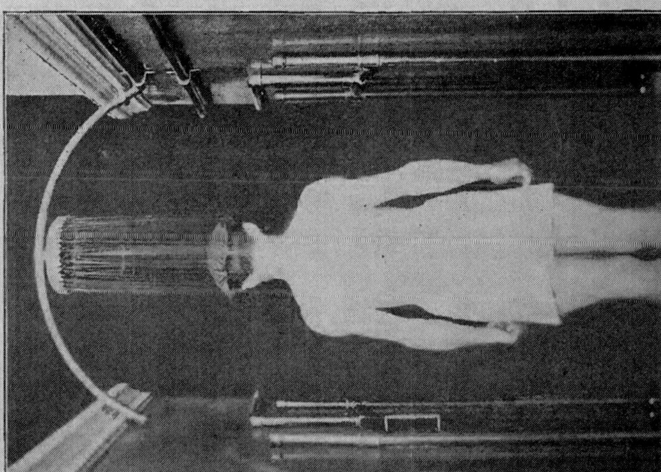

FIG. 37. RAIN DOUCHE (p. 472).

especially useful in cases in which the skin is very inactive, or is relaxed, as indicated by *profuse and frequent sweatings.* It renders valuable service in the sweatings which are characteristic of the climacteric period, and which are frequently encountered in neurasthenic cases, both men and women. When employed for this purpose, the hot application should be at as high a temperature as can be borne (115° to 125°), duration, 1 to 2 minutes; and the cold application should be short (2 to 6 secs.), and of as cold water as is obtainable—from 55° to 65° if possible. Patients generally require considerable training to enable them to tolerate with benefit the lowest temperature mentioned.

The Scotch douche is one of the best of all means of energizing relaxed or *paralyzed muscles.* Short and very hot applications are powerfully restorative in cases of *muscular fatigue,* while cold applications increase muscular irritability and contractile power. By a combination of these two measures, we have the most effective means known for the invigoration of weakened muscular structures.

The Scotch douche is of great value, not only in actual *paresis* or *paralysis,* but in the cases of neurasthenics and dyspeptics who suffer constantly from *malaise* and a sensation of muscular fatigue and an actual inability to exercise on account of the extreme exhaustion following. In such cases the Scotch douche, consisting of a rain douche at 106° for 1 minute, followed by a general fan or broken jet and full jet or percussion douche to the spine and legs at 60°, for 20 to 30 seconds, is a most admirable measure, producing, almost immediately, noticeable good effects.

The localized Scotch douche is of very great service in **1040**
cases of *lumbago, crural neuralgia, sciatica, enteralgia, gastralgia, uterine* and *ovarian neuralgia, pleuritic pains, intercostal neuralgia, gastric ulcer, "spinal irritation,"* and *chronic "backache."*

This procedure is often of exceeding value in the treatment of chronic cases requiring general tonic treatment while suffering from painful local affections of the sort mentioned, and in connection with the neutral douche in *insomnia* and other affections requiring sedative effects. In *cerebral congestion*, the Scotch douche to the legs is an invaluable derivative measure, and should precede the general cold douche in cases of *cerebral congestion*, *hepatic* or *splenic congestion*, *hyperpepsia*, and severe *visceral congestions* of all sorts. It is also a valuable measure in *asthma*, especially the form known as *nervous asthma*, in which the Scotch douche to the legs will often cut short an attack with most satisfactory promptness.

Bougarel utilized the Scotch revulsive douche to the feet in *nasal catarrh* and *bronchitis*, as well as in *asthma*.*

Glatz † maintains that there is no better means for combating *chronic muscular rheumatism* than the Scotch douche, and that it is invaluable in the treatment of *sciatica*,—statements which the author has been able to verify in a multitude of cases.

THE REVULSIVE DOUCHE.

1041 The revulsive douche is simply the Scotch douche employed in such a manner as entirely to suppress the thermic reaction which follows the ordinary cold douche. The principles underlying the application are precisely the same as those which have been fully explained under the heading "The Revulsive Compress" (**1341**). The hot douche is at first administered at a temperature as high as the patient can bear, the temperature being gradually increased as tolerance is established until it reaches a maximum of 122° or even 130°, when the area to which the application is made is small. The duration of the application should usually be 2 to 4 minutes, or

* Bougarel, *Ann. de la Soc. d'Hydrol Med.*, Paris.

† Glatz, "L'Hydrotherapie Tonique et Revulsive," Cong. Period, internal, d. sc. med. Compt. rend. Geneve, 1878, page 524.

until the skin acquires a dusky-red or cherry color. The cold application is then administered for 2 to 15 seconds, according to the temperature of the water employed, and the degree of irritability of the parts. Very irritable conditions require very brief cold applications. With water at 50°, 3 or 4 seconds will usually be sufficient; at 60° to 70°, from 5 to 30 seconds will be required.

As the purpose of the cold application is to remove the heat which has been absorbed by the skin during the hot douche, and thus to convert the paralytic dilatation of the vessels into an active dilatation by securing the circulatory reaction of cold without the thermic effect, if the cold application is continued too long, thermic reaction will be produced, and the effect of the application will be spoiled. The exact length of the cold application may be regulated by watching the color of the skin.

When the change from passive to active dilatation occurs, it is indicated by a change in color from dusky-red to scarlet. In most cases no serious harm will result if the cold application be carried a little farther than necessary, as the thermic reaction will be too slight to produce any noticeable effect; but decided chilling of the surface produces, especially in those cases in which severe pain is present, a very unpleasant aggravation of the patient's sufferings. Considerable practice is required to administer the revulsive douche with skill.

For a precise application of this douche it is necessary to employ a pressure gauge as an indicator of the amount of mechanical energy brought to bear in the case. The physician skilled in hydriatry is not, however, necessarily dependent upon the pressure gauge when the application is administered under his own eye, which is the almost universal practice in the scientific hydriatic establishments of Germany and France.

To the well-trained hydriatrist the immediate effect of the application is the best possible means of regulating the procedure. As a rule, the pressure ought to be strong enough to produce prompt reaction. In general, the reaction should begin to appear before the application has ended. The pressure can of course be perfectly regulated when the horizontal jet is employed, by placing the tip of the finger over the end of the nozzle, thus breaking the force of the stream more or less.

In the employment of the author's percussion douche the force of the stream may also be regulated at the nozzle by the small valve which controls the air current. When employed for relief of pain, the fan douche should be used.

1042 **Physiological Effects.**—The revulsive douche is perhaps the most powerful means of producing vascular revulsion. The nervous impressions made may be less profound than those which result from the cold or alternate douche, but the circulatory effect is intense and lasting. The temporary congestion produced by the hot douche is rendered much more permanent or prolonged by the procedure described, as the circulatory reaction of cold fixes the blood in the skin, this effect becoming more and more pronounced as the treatment is repeated from day to day. The physiological effects of the procedure are thus confined almost exclusively to the circulatory system, and if not wholly mechanical, are certainly to a large extent due to the storing of blood in the skin and the drawing of blood from internal parts.

The revulsive douche unquestionably quickens the movement of blood throughout the whole body when employed either as a general procedure or through associated parts when the application is confined to reflex cutaneous areas.

The revulsive douche differs radically from the alternate douche, in that the latter is especially potent as a means of quickening metabolic and other vital activities; whereas the revulsive douche, by eliminating thermic reaction, has no effect upon metabolic processes other than such modifications as result from circulatory changes.

1043 **Therapeutic Applications.**—The general effect of the revulsive douche is precisely the same as that of the Scotch douche, except that it is less exciting to the general nervous

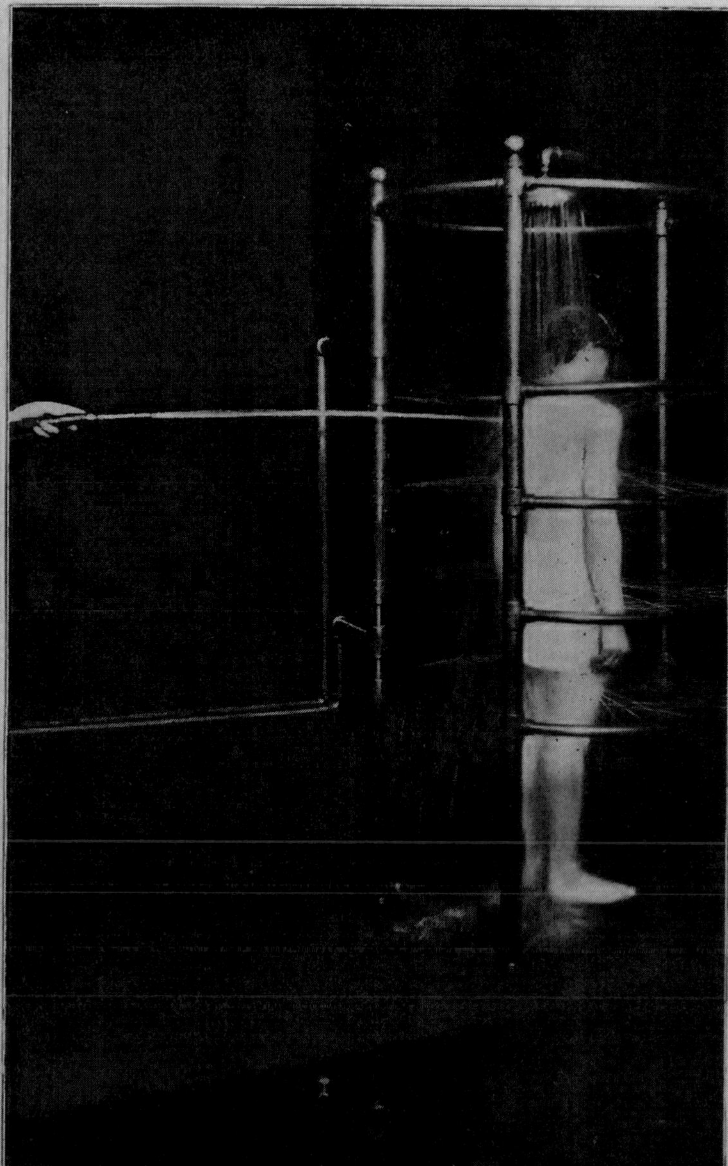

FIG. 38. COMBINED RAIN DOUCHE, HORIZONTAL JET, AND MULTIPLE CIRCLE DOUCHE (p. 473).

system, and is not to so great an extent productive of metabolic changes, owing to the absence of thermic reaction. The atonic reaction of heat, as well as the tonic reaction of cold, are both prevented by the antidotal influence above described. The effect is practically nothing more than a dilatation of the surface vessels exercising a derivative effect upon the deeper structures of the body, but without producing the preliminary congestion of the internal structures which precedes the reaction when the cold douche alone is employed. This renders the revulsive Scotch douche an exceedingly valuable measure for use in cases of *cardiac insufficiency*, *cerebral hyperemia*, *chronic gastritis*, *chronic gastro-intestinal catarrh*, *chronic congestion of the liver and spleen*, *acute and subacute nephritis*, *hyperemia of the spinal cord*, *acute congestion and inflammation of the uterus and its adnexa*, and *subacute rheumatism*. By careful observance of the technique described it is possible to employ the douche with great advantage in the cases here mentioned, in which the cold douche must necessarily be interdicted, and in many allied conditions.

The revulsive douche is a valuable measure in cases of both *profuse sweating* and *excessive dryness* of the skin. Its effect is to produce an increase of tone in the tissues of the skin, and thus to bring about normal cutaneous activity. In *dysmenorrhea* with scanty flow it may be applied to the hips, thighs, and legs. The same measure is useful in *congestive headache* and *pulmonary congestion*, provided care be taken that the jet does not fall upon any portion of the body above the umbilicus. The revulsive douche to the legs is also useful in cases of *hyperpepsia*, the hot douche being at the same time applied to the epigastrium and the spine opposite. In *gastric catarrh*, *gastralgia*, or in the acute crises of *locomotor ataxia*, it may be employed in the same manner as for hyperpepsia.

The revulsive douche affords great relief as a local application to the painful joints of *acute* and *chronic rheumatism*, also in *myalgia*, *dermalgia*, *intercostal neuralgia*, *pleuro-*

dynia, and the lightning pains of *locomotor ataxia*. In cases in which the douche (fan) is used for the relief of pain, the pressure must be light, not more than 3 to 15 pounds.

THE ALTERNATE DOUCHE.

1044 The alternate douche resembles the Scotch douche in that it employs both hot and cold water; it differs from it in that the Scotch douche consists of a single application of water at each temperature,—first hot, then cold,—while in the alternate douche hot and cold water are repeatedly applied in alternation. The alternation may be repeated as many times as is considered desirable in the particular case. The alternate douche also differs from the Scotch douche in that the hot application as well as the cold is short. Ordinarily the applications of heat and of cold are of equal length, each of about 15 seconds' duration. It is obvious, however, that there is opportunity for an infinite variety of modifications in this regard. The longer the hot application and the shorter the cold application, relatively, the less pronounced and characteristic will be the excitant effects produced. The temperatures employed must be suited to the individual case. The greater the extremes of temperature and the more sudden the transition, the more decided will be the excitant effects.

1045 **Physiological Effects.**—The alternate douche is perhaps the most exciting of all hydric procedures. It combines with the primary excitant effects of heat the secondary excitant effects of cold, and through the removal of the heat accumulated by the skin during the hot application by means of the preceding cold application, the susceptibility of the skin is renewed, and its reflex activities maintained, and thus the excitant effect of the hot application is intensified and extended.

With persons who are very sensitive to thermic applications, and especially to sudden changes, the alternate douche may be modified in a variety of ways, the most important of which may be indicated as follows:—

1. Beginning with a lower temperature for the hot application, and a higher temperature for the cold application, thus lessening the extremes of temperature employed, and by progressive graduation, from day to day increasing the extremes, raising the temperature of the hot application and lowering the temperature of the cold, the most powerful effects may after a time be realized.

2. Graduating the procedure during the application, beginning at a temperature near that of the body, raising to the highest limit, then gradually lowering to the lowest extreme, repeating this as many times as necessary to produce the effect desired.

3. Increasing the relative time of the hot application, or lessening the time of the cold application, thus diminishing the thermic effect.

Therapeutic Applications. — The alternate douche is to 1046
be employed in cases in which powerfully excitant effects are desirable; that is, in cases of *old exudations*, *enlargement of the liver*, the so-called "*liver of dyspeptics*," *enlarged spleen*, and *stiffened joints* in which active inflammatory processes have ceased. It may also be employed wherever increased functional activity is desired, as in cases of *atony of the genito-urinary organs*, unaccompanied by irritability, in *paresis or paralysis* of a group of muscles, in certain inveterate cases of *sciatic neuralgia* in which the pain is due to chronic inflammation of the nerve sheath, and in *pleuritic effusions* and *dropsical accumulations* in other cavities, in the joints, or in the tissues, as in swellings of the limbs due to *anemia*, *chronic Bright's disease*, *erythema nodosum*, and the muscular soreness and rigidity left behind by an attack of *muscular rheumatism*. The local alternate douche should be systematically employed two or three times daily as a means of preventing *bed-sores* in low fevers, to prevent *sloughing* after prolonged exposure to the X-ray, in *chilblains*, in

chronic ulcer of the leg, and in *eczema* with thickening of the skin. Indeed, this is a procedure of wide applicability and utility.

The localized alternating douche is exceedingly valuable in cases of *hypopepsia* (the epigastric douche), *constipation* (lumbar and abdominal), *amenorrhea* (lumbar spine, thighs, and feet), *chronic renal insufficiency* (the lower third of the sternum), *neurasthenia* (dorsal), *cold feet and legs.* It may be applied internally to the prostate in chronic enlargement of this organ, to the rectum in cases in which normal sensibility is lost, and to the stomach by means of the stomach-tube in cases of *dilatation of the stomach* with motor insufficiency.

The general alternate douche is useful for dryness and inactivity of the skin, a condition commonly present in *diabetes mellitus* and many cases of *chronic dyspepsia.*

The alternating douche is especially indicated in cases in which local stimulation is required. The extreme temperatures necessary to secure the best effects render it unsuited to general application.

THE RAIN DOUCHE OR SHOWER BATH.

1047 In this form of douche (Fig. 37) the water is projected through a "rose," or perforated disc, falling upon the patient in a number of fine streams. When the disc is placed above the patient, the procedure is termed the *rain* or *shower douche;* when held in the hand or fixed beneath a seat, it is termed a *spray.* In the rain douche the size of the openings is usually somewhat larger than in the movable hand spray, and the disc is also larger and the apertures more numerous.

In administering the rain douche, the same general principles apply as in the use of the horizontal jet. The procedure is somewhat more vigorous than the jet, as both the quantity of water falling upon the patient at each instant and the amount of surface exposed to contact with the water are greater. The pressure is less, hence the mechanical effect is less and the reaction more difficult, so that great care must be observed to prepare the patient for the application by a preliminary heating, and to take all necessary precautions to secure reaction afterward.

The shower bath was much used by Priessnitz and in the numerous water-cures which were established upon essentially the same plan as that at Graefenberg, in various parts of the United States and England during the first half of the present century. Bell, of Philadelphia, in his admirable work on "Baths" (1850) mentioned the shower bath, and it was also described by Dr. Joel Shew and other early writers on hydrotherapy in this country.

The author has been familiar with the rain douche or shower bath for over forty years, having been introduced to it while a boy in his father's house, where it was a part of the household furnishing, and its use one of the routine duties of each member of the family; and during an experience of more than twenty-five years with this douche in the treatment of chronic invalids of all classes, he has come to regard it as an indispensable part of a completely equipped establishment for the scientific use of water as a curative agent.

The accompanying cut (Fig. 38) represents one of the large rain douches constructed under the author's direction for use in the Battle Creek Sanitarium. The apparatus is also arranged for giving the multiple circle spray, or so-called needle bath, and the horizontal jet. The apparatus is supplied by two inch pipes, and gives a shower of sixty streams through as many openings with diameters of one sixteenth of an inch. The horizontal jet supplies an inch stream under a pressure of 45 pounds.

On account of the powerful impression made upon the shoulders and the upper part of the trunk, the skin covering these parts being in intimate reflex relation with the brain and heart, the disc of the rain douche should be placed not more than two or three feet above the head of the patient. In general, the perforations should be large enough so that the water will fall with no great force aside from that given to it by gravity. As a further precaution, to prevent too great concentration of the effect upon the organs of the chest, it is well to begin the application by allowing the water to fall first upon the feet, first one and then the other being held in proper position for this purpose for a few seconds each, the water then being allowed to fall upon the hands, arms, shoulders, back, and, lastly, upon the chest and abdomen. Or, the same end may be attained by administering to the feet and legs a horizontal jet at the same time that the rain douche falls upon the upper part of the body.

The head should always be covered, in the rain bath, by a thick towel folded to several thicknesses, or by a rubber cap. The patient should keep in lively motion during the application, flexing the limbs by raising the feet alternately, turning around first in one direction then in the other, and rubbing the chest with the hands. At the beginning of the application the hands should be applied to the chest to protect it, and especially the precordial region, from the impact of the water. This exercise aids reaction, and thus mitigates the effect upon the heart and lungs.

The combined cold horizontal douche and the vertical rain douche are certainly the most energetic excitants of all hydrotherapeutic measures. Cases are not infrequently encountered in which the effect of this vigorous combination can not be tolerated, and it is not ordinarily required.

1048 **Physiological Effects.**— The cold rain douche is one of the most exciting of all hydriatic procedures. A large amount of cold water under moderate pressure falls upon the most highly sensitive and reflexly active portions of the cutaneous surface, causing a perfect cyclone, so to speak, of nerve impulses to be sent in upon the cerebrospinal axis; and, naturally, most extensive reflex actions are set up. At first, the respiratory movements are almost suspended; the breathing is in quick, gasping efforts, the heart is powerfully excited, the blood pressure is raised, and all the phenomena resulting from other general external applications of cold are presented in an intense degree. General metabolic activity is stimulated; the brain and nervous system are intensely aroused, and all the vital movements are accelerated. According to the observations of Schüller, the powerful respiratory movements produced by the cold rain douche must exercise a salutary effect of the highest importance in stimulating the lymph currents of the brain and spinal cord, and in aiding the hepatic and portal circulations.

The sudden inrush of blood from the surface causes dilatation of the vessels of the brain, but the brain is to some extent protected by the powerful vasomotor reflexes sent inward from the face, neck, and upper cervical regions.

In the majority of cases in which the cold rain douche is employed, a preliminary heating should be applied. This measure is, on this account, exceedingly convenient, for the reason that the heating and cooling may be effected by the same apparatus. When required, the rain douche at 100° to 104° is applied for 1 to 3 minutes before the cold application.

The *cool* rain douche (75° to 65°) is an excellent training measure for persons who are so sensitive as to prohibit the employment of water at a lower temperature, also for gradual cooling after a sweating bath.

The effect of the *hot* rain douche is likewise powerfully 1049
exciting, causing intense cerebral congestion, and first slowing, then quickening, of the heart, which continues for some time after the bath. The duration of the hot shower should be from one-half minute to 2 minutes; temperature, 100° to 112°.

The *neutral* rain douche (92° to 97°) causes immediate 1050
contraction of the cerebral vessels (Schüller), and produces a general calm in the storm of nerve reflexes continually playing between the periphery and the brain and cord. Its effects are essentially the same as those of the neutral immersion bath (**1130**), but are much more quickly attained.

The usual duration of the neutral shower bath is from 3 to 5 minutes.

1051 **Therapeutic Applications.**—The rain douche has the disadvantage of being far less perfectly controllable than the horizontal jet or the spray, which may be regulated to a nicety during administration by one skilled in their use. The *cold* shower is practically a fixed procedure, and hence is not adapted to feeble persons. The *neutral* and *graduated* rain douche have a much more general application than the cold or hot douche in this form. However, the rain douche is an exceedingly useful measure at all temperatures.

The cold shower fell into discredit in this country more than forty years ago, because of its excessive and unwise use by empirics as a panacea, and by the laity as a daily morning bath for prophylactic and hygienic purposes. Within the last twenty years, however, this measure has been steadily returning to favor, and at present every well-furnished private bathroom is supplied with a fairly good rain douche apparatus. The accompanying cut (Fig. 39) shows a style of shower bath such as may be obtained at any large plumbing establishment of this country or Europe.

1052 The cold shower may be used with advantage as a tonic measure for *anemics* who are fairly strong, also in *obesity* where the heart is not seriously involved, and with the *chlorotic* and *plethoric*. It should be preceded by some appropriate heating procedure, as the heating pack, the dry pack, or a sweating process of short duration.

The short cold rain douche (60° to 70°, for 5 to 30 secs.) is to be employed in cases in which moderate stimulation is required, with little withdrawal of heat, as in *anemia* and *chlorosis* with emaciation, and in *neurasthenia* and *dyspepsia* when the height-weight coefficient is low. When considerable heat elimination is required, the douche is prolonged to 1 or 2 minutes. This procedure is especially useful in *phlegmatic neurasthenics, sedentary persons* in whom the general metabolic activity is diminished, in *obesity*, and in all cases

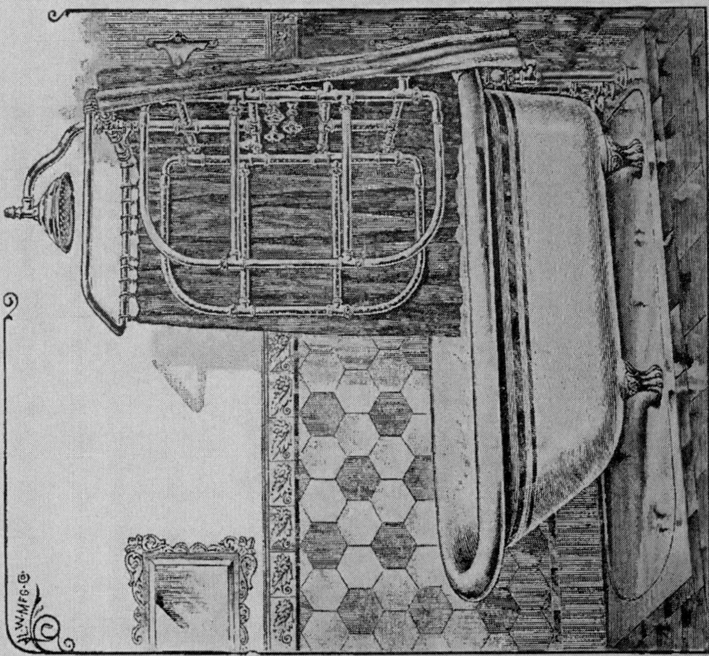

FIG. 39. COMBINED DOUCHE APPARATUS AND BATH TUB (p. 476).

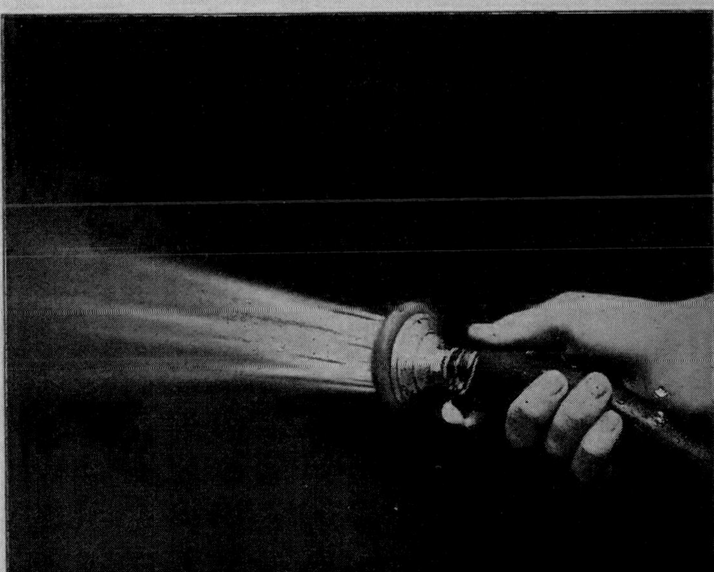

FIG. 40. HORIZONTAL RAIN DOUCHE OR SPRAY (p. 479).

in which after a long sweating process a gradual and very thorough cooling is necessary to prevent continued perspiration.

The cold shower may be combined with the Russian bath with good effects. By standing in the hot vapor, the patient tolerates the cold shower much more readily than when exposed to the chilling effect of evaporation and currents of cool air. Still better effects may be obtained from the combination of the shower and the electric-light bath, as shown in Fig. 139 (page 709).

While the *cold* shower bath perhaps offers some disadvantages over the jet or spray douche, the *warm* or *neutral* shower presents distinct advantages. As a hygienic measure, it offers a most agreeable and rapid method of cleansing the whole surface of the body, a most important consideration when large numbers of persons are to be bathed in a short time, as in military barracks, charitable institutions, schools, and public baths. The warm shower bath has long been extensively used in prisons, reformatories, and other public institutions as a convenient form of bath for cleanliness.

The author a few years ago (1893) introduced this bath into a charitable home under his direction located in Chicago, (the Chicago Medical Mission) especially designed for the benefit of waifs, tramps, discharged prisoners, and other classes of homeless men. Of the one hundred thousand and more men who have made use of the bath in this institution, a large proportion have testified to the benefit derived from its use, not only as a means of cleansing the skin, but as a tonic and invigorating measure. In dealing with this class of persons, the neutral or warm bath followed by a cold shower bath has incidentally been found to be a most effective means of sobering men under the influence of alcoholic liquors. The cold rain douche of 1 to 3 minutes' duration is generally sufficient to restore the mental equilibrium and muscular coordinating power of a man so fully under the influence of alcohol as to be unable to walk or even stand without support.

1053 The *neutral* rain douche (93° to 96°) is one of the most effective measures which can be employed for the relief of *insomnia* due to irritability of the cerebrospinal nervous system, *cerebral congestion*, and *general nervous excitability*. The application should be made with little force, special attention being given to the legs and back. The application of the broken jet, with light aspersions at intervals of a few seconds to the back of the neck and the occipital region of the head, during the rain douche, has a remarkably soothing and soporific effect.

The action of the neutral douche is quicker than that of the neutral immersion bath, and in some cases its application may be preferred. A neutral rain douche of 3 to 5 minutes' duration often produces the same quieting effect obtainable from a neutral immersion bath of 40 to 60 minutes. The neutral rain douche may be used in cases in which patients complain of the necessary length of the full bath. The latter, however, is preferable for many cases requiring the sedative effect of a neutral temperature, owing to the recumbent position, which permits the patient to fall asleep in the bath.

The neutral rain bath may be used to great advantage in cases of *mania* with cerebral congestion. Care should be taken to protect the head by a thick cold compress after a previous thorough cooling. This method is of course applicable only to cases in which the patient may be readily controlled.

1054 The *hot* shower serves a useful purpose as a ready and convenient means of heating the skin in preparation for a cold jet or spray. The duration may be from one-half minute to 2 minutes when used for this purpose, or long enough to heat the skin and cause the patient to long for the refreshing effect of the cold douche or spray. Care must be taken to protect the head by a rubber cap or a thick towel well saturated with ice-water, and the hot water must not be allowed to fall directly upon the head.

THE HORIZONTAL RAIN DOUCHE OR SPRAY.

This form of douche (Fig. 40) is identical with the horizontal jet in its mode of application, with the exception that, instead of a single jet, the water issues from a perforated head in a considerable number of small streams. The diameter of the head is commonly about three inches, and the size of the perforations one millimeter (Fig. 41). 1055

Method.—The horizontal rain douche or spray is applied in precisely the same manner as the horizontal jet, the directions and observations relating to which need not be repeated here.

Physiological Effects.—The spray douche produces effects analogous to those of the horizontal jet, but less intense, for the reason that the impression made is so generalized, and the several streams are so small in size, that the mechanical effect is very much less than that of the horizontal jet. 1056

The horizontal jet, when broken, may be made to produce much the same effects as the spray; while the spray, applied at high pressure, may produce effects essentially the same as those of the broken horizontal jet or the full jet at lower pressure.

Therapeutic Applications.—The spray is to be used in cases in which the mechanical effects of the douche are required as a means of encouraging circulatory reaction, and yet the horizontal jet is for some reason regarded as too severe a measure to be safely employed. It is indicated in any case in which the broken jet is applicable. The broken jet is most conveniently employed in cases in which the full jet may be received with advantage upon some portions of the body, while the broken jet alone is admissible upon other parts. When no portion of the body can safely receive the full or horizontal jet, the spray douche may be advantageously employed. 1057

The hot spray is especially indicated in the treatment of *neuralgia* with *hyperesthesia* of the overlying skin, *swol-*

len, *painful rheumatic joints*, *spinal neuralgia*, and *spinal irritation* with *hyperesthesia;* at *neutral* temperature, with little pressure, for the relief of the lightning pains of *locomotor ataxia; very hot* (106° to 120°) in alternation with very cold water, for producing powerful revulsive or derivative effects, as an application to the feet and legs for the relief of *asthma*, for the Scotch douche (**1037**), and in cases in which the douche is indicated, but the horizontal jet douche is found too exciting.

The spray has the advantage over the vertical rain douche in that it is very readily adjustable to all parts of the body. It does not affect disproportionately the upper part of the body, and especially the chest, as does the vertical douche. It may be made a very exciting procedure, although at its maximum of intensity it is much less exciting than is the full horizontal jet.

The *neutral* spray is an excellent measure for *insomnia.* For this purpose it should be continued for 4 or 5 minutes at moderate pressure (10 to 15 lbs.), special attention being given to the back and legs.

THE ASCENDING DOUCHE.

1058 This ordinarily consists of a jet or spray directed upward from a nozzle placed near the level of the floor (Fig. 42). It is chiefly useful for applications to the soles of the feet, the perineum, and the anal region.

The ascending douche is usually applied at a very low temperature (60° to 45°), with a duration of half a minute to one minute. It is especially valuable in cases of *atony* of the *bladder* without dilatation, and in cases of *weakness* of the *genital organs* not accompanied by irritation or pain. It is evident that in cases of chronic dilatation of the bladder the cold douche will prove of no value, as the muscular walls of the organ are so relaxed as to be unable to respond to the stimulus of the douche. The *cold* ascending douche is also

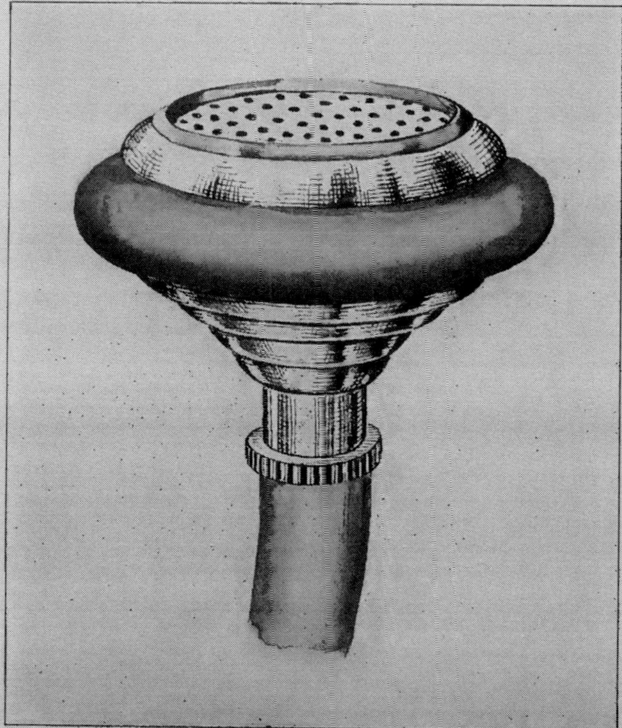

FIG. 41. SPRAY NOZZLE (p. 479).

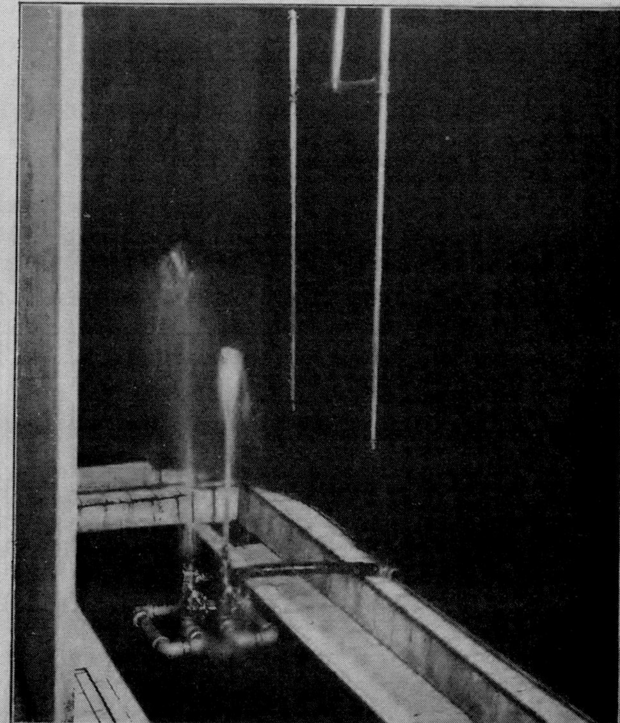

FIG. 42. ASCENDING DOUCHE (p. 480).

of great service in cases of *hemorrhoids*, *constipation*, and *uterine* and *rectal prolapse*.

The *short cold* ascending douche is very useful in rectal prolapse and anal insufficiency, also in flatulence due to constipation.

The *neutral* ascending douche is applicable when hyperesthesia with excessive irritability of the bladder and genital organs exists.

The *warm* ascending douche is very useful as a means of relieving the pain of anal fissure and irritable rectum.

The *hot ascending* douche is one of the most efficacious remedies for the relief of *pruritus ani* and *pruritus vulvæ*. When employed for this purpose, the temperature should be as high as can be borne.

The *alternate* ascending douche is to be employed in cases of *vesical paresis*, *chronic hypertrophy* of the *prostate*, and exudates resulting frum inflammation of the testicles or cord.

The *revulsive* (**1041**) ascending douche may be used in most affections of the genito-urinary organs and rectum, accompanied by pain.

THE CALIPER DOUCHE.

This apparatus,* which was devised by the author, and is **1059**
in daily use at the Battle Creek Sanitarium, consists, as shown in the accompanying cut (Fig. 43), of two semicircular tubular arms, joined to a support at one end in such a manner that the opposite ends can be separated for the admission of the patient within the circle. Being portable, the apparatus may be adjusted to any portion of the body, as the chest, the neck, the waist, the hips, and one or both legs.

The arms are perforated on the inner side, the openings all pointing slightly downward and toward the center, so that when in use, the water is directed upon a narrow circular area·

* Since the above was written, the author has learned that a similar device had previously been made by a Chicago plumber, but so far as known, no practical use was ever made of it.

31

of the skin. Two forms are in use, one in which the tubes are perforated with small openings, the other in which a narrow slit extends from one end to the other of each circular tube. The latter form allows the water to issue in a thin, unbroken sheet, instead of a large number of small streams.

This apparatus is exceedingly convenient for localizing the douche upon a certain area of the body, in cases in which prolonged applications of this sort are desirable.

The caliper douche serves the same purpose as the spray sitz bath so much used in France, when adjusted for application just above the hips, with the patient in a sitting position. The ascending douche may be applied to the anus and the perineum at the same time, thus influencing at once all the voluntary and involuntary muscular structures involved in defecation, and affording one of the most valuable means of combating constipation.

The caliper douche is especially useful for the application of the *cold* douche to relieve *constipation*, *hypopepsia*, *amenorrhea*, and *flatulence* of the stomach and bowels, for which purposes it is applied to the trunk at the different levels indicated.

The *hot* caliper douche is of equal value in cases of *hyperpepsia*, *hyperesthesia* of the lumbar ganglia of the abdominal sympathetic, some cases of *menorrhagia*, *chronic intestinal catarrh* with *diarrhea*, *chronic gastritis*, and *infectious jaundice*.

THE CIRCLE DOUCHE.

1060 The device employed in this douche (Fig. 44) consists of a hollow ring perforated in such a manner that the streams of water emitted converge on a line passing vertically through the center of the circle. In use, the ring, connected with the douche apparatus by a rubber tube, is passed over the head. By directing movements the water may be made to pass chiefly over the front and back, or over one shoulder or the other, passing down over the entire body. The circle douche may be administered to an arm or leg by passing the limb

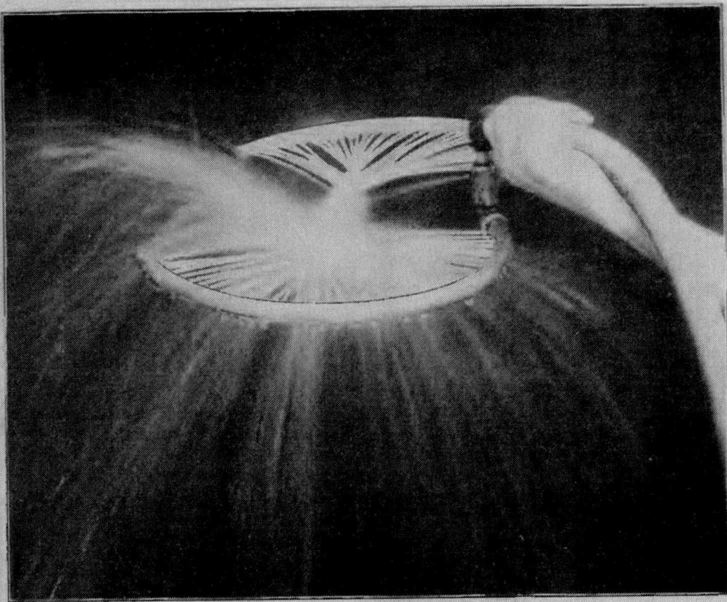

FIG. 43. CALIPER DOUCHE (p. 481).

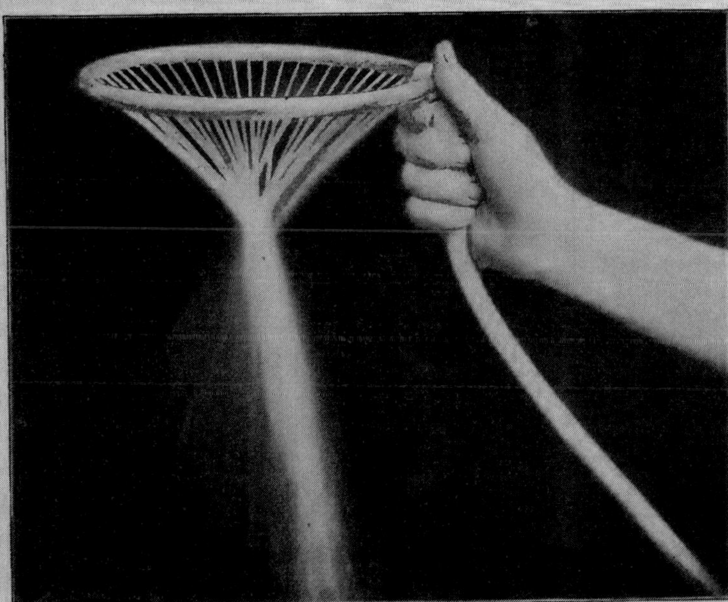

FIG. 44. COLLAR DOUCHE (p. 492).

through the center, and moving the ring back and forth. The circle douche is a very convenient instrument for home use in a common bath-tub, as the convergence of the streams renders it possible to employ it without wetting the walls or furniture of the room. It has the disadvantage, however, that when utilized for general purposes, it produces too strong reaction to the head, especially if very strong pressure is employed.

The circle douche appliance may be used for administering the circle douche to an arm or a leg, and with excellent results, when a localized effect in these parts is for any reason desirable.

THE FAN DOUCHE.

This consists of a horizontal jet from a nozzle of such 1061
form that the water issues in a broad, thin stream (Fig. 45). The friction at the narrow orifice through which the water is projected greatly diminishes the pressure.

In the absence of a special nozzle the fan douche may be produced by holding a piece of metal or wood with a smooth surface against the stream of a jet douche, close to the end of the nozzle.

Physiological Effects.— The weight of the thin blade of 1062
water falling upon the skin is very slight, so that the mechanical effect of the fan douche is reduced to a minimum.

The physiological effects of the fan douche are essentially the same as those of other forms of the douche, but less intense than the full jet, or the rain or spray douche.

Therapeutic Applications.—The fan douche is generally 1063
employed in the same class of cases in which the rain douche is indicated. It has a wider and more varied application than almost any other hydriatic procedure.

This form of douche is used in cases in which strong percutient effects are undesirable, as in the application of very cold water to sensitive surfaces, over painful nerves, hysterogenous zones, inflamed structures, and such especially sensitive portions of the body as the precordial region, the genitals, and the head and neck.

The *cold* fan douche may be employed to great advantage in the following cases: Over the course of the paralyzed nerve trunk in *paralysis;* to the dorsal region in *neurasthenia* with marked muscular weakness and general feebleness; to the dorsal and epigastric regions in *hypopepsia;* over the stomach, bowels, and bladder in *enteroptosis* and *atony* of the organs named.

The *alternating* fan douche is useful in *rheumatism* with *exudates*, but accompanied by little pain.

The *revulsive* fan douche renders invaluable service in *lumbago, sciatica, painful joints, neuritis;* to the spine in *spinal irritation;* to the feet and legs in *asthma;* over the liver in inactivity of this organ; and in *chronic icterus*.

When pain is not present, the cold douche may be substituted in applications to the hepatic region.

The *hot* fan douche is exceedingly valuable in *neuralgia* over an affected nerve, and to the dorsal and epigastric regions in *hyperpepsia*, and over the affected organ in cases of visceral pain, whether due to neuralgia, congestion, or inflammation.

The *neutral* fan douche renders signal service when applied to the limbs as a relief for the lightning pains of *locomotor ataxia*, and to the spine and back of the neck in *insomnia*.

The *short cold* fan douche to the upper part of the dorsal region and the neck stimulates the respiration and circulation, and is often useful in certain cases of *asthma*.

The fan douche at a temperature of 80° to 90° (50 to 60 secs.) is useful in the treatment of irritable neurasthenics who can not endure the douche in any other form. Employed in this way, a good circulatory reaction may be produced without much excitation of the central nervous system, and a sedative effect may thus be secured without the incon-

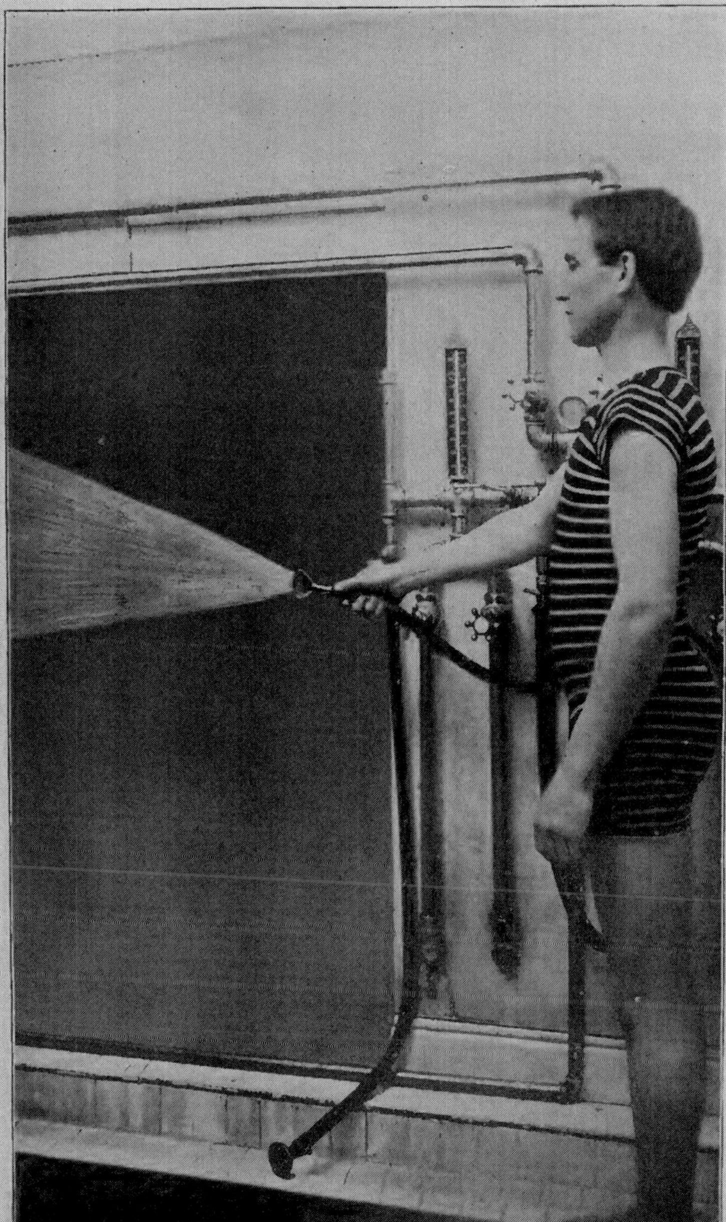

FIG. 45. FAN DOUCHE (p. 483).

veniences accompanying the cold douche. The cold jet or spray, even the percussion douche, may be employed later.

The fan douche has the advantage over other baths having approximately the same temperature, in that equal effects are secured by applications of much shorter duration.

THE FILIFORM DOUCHE.

This is a form of horizontal jet in which the water 1064
issues from an exceedingly small opening. It was devised by de Lauré. In France the filiform jet is produced by a nozzle terminating in a piece of agate perforated by a capillary opening through which the water is forced with such great pressure that it becomes a cloud a short distance from the apparatus. The duration is from 1 to 10 minutes.

Physiological Effects.— The effects of the filiform douche are those of strong counter-irritation, suggesting the effect of mustard. It is capable of producing most powerful irritation of the skin, even bleeding through rupture of the small vessels. Exceedingly strong circulatory reaction is produced with little or no thermic activity.

Therapeutic Applications. — Bernard* extols the filiform douche as a means of producing powerful counter-irritation for the relief of pain. He describes the effect of this douche as being very painful for the first two minutes, but after that period producing very agreeable sensations. This procedure is usually reserved for rebellious cases, as obstinate *sciaticas*, and other forms of neuralgia which do not yield to ordinary measures. It has been used successfully in *hemicrania*, *diphtheritic* and *hysterical paralysis*, *chronic rheumatism*, and *lumbago*. The first applications must be very brief. Gradually, as tolerance is established, they may be extended to 8 or 10 minutes.

---

*P. Bernard, *Ann. de la Société d' Hydrol.*, 1894, p. 147.

THE FOG DOUCHE.

1065 This douche, known by the French as the *douche d'eau pulvérisé*, is produced by the same device as that employed for the percussion douche. A current of air under pressure is admitted to the nozzle of the douche apparatus at such a point that the water is made to issue from the orifice of the nozzle in the form of a fine mist driven with great velocity. The percussion douche is produced in precisely the same way, except that a smaller amount of air is admitted. The refrigerant effect of an application of this sort is very great, while the percutient or mechanical effect is less than that of the percussion douche proper (Fig. 46).

Therapeutic Applications.—The fog douche is a most excellent measure to be substituted for the Scotch douche, used in combination with the vapor douche in cases in which refrigeration without mechanical effect is desired, especially in general *hyperesthesia* of the skin, *spinal irritation*, *painful joints*, and *sciatica* with tenderness of the tissues. The Scotch douche to the legs, produced by means of the vapor bath combined with the fog douche, produces most powerful derivative effects in favor of the brain and other organs of the upper portion of the body.

THE MASSAGE DOUCHE.

1066 This is a mixed procedure, in which the kneading movements of massage are executed at the same time that a stream of water is allowed to play upon the surface (Fig. 47). The kneading movement consists of strong intermittent pressure with the palms of the hands, as in palmar kneading and kneading with the thumb and fingers. The movement should be so applied as to affect the blood-vessels of the muscular structures as well as those of the subcutaneous tissue.

The parts to which the massage douche is especially applicable are the back, the limbs, and the abdomen. Particular attention is given to the joints when stiffened by chronic rheumatism. Two attendants are required to secure the best effects, one applying the douche while the other manipulates the parts.

Physiological Effects.—The massage douche, water at a 1067
low temperature being employed, is without doubt the most powerful of all hydriatic procedures, especially with the use of the horizontal douche at high pressure, or the percussion douche.

The massage douche adds to the thermic and mechanical effects of the ordinary douche the mechanical effects of massage, thus bringing to bear at the same time and place two most powerful procedures. The ordinary douche acts directly upon the skin only, producing effects in the deeper structures by reflex nervous action and by retrostasis, or mechanical displacement of the blood inward. The douche renders the skin anemic, while it produces collateral hyperemia of the muscles. In the reaction which follows, the skin becomes hyperemic, while the blood supply of the muscles is to an equal extent diminished. By the combination of massage with the douche this reaction of the circulation in the muscles is stimulated, thus at first creating collateral hyperemia and the stimulation of heat production which results from the increased supply of blood and heat to the thermogenic tissues located in the muscles.

On the other hand, by hastening the return of blood to the skin and intensifying the cutaneous hyperemia, the secondary effect of the combination of massage with the douche is to increase the cooling process, thus offsetting its influence in stimulating heat production.

The intimate connection of general metabolism with heat production renders the massage douche a most powerful tonic and alterative measure. It is, indeed, but one of the diversified forms of the ordinary douche the various therapeutic effects of which it intensifies; and by acting upon the deeper structures, it may be said to carry the effect of the douche inward as far as the internal structures can be influenced by external manipulations.

The massage douche may be employed with either very hot or very cold water, and at all intermediate temperatures. The most important applications are in connection with the very cold douche at high pressure, or the percussion douche, the very hot douche (104° and upwards) and the neutral douche (92° to 98°).

The effects of the *hot* massage douche are powerfully revulsive, by adding to the profound circulatory reaction following the ordinary hot douche the active congestion of the deep muscular and cellular structures. The hot douche congests the skin only; while the hot massage douche congests the entire soft parts of the limb to which the application is made.

The effect of the hot massage douche upon the local temperature is somewhat peculiar. A certain amount of heat is of course absorbed from the water, and at the same time the manipulation of the muscles and increased flow of blood through them stimulates heat production. Both these influences, however, are antagonized and their effect quickly annulled by the atonic thermic reaction following the application, and the rapid loss of heat from the widely dilated vessels.

Both the hot and the cold massage douche produce a more intense circulatory reaction in the part to which the application is made than does the ordinary douche, either hot or cold. The effect of the cold douche without massage is to produce anemia of the skin with collateral congestion of the muscles, but without materially influencing the total amount of blood supplied to the part; while the hot douche produces hyperemia of the skin with a corresponding anemia of the muscles, likewise without great influence upon the total blood supply. In both cases, however, the combination of massage with the hydric application, by independently stimulating the circulation of the blood-vessels of the deeper structures, has the effect to increase to a marked degree the total blood supply. It is this fact which gives to the massage douche its powerful derivative effects. Indeed, it may be justly said that there is no other known means by which such powerful revulsive and fluxion effects may be produced as by the massage douche.

The massage douche employed at *neutral* temperatures or a temperature near the neutral point, produces little or no thermic effects, but does produce most decided circulatory reaction, not only upon the surface, but in the deeper structures as well. Thus its action is almost wholly local. The douche at a neutral temperature annuls the effect of the massage as a cutaneous irritant by lessening the sensibility of the nerves of the skin, thus giving to this form of the application peculiar properties, and adapting it to meet special therapeutic indications.

Therapeutic Applications.—The *cold* massage douche is **1068**
the most powerful alterative and tonic of all hydriatic procedures. It at the same time has the decided advantage of being much more easily tolerated than the ordinary cold douche. The shallow bath can be tolerated by persons who can not endure the cold immersion, for the reason that the constant friction of the skin maintains the surface circulation, and prevents chilling of the cutaneous nerves to such a degree as to produce injurious internal congestion, shivering, and thermic reaction. The Brand bath is by the same means rendered tolerable and beneficial in cases in which the immersion bath without friction would produce dangerous and even fatal effects. During the application of the vigorous kneading which accompanies the massage douche, the ordinary unpleasant impression produced by a stream of cold water is lessened to such a degree as to be easily tolerable. The cold massage douche may thus be employed with persons who are keenly susceptible to cold impressions, and may also be of service as a means of training them to the use of cold water in other ways.

In many cases the *tepid* douche may be employed with the best effects, the temperature being lowered from day to day as tolerance is established. The general cold massage douche will naturally be employed with persons of good strength, and particularly in cases in which emaciation is not present, and is especially useful in cases in which spoliative effects are desirable, as in obesity, fleshy rheumatics, and diabetics in whom there is no loss of flesh.

The massage douche to the lower extremities furnishes a useful means of producing derivative effects in favor of the head and chest. It has the advantage over the ordinary cold douche that the local anemia and the resulting retrostasis and increased congestion of the already overfilled vessels of the head or chest are lessened in duration and in degree by the stimulating effect of the massage upon the whole circulation of the parts.

The cold massage douche also possesses great value as a means of stimulating the circulation in joints which have been the seat at some previous time of inflammatory processes which have left behind exudation products with rigidity of the joint structures and limited movement, but in which pain and other indications of congestion are absent. The powerful fluxion effects produced by the massage douche in these cases is a most efficient means of producing an increased flow of healthy blood through the parts, thus bringing to bear upon them the healing influence of the vital fluid, the most potent of all curative means. In cases of this sort the application should not be confined wholly to the joint, but should extend to the soft structures of the limb, both above and below the joint. In the case of the knee, for example, the muscles of both the calf and the thigh should be manipulated in alternation with the joint itself. The effects of the massage douche to the joint may be extended by applying the heating compress, to be changed as often as dried, and to be worn until the application of the next douche.

The local cold massage douche is equally efficient as a means of stimulating the removal of old *inflammatory exudates* in other accessible parts as well as the joints.

The cold massage douche likewise renders great service in cases of intractable *lumbago* and *sciatica* in which the parts are not sensitive to pressure.

The *hot* massage douche may be advantageously applied to the joints in connection with a cold application of some sort for the purpose of heightening the effect of the latter or rendering the joint less sensitive to thermic and mechanical stimulation. The analgesic effects of the hot massage douche are likewise effective in cases of *sciatica* in which cold applications prove too stimulating.

The *neutral* massage douche to the legs, with strong pressure, is an excellent derivative measure for use in cases of *insomnia* in which the neutral douche alone applied to the legs or to the whole surface fails to accomplish the desired result.

Contraindications.—The contraindications of the cold massage douche are essentially the same as those mentioned in relation to the ordinary cold douche (**1023**). It may be mentioned, however, that by making the application partial in character,—that is, confining it to a small area, as a single limb, until a good reaction has been produced, then extending to another part, and so on until the whole body has been gone over,—the untoward effects resulting from a general cold douche may be obviated without sacrificing any of its good effects. When employed in this way, the cold massage douche produces effects similar to those of cold friction or the cold towel rub, but very greatly intensified. The cold massage douche should not be applied to joints when inflamed, congested, or painful to pressure. In certain cases, however, the application may be made to the soft parts above the joints, as a means of producing powerful derivative effects. **1069**

LOCALIZED DOUCHES.

One of the most valuable uses of the douche (jet, spray, **1070**
percussion, fan, filiform) is in applications to certain well-defined, cutaneous areas with special reference to the internal organs connected with them. The douche is also sometimes localized in the treatment of certain superficial parts without

reference to internal parts which may be reflexly influenced. The names by which the principal of these localized douches are designated are the following: *Cephalic, dorsal, lumbar, thoracic, shoulder, sternal, epigastric, abdominal, hypogastric, douche to feet, plantar, anal, perineal.*

Physiological Effects.—The effect of localized douches depends not only upon the duration, temperature, pressure, and mass of water employed, but upon the particular surface to which the application is made. The fact that every portion of the cutaneous surface is reflexly related through the central nervous system with some special internal vascular area, has elsewhere been sufficiently dwelt upon (**353-382**); it is only necessary here to call attention to the fact that a certain number of clearly defined reflex arcs have been worked out by various investigators, and it is with these that localized douches are chiefly concerned.

Without undertaking to review the general principles which have been previously explained, it may be said, briefly, that —

1. *Short applications* of cold water with strong pressure *are strongly exciting*, producing powerful circulatory reaction with dilatation of the blood-vessels and increased activity of the small arteries, veins, capillaries, and lymphatics, both in the cutaneous surface to which they are applied and in the internal vascular area reflexly connected with it.

2. *Prolonged cold applications without pressure produce contraction* of the small arteries, capillaries, veins, and lymphatics of the cutaneous area to which the application is made, and of the reflexly associated internal vascular areas.

3. *Hot applications produce analgesic effects.*

4. *Neutral applications* to these areas *produce local and reflex sedative effects.*

5. *Alternate applications produce* most powerful and valuable *exciting and fluxion effects.*

6. *Revulsive applications produce powerful derivative and analgesic effects* by causing collateral hyperemia of the skin.

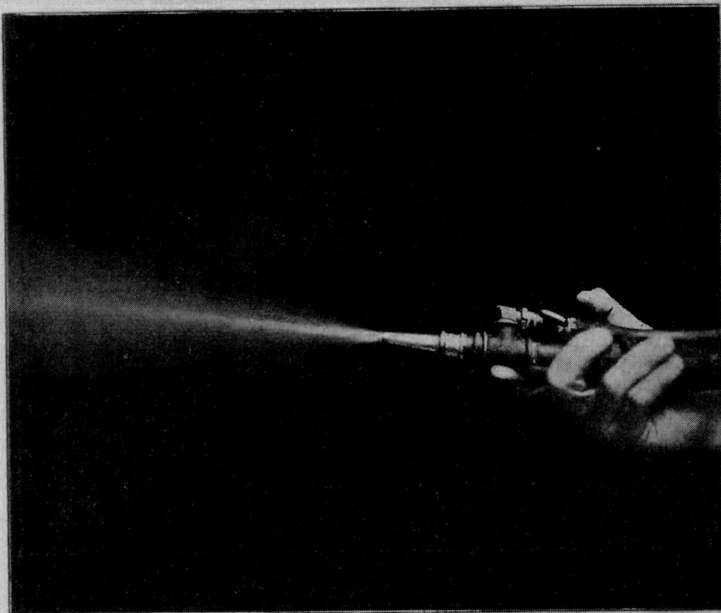

FIG. 46. FOG DOUCHE (p. 486).

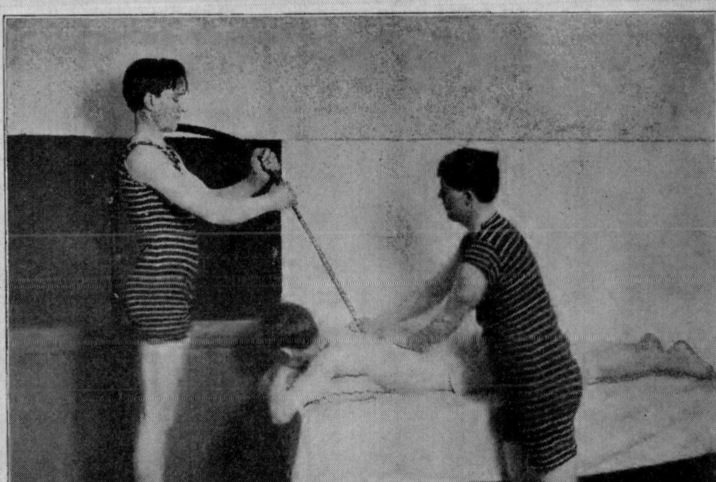

FIG. 47. MASSAGE DOUCHE (p. 486).

THE CEPHALIC DOUCHE.

The cephalic douche, or the application of a stream of water to the head, is a procedure whereby the central nervous system is powerfully influenced (Fig. 48). 1071

Method.—There are two methods of applying the cephalic douche. In one the patient lies on his face, the head projecting over the end of the couch, and depressed sufficiently so that the stream of water poured upon the back of the neck runs down over the head. Cold water may be poured from a dipper or pitcher held at a distance of a few inches to two or three feet above the patient's head; or if preferred, the patient may sit in a tub of water at a temperature of 100° to 102° while water is poured upon the top of the head and allowed to run down the back of the neck. It is an excellent plan to pin a towel about the head in such a way as to protect the ears and shoulders, and direct the stream of water upon the neck and spine. The pressure must always be slight. The fan douche may be used, but not the full jet.

In the general neutral douche for insomnia, the broken jet may be allowed to play upon the back of the head and the neck with gentle aspersions for a few seconds at the end of the application.

Physiological Effects.—A short cold application to the head causes dilatation of the blood-vessels of the brain. 1072
Prolonged cold applications cause contraction, especially if the application be continued long enough to produce chilling (Schüller).

Therapeutic Applications.—The *cold* cephalic douche is 1073
well-nigh obsolete, being rarely employed except in connection with typhoid or some other grave fever, in which the cold bath is used. In these cases, affusion to the head or the fan douche to the head is a means of highest value to rouse the activity of the brain, and through it to quicken all the bodily activities. In these cases the cephalic douche is administered in connection with the cold immersion friction

bath (Brand, **1150**), and is repeated at intervals of five minutes during the bath. The temperature should be a few degrees lower than that of the general bath (60° to 50°).

Great care must always be taken in the application of douches or affusions to the head. A *short cold* application excites the brain, and is useful in *melancholia*, in *cerebral anemia*, and in *sunstroke with pallor*. It is especially applicable in cases of *melancholia with stupor*, in which the cerebral anemia is usually very marked. The *prolonged cold* douche to the head is one of the most powerful of all depressing measures; unless very short, the effect may be too profound; hence the cold affusion is safer.

Long cold applications to the head are exceedingly depressing, but may be used in fever, in *cerebral congestion*, and in *sunstroke with congestion* of the skin.

Affusion, the ice compress, and the evaporating compress are usually more convenient for application to the head than the douche, and safer because less likely to be overdone.

A cold douche to the back of the neck stimulates the respiratory centers. If too cold or too prolonged, suffocation or arrest of the heart may result. The hot or cold compress, alternate compresses, or sponging are milder measures which produce similar effects, and are in general to be preferred.

A short *tepid* douche to the head or a tepid affusion will allay cerebral excitement. It may be usefully employed in *insomnia*, *maniacal excitement*, and *cerebral irritation*. The temperature should be from 80° to 92°, duration from 3 to 5 minutes. Affusion is to be preferred to the douche in most cases.

The *neutral fan* douche to the occipital region and the back of the neck, in connection with the general neutral douche, is a remarkably useful measure in procuring sleep in *insomnia*.

Hot affusions to the head are useful in *syncope* and *collapse*, and in cases of *migraine* with low arterial tension, but should be employed with great caution.

In cases of *cerebral anemia*, *alternate* applications may be employed instead of the short cold douche, the hot douche, or hot or cold compresses.

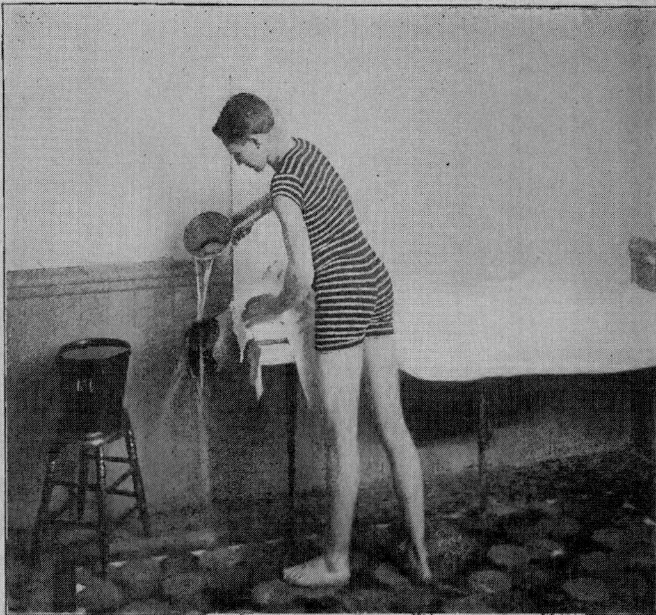

FIG. 48. CEPHALIC DOUCHE (p. 493).

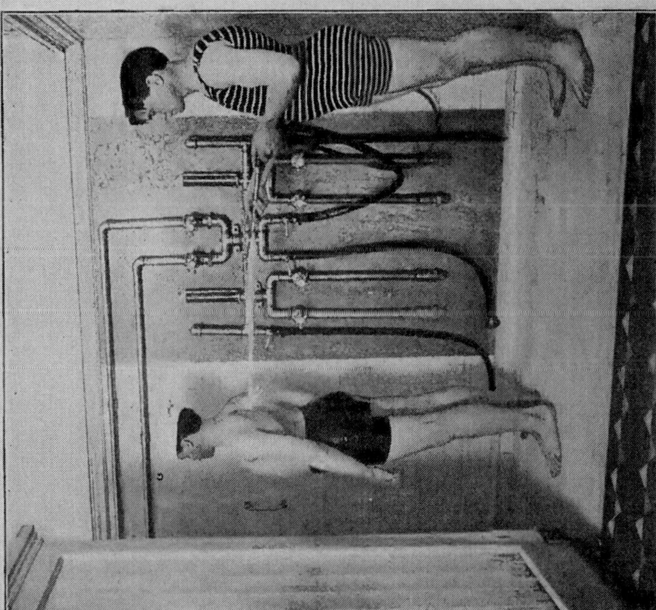

FIG. 49. DORSAL DOUCHE (p. 495).

Applications to the head should be managed with great care, and should at first be employed in a tentative manner, the effects being carefully noted.

THE DORSAL OR SPINAL DOUCHE (Fig. 49).

In this procedure either the full or the broken horizontal 1074
jet, the percussion douche, the fan douche, or the spray may be employed. The skin of the back is less sensitive than that of most other portions of the body, and hence intense applications may be made without unpleasant excitant effects in most cases in which percutient effects are at all admissible.

The stream of water should not be confined to the median line, but should be allowed to play rapidly up and down over a surface extending three or four inches on either side of the spinal column. As a rule, the pressure employed should be as great as the patient can bear. The percussion douche should be employed when available.

Physiological Effects.— The purpose of the dorsal douche 1075
is to influence the central nervous system, and through its effects upon the vasomotor nerves to influence the system at large. That most pronounced effects are obtainable by this procedure is clearly evidenced by the sense of buoyancy and increased energy experienced as the result of a vigorous application, especially of the cold percussion douche, in cases of either temporary or chronic nervous exhaustion.

Therapeutic Applications.— The *tepid* douche calms excitability of spinal origin, as in *hysteria* and *spinal irritation*, *hyperesthesia* of the *lumbar ganglia* of the abdominal sympathetic connected with *irritation* of the *splanchnics*, *irritability* of the *bladder* of spinal origin, and *irritability* of the *genito-urinary center;* and relieves *incontinence* in children.

The *cold* dorsal douche should be employed in *spinal anemia*, in functional *locomotor ataxia*, in *motor insufficiency of the bladder* resulting in *urinary incontinence* or *retention*, in *nervous vomiting*, in *diminished renal activity*, and in *melancholia*, but must be carefully avoided in cases of insanity of organic origin and all forms of structural disease of the spine. The cold percussion douche to the spine produces a most wonderfully beneficial effect in cases of *chronic neurasthenia*. By the daily application of this procedure the patient sees himself steadily lifted up to a higher level, his mental and nervous tone improving, the trembling, languor, mental confusion, and indecision disappearing; indeed, the effect of a single application is so pronounced that the patient himself at once recognizes the benefit derived from this simple procedure. Great care must be taken to avoid overdoing the application. The result will be headache, depression, and nervousness following a feeling of buoyancy.

The very *hot* dorsal douche should be applied in *gastralgia*, in connection with the hot douche to the hypogastrium; and the *warm* spinal douche (92° to 98°) is of great value in *locomotor ataxia* with lightning pains, and in *spinal sclerosis*.

The *Scotch* douche to the back may be employed in *lumbago*, in cases of *diabetes insipidus*, in the *irritation* of the *renal plexus* of the sympathetic so often encountered in *movable* or *floating kidney* in connection with *enteroptosis*, and in *neuralgia of the kidney*.

THE LUMBAR DOUCHE (Fig. 50).

1076 Either the full, the broken, the percussion, or the fan douche may be applied to the lumbar region; and, except in cases of painful affections, full pressure may be employed. Powerful reflex effects are produced by the lumbar douche upon the organs of the lower abdomen, the pelvic viscera, and the lower extremities.

The *cold* lumbar douche is especially useful in cases of *constipation*, in *motor insufficiency of the bladder* resulting in *incontinence* or *retention*, in *amenorrhea*, in *renal insufficiency*, and in *infantile uterus*, or *delayed development* of the

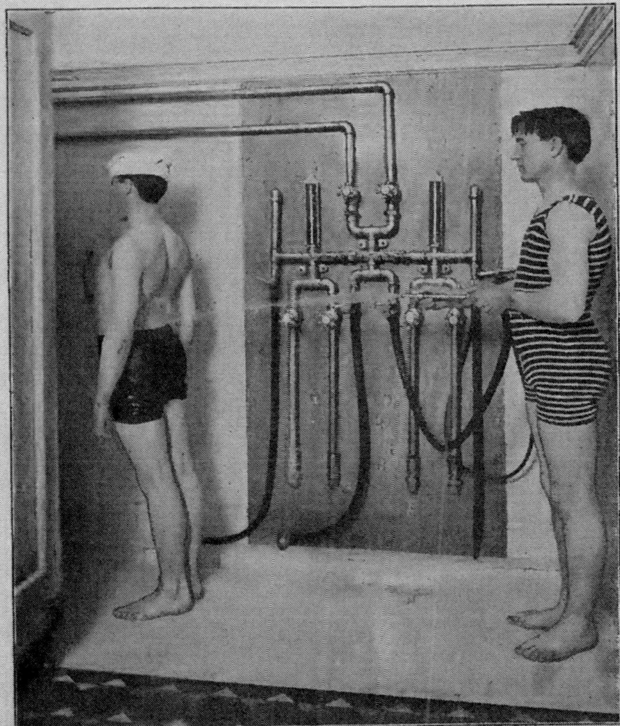

Fig. 50. LUMBAR DOUCHE (p. 496).

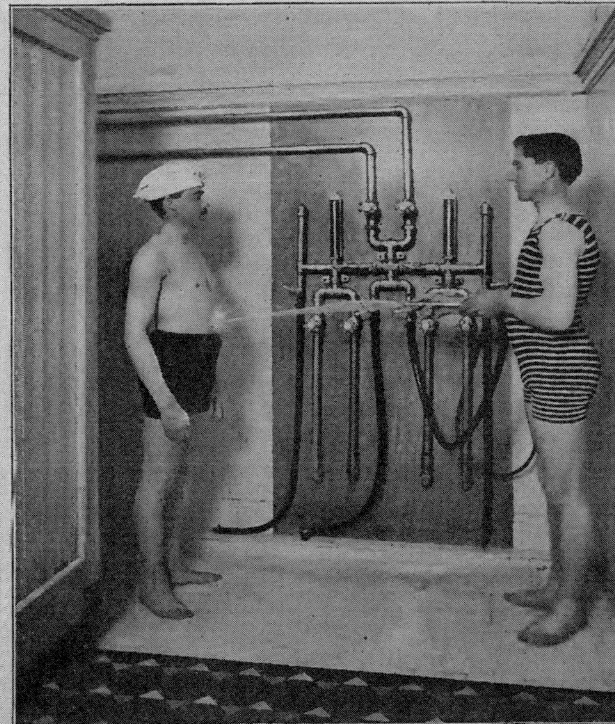

Fig. 51. ABDOMINAL DOUCHE (p. 500).

pelvic viscera or functions. It should be borne in mind that a douche to this region, to obtain the effect above described, must be administered with a considerable degree of pressure, at a low temperature, and very short.

The *Scotch* lumbar douche is a most excellent remedy in ***neuralgia of the uterus and ovaries***, in ***renal congestion***, in ***urinary retention*** due to spasm of the neck of the bladder, and especially in ***lumbago***. It is a sovereign remedy also for the ***backache*** so common in women suffering from pelvic displacements, although of course in these cases its effects are chiefly palliative. But when employed in connection with the use of the abdominal supporter, relief is nearly always prompt and permanent, when no inflammation exists.

In connection with the Scotch fan douche to the lumbar region for the relief of congestion, revulsive applications should be made to the feet and legs. Sometimes a better effect is obtained by applying the revulsive douche to the shoulders and upper part of the back.

THE SHOULDER DOUCHE.

Either the full or the broken jet may be applied to the **1077** shoulders, special care being taken to avoid the neck and the chest surfaces. A very short *cold* application to the shoulders and arms, followed by a hot application at 113° to 120°, produces strong derivative effects in favor of the pelvic viscera. When employed for this purpose, the cold application should be made with the percussion douche. The *hot* or the *Scotch fan* douche generally affords prompt relief in cases of rheumatic pains in the shoulder joints.

THE THORACIC DOUCHE.

In this procedure, the application of the douche is con- **1078** fined to that portion of the trunk above the diaphragm, or practically the area of the skin covering the ribs, sternum, and vertebræ. The application should include not only the throat, sides, and back of the chest, but the tops of the shoulders as well. The broken or the fan douche should be employed. The full jet is likely to produce too powerful an impression.

Physiological Effects.— A *short cold* application, with high pressure, made to this region increases the amount of blood not only in the dermal and muscular coverings of the chest wall, but within the lungs and pleura.

Prolonged cold applications, with little pressure (65° to 80°, 6 to 10 lbs., 1 to 3 min.), contract the blood-vessels, and lessen the amount of blood in the lungs and other organs contained within the chest cavity.

A *short, very cold* douche to the breasts stimulates the circulation in the pelvic viscera, and causes contraction of the uterine muscle (50° to 45°, 4 to 10 secs.).

Prolonged cold applications to the breasts with little pressure cause contraction of the blood-vessels of the uterus, and thus relieve uterine congestion (75° to 65°, 1 to 3 min.). The application of the cold douche to the lower third of the sternum causes contraction of the vessels of the kidney, and increases the flow of the urine. Applied over the heart, the douche powerfully excites cardiac activity.

Prolonged application, with little pressure, slows and energizes the heart.

THE EPIGASTRIC DOUCHE.

1079 The broken jet, the fan douche, or the spray should be employed rather than the full jet in the application of the epigastric douche.

Therapeutic Applications.— The *cold* epigastric douche is of the greatest value in the treatment of *hypopepsia*, *apepsia*, *gastroptosis*, *dilatation* and *atony* of the stomach, and in gastric *flatulence*. It stimulates both the glandular and the muscular activities of the stomach through its influence upon the plexuses of Meissner and Auerbach.

The *very hot* epigastric douche (115° to 122°) is equally valuable in cases of *hyperpepsia*, *gastrorrhea*, so-called *gastric rheumatism*, *gastric crises*, *gastralgia*, *subacute gas-*

tritis, *gastro-duodenitis*, or *gastric* and *duodenal catarrh*, *infectious jaundice*, and the distressing pain accompanying *chronic ulcer* of the stomach.

The *tepid thoracic* douche (fan) without pressure relieves nervous asthma when applied to the back and sides of the chest, and quiets palpitation from irritability of the heart when applied over the cardiac region. It is rare that very cold water can be employed at first in these cases; hence it is better to begin with a temperature of 80° to 92°, lowering the temperature at successive applications if the patient is found able to tolerate colder water.

The Scotch douche may be employed with excellent success for the relief of *intercostal neuralgia*, *pleurodynia* from chronic pleuritic adhesions, *brachial neuralgia*, and *reflex irritations* arising from *hyperesthesia* of the solar plexus.

In all painful affections of the stomach the *Scotch* douche generally affords marvelous relief. The hot applications should be at as high a temperature as can be borne (120° to 125°), and the cold application should be very cold and very short, 50° to 60°, for 6 to 12 seconds. When pain is produced by slight pressure of the hand upon the epigastrium, the douche should be applied with the least pressure possible. *Hyperesthesia* of the solar plexus, a condition usually present as a fundamental cause of *intercostal neuralgia*, *pain between the shoulders*, *spinal irritation*, so-called *painful dyspepsia* and *nervous asthma*, is wonderfully relieved by the Scotch epigastric douche.

THE HYPOGASTRIC DOUCHE.

This application, in which only the broken jet, the fan, 1080
or the spray douche may be employed, is confined to the hypogastric region. For its application the patient sits upon a stool with the knees separated, the head erect, and the trunk inclined backward.

Physiological Effects.—Through the influence of this procedure, most powerful reflex effects may be produced upon the organs of the lower abdomen and pelvis. It acts especially upon the bladder, the uterus, and the ovaries.

Therapeutic Applications.— The *cold* douche to the hypogastrium, with little pressure, and continued for a half minute to one minute, causes contraction of the bladder and the uterus, and of the vessels of all the pelvic viscera; hence this procedure is of great value in conditions of both *active* and *passive congestion*, and in all chronic morbid conditions of the pelvic viscera in which congestion is a prominent factor, such as so-called *chronic inflammation* of the *uterus*, and *endometritis*. It is likewise very useful in *subinvolution*, in *displacements* due to relaxation of the supporting structures, in *atony* of the *bladder*, and in *enteroptosis* due to weakness of the abdominal muscles.

The *revulsive Scotch* douche to the hypogastrium affords prompt relief in *neuralgia* of the *uterus*, the *bladder*, or the *ovaries*, in *uterine pain* due to contraction of the cervix, in *vaginismus*, *vesicle tenesmus*, and in *hyperesthesia* of the sympathetic ganglia of the pelvis, as shown by pressure upon the lumbo-aortic plexus and the sympathetic nodes of the pelvis.

THE ABDOMINAL DOUCHE (Fig. 51).

1081 This local application of the douche is properly confined to the anterior abdominal surface. It influences the small intestines, the colon, and the lumbar ganglia of the abdominal sympathetic. Through these nerve centers important general effects are produced.

A *cold* douche applied to the abdomen is highly useful in *constipation*, especially when it is due to *dilatation* of the *colon*, and *enteroptosis*.

The *cold abdominal* douche is of service in *atony* of the *bladder*, in *enteroptosis* due to relaxation of the abdominal muscles, and in *pelvic displacements* due to atony, when not accompanied by uterine or ovarian congestions.

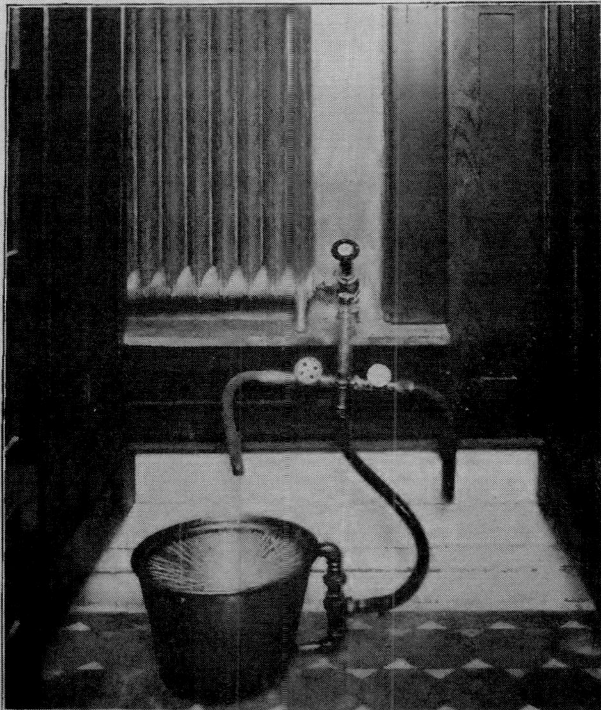

Fig. 52. PLANTAR DOUCHE APPARATUS (p. 502).

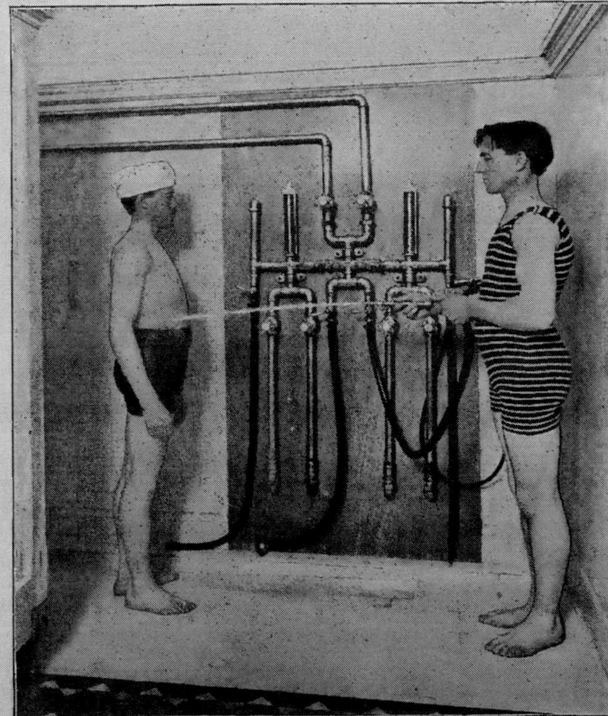

Fig. 53. HEPATIC DOUCHE (p. 510).

The *warm* or *hot* douche should be employed when *pain* or *irritability* exists in the *bladder*, the *uterus*, the *ovaries*, or other pelvic viscera.

The *Scotch* douche is most valuable for the relief of the pain due to *irritation* of the *splanchnic nerves* or of the *lumbar ganglia* of the abdominal sympathetic, a condition recognized by pressure upon the ganglia situated about two inches to the right and the left of the umbilicus, on the inner surface of the posterior wall of the abdominal cavity.

The Scotch douche gives excellent results in *chronic diarrhea*, *chronic dysentery*, and *enteralgia*.

DOUCHE TO THE FEET.

In this application the broken jet or the spray is com- 1082
monly employed, as the fleshy covering of the foot is so thin as to make the percussion douche or even the full jet too painful to be borne in most cases. The stream is directed upon the feet and ankles, the patient sitting in such a position that the largest amount of surface may be readily reached. It is the usual practice to apply the *cold* douche to the feet for a few seconds at the end of general applications of the douche, for the purpose of producing a certain amount of revulsive effect in this region of the body. In very susceptible persons the douche may be applied to the feet only, until the patient has been trained to bear a more general application. This is especially necessary in cases of patients subject to painful affections of the head or nervous affections of the chest and heart, as in *cerebral hyperemia*, *nervous asthma*, *palpitation* of the heart of sympathetic origin, *pulmonary congestion*, *exophthalmic goiter* and *chronic migraine*. By taking the precaution to allow the stream of cold water to fall upon the feet at the beginning or end of the general cold douche, the headache which often follows the douche (sometimes called the "hydropathic headache") may generally be prevented.

The *cold spray* douche prolonged until the skin is reddened, produces contraction of the cerebral vessels, and hence exerts a most useful derivative effect in cerebral hyperemia.

The *Scotch* douche and the *very hot* douche may be applied to the feet with advantage as a means of relieving cerebral congestion.

THE PLANTAR DOUCHE.

1083 The plantar douche consists in the application of water under strong pressure to the soles of the feet. Either the single jet or the spray douche may be employed. The author has for many years used the apparatus shown in the accompanying cut (Fig. 52), which he had especially constructed for the purpose. It consists of a copper tub with double bottom, the uppermost one of which is perforated over a surface equal in area to that of the average foot, and with an outline adapted to the foot. Several openings around the side permit the ready escape of the water. A perforated pipe placed around the side of the inner surface of the vessel at a higher level permits the application of water to the upper surface of the foot when desired.

The *cold* plantar douche, continued for one half minute to 2 minutes, or until strong reaction occurs, produces powerful reflex impressions upon the organs of the abdomen and pelvis. Both the blood-vessels and the muscular walls of the hollow organs of the pelvis and the abdomen are brought into strong contraction by this procedure.

Burgonzio has also shown that the vessels of the brain may be caused to contract by this application, rendering it useful in *chronic headache* from congestion. The duration of the applications for this purpose should be one and one-half to 2 minutes.

The cold plantar douche may likewise render service in *anemia* of the brain, in which case the application should be much shorter (4 to 10 sec.). This douche affords one of the very best means for overcoming habitual *coldness* of the *feet*, a condition which is exceedingly common in *gastric neurasthenia*, in *hyperesthesia* of the *lumbar ganglia*, and especially in *enteroptosis*. It is chiefly in these cases of vascular spasm due to reflex irritation, that the plantar douche is useful as a means of warming cold extremities. It is not applicable when the coldness is due to general feebleness of the circulation. In cases of the latter sort, general cold frictions, the cold precordial compress, the general Scotch douche, and other measures for stimulating the circulation are required.

The cold plantar douche renders valuable service in *hematuria*, *atony* of the *bladder*, *incontinence* of urine in old men, in *spermatorrhea* from relaxation of the ejaculatory ducts, in *neurasthenia*, the result of excessive cerebral activity, in cases in which the *urinary secretion* is *scanty*, and in *chronic epistaxis* not due to ulceration of the nasal mucous membrane.

THE PERINEAL DOUCHE.

In this douche the application is confined to the cutane- 1084
ous region in front of the anus or the perineum, its purpose being to affect the organs of the pelvis, especially the rectum, the prostate, the vesiculæ seminales, the deep urethra, the ejaculatory ducts, the testicles, and the bladder, in men; and the rectum, the uterus, the ovaries, the Fallopian tubes, and the bladder, in women. The perineum has an exceedingly rich vascular and nervous supply, and strong reflex effects may be produced by suitable applications to this region. The application is made with the ascending douche, as much pressure being used as is possible without pain.

Therapeutic Applications.—The *very cold* perineal douche is 1085
useful in *constipation*, *atony* of the *bladder*, *chronic urethritis*, *prostatorrhea*, *prostatitis*, *hypertrophy* of the *prostate* with *induration*, *spermatorrhea* with *atony* of the *ejaculatory ducts*, and especially the diurnal form of the disease, *inflammation* of the *uterus*, *subinvolution* of the *uterus* with relaxation of the supporting structures of the uterus and *displacements*, as well as other chronic disorders of the pelvic region characterized

by lowered tone. It must be remembered, however, that this application should never be employed in cases in which pain is a marked symptom, as the powerful thermic reaction set up is likely to increase the pain; spasmodic affections, as *vesical, rectal,* or *vaginal tenesmus*, are also aggravated by cold applications. The duration of the cold application should be 2 to 3 minutes.

1086 The *very hot* perineal douche is useful in most affections of the prostate, the rectum, the uterus, the bladder, and associated organs. It is especially valuable in cases of *spermatorrhea* with great *irritability* of the *deep urethra* and *hyperesthesia* in the region of the *vesiculæ seminales* and *ejaculatory ducts*. The duration of the hot perineal douche should be 1 to 3 minutes (115° to 122°). The hot perineal douche is very useful as a means of relaxing a *rigid perineum* in preparation for childbirth when rigidity of the perineum is known to be present. Little pressure should be employed in these cases. *Vaginal, rectal,* and *vesical tenesmus* are relieved by the hot anal douche with moderate pressure.

It is generally useful to terminate the application with cold for 2 or 3 seconds.

THE ANAL DOUCHE.

1087 This application, administered by means of the rising or ascending douche, allowed to fall upon the anus, is of great value in the treatment of hemorrhoids, especially in external hemorrhoids and in the mixed variety, in which the internal and external structures are both involved, and joined by extension of the morbid process across the anal margin.

Galtz produced evacuation of the bladder in dogs having paraphlegia from division of the spinal cord, by placing a sponge saturated with cold water against the anus.

The *cold* anal douche is of special service in the treatment of *constipation*, reflexly exciting normal peristaltic movements, and is especially useful in restoring normal sensibility of the rectum which has become lost by neglect to answer promptly the calls of nature, resulting in an abnormal accumulation of hardened fecal matters in the rectum, and consequent constipation. It is also of great service to persons who have suffered from the unwise application of surgical procedures to this portion of the body, resulting in *weakening of the anal muscle* to such an extent as to prevent the proper retention of fluid fecal matters and gas. By the use of this simple measure such few fibers of the sphincter as may remain intact may be stimulated to vigorous action.

The cold douche may be advantageously employed in cases in which internal hemorrhoids have become inflamed, and are prolapsed.

The very cold anal douche will generally cause a contraction of the hemorrhoids to such an extent that they may be easily replaced.

The *very hot* anal douche is useful in cases of *rectal ulcer* and *fissure*, *vaginismus*, and *spasm* of the *sphincter muscle.*

This application is contraindicated in cases of *ovarian neuralgia*, *enteralgia*, *vesical irritability*, and other painful affections of the pelvic and abdominal viscera.

VISCERAL DOUCHES.

By the general term "visceral douche" it is intended 1088
to designate a douche administered in such a manner as to influence an internal organ. It should be understood, however, that, with one or two exceptions, it is impossible to make an application directly to the organ itself, but that the desired effect is obtained through the medium of an application to the cutaneous area or areas reflexly associated with the organ, the condition of which it is desired to influence.

General Physiological Effects.—The visceral douche oper- 1089
ates through the sympathetic or vasomotor centers and nerves upon internal associated organs. There are good grounds for believing that in many instances the good effects experienced are the result of a collateral anemia or hyperemia

produced in the affected parts by retrostasis or the opposite action, as the case may be. The active fluxion in internal parts set up by exciting applications of the douche upon the surface is also a powerful factor in the therapeutic results produced by these simple but wonderfully potent procedures.

The *visceral douche* differs from the *localized douche* in that the latter involves but a single circumscribed area, while the former often involves a number of areas, which, though in some instances widely separated anatomically, are intimately associated physiologically through a common relation with the internal viscus which it is desired to influence.

The principal visceral douches may be designated as follows: *Cerebral, cerebrospinal, pulmonary, cardiac, gastric, enteric, hepatic, splenic, renal, genito-urinary.*

In the description of these several forms of douche it will be unnecessary to repeat such details of method as have already been given in connection with the several forms of localized douches; it is sufficient to indicate the surfaces which are to be acted upon, with suggestions respecting the therapeutic indications.

THE CEREBRAL DOUCHE.

1090 The cerebrum is influenced by applications to the head itself, to the back of the neck, the face, the hands, and the soles of the feet. Next to the applications to the head itself, the most powerful impressions may be made by applications to the soles of the feet, the so-called "plantar douche." A *prolonged cold* application to these surfaces produces powerful contraction of the blood-vessels of the brain by reflex action. In applications to the plantar region the thermic effects of extreme cold are supplemented by the percussion effects of water at high pressure. Powerful circulatory reaction is produced in the feet and lower extremities, especially if the application be extended to the feet and legs, thus producing a derivative effect in favor of the brain, in addition to the reflex influence exerted.

Short cold applications to the face, neck, and scalp are quickly followed by reaction, with dilatation of the cerebral vessels, and increased activity of all the cerebral functions. This is also true of general cold applications.

Prolonged cold applications to the reflex surfaces named produce more permanent contraction of the vessels, and secure relief when *cerebral congestion* is present, especially if the applications are renewed every few minutes so as to repeat the reflex effect upon the vessels.

Warm applications to the face, neck, and scalp tend to congest the brain.

Very hot applications, on the other hand, cause temporary contraction, and relieve *congestion.*

Neutral applications (92° to 94°) to the occiput and the back of the neck relieve *cerebral excitability.*

Very cold or *very hot* applications to any portion of the dermal surface produce an exciting effect upon the cerebrum.

THE CEREBROSPINAL DOUCHE.

The purpose of this douche is to influence the whole 1091
cerebrospinal system, and through it the body at large. All the spinal nerves send out branches, which are distributed to the skin covering the back; so that by applications made to the dorsal surface of the trunk, in addition to the applications which have been described under the head of "the cerebral douche," all the cerebrospinal centers may be acted upon. The method consists essentially in that described for the cerebral douche, with the addition of an application to the back. The several steps of the procedure are as follows: —

1. Affusion, or douche without pressure, to the head, as described for the cerebral douche.

2. The application of the douche to the feet for 15 or 20 seconds, at a temperature as low as possible, usually at least as low as 60° to 50° F.

3. The percussion douche to the spine from 20 to 30 seconds, the stream being rapidly moved up and down and across the back in every direction.

4. The broken jet to the dorsum and soles of the feet for 30 to 60 seconds.

The cerebrospinal douche is indicated in cases of neurasthenia with cerebral congestion. Care should be taken to see that the patient's skin is warmed before the application of this douche, so that the internal congestion, including congestion of the brain, which always occurs when the surface is chilled, may be avoided. The electric-light bath, the vapor bath, the hot-air bath, or the warm rain douche (care being taken to protect the head) are all excellent means of heating the skin preparatory to the cerebrospinal douche. In patients who chill easily, the spray douche at 102° to 104° may be applied for 1 minute to the feet and spine, before the cold application to these parts.

The *tepid* or *neutral* cerebrospinal douche is useful in cases of *spinal sclerosis*, *general feebleness*, *sexual dementia*, *exhaustion* from *alcoholism* and other forms of dissipation, as well as in an *enfeebled condition* resulting from loss of sleep and prolonged mental anxiety.

In certain cases, as in *irritable* and *feeble neurasthenics* with *cerebral congestion*, the neutral douche to the back of the neck may be combined with the cold percussion douche to the spine and feet. In cases of *cerebral anemia* associated with chronic nervous exhaustion, the prolonged cold douche to the spine, legs, and feet may be advantageously associated with the warm douche or affusion to the head.

THE PULMONARY DOUCHE.

1092 The pulmonary circulation may be influenced by applications made to any portion of the cutaneous covering of the chest, but especially to the vertebra prominens. Askatchensky showed that a *cold* application to the hands is capable of controlling epistaxis, and the writer has clinically shown that

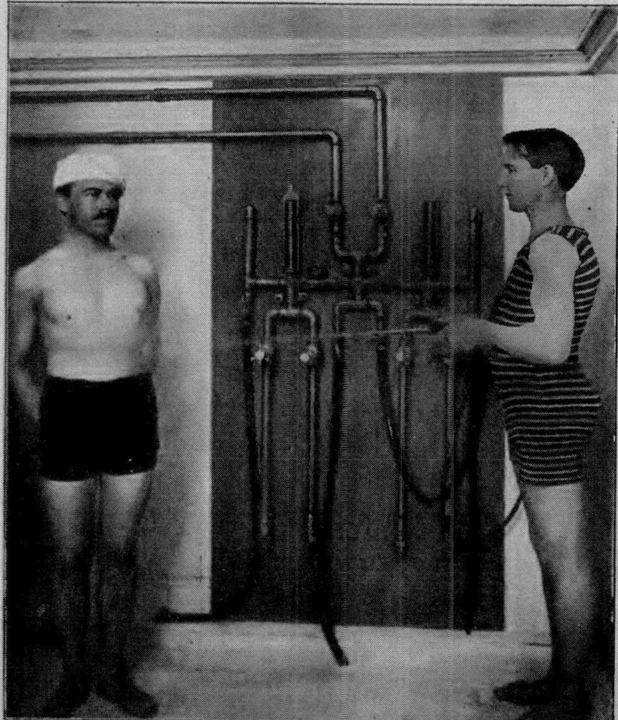

FIG. 54. SPLENIC DOUCHE (p. 511).

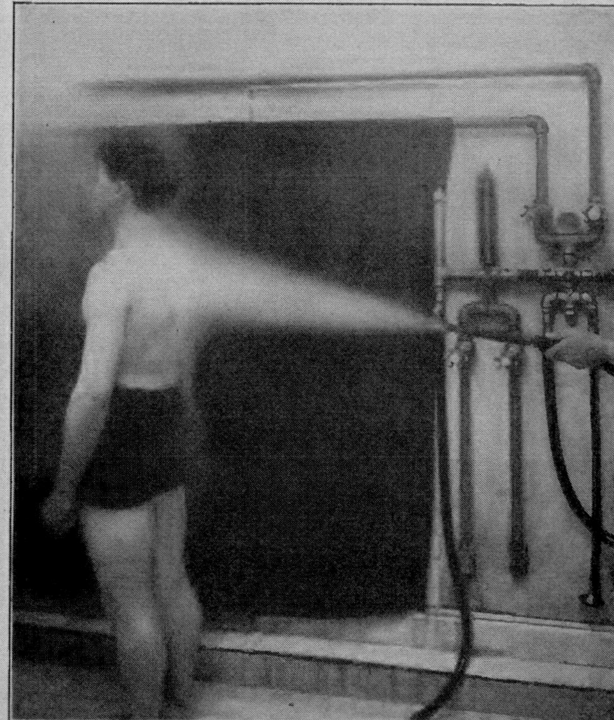

FIG. 57. VAPOR DOUCHE (p. 515).

pulmonary hemorrhage may likewise be favorably influenced by this procedure. That *very cold* applications to the hands and feet, with strong pressure, are also capable of influencing the pulmonary circulation to a marked degree, has been shown by the experiments of Vasilieff. Winternitz has noted a similar relation between the thighs and the lungs. The application should be considerably prolonged, and with little pressure. The procedure in the pulmonary douche should be as follows: —

A rapid percussion douche, or horizontal jet with strong pressure, at 60°, to the arms and shoulders; then the broken jet to the front and sides of the chest; ending with the percussion douche to the back and vertebra prominens; the duration being from 10 to 15 seconds to each part. The *neutral* douche to the back of the chest is of value in cases of asthma, especially if accompanied by the *Scotch* douche to the feet and legs.

The pulmonary douche has a somewhat limited sphere of usefulness, but may be employed in cases which require either quieting or exciting of the respiratory movements. Thus the *hot* pulmonary douche applied to the back may be used with advantage in asthma; while the *cold* douche is equally useful for sedentary neurasthenics who need increased pulmonary activity to supply an increased amount of oxygen and to encourage the portal circulation.

THE CARDIAC DOUCHE.

A *cold* douche, with slight pressure over the heart, first 1093
quickens, then slows, its action, increasing arterial tension. Prolonged application of cold to the hands has the effect to slow and energize the heart. Only the broken or the fan douche should be employed in applications over the heart. The douche is less useful as a local measure for influencing the heart than is the ice-bag or the cold compress.

THE GASTRIC DOUCHE.

The *very hot* douche (115° to 122°) applied over the 1094
epigastrium and the spine opposite often gives relief in

painful affections of the stomach. It has the effect to diminish the secretion of gastric juice; hence is applicable in *chronic gastritis*, *gastric ulcer*, *gastralgia*, *gastrorrhea*, *gastroduodenitis*, *infectious jaundice*, *hyperesthesia* of the *solar plexus*, and especially in *hyperpepsia*.

A *cold* douche applied to the same areas increases the production of HCl, and increases the muscular tone of the stomach. It is of especial service in *apepsia*, *hypopepsia*, *dilatation* of the *stomach*, and *gastric flatulence*.

The *Scotch* douche is in some cases more successful in relieving pain than the hot douche. The hot application should be prolonged to 3 or 4 minutes. The duration of the concluding cold application should not be more than 15 to 20 seconds. The fan or broken jet should be used, and with little pressure.

THE ENTERIC DOUCHE.

1095 The blood-vessels of the muscular walls of the small intestines are powerfully influenced by applications to the umbilical region, the hypogastric region, the lumbar region of the spine, and the feet. A cold douche to these parts powerfully stimulates peristalsis, and increases the tone of the muscular walls. A short application with considerable pressure increases the secretion and vascular activity, while more prolonged applications with little pressure lessen *congestion* when present.

The Scotch douche relieves painful affections, such as *enteralgia*, *colic*, and the pain of *chronic peritonitis*. In applying this douche for *constipation*, the cold application should be made first to the feet, then to the lumbar region, then to the umbilical and hypogastric regions, and lastly another short application to the feet, with strong pressure.

THE HEPATIC DOUCHE (Fig. 53).

1096 Administered with proper care, there is no therapeutic measure which secures better or more definite results than does the hepatic douche. Lying close to the surface, and having an exceedingly vascular structure, the liver may be most profoundly affected by a douche properly administered; but for this reason, great care must be employed in applications of this sort. The douche is applied over the region of the liver; that is, the lower part of the right chest and the epigastrium. The fan douche or the broken jet at a low temperature is employed for excitant effects.

To relieve *congestion*, the application should be cold and with moderate pressure (65° to 75°, 15 to 20 lbs, 5 to 10 min.); and the internal reaction should be suppressed by a general douche to the whole surface immediately following the hepatic douche, or by some other of the several means elsewhere described. If considerable pain is present, the general douche may be employed first, the local application following immediately. In cases of *chronic enlargement* of the *liver*, the alternate douche should be employed. In *acute congestion* of the *liver* accompanied by pain, the tepid douche should be used. In cases of extreme *pain*, as in *gall-stones*, *infectious jaundice*, and *inflammation* of the *liver*, the Scotch douche is indicated. The hepatic douche is of especial value in the disorders of the liver encountered in hot countries, particularly those resulting from malarial infection.

THE SPLENIC DOUCHE (Fig. 54).

By means of the fan douche or the broken jet an applica- 1097
tion of cold water of moderate pressure is made over the lower portion of the left chest, the cutaneous surface overlying the spleen.

The cold or alternate douche constitutes the most effective of all means for combating an enlarged spleen, especially in cases in which the hypertrophy is due to chronic malarial infection. Not infrequently, a considerable degree of diminution in the size of the spleen may be recognized immediately after an application of this sort. In general, the observations made in reference to the hepatic douche apply equally well to the splenic douche.

If pain or tenderness is present, the *very hot* or *Scotch* douche should be employed. In the administration of the splenic douche, short applications should be made to the feet both before and after the application to the spleen. In cases in which the general cold douche can be tolerated, it is well to make such an application in connection with the splenic or hepatic douche; but in cases of congestion of these organs care should be taken to make a short cold local application first, so as to avoid an increase of the congestion by the inrush of blood produced by the general application.

THE RENAL DOUCHE.

1098 The kidneys are influenced by the douche to the lumbar region, as also to the cutaneous surface covering the lower third of the sternum. The interesting fact that the sternal area is reflexly connected with the kidneys, was first pointed out by Beni-Barde, of Paris. Prolonged *cold* applications with little pressure to these areas produce contraction of the vessels of the kidneys, especially influencing the small vessels of the parenchyma of the organ, thus increasing the pressure in the glomerules, and so favoring the outflow of urine. This interesting explanation of the action of the cold douche upon the kidney was first offered by Bottey, and makes clear how the urinary excretion is increased by the action of the cold douche, while at the same time congestion is relieved. The renal douche is especially serviceable in the treatment of *renal congestion*, which is frequently associated with *chronic alcoholism* and *malarial infection.* It also serves a useful purpose in *diabetes* and in some cases of *Bright's disease;* but when albumin is present in the urine, the *Scotch* douche should be substituted for the cold application.

In *painful affections* of the *kidneys*, as in *pain* due to *movable* or *floating kidney*, *hydronephrosis*, *neuralgia*, and *renal calculus*, the *very hot* douche or the *Scotch* douche applied to the lumbar region is indicated.

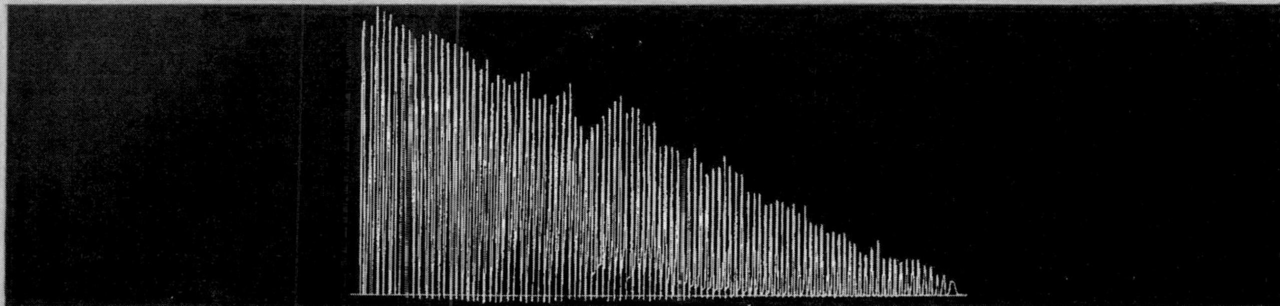

Fig. 55. Normal Fatigue Curve of Man Aged Twenty-four Years. Total work, 6.703 kgm. (p. 514).

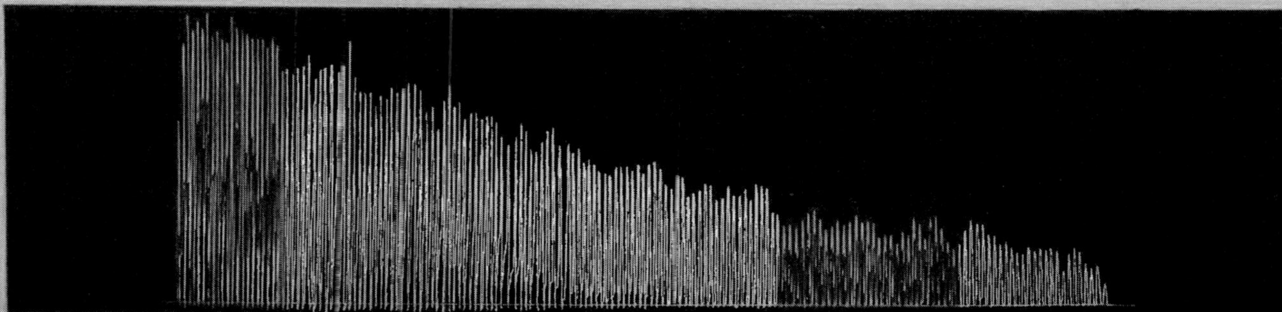

Fig. 56. Fatigue Curve of the Same Subject after a Cold Douche. Total work, 9.805 kgm. (p. 514).

THE GENITO-URINARY DOUCHE.

The uterus, the ovaries, and the bladder in women, and 1099
the prostate, the bladder, and the testicles in men, are powerfully influenced by the application of heat to the lumbo-sacral and hypogastric regions, and to the inner surfaces of the thighs in both sexes, and to the breasts in women. There is also marked evidence of a close relationship between the feet and the pelvic viscera. In the application of the genito-urinary douche the stream of water is allowed to fall first upon the feet, then upon the lumbar region, then upon the inside of the thighs, and finally upon the breasts and hypogastrium. Strong pressure may be used in applications to the lumbar region and the feet, but the broken jet or the fan jet only should be applied to the breasts and the hypogastrium, and with little pressure.

The *short cold* genito-urinary douche is applicable in cases of *amenorrhea*, *relaxed abdominal muscles* and *uterine deviations*, *subinvolutions*, *seminal weakness* in men, especially the form known as *diurnal emissions*, *enlarged prostate* in men, and *atony* of the *bladder* in both sexes. The cold douche should never be employed in painful or spasmodic affections of the pelvic viscera. In the last-named disorders, such as *vesical tenesmus*, *vaginismus*, and *coccygodynia*, *ovarian neuralgia*, *uterine neuralgia*, and, in men, *neuralgia of the testicles* and *spermatic cord*, the *very hot* or the *Scotch* douche may be employed with advantage.

THE ARTICULAR DOUCHE.

This douche and the one following differ from others of 1100
this class only in the fact that the internal parts concerned are outside the abdominal cavity. The fan, the broken jet, or the spray may be employed with advantage in many affections of the joint, though in painful affections of this kind the *Scotch* douche is preferable. The *prolonged cold* douche with little pressure may be used to advantage for antiphlogistic effects in cases in which heat or swelling are present.

The position of the patient while receiving the application may be either sitting or standing, whichever will render the affected part most easily accessible. By producing hyperemia of the skin by means of the hot douche, collateral anemia of the joint may be produced in conditions of congestion and inflammation. On the other hand, when it is desirable to congest the joint as a therapeutic measure, an anemic condition may be readily produced by a prolonged cold application to the knee with little pressure.

Therapeutic Applications.— In chronic affections in which exudates exist, with limitation of movement, absorption may be promoted by the *alternate* douche. Extreme temperatures and as high pressure as can be conveniently borne must be employed. The alternate douche is of course contraindicated by local pain or tenderness. The *short, very cold* douche produces powerful alterative effects, and is of value in cases in which the joint structures are relaxed.

THE MUSCLE DOUCHE.

1101 By means of the douche at different temperatures applied to the skin overlying a muscle or group of muscles, almost absolute control may be exercised over the circulation and functions of the part. This control depends upon the principles of fluxion considered elsewhere (698). The douche may accordingly be utilized with advantage in most affections of the muscles. When *inflammation* exists, the prolonged *cool* douche with little pressure may be employed at intervals of two or three hours, or until the acute stage is past; later, for the relief of pain, the *Scotch* douche may be used. For relieving the pain of *muscular rheumatism*, the Scotch douche or the *hot* douche may be advantageously utilized, also in painful conditions of the muscles accompanying so-called *muscular strain*, and in the condition known as *secondary fatigue.*

The *cold* douche applied over a muscle wonderfully increases its working capacity, as shown by the tracings easily obtainable with Mosso's ergograph (Figs. 55, 56). This effect is produced, however, only with the short cold douche at high pressure (50° to 65°, 3 to 6 secs., 25 to 40 lbs.). The prolonged douche at low temperature, without pressure, is capable of completely annihilating muscular excitability. The *hot* douche and the *Scotch* douche diminish muscular excitability, and render valuable service in the treatment of contractures and muscular spasm, as well as in painful conditions of the muscle.

THE VAPOR DOUCHE.

This douche (Fig. 57) consists of a jet of steam projected 1102
upon the patient in a manner precisely analogous to that in which water is employed in the horizontal jet douche. The apparatus should be so constructed that hot water can never be ejected from the nozzle, and the controlling valve so arranged that the maximum amount of steam admitted to the nozzle shall not be sufficient to carry an injurious amount of heat to a distance of more than a few inches from the nozzle. The temperature of the application may be perfectly regulated by the distance at which the nozzle is held from the surface of the body.

The advantage of the vapor douche is that it produces the most powerful thermic effects with practically no percutient effects, which renders it extremely useful as a means of producing revulsion in cases of neuralgia, as in *sciatica*, *lumbago*, *spinal neuralgia*, and also in cases of *painful joints*, *muscular* and *articular rheumatism*, and joints affected by *fibrous ankylosis* and *local* or *general hyperesthesia*. A most excellent revulsive measure consists in alternate applications of the vapor douche in connection with the cold percussion douche. The vapor douche is one of the most effective means of heating the skin preparatory to or in connection with a cold rain douche or a horizontal jet.

THE AFFUSION, PAIL DOUCHE, OR POURING BATH.

This bath (Fig. 58) resembles the douche in that the 1103
water falls upon the body in a stream. It at the same time

resembles the immersion bath in that the water is simultaneously applied to a large portion of the entire surface, and with very slight mechanical effect. As a pail is often used in administering this bath, it is frequently called the "pail pour." Like the douche, the application may involve the whole or any portion of the surface.

Method.—The requisites are, a tub, which may be an ordinary wash-tub if the patient is able to stand, or if it is preferable to sit, a full-bath tub. If the patient is unable either to sit or to stand, he may lie upon his face on a cot or stretcher, over which a large piece of rubber has been spread. The head of the cot should be so raised that the water will run off its lower end into a tub properly placed for the purpose.

Several pails of water (three to ten) should be conveniently placed for use; a wet towel for the head, a Turkish towel, and a large linen or Turkish sheet are also required. The temperature of the water employed may vary from 50° or 60° to 105° or 110°, according to the effect desired. The application may extend to the whole body or to a portion only. When employed as a general application, the sitting position in a full-bath tub is usually to be preferred.

Before the bath the patient's head, face, and neck should be thoroughly cooled with water a few degrees lower than that to be employed in the affusion. A towel wet in very cold water is then wrapped about his head; he seats himself, with legs extended, in an empty full-bath tub with the plug left out; the requisite number of pails of water are then quickly poured over him. The water should not be simply poured upon the patient, but should be dashed upon him from as great a height and distance as arrangements will permit. The attendant, grasping the pail to be emptied upon the patient, gives it a little swing backward, then tilts it in such a way as to empty its contents upon the patient as the pail swings forward and upward (Fig. 58). The patient sits with his hands folded over his chest in such a manner as to protect the precordial region. The first pailful of water is thrown upon the folded hands; the

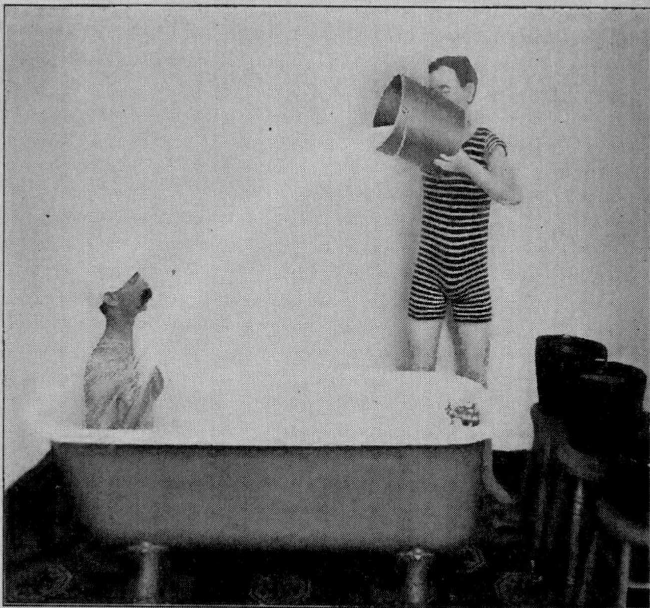

FIG. 58. AFFUSION (p. 515).

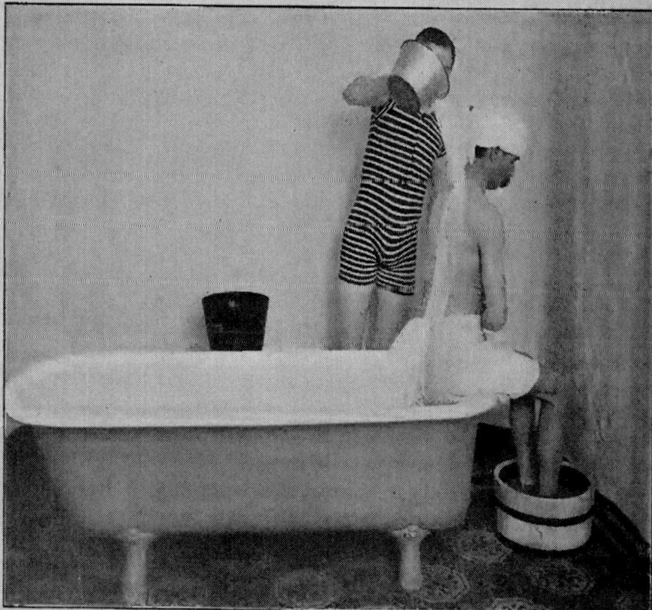

FIG. 59. LOCAL AFFUSION (p. 517).

next is dashed upon the upper part of the back. The front and back of the body are thus treated in alternation until the required number of pails of water have been employed. After the last pail is emptied, the attendant vigorously rubs the trunk and limbs of the patient for 20 to 30 seconds, then removes him from the bath, wraps the sheet about him, and rubs him dry. Special attention should be given by the attendant to the back, legs, and feet, while the patient, if able, is rubbing the arms and the anterior portions of the trunk.

Local affusions are made to the spine, head, extremities, and other parts. When it is desired to confine the application to the spine, the patient sits on the edge of a bath-tub while the water is allowed to flow from as great a height as the pail can be held by the attendant, down the whole length of the spine.

When the application is to be made to the arm, leg, or foot, the part is simply held over the bath-tub and the water poured over it from the desired height. The quantity of water employed, the temperature, the duration of the application, and the size of the stream must be regulated to suit the patient and the conditions present. Numerous effects may be obtained by variation of the several factors named (Fig. 59).

In patients who dread the contact of cold water, and in whom reaction does not readily occur, the feet may be immersed in water as hot as can be borne. If too feeble to stand, the patient may sit in a chair while affusion is applied, or in case of great feebleness, he may lie in a horizontal position upon a cot covered with rubber cloth, so arranged that the water will run off at the bottom, being caught in a tub or some other proper vessel.

In the treatment of chronic cases it is best to prepare the patient for this bath by heating the skin by means of fomentations or hot bags to the spine and limbs, while his body is wrapped in warm blankets, or by the vapor bath, the electric-light bath, the wet sheet, the hot-blanket pack, the hot bath, and other appropriate means.

The author has had constructed a pail, shown in the accompanying cut (Fig. 60), which has been found very convenient for the administration of this bath. When the water is poured from one side of this pail, a broad, thin stream is obtained; when poured from the opposite side, it flows in a solid column somewhat smaller than the arm.

The affusion may be employed as a substitute for the douche when the latter is not available. It may also be combined with various other baths, as the Brand bath (**712**), the dripping sheet (**1216**), and as a cooling process after hot baths.

Physiological Effects.—The French divide baths into two classes, according to whether the water employed is in motion or quiescent. Affusion is the simplest form of the bath in which the water employed is in motion, and may be regarded as a sort of transition from the full or immersion bath to the douche, the favorite hydriatic procedure of the French hydrotherapeutists.

Both the thermic and the circulatory reactions are very pronounced as the result of an affusion bath at a temperature of 55° to 75°, and as a result, the evidences of tissue change are marked.

The effects upon a healthy person are chiefly the following: Cardiac and pulmonary excitation, with an increase of CO_2 excretion; slowing of the pulse and increase of arterial tension; increase in the amount of cutaneous excretion; increased assimilation of albumin; improved oxidation of nitrogenous wastes; slight lowering of the temperature. The circulatory effects of the cold affusion are essentially the same as those of the douche, except that they are less pronounced, as the mechanical effect is less.

The *hot* affusion is at first powerfully exciting, but is quickly followed by atonic reaction. The *neutral* affusion, if so managed as to secure as little mechanical effects as possible, is quieting or sedative. The *prolonged* local *cool* affusion (15 to 60 min.) is a measure of value in combating subacute inflammation in large joints, through its powerfully sedative effects. The temperature should be 70° to 80°. This application has the advantage over the cold compress in that the temperature of the application is constant, so that reaction is altogether suppressed, and thus the desired sedative effects are more quickly and decidedly developed.

The *neutral* pour to the spine is a powerful sedative to the nervous system. It is highly useful in cases of locomotor ataxia accompanied by lightning pains, or when the disease is making rapid advancement. The *hot* local pour is powerfully revulsive. The local alternate pour is a strongly excitant measure, and may be employed in such a way as to produce the most powerful revulsive effects.

Therapeutic Applications.—This is one of the oldest of 1104
hydriatic procedures. It was employed by Hippocrates in the treatment of *syncope*, *puerperal fever*, *delirium*, and in *swollen joints*, as well as in other affections, and at different temperatures.

Sir John Chardin, the noted English traveler, found it in use for fevers in Persia in the seventeenth century; and it is said to be still a custom in Persia to keep pails of cold water standing upon the street corners during a cholera epidemic. The natives so thoroughly understand the use of water in these cases that when a man falls with cholera, the cold water is immediately poured over him by the bystanders, who afterward rub him vigorously until thorough reaction is produced.

This hydriatric procedure was introduced to the medical profession of England by Dr. Wright more than one hundred years ago. Dr. James Currie, of Liverpool, became acquainted with Dr. Wright's practice, and introduced it into the infirmary of which he had charge, where he made a careful study of its physiological and therapeutic effects. It may be said, in fact, that scientific hydrotherapy began with the study of this bath by Currie, who made careful use of the thermometer for the purpose both of regulating the temperature of the water employed and of determining its effect upon the patient.

Currie proved that the affusion bath is a most excellent means of reducing the temperature in fevers. He also observed, as recorded in his "Medical Reports,"[1] that a tepid affusion is more effective in reducing temperature than a very cold application. Some modern writers who have called attention to this same effect seem not to be aware of this observation by Currie, though all who have had any considerable amount of experience in the use of water in fever, must have noted, as did Currie, that the temperature not infrequently rises after a short cold bath to a point higher than before the bath.

Currie was also the first scientific physician to call attention to the great value of affusion as a means of combating the morbid process in infectious fevers. He noted that the most important effect produced by the application was its tonic influence, whereby the vital resistance of the patient may be increased.

1105 General affusion is of very great value, especially in fever cases in which pulmonary or cerebral congestion or cardiac weakness is a prominent symptom. Applied to the whole surface of the body, and especially to the chest and shoulders, cold affusion furnishes a powerful means of stimulating the nervous mechanism of the heart, and may well replace the drugs recommended for this purpose. Similar effects may be produced by heat and cold to the spine, and by cold wet rubbing, as elsewhere described; but the effects thus produced are less vigorous than those of the affusion bath. Affusion is an essential feature of the Brand bath, water at a lower temperature than the water of the bath being poured upon the back of the patient's head at intervals during the bath (**712**). Employed in this way, it lessens the delirium, and greatly improves the heart's action in continuous fevers.

The stimulation of the respiratory movements induced by the pouring of cold water over the chest is a most powerful

[1] Currie, "Medical Reports," page 64.

means of combating the tendency to *hypostatic congestion*, a very grave complication in fevers of severe type. In the management of low fevers, affusion may be employed in conditions of *depression* in which the prolonged cold bath would seem to be contraindicated. In cases of this sort, the patient should be prepared for the bath by a hot-blanket pack, a fomentation to the back, or by the application of heat in a tub of water at 100° to 102° for 2 or 3 minutes, until the skin is warm, when he may be removed from the warm bath, and cold water poured upon the head and shoulders.

In *capillary bronchitis* in children, when the air-passages are clogged with mucus and the respiratory centers so overwhelmed by the retained CO_2 that there is insufficient power to expel the accumulation, cold affusion to the chest, by stimulating the respiratory center, and thus provoking powerful breathing movements, renders valuable service.

In the case of young children suffering from *capillary bronchitis* or *broncho-pneumonia*, the patient may be seated in a tub partially filled with water at 102°, and cold water poured over the chest and shoulders. After two or three pailfuls of water have been thus poured upon the patient, a Turkish sheet and warm blankets should be quickly wrapped about him; he should be thoroughly dried, and the surface circulation stimulated by rubbing.

The combined hot full bath and cold affusion may be used in the various forms of *collapse* as well as in *prolonged* cases of *fever* in which the skin is cyanotic. The last-named measure is of great service in the treatment of *cerebrospinal meningitis*. The patient should be placed in a hot full bath at 100°, and while in the bath very cold water may be poured over the head, hot water being added to the bath as required to maintain the temperature.

Cold affusion is one of the most efficient means of combating the cardiac and general vascular depression present in alcoholism. Nothing will more quickly arouse the patient from a drunken stupor than affusion with a half dozen buckets of water at 60°. This application should not be made without a preceding hot application if the skin is cold or the temperature subnormal, and must be followed by rubbing and other means necessary to secure complete reaction.

A *very short hot* affusion following a cold bath has been shown to increase its antipyretic effect by atonic reaction, whereby heat production is diminished.

Affusion, preceded, when possible, by a short hot application, is one of the most powerful of all means for rallying the vital forces in case of *collapse*, *surgical shock*, *asphyxia*, and even in *drowning*. It should be noted, however, that the skin is often quite cold in cases of this sort, and that the cold application must be at a temperature considerably below that of the skin, in order that the revulsive effect may be produced.

In cases in which the elevation of the body temperature is due to some local infection, the *tepid* affusion is to be preferred, as also in other febrile cases in which the patient is very young or very feeble.

Currie's greatest successes with the use of the cold affusion were in the treatment of *scarlet* and *typhus fevers;* but this measure is equally effective in chronic as in acute affections. In private practice it may take the place of the douche, which requires a special apparatus and a hydriatic establishment for its successful administration.

1106 **Contraindications.**—Cold affusion must be avoided in cases of *cardiac disease* with *degeneration* of the *heart muscle*, in *asthma*, in *hemorrhagic* cases of tuberculosis, and in cases of *typhoid fever* complicated with *myocarditis*, *acute nephritis*, *intestinal perforation*, *peritonitis*, and in *hemorrhages* from *uterine fibroids*. It need not be avoided in cases of typhoid fever in which slow hemorrhage occurs from congestion, but the patient must be managed carefully in such cases.

THE IMMERSION BATH.

1107 This bath (see also **712**) presents itself in the different forms of the full bath, the plunge bath, and the swimming or surf bath in fresh or salt water. Bathing in natural sources, as in the sea and in fresh water lakes and rivers, is a most healthful exercise and a powerful prophylactic, and may be employed with advantage by semi-invalids, although this form of bathing can not be controlled with the accuracy necessary to secure definite and reliable therapeutic results.

THE COLD PLUNGE.

This bath (Fig. 61) requires a water-tight tank to which 1108
water of a proper temperature is regularly supplied. The depth is ordinarily about five feet. The temperature is varied in different establishments from 48° to 68°.

Method.—The plunge bath should never be entered when the skin is cold or a chilly sensation is present. The body should be well warmed before the bath is entered, either by a hot bath of some kind, or by the accumulation of heat in the wet-sheet pack, the dry pack, or by exercise. The head, face, and neck should be thoroughly bathed with very cold water before the bath is entered.

It is best to enter the bath suddenly, as the sensation of cold is thus far less noticeable than when the bath is entered gradually. The duration of the bath may vary from 2 or 3 seconds to 1 or 2 minutes.

The patient should rub himself vigorously while in the bath; or if the space is sufficient, should exercise by swimming movements. Successive dipping under the water is also advantageous, the head and shoulders being completely immersed each time.

As soon as the patient emerges from a bath, he should be wrapped in a Turkish sheet and vigorously rubbed by two attendants, himself assisting. When dry, he should dress at once, and exercise moderately for half an hour, or if too feeble to do this, massage or manual Swedish movements should be administered to insure good reaction.

In taking the cold plunge bath, as in other forms of the cold immersion bath, the patient should leave the bath during the first reaction, that is, while the surface circulation is good and the sensation of warmth pervades the skin, and before chilly sensations have begun to be experienced. If he remains until the secondary chill occurs and the skin begins to assume a bluish appearance, thermic reaction is almost certain to be excessive, often resulting in fainting and subsequent intense congestion, with headache, visceral pain, and possibly inflammation of internal parts.

The effects of the plunge bath are most excellent if good reaction is secured, but highly depressing when reaction does not occur. Headache, malaise, nervousness, and depression are indications of defective reaction or an excessive application; that is, too long a time spent in the bath.

1109 **Physiological Effects.**—The plunge bath is a powerfully exciting and alterative measure; the whole surface of the body being suddenly brought into contact with water at a low temperature, a most profound impression is made upon the central nervous system. The heart and the circulation are also powerfully influenced. The sudden inrush of blood from the surface causes an intense congestion of all the internal viscera, a fact which should never be forgotten, as it renders this bath inapplicable in quite a large number of cases.

The effect of the bath is at first a slight elevation of the internal temperature in consequence of the sudden checking of heat elimination. After reaction occurs, there is a slight falling of the temperature, but respiration, heart action, and all the vital functions are quickened by the profound nervous impression made. The blood pressure is raised, the circulation of the brain is stimulated, respiratory movements produce vigorous fluxion of the blood and lymph through the cerebrum, so that the mind, if previously clouded, becomes clear, and all the intellectual functions are facilitated. The sudden contact of cold water with the general surface likewise stimulates the action of the kidneys and the liver, excites peristalsis, causes contraction of the hollow viscera, and arouses all

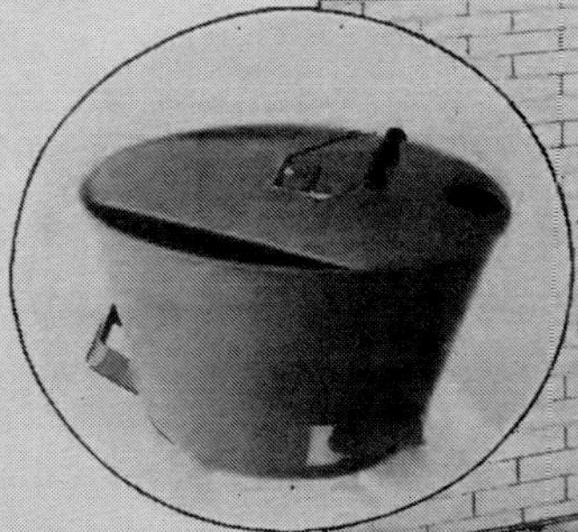

Fig. 60. AFFUSION PAIL (p. 518).

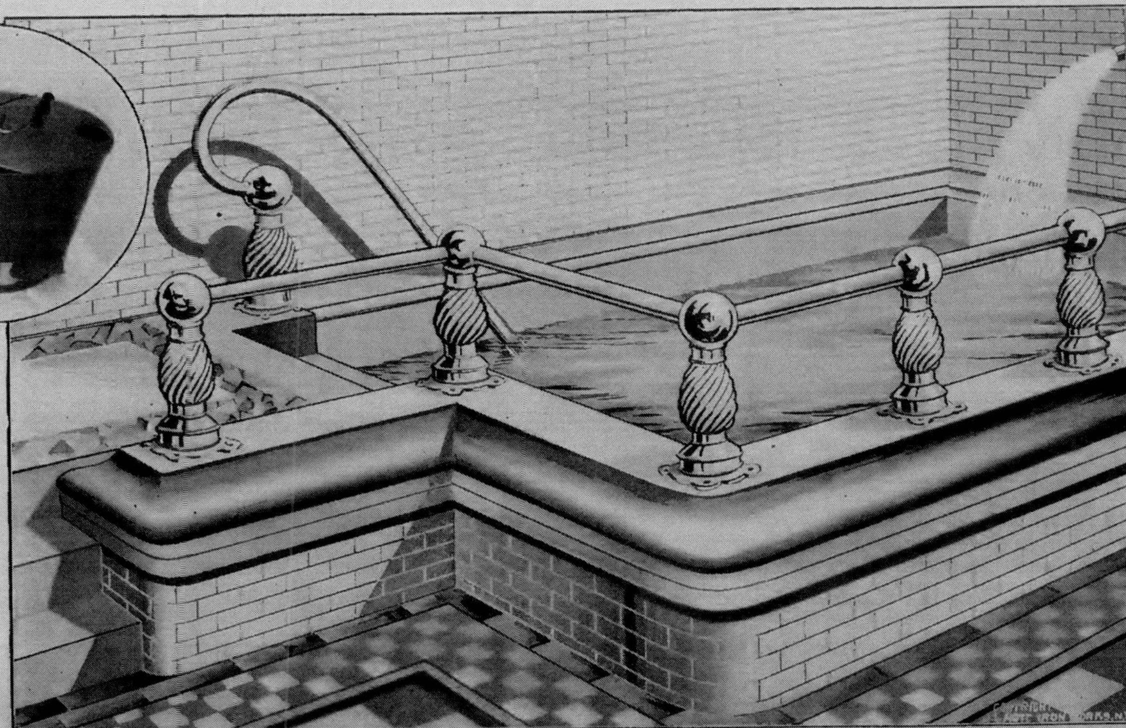

Fig. 61. PLUNGE BATH (p. 523).

the vital functions. Indeed, the cold plunge produces a more powerful thermic reaction than any other form of bath.

Therapeutic Applications.—The cold immersion bath is 1110
especially indicated in cases requiring powerful stimulation of metabolism, and especially in the class of cases designated by Bouchard under the general term "slowed nutrition," in diabetes without emaciation, in obesity, and for persons in ordinary health, requiring simply vigorous recuperative measures to repair the damages arising from sedentary employment and lack of exercise. The plunge bath is useful in cases in which the cold douche can not be employed in consequence of its percutient effects. It is a much more vigorous application than the half bath, producing very powerful refrigerant effects, with correspondingly strong thermic reaction and metabolic changes. It may be properly used after any sweating procedure, as the sweating pack, the electric-light bath, the vapor, the Turkish, the Russian, the hot air, the hot immersion, and other similar procedures. In the Turkish bath establishments of Constantinople and Cairo, visited by the writer, there are tanks of hot water in which the patients immerse themselves, or sit upon the edge with the legs immersed, laving the water upon their bodies. Some European establishments provide a hot plunge in addition to the cold, but it is very little used. The cold plunge bath, being a most vigorous procedure, should not be prescribed without a full knowledge of the patient's condition.

Contraindications.—The routine use of the plunge bath so 1111
common in connection with Turkish bath establishments is highly dangerous. Many persons can not take the plunge bath without running the risk of serious injury. The short cold plunge should be avoided in all cases in which there is an elevation of temperature, as the bath has a decided tendency to produce temperature elevation, the body temperature being sometimes found one or two degrees above normal several hours after the bath, owing to the great increase of heat production resulting from the thermic reaction.

This bath is contraindicated in pernicious anemia, anterior sclerosis, cardiac weakness, great exhaustion from either physical or mental labor, loss of sleep, great emaciation, Bright's disease with albumin in the urine, and in diabetes with rapid loss of flesh. It is also dangerous for persons having a tendency to pulmonary hemorrhage, or hemorrhage of the stomach, as in gastric ulcer and hepatic sclerosis.

THE FULL OR IMMERSION BATH.

1112 This bath (Fig. 62) was first scientifically studied by Currie, who recommended the cold immersion bath as a means of prolonging the effects obtained by cold affusion, and especially as a measure to be applied in intermittent fevers as soon as the second or hot stage is developed, asserting that "the judicious and resolute application of cold might supercede all other remedies in fevers of this class." *

Method.—The full bath is administered in an ordinary bath-tub, which may be made of wood, copper, zinc, porcelain, or enameled iron; or a bath-tub may be improvised in a number of ways. Portable tubs convenient for dwellings not provided with plumbing may be easily constructed. The first requisite is a frame of wood resembling in shape the top of an ordinary bath-tub. To this support, rubber sheeting is attached in such a way that when the ends of the frame are placed on chairs or other supports, the sagging sheeting just touches the floor (Fig. 63). Water may be conducted into the tub by means of a rubber hose attached to the water faucet. Well-oiled or painted ducking may be used in place of the rubber sheeting.

Perhaps, on the whole, the cheapest way, when it is necessary to improvise a tub, is to make one of ordinary lumber —whitewood, basswood, or pine boards, an inch and a half thick, and planed smooth on both sides. The tub should be about six feet in length, two feet in width, and a foot and a half in depth. The cracks may be caulked with oakum.

*Currie's "Medical Reports."

Such a tub can be made by a good carpenter in a few hours, and if kept well painted inside, may be used for a long time. When necessary for use for a fever case, the tub may be placed near the bed and filled with water. The temperature of the water may be regulated by adding either hot or cold water as needed. The prolonged cold bath will require the addition of ice or very cold water. The temperature of the hot bath, that is, a bath above the temperature of the body, may be readily maintained by the addition, from time to time, of jugs or bottles filled with boiling water, which does away with the necessity of so much dipping out and in of water. The patient's head while in the bath should be supported by an air pillow, or other suitable means.

For an alkaline full bath, add a half ounce of salsoda for each gallon of water.

Full baths may be conveniently classified according to their **1113**
temperature as ***cold*, *neutral*, *hot*, *graduated***, and ***alternate*.**

THE COOL OR COLD FULL BATH.

The temperature of this bath may be from 50° to 75°; **1114**
duration, 4 seconds to 20 minutes. Before entering the bath the patient's head, neck, and chest should be well wet with water at a temperature ten or twelve degrees below that of the bath, the head while in the bath being protected by a towel wet in very cold water. The bath should be entered as suddenly as possible, so as to generalize the impression made. Vigorous rubbing by the patient himself or by one or more attendants should be applied during the entire duration of the bath.

As in the case of the plunge bath, the patient should leave the bath during the first reaction, and should never remain until the second rigor occurs.

Currie's method of administering the cold bath was quite unique. The temperatures employed ranged from 54° to 59°. The patient was placed on a sheet, with which, by the aid of several attendants, he was lowered into the bath and allowed to remain for five seconds, then lifted out until reaction began, as shown by slight reddening of the skin, then dipped again, the operation being repeated from three to five times. After the last dip he was rubbed vigorously. Currie found this method especially successful in the treatment of infectious fevers, for which purpose he considered it a specific more than a century ago (1797). It is evident, however, that the beneficial effects he obtained from this bath could not to any considerable degree be attributed to the temperature reduction, but must have been derived from the stimulating influence of the application upon the general vital processes, whereby the vital resistance of the patient was increased.

It is interesting to note that Currie was familiar with the fact that the cold bath gives rise to an elevation of the temperature,* when of short duration (1 to 5 min.). This elevation of temperature is especially marked when the friction, which should always be applied during the bath, has been omitted.

When the bath is prolonged beyond a mere dip in cold water, it is a good plan for the patient to sit up in the tub, rubbing his chest, legs, sides, and arms, dipping his hands constantly in the water, and every three to five seconds leaning backward until the body is immersed to the neck.

1115 **Physiological Effects.**—The effects of this form of immersion upon a healthy person are essentially the same as those of the cold plunge bath, but a little less intense. The thermic reaction after the cold full bath is greater than after any other bath. The temperature curve shows first a depression amounting to one or two degrees, continuing for two or three hours after the bath, but finally followed by a return to normal, or even an elevation of a degree or more. The temperature rise may be followed by sweating, as after a malarial chill and fever. By a frequent repetition of the cold bath a veritable hydropathic fever may be induced.

---

*Currie, "Medical Reports," page 154.

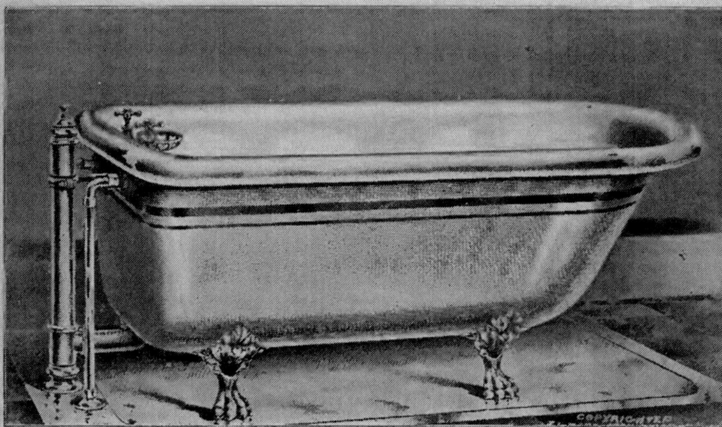

FIG. 62. IMMERSION BATH TUB (p. 526).

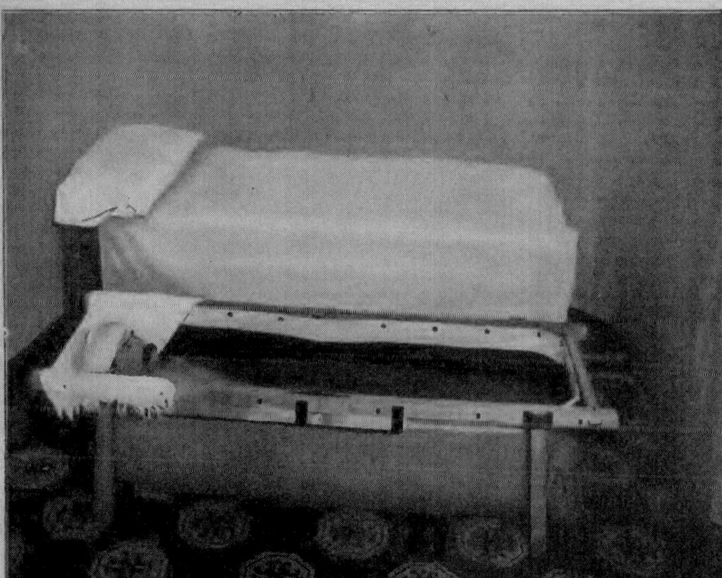

FIG. 63. IMPROVISED IMMERSION BATH (p. 526).

According to Maggiori and Vinaj* the cold immersion bath nearly doubled the muscular capacity of the middle finger of the left hand, while the neutral bath produced no effect at all, and the warm bath at 104° for 6 minutes decreased the work from 5,000 to 900 kilogrammeters (Exp. 58).

The perturbing and alterative effects of the cold immersion bath are greater than those of the douche and half-bath, for the reason that the system is left almost wholly to its own resources to produce reaction; hence this bath is unsuited for very feeble patients, or those whose reactive powers are not vigorous. The immersion bath is less valuable as a tonic than baths in which the application is accompanied by mechanical movements, as friction or percussion; but that it powerfully stimulates metabolism is shown by the observation of Lepine,† who found that the immersion of a fasting dog for 15 minutes in water at 40° more than doubled the amount of urea.

Therapeutic Applications.—The immersion bath may be 1116
used in cases in which the plunge bath is not readily accessible. It is also admissible in cases in which the plunge bath can not be safely employed on account of its excessively exciting effects, as with certain neurasthenics, or when the patient is too feeble to take the plunge bath because of inability to assist himself to the extent necessary. The prolonged cold full bath not accompanied by friction is one of the most depressing of all hydriatic procedures, and is seldom indicated. When a general cold application is required, the wet-sheet pack, the shallow bath, the douche, or some other form of bath in which the mechanical effects of friction or percussion are added to the powerful thermic effects of the cold as an aid to reaction, will, with but very rare exceptions, be found preferable.

The cold bath was once used as an antipyretic measure,

* *Blätter für Klin. Med.*

† *L' Union Médicale*, 29, 1880, p. 722.

but has long since been abandoned in favor of the so-called "Brand bath," to be described later, which is generally meant whenever the term "cold bath" is employed in current medical literature as used in connection with the treatment of febrile disorders. That the cold bath may render valuable service in the treatment of fevers has been abundantly proved by clinical experience; and it is not necessary to appeal to modern statistics to find proof of the marvelous efficiency of the cold bath in the treatment of febrile maladies. Currie describes an epidemic of typhus which occurred at the military prison located at Stapleton, England,* where a large number of French prisoners were confined. There were, in all, 815 cases. All were treated by the cold affusion, with a result of only forty-one deaths, a little less than five per cent., which for typhus fever is certainly an unusually fortunate record. The mortality was almost wholly confined to persons who were debilitated by age, dissipation, or exposure. We find no equally favorable statistics in the record of modern military practice. The usual enormously high mortality, in the light of present knowledge, would certainly seem to indicate an unnecessary waste of human life.

The cold full bath is indicated, and may be most appropriately employed, in cases of obesity without marked cardiac degeneration, and in cases of slowed nutrition when the general strength is fair. It creates an appetite and improves the digestion in appropriate cases, but is so much inferior to other hydric procedures equally useful for the same purpose that it is seldom used.

Employed as a means of cooling after a vigorous heating procedure, it may render excellent service.

The cold full bath is a useful measure as a means of toning the skin after a prolonged hot bath, and may be advantageously employed in some cases in alternation with the hot immersion bath as a means of exciting the sympathetic centers and encouraging the production of hydrochloric acid in cases of hypopepsia. For persons enjoying fairly good health, a dip

* Currie, "Medical Reports," 4th edition, p. 388.

into a tub full of cold water is an excellent morning bath. It creates an appetite, accelerates the circulation, arouses the nervous system, and produces decidedly exhilarating effects in those who have become accustomed to its use. When employed for this purpose, the duration of the immersion should not be more than 3 to 15 seconds. The patient should rub himself vigorously while in the bath, and should dry himself quickly and thoroughly afterward. He should then take moderately active exercise for 15 to 20 minutes, such as walking, or general exercises in the gymnasium. The daily use of the cold immersion bath in the manner suggested is one of the most effective means of fortifying the system against disease, both acute and chronic.

Contraindications.—These are essentially the same as 1117
for the plunge bath, though the cold full bath may often be tolerated when the cold plunge would be inadmissible. It is contraindicated for young children and very aged persons. The cold full bath should be avoided during gestation and in febrile conditions due to acute inflammation of some internal organ, as in acute peritonitis or gastritis, enteritis, inflammatory conditions of the uterus or ovaries, and other visceral inflammations.

Another morbid condition which should have mention as a contraindication to the cold bath, is hematuria. This condition, when present, indicates disease of either the bladder or one or both kidneys, a condition likely to be enormously increased, perhaps to a dangerous stage, by the retrostasis necessarily resulting from the cold bath. The short hot bath, followed by cold friction, wet-sheet rubbing, and the cold compress, exchanged at intervals of an hour or two for fomentations to the loins, are suitable measures for cases of this sort.

The Cold Full Bath as a Hygienic Measure.

The cold full bath may be advantageously em- 1118
ployed as a measure of hygienic routine by persons of fairly robust constitution. The author does not recommend plunging into rivers and lakes in the winter-time through a hole in the ice, a practice highly lauded by certain writers, and under-

taken by many to their sorrow, a quarter of a century ago. Such a measure is dangerous and quite unnecessarily heroic, as all the good effects obtainable from the cold bath may be secured by its use in a more rational and convenient way.

A good method of employing the cold bath as a morning tonic is this: Fill the tub sufficiently full of water to allow complete and instantaneous submergence of the entire body except the head. Immerse as quickly as possible after cooling the head. The duration of the bath must be very brief, not more than 5 to 10 seconds. Rub vigorously while in the bath, and after emerging rub with coarse towels until the body is warm and dry. Exercise till reaction is complete. The best time for the bath is immediately after rising from bed, and while warm and feeling a relish for the contact of cold water. Used thus, this bath is a powerful means of promoting vital resistance and maintaining the integrity of the body.

A remarkable testimony to the hygienic value of the daily cold bath is noted by Currie in his "Medical Reports" (4th edition, p. 378). Quoting Dr. Wright, he says: "I agree with Dr. Falconer, of Bath, in thinking that the cold affusion will secure persons from taking the plague itself, though exposed to its contagion."

Surgeon Mc Gregor, formerly superintendent surgeon of the English army in Egypt, confirms this view by a very interesting observation. While he was in charge of the "Blues," a famous old regiment then located at Canterbury, an epidemic of typhus fever, generally complicated with pneumonia, broke out. The disease developed so rapidly that in a short time one fifth of his regiment were on the sick-list, and there were thirty-three cases of fever, with daily accessions to the number. At this juncture it occurred to McGregor, a disciple of Currie, who was familiar with the use of the bath in the treatment of cases of fever, that the cold bath might be used for prophylactic as well as curative purposes. Accordingly, to use his own words, "About the 12th, at my earnest recommendation, all the regiment out of the hospital were marched three times a day to the riverside, and every man was made to bathe. The good effects of this were speedily manifest; the number of new fever cases decreased daily, and those that did appear wore a milder aspect. Many, indeed, yielded to the common treatment; in some cases an emetic, and in others the cold bath, at once cut short the disease. We lost no case in October. Indeed, it was evident to all that after the general bathing of the regiment, the contagion stopped; the few cases that occurred after this were stripped of all the alarming and dangerous symptoms with which the disease broke out. In all, there were sixty cases of fever occurring from July to the 21st of October, on which day the last case appeared. We lost six of this number." *

The immunity evidently conferred by the tri-daily bath was certainly more than a coincidence. It would seem eminently reasonable to suppose that if the cold bath aids recovery by stimulating the vital forces and increasing the vital resistance, and to such a degree that the patient already thoroughly infected with the disease is brought to a safe recovery, the application of the same measures before the contraction of the disease ought so to fortify the system as to enable it to successfully withstand the influence of the infectious element to which the malady owes its origin. The principle involved in this suggestion is one well worthy of the most thoughtful consideration. If the principle holds in relation to a single malady, it is equally sound in relation to all others which depend upon either infection or any other external cause, of course excepting accidents.

The Cold Bath an Antidote for Alcoholic Intoxication.

It is a well-known fact that intoxicated sailors 1119
are often suddenly sobered up by falling into the sea. The excitant effect of the contact of the cold sea water with the temperature nerves of the skin reacts upon the brain and spinal cord with such intensity as to arouse to activity the alcohol-narcotized centers. The author has long

* Currie's "Medical Reports," p. 394. † Curiosities of Common Water, 1793.

been familiar with this fact, and has made very frequent use of it in overcoming the acute effects of alcohol poisoning. He has frequently seen a man so profoundly under the influence of liquor as to be unable to stand alone, who could not speak distinctly or coherently, completely sobered within four or five minutes by the employment of the hot and cold shower bath.

Dr. Robertson, of Barbadoes, reported in the early part of the present century an interesting case which illustrates very forcibly the powerful influence of cold water in antagonizing the acute effects of alcoholic poisoning. The temperature of the water employed, as determined by Dr. Robertson, was 76° to 80°. We quote as follows from page 201 of Dr. Currie's "Medical Reports," to which we are indebted for the account of this interesting case:—

"A gentleman of this island, whose name was Weeks, a great votary of Bacchus, was in the practice, from fifteen to twenty years, of plunging into cold water when he rose from his bottle, and of actually going to sleep in a trough full of water, with his head supported on a kind of wooden pillow made for the purpose, above the surface. When he dined abroad, and had not the convenience of his own trough, he used to strip off coat, waistcoat, and shirt, and sit exposed in the open air, and in that situation go to sleep, whether it rained or not. And sometimes he went and bathed in the nearest adjoining pond, to which he generally required assistance to be conveyed. The effect of this practice was, that instead of experiencing debility, lassitude, headache, and nausea on awakening, he found himself cheerful and refreshed, and free from all the effects of intoxication. In the year 1789, dining one evening abroad, he got alternately drunk and sober three several times before midnight, each time recovering his sobriety by immersing himself and sleeping in cold water; and on awakening, returning to the company. The last time, after supper, he was so immoderately intoxicated that he insisted on his companions' undressing him and carrying him to the pond. They carried him accordingly in a chair, and set him up to the chin in water, where he continued upwards of an hour, a person supporting him. I have this last circumstance from a gentleman of the party, whose veracity may be entirely depended upon.

"At home, however, he used, as I have already mentioned, a trough made for the purpose, with a bench in it as a pillow, having been nearly drowned when sleeping in his pond, from the negro who was appointed to watch him having himself fallen asleep. In this watery bed he would sleep, one, two, three, or even more hours, experiencing always the greatest refreshment. His wife and family, when they wished him to change his quarters, used to draw out the plug and let the water run off, when he would awake, and humorously complain of the loss of his bed-clothes. At length this expedient began to lose its effect in arousing him, and one time he continued to sleep in his empty trough. In consequence of this he was seized with extreme rigors and chills, followed by a severe attack of rheumatism, which affected him a long time, and made him desist from this practice in future. But to the end of his life he was in the habit of sitting with his clothes open, and sometimes quite naked, exposed to the wind and rain."

THE GRADUATED BATH.

This bath, the advantages of which have been urged by **1120**
Ziemssen, Bouchard, and others, is a form of the full bath especially adapted to the treatment of fevers. The method consists essentially in a full bath the temperature of which is gradually lowered.

Method.—The patient enters the bath at a temperature from nine to ten degrees below that of the body, and the temperature of the bath is lowered at the rate of two degrees a minute to 77°, continuing at this point until shivering and chattering of the teeth occur (Ziemssen).

The principle of graduation thus suggested by Ziemssen is

a valuable one, but the temperature of the bath is so rapidly lowered that the discomfort to the patient is almost as great as in the method of Brand. Bouchard aims to avoid the nervous shock and suffering of the patient by the following method, as described in his work.* The initial temperature of the bath is three or four degrees below the temperature of the patient. For example, if the patient's temperature is (per rectum) 104°, the bath will begin at 100° F. At this temperature the patient is comfortable, and experiences no shock. The water is cooled at the rate of two degrees Fahrenheit, or 1° C. (1.8° F.), every five minutes until the temperature of the bath is reduced to 86°, never lower. The patient should be continuously rubbed after the temperature of the water has been lowered sufficiently to produce chilly sensations. This prevents chilling and shivering, and the consequent increase of heat production.

The advantages of the graduated bath of Bouchard are that it does not produce vascular spasm, arterial pressure is not raised, and the lowering of temperature is greater than in the cold bath. In fevers, the bath is administered every three hours; so that when a patient's temperature rises to 104° or above, it may be necessary for him to spend half of his time in the bath. The temperature is usually reduced about one degree, though sometimes it falls as much as three or four degrees.

A formidable objection to the cold bath is the nervous shock which it produces, the dread the patient experiences, the discomfort, the cyanosis, which latter symptom often gives a case a very grave appearance, although the danger may not be so great as it appears. It must also be remembered that in persons whose hearts are organically diseased, and especially when the arteries are weakened by arteriosclerosis, the very cold bath can not be employed without great danger. The graduated bath is free from these objections, and is hence a most valuable hydrotherapeutic measure.

* "Leçons sur les Auto-Intoxications," Paris, 1887, p. 230.

Physiological Effects.—The special physiological effect of the graduated bath is to reduce the body temperature, which it accomplishes in a most efficient manner, though perhaps less rapidly than by the cold bath with friction. The graduated bath for 30 minutes is equivalent, as an antipyretic measure, to a cold bath at 70° for 10 minutes, and its effects are more permanent. 1121

A marked advantage of the graduated bath is that it promotes thermic reaction to a much less degree than does the cold bath, hence has not so great a tendency to increase heat production, while it is equally efficient as a means of increasing heat elimination.

The graduated bath may be managed in such a way that no shock whatever is produced; so that it is much more agreeable to sensitive patients and those who dread cold applications.

The intensity of the bath depends upon the length of time it is continued and the degree of temperature to which the water is lowered. As the temperature of the bath is gradually lowered, opportunity is afforded for observing the effect upon the patient, so that the bath can be stopped at the point at which the most favorable results are noted; that is, the cooling may cease at any temperature desired, the bath being then continued at a fixed temperature, which may be tepid, cool, or cold, as is most desirable.

Therapeutic Applications.—The graduated bath is, in the author's opinion, the most efficient method of reducing temperature in fevers. By its aid all the effects can be secured which are obtainable from any other form of the bath. It can be easily managed in such a way as to produce the temperature-reducing effects of the tepid, cool, or cold bath, by ceasing to add cold water at the proper point, and may be graduated to a nicety to suit the varying conditions of individual cases. 1122

The principle of the graduated bath is an exceedingly important one, and may be applied to other procedures as well as the full bath. It may be remarked also that in the employment of the cold bath and cold friction, the bath may be graduated by giving the first bath at a temperature eight or ten degrees below that of the body, and lowering each successive bath.

If in a fever case indications are present which point to the necessity for cold applications for *general tonic effects*, *to increase vital resistance*, or *to energize the heart*, these may be met by the cold friction, the cold towel rub, the rubbing wet sheet (in bed), the ice-bag over the heart, and a variety of measures which may be much more conveniently, safely, and comfortably employed than the Brand bath.

THE TEPID IMMERSION BATH.

1123 The method of administering the tepid bath is essentially the same as has been described for the cold immersion bath (**1112**). The temperature is from 80° to 90°. The tepid bath is generally administered at a temperature ten to twelve degrees below that of the body. Care should be taken to see that the water covers the shoulders, in order to prevent pulmonary congestion. The usual time of the tepid bath is about 30 minutes, but by employing general friction it may be continued for many hours (at 88° to 90°).

1124 **Physiological Effects.**—The tepid bath slows the pulse, lowers the temperature of the body by the abstraction of heat, but produces little or no thermic reaction, and hence does not give rise to increased heat production. The circulatory reaction takes place slowly, the preliminary contraction being slowly developed and the subsequent dilatation equally slow. The effect of the bath in reducing temperature will depend upon the relative temperature of the patient, the duration of the bath, and the degree to which the bath approaches the lower limit of the range of tepid temperature, or near 80°.

1125 **Therapeutic Applications.**—The tepid bath was much used by Hippocrates in the treatment of fever, and has been in modern times extolled by Dujardin-Beaumetz and Bouchard.

Riess treated several hundred cases of typhoid fever with the continuous tepid bath at 88°. The patients were kept in the bath from eight to fifteen hours, or until the temperature fell to the normal, or nearly so. The temperature usually began to rise again soon after the patient was removed from the bath. As soon as it reached 101°, the application was repeated. In some instances the patient was obliged to spend almost his entire time in the bath in order to keep the temperature near the normal point. For a continuous bath of this sort it is necessary that the patient be made comfortable by suspension in a sheet, the ends of which are secured to the sides of the bath-tub. The statistics furnished by Riess showed that the duration of the disease was very perceptibly diminished by the continuous tepid bath.

The tepid bath given for half an hour or an hour is to be preferred to the very cold bath in *pneumonia*, also in low stages of *typhoid fever* in which the patient has not had the advantages of cold water treatment in the early period of the malady. Care should be taken to protect the head with cold water in the tepid bath as well as in the cold bath, and friction should be applied when there is the slightest tendency to chill. Friction must be more energetic in the tepid than in the cold bath, for the reason that the thermic impression is feeble, so that the circulatory reaction depends almost wholly upon mechanical effects.

The tepid bath may sometimes be used as a training for cold applications. It is also a very useful measure in connection with electricity in the electro-thermal bath.

THE HOT IMMERSION BATH.

This is an ordinary full bath administered at a tempera- 1126
ture of 98° to 104°. At temperatures above 104° the bath is properly termed "very hot," but the effects of the full bath at temperatures ranging between 100° and 113° differ in degree only, not in kind. It is the purpose to consider under this heading the effect of the immersion bath at any temperature above that of the body.

Methods.—The time of the hot bath varies from 2 or 3 minutes to 15 minutes, according to the temperature and the case. It must never be very greatly prolonged, for the reason that baths at any temperature above that of the body cause a rapid accumulation of heat and rise of temperature. In the administration of the bath at a temperature considerably above that of the body, the beginning temperature should be 100°, it being gradually raised by the addition of hot water to the maximum temperature desired. By this means the skin becomes gradually accustomed to the heat, and a much higher temperature will be tolerated than if the patient enters the bath at the maximum temperature. The cerebral excitation is also less.

1127 **Physiological Effects.**—The hot or very hot immersion bath is a powerfully exciting measure. During the application the general nervous system, the heart, and the blood-vessels, as well as the system generally, are strongly excited by the powerful thermic impressions transmitted inward and by the profound vascular impression made through the dilatation of the surface vessels. Heat production, the oxidation of nitrogen, or the production of urea and metabolism in general, are quickened under the influence of the elevated temperature. The skin is intensely congested by the paralytic effect of the heat upon the vasoconstrictors. A very short primary contraction of the vessels occurs when the temperature of the application is very high (113° or above), but the characteristic effect upon the cutaneous circulation of hot general applications is to paralyze the small vessels. The cutaneous glands are excited to activity, the skin is reddened and bathed in perspiration.

The study of the effects of the hot immersion bath upon the circulation by means of the instruments of precision devised by Oliver, of England, for determining arterial pressure and measuring the caliber of the arteries, affords interesting results. The author has found the use of these instruments somewhat difficult, requiring considerable practice in order to secure uniform results. They are the best yet made for the purpose, however, and afford reliable data when carefully used. The general result of many experiments, as reported by Oliver, is that a hot application — that is, a bath at 100° to 105° — causes contraction of the radial artery, by reason of the extreme dilatation of the small vessels; it is also indicated by the marked enlargement of the submerged parts, which may amount to more than six per cent. When the temperature of the bath was slightly below that of the body, the radial artery was at first enlarged, but later contracted with the dilatation of the surface vessels. The cold bath caused strong contraction of the radial artery, its diameter being reduced by a bath of 40° from 2.2 mm. to 1.3 mm., with a corresponding increase of tension. This effect lasts, of course, only until reaction begins.

These experiments are of great practical interest in showing that the effects of applications to the surface are not upon the small cutaneous vessels only, but involve the large arterial trunks lying deep in the tissues, at least when large areas of the skin are acted upon.

Much useful information respecting the effects of the hot immersion bath has been gathered from a study of this bath in the public baths of Japan (Fig. 64). Professor Bältz has had an excellent opportunity, during many years' residence in Japan, for a thorough study of the effects of these baths, since in that country it is the general custom to take a hot bath almost daily. In Tokio alone there are given about 400,000 hot baths daily, the price being so low as to be within the means of the very poorest, — one-half to one cent. Bältz himself has for many years taken a hot bath at least twice a week, and in summer, after great exertions in mountain-climbing, often twice a day.

The Japanese usually take the bath at 115°, sometimes hotter; while Europeans living in Japan take it at 104° to 109.4° F. Before going into the bath, the head is rubbed with hot water, whereby the blood-vessels of the head are at once relaxed, and anemia of the brain is prevented. The duration of the bath is 5 to 20 minutes, according to the temperature. When the sensation of heat is very great or strong palpitation of the heart is experienced, the bather leaves the bath at once.

The first effect upon going into the hot bath is a goose-flesh contraction and blanching of the skin for a few seconds, followed by a gradual relaxation of the cutaneous vessels with reddening. The pulse is at first slow, then gradually quickens. The respiration is only slightly influenced at the beginning; later it is manifestly changed, especially in the case of men, to the thoracic type. The body temperature, measured under the tongue, shows a gradual rise to 104° F., and even above. This rise is produced not only by the retention of heat, but also through its direct absorption. The rise appears very quickly, often within six minutes. After leaving the bath, the temperature rise generally continues to the amount of .6° to 1° more; and does not return to the normal until from one to two hours have passed. The arteries relax, and the temporal artery becomes tortuous, as in arteriosclerosis. The pulse is full, and the pulse-curve high. Remaining in the bath after the proper temperature is reached causes dizziness and nausea. The albumin metabolism is, according to this observer, not increased in the hot bath, as previously supposed. Before leaving the bath, the bather generally pours cold water over himself to prevent continued sweating.

It is generally supposed that after a hot bath one takes cold very easily. Dr. Bältz claims, on the contrary, the very opposite, namely, that it is impossible to take cold; that taking cold occurs only after a tepid or warm bath whose temperature is the same or lower than that of the body. The very hot bath produces paralysis of the skin vessels, which continues for some time, and prevents the vessels' reacting to cold. The opinion that the very hot bath produces diminished resistance is disproved by daily experience in Japan.

The author has obtained interesting information concerning the Japanese baths from a friend, Dr. Swartz, who was for many years a medical missionary in Japan, and through long residence in the country and frequent attendance at the baths, became able to enjoy them at as high a temperature as the Japanese. Dr. Swartz testifies that the effect of the bath is decidedly stimulating, and that no depressing effects whatever follow its use. Some persons cool off the skin by means of the cold bath after coming from the hot bathing tanks, but natives may frequently be seen running through the streets quite nude, even in very cold weather, without any cooling application; and yet it is asserted that they do not take cold.

The effects of the bath at this very high temperature are in many respects identical with those of the cold bath. This is true, however, only during the application. After the hot bath, certain atonic effects are apparent. Perspiration, quickening of the pulse, and reddening of the skin continue for a varying period; but sooner or later contraction of the cutaneous vessels occurs, accompanied by dilatation of the internal vessels. The heat production, which was temporarily increased, is now lessened, and the phenomena of atonic reaction appear.

That the Japanese native does not take cold after this extremely hot bathing, is probably due to the fact that the temperature of both the skin and the blood is at so high a point that ordinary and even extraordinary exposure does not suffice to produce a chill either by lowering the temperature or by cooling the peripheral nerve filaments. The cutaneous vessels remain dilated for a long time after these extremely hot baths, as the result of paralysis of the vasoconstrictors. The cooling occasioned by evaporation takes place very slowly; consequently the contraction of the peripheral vessels and the resulting intense visceral congestion which introduces the train of phenomena accompanying the condition known as a "cold," does not take place.

1128 **Therapeutic Applications.**—The hot immersion bath is perhaps most useful as an eliminative or spoliative procedure. The bath at 104° to 110° for 10 minutes, followed by a dry pack, is a most efficient sweating procedure. This bath may be advantageously employed in *dropsy*, when excessive loss of tone of the heart and blood-vessels, as indicated by general cyanosis, is not present. It must be remembered, however, that in dropsy, when due to cardiac disease, the heart is not able to bear the sudden shock of cold water, and consequently the greatest care must be taken in cooling off the patient after the hot bath. He should be wrapped in a Turkish sheet, covered with a blanket, and allowed to cool off gradually in a room at a temperature of 65° to 70°, or he may be rubbed with the moist hand, or even tepid sponging may be practiced when the skin is very hot and the tendency to perspiration strong. To avoid chilling by evaporation, only a small portion of the body should be uncovered at a time during the sponging or rubbing. In treating patients who chill very easily it may be necessary to do the rubbing beneath the blanket. Very high temperatures should be avoided in the hot immersion bath, because of the tendency to excitation of the brain and heart. A temperature of 120° is dangerous to life, and a bath at 110° should not be continued more than 10 or 15 minutes.

The hot bath is also a powerful derivative. Bältz considered it a specific in the *capillary bronchitis* and *bronchial pneumonia* of children, but found it of no benefit in croupous pneumonia. It operates in these cases as a derivative measure, relieving the overfilled vessels of the lungs by congesting the vessels of the skin and the muscles. Its effect is manifested very quickly. The breathing at once becomes easier, and the cough ceases. The temperature of the bath in such cases should be 104° to 106°; its duration from 5 to 15 minutes. As soon as strong reddening of the skin appears, the patient is removed from the bath. Such a bath may be applied to children two to four times in the twenty-four hours,

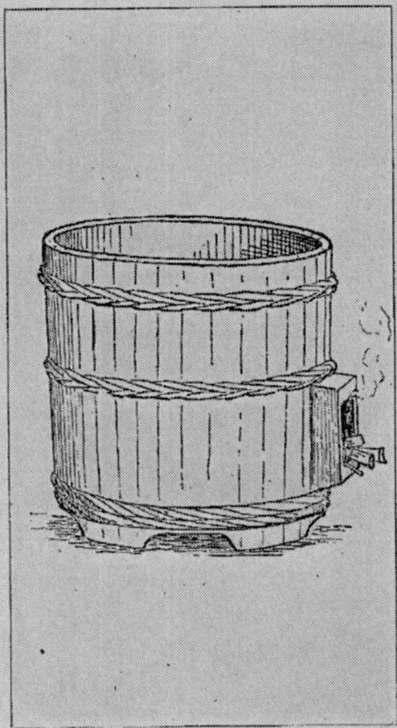

Fig. 64 *(a)*. JAPANESE BATH TUB CONTAINING HEATING OVEN (p. 541).

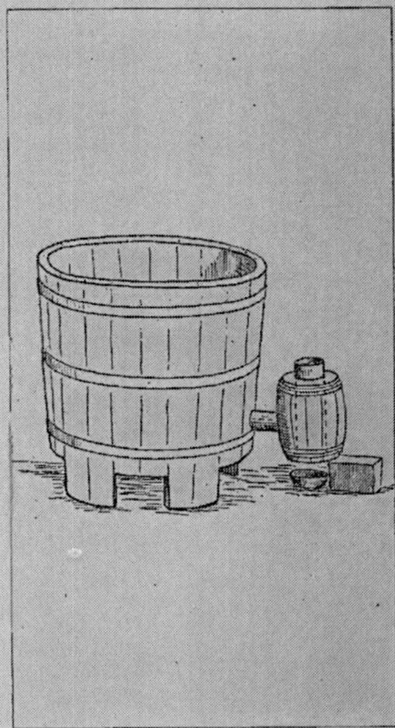

Fig. 64 *(b)*. JAPANESE BATH TUB WITH EXTERNAL HEATING CHAMBER (p. 541).

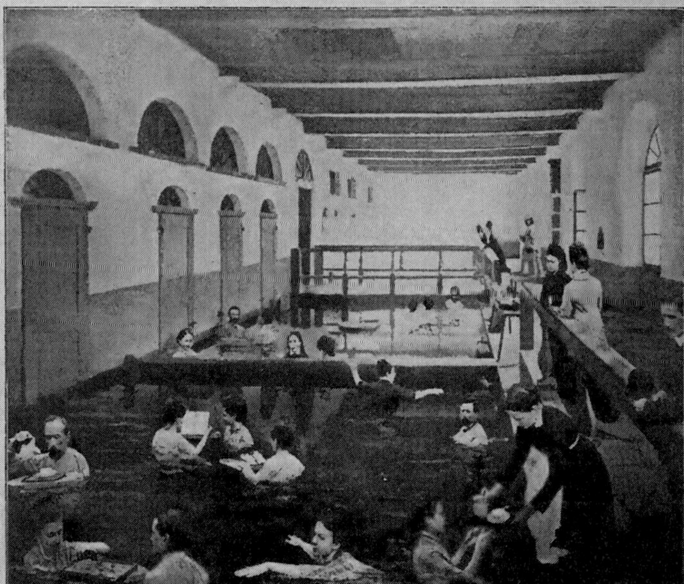

Fig. 65. BATHING AT LEUKERBAD, SWITZERLAND (p. 552).

as seems to be indicated. In cases in which the temperature is very high, the child may be placed in the bath up to the epigastrium while cold water is poured over the upper part of the body.

The hot immersion bath has proved itself a very valuable measure of treatment in *cerebrospinal meningitis*. The temperature should be 103° or 104°; duration from 10 to 15 minutes, the application to be repeated every three or four hours. The head should be protected by a compress saturated with ice-water, which should be frequently renewed, or by cold irrigation or a cold coil.

In *amenorrhea* or in *suppressed menstruation* this bath should be administered at 101° to 105°; duration half an hour or more, at the time menstruation is due. It may be repeated twice a day for two or three days in succession. There is no more effective measure for *dysmenorrhea* with scanty flow, a temperature of 102° to 112° being employed for 15 minutes. The hot bath may also be administered in *painful menstruation* when the flow is profuse; but when employed in such a case, it should be of short duration, not more than 3 or 4 minutes, at a temperature of 105° to 110°, and should be immediately followed by the hot vaginal douche at 104°.

In *chronic bronchitis*, a very hot bath, 5 to 7 minutes in duration, accompanied by rubbing with the friction mitt, relieves congestion of the mucous membrane; and when the disease is complicated with asthma, generally affords prompt relief from the distressing paroxysms. The patient should be carefully cooled after the bath, and oil should be rubbed upon the skin.

The hot bath at 102° to 106° may be very profitably employed in *chronic rheumatism* and *obesity*, being used daily, or every other day, for 10 to 15 minutes. Rubbing during the bath increases the beneficial effect in rheumatism, by aiding circulatory reaction. Massage of the joints may be practiced with great advantage during the hot bath.

Lasèque* in his work upon "Hot Baths" recommends the bath at a temperature of 113° in rheumatism.

The hot bath should always be followed by a cold application, which in cases of obesity should be very vigorous and prolonged, as cold immersion or a cold shallow; but in rheumatism the prolonged tepid or Scotch douche or cold friction should be employed instead.

In the *acute nephritis* of scarlet fever the Scotch douche affords the best means of relief from the renal congestion. The temperature should be from 106° to 110°; duration, 10 minutes. It may be repeated two or three times in twenty-four hours when the symptoms are urgent.

The daily hot bath affords relief from the intolerable *itching* of *jaundice*, and aids the skin as well as the kidneys in ridding the system of the bile pigment with which the tissues are poisoned. *Gastric* and *intestinal colic* are quite promptly relieved by the bath at 110° for 10 to 15 minutes, but in *cholera* the cold friction bath succeeds better.

The relaxing effect of the hot bath is highly valuable as a palliative measure in cases of *gallstones* and *renal colic*. The effects of the bath may be increased by gentle massage employed at the seat of pain in such a way as to aid the movement of the calculi through the proper channel.

The intolerably depressing pain of *cystitis* yields promptly to the very hot bath, but is greatly aggravated by cold; so that gradual cooling at a neutral temperature is required. Other measures must of course be employed to remove the causes of the pain.

In *muscular rheumatism*, the hot bath relieves pain by encouraging the elimination of the toxins to which the pain is due, as well as by direct revulsive or derivative effects.

The hot bath is an excellent means of preparing the skin and the system at large for a cold bath in cases in which such a preparation is necessary. The hot bath may be equally well employed in cases in which an overdose of cold water

* Lasèque, *Arch. Gen. de Med.*, 1874, p. 132.

has been inadvertently applied. It is well to remember that heat is a perfect antidote for cold, while cold is an equally perfect antidote for excessive applications of heat, provided no structural change has taken place.

In *delirium tremens* a short hot bath followed by cold friction or a cold shower bath renders valuable service.

In the beginning of *measles*, *scarlet fever*, and other eruptive disorders, the hot bath often renders great service by encouraging the development of the eruption.

In *typhoid fever*, when the patient is in a low state, and in cases in which the circulation is sluggish, as indicated by cyanosis, and when the nerve centers are depressed by the profound toxemia present, the hot bath at 102° to 106° may be advantageously employed for 3 to 5 minutes. It should be followed by cold affusion, two or three gallons of water being poured over the back and chest, with the patient sitting up in the tub, or by general cold friction with the friction mitt. The same measure is equally valuable under similar conditions when occurring in *measles*, *smallpox*, *diphtheria*, and other febrile disorders.

Galen recommended the warm bath followed by rubbing with cold water as a means of lowering the temperature in *fever*.

In *infantile convulsions* the hot bath for 3 to 5 minutes, followed by affusion consisting of a quart or two of water poured over the patient's head and spine, is a powerful life-saving means. Immediately after the affusion the child should be wrapped in warm blankets, so as to produce quick reaction.

The very hot bath may also be used with very great advantage in *asphyxia* of the newborn. The child should be dipped in hot water for 15 to 20 seconds, then cold water dashed over it, while artificial respiration is practiced.

Tarnier recommends the hot bath (100° to 104°) for 40 minutes as a successful means of combating the profuse vaginal discharge which so often occurs in nursing mothers of feeble constitution. The continued and obstinate bloody discharge which often occurs under the same conditions likewise yields to this measure. A brief application of cold friction should follow the bath.

1129 **Contraindications.**—The hot bath must be avoided in cases of organic disease of the brain or spinal cord, as *tabes, sclerosis,* and *myelitis;* in cases of *cardiac weakness* and *cardiac hypertrophy;* in *arteriosclerosis;* and in threatened or existing *cerebral apoplexy.* If employed at all in cases of *chronic nephritis,* it should be with the greatest care and precaution to prevent subsequent chilling, and resulting visceral congestion with an increase of renal inflammation.

It should be remembered, also, that in the employment of the hot bath the body temperature is rapidly increased. Hot baths are naturally contraindicated in febrile disorders, except in certain adynamic states; and even then the hot immersion bath will rarely be called for, other procedures being preferable and safer. If for any reason it seems necessary to employ the hot bath in a febrile case, the application must necessarily be very brief (3 to 4 minutes), to avoid undue elevation of temperature.

THE NEUTRAL BATH.

1130 This is simply a full bath at the temperature of 92° to 97°, administered in the usual manner. For a discussion of the general properties of the neutral bath, see paragraph **717**.

Method.— Friction should not be administered, unless it be very gentle rubbing when the patient first enters the bath, if he feels a slight inclination to chill. Chill will not occur, however, if the temperature of the bath is properly adjusted to the patient's conditions. The average temperature of the bath should be 94° or 95°. When the patient is feverish and the skin hot and flushed, even though there be no rise of temperature, the temperature of the bath may be 92° or 93°. If the patient is thin and bloodless, with small heat-making capacity, the temperature of the bath should be 96° or 97°.

All mechanical effects should be avoided after as well as during this bath, as its purpose is to secure calmative or sedative effects. The duration of the bath when applied for relief of insomnia should be from 15 minutes to one hour. When used for the reduction of temperature, however, it may be continued for a much longer time, as three to four hours: and in certain cases of *acute mania, obstinate insomnia*, or *fever*, it may be continued for several hours consecutively, at a temperature of 92° or 93°. In certain traumatic cases, it may even be continued for weeks or months, the patient being removed only for urination and defecation **(1136)**.

Physiological Effects.—Kuhn, of Niederbronn,* first scien- **1131**
tifically described the interesting characteristics of the neutral bath. He considered a bath as neutral when of such a temperature that it abstracts from the part immersed exactly the same quantity of heat that the part naturally receives from the blood. The neutral point, according to this authority, is the physiological zero. Below this point water is absorbed; above, it is exhaled. Both the absorption and the exhalation increase in proportion as the temperature of the body varies from the neutral point. This is usually 93° to 94°. This point marks, then, the limit where absorption ceases and exhalation begins. He also noted that fresh water, in determining the more or less rapid imbibition of water by the skin, promotes the cutaneous reaction which plays so important a rôle in hydriatic treatment. The reaction in this case is increased according to the coldness and purity of the water. Cold or cool baths, by introducing cool water into the blood mass, render the blood more aqueous, diminishing its density, and thus acting as a sedative. The purer the water, the more calming are the effects of the bath on account of the greater amount of water absorbed. The neutral point is not fixed. It is solely and entirely regulated by the individual sensation. There is a certain equilibrium between the heat subtracted and the heat produced in normal conditions. It varies a little

*Monograph, Paris, 1854.

according to the constitution of individuals, and the disease, and especially with the refrigerating power of the surrounding medium; that is, it is always more elevated when the water is charged with salts than with pure water. In other words, salt-water baths can be taken at a lower temperature than fresh-water baths, since the former stimulate heat production more than do the latter at the same temperature.

The neutral bath diminishes the pulse-rate, but does not modify the respiration. Exhalation by the skin is suspended, so that water accumulates in the tissues. It is in this way the cutaneous nerves become supersaturated with water, rather than by absorption of water from the bath. At the neutral point, there is then practically no movement of fluids either inward or outward. The urine is greatly increased in quantity; while its acidity is decreased; it may even become alkaline.

The temperature and mode of administration of the neutral bath are such that neither thermic nor circulatory reaction is produced. The bath may consequently be prolonged for an almost indefinite period without producing exhaustion or any other untoward effects. When the bath is prolonged for a considerable period, the patient should be suspended in a sort of hammock consisting of a sheet let down into the tub and secured to the edges, and should be made comfortable by means of an air pillow. The temperature of the neutral bath may be maintained uniform by placing covers over the tub, and adding jugs or bottles filled with hot water as often as may be necessary; or a portion of the water may be removed from time to time, and replaced with water at a higher temperature. When the temperature of the surrounding atmosphere is such as to prevent cooling, so that the bath is warmed by the heat of the body, it may be necessary to add cooler water occasionally to prevent elevation of temperature, whereby the bath would cease to be neutral in its effects. This bath depends for its good effects entirely upon the careful adjustment of the temperature within the limits named, 92° to 97° F.

The physiological effects of this bath are to lessen nerve sensibility, and Kölliker, Hyman, and Krebs have shown that the absorption of water by the nerve filaments accomplishes this. That an anemic or bloodless skin is more sensitive than a congested skin has long been a matter of observation, but it is only recently that the actual demonstration has been afforded by the experiments of the investigators named. The protection afforded the central nervous system against reflex irritation of all sorts by a perfectly neutral medium contributes to the sedative effects of the neutral bath.

The neutral bath is the most purely sedative procedure afforded by the whole range of hydriatic measures. The neutral douche produces very similar results. Its influence is strongly derivative through the circulatory reaction induced by the mechanical effects. The neutral bath excites activity of both the skin and the kidneys to a marked degree.

The neutral full bath, as well as other baths near or above the body temperature, is followed by a decided lowering of the surface temperature. The internal temperature remaining normal, it is evident that there must be a decided reduction in the rate of heat production. The surface temperature sometimes falls as much as six degrees, which would indicate a lessened heat loss amounting to nearly 25 per cent. and a corresponding decrease of heat production. In the case of the neutral bath, this effect is not due to atonic thermic reaction, as when an application above the temperature of the body is made to the skin, but must result simply from the cutting off of those reflex influences due to contact with the skin of air at a temperature below that of the body, thus annulling one of the important factors in maintaining the activity of the thermogenetic processes in the muscles. This effect of the neutral bath necessitates special care to avoid chilling of the patient by exposure to cold air. The patient should generally recline for an hour after the bath, covered sufficiently to prevent chill, but without overheating.

1132 **Therapeutic Applications.**—At the quaint and interesting old bathing resort at Leukerbad, Switzerland, which the author visited in 1883, he found still in use the system of immersion in water at a neutral temperature which has there been employed during several generations in the treatment of a large class of chronic disorders, including skin affections of various kinds. The patients enter the bath about 6 or 7 o'clock in the morning, without breakfast, and remain immersed up to the chin until about 1 P. M. The accompanying cut (Fig. 65) represents scenes such as may be daily observed.

Riess applied the neutral bath in a large number of cases of organic disease of the brain and cord, including *paraplegia, locomotor ataxia, chronic inflammation* of both *brain* and *cord*, especially in *meningitis*, in *rheumatism deformans*, and in various other chronic affections. His success was so great as to give good reason for the belief that this procedure presents valuable therapeutic value in cases of this sort. The author's experience with the continued neutral bath has been sufficient to convince him of its great value.

It is interesting to note that Currie* had a thorough appreciation of the value of the neutral bath, which he employed at 90° to 95°. He recommended it "when the strength is wasted by fatigue and perspiration." He remarked, "In the degrees in which it does not quicken the circulation, the warm bath is soothing and sedative, especially when the immersion is prolonged; and it is the temperature from 90° to 95° that is so singularly restorative for fatigue."

The neutral bath, continued for thirty to sixty minutes, or even longer, renders great service in *general dropsy*, whether due to cardiac or renal disease, especially in cases in which more vigorous measures can not well be employed. It also renders valuable service in chronic sciatica accompanied by severe pain, as a means of continuing the good effects obtained in the use of other measures, such as the Scotch

*Currie's "Medical Reports," pp. 194–196.

douche, the prolonged fomentation, the revulsive compress, massage, electricity, and other well-known means.

In *insomnia* there is practically no single measure of treatment so valuable as the neutral bath. For this class of patients the bath should be administered at bedtime. The patient often becomes drowsy in the bath, and may fall asleep. He may be allowed to sleep in the bath for several hours if it is found that removal counteracts its hypnotic effect, which is not infrequently the case. The sleeping patient must be carefully watched, however, to see that the head is not submerged. 1133

On removal from the bath, in cases of insomnia, great care should be taken to avoid chilling of the surface by evaporation. The patient should be instantly wrapped in a Turkish sheet and woolen blankets, and should be dried by gentle patting of the sheet or blanket, and without rubbing either with the sheet or with the dry hand, being afterward placed in bed as quickly as possible, and his surroundings made in every way conducive to sleep, so that the good effects of the bath may not be lost by excitation of the nervous system by unfavorable conditions.

It will be interesting to recall the fact that Hippocrates well appreciated the neutral bath as a means of inducing sleep.

In *multiple neuritis*, *apoplexy*, and in the treatment of the *alcohol*, *opium*, *cocaine*, and *chloral habits*, the sedative effects of the neutral bath are of immense service. In cases of this sort it is generally necessary to employ a temperature of 95° to 97°. The influence of a difference of two or three degrees, or even of a single degree, is quite surprising to a person who is not thoroughly acquainted with the singular potency of hydriatic measures, when employed with exactness.

Vigoroux* recommends the neutral bath for one to three hours for *neurasthenics* and *rheumatics*. This author strongly condemns the cold douche in these cases, as he finds the

* Vigoroux, "Neurasthénie et Arthritisme," p. 308.

urine of neurasthenics, as of rheumatics, acid, which denotes deficient oxidation, notwithstanding the total amount of the products of excrementitious waste is deficient.

When there is a tendency to *heart failure* in the use of the warm bath, in cases of cardiac insufficiency, or after the withdrawal of opium or other drugs, this inconvenience may be wholly overcome by the use of the ice-bag over the heart during the bath. An application to the head and neck is also necessary in cases of this sort when a temperature approximating that of the body is employed. The value of the neutral bath in the affections mentioned is largely due to its action upon the kidneys, the activity of which it encourages to a high degree, while at the same time it quiets the irritated brain and cord. This purification of the blood through increased renal and cutaneous activity improves general vital action, and gives this bath decided restorative as well as sedative effects.

The neutral bath is of great value in *chronic diarrhea*, *peritonitis*, and other chronic affections of the abdomen, and especially those in which the patient is in a condition to interdict the employment of very hot or very cold baths. In such cases it may be employed daily for 15 to 30 minutes. It is also of value in cases of *toxemia*, which is so commonly present in *chronic dyspepsia*, and in *pruritus* without eruption, either with or without jaundice, also in the several forms of *urticaria*.

The neutral bath is often employed in connection with electricity. The author has for more than twenty years made extensive use of this bath as a means of making general applications of the galvanic, faradic, and sinusoidal currents. This subject will be treated more fully under the head of Electro-Hydric Baths (**1457**).

1134 The neutral bath may be employed as an antipyretic and antifebrile measure in *continued fevers*, and is especially serviceable for infants, old persons, and others with a feeble constitution, or in cases which have been neglected in the early stages until the patient has reached so low a state that the cold bath is interdicted because the nerve centers have not enough vitality left to react to so heroic a measure. When employed for this purpose, the temperature of the bath at the beginning should be 98°, and should be rapidly lowered to 92° or even 90°, when it should be prolonged for half an hour to two hours. The length of the bath should be not more than 10 minutes for very aged persons, and 5 to 10 minutes for infants, but should be repeated every two hours, or whenever the temperature reaches 100° to 102°.

The neutral bath is especially indicated in disorders of the nervous system and of the heart and blood-vessels. Arteriosclerosis gives rise to deterioration in the central nervous system as well as elsewhere. From deficient flushing of the parts with healthy blood, tissue deterioration begins; and the disorder is then rapidly intensified by the accumulation of tissue poisons in the part, and degeneration of the blood-vessels takes place with great rapidity. Long-continued contraction of the blood-vessels gives rise to a disturbance in the nutrition of their walls, which finally results in relaxation and paralysis, and the local disorder becomes fixed.

Either very cold or very hot applications must be avoided in cases of chronic disease of the central nervous system, because of the diseased condition of the vessels, which are overworked, and liable to rupture under the strain of the sudden inrush of blood in the general retrostasis accompanying applications to the whole surface, and in the collateral hyperemia resulting from very cold applications to the back. As a rule, a temperature below 70° or above 110° is not useful in the treatment of organic nervous disorders. Partial cold friction may be employed in these cases, but general applications should be at temperatures not far removed from the body temperature, or 85° to 104°.

Contraindications.—About the only contraindication for 1135
the neutral bath is the presence of some morbid condition to which the application of water may be inappropriate or inju-

rious. In certain cases of *eczema* and some other forms of skin disease, water aggravates the symptoms. Also in great *cardiac weakness*, and in certain cases of *neurasthenia*, the neutral bath is depressing, and must be avoided, or at least employed with exceeding care and caution, and accompanied by supplementary procedures, such as cold friction, the wet-sheet rub, and the cold precordial compress over the heart.

THE CONTINUOUS BATH.

1136 The continuous bath (Fig. 66) is simply a neutral bath prolonged for many hours, days, weeks, or months, as the case may require.

Method.—A suitable bath-tub must be provided, and should be placed in a well-ventilated and convenient apartment with suitable arrangements for changing the water as may be required for cleanliness and regulation of the temperature. The ordinary bath-tub, without accessories, will not answer the purpose, for the reason that the patient soon becomes weary with the effort to support himself, or is inconvenienced by the pressure of his tissues against the hard metal or porcelain surfaces of the tub. The arrangement should be such that the patient may be as fully as possible at ease. This requires that he should be suspended by some arrangement resembling a hammock. A closely woven hammock, covered with a blanket, may be used for the purpose, or a strong linen sheet may be employed. The hammock may be suspended from hooks attached to the walls of the room, being allowed to sag into the bath-tub sufficiently to submerge the patient. The sheet may be supported in proper position by means of a frame with pegs or holes properly adjusted to the top of the tub. By means of strong tapes attached to the sheet, it may be fastened to the frame in such a way as to maintain the patient's body in the most comfortable and restful position.

In emergency, and while better arrangements are being perfected, the patient may be made comparatively comfort-

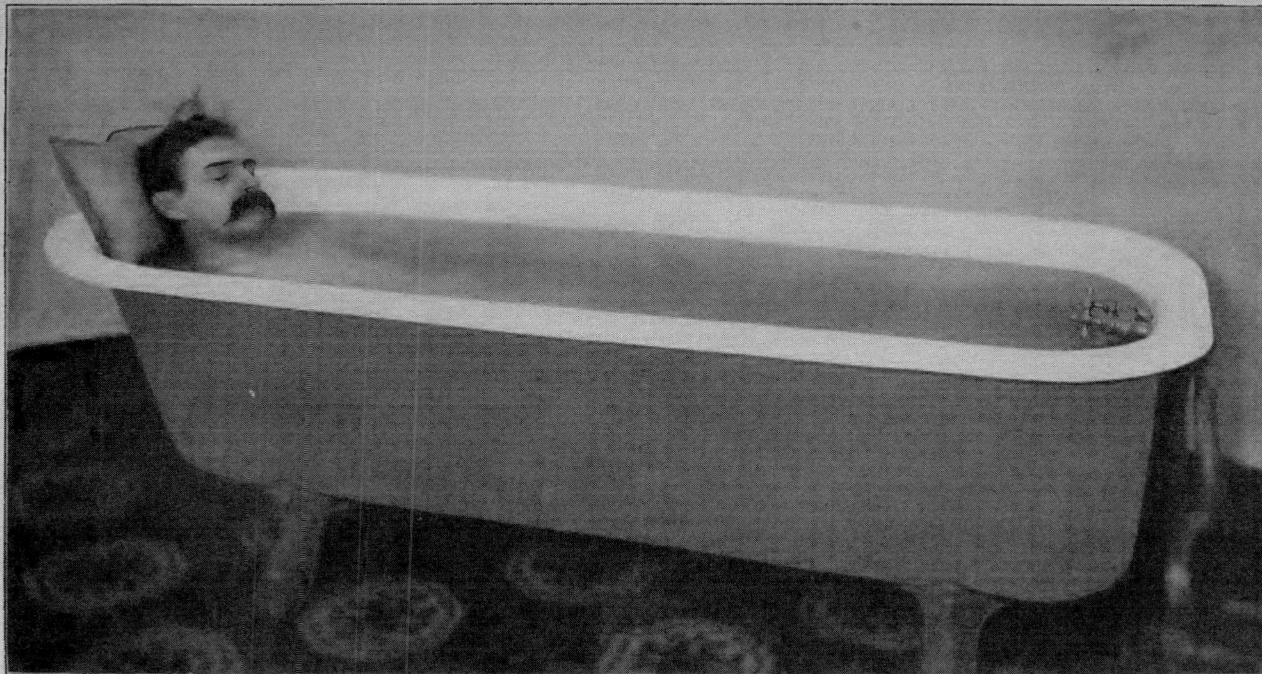

Fig. 66. CONTINUOUS BATH (p. 556).

able by means of one or more blankets folded and placed in the bottom of an ordinary bath-tub, or better still, by means of air pillows filled with water of the same temperature as the bath, or several large water-bags placed in the bottom of the tub so as to support the hips, shoulders, and heels. Pillow-cases filled with excelsior, such as is used for mattresses, or curled hair, may be employed in the same way. The head should be properly supported, and care should be taken that the shoulders are constantly covered with water to prevent chilling by evaporation and the consequent pulmonary congestion which is almost certain to result from prolonged cooling of these important reflex areas.

The temperature of the water should be 94° to 95°, the average neutral temperature. On first entering the bath, the patient may be very gently rubbed for one or two minutes, to prevent the preliminary contraction of the cutaneous vessels which sometimes occasions at first a slight disturbance of the general circulation. The temperature of the bath may be maintained by dipping out a portion of the water from time to time, and adding either hot or cold water, as may be required to bring the temperature to the neutral point. By covering the bath, cooling by evaporation may be prevented, and the necessary reduction in temperature may be readily effected by putting into the bath bottles or jugs filled with ice-water. A jug containing three quarts of ice-water will lower the temperature of a forty-gallon bath one degree.

The duration of the bath will differ according to the character of the case. When employed for temperature reduction or to control delirium, pain, peripheral hyperesthesia, nervous excitability, or mania, a few hours (at most ten or twelve hours) will usually suffice to accomplish the result desired. In continued fevers, and in organic affections of the brain and spinal cord, for which the bath may be employed, it is sufficient in most cases to keep the patient in the bath during the greater part of the day, allowing him to rest in bed at night. But in cases of extensive burns, bed-sores, and certain forms of skin disease, it is often necessary to make the bath absolutely continuous, removing the patient only long enough at proper intervals to allow opportunity for evacuation of the bowels and bladder. In a few instances, the bath has been continued for an entire year, and even longer. There is no reason why life might not be prolonged indefinitely in this bath so far as the normal performance of all the vital functions of the body is concerned, as the bath interferes with no vital process. The water of the bath should be entirely changed every twenty-four hours.

1137 **Physiological Effects.**—Riess, who made a careful study of this bath in the city hospital of Berlin, in the years 1874 to 1876, maintained that the physiological effects of the bath are negative, affecting neither pulse, temperature, nor respiration. More recent observations have, however, shown that the pulse is slowed by the bath, and that other bodily functions are affected, if not profoundly, at least to a noticeable and important extent. As in the neutral bath, the cutaneous nerves imbibe moisture, not through the absorption of water from the bath, but by retention of water through the suspension of perspiration. The urine is noticeably increased in quantity, and becomes less acid or even alkaline. The higher the temperature of the bath, the greater the alkalinity, as shown by Jardet. At the neutral temperature there is practically no absorption of water nor of substances contained in the water. There is only suspended perspiration.

1138 **Therapeutic Applications.**—Hebra was one of the first among scientifically trained physicians to make use of the continuous bath.* When studying skin diseases in Vienna with Hebra, Jr., and Professor Kaposi, Hebra's successor in 1883, the author found the continuous bath in systematic use. One patient then in the hospital had been in the bath more than a year. Hebra reported five hundred cases,—of *variola*, *pemphigus*, *burns*, and *gangrene* of the *skin*,—and showed that most excellent results were obtainable by this therapeutic procedure.

*Hebra, *Wien. Med. Woch.*, 1877, also 1865, pp. 893, 920, 940.

Passavant, of Frankfort, reports most gratifying success in the treatment of extensive burns with the continuous bath. According to his experience, pain is almost instantly relieved by immersion in the neutral bath, the patient remaining comfortable so long as submerged.

Riess,* of Berlin, made a special study of the influence of the continuous bath upon internal maladies of various sorts, as well as in the treatment of typhoid and other fevers. In the treatment of over eight hundred cases of typhoid fever he secured a death-rate of 8.5, a much better record than that shown by the statistics of any other hospital in the city. He employed a temperature of 88° in fever cases, and administered the bath whenever the temperature rose to 102°, keeping the patient in the bath continuously until the temperature was brought down to 100°, and returning him to the bath as soon as the original temperature was reached. The continuous tepid bath presents the following advantages over the cold bath, as shown by Riess, together with some possible disadvantages: —

1. It is less disagreeable to the patient; indeed, it occasions him no inconvenience, and is generally welcomed, while the cold bath is received only under vigorous protest.

2. It involves no risk of injury to the heart in cardiac weakness, nor to the brain in arteriosclerosis, and can be used in many cases in which the cold bath must be interdicted.

3. It affords more prompt relief to cerebral and nervous symptoms, these features, when present, disappearing almost altogether with the first bath.

4. Cyanosis and other evidences of disturbance of the circulation do not occur.

5. The temperature is reduced slowly, hence temperature reduction is more permanent, there being no increased heat production by thermic reaction.

6. The duration of the disease is decidedly shortened, the

---

* Riess, *Arch. für Klin. Med.*, 1889, 1890.

average stay in the hospital, with Riess's eight hundred cases, being less than eighteen days.

7. All the symptoms of the disease are mitigated to a marked degree.

8. The labor of caring for the patient is greatly lessened, which is a boon to the patient as well as to the attendant.

It is true that the continued bath does not afford that degree of cardiac stimulation or excitation of vital resistance which is developed by the cold bath; but this is largely compensated for by the increased activity of the kidneys and skin which is secured by the continuous bath, a fact of primary importance, since the symptoms of cardiac weakness which are often so pronounced in continued fevers, are to be properly attributed not so much to actual exhaustion of the heart as to the profoundly depressing effects of the toxins characteristic of the special malady present and the retention of tissue wastes resulting from diminished oxidation. When desired, however, any required degree of cardiac or general vital stimulation may be secured by the occasional application of the Brand bath, when not contraindicated, or by the cold friction, the cold-towel rub, or the cold wet rubbing sheet in bed.

The large clinical experience of Riess showed that the continuous bath possesses powerful curative virtues in all affections of the brain and the spinal cord which are at all curable, as in cases of exudate from inflammations, as in *meningitis*, and mitigates the symptoms to a wonderful degree even in the most intractable and incurable cases. The measure proved decidedly beneficial in cases of *spinal sclerosis*, *locomotor ataxia*, *paraplegia*, *hemiplegia*, *apoplexy*, and *chorea*. It was found equally helpful in the treatment of *intractable sciatica* and *cutaneous hyperesthesias*, affecting a cure in cases which had resisted all other measures. In *delirium* and *mania*, it exercised a phenomenal sedative effect, was highly beneficial in *dropsy* and in *chronic diarrhea*, and afforded excellent results in *chronic rheumatism*. No remedy has been found more useful in *bed-sores*. Its results in other functional nervous disorders suggest its possible value in *epilepsy*.

Dauchez* reports complete relief from *hysteria* with extremely grave gastric symptoms. The patient was immediately relieved by the tepid bath in four to eight hours, and in three weeks was well.

The principal patrons of Leukerbad, Switzerland, where the neutral bath is administered to many scores of persons in great tanks for several hours a day, are *irritable neurasthenics, rheumatics,* and persons suffering from *psoriasis* and *eczema.* That many are cured is evident from the fact that these famous old baths still retain their popularity, notwithstanding their comparative inaccessibility, and the powerful competition of the more fashionable resorts in Germany and Bohemia. When the author visited these baths, some seventeen years ago, although the season had yet scarcely opened, multitudes were already flocking there, to avail themselves of what they supposed to be the specific virtues of the mineral ingredients of the bath, by which, however, they were not at all likely to be benefited, since at the temperature at which the baths are given (95° to 98°) the movement of fluids is toward the surface of the body, so that absorption can not take place to any appreciable degree.

The partial continuous bath, which renders such signal service in certain surgical cases, will receive attention elsewhere in this work **(1303)**.

Hebra employed the continuous neutral bath for many days, and even months, in hundreds of cases of *skin diseases,* especially in *pemphigus* and *extensive burns.* When the continuous neutral bath is to be employed, the precaution should be taken to rub the skin with vaseline at least once a day, to avoid unpleasant effects from the prolonged maceration of the skin in water.

In employing the continuous bath, care should be taken

**Bull. Gen. de Therap.*, 1884, p. 153.

to apply oil or vaseline to the surface of the body to avoid excessive maceration of the skin.

The continuous bath is certainly a hydriatic procedure of great value, and one worthy of more attention than it has received from the profession in this country.

THE EFFERVESCENT BATH.

1139 This consists of a full bath the water of which contains chloride of calcium, carbonate of soda, and carbonic acid gas. The effervescent bath is administered at the famous resort of Nauheim, Germany, by the aid of natural mineral water which is heavily charged with carbonic acid gas and contains in solution a large amount of chloride of calcium. The author was, through the courtesy of Dr. Schott, afforded an excellent opportunity of studying this bath and its effects at the principal bathing houses at Nauheim; and, having for a number of years made use of the artificial Nauheim bath in a similar manner at the Battle Creek Sanitarium, he feels confident that just as good effects are obtainable from the artificially prepared bath as from the natural mineral water of Nauheim.

1140 An artificial effervescent or Nauheim bath may be prepared by adding to ordinary water carbonate of soda, chloride of calcium, chloride of sodium, and hydrochloric acid, in proper proportions. The effects obtained from a bath thus prepared are practically identical with those obtained from the use of the natural Nauheim water.

Method.—The bath is given in three grades, the intensity and stimulating effect of which are progressively increased with the increasing proportion of the chemical substances which they contain. The composition of these several grades is as follows for a bath of forty gallons:—

1. Chloride of sodium, 4 lbs.; chloride of calcium, 8 lbs.; sodium bicarbonate, $^1/_2$ lb.; to which is added commercial hydrochloric acid (25 per cent.), $^3/_4$ lb.

2. Chloride of sodium, 8 lbs.; chloride of calcium, 12 lbs.; sodium bicarbonate, 1 lb.; commercial hydrochloric acid, 1½ lbs.

3. Chloride of sodium, 12 lbs.; chloride of calcium, 20 lbs.; sodium bicarbonate, 2 lbs.; commercial hydrochloric acid, 3 lbs.

When a copper tub is employed, the amount of bicarbonate of soda must be increased about one fourth, to protect the copper from the action of the hydrochloric acid.

In the preparation of the bath, the chloride of sodium, chloride of calcium, and bicarbonate of soda are first dissolved in the water, and the hydrochloric acid, the quantity of which should be fifty per cent. greater than the bicarbonate of soda, is then added. The effervescence may be produced rapidly or slowly, as desired.

For slow effervescence, place the bottle containing the acid, with stopper removed, at the bottom of the bath, laying it down upon the bottom, and moving it around from time to time. The bath will be ready in two or three hours. For rapid effervescence, invert the bottle without removing the stopper, place the mouth of the bottle just below the surface of the water, withdraw the stopper, and move the bottle about over the surface of the bath, so as to distribute a uniform layer of acid. By this means, the bath may be prepared in five minutes. Its temperature should be 92° F.

Hydrochloric acid may be dispensed with by employing 1141
the substances indicated in the formula given on the next page, the intensity of the application being regulated by the number of powders used, one, two, or three powders being employed, according to the effect desired. The powders are graduated in such a way as to give three degrees of cutaneous stimulation, according to the strength of the solution formed by dissolving them in the water of an ordinary full bath. No harm is done to tin-lined copper tubs.

FORMULA FOR ONE POWDER.

℞

Sodium carb. (sal-soda)	1½ lbs.
Sodium bicarb	½ lb.
Calcium chloride	3 lbs.
Sodium chloride	2 lbs.
Sodium bisulphate	1 lb.

Mix and dissolve the first four ingredients; then add slowly the sodium bisulphate, which should be kept by itself. It is not desirable to produce very marked effervescence, but rather to secure the saturation of the water of the bath with CO_2.

The carbonic acid gas is produced by this formula very slowly, so that it is nearly all absorbed by the water, thus making the method an economical one. It should be remembered that it is the CO_2 dissolved in the water, and not that which escapes by effervescence, that produces the desired effect upon the skin.

Generally the bath should be taken two or three days in succession each week, then one day's respite be allowed. With persons in good strength, four or five successive baths may be given.

1142 **Physiological Effects.**—In the effervescent bath the thermic and circulatory reactions produced by an ordinary water bath at the same temperature is supplemented by powerful reflex vasomotor effects resulting from the irritation or stimulation of the skin by the carbonic acid gas, the chloride of calcium, and the chloride of sodium in solution in the water. Chloride of calcium and CO_2 are by far the most active of the several chemical substances present. These substances stimulate the cutaneous circulation to a high degree without provoking thermic reaction, and in this way a powerful derivative or revulsive effect is produced. The viscera are relieved of congestion; the activity of the peripheral vessels greatly lessens the labor of the heart, and secures a better distribution and more active movement of the blood throughout the body; the skin is stimulated to increased activity, thus lessening the labor of the kidneys.

Therapeutic Applications.—The increased activity of the 1143
surface circulation, through dilatation of the cutaneous blood-vessels, produces a powerful derivative and revulsive effect upon the viscera. In this respect the effervescent bath at a neutral temperature accomplishes the same result as does the very hot bath or the Scotch douche, and has the advantage that the extreme temperature is avoided, a matter of great importance in cases of *cardiac weakness* with *dilatation*, and in *chronic nephritis*, since in both these cases very hot and very cold baths must be avoided. In *weakness of the heart*, hot baths are contraindicated because of the harmful excitation first produced and the secondary depressing effect. Cold baths are equally damaging because of the increased labor brought upon the heart by the contraction of the cutaneous vessels before reaction appears. In cases of *renal disease*, the diseased organs are likely to suffer serious injury from the temporary congestion resulting from the contraction of the surface vessels.

An ordinary water bath at a neutral temperature is incapable of calling into activity the reflexes essential for decided revulsive or derivative effects. By the warming of the skin through the strong circulatory reaction produced, a lower temperature is tolerated without shivering, and thus a decided tonic effect upon the heart and vessels is realized from the neutral bath, a fact of much importance in the treatment of cases of cardiac insufficiency with dilatation. The author has for more than a quarter of a century been decidedly opposed to the use of mineral waters of all descriptions, as wholly unscientific in principle; but from his personal experience at Nauheim, he feels compelled to admit that, in this one instance at least, the presence of mineral salts in the water effects certain advantageous results worthy of recognition; and the effervescent bath has given, in his hands, most excellent results, even in some very extreme cases of cardiac disease with dilatation. Dropsy soon disappears, the heart lessens its volume, sometimes to the extent of one fourth its size during a single bath, and all the symptoms improve, many times to the extent of complete disappearance. Equally good results are obtained in renal affections. Not infrequently albumin disappears entirely from the urine, and dropsical and other symptoms also disappear, so that the patient is brought to a condition of comparative health. Graduated manual Swedish movements and a special dietary must be employed in connection with the baths.

Schott,* who has made a study of the Nauheim baths for more than twenty years, claims them to be very efficient in the cure of cardiac and renal cases. He has even seen old valvular murmurs disappear entirely under treatment by these baths.

In illustration of the power of the effervescent bath to influence the dilated heart in a favorable way, several illustrations are presented herewith, showing the diminution in size which may be secured by this means, and that often in a remarkably short space of time (Figs. 67, 68, 69). The author has seen the area of cardiac dulness diminish nearly an inch in diameter after an effervescent bath in a case of marked cardiac dilatation and loss of compensation.

1144 **Precautions.**—In the employment of the effervescent bath, care should be taken to avoid exhausting the patient, especially in cases of cardiac disease. The breathing of the patient should be quiet when the bath is entered. If considerable dyspnea is present from walking to the bath, the breathing should be allowed to become tranquil before the bath is administered. The chest should be wet before entering the bath, and the limbs should be well rubbed during the process. With very feeble patients, this bath should be administered only every other day. To those a little stronger it may be given two or three days in succession, but even the strongest

* *Blätter Klin. Woch.*, 1880, 17, 35, 7-9, 372, 4. *Medical Record*, March 11 1899, p. 345.

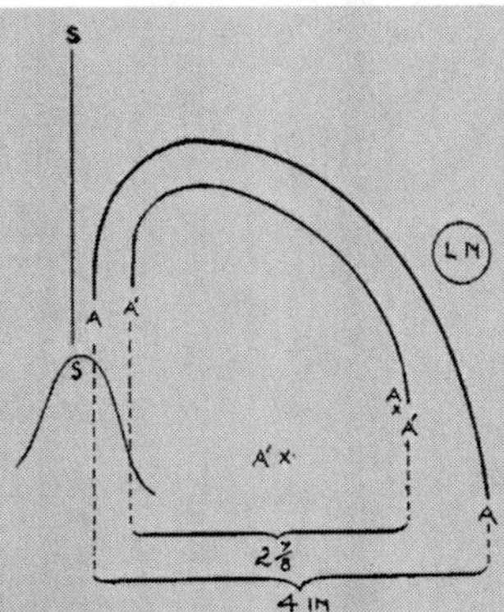

FIG. 67. Outline of Dilated Heart, (*a*) before Treatment; (A′) after Treatment (p. 566).

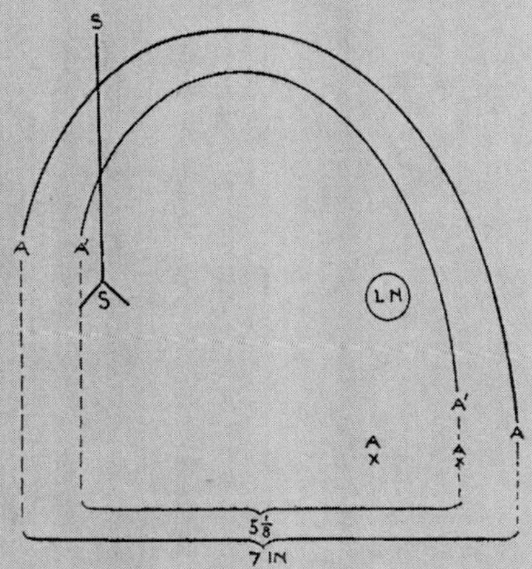

Fig. 68. Outline of Dilated Heart (A) before and (A′) after Effervescent Bath (p. 566).

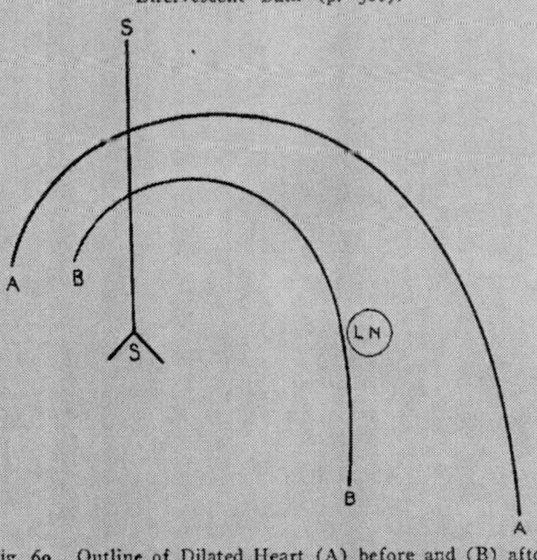

Fig. 69. Outline of Dilated Heart (A) before and (B) after Effervescent Bath (p. 566).

patient should not take more than three baths in succession without a day's interval.

At the beginning and before the patient's susceptibility is known, it is best to start with the mildest bath, increasing the quantity of the chemical ingredients as he becomes accustomed to the measure. In the case of very sensitive persons, the temperature may be made a little higher (94° or 95°). It is important that the patient should not become chilled during the bath.

THE SURGE BATH.

This bath is given in a rocking tub (Fig. 70). The tem- 1145
perature of the water employed should be from 60° to 75°. The effects are intermediate between those of the ordinary full bath at the temperature named and the sea bath. Reaction occurs more quickly than in the ordinary full bath, allowing the use of a temperature from five to eight degrees lower.

Therapeutic Applications.—The surge bath at 60° for 15 1146
or 20 seconds is a powerfully tonic measure, well adapted to robust patients. The bath should be used following a heating bath of some sort, as the wet-sheet pack, an electric-light bath, a hot shower, or some similar procedure.

SEA BATHS.

The sea bath is a measure of great value from both a 1147
hygienic and a therapeutic standpoint. Under this head we may consider the swimming bath, and baths taken in natural bodies of water, whether in lakes, rivers, or the sea.

Method.—The sea bath may be a simple immersion, or a swimming bath in which the effects of the bath are combined with exercise. The length of the bath must depend upon the temperature of the water, and upon the individual's susceptibility, or whether he has been accustomed to the baths. Ordinarily, the duration of the bath at first should not be more than 3 to 5 minutes. Later, it may be increased to 20 or 30 minutes, but should seldom be longer than this. The effects of the sea bath are essentially those of the full bath at a slightly higher temperature. The saline constituents of sea water encourage circulatory reaction, as does also the exercise which is commonly taken with the bath.

1148 **Therapeutic Applications.**—This bath is especially useful as a tonic or restorative measure, for which purpose it is employed by many thousands of people who visit seaside resorts during the summer season. Many persons are injured by the sea bath through neglect of the common rules which should always be observed with reference to cold bathing. The following precautions are especially important:—

1. The bath should not be taken within an hour before or after eating a meal.

2. The bath should not be taken when a person is exhausted from either mental or muscular effort, or through loss of sleep, or if he is nervously weak from any other cause.

3. On first entering the water, a slight chill occurs, which, however, quickly disappears as reaction sets in. The bather should not remain in the water until the second chill appears, as the reaction from the second chill will be imperfect, and the result will be languor, lassitude, stiffness in the muscles and joints, and depression with possibly various nervous symptoms. Gentle rubbing must be continuous to prevent chill.

4. When the bather emerges from the water, he should receive a spray or shower douche at a temperature ten or fifteen degrees below the temperature of the sea, and should afterward be thoroughly dried and vigorously rubbed. The cold douche following the bath should be of short duration, not more than 3 or 4 seconds.

5. The bather should dry quickly, and afterward exercise with moderate vigor for 15 or 20 minutes, or until the circulation is thoroughly established.

If the bath is succeeded by cold feet or hands, headache, chilliness, lassitude, sleepiness, or other unpleasant symptoms, it is probable that it was too long continued, or that some of the foregoing rules have been violated.

MUD BATHS.

In this bath, the patient lies in a tub surrounded with mud of about the consistency of thick gruel or mush. The muds used for this purpose usually contain saline and alkaline substances, which act upon the skin, stimulating the peripheral circulation. The effects of course vary somewhat according to the ingredients of the particular mud employed. The mineral substances are not absorbed from the mud, as is generally supposed, but simply act upon the skin. The effect is consequently in some cases similar to that of the effervescent bath. 1149

Therapeutic Applications.— The mud bath is most often employed in cases of rheumatism and gout. Many persons are doubtless helped by its use, but the benefit received is not greater than might be obtained from the scientific use of water without the mud.

THE BRAND BATH.

This bath (Fig. 71), which is generally meant when a cold bath is spoken of in the treatment of typhoid fever, differs from the ordinary cold bath in several particulars. The routine procedure as employed by Brand and his disciples in the treatment of continued fever cases is as follows: — 1150

Method.— The bath-tub, containing water at a temperature of 65° to 70°, is placed near the bed. The patient is lifted from the bed into the tub as quickly as possible, the face and head having been previously cooled by the application of water at 50°. Care should be taken to immerse the patient to the neck. Exposure of the shoulders is likely to give rise to pulmonary complications. The head should be protected by a towel wet in ice-water and wrapped about the head in such a way as to form a sort of trough leading down the back of the head. On entering the tub the patient is rubbed vigorously for two or three minutes, then sits up for a few seconds while two or three gallons of water at 50° are poured upon his head and allowed to run down the back of his neck. He then lies down again, and the rubbing is repeated. At the end of five minutes the affusion to the head is repeated, and the rubbing continued.

If there is weakness of the heart, the cold water should also be poured upon the front of the chest. The rubbing of the patient should be continued during the whole bath. When the patient first enters the bath, he often experiences extremely unpleasant sensations. Respiration is gasping and difficult. This inconvenience is at once relieved when the cold water is poured over the head. The bath is continued from 10 to 20 minutes. If employed for infants or old persons, the bath should be very short. If the skin becomes cyanotic, or if marked shivering or chattering of the teeth occurs, the patient should be quickly removed from the bath, snugly wrapped in a sheet, and covered with a blanket. A hot bottle should be placed at his feet if cold, and the limbs should be rubbed. Reaction soon takes place, and the skin is reddened by the increased movement of blood through it. The patient's temperature falls from half a degree to two or three degrees. The bath is usually repeated at the end of three hours or sooner — whenever the rectal temperature reaches 102°. The author prefers not to allow the temperature to rise above 101.5° before administering an antipyretic bath of some sort. This rule may be easily adhered to during the whole course of the fever, except, possibly, during the developmental stage of the disease, when the temperature is rising.

Although this bath is a most effective and valuable therapeutic procedure, and one which is much used, its rationale is comparatively little understood; it will therefore be worth while here to devote space to a special consideration of its physiological and therapeutic effects, that there may be a thorough appreciation of their bearing upon the management of febrile disorders.

It is certainly a mistake to govern the employment of hydric procedures altogether by the temperature in febrile

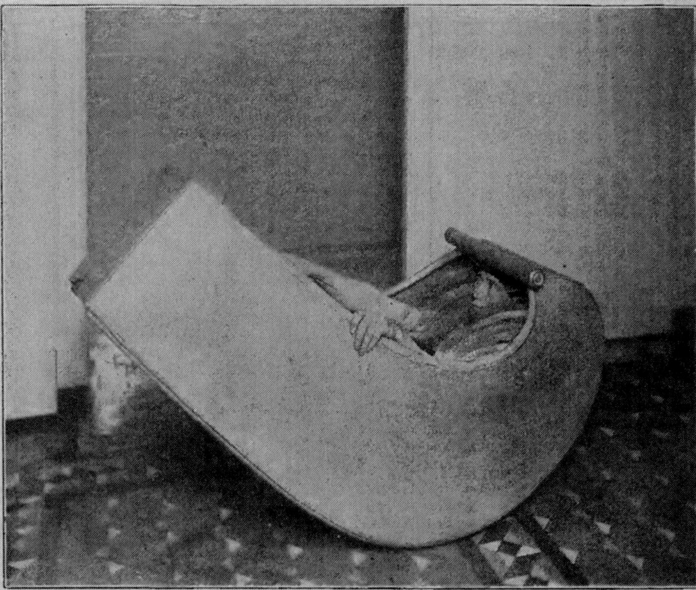

FIG. 70. SURGE BATH (p. 567).

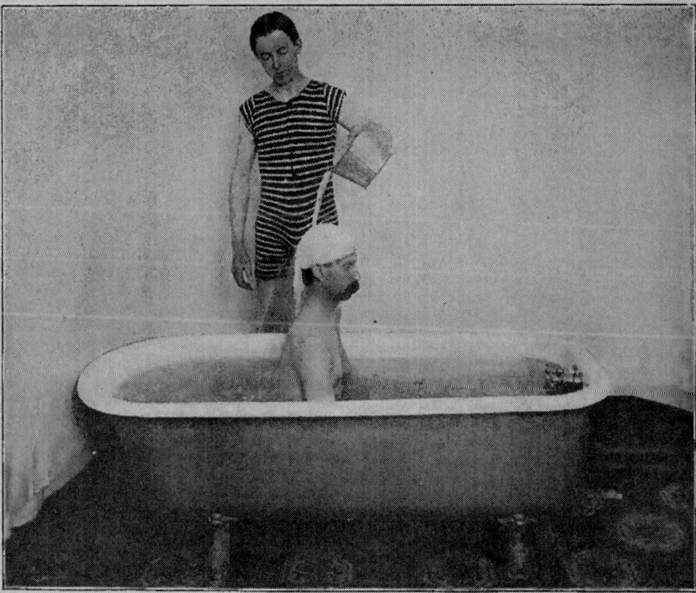

FIG. 71. BRAND BATH (p. 569).

cases. In typhoid fever, it might not be wise to use the cold bath when the temperature is below 102°, but hydric procedures of some sort may be applied; hence the author does not think of confining himself to the use of the Brand bath alone in the treatment of this disease, notwithstanding his high opinion of its value. The most important purpose gained by the use of this application is not the reduction of temperature, but the increase of vital resistance and the elimination of toxins, as Winternitz long ago pointed out.

In rare instances of typhoid fever, the temperature scarcely rises above normal during the whole course of the malady, and yet a fatal issue has sometimes occurred in these cases. This fact alone is sufficient indication of the necessity for the employment of other means than the thermometer as a guide in the direction of therapeutic agents. In cases in which the temperature remains comparatively low because of some peculiarity of the patient's constitution or some unknown factor, there may be as great need as in any possible case for the general vitalizing and tonic effect of cold, which, however, may be obtained by the employment of measures far less vigorous than the Brand bath. It is certainly a patent error to say that if a patient's temperature does not reach 102° or more, there is no call for a bath. The bath is needed for cleanliness, for tonic effects, and to energize and sustain the heart. Cold friction, the cold-towel rub, the tonic wet-sheet pack, and even the half-bath at a moderate temperature, are all measures which may render invaluable service in so-called mild cases of typhoid and other fevers, and should have their place in the therapeutics of febrile disorders.

Physiological Effects.—Applied in the manner indicated, 1151
the effects of the Brand bath are as follows:—

1. General vital resistance is increased.
2. The nerve centers are energized.
3. Muscle tone or excitability is increased.
4. Activity of the kidneys, liver, and skin is increased.

5. The amount of oxygen received and CO_2 exhaled during the bath is nearly three times the normal amount, showing great increase of oxidation.

6. There is marked increase in the blood pressure.

7. The pulse is slowed.

8. The heart is energized.

9. The number of blood-corpuscles in the circulation is increased, especially white corpuscles.

10. The circulation is improved in a number of ways; viz.:—

(*a*) By the primary contraction of the cutaneous vessels and subsequent dilatation, vigorous fluxion is produced in the internal viscera and vessels, which are first made to contract, then to dilate; and then, as dilatation of the skin vessels increases, contraction again takes place, thus wonderfully stimulating the movement of the blood through the body, and correcting any condition of stagnation or hyperemia which may exist in the lungs, liver, spleen, brain, or elsewhere.

(*b*) The excited respiratory movements act in a powerful manner in increasing the movement of blood and lymph in the central nervous system and the abdominal viscera, the diaphragm acting as a blood-pump as well as aiding the processes of respiration.

The friction applied aids the reaction by dilating the vessels of the skin, prevents shivering, and assists heat elimination. The rubbing must not be too violent, as vigorous rubbing will have a tendency to excite heat production. It must be applied with just enough vigor to warm and redden the skin. Strong shivering gives rise to marked increase in heat production. When shivering is prevented by friction, the refrigerant effects of the bath are greatly increased at the same time that the internal congestion is prevented, and the patient is able to endure the bath very much longer, and a more pronounced antipyretic effect is produced.

Cold affusion practiced at intervals during the bath causes contraction of the cerebral vessels, accelerates the movement of the lymph and blood throughout the brain and cord, and thus energizes the nerve centers to a remarkable degree. By the application of cold water to the chest, the respiratory and cardiac centers are also powerfully stimulated.

Therapeutic Applications.— How these effects may be usefully employed in typhoid and all continued fevers will be readily appreciated after considering the conditions and indications present in these disorders. The indications in typhoid fever and most other continued fevers may be briefly stated as follows:— **1152**

1. To sustain vital forces, and increase vital resistance.
2. To destroy and eliminate bacterial toxins and tissue poisons.
3. To increase respiratory activity.
4. To increase oxidation.
5. To augment the activity of the liver.
6. To facilitate the work of the kidneys.
7. To encourage the functions of the skin.
8. To energize the heart.
9. To raise the tone of the peripheral vessels; that is, to energize the peripheral heart.
10. To regulate and increase the movement of the blood through the vessels, preventing visceral congestion and functional failure.
11. To encourage blood formation, and to improve the quality of the blood.
12. To lower the temperature of the body.
13. To ameliorate the sufferings of the patient.
14. To prevent complications.

Let us consider each of these indications somewhat at length.

1. It is not by the high temperature, nor by the patho- **1153**
genic organisms which invade the body, but by the poisons produced by these organisms and by the toxins generated within the body itself, that life is destroyed. These poisons kill by their effect upon the nervous system,— a pernicious

influence which is manifested by headache, delirium, insomnia, weakness, stupor, coma, ataxia, and various other symptoms which point directly toward the great centers of life, the ganglia of the brain and cord. Space does not here permit the detailing at length of the various ways by which the organism defends itself against these toxins, which have been so admirably pointed out by Charrin in his work, "Le Defenses Naturelles de l'Organisme." But a modern study of febrile disorders has shown clearly that the most important thing to be accomplished in dealing with this class of cases is to aid the body in its battle against death by toxemia through support of the organism in every possible way; hence, any measure which increases vital resistance, which replenishes the life forces, which antagonizes the depressing and other toxic influences of the poisons present must be of paramount importance. The fever patient has no appetite because digestive ability is lacking; little or no hydrochloric acid is found in the gastric juice; the secretion of the salivary glands, the pancreas, liver, and other digestive glands is likewise lessened or impaired in quality, and all the nutritive processes are nearly paralyzed. The assimilative activity of the tissues is also weakened as much as is the digestive power of the alimentary canal and accessory organs.

The cold bath rouses to activity the nearly paralyzed nerve centers by the powerful sensory impressions sent inward from the skin; it relieves the congested brain of surplus blood by the powerful fluxion induced, cleansing it from the accumulated poisons by increased movement of fluid in the lymphatics of the brain, and secures conditions favorable to sleep, thus giving the nerve centers a chance for rest and recuperation. And it does more: it increases the activity of the gastric glands, thus encouraging the production of hydrochloric acid, thereby securing both an appetite and the ability to digest the food taken. With improved nutrition, the resisting power of all the cells of the body is increased. This is shown by the clean tongue, the absence of sordes, and the disappearance of fetor in the breath. The bodily forces, thus encouraged, are enabled to maintain the battle against the invading parasites until their life period has run out, or the body, by physiological changes, is rendered an unfavorable habitat for them.

2. In typhoid fever the body is exposed to the noxious influence not only of typhotoxin, a product of the specific germs which characterize this disease, but also other toxins produced by the colon bacillus, and various microbes which thrive in the alimentary canal. Roque and Wile have shown that the quantity of toxins found in the urine of typhoid fever patients is double the normal. The application of the cold bath decreases the toxicity fivefold until convalescence is established. The advantage to the system of thus getting rid of this enormous amount of toxic material can not be overestimated. 1154

The cold bath, by increasing the movement of the blood, and thus stimulating the activity of the entire organism, encourages not only the destruction of germ poisons by those glands which are charged with this special duty, but also their elimination through the various channels which furnish outlets for both physiological and pathological poisons.

3. The increase of respiratory activity reflexly produced by the bath secures a vigorous movement of blood in the pulmonary vessels, thus combating stagnation and preventing hypostatic congestion with its resulting evils. Accumulated mucus is expelled from the small tubes, and the volume of air passed into the lungs is increased to two or three times the ordinary amount. 1155

4. One of the best-known effects of cold applications to the surface is the thermic reaction (460), by means of which there is an increase in all the metabolic processes, and especially in the oxidation processes. This is very important, as in the grave forms of fever there is generally a marked decrease of oxidation. The leucomains, or accumulated typhotoxins, are imperfectly oxidized; and not being reduced 1156

to the perfectly soluble form necessary for elimination, they accumulate in the blood. The retained excretions and accumulated specific poisons, as has been shown by Robin, sometimes augment the amount of extractives from four to twelve per cent., or over three times the normal amount. In ordinary cases of fever these substances have been shown to increase more than fifty per cent. The increased oxidation produced by the cold bath renders these substances soluble, and thus facilitates their elimination, while the increased movement of blood brings them in contact with the organs capable of further changing or removing them. That the increased amount of oxygen introduced by the deeper respiration resulting from the cold bath is utilized, is shown by the fact that the respiratory quotient remains the same; that is, while the amount of oxygen absorbed is three times the usual quantity, the amount of CO_2 eliminated is proportionate to the oxygen absorbed.

1157 5. The liver plays an exceedingly important rôle in fever cases. It is the organ upon which, more than upon any other, perhaps, depends the life of the fever patient. The liver is a sentinel standing at the door of the circulation. The toxins which enter the portal vein from the alimentary canal, as well as those which are in circulation in the blood, when brought to the liver, are held back and destroyed by it to such an extent that by comparison of the blood of the portal vein and that of the hepatic vein, its toxicity is found to have been diminished one half by passing through the liver, as has been proved by Rogers and others. In fever, its functions as a regulator of nutrition, as an excretory organ, as a blood organ, and as a destroyer of toxins, are all in large measure held in abeyance, as is readily shown by the glucose test for hepatic insufficiency. The system is so flooded with poisons as to overwhelm the liver; it becomes congested, its vessels are distended with stagnated blood, its tissues filled with paralyzing poisons, and local pathological processes not infrequently result, as shown by the enlargement so frequent in febrile cases, and the degeneration which is so prominent a feature in the post-mortem changes observed after death from typhoid and other fevers. These degenerative processes, once supposed to be due to the elevated temperature of the blood, are now known to be due to the influence of the toxins with which the blood is filled.

The cold bath, by the strong fluxion of blood which it sets up, empties the vessels of the stagnated and half-paralyzed liver, energizes to renewed activity the poison-benumbed ganglia which control it, arouses to its work the hepatic cell, thus renewing all the functions and maintaining the integrity of this most important viscus, which has been aptly described as a "shut door," preventing the entrance of poisons into the general circulation so long as it retains the full use of its powers.

6. One of the most marked effects of the cold bath is its 1158
influence upon the kidneys. The volume of the urine is sometimes increased two or three times. The kidney, as well as the liver, suffers from the constant contact of the toxins with which it has to deal, as shown by the renal degeneration often found after death from febrile diseases. So long as the kidneys and liver can be kept doing their duty as blood purifiers, the organism has a good chance to hold its own in the battle for life. The cold bath assists the functions of these organs as no other measure does.

7. The dingy, dry, inactive skin of the fever patient, under the influence of the cold bath soon becomes white, moist, and active. The improvement of the cutaneous circulation may be noted from day to day. Nothing could be more marked than the contrast between a fever patient who has been subjected to daily bathing and one who has not enjoyed the advantage of this wonderful regulator of the vital processes. The skin of the latter is dry, leathery, tawny, inactive as parchment, while that of the bathed patient is clear, supple, moist, elastic, lively, and responsive to the thermal and mechanical agents applied for the purpose.

of aiding heat elimination, arousing the nerve centers, and awakening vital resistance. The skin has been shown by Bouchard and others to be an important outlet for highly toxic substances, which are generated in the body under morbid conditions as well as in the physiological state. The marked stimulation of the skin by the contact with cold water, and the friction to which it is subjected, adds a powerful factor to the defenses of the body against the toxins which are poisoning the nerve centers, in addition to the service rendered through the internal reflex actions set up by the impressions made upon the cutaneous nerves, whereby the liver, the suprarenal capsules, and other poison-destroying glands are brought to a high degree of activity.

1159 Brunner has shown * that the active skin is capable of eliminating germs in vast numbers; while Herz has shown that the dry skin transmits very little heat outward; and Leyden, that one of the most important indications in typhoid fever is to encourage the elimination of water, which, as he has demonstrated, accumulates to an abnormal extent in the tissues in this disease. Weyrich has shown that friction of the skin may increase the elimination of water fifty per cent. The moist friction of the cold bath and the increase of skin activity created by it thus meet at one and the same time three important indications presented in typhoid and other infectious fevers; viz.: (1) Increased elimination of moisture through improved blood supply; (2) increased elimination of heat through conduction and evaporation of the moisture of the skin, not only immediately after the bath, but subsequently, as the result of the increased blood supply; (3) increased cutaneous activity and elimination of germs.

1160 8. The cold bath aids the heart to a degree which is unapproached by alcohol, digitalis, strychnia, or any other known agent. It renders a still more valuable service in its influence upon the blood-vessels. The low tension often

---

* Brunner, *Berliner Klinische Wochenschrift*, 1891, page 505.

present in grave febrile conditions is not due alone to the depressing influence of the toxins upon the cardiac centers and the interference with the nutrition of the muscular structures of the body, but is largely, perhaps chiefly, due, as shown by Romberg,* to the loss of tone in the peripheral vessels and the weakening of the vasomotor centers of the medulla. This is indicated by the cyanotic appearance of the face, the blue lips and nails, and the general turgid appearance of the skin.

The condition of the blood stream under these conditions may be compared to that of a stream of water leaving the hose of a fire-engine from which the nozzle has been removed. The machinery itself may be in no way interfered with, but owing to the removal of the resistance against which it has been working, and which acts as a means of regulating its action, the pump "runs away," as the engineer says. The wear and tear to the engine is tremendous, but its cylinders do not fill with water, and the lessened quantity of water pumped is raised only a few feet, and runs away with little force to low levels where there is no resistance.

The same thing happens with the heart when general vasomotor relaxation occurs. An important element in heart regulation is lost. The steadying influence of well-filled vessels and a solid column of blood to work against being no longer in operation, the heart flies away in rapid, ineffective movements, and the blood stream flows off in the shortest circuits instead of filling the whole system. The natural result is congestion of the great vascular internal viscera, the liver, lungs, and kidneys, as well as the brain and spinal cord.

Under these circumstances the heart may be compared, as Hare has suggested, to a locomotive which has steam up, and is in a condition to do a tremendous amount of work, but because of the slipperiness of the track makes no headway in pulling the train, its wheels only flying around like a spinning

---

* *Berliner Klin. Woch.*, 1895.

top, doing no effective work. A little sand on the track, however, changes the whole situation by affording the resistance necessary to regulate the action of the engine. The wheels move slowly and steadily, the steam cylinders have time to fill, and the energy in the steam is utilized.

These illustrations are not wholly exact, since in the case of the pump and the locomotive the machine may remain wholly intact, while in the case of the heart this is not true. The heart depends for its energy upon the constant filling and flushing of its vessels. When the blood pressure is low, its nutrition suffers in consequence. Blood accumulates in the dilated vessels, so that the volume passing through the heart is diminished; the whole blood stream is slowed; it becomes filled with waste products, and may be compared to a stagnant or sluggish stream of water in which filth accumulates. In consequence of this slow movement, the action of the liver, kidneys, skin, lungs, and other poison-destroying organs is interfered with, and the heart is worn out by its constant ineffective work. Its period of rest may be diminished perhaps one third or more. Under these defective conditions for nutrition and rest, its energy rapidly fails, so that a vicious circle is formed. The low pressure weakens the heart, and the weakened heart still further decreases the pressure. In this condition, without relief of some sort, the patient must rapidly sink into collapse, followed by complete syncope and death from so-called heart failure. The cause of the failure is not, however, primarily with the heart, but in the vessels, as suggested by Romberg, and further demonstrated by Paessler.* The importance of the researches of Romberg and Paessler can scarcely be overestimated, for they show us at once the folly of seeking to correct the morbid condition known as cardiac weakness or failure, when present in acute febrile disorders, by the administration of drugs to excite or stimulate the heart. To do this is like putting on more steam

*"Kongress für innere Medicin," Weisbaden, 1896, pp. 256, 266.

pressure when the pump is running away or the locomotive wheels slipping on the track. Nature has provided us with a most admirable remedy in an external agent; viz., cold, which strikes at the root of the evil, and is attended by no ill effects. It is only necessary that these facts should become known to the medical profession to secure for cold water the universal recognition which intelligent men are always ready to accord a great truth that has for its basis a fundamental law of nature.

9. Cold applications to the skin cause contraction of the 1161
small arteries throughout the body, and this instantly raises the blood pressure. Cold excites the activity of the heart also, so that at first it beats not only with more vigor but with greater frequency. As a result, the blood-vessels are rapidly filled, blood pressure is raised, and the liver, kidneys, and other excretory organs are flushed with blood and encouraged to do their normal work, thus rapidly diminishing the amount of poison taken into the blood. The nutrition of the heart is also improved; and with the higher tension its movements are slowed, so that its periods of rest are increased; while at the same time the small vessels, constituting the peripheral heart, by their increased activity, accelerate the movement of blood, thus lessening the work of the heart. While by this combination of factors the heart's work is decreased, the energy of its action is increased, as is also its power to work, *by the improved conditions under which it labors;* so that, instead of a vicious circle, there is soon organized a group of influences which steadily improve the condition not only of the heart but of all the tissues, thus enormously increasing the power of the body to resist the disease and expel the invading organisms and their toxic products.

10. The increased movement of blood throughout the 1162
body, and especially the fluxion of the visceral vessels, occasioned by the several vascular movements set up, — first brief contraction, then a longer dilatation from retrostasis of the blood from the skin, and lastly a considerably prolonged con-

traction due to the filling of the surface vessels when reaction occurs,—antagonize in the most powerful way the tendency to visceral congestion with stagnation of blood, failure of local nutrition and function, and the multiple mischiefs flowing out of the disturbance of the activity of the organs essential to the maintenance of organic life.

1163 11. The effect of the cold bath upon the blood must certainly exert a potent favorable influence in febrile disease. As has been shown by Winternitz and various other observers, the number of corpuscles in circulation in the blood may be at once increased by the cold bath to the extent of twenty-five per cent., or even more; and Thayer* has shown that this effect follows the administration of cold baths in typhoid fever as well as in health.

In fever the number of corpuscles is greatly diminished, consequently the oxygen-carrying power of the blood is proportionately diminished. The area of the corpuscles circulating in the blood of a healthy person is about 3,100 square yards. With the reduced blood count of fever, this oxygen-absorbing area may be reduced to 2,000 square yards or less. If this area can be increased two thirds, or brought up to nearly the normal amount, the oxygen-absorbing power, and consequently the oxidizing power of the blood, may be proportionately increased. It is interesting in this connection to recall the fact that the white corpuscles are increased in number to a greater extent than are the red corpuscles by cold applications. The leucocytes play an important rôle as defenders of the body, in destroying microbes, while the serum destroys bacterial toxins. From these facts it is readily apparent that the action of the cold bath in increasing the number of corpuscles in circulation serves a most important purpose in sustaining the body in its conflict. What other agent known to man is capable of rendering such service as this? *Antipyrine and antipyretics of all sorts diminish the*

---

* *Johns Hopkins Hospital Bulletin*, Balt., 1893, IV, 37-40.

blood count instead of increasing it, and thus greatly lessen the oxidizing power of the blood.

12. Liebermeister * has shown that heat production is 1164
increased in fever, while Winternitz has demonstrated that heat elimination is decreased, at least in many cases. It is apparent that the greatest degree of elevation of temperature would be produced by the co-existence of increased heat production with diminished heat elimination. The cold bath renders an important service in reducing the temperature, although this is not by any means the most valuable of its effects. The elevation of the temperature in fever is without doubt a conservative or protective action by the vital forces, it having been clearly shown that the elevation of temperature accompanying infectious disorders serves a most useful purpose in establishing immunity, by rendering the body an unfavorable habitat for the invading parasites.

However, the importance of lowering the temperature in fever, even one or two degrees, or a fraction of a degree, is shown by the investigations of Maurel,† according to which the white blood-corpuscles are destroyed at a temperature of 109° to 111° within an hour, and are able to survive at a temperature of 107.6° to 109.4° for only three hours. When it is remembered that the internal temperature of the body is two or three degrees higher than the axillary temperature, it is evident that whenever the patient's axillary temperature reaches 105° to 106°, his life is in imminent danger. The lowering of the body temperature one or two degrees in such a case may be the immediate means of saving life.

Another consideration of importance is the fact that elevation of body temperature gives rise to increased oxidation of nitrogen, causing rapid wasting of the muscular, nervous, and glandular structures of the body. This weakening of vital structures is one of the chief sources of danger in febrile diseases. Here is a frequent cause of cardiac failure, and of

* Liebermeister, *Deutsch. Arch.*, 1868, v. V, p. 217.

† *La Semaine Médicale.*

many other grave conditions which accompany ataxic and adynamic febrile states.

The cold bath lowers the temperature of the body not simply by abstracting heat or by dilating the surface vessels, but by aiding in the removal of the conditions which give rise to the elevation of temperature; in other words, it strikes at the causes of the condition, and is hence not merely a symptomatic remedy. The cold bath is thus not only a powerful antithermic agent, but is antifebrile as well, which is more than can be said of any of the medicinal antipyretics; for, while they do lower the temperature, *they do not shorten the duration of the malady, nor lessen its fatality.* While lowering the temperature, they at the same time lessen the vital resistance, stupefy the nerve centers, and weaken the defenses of the body. The cold bath, on the other hand, arouses the dormant nerve centers, energizes all the vital functions, and improves oxygenation and metabolism at the same time that it abstracts superfluous and harmful caloric.

1165 13. Another most important service which the cold bath renders the fever patient is the amelioration of his discomforts. Medical men who have been subjected to this method of treatment while suffering from typhoid and other fevers, have unanimously testified to the comfort which it secures. The application itself is by no means a pleasant procedure; but the relief which it affords, the sense of well-being which it creates, with the decidedly favorable modification of all the morbid conditions characteristic of febrile maladies, speaks so strongly in its favor that intelligent patients readily submit to it, and after the first few baths welcome the arrival of the hour for the treatment.

It is true that nervous, excitable, and illy controlled individuals sometimes resist the treatment, while ignorant friends urge vigorous protests against what seems to them unnecessarily severe and cruel treatment. Their prejudices must be overcome by gentle management and a little tact, which seldom fails to secure their co-operation. The brown, thickly coated, swollen, and parched tongue, the sordes-covered lips and teeth, the catarrh of the stomach and bowels, the tympanitis, flatulence, exhausting diarrhea, headache, mental stupor, nervousness, apprehension, the cadaverous, ocher-colored appearance of the patient are almost never seen when the cold bath has been administered from the very beginning. Indeed, the picture of the disease is so completely changed that one would scarcely recognize it from the typical description in the text-books. If all patients could be taken in hand with thorough hydriatric management within two or three days after the beginning of the attack, or at least before the fifth day, in typhoid fever, the disease would rarely appear in other than its mild form.

14. Lastly, it may be said in behalf of the cold bath as a 1166
remedy in typhoid fever, that its thorough use early in the disease rarely fails to prevent grave complications of any sort, such as pneumonia, myocarditis, nephritis, perforation, intestinal hemorrhage, and the various paralyses and other distressing sequelæ so notoriously frequent in typhoid fever when managed in the usual way. The same is true as regards all the infectious fevers. The prejudice sometimes encountered against the use of cold water, based on the supposition that it increases the liability to pneumonia or other complications, is wholly without foundation. The very opposite, in fact, is true.

In regard to the results of the cold bath in typhoid fever 1167
and other infectious febrile disorders in relation to the saving of lives, a long chapter might be written. A very few statistical facts must here suffice: The ordinary mortality in typhoid fever, as shown by the statistics of our large cities, is 25 to 30 per cent., and a still larger percentage of mortality is not infrequently reported. Brand has collected a series of 1,223 cases in which the cold bath was intelligently employed from the beginning, the treatment having been instituted within the first week. Of these only twelve died, or less than 1 per cent. The mortality in a series of 5,000 cases,

including many in which treatment was not thoroughly applied, was less than 4 per cent. Osler,* of the Johns Hopkins Hospital, reports a very great reduction in mortality from typhoid fever by the adoption of the cold bath treatment. In the experience of the author and his colleagues, which includes several hundred cases of this disease treated by the cold bath and analogous procedures, the mortality has been less than 3 per cent. In pneumonia, the mortality has been reduced more than one half. Schill reports 110 cases of scarlet fever, with no deaths. Remier treated 3,000 cases of scarlet fever with cold baths followed by rubbing, and with a very low mortality rate.† Equally satisfactory results have been obtained in the treatment of smallpox and other infectious fevers.

The Question of Alcohol with the Cold Bath.

In Germany and France it is the almost universal custom to administer alcohol to the patient just before putting him in the cold bath. Some practitioners, as Winternitz, administer but a very small amount, as a single mouthful of wine; while others give brandy in considerable quantities. A few American practitioners also employ brandy freely with the cold bath. The unwisdom of this practice will be apparent on due consideration of the following facts: —

1168 1. One purpose in administering the cold bath is to secure a true stimulant or tonic effect by arousing the vital energies, especially through excitation of the nerve centers of the vasomotor, sympathetic, and cerebrospinal systems. Alcohol was once supposed to be capable of effecting this, and was used for this purpose in typhoid fever and various other morbid conditions accompanied by depression of the vital forces. At the present time, however, it is well known, and with practical unanimity admitted, that alcohol is neither a tonic nor a stimulant, but a narcotic; that it depresses and does not excite; that it lessens, and does not increase, the activity of

* "Johns Hopkins Hospital Reports," p. 321.

† Thomas, *Journal of the American Medical Association*, 1896, p. 1332.

the nerve centers; and that this is true of small as well as large doses, as has been shown by the researches of careful investigators. In evidence of the foregoing may be cited the following statements from medical men recognized as authorities throughout the civilized world: —

Harnack says: "It should also never be forgotten, that, even in small doses, *the paralyzing action of alcohol is exercised most rapidly and energetically upon the tonus of the blood-vessels — the importance of which tonus for the regularity of the circulation and the cardiac energy is well known.*"

Victor Horsley, an eminent English surgeon, speaks thus respecting the influence of alcohol upon the heart: "Surgeons of former days used alcohol extensively to combat shock, but *the old theories of shock have been proved erroneous, and alcohol has consequently become unnecessary. It will be less and less used in the future, and the discredit into which it has fallen is justified.*"

Hermann Frye, by the use of Mosso's ergograph, showed that "*in the unfatigued muscle, alcohol lessens the extent of its maximum contraction*, owing to a lessening of the peripheral irritability of the nervous system."

The heart is a muscle, and consequently alcohol can not be expected to increase its working power; and when laboring under the influence of toxic agents, as in a febrile state, it is clearly evident that the effect of this agent must be distinctly and altogether pernicious.

Chantemesse * calls attention to the diminished toxicity of the urine in many cases of typhoid fever, the toxins being retained in the body during the fever, resulting in an enormous increase of the toxicity of the urine during convalescence. This fact is of great importance in connection with the use of antipyrine and alcohol, which lessens the activity of the kidneys, and so causes still further retention of toxins.

The use of hot coffee, tea, or other medicaments in con-

---

* Bouchard's "Traité de Médecine."

nection with hydriatic procedures is also to be in every way deprecated, as a sort of mixed and antagonistic therapeutics, for which no good scientific reason can be assigned. Coffee, like alcohol, is a narcotic. It lessens the susceptibility of the nerve centers to stimulation by the thermic impressions made upon the skin, and thus lessens the effect of the applications made, as shown in relation to alcohol. When it is desirable that these impressions should be mitigated, this may be accomplished much more effectively and consistently by raising the temperature of the application, or by preparing the skin for the application of cold water by a preceding hot application, either local or general.

In a series of physiological experiments conducted by the author in 1893, and reported at the meeting of the American Medical Temperance Association held at Milwaukee in May, 1893, it was clearly shown that nervous, muscular, and glandular activities are all diminished to a noticeable degree by the ordinary medicinal doses of brandy and other stimulants.*

It is clear, then, that those who administer alcohol before the cold bath, by so doing antagonize the therapeutic activity of the measure, since so far as the alcohol has any effect whatever, it is to depreciate or neutralize the very effect which it is designed to secure by the cold application.

1169 2. The effect of alcohol is to cause dilatation of the peripheral vessels. This it does by paralyzing the vasoconstrictors.

As already stated, paralysis of the peripheral vessels and of the vasomotor centers of the medulla, as shown by Romberg and Paessler, are the real causes of heart failure; hence alcohol, in its effect upon the vasomotor centers and nerves, can only aggravate the very condition for the relief of which it is administered. Alcohol at the same time exercises a like effect upon the accelerator nerves of the heart, which are both anatomically and physiologically associated with the vaso-

* See *Medical Temperance Quarterly*, July, 1893.

constrictors, as Waller has so clearly pointed out. By this means, while the heart's action seems to be freer, the movement of the blood through the systemic circulation is slowed, as is shown by the stasis in the peripheral vessels, which is clearly indicated by the dusky hue of the skin in a man under the influence of alcohol. The influence of alcohol is in this respect somewhat akin to that of the warm bath. The effect of a cold application, however, is the very opposite; viz., the stimulation of the vasoconstrictors. At first this effect is so pronounced that the blood-vessels are almost completely emptied of their contents, and the skin becomes blanched in appearance.

As reaction sets in, the caliber of the blood-vessels is increased, but stimulation of the vasoconstrictors continues in that wonderful rhythmic activity of the small vessels, the peripheral heart, whereby the blood is steadily pumped from the arterial into the venous system, resulting in a bright red flushing of the skin, which indicates an increased flow of the blood through the periphery and an increased rate of movement throughout the whole circulatory system.

3. It is not maintainéd that no preparation for the cold 1170
bath is needed, but rather that there is a far better method than by the use of alcohol. The ideal preparation is to be found in the application of heat. If alcohol in any way aids reaction, it is not by augmenting the activity of the nerve centers, but by encouraging the relaxation of the surface vessels. But this can be accomplished far better by either a general or a local application of heat, as a foot bath, fomentations to the spine, or when convenient, a general application of heat, such as a hot full bath for one or two minutes, a hot-blanket pack, a hot shower, or even hot water drinking or a hot enema, or wrapping the patient in warm woolen blankets for a half hour or so, with hot bags about him. All these are measures whereby the preparation for the cold bath may be accomplished far more efficiently than by any form of medication.

Heat is a natural preparation for cold. The application of heat to the surface vessels is a physiological stimulus whereby the centers are aroused to activity, and the thermic nerves rendered in the highest degree capable of responding to the reflex stimulus which the cold applications communicate to the skin, and through it to the nerve centers.

1171 4. While it is true that the patient *seems* to bear the cold bath better when alcohol is administered, this fact is the strongest kind of argument against the use of alcohol in this connection; for the only way in which alcohol can diminish the shock or lessen the discomfort of the patient in the application of cold water, is by lessening nervous sensibility through its narcotic effect; and just so far as this is accomplished, the effect of the bath is neutralized and its efficacy lessened, for the reason that the whole effect of the cold application depends upon the thermic impression made upon the skin. Thus, *so far as this impression is diminished, the effect of the bath itself is diminished; the combination of such antagonistic measures as alcohol and cold water can not be regarded otherwise than in the highest degree unphilosophical, and from the standpoint of rational therapeutics, absurd.* The practice is one which appeals strongly not only to the prejudices of the laity, but to the predilections of quite too large a proportion of physicians; but not one scientific fact or even plausible apology can be brought forward in support of this practice.

After twenty-five years of extended experience in the use of baths of all temperatures, the author feels justified in taking a most uncompromising stand against the use of alcohol in any form in connection with hydriatic procedures. If there are any two agencies in the world which are absolutely irreconcilable, they are alcohol and water. Their application in conjunction gives, not the sum of two co-operating or complementing agents, but the difference between two neutralizing and antagonistic measures. In any case in which alcohol may seem to be indicated as a means of preparing the patient for the application of a cold bath, heat may be employed to far better advantage, with the certainty of better results, and with absolute physiological consistency.

It is important that a further word be said regarding the employment of the cold bath. The idea that no very decided effects can be obtained from the use of water without resorting to a very low temperature, is certainly an error. The utility of the cold and the very cold bath has certainly been very greatly overrated. In France, Beni-Barde and others have long been contending for the employment of less heroic measures in hydrotherapy, and the more general recognition of the utility of wider ranges of temperatures for hydriatric applications.

A long experience in the practical use of hydrotherapy in the treatment of all classes of ailments, acute and chronic, has convinced the author that very cold general applications, especially if prolonged, are rarely needed, and that far better effects can be obtained by the use of temperatures which do not occasion the patient so much discomfort nor give rise to such apprehension as to constitute a nervous shock either to him or to his friends. The author has never found it necessary to exclude the patient's friends from witnessing any treatment applied because of the alarming or distressing symptoms occasioned by it, and considers that it is entirely unnecessary that any such treatment be employed. Indeed, a measure so violent in character that constant vigilance must be employed to prevent collapse or heart failure can not be regarded as safe to be commended for general use. Putting a patient into a very cold bath and keeping him there until his teeth chatter and there is painful shivering with perhaps cyanotic skin, is a measure which would better be relinquished for other safer and quite as potent procedures, which the science of hydrotherapy is abundantly able to supply.

It is true that by constant rubbing of the patient during the bath and by the strictest attention to the pulse, the color of the surface, and the condition in general, any serious effects from cold applications of water may generally be avoided; but it must be considered that if the desired results can be obtained by the employment of less violent measures, they are certainly to be preferred.

1172 In this connection it should be mentioned that Jacques, of France, reported, in 1839, 313 typhoid fever cases, with only four deaths, treated by means of the cold enema, cold water drinking, and the cold abdominal compress changed every 10 to 30 minutes, while 349 cases treated at the same period by ordinary methods gave a mortality of 91 deaths,* a statistical showing which is scarcely outdone by the most favorable results reported for the Brand treatment.

Scientific therapeutics gives no countenance to routine methods in the treatment of any malady, whether by the use of water or medicinal agents, and the author feels certain that a better acquaintance with the versatile resources of hydrotherapy will lead many practitioners who have regarded cold baths as almost the sole method to be employed in the treatment of infectious fevers, to adopt a much more comprehensive hydriatic armamentarium.

1173 The following excellent suggestions concerning the hydriatic treatment of fevers are from Winternitz, the highest living authority on all subjects pertaining to hydrotherapy:—

1. Give the first bath at a temperature of 75° to 85°, diminishing the temperature of each bath one degree until 65° is reached.

2. During the bath pour over the head and spine water at a temperature two to five degrees lower than the water of the bath. The effect of this will be not only to cool the head but also the bath, and thus secure better reaction.

3. The duration of the first bath should be 3 or 4 minutes. The time may be extended with succeeding baths until the duration is from 10 to 12 minutes. If the first bath is given at as high a temperature as 88°, the duration should be longer, as longer time is required for temperature reduction.

*Bernard, "Leçons sür la Chaleur Animale," Paris, 1876.

4. The number of baths should be three or four daily.

5. The abdominal compress should be worn during the night. It should not be too cold nor too frequently changed, to avoid excessive excitation of the nervous system. The temperature should be ordinarily about 60°, and the compress should be changed about once in 40 to 60 minutes.

6. When the maximum daily temperature begins to decline, the temperature of the bath should be raised to 84° to 88°.

7. Avoid too severe friction on account of excessive stimulating effects.

8. The patient should be left in the bath until the axillary temperature, as felt by the hand, is the same as that of the rest of the body. This is a good indicator of the effects of the bath in lowering temperature.

9. The patient should be immediately removed from the bath at the first symptom of secondary chill. If he is threatened with collapse, a very short bath should be administered every hour until the collapse is no longer threatened.

It is almost needless to add that the application of the cold bath or an equivalent hydric measure should begin at the earliest possible period in the disease, or as soon as decided febrile symptoms make their appearance, both in typhoid and other more infectious maladies, when not contraindicated.

The author employs the bath whenever the temperature reaches 101.5° F., repeating it as often as once in three hours if necessary. Natural and refreshing sleep should not be interrupted for the bath unless the temperature is high and rising rapidly; but the comatose sleep indicating profound intoxication may be interrupted with advantage by the administration of the bath, which will often be followed by normal refreshing sleep for an hour or more.

Contraindications.—Collapse, sub-normal temperature, inability to react, threatened pulmonary or intestinal hemorrhage, hematuria, shivering, sweating, old age, infancy.

The Brand bath is likewise contraindicated in the eruptive fevers, as smallpox and measles. In the author's opinion its use is unwise in *pneumonia*, and in other disorders in which intense inflammation is present in an important internal organ, as in acute *hepatitis*, *salpingitis*, *ovaritis*, *meningitis*, acute *gastritis*, *enteritis*, and especially in the various forms of *nephritis*, either acute or chronic.

THE SHALLOW BATH.

1174 In this procedure (Fig. 72) the patient is rubbed while sitting in a tub partially filled with water. The requisites are, a tub with four or six inches of water of the proper temperature, a sheet, two or three towels, and a large dipper.

Method.—The patient, having been properly prepared,—the feet warm, the general circulation well established by exercise or previous warming in bed or by a warm bath, the head protected by a towel wet with water at 60°,—seats himself in the tub with the legs extended, and immediately begins vigorous rubbing of his arms, chest, and abdomen, while the attendant rubs the back and sides with both hands for 20 seconds, then dips water from the tub and dashes it upon the back for 10 seconds, then rubs 20 seconds, then the patient lies down in the bath while the attendant rubs his legs for 10 seconds. This occupies just one minute. For a two-minute bath, the above is repeated; for a bath of three minutes, the procedure is repeated a third time.

At intervals of one minute the patient should lie down in the bath, so that the whole body except the head is submerged for 5 to 10 seconds, the attendant rubbing the legs vigorously in the meantime.

When employed for tonic effects, the temperature of the water should be 75° to 65°, and the length of the bath 1 to 3 minutes. For the reduction of temperature in febrile cases, the temperature should be 85° to 70°, and the duration 6 to 15 minutes.

Care must be taken to adjust the temperature of the bath

exactly right, for when the temperature is too high, the skin is left in an anemic, pale, and relaxed condition. If too low a temperature is used, excessive congestion of the internal viscera may be induced through weakness of the walls of the blood-vessels, which, being unable to contract with sufficient vigor to throw the blood back to the skin, reaction may fail, and the effects of the bath be spoiled, by exhaustion of the vasomotor centers through a too prolonged application.

The depth of the water in the shallow bath is ordinarily not more than six inches; if deeper, it interferes with the rubbing. When the depth of the water is sufficient to reach the umbilicus, the bath is termed a *half-bath*. The points in which the shallow bath differs from the half-bath are chiefly, (*a*) the longer continuance of the latter; (*b*) the rubbing may be dispensed with unless the temperature is low; (*c*) the temperature is usually cool, neutral, or hot.

The effects of the shallow bath are intensified and somewhat improved if two attendants are employed, one rubbing the legs while the other rubs the back and sides.

A useful mode of applying this bath is in combination with the immersion bath — the shallow bath at 70°, the immersion at 60°, the water having been previously prepared in two tubs at the temperatures indicated, and the patient warmed by the hot-blanket pack, the vapor bath, or the electric-light bath. The patient is first immersed for three to five seconds in the full bath, then placed in the shallow bath, which, having a temperature ten degrees higher, produces a warm and comfortable sensation. The patient feels no disposition to chill, and by the aid of rubbing he is rendered so comfortable that the bath may be continued for a considerably longer period than when administered without the preparation suggested.

A fairly vigorous patient can administer the shallow bath to himself, sitting in a tub containing a few inches of cold water, and applying the water to various parts by means of a long towel folded lengthwise and dipped in water, one end being grasped by each hand, whereby the towel may be drawn back and forth in a sawing motion across the back and other portions of the trunk. It may be used in this manner daily as a hygienic measure with great benefit.

The *standing shallow* (Fig. 73) is a modification of the bath in which the patient stands in a tub containing water at 75° to 80°. The patient is rubbed by two attendants, one on each side. The water is poured over his spine, chest, and shoulders, at intervals of 15 or 20 seconds. In rubbing the legs, the attendant's hands are constantly dipped in the water, and very vigorous friction is applied, duration 1 to 3 minutes.

At the conclusion of the bath, a pailful of cold water (60° to 55°) is poured over the patient, thus insuring good reaction. He is then quickly dried and vigorously rubbed, after which he should engage in moderate exercise until good reaction is secured.

The standing shallow is a sort of transition from the dripping sheet to the douche. The best time for giving it is in the morning as the patient comes warm from the bed, unless it be preceded by a hot bath. It is necessary that it should be applied when the skin is well heated.

1175 **Physiological Effects.**—The term "half-bath," devised by Priessnitz, is really a misnomer, as in this procedure the application involves the whole surface of the body. It combines the effects of the rubbing wet sheet, the affusion, and the immersion bath, producing powerfully alterative and tonic effects by reason of the repeated and ever-varying thermic and mechanical impressions made upon the skin.

The cold shallow bath stands next to the douche in power and efficiency as a tonic hydriatic procedure. That the shallow powerfully stimulates metabolism was clearly shown by the experiments of Pospischil, who found the flow of respiratory air to be increased nearly 300 per cent. during the bath, while the respiratory quotient remained the same; viz., 67. The favorable influence of this bath upon the general

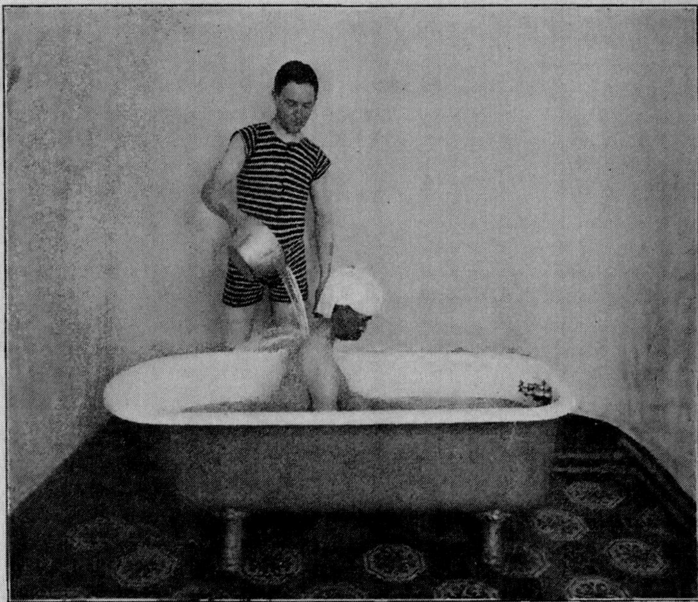

FIG. 72 *(a)*. SHALLOW BATH — First Step (p. 594).

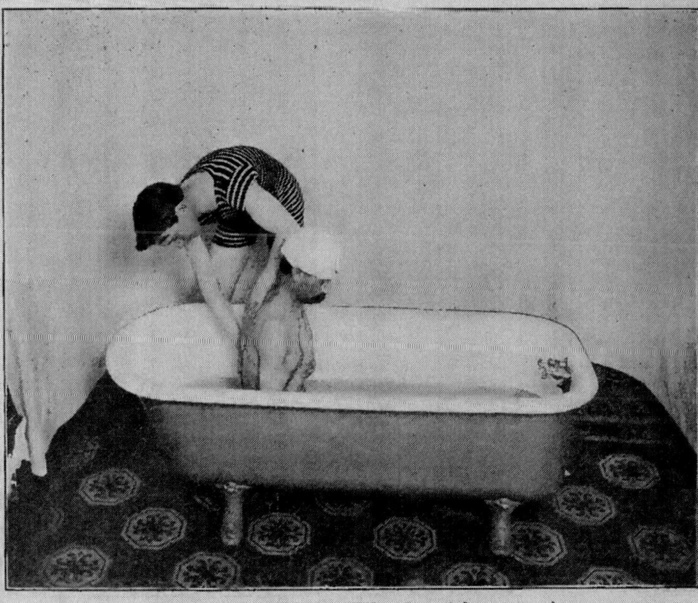

FIG. 72 *(b)*. SHALLOW BATH — Second Step (p. 594).

condition of the patient and its power to increase vital resistance is clearly indicated by its effect in increasing muscular capacity, as has been repeatedly and clearly shown (Exp. 59).

Employed at a temperature of 80° to 85°, the shallow or half-bath is a quieting or sedative measure. The higher the temperature, the more vigorous the rubbing necessary to produce good circulatory reaction, as the intensity of the thermic impression is lessened.

Therapeutic Applications.—The shallow bath is one of the 1176
most generally useful of all hydriatric procedures. It may be used as a substitute for the douche when the latter is not available, and when a procedure less powerful than the douche is desirable, though essentially the same results may be obtained by increasing the length of the application and the frequency of its repetition.

The impact of cold water upon the skin, the thermic impression, together with the strong friction applied by the attendants, and the exertion made by the patient in rubbing himself, together constitute a powerful combination of potent factors for dilating the surface vessels, and thus antagonizing the *anemia of the skin* present in the vast majority of *chronic diseases* and in most *infectious fevers* as a result of the toxic influence of the retained excretions and the specific poisons of bacterial origin.

The temperature of the shallow bath, when administered for anemia, should ordinarily be about 75° to 60°. The application should be short (1 to 2 min.). For very feeble and irritable patients, the duration of the bath at first application should be not more than from 15 to 30 seconds, a simple dip in the cold water.

The bath may be usefully employed in *anemia*, in *organic affections* of the *spine*, as *chronic myelitis*, *meningitis* with *exudate*, and *ataxia* with *paralysis* but without marked pain. The temperature of the application in such cases should be 70° to 80° and the duration 6 to 10 minutes.

The shallow bath may be used not only as a principal procedure, but also as a tonic measure following a sweating application. It is much better tolerated than the douche by persons suffering from *cardiac troubles* and *asthmatic affections*. It may also be employed in place of the Brand bath as a means of *lowering temperature* in patients whose temperature is not very high and who are not very weak. When the antipyretic effect is desired, it is wise to introduce the principle of graduation, by beginning the bath with a temperature of 92° to 95° and lowering it by pouring water upon the patient and lowering the temperature of each pailful until 70° to 75° is reached. The patient must be rubbed vigorously enough to prevent chilling. If severe chill occurs, he should be removed from the bath at once, rubbed dry, and put to bed, wrapped in warm blankets.

The shallow bath is an excellent means of antidoting the depressing effects of heat after a prolonged spoliative application, as the electric-light bath or the vapor bath employed in cases of obesity, the sweating pack, or any other prolonged heating process which leaves the patient in a depressed condition. For this purpose it answers very satisfactorily as a substitute for the douche, and is of great service in cases in which the latter is contraindicated, or when a douche apparatus is not accessible.

The shallow bath is an excellent bath for use in neurasthenia, especially *gastric neurasthenia*, also in *hypopepsia, chronic constipation, diabetes, uric acid diathesis*, and a large class of disorders due to uric acid accumulation, when neuralgia and local inflammatory processes are not present to any marked extent.

Röhrig has shown that a considerable increase of perspiration causes constipation, a result frequently noted in hydriatic establishments in patients who are taking a course of sweating baths for the reduction of flesh, or other spoliative or eliminative purposes. The shallow bath is of special service in these cases as a means of counteracting the constipating effect of the sweating processes, as well as in ordinary cases

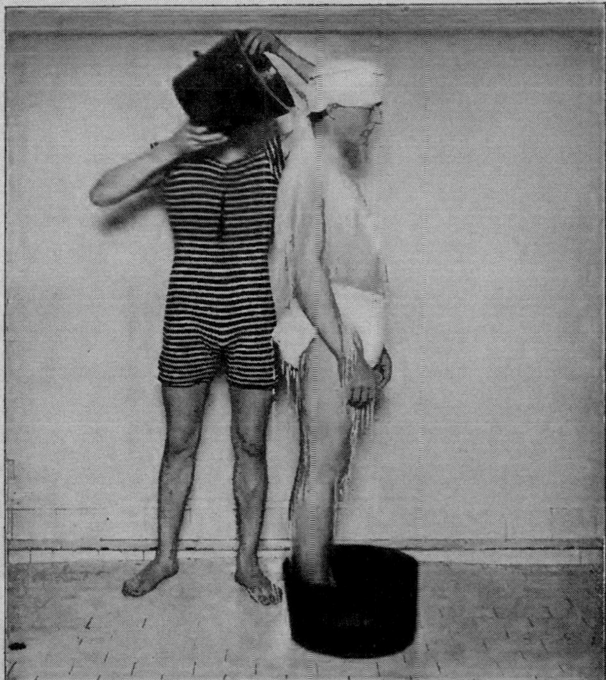

FIG. 73. (*a*) STANDING SHALLOW – First step (p. 596).

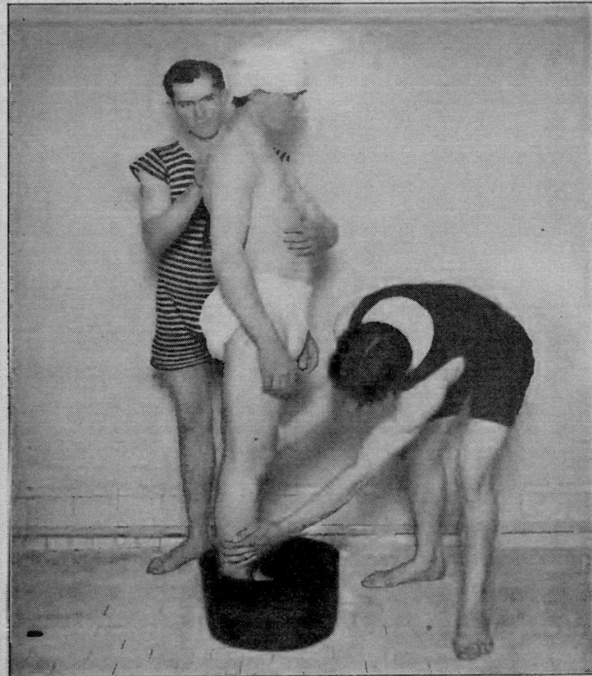

FIG. 73. (*b*) STANDING SHALLOW (p. 596).

of constipation in which the disorder is the result of deficient intestinal secretion. This effect must of course be encouraged by the copious drinking of cool or cold water at the proper hours (1375).

When employed for the relief of constipation or congestion of the liver or spleen, the water should be dashed upon the umbilical region or upon the surface overlying the liver or the spleen as may be indicated.

In Germany the shallow bath is much used as a method of preventing threatened chill in *intermittent malarial fever*. The author can testify to its merits as a means of aborting the malarial paroxysm, but he prefers to precede the application by a preliminary heating by means of a hot immersion, a hot-blanket pack, an electric-light bath, a vapor bath, or a vapor douche. When given for preventing the malarial chill, the bath should be very short and very vigorous, duration not more than 30 to 60 seconds. The patient should be immediately afterward wrapped in warm woolen blankets and surrounded with bags or bottles filled with hot water or other means of heating, and kept in bed until two hours after the time of the expected chill has passed.

The *hot* half-bath produces powerful revulsive and anal- 1177
gesic effects in relieving pain. The shallow bath is seldom employed except for cold applications, but the hot shallow bath may be used in place of the hot sitz for the relief of *pelvic pain*, also for the relief of *sciatic* and *crural neuralgia*, and in some cases of *rheumatic pains* affecting the joints of the legs. It allows a better position of the limbs than the sitz bath, the circulation through them being less interfered with than when they are flexed, as in the sitz bath, and pressure upon great nerve trunks is avoided.

Contraindications.—The shallow bath is contraindicated 1178
in cases of chronic congestion of the heart, brain, or spinal cord. With great care it may be used in *pneumonia* and *pleurisy*, but it is not needed in these disorders, and may better be avoided. Its use is contraindicated in fever cases compli-

cated with *myocarditis*, in *perforation*, *collapse*, *peritonitis*, and *hemorrhage* from injury to the vessels, also in acute *pelvic inflammation* or congestion, in all *suppurating processes* in the pelvis, in cases of *ovarian neuralgia* and neuralgia of the *sciatic nerve*. Neither should it be used in cases of *menorrhagia* or *profuse menstruation* or *metrorrhagia* from *bleeding fibroids* or *cancer*. It must be sedulously avoided in all forms of acute inflammation when deeply seated, as in *cystitis*, *enteritis*, *gastritis*, *nephritis*, *myelitis*, or *meningitis*, *prostatitis*, *ovaritis*, and *salpingitis*.

THE WET-SHEET PACK.

1179 This extremely useful and widely applicable hydriatic procedure, generally accredited to Priessnitz, was invented and first used by Lucas, in 1750. It consists in enveloping the body with a wet sheet, and preventing evaporation by careful protection with dry wrappings.

Requisites.— One large double blanket, one single blanket, two large sheets, one of which should be linen, a large linen towel, two or three gallons of water at a temperature of 60° to 70°. Water at a higher or lower temperature may be used when indicated, but is seldom required.

Method.— The pack may be applied in various ways, but the following method, which is employed by Winternitz, and was kindly demonstrated to the author by Dr. Strasser, assistant to Professor Winternitz, and lecturer at the Polyclinic in Vienna, is the most satisfactory: —

1. A sheet is folded once lengthwise, and laid across a couch near its head. The upper edge of the sheet should cover the lower third of a thin cotton or hair pillow placed at the head of the couch (Fig. 74).

2. Next, the double blanket is spread out, and placed across the couch so that one end hangs over the side opposite the attendant about two feet, the upper edge falling about two inches below the upper edge of the dry sheet (Fig. 75).

3. The linen sheet should now be wrung out by two persons' grasping the sheet at each end and twisting it in opposite directions until it is as dry as possible. The sheet is then spread out upon the blanket, the lower end falling an inch or two below the upper edge of the blanket (Fig. 76).

4. The patient lies down upon the sheet in such a way that the upper edge of the wet sheet projects three inches above the shoulders.

5. The patient raises both arms above his head while the attendants draw one side of the sheet across the body, turning it well up under the arms and tucking it in closely all along the side of the body. From the hips down, the edge of the sheet is tucked snugly around the leg of the corresponding side, leaving the other leg uncovered (Fig. 77). The patient lowers his arms and holds them close by his side while the other side of the sheet is passed over and tucked in. A fold is made in the sheet over each shoulder so as to make it fit the neck closely, care being taken not to constrict the vessels. The body is thus completely and closely enveloped by the sheet (Fig. 78).

6. The farther edge of the blanket is now drawn across the patient and tucked under the shoulder, the side, and around the legs, with great care. A fold is made over the farther shoulder, so as to make the blanket fit closely about the neck (Fig. 79).

7. The attendant now seizes the long end of the blanket, and pulls upon it in such a way as to bring the coverings in close contact with the body everywhere. The loose end is then thrown over and tucked around the patient, being wound about him two or more times like a winding-sheet. He is thus enveloped like a mummy (Fig. 80).

8. The blanket is next doubled under at the foot, and the dry sheet at the head is brought around with a neat fold over each shoulder, and tucked under the shoulders so as to protect the skin of the face and neck from contact with the blanket, and completely to exclude the air (Fig. 81).

9. For additional warmth, a woolen blanket is folded once, laid lengthwise upon the patient, and tucked under the shoulders and sides and about the legs. Two or more blankets may be applied at first, if necessary, one or more to be removed later.

When the pack is administered in this way, the patient will rarely complain of long delay in "warming up." Chill in the pack is usually due to the fact that at some points the wet sheet is not in perfect contact with the surface, and as a result, evaporation takes place with cooling, instead of accumulation of heat and vigorous reaction. The cooling effect thus started in small areas extends to the whole surface, and the patient is made exceedingly uncomfortable. But when the cold sheet is brought everywhere in close contact with the skin, reaction occurs immediately, and the disagreeable effects resulting from prolonged chilling are avoided.

In cases of very feeble or very nervous persons, one or both arms may be left out of the wet sheet, but should be included in the blanket, to avoid chilling.

Care should be taken to see that the patient's feet and the whole surface of the body are warm when the pack is applied. If the feet do not warm up readily in the pack, they may be left out at the first application, and until reaction is improved.

Kussmaul recommends the wet-sheet pack in acute nephritis. When used for this purpose, it should be applied immediately after a vigorous heating of the skin by means of the hot-blanket pack or short hot immersion bath, that reaction may take place immediately. The sheet should be wrung very dry, and the patient should be well and very carefully enveloped, and allowed to sweat freely.

Rendu prefers the wet-sheet pack to the Brand bath as a therapeutic measure in acute febrile disorders, not only because it aids the elimination of the toxins present in the disease, but because of its quieting effects upon the central nervous system, while it at the same time develops vital resistance.*

* *Revue d'Hygiene Therapeutique*, June, 1893, p. 164.

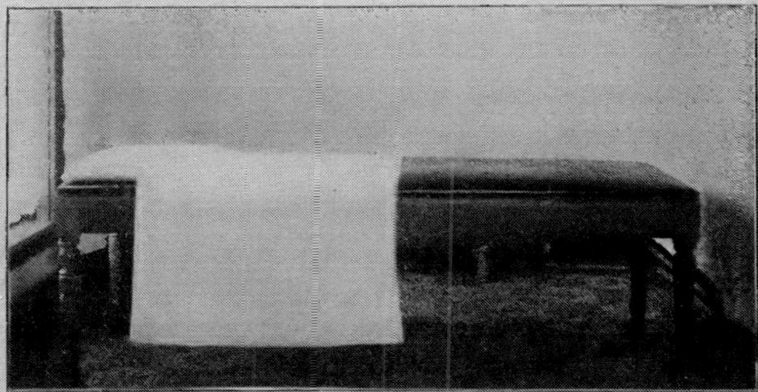

Fig. 74. WET-SHEET PACK — First Step (p. 601).

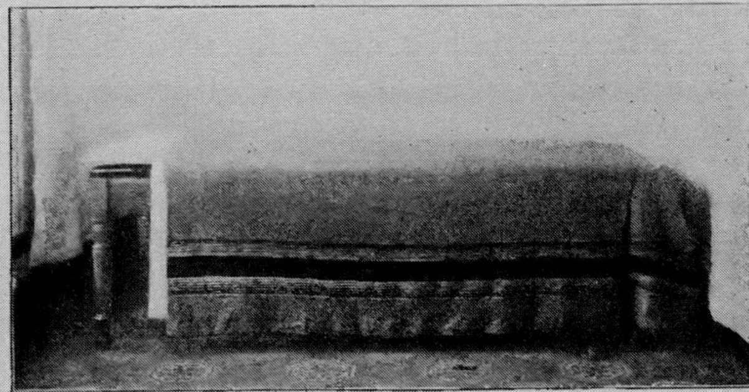

Fig. 75. WET-SHEET PACK — Second Step (p. 601).

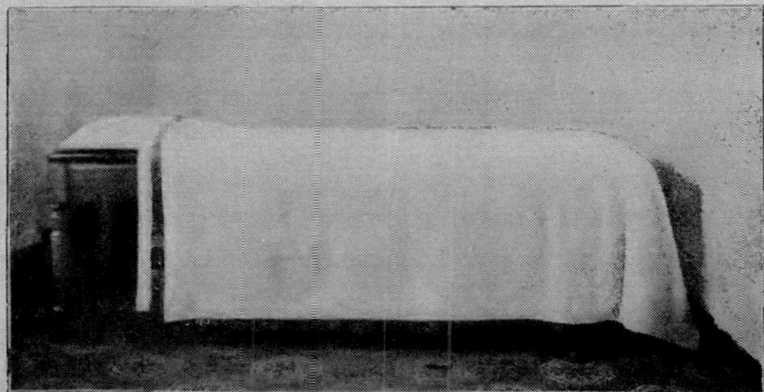

Fig. 76. WET-SHEET PACK — Third Step (p. 601).

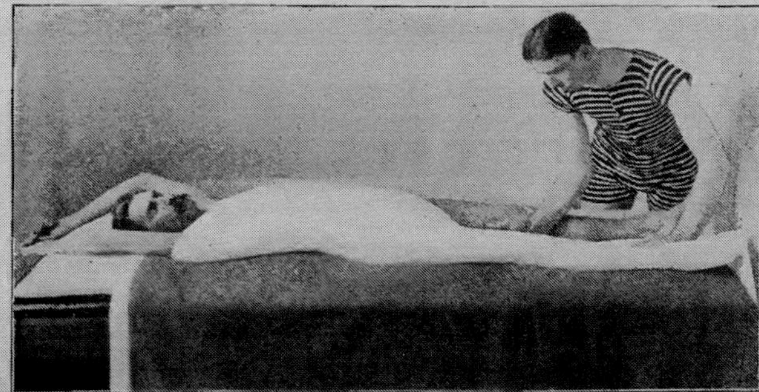

Fig. 77. WET-SHEET PACK — Fourth Step (p. 601).

Rendu* also especially praises the pack as a measure for the treatment of pneumonia, because of its value as a means of preventing cardiac failure and collapse.

It is less disturbing to the patient, much more convenient to use, does not require a bath-tub, which is not always ready at hand; hence can be used anywhere, and may be graduated to any degree of intensity required.

The cold wet-sheet pack employed in the manner directed has another advantage over the cold bath in that its effects are more durable, being somewhat slowly developed.

Winternitz has clearly shown that the cooling pack is much more effective as a means of reducing temperature than the Brand bath, the gradual lowering of temperature being more decided and more durable than after the cold bath.

In the use of the wet-sheet pack as an antipyretic, it will be observed that the sheet is warmed up more slowly with each successive application; consequently, the duration may be increased from three to five minutes at each successive renewal. The sheet need be changed only when it is shown by actual examination to have acquired nearly the temperature of the body. So long as the temperature of the sheet is lower than that of the body, a good cooling action is taking place.

In the dripping sheet, shallow bath, and many other hydriatic procedures, reaction is increased by friction; but in the wet-sheet pack, friction can not be employed; as a substitute, in cases in which reaction does not readily set in, warm bottles may be placed at the feet and sides of the patient. This is undesirable, however, as a routine method; the bottles should be used only when actually necessary. A better plan is to press and rub the limbs outside the coverings.

The head should be thoroughly cooled by wetting the scalp, face, and neck with cold water before the patient goes into the pack, and a towel, or better, a cheese-cloth napkin, saturated with cold water should be placed upon the face and

* Rendu, *Journal de Med. et de Chirurgie Pratiques*, 1893, p. 209.

wrapped around the head, or the neck, if the patient will not permit the wetting of the hair. The towel should be changed at intervals of 10 to 15 minutes during the pack. The duration of the pack will depend upon the effect desired. For tonic effects the usual length of the application should be 20 minutes, or until the patient feels a general glow induced by the return of the blood to the skin and a sensation of comfort and well-being, which marks the beginning of reaction. If *exciting* or *heating* effects are desired, the patient should remain in the pack until perspiration begins. If the effect desired is *elimination*, then the pack may be continued for one to two hours or even longer, or so long as sweating continues, if the strength of the patient will permit. If a sufficient supply of blankets is not at hand, the accumulation of heat may be assisted by enveloping the patient in a rubber sheet outside the other wrappings. When this plan is adopted, the rubber sheet must be spread upon the bed or couch between the folded dry sheet and the blanket.

1180 **Physiological Effects.**— When the wet sheet first comes in contact with the surface of the body, a decidedly chilly sensation is produced, which lasts for 5 to 20 minutes, when a febrile process is not present; when the skin is hot and the temperature high, no disagreeable sensation is produced. As reaction sets in, the chilliness disappears, and gives place to a sensation of comfort and well-being. Nervousness, when present before the application, is somewhat aggravated during the first few minutes after the patient enters the pack, but soon disappears, and a sensation of delicious calm pervades the system, and in many cases the patient falls asleep.

Schüller, in his experiments upon rabbits, noticed that the vessels of the brain, which were dilated at first, as soon as the general reaction set in, began to contract, the brain substance steadily shrinking, while the dura bulged more and more through the accumulation of lymph. This condition is one most favorable for the production of sleep and repair of the brain structure. It is the condition present during

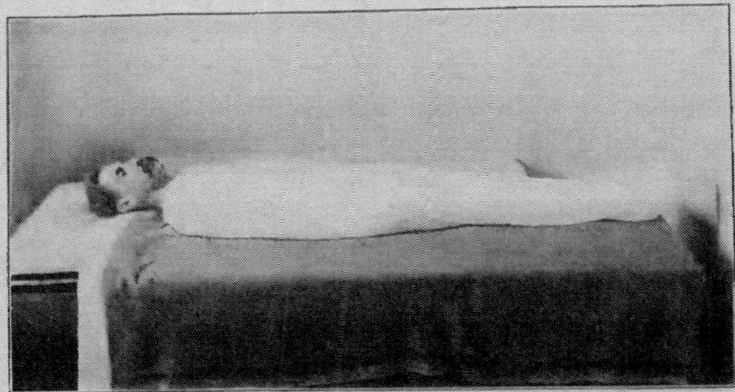

FIG. 78. WET-SHEET PACK — Fifth Step (p. 601).

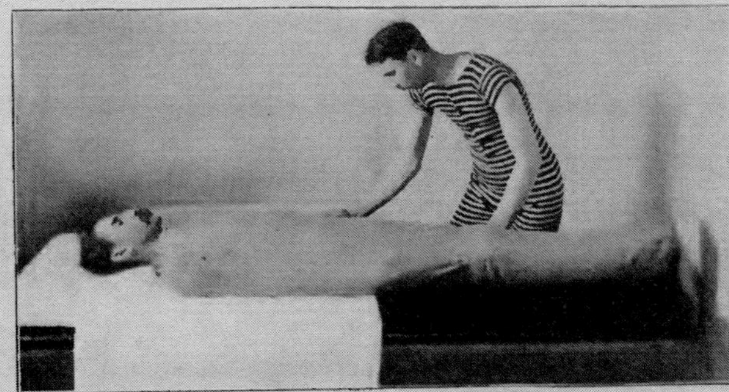

FIG. 79. WET-SHEET PACK — Sixth Step (p. 601).

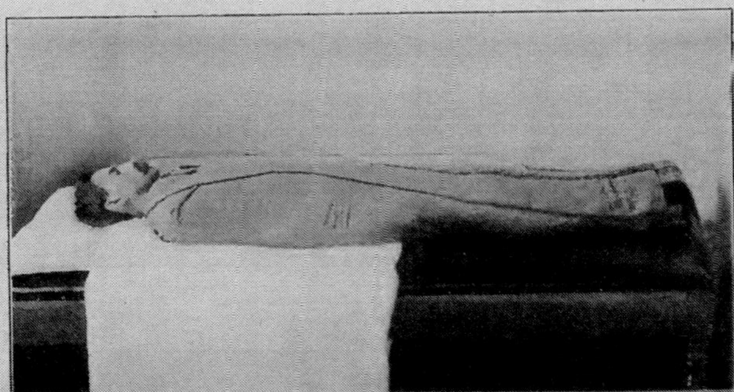

FIG. 80. WET-SHEET PACK — Seventh Step (p. 601).

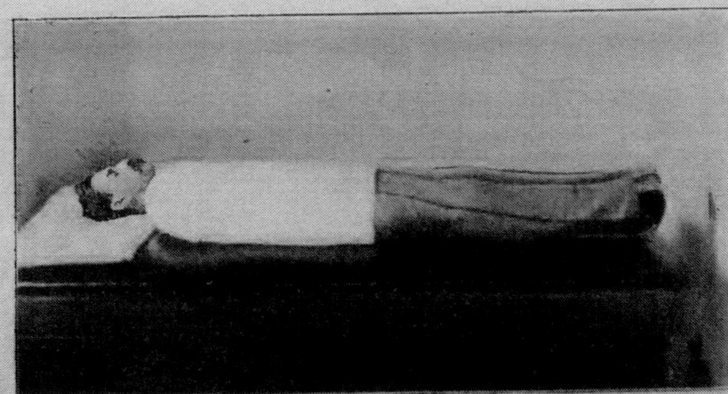

FIG. 81. WET-SHEET PACK — Eighth Step, Application Completed (p. 601).

physiological sleep. Later, as the heat thrown off by the skin, which is greatly increased in amount by the dilatation of the surface vessels, warms up the wet sheet, the heat accumulates in the covering about the patient, and the temperature of the blood is raised sufficiently to induce general perspiration, the beginning of which is indicated by the moistening of the brow.

If the pack is continued for several hours, perspiration will continue, growing more and more profuse for one or two hours, and possibly longer in some cases, but sooner or later the activity of the sweat-glands will cease, their energy seeming to be exhausted. Sweating may be increased and prolonged by making the patient drink freely.

From the foregoing it will be recognized that the effects produced by the wet-sheet pack are exceedingly varied, a series of distinct groups of effects presenting themselves in regular succession. The actual effects produced will depend, then, upon the length of the application, or at least upon the degree of development reached. In some persons the march of the phenomena is more rapid than in others.

The time occupied in the development of the various phases of the procedure may be divided into four periods, which are characterized as follows: (1) Cooling or antipyretic, (2) neutral, (3) superheating, (4) sweating. These several periods are the natural result of the progressive accumulation of heat, for which provision is made by the close wrapping of the patient, and which necessitates the exercise of very great care in so adjusting the wrappings about the neck and the feet as to prevent the escape of the warm air and vapor developed by the heat of the body. The amount of heat generated by a person of average size in the course of an hour is very considerable, amounting to 450 heat units, or sufficient to raise 45 pounds of water ten degrees in temperature, or to elevate the temperature of the entire body of a patient weighing 150 pounds three degrees, if this heat should be all retained. The greater part of this thermic energy is expended in warming up the wet sheet and its coverings and in evaporating the moisture of the sheet. As soon as the coverings are raised to the temperature of the body, the heat begins to accumulate; and as soon as it has accumulated sufficiently to elevate the temperature of the blood .7°, perspiration begins (Bouchard).

1181 During the *first* or *cooling* stage, heat is rapidly abstracted from the body, and powerful thermic reaction is induced. Circulatory reaction is slow, for the reason that there are no mechanical aids to dilatation of the surface vessels, such as the friction of the rubbing sheet and the shallow bath, and the percussion effects of the douche. The pack in this respect differs from nearly all other general hydriatic procedures. The body is left wholly to its own resources, hence the importance of the proper preparation of the patient before the bath, so that his powers of calorification and circulatory reaction may be equal to the demand made upon them. This is the reason why heating processes of some sort—exercise, vigorous rubbing, or the hot bath—are almost indispensable as a preparation for the cold wet-sheet pack, unless the patient is in a febrile state. Priessnitz, who, though without scientific education, was certainly blessed with remarkably acute intuition, usually administered the wet-sheet pack before the patient arose in the morning, while the skin was warm with the heat accumulated during the night.

The effects produced during the cooling or refrigerative stage of the pack are intensely alterative in character. All the organic processes are excited in connection with the intense thermic reaction induced, and an exceedingly powerful appeal is made to every nerve center in the body. The whole system rallies to resist the invasion of the depressing agent, cold; and if the pack is arrested during or at the end of this stage, or when reaction begins, the general effect produced will be tonic, and will be essentially the same as that of a cold bath of the same temperature, provided, of course, that reaction is fully developed by exercise, rubbing, or other means, after the conclusion of the process. If the process is arrested as soon as the reaction begins, that is, at the end of 8 to 12 minutes, a freshly cooled sheet being applied, the effect is powerfully antithermic and antifebrile.

The *second*, or *neutral*, stage of the pack begins when the 1182
temperature of the wrappings and the warm moist air surrounding the patient reaches a point approximating that of the body, or 92°. The effect during this period is essentially the same as that of the neutral bath. It is quieting, calmative, and productive of a disposition to sleep. Renal activity is excited. When the pack is ended with this period, no other effects are produced.

When prolonged to the *third* period, that of *superheating*, 1183
the body temperature is slightly elevated as heat elimination is more and more interfered with, and the excitant effects of a temperature above 98° make their appearance, the face becoming flushed, and the brain intensely congested, unless the head is cooled by a cold compress to the head and face, frequently renewed. When the pack is prolonged, and perspiration does not promptly make its appearance, the patient experiences the same weakness and languor which result from a prolonged bath at 100° to 102°.

As excitation resulting from the accumulation of heat increases still further, the skin becomes more and more active, until the perspiratory glands are so excited that visible perspiration appears upon the brow, marking the beginning of the *fourth* stage, that of *excitation*, or the *sweating* stage. During this stage a prodigious amount of vital work is performed, not only by the skin, but by the nerve centers and internal viscera associated with it. Every cell in the body is stimulated to increased activity by the elevation of temperature and the powerful thermic impressions made upon the whole cutaneous surface. Under the influence of the elevated temperature, the elimination and destruction of tissue toxins take place with augmented rapidity; the heart beat is accelerated, the activity of the peripheral heart is likewise increased, and the movement of blood in the vessels is augmented, resulting in increased activity of all the eliminative processes; there is increased oxidation of albumin, and increased elimination as well as more perfect oxidation of nitrogenous wastes. Thus the sweating pack is a powerful spoliative or reducing measure.

It should be noted that the pack may not only be arrested at the end of the several stages, but that any stage may be prolonged for almost any desired length of time. For example, the first stage may be prolonged either by removing a portion of the covers so as to permit evaporation as the sheet is warmed, or by renewing the sheet, as has been described.

Instead of the long woolen blanket applied like a winding-sheet, the author prefers for the *cooling* pack two single blankets, which are laid across the couch in such a way that the patient lies in the center. In wrapping the patient, the two angles are each brought across and disposed in like manner. An extra folded blanket may be added for warmth. This plan facilitates renewal of the sheet.

The second, or neutral, stage may be prolonged by withdrawing most of the covering as soon as reaction has well set in, so that the loss of heat by evaporation will not be interfered with sufficiently to cause the temperature to rise above that of the body. Care must be taken constantly, however, to see that the body is uniformly protected; the sheet must not be loosened so as to allow local air currents to be established, as this would produce local chilling and effects which might in some cases be really serious.

The third stage may be prolonged by withdrawing a small portion of the covers, as by taking off the outside blanket, and by bathing the head and face almost continually with cold water so as to produce a slight refrigerant effect, by cooling the brain. A cold towel may also be wrapped about the neck. Thus the extreme excitant effects of the pack may be checked and sweating delayed.

The fourth, or sweating, stage may be prolonged almost indefinitely by making the patient drink every half hour a glassful of water, either hot or cold, or some suitable beverage prepared with water and fruit-juice. The head should not be cooled excessively, and extra blankets may be applied, if necessary to increase accumulation of heat. In cases in which the skin is very inactive, so that perspiration is long delayed, several hot-water bottles may be placed about the patient inside the dry blankets, and he may be made to drink copiously of hot water or hot lemonade.

Therapeutic Applications.— From the foregoing it will be 1184
readily seen that the wet-sheet pack is an exceedingly useful hydriatic procedure, and that it is capable of ready adaptation to a great variety of conditions. If a *tonic effect* is desired, the pack may be interrupted soon after the beginning of the second stage, or when reaction is well established. Employed in this way, the pack may be made useful in a great variety of conditions; but it is far less valuable for securing tonic effects than the douche, the half-bath, the wet-sheet rub, and other procedures of briefer duration, and in which the thermic irritation is supplemented by the mechanical stimulus of friction, and the percussion effect of the douche.

The *tonic* pack is indicated in all forms of wasting disease, as in *anemia*, *tuberculosis*, *convalescence* from *fever*, and *chronic toxemia* connected with dyspepsia, as well as in *chronic disorders* of the *liver*, and especially in the *toxemia* of *chronic malarial infection*. Its value in the treatment of *infectious fevers* is largely due to its tonic effects.

The pack may be employed in many cases in which the shock of the cold bath could not be well borne by the patient. Employed for tonic effects, the wet-sheet pack, continued well into the second stage, is of great value in *anemia*, *chlorosis*, *diabetes*, *nervous dyspepsia*, *neurasthenia*, *scurvy*, *chronic gastritis*, *hypopepsia*, *constipation*, and *general paresis*. The tonic pack also renders most valuable service in the intervals of *intermittent* and *relapsing fever*.

1185 The *neutral* pack, that is, the wet-sheet pack, continued until the end of the second stage, is of much value in a great variety of cases, being especially useful in *insomnia*, *acute mania*, *melancholia*, *neurasthenia* with nervousness and depression, and in cases of *cerebral irritation* of whatever origin. The neutral pack is an excellent measure of treatment in the class of cases mentioned, since it is not only tranquilizing but tonic in its effects. The excitation resulting from the tonic effects of the first stage is calmed by the tranquilizing influence of the second period, which is terminated before the development of depressant effects, thus adapting this measure to the class of patients with whom purely tonic measures, such as the cold rubbing wet sheet and the douche, produce unpleasant effects by exaggerating symptoms due to irritability of the nerve centers.

Schüller's experiments showed the wet-sheet pack to be one of the most effective of all means for quieting the general nervous system, which it accomplishes by lessening the blood supply of the brain, slowing the respiration and heart beat, lessening the reflex irritability and activity of the cerebral ganglia, increasing the quantity of lymph in the brain, and thus supplying a condition essential for sleep.

The wet-sheet pack is of special service in the *insomnia* and *delirium* of *typhoid* and *typhus fevers*, and in *pneumonia*. The author has more than once seen a delirious fever patient who had not slept for several days, while in a pack fall into a tranquil slumber from which he awoke refreshed and quiet.

The neutral pack is of almost equal service in the treatment of *epilepsy*, *chorea*, and *tetany*.

1186 The *heating* pack, that is, the cold wet-sheet pack continued until the end of the third stage, is perhaps most useful as a preparation for tonic applications, such as the shallow bath, the cold douche, the pail douche, the wet-sheet rub, and the cold immersion in cases in which powerful derivative measures are required. If interrupted before the exciting effects are pronounced, it may be usefully employed in *cerebral congestion*, *hepatic* and *splenic congestions* from chronic malarial infection, *constipation* accompanied by *hemorrhoids*, *abdominal dropsy*, and as a means of developing the eruption in eruptive fevers. For the last-named purpose this procedure is unexcelled, producing powerful cutaneous stimulation.

The pack is also of especial service in the early stage of *eruptive fevers*, when the skin is hot, dry, and congested, and before the eruption has fully appeared. It not only relieves the patient's discomfort by lessening the cutaneous congestion, but evidently aids, as above pointed out, in developing the eruption. Hence its value in measles, scarlet fever, and smallpox.

The *sweating* pack, or fourth stage of the process, is a 1187
highly spoliative and eliminative measure.

The efficiency of the wet-sheet pack as a means of stimulating the elimination of poisons is well shown in persons addicted to the tobacco habit. In such cases the sheet often smells strongly of nicotine after having been wrapped about the patient for an hour, even a week or two after he has discontinued the use of the weed.

Indeed, the wet-sheet pack is one of the most useful of hydrotherapeutic procedures, as it combines at once very powerful effects, great convenience and universality of application, and remarkable flexibility for modification to suit different pathological conditions. It is a powerful means of influencing the general nutrition through its effects upon the sympathetic nervous system, and through it upon all the processes of secretion, circulation, assimilation, and excretion. While less perturbing than the douche, it is still capable of producing in a more gradual, gentle, but none the less effective manner, most profound impressions upon the whole vital economy.

In the absence of more ready means of heating the skin, the wet-sheet pack, continued until the skin becomes well warmed, or until very gentle perspiration shows upon the face, is an excellent preparation for the cold douche or other cold application. The electric-light bath, the vapor bath, fomentations to the spine, the hot-air bath, and other heating measures are, however, generally more convenient than the wet-sheet pack as a means of accumulating heat in the skin; and there is danger, especially in the case of feeble patients, that the prolonged character of the application may excessively fatigue the patient or exhaust the nerve centers.

One of the characteristic physiological effects of the wet-sheet pack is increased activity of the mucous membrane. This effect is produced only when the application is carried to the stage of reaction. Thus used, the pack is invaluable in cases of chronic constipation and hypopepsia. It is equally valuable in many cases of *chronic bronchitis*, with dry cough, and in *chronic pneumonia* and *pleurisy*.

By its *derivative* effect the wet-sheet pack removes visceral irritation and congestion, and its beneficent influence is indicated by the fact that the patient from day to day gains in power to warm the sheet, thus showing that his power to react is increasing, and that the blood is being strongly diverted toward the skin. When the visceral congestion and irritation are removed, as indicated by the disappearance of symptoms directly due to these conditions, the wet-sheet pack may be exchanged for a more highly tonic measure, as the shallow bath, or the cold or Scotch douche. As a derivative measure it is of great service in *intestinal catarrh*, *congestions* of the *spleen* and *liver*, and in *cerebral hyperemia.*

The leathery, dry, hide-bound skin of the chronic dyspeptic becomes clear, supple, and active under the influence of the wet-sheet pack employed tri-weekly, followed by oil rubbing. For the most rapid effects, the pack should, in these cases, be carried just to the point of beginning reaction; but perspiration should not be induced unless the patient has a considerable amount of flesh; and then great care must be taken to avoid too long continuance of the pack, as when thus used, it is a very exciting measure, and the majority of patients suffering from chronic indigestion have but little recuperative power and small capacity for tissue production.

In *jaundice* the wet-sheet pack affords an excellent method for relieving the extreme itching and irritation which usually accompany this condition, at the same time aiding in the elimination of morbid elements from the blood. In these cases the pack may be carried to the point of slight perspiration, if irritation is not thereby induced. In cases in which the itching is very pronounced, care should be taken to avoid perspiration; the pack must terminate at the end of the neutral stage, which may be prolonged if desirable (page 608).

Contraindications and Precautions.—The cold wet-sheet 1188
pack can not be employed for patients whose vital resources are so small that they are unable to react without the aid of friction or other mechanical means. It must also be avoided in eruptive disorders of the skin, and in the exanthemata after the eruption occurs, being too strongly exciting to the skin.

It is possible to use the pack in many cases in which it would otherwise be contraindicated, by previously subjecting the patient to some mild heating procedure, as a short hot immersion bath (3 to 5 min., at 104° to 110° F.), the electric-light bath, fomentation to the spine, hot water drinking, a short hot sitz bath, or a hot blanket pack.

By the aid of special precautions the pack may be employed without difficulty in cases in which untoward effects might otherwise be produced. Parts that are sensitive to cold may be covered with a dry cloth. Parts requiring special protection are: the spine in spinal irritation; the chest in asthma; the heart when very excitable; sensitive surfaces in neuralgia; and in certain cases, the genitals.

For example, in cases of so-called spinal irritation or spinal neuralgia, in which the contact of cold water with the skin produces severe pain, the spine may be protected by a strip of flannel six or eight inches in width and of the proper length. This should be laid in the proper position on the sheet just before the patient lies down to be enveloped.

In asthmatics, in whom cold applications to the chest produce paroxysms of dyspnea, the chest should be protected by a piece of flannel of proper size and one thickness.

In cases accompanied by hyperesthesia of the skin covering the abdomen, similar precautions may be employed, the dry flannel being placed over the abdomen. If the feet do not react well, they may be left out of the sheet, and warmed by means of rubber bags or bottles filled with hot water, or other similar means, or by rubbing before the pack. It is not necessary that the feet be included in the pack in order to secure the general results desired.

When applying a cold pack in cases in which a nervous state of the heart or lungs exists, place a dry towel over the chest before wrapping the patient in the wet sheet.

In the case of very feeble patients, a training for the pack may be practiced, by beginning with a narrow trunk pack, daily extending it in both directions until the whole body is involved. Or, with very feeble patients, the treatment may be begun by placing a single towel wrung quite dry out of cold water over the front of the body, enveloping the whole body with blankets. The next day a wet towel to the back may be added, then one to each of the lower extremities, and later to the upper extremities, until finally the entire body may be enveloped in the sheet.

In the use of the wet-sheet pack, headache, nervousness, fainting, vertigo, indicate that the pack has been continued for too long a time, and the circulation has been unduly excited.

A curious phenomenon which sometimes accompanies the application of the wet-sheet pack, is the appearance of a rose color, accompanied by a fetid odor, and sometimes a mucilaginous secretion. The cause of this phenomenon is not fully explained, but may be due to bacterial action.

The majority of patients who are benefited by the pack fall asleep within a few moments after reaction begins. The patient may be allowed to sleep during the pack; but the

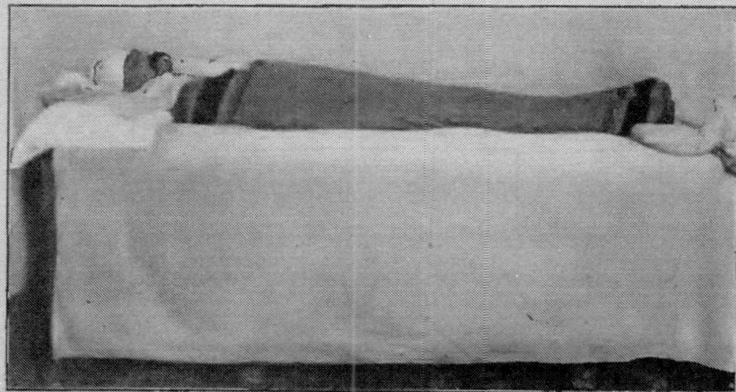

FIG. 82. METHOD OF PROTECTING SHOULDERS OF FEEBLE PATIENTS (p. 616).

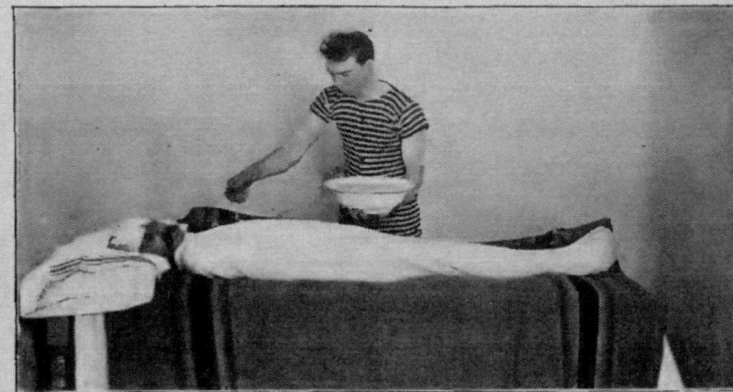

FIG. 83. SHOWER PACK (p. 617).

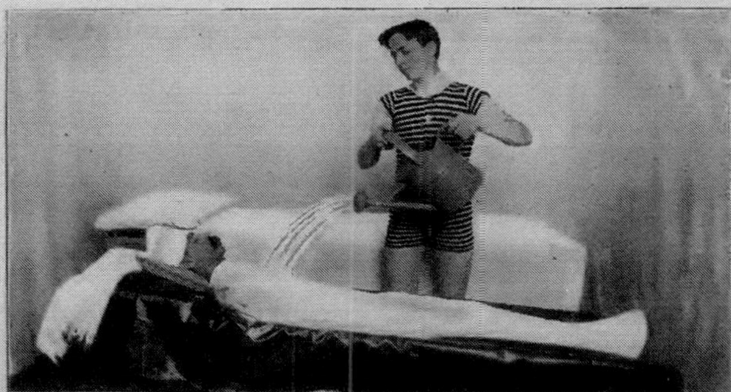

FIG. 84. SHOWER PACK (p. 618).

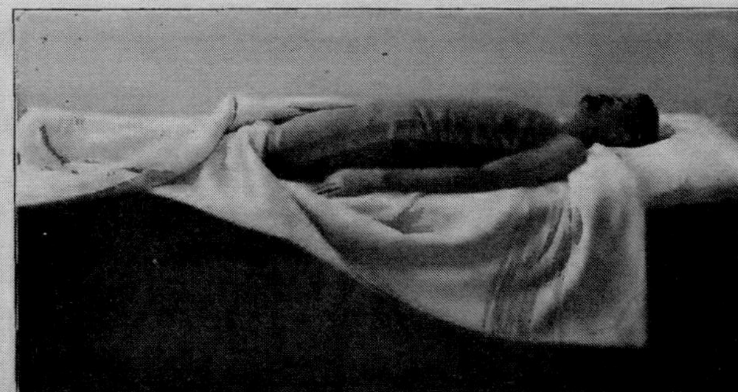

FIG. 85. HALF PACK (p. 622).

application should be terminated when the proper effects have been produced. Sometimes in cases of acute mania with insomnia, or even in ordinary cases of insomnia which do not yield to other measures, the patient may with advantage be allowed to remain in the pack for several hours if he continues to sleep, but care must be taken to remove a sufficient amount of the coverings so that he shall not be overheated, and also on the other hand equal care must be observed against chill. It is generally necessary to cover the legs and the feet somewhat more warmly than the trunk. The tendency to overheating may also be combated by cold applications to the head. If applications to the face and forehead are not sufficient, the scalp may be moistened. It is not generally necessary to use the ice-cap or ice-water. The head compress should be omitted when it causes chilliness.

A graphic proof of the tonic effect of the wet-sheet pack concluded at the first stage of the procedure is afforded by the ergograph of Mosso, which shows a decided increase in muscular capacity as the result of the tonic application of the pack (Exp. 60).

THE COOLING PACK.

If it is desired to employ the pack as an *antipyretic*, it 1189
should be applied in the ordinary way (page 608), but must be interrupted before the end of the first stage; that is, before the refrigerant effects are obliterated by the accumulation of heat. The procedure must be repeated as soon as the sheet is warmed by applying a sheet freshly wrung from water of the proper temperature. Any degree of antithermic effect desired being secured by repeating the renewal. To secure the most pronounced antithermic effects, water at 60° to 70° should be employed. There is no advantage in using water at a lower temperature. Colder water stimulates heat production to such an extent as to antagonize the effect desired. The sheet should be left very wet; and if the tem-

perature is high and the skin very hot, two sheets instead of one may be used, so as to prolong the refrigerant effect.

The patient should be covered with only two thicknesses of blanket, so as to allow slight cooling through a moderate amount of evaporation; but care should be taken to prevent the entrance of air about the neck so as to avoid undue chilling of this part, whereby congestion of the lungs and possibly acute bronchitis or even pneumonia may be produced. Fig. 82 shows a method of protecting the shoulders.

Rub the limbs vigorously for a few seconds after the application of each new sheet before wrapping the woolen blankets about the patient. This will ensure reaction and encourage heat elimination. When the patient's temperature is high and the skin very hot, it may be necessary to renew the wet sheet at the end of five or six minutes. The duration of each successive application is from five to eight minutes longer than the preceding. The first sheet may be applied at 60° to 65°, and each successive sheet 2° or 3° higher. The renewal of the wet sheet may be avoided by opening the wraps and rubbing the sheet with ice, continuing until the sheet is sufficiently cooled.

If there is prolonged chilling, or if the patient's teeth chatter, the woolen blanket should be opened, and the patient vigorously rubbed between the sheet and the blanket. As soon as the shivering ceases, he may be wrapped up again until he becomes warm. The cold wet-sheet pack managed in this way is an excellent substitute for the cold bath.

Therapeutic Applications.— The cooling pack is indicated in all cases of febrile disease, and especially in *typhoid fever*, *typhus*, *erysipelas*, *febricula*, *dengue*, *malarial fevers*, *yellow fever*, the *plague*, *acute bronchitis*, and *influenza*.

THE COLD SHOWER PACK.

1190 When antipyretic effects are desired, instead of removing the sheet from the patient for rewetting, the same results may be accomplished, though not quite so rapidly, by opening the sheet and sprinkling the body as well as the sheet with cold water (Fig. 83). The patient should be made to turn first on one side and then on the other, so that the whole body may be exposed to the cold application. A better method still is to place the patient upon a cot covered with rubber cloth so arranged in relation to a tub placed at the foot of the cot that any surplus water may be caught as it runs off (Fig. 84). Water may be turned over the patient from a sprinkler or any convenient vessel. By this means the cooling effect of the sheet may be continued, and may be made almost as intense as the cold bath. The temperature employed should be from 60° to 65° F. If the patient does not well tolerate very cold water, a temperature of 70° to 80°, or even 85°, will be found efficient if the application is prolonged.

Nearly twenty-five years ago the author made use of this form of pack as an antithermic means in the treatment of some fifty cases of typhoid fever in an epidemic of this disease. Every case recovered, although the type of the disease was in several cases very grave.

Therapeutic Applications.—The practical applications of the shower pack are the same as those of the cooling pack (**1189**). It need only be added that the shower pack, being a measure which may be made almost as powerfully antipyretic as the Brand bath, is especially suited to cases in which the temperature is persistently high, and does not yield to more moderate measures.

Contraindications.—These are the same as those pointed out for the Brand bath.

THE SWEATING PACK.

When it is desired to produce powerful eliminative effects **1191**
by means of the wet-sheet pack, the application may be made in the manner already described (**1179**), with the exception that more covers are employed, to encourage reaction, and it is generally wise to place hot bags at the patient's feet and sides. He should take a glassful of hot water before the

pack, and two or three glasses while in the pack. In cases in which perspiration is not easily induced, the pack may be preceded by a hot bath for 3 or 4 minutes. The temperature of the bath should be from 105° to 110°. The patient's skin should be so well heated that he will anticipate the contact of the cold sheet with pleasure. There should not be the slightest delay between the hot bath and the cold sheet. The hot-blanket pack may be used in case of the hot bath when the latter is not convenient.

When it is desirable to prolong the perspiration, the patient may be removed from the wet-sheet pack after the activity of the skin is well established, to be at once wrapped in dry blankets surrounded by bottles or rubber bags filled with hot water. He should be induced to drink at intervals of 10 to 15 minutes a half glass of hot water or weak hot lemonade. Rubbing the limbs and trunk outside the wrappings will stimulate perspiration. The patient may increase heat production by contracting and relaxing the muscles without changing the position of the limbs.

Therapeutic Applications.— This procedure is one of the most powerful of spoliative and eliminative measures. It is invaluable in *jaundice*, *dropsy*, *syphilis*, and most other maladies in which eliminative effects are indicated. It may be employed with very great advantage in cases of *obesity*, *rheumatism*, *gout*, *dyspepsia*, *chronic toxemia*, *neurasthenia* with inactive skin, *chronic nephritis*, enfeebled chronic invalids whose habits have been sedentary, *alcoholics*, victims of the *tea* and *coffee habit*, and *tobacco users*, especially smokers, and in *malarial fever*, *catarrhal jaundice*, *septicemia*, *ascites*, *amyloid liver*, *Bell's palsy*, *acute* and *chronic myelitis*, *leptomeningitis*, *epilepsy*, *neuralgia*, *migraine*, *tetany*, and *Raynaud's disease*.

Any degree of depletion or eliminative effect desired may be produced by prolonging the sweating process.

A cold application should always follow the sweating pack. In rheumatism, neuralgia, Bright's disease, and feeble heart,

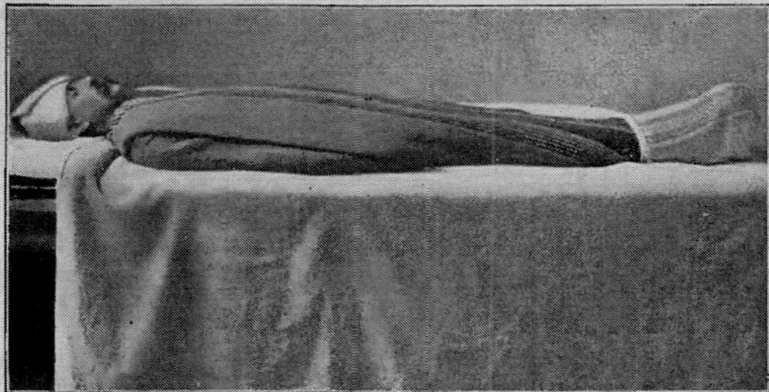

Fig. 86. HOT-BLANKET PACK (p. 623).

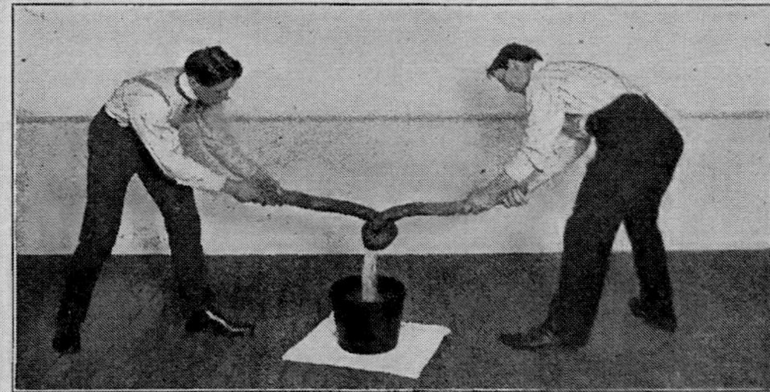

Fig. 87. WRINGING BLANKET FOR HOT PACK (p. 624).

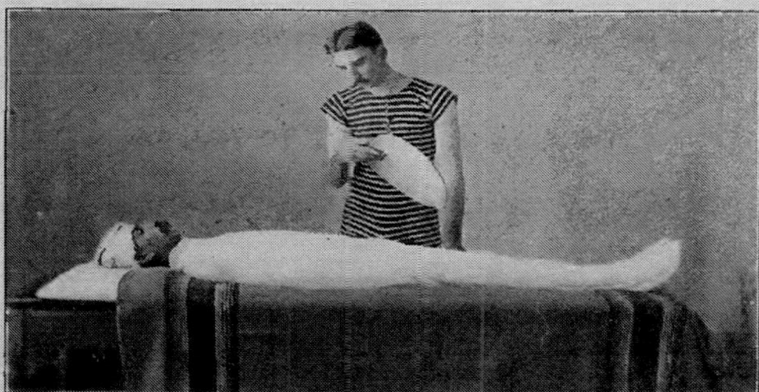

Fig. 88. EVAPORATING WET SHEET (p. 625).

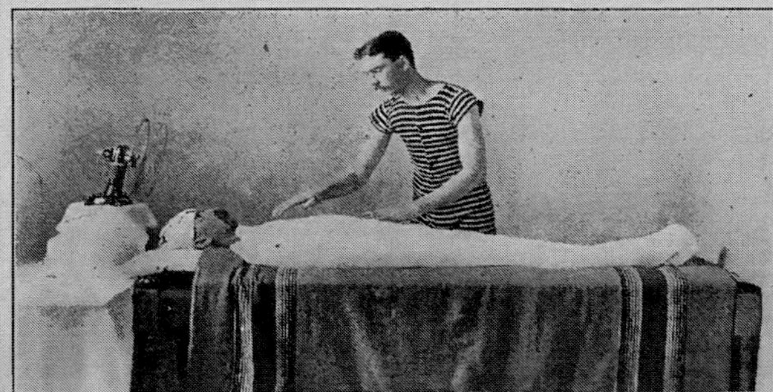

Fig. 89. EVAPORATING SHEET — Employing Electric Fan (p. 626).

cold wet friction may be employed safely, even when more vigorous measures are contraindicated.

Contraindications.— The sweating pack must be avoided in eruptive disorders, in the exanthemata after the eruption appears, in advanced cases of *cardiac* or *Bright's disease*, in *anemia*, feeble *neurasthenics*, *diabetics* with *emaciation*, *rheumatic gout*, general *cutaneous hyperesthesia*, and in febrile states in which accumulation of bodily heat is decidedly contraindicated.

THE DRY PACK.

In this application the patient is completely enveloped in 1192
dry blankets, the head only being excluded, the purpose being to lessen heat elimination, and thus produce an accumulation of bodily heat, and in some cases to induce perspiration.

Requisites.— A bed or couch with a comfortable mattress, a number of dry woolen blankets, bottles or rubber bags for hot water, hot sand bags, or other convenient means of applying dry heat to the body.

Method.— The pillow and several woolen blankets are arranged upon the bed or couch, as directed for the wet-sheet pack. The patient, divested of his clothing, lies down, and the blankets are quickly applied as directed for the wet-sheet pack, care being taken to tuck the edges in well about the head and feet, so as to avoid the circulation of air. If the patient is very feeble, very cold, or deficient in ability to generate heat, several hot-water bottles or bags may be placed at the feet and sides next to the first blanket, beneath the other coverings. The patient should drink one or two glasses of water before entering the pack, and while in the pack half a glass of hot or cold water should be swallowed every 15 or 20 minutes. The temperature of the room should be not less than 70°. If simply an accumulation of heat is desired, the patient should be removed from the pack before perspiration begins. If diaphoresis is sought, the application may be continued for two to five hours, or as long as necessary.

The dry pack may be applied to a portion of the body only, as the trunk, the lower half of the body, one or both legs, the knee, ankle, or elbow joint, or a paralyzed limb.

If used as a means of preparing the skin for a cold application, by storing up in it a quantity of bodily heat, the result sought may be facilitated by vigorous rubbing of the limbs outside the coverings.

In certain countries a dry pack is administered by enveloping the patient in dry hot sand. The effect is the same as though blankets were wrapped about the patient. Ruschpler introduced the methodical use of the sand bath in 1831. It is still employed in Germany. The temperature of the sand is from 118° to 122° F.

1193 **Physiological Effects.**— The effect of the dry pack is first to secure an accumulation of heat by lessening the heat elimination, and in extreme cases to augment the heat of the body by the application of artificial heat through the aid of hot-water bottles, hot bags, the drinking of hot water, etc.

The natural result of this accumulation of heat is to increase the temperature of the blood. The body temperature often rises two to four degrees. The elevation of temperature is doubtless due not only to the accumulation of heat, but to an increase of heat production, the natural result of the continuous exposure of the body to a high temperature.

With the elevation of body temperature, perspiration is induced. Before perspiration begins, the face is often flushed, the patient experiences an uncomfortable sensation of fulness in the head, and the pulse rate is decidedly increased. With the beginning of perspiration the patient becomes more comfortable; but the dry pack, as a sweating process, is by no means the most agreeable of thermic applications.

1194 **Therapeutic Applications.** — The dry pack is especially indicated in *shock*, *collapse* after hemorrhage, anesthesia, or a severe surgical operation. It is also of great value in the treatment of the cold stage of *intermittent fever*. It is useful in all cases in which there is a subnormal temperature.

In cases of *paralysis*, applications of the dry pack, sometimes general, but more frequently local, as in *paraplegia* and *hemiplegia*, may be used to great advantage.

In the absence of better means, the dry pack may be used as a preparation for the cold douche and other cold procedures. Care must be taken, however, to make the cold application instantly on the removal of the patient from the pack; otherwise a slight chill will be produced, and the effect will be spoiled. The dry pack may also be used with advantage for "breaking up a cold," for which purpose it is often very successful when applied within a few hours after the exposure. In cases of *collapse*, *arteritis*, or *phlebitis* in *typhoid*, in *septicemia*, *malarial* and *typho-malarial fever*, *malarial neuralgia* and in *obesity*, the dry pack is useful.

In *chronic rheumatism*, when the patient is not able to secure the advantages of the hot-air, vapor, Turkish, electric-light, or hot immersion baths, the dry pack may be employed with advantage. It may also be used in chronic rheumatism for continuing the effect of the hot bath, the patient being immediately after the bath wrapped in dry warm woolen blankets, and left to continue perspiring for an hour or two.

The dry pack is frequently employed as a means of promoting reaction after a cold bath in feeble patients.

Contraindications and Precautions.— 1. In the application 1195
of the dry pack, the fact that heat elimination is diminished should be borne in mind. If the application is continued too long, or if too great an amount of heat is applied, the body temperature may rise to an injurious degree. This is especially true in its use to abort a malarial chill.

2. When employed for the relief of chronic rheumatism, or for sciatica and other neuralgias involving large nerve trunks, the dry pack can not be followed by extremely cold applications without running the risk of producing severe pain and other inconveniences. In cases of this sort, the wrappings may be removed gradually, so that the patient may be cooled off by degrees, or partial cold friction may be employed.

3. When employed in cases of paralysis, the application should not be continued so long as to induce profuse perspiration. When the normal heat of the skin is restored, a portion at least of the wrappings should be removed.

4. When employed to produce perspiration, the dry pack should not be used more frequently than once or twice a week, except in cases of obesity.

5. The dry pack is contraindicated in cases of chronic *cerebral congestion*, *irritable heart*, *eruptive disorders* of the skin, and in cases in which patients are extremely nervous or excitable. It can seldom be employed to advantage with children as a means of inducing perspiration, and except when used to combat *collapse* or abort a *malarial paroxysm*, is not very frequently called into use, as the hot-blanket pack and other heating procedures are more convenient.

THE HALF-PACK.

1196 This procedure (Fig. 85) is precisely the same as the wet-sheet pack (**1179**), with the exception that it is confined to the trunk of the body and the hips, the arms and legs being excluded from the application. It may be confined to the trunk only, and is then called the trunk pack.

The same materials are needed for the application, the only difference being in their disposition; the same temperatures are employed, and the remarks made with reference to physiological effects and therapeutic indications are equally applicable. It may be added simply that the half-pack is attended by less inconvenience to the patient, while its therapeutic efficiency is almost as great as that of the full pack.

The half-pack is of special value in *insomnia* and the *nervous affections* growing out of indigestion with resulting irritation of the abdominal sympathetic. When employed for insomnia, the pack should be applied at bedtime, and may be kept in place during the greater part of the night if necessary to enable the patient to sleep.

The contraindications are the same as for the pack (**1188**).

THE HOT-BLANKET PACK.

The hot-blanket pack (Fig. 86) consists in the envelop- 1197
ment of the body in a woolen blanket wrung out of water as hot as can be endured by the patient without pain or injury.

Requisites.—A couch or bed with a good mattress, a small hair or cotton pillow, four or five woolen blankets, a rubber blanket, two or three bottles or rubber bags filled with hot water.

Method.—The pillow is laid upon the couch, the rubber blanket is first spread out, the upper edge overlapping the pillow, and all but one of the woolen blankets are spread out smoothly, one after the other, in such a manner as just to cover the pillow. Another blanket, having been placed in water at a temperature of about 160°, is then wrung out. The most convenient manner of wringing out blankets is shown in Fig. 87. The blanket should be rapidly wrung as dry as possible. After wringing, it is spread out upon the dry blanket as quickly as possible, and the patient, having previously disrobed, lies down at once in the center of the blanket and is quickly enveloped as directed for the wet-sheet pack (**1179**). Hot water bottles or bags are placed at the feet for additional heat.

Physiological Effects.—The hot-blanket pack is an excit- 1198
ing and heating measure of great power. It communicates heat to the body, diminishes heat elimination, and increases heat production. Its application excites the circulation, increases the pulse-rate, raises the temperature two to three degrees, and when sufficiently prolonged, induces profuse perspiration. It differs from the sweating wet-sheet pack in that its action as an exciting procedure is direct, whereas the wet-sheet pack is primarily sedative, the exciting effects being secondary, as the result of the reaction.

The hot-blanket pack is followed by an atonic reaction through which the circulation is slowed, nerve tension lowered, and the activity of the vital processes diminished. Its frequent repetition produces depression of nerve tone, lowers vital resistance, and enfeebles the circulation.

The effects of the hot-blanket pack differ from those of the dry pack in that the application of the dry pack is not followed by atonic reaction, the heating being gradual.

The hot-blanket pack, after the first moment, is essentially a vapor bath. The loose meshes of the wrappings are filled with warm vapor, which is retained by the rubber sheet. The effects are essentially the same as those of a vapor bath.

1199 **Therapeutic Applications.**—The hot-blanket pack is especially useful in cases in which the temperature is subnormal, as in cases of *collapse*, *surgical shock*, etc. It is useful in all cases for which the dry pack is indicated, and is generally to be preferred to the dry pack except in the cold stage of intermittent fever, when the dry pack is preferable, because of the danger of provoking chill through the evaporation which takes place from the moistened skin when a hot-blanket pack is administered.

The hot-blanket pack is a valuable procedure in cases of *acute Bright's disease*, in the *albuminuria* of pregnancy, in *eclampsia*, in *convulsions* of children with pallor, to induce perspiration in *subacute rheumatism*, in *chronic toxemia*, in *infectious jaundice*, in nephritis complicating *typhoid*, *scarlatina*, *yellow fever*, *measles*, and other *infectious fevers*, in *influenza*, *malarial* and *uremic coma*, *malarial hematuria*, *septicemia*, *muscular rheumatism*, *dengue*, *collapse* of *cholera* and *cholera morbus*, *peritonitis*, *renal calculus*, *acute myelitis*, and as a derivative in *lobar pneumonia*.

The hot-blanket pack is also useful as a preparation for cold applications, especially in adynamic febrile types, when the skin is cold, to insure good reaction, and thus aid heat elimination. It is almost equally useful in cases in which heat production is much increased as a means of lessening thermogenesis by atonic thermic reaction. In the first class of cases, the duration of the application should be just long enough to warm the skin; in the second class, the application should not continue more than from 2 to 4 minutes. In all cases the temperature should be as high as the patient can bear without burning.

Contraindications and Precautions.— Most of the suggestions made in relation to the dry pack are applicable here.

1. Extreme care must be taken to prevent increase of body temperature, especially when employed as a means of increasing heat elimination in fevers. The body temperature must be taken in the mouth, before, during, and after the application.

2. Care must be taken not to burn the patient by wringing the blanket out of water at too high a temperature. This is especially likely to occur in cases of paralysis in which there is found not only diminished sensibility of the skin, but lowered vitality of the tissues, and hence a double risk of injury from the application of too high a temperature. This danger is also very great in cases in which the circulation is greatly slowed in consequence of the administration of an anesthetic for surgical purposes and in cases of collapse in cyanosis and anasarca.

3. It must not be forgotten that the hot-blanket pack, like other general hot applications, although primarily stimulating, is ultimately exhausting and depressing; hence it must be carefully employed, especially in the case of chronic affections. It affords so much comfort in many cases that patients often call for its too frequent repetition.

Recent observations afford ground for the belief that disease germs are eliminated in great numbers by the skin, especially during very vigorous perspiration. This fact renders this procedure useful in all the acute infections.

THE EVAPORATING SHEET.

The evaporating sheet (Fig. 88) is one of the simplest of 1200
cooling procedures. It consists in wrapping the patient in a sheet wrung out of hot or cold water, as the indications may require, and allowing cooling by evaporation. The sheet should be wrung moderately dry, and should be applied next

the skin. The cooling is the result of the absorption of heat due to the evaporation of the water contained in the sheet.

Physiological Effects.—The evaporation of one pound of water will absorb about one thousand heat units, which for a patient weighing 160 pounds, would amount to a lowering of the body temperature six degrees. Such an effect is never produced, however, for the reason that heat production is constantly going on, and is replacing the heat loss at the rate of 7.2 units per minute or more. With a febrile temperature of 103°, spontaneous evaporation takes place at a very rapid rate from the surface of the sheets wrapped about the body; and when the evaporation is aided by means of vigorous fanning, as with a current of air from an electric fan (Fig. 89), most powerful refrigerative effects are produced. The patient should be gently rubbed continuously.

Therapeutic Applications.— The evaporating sheet is a useful measure in certain cases of fever. Either the cold or the hot evaporating sheet may be used, according to the indications present. The hot evaporating sheet is, however, most commonly employed. It is especially useful in adynamic cases, or where the patient is very nervous, depressed, apprehensive, and distressed at the thought of contact with the cold water. The hot evaporating sheet should be wrung very dry out of very hot water; the attendant should wrap the sheet about the patient very quickly, so that a strong impression of heat may be made upon the skin. As the evaporation takes place, the sheet will be rapidly cooled, and heat should thus be removed from the body.

The first impression of the hot sheet lessens heat production by reflex influence and dilates the surface vessels. While the vessels remain dilated, heat elimination takes place at ten times the ordinary rate (Conrad Klar). At the end of 3 to 5 minutes, the vessels become contracted so as greatly to lessen the rate of heat elimination, and hence the application should be renewed at short intervals (1 to 3 min.).

Evaporation is on the whole not a desirable or valuable mode of refrigeration except in cases in which there is very excessive activity of the surface circulation, with abnormal heat and no tendency to chill. Slow cooling of the skin by evaporation causes a contraction of the surface vessels which is not followed by reaction, and which is accordingly not only accompanied but followed by congestion of internal parts. Therefore this method of cooling is rarely indicated.

The cold sheet should be resorted to only in cases in which the surface congestion is so excessive that the contraction occasioned by cooling will be only sufficient to establish a normal condition of the vessels, and without inducing retrostasis of blood and congestion of the viscera. Active cutaneous circulation should be maintained by rubbing.

WET-HAND RUBBING.

This procedure (Fig. 90) consists simply in rubbing the 1201
cutaneous surface with the wet hand.

Method.— Water at 40° to 75°, with plenty of Turkish towels, a Turkish sheet, and a woolen blanket, are the only requisites for this bath. In beginning the application the attendant stands with his side to the couch, facing the patient, dips both hands into the water, then applies them, one to each side of the patient's face, covering as large an area as possible. Friction is made from the median line outward, the tips of the fingers sweeping over the brow and describing a sort of semicircle along the cheeks to the under side of the jaw. Repeat the movement three to six times. In men, wet the hair by shampooing with wet fingers or a wet towel.

Before wetting the face, a dry Turkish towel should be folded about the head in such a way as to protect the ears, and if the patient is a lady, the hair also, a precaution which will be much appreciated by nervous patients (Fig. 91).

Next the application is made to the chest, both hands being employed, first the upper part, then the sides of the chest being rubbed vigorously, then the abdominal surface. After the entire chest has been gone over three or four times with quick, short movements and considerable pressure, the towel is thrown over the chest and the surface dried quickly, the rubbing being continued until the surface is reddened. The face and head are not to be dried until the end, as it is desirable that these parts be cooled by evaporation.

The prolonged application to the head is to protect from congestion; the application to the chest before proceeding to other portions of the body is to stimulate the heart and lungs to increased activity, thereby promoting reaction.

The arms, first one, then the other, next receive attention. The attendant grasps the patient's hand with his left hand, while with the right he vigorously rubs the arm with long rapid strokes reaching from the shoulders to the wrist, his hand being kept cold and moistened by dipping in the basin after every four to six strokes. If the patient is fairly vigorous, he may hold his arm perpendicular while the attendant rubs with both hands.

On finishing the arm, the attendant rubs the hand between both his own, and ends with one or two smart blows upon the palm with the flat of his hand. The arm is quickly enveloped with a Turkish towel (Fig. 92), the patient holding one end, and is rubbed until the reddening of the skin indicates the establishment of reaction. The blanket is then drawn over it, and the other arm is treated in like manner.

Next give attention to the abdomen. Apply the friction first transversely, the rubbing being done alternately with the two hands, then in a circular manner, following the course of the colon. The thighs are next treated, but one being uncovered at a time. Then follows the treatment of the legs and feet, each of which should be rubbed until the circulation is well established.

The patient should now turn upon his face, and fold his arms beneath his forehead, thus drawing the shoulder-blades upward and outward, so as to flatten the dorsal surface as much as possible. The attendant then dips his hands and applies them first to the back and sides of the neck, extending the fingers around so as to reach the front of the

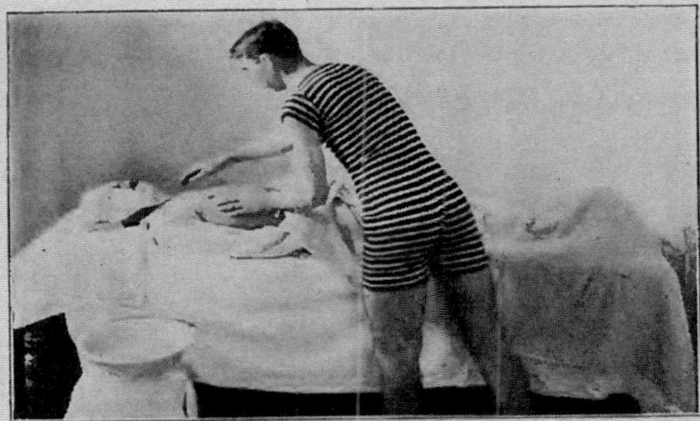

FIG. 90. WET-HAND RUB (p. 627).

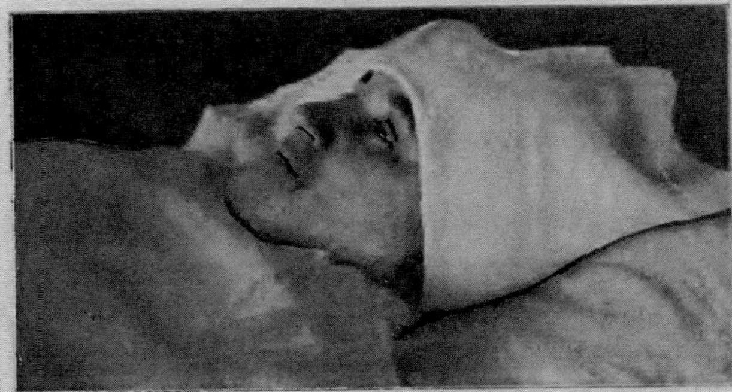

FIG. 91. WET-HAND RUB — Protection of hair and ears (p. 627).

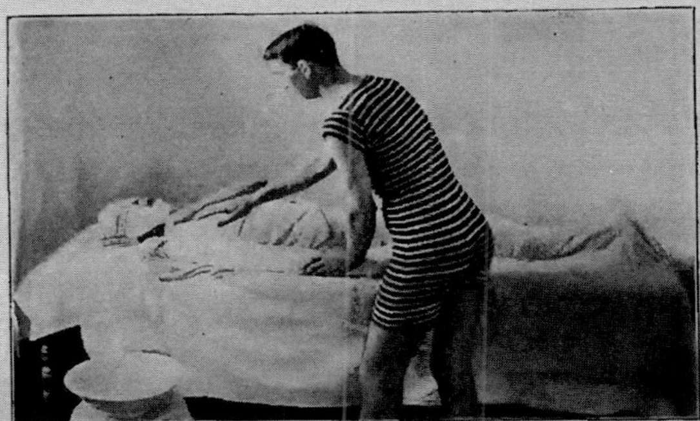

FIG. 92. WET-HAND RUB — Drying Arm (p. 628).

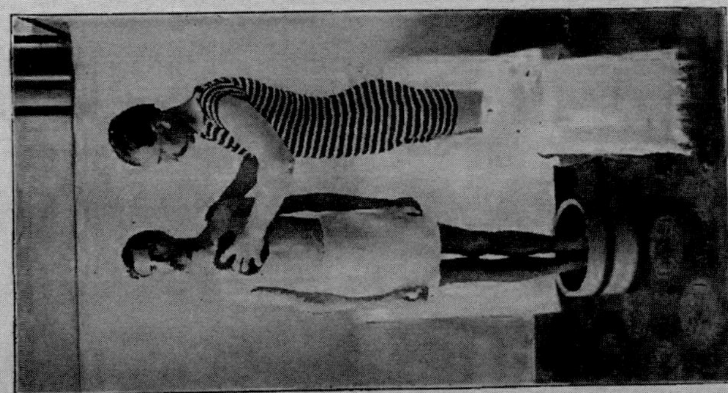

FIG. 93. SPONGE BATH (p. 634).

neck. The upper part of the back, the shoulders, and the outer portion of the upper arm should next receive attention, then the middle and lower parts, and the sides of the trunk. Lastly, apply to the whole length of the spine a few vigorous strokes. As fast as any part is dried, it should be covered.

The treatment concludes with an application to the feet of water at the same temperature as that applied to the head. The ankles and dorsum of the feet should be vigorously rubbed, and the sole percussed with energy, but not rubbed, on account of the unpleasant tickling sensation induced.

Not more than 5 to 15 seconds should be occupied in rubbing any part with the wet hand before the application of the towel. If the rubbing is insufficient to produce reddening of the surface, light spatting or percussion should be applied after drying. Good reaction should be secured in each area treated before proceeding to another portion of the surface.

The skin must be warm at the time of the application. An excellent hour is before rising in the morning.

The temperature employed and the duration of the treatment must depend upon the individual case. The temperature most frequently employed is from 65° to 75°, or the ordinary living-room temperature. Generally the hands of the attendant are simply dipped into water so as to moisten their surfaces, no more water being applied than is naturally carried by the moist hand. In certain cases, however, as when this procedure is employed as a general antipyretic or antifebrile measure, a larger quantity of water should be employed. The bed of the patient in such cases should be protected by a rubber blanket and the patient should be wrapped in a Turkish sheet. Instead of simply dipping his hand into the water, the attendant cups his hand in such a manner as to dip up all the water possible. This is quickly thrown upon the portion of the surface under treatment at the moment, which is at once vigorously rubbed. This alternate deluging and rubbing of the skin may be repeated from one to half a dozen times. In certain cases hot instead of cold water is employed.

1202 **Physiological Effects.**—Wet-hand rubbing is an efficient means of producing strong circulatory reaction with moderate thermic reaction by the combined influence of cold and friction. The reaction is still further encouraged by rubbing with the dry towel, and afterward applying friction and percussion with the hand.

The physiological effects of wet-hand rubbing are mixed in character, owing to the mixed nature of the application, the friction giving rise to mechanical effects, while the hydric effects proper are purely thermic. Employed at a temperature considerably below that of the skin, the application energizes both the cardiac and the respiratory functions, and thus a mild general tonic effect is produced. The friction as well as the cold impression increases blood pressure. The activity of the peripheral heart is increased, while the central heart is energized, often to a remarkable extent. By the employment of ice-water, the tonic effects may be considerably intensified, while on the other hand, by the employment of very hot water or even that at a neutral temperature, quieting effects are produced, with relief of pain when this symptom is present.

It is interesting to note that *while hot applications generally produce lowering of blood pressure, when the application is accompanied by moderate friction, there may be a moderate increase of tension.*

1203 **Therapeutic Applications.**—The cold wet-hand rub combines tonic, restorative, and derivative effects. The intensity of the effects produced depends upon the temperature of the water and the vigor of the friction. The colder the water, and the more vigorous and prolonged the friction, the more intense the effects. The feeble neurasthenic patient experiences, after an application of cold wet-hand rubbing, a delightful sensation of increased vigor, and relief from malaise and mental and nervous weakness.

Wet-hand rubbing may be made a most useful means of *reducing the temperature* and *increasing vital resistance* in febrile cases where the patient is too feeble to endure the application of the cold bath or the cooling pack, or under circumstances prohibiting these antipyretic measures. The lower the temperature of the water used, the more freely it is applied to the parts which are being rubbed, the longer the application, and the more frequent its repetition, the greater will be the antithermic or antifebrile effect produced (40° 65°). This means of reducing temperature is very appropriate for children and aged persons, and in cases of typhoid and other continued fevers in which the cold immersion bath can not for any reason be employed, as in cases of *intestinal perforation*, *myocarditis*, *nephritis*, *collapse*, and other complications.

Wet-hand rubbing with water at a temperature of 85° to 95° is a quieting measure of value in *feverishness* due to nervous excitability rather than to actual elevation of temperature. When employed for this purpose, the rubbing should be very gentle, and the passes should be in the form of stroking, the direction being, so far as possible, from the center toward the periphery. The surface may be left moist or may be dried by simply covering with a towel and gently passing the hand over the surface. The effort should be to avoid both thermic and circulatory reaction or stimulation of the heart.

Wet-hand rubbing is a measure of less power than the rubbing wet sheet, cold friction, and most other tonic applications, and hence its use is naturally limited to cases in which other more vigorous and more efficient measures can not be employed. It is well adapted to *very feeble neurasthenics* who dread water and have but little power to react. The warmth of the hand of the attendant, the rubbing, and the small amount of water employed when used for tonic effects, all tend to promote reaction, so that it may be said that there is no patient too feeble to admit of the application of this measure. Even very weak patients allow the application of ice-water when applied to the surface by the medium of the hand, though water at a much higher temperature would not be tolerated if applied by means of a sponge, towel, wet sheet, or any other vehicle. In very feeble, nervous, and excitable patients, the application should be made at first at a temperature of 70° or even 80°, and lowered one or two degrees each day until water at a temperature of 50° or even lower can be tolerated.

By this means the patient may be gradually trained to receive at first tepid, then cool, and finally cold water; then other procedures, as the cold friction, the towel rub, the rubbing wet sheet; and later the half-bath, the cold shower, and the horizontal douche, may be employed.

Wet-hand rubbing is especially indicated in the cases of very feeble invalids who, being entirely unaccustomed to cold water, have a dread of its application, which might almost be termed a species of hydrophobia.

Wet-hand rubbing is useful in *fever* cases in which the circulation of the skin is deficient, as shown by pallor, coldness, and *cyanosis*, as a preparation for more vigorous antipyretic measures. Each part must be rubbed until red. It may be appropriately employed whenever it is desirable to encourage cutaneous reaction, either alone or following a hot bath of some sort. This measure is especially useful in *chilblains* (40° to 50°).

For very feeble patients wet-hand rubbing may be applied to the back only. Very cold water applied to the back in this way is an excellent tonic. Cold wet-hand rubbing is also useful in aiding the circulation in the lower extremities in dyspeptics and neurasthenics troubled with cold feet and legs. In these cases the circulatory disturbance is not due to weakness of the heart, but to vasomotor spasm in the cold parts. Rub first with ice-water, then with warm flannels until red and warm.

There is no procedure of more general value than this simple measure. It is applicable to almost every form of acute and chronic disease. It is of special service in all forms of chronic disease accompanied by *anemia* or *low nerve tone* and *feeble vital resistance*, the number of which is too great to mention. It may be so graduated as to constitute the most mild and gentle measure possible, or a most vigorous and thoroughgoing hydriatic procedure.

Vigorous rubbing of the surface with the hand while cold water is poured upon the patient from the height of a few feet, is the most efficient means of combating sunstroke. This method was first used by Paulus of Ægina, A. D. 660 (Winternitz). It has been advocated in recent years by a number of writers on hydrotherapeutics.

Wet-hand rubbing is constantly employed in combination with many other baths. For instance, in the application of heating compresses, if the patient does not react promptly, the surface should be first rubbed with the hand dipped in cold water. Rubbing the chest with cold water is a valuable means of accelerating the heart's action before a general cold application, and thus increasing the patient's ability to react. Rubbing the face, head, and neck with cold water is the usual preparation for cold baths of all kinds.

Wet-hand rubbing is employed in connection with the shallow bath and the shallow foot bath, and rubbing with the hands is practiced in connection with nearly all cold baths excepting packs, compresses, and the different forms of the douche. In general, cold friction applied locally is an excellent means of protecting an internal part against congestion from the cold douche. The water employed should be very cold, and the application should be made to the cutaneous area in reflex relation with the internal part which it is desired to protect; as, for example, if it is desired to protect the liver, the application should be made over the region of the liver just before the douche. The stomach, bowels, chest, and heart may be protected in like manner.

Contraindications. — Wet-hand rubbing should not be employed for the reduction of temperature in *smallpox*, *scarlet fever*, or other *exanthemata*. It is also contraindicated in *eczema* and other non-inflammatory types of eruptive diseases of the skin.

THE SPONGE, ABLUTION, OR TOWEL BATH.

1204 This (Fig. 93) is a general hydriatic measure consisting of an application of water to the surface by means of a wet sponge or towel.

Requisites.—A basin of water at the proper temperature; a large bath-sponge or coarse towel; Turkish towels; a foot tub if the patient is able to stand erect.

Method.—The foot-bath tub should contain water at a temperature of 104° to 110°. With the patient standing in the foot bath bending forward, his head, face, and neck are thoroughly and repeatedly drenched with cold water (50°) by means of a saturated sponge or towel. The attendant then applies the saturated sponge (60° to 70°; average 65°) first across the chest and abdomen, then the back, the arms, and the legs. The sponge should be applied with moderate pressure, and should be rewet as often as emptied of water. The whole surface of the body should be gone over very rapidly.

The sponging being completed, a dry sheet is thrown about the patient, who steps out of the foot bath, and holds his feet in alternation over the foot bath each two or three seconds, while cold water is poured over them. The patient is quickly rubbed dry, assisting himself as much as possible in the rubbing so as to encourage reaction by exercise. After the bath the patient should take moderate exercise, or if unable to do so, dry friction should be applied (**1221**).

The patient whose strength is at least moderately good may administer this bath to himself by means of a towel, following as nearly as possible the order just indicated as regards the application. The application to the back may be easily made by grasping the towel by its ends, throwing it over a shoulder, and making a seesaw movement.

To a patient who is unable to stand, this bath may be

administered in bed (Fig. 94). Care should be taken that the feet are not cold, and that the whole surface of the body is warm. The application is made when the patient is reclining in essentially the same manner as when in the standing position. A rubber blanket must be placed beneath him on the bed, and so arranged that the surplus water may run away into some proper receptacle, to prevent wetting of the bedclothing. The rubber sheet should be covered by a Turkish sheet, which for simple sponging with a well-wrung sponge may be sufficient. The patient having been undressed and covered in the bed, the attendant begins the application by first sponging the face and neck, then the following parts in succession: One arm, the other arm, the chest and abdomen, the front side of the legs, the back, the back side of the legs. No portion of the body should be exposed to the air except the portion under treatment, and this should be covered as quickly as possible after drying. Not more than 3 to 5 seconds should be employed in the sponging of each part, the same length of time in rubbing the parts with the hands, and 5 to 10 seconds in the drying and rubbing of each part.

The temperature of the bath and its duration depend upon the effect sought. If the desired effect is the reduction of temperature and the stimulation of vital resistance, water at a temperature of 60° to 70° should be employed, and a basin of water should be placed near the bedside so that as much water as possible may be lifted in the towel or sponge and applied to the patient. Each part should be sponged and rubbed thoroughly so as to induce good reaction; and after the whole surface has been gone over, the application may be repeated as many times as is necessary to secure the effect desired. When employed for tonic effects, the amount of water should be small, the temperature low (50° to 35°), and the rubbing and spatting vigorous.

The whole body should be kept warmly covered, except the part being rubbed, in all cases other than those in which reduction of temperature is the object sought, and even in these cases so much exposure should not be allowed as to prevent reaction by the disturbing effects of evaporation.

The patient, if feeble and with defective circulation, should be prepared for the bath by an accumulation of heat in the skin in any convenient manner, as by the dry pack, that is, wrapping with warm blankets with a hot bag to the spine and feet; by a hot-water bath; by hot-water drinking; or by a fomentation over the abdomen.

1205 **Physiological Effects.**— The physiological effects of the sponge or towel bath, or ablution, as the application is sometimes termed, are essentially the same as those of wet-hand rubbing, and depend upon the same conditions. The difference is simply that this application is more vigorous; a larger quantity of water is employed, more heat is abstracted from the body, the general thermic and circulatory reactions are more intense, and the application is in every way a more vigorous one than the simple rubbing of the surface with the wet hand. The procedure is also somewhat more strongly refrigerant, and hence better adapted for use in febrile conditions. Very hot and very cold applications contract the vessels of the limited area to which the application is being made, but this is so small compared with the whole cutaneous surface that no perceptible retrostasis toward the viscera occurs, as in the cold immersion, the cold douche, and many other forms of cold application; while by successive applications to different parts of the surface, the whole body is gradually brought into a state of vigorous reaction. This is one of the chief characteristics of the bath, and constitutes its leading distinguishing feature.

1206 **Therapeutic Applications.**— The therapeutic effects of the sponge bath are likewise essentially the same as those of wet-hand rubbing. It is simply a somewhat more vigorous application, which may be employed for the production of tonic, antipyretic, analgesic, calmative, and other therapeutic effects, both general and local. It is one of the most use-

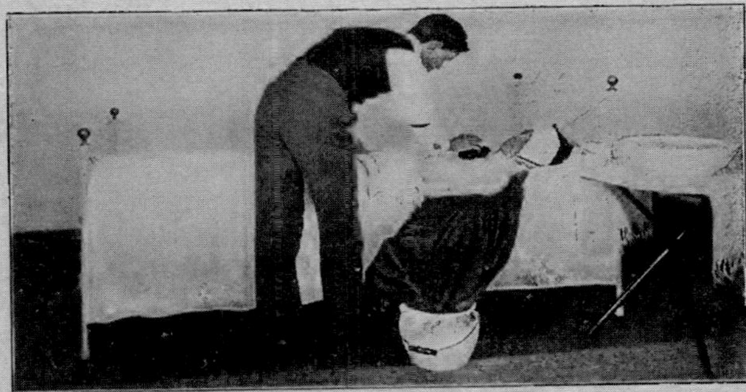

Fig. 94. SPONGE BATH IN BED (p. 635).

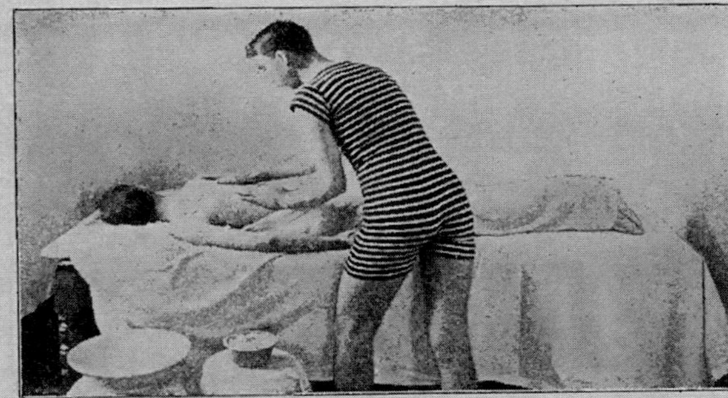

Fig. 95. SALT GLOW (p. 641).

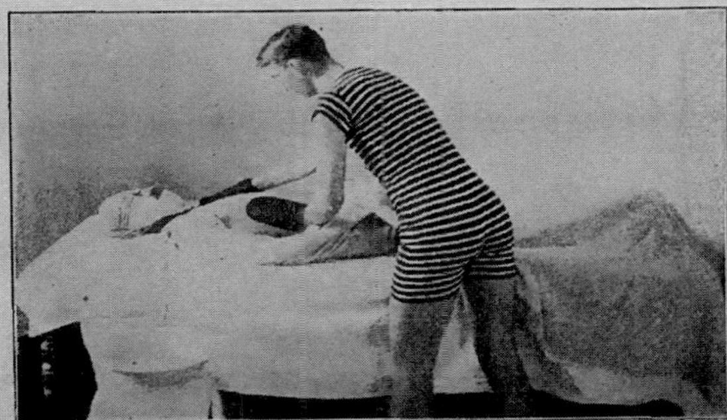

Fig 96. COLD MITTEN FRICTION (p. 642).

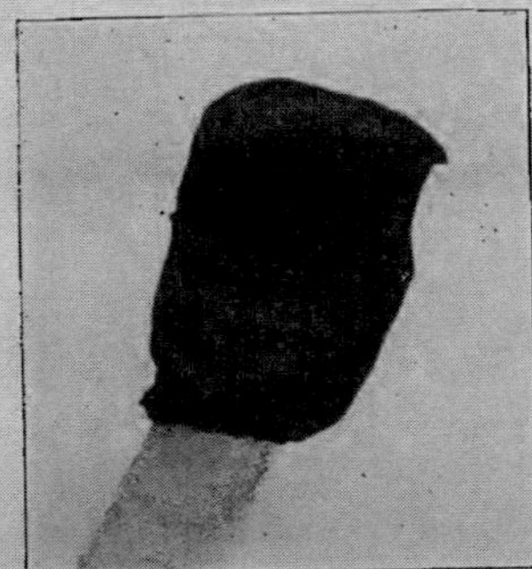

Fig. 97. FRICTION MITT (p. 643).

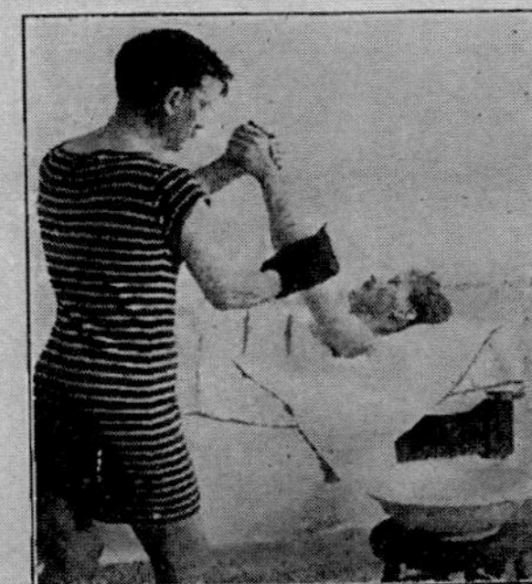

Fig. 98. COLD MITTEN FRICTION TO ARM (p. 644).

ful of hydric applications because readily available under almost any circumstances demanding the employment of water as a therapeutic means.

The *cold* ablution or sponge bath is highly advantageous in all cases in which the skin is anemic, as in *chlorosis*, *myxedema*, *anemia*, cases of *cardiac* and *renal dropsy*, and in all cases to which cold friction and cold towel rubbing are applicable. Skilfully applied, it is a good refrigerant measure, but when used to reduce fever, it must often be employed almost continuously for several hours in succession, or until the desired effect has been obtained. The work should be done so briskly and energetically that good cutaneous circulation is maintained, and shivering prevented. The beginning of pronounced shivering is an evidence that the full effect of the bath as an antipyretic has been obtained. The cool sponging should be continued in fever cases until shivering or other evidences of secondary chill appear, notwithstanding the most active efforts to postpone the same by rapidly going over the whole surface, first with the very wet sponge, then rubbing with the hands and drying with the towel, and finally rubbing with the warm hand, then repeating the process.

The cold sponge bath is useful in *adynamic febrile states*, as in typhoid fever, when the extremities are cold. The water employed should be quite cold (50° to 60°). The sponge should be wrung quite dry, and should be rubbed quickly over the limbs, which should then be rubbed vigorously with the warm hands until reaction occurs. The success of this measure depends upon using very cold water and making the application very short and vigorous.

Currie called attention to the value of the sponge bath in mild cases of fever in children and in very feeble patients, and also pointed out that this measure may be advantageously employed in cases of general fever due to some internal inflammatory process in which the cold bath can not be safely used on account of the condition of the blood-vessels of the affected part.

This bath is an excellent one for self-application when the patient is able to administer the treatment to himself at home. It may be employed every morning, on rising, with advantage. As the patient becomes accustomed to the application of cold water, more vigorous measures, such as a sponge or towel bath, a cold friction bath, or cold immersion, may be employed.

Hot sponging is sometimes advantageous in fever as a means of reflexly lessening the tendency to heat production; the water employed should be very hot (130° to 140°), and the application should be very rapidly made.

Local ablutions are valuable in many conditions, as in hot sponging of the spine for the relief of so-called *spinal irritation*, *headache*, *intercostal neuralgia*, *sleeplessness*, and the general nervousness so often encountered in *neurasthenia*.

The general hot sponge bath is of value in relieving the *night sweats* of consumption. The water should be applied as hot as can be borne, especially over the chest and abdomen.

The *hot alkaline* sponge bath is of service in *urticaria*. In this the application should likewise be made as hot as the patient's skin will bear; that is, 130° to 140°. The water employed should be rendered alkaline by the addition of a teaspoonful of soda for each pint of water. Very hot sponging is highly useful as a means of relieving itching of the skin when not accompanied by eruption.

When warm or hot water is employed, vigorous rubbing after the bath is not required. If a towel is used to dry the parts, it should be simply laid upon the surface and gently rubbed or patted with the hand outside. Wrapping the patient in a Turkish sheet is the best method of drying.

The very hot sponge bath is much employed for *hemostatic effects*. The application may be made directly to the bleeding surface, as in capillary oozing, for which it has rendered most efficient service in abdominal surgery, or through the remote effect of the stimulus of heat upon the vasomotor nerves, as in the stoppage of nosebleeding by sponging the face with very hot water. When used for hemostatic effects, very high temperatures must be employed,—from 140° upwards. When directly applied, the sponge must be only half wrung, and must be held with firm pressure in close contact with the bleeding surface, but great care must be taken to avoid injury to the parts.

Recent results show that local septic processes may often be checked by the application of water at a temperature of 180° to 212°, by means of a saturated sponge held for a few seconds in contact with the suppurating surface. Care must be taken to avoid injuring the healthy tissues adjacent. The object sought is not simply destruction of the pyogenic microbes, but a slight cooking of the devitalized and degenerated tissues upon the pyogenic surface, and a powerful stimulation of the circulation and the nerves of the part.

The *tepid* sponge bath is a very grateful application in feverish conditions, especially in cases in which the temperature is not sufficiently high to admit of more vigorous measures. If the skin is kept moist by frequent sponging, evaporation is promoted and the patient is thus cooled without producing the thermic reaction and consequent elevation of temperature likely to result from cold sponging. The purpose of tepid sponging is simply to restore the natural cooling process which has been interrupted by suspension of perspiration.

The *neutral* sponge bath at a temperature of 90° to 98° is a quieting, sedative measure of great service in nervous states accompanied by feverishness without elevation of temperature. It is also useful in mild *febricula*, and in fevers in which the temperature is only slightly above normal, and in which the skin is flushed and dry.

Alternate sponging of the spine is a powerful excitant of the cardiac and respiratory centers, and may be employed with wonderful advantage in cases of *opium poisoning*, *asphyxia* from coal gas, and in cases of *toxemia*, in which the heart's action is greatly weakened. This application is also valuable for its remarkable tonic effects upon the central nervous system; for the relief of *headache* and the *pains* at the back of the head and neck of which neurasthenics often complain, there is no better palliative than hot and cold sponging to the cervical and dorsal spine. When used for such excitant and revulsive effects, two sponges are employed, with one of which hot water is applied, with the other cold, the two being used in alternation. Ice is sometimes used in place of the cold sponge.

Sponging the parts with either hot or cold water is an exceedingly valuable measure for *sprains* and *bruises*. The water employed should be either very hot or very cold, or *revulsive* hot and cold applications may be made (130°, 2 min.; 60°, 20 secs.) If the sprain is recent, having occurred within a few hours, the ankle and foot should be sponged with water as hot as can be borne, the temperature being raised as the skin becomes tolerant. In cases of neglected sprain, in which the parts have become swollen and acutely inflamed, sponging with ice-cold water, gently passing the sponge over the part and squeezing the water upon it, may be employed for an hour or two at a time several times a day until the acute stage of the inflammation is passed, or during twenty-four or forty-eight hours. In the interval between the applications, the cooling compress should be applied.

Alternate hot and cold applications may be applied to joints in which exudates have occurred as the result of *rheumatism*, *sprain*, or *traumatic arthritis*. Alternate applications are not useful in cases in which the parts are very painful. Neither cold nor alternate applications of this sort should be made to joints which are the seat of a tubercular process.

1207 **Contraindications.**—The cold sponge bath should be avoided in cases of fever accompanied by cyanosis with coldness of the surface. In such cases, cold friction following a hot application is indicated. The surface must be warm and the movement of blood active in the skin to secure good reaction to a cold application. It must also be avoided in feeble cases when the patient is perspiring. This precaution does not apply when perspiration is the result of exercise without exhaustion or after a sweating process.

Sponging, as well as other procedures accompanied by friction, is generally inapplicable to cases in which the skin is irritable, as in cases of cutaneous disease and the eruptive fevers.

THE SALT GLOW.

In this procedure (Fig. 95), salt of medium fineness and 1208
slightly moistened is applied to the surface of the body with friction movements, the amount of pressure being adjusted to the patient's sensation. With very thin-skinned persons, abrasion and irritation of the skin may be very easily produced. Persons of dark complexion, whose skins are usually thick, bear more vigorous applications than blondes.

The patient prepares for the treatment by lying down upon a slab or bed covered with a sheet, having previously been divested of his clothing. The sheet is drawn over the patient to prevent chilling. One part after another is then exposed and rubbed with the moistened salt, two or three pounds of which should be conveniently at hand in a basin. When this treatment is given in an institution, the patient may sit upon a stool, lie upon a slab, or stand upon a low stool, while receiving the application, in a room especially arranged for the purpose, and at a temperature sufficiently high to prevent chilling.

After the application, the salt which adheres to the surface is removed by the cold affusion, shower, or spray. The patient is quickly dried and rubbed in the usual manner. It will be noticed that the skin is hard and almost as smooth as marble after this application. In cases of feeble patients, a dash of hot water or a warm shower should be given just before the final cold application.

Physiological Effects.—The salt glow is an admirable means of producing circulatory reaction, without thermic reaction if the temperature employed is not very much below that of the surface of the body. The salt acts as a chemical irritant to the skin, in addition to the mechanical stimulus produced by the rubbing of the sharp crystals in contact with the surface of the body.

The salt glow produces to an intense degree the circulatory stimulation of the brine bath, the sea-water bath, the effervescing bath, and the saline sponge, and with little thermic effect, provided the temperature of the salt when employed is not much below that of the body. By moistening the salt with ice-cold water, it is possible, however, when desirable, to produce most powerful thermic effects in addition to the circulatory reaction produced by the chemical effect of the salt and the friction.

Therapeutic Applications.—The salt glow is a tonic measure of high value, and also produces valuable derivative effects; it is especially valuable in feeble patients whose heat-making powers are small, and in whom thermic reaction does not readily occur, or if it does, the cold bath still has the effect to exhaust the patient and produce loss of heat. The salt glow is valuable in cases in which the skin is very inactive, a condition commonly found present in *chronic indigestion.* It may be usefully employed in cases of *Bright's disease*, and in *diabetics*, conditions demanding increase of skin activity, but contraindicating the cold bath.

The salt glow must be avoided in *eczema* and most other forms of skin disease, and must not in any case be used so frequently as to produce cutaneous irritation. This measure is rarely of use in any form of acute disease.

COLD FRICTION.

1209 By the term "cold friction" (Fig. 96) is designated a procedure which consists in the application to the surface of the body of a series of partial wet rubbings, one part after another being taken in systematic order until the whole cutaneous surface has been brought into vigorous reaction.

Requisites.—A vessel containing a few quarts of cool, cold, or very cold water; ice-water may be employed in many cases. A mitt (Fig. 97) consisting of rough material of some sort,—ordinary rough linen or Turkish toweling is not desirable. Coarse mohair answers fairly well for the purpose; but the best fabric is a closely woven woolen cloth resembling hair-cloth, but slightly rougher to the touch, which is manufactured in Egypt and Turkey, where the author became acquainted with it in the Turkish baths of Cairo and Constantinople. It is there used for a sort of preliminary shampooing applied after the sweating process is completed and before the application of soap. This material possesses just the right degree of roughness, stimulating the skin without irritating it, and is so closely woven that it may be made to hold just the right amount of water for the purpose for which it is designed. A Turkish sheet and one or two towels are also required.

Method.—The patient is undressed, and lies upon a bed or a massage couch wrapped in a Turkish sheet. First of all, the head, face, and neck should be wet with cold water. If the hair is not wet (ladies often object to this), a napkin wet with cold water should be placed over the face. The vessel containing the cold water is placed at one side, near the head of the couch; the attendant places the mitt upon the right hand, and then uncovers a small portion of the patient's body, preferably the front of the trunk. He then dips the mitt into the cold water, and proceeds to rub the surface until reddened, redipping the mitt one or more times, covering the whole surface rapidly. Care should be taken to secure reaction in each part before proceeding to the next. Then with his left hand the attendant extends the arm and treats it in like manner, drying rapidly and covering. The other arm is then treated, and then in succession, the legs, and back, the hips, and back of the legs, and lastly the feet. The soles of the feet should be spatted, not rubbed (Fig. 98).

This application is graduated by the temperature and the degree of saturation of the mitt,—"moist mitt," "wet mitt," and "filled mitt." The mitt is first saturated with water, then well wrung, and slipped on the hand. For the (*a*) "moist mitt" the palmar surface is merely touched to the surface of the water; for the (*b*) "wet mitt," the hand covered by the mitt is quickly dipped in the water two thirds its length, then shaken to remove surplus water; for the (*c*) "filled mitt" the whole mitt is immersed and filled with water, and quickly carried to the part to be treated; the water flows out while the surface is being rubbed, and the effect is thus almost as vigorous as that of the half-bath, only that it is partial in its application, and hence may be employed in cases in which the shock of a cold application to the whole surface simultaneously would be injurious.

By this means it is easy to bathe a fever patient with ice-water or water at a temperature of 35° to 45° without the production of shock or other undesirable effects, while securing the tonic effect upon the heart and the increase of general vital resistance, which are the most desirable effects.

In cases in which cold is positively contraindicated, hyperemia of the skin may be induced by hot mitten friction, using water at as high a temperature as possible.

This method, which the author has systematized and introduced within the last year (1899), he has found among the most useful of all cold applications, both as a tonic and as an antipyretic. One of the great advantages of the method is that it lends itself so readily to all the various conditions arising in the treatment of pathological states.

1210 **Physiological Effects.**—The act of rubbing the surface produces mechanical effects similar to those from the impact of water under pressure, as in the douche, although the effect is certainly much less pronounced than that of water at the same temperature in the form of the douche; however, a much lower temperature may be employed with cold friction than with the cold douche (32° F.), and hence the reaction induced may be even more powerful, and indeed, according to the author's observation, is more quickly secured, than with the cold douche. Indeed, there is no form of douche, except the author's percussion douche, which produces so vigorous and prompt reaction as does the cold friction applied with a mitt of proper texture. Reaction occurs with great rapidity in this procedure for the reason that the delay which commonly follows the thermic impression of cold before reaction begins, is prevented by the application of vigorous friction simultaneously with the thermic impression. Circulatory reaction is also stimulated to a high degree, and a large amount of blood is rapidly brought to the skin.

The stimulation of the peripheral nerves induced by cold friction produces most profound reflex effects upon the nervous system, the heart, the glandular structures, and indeed the whole organism. It is a most powerful tonic; hence a regulator of nutrition and a potent vital stimulant.

The friction mitt may be advantageously employed in the rubbing sitz, the rubbing shallow, or the Brand bath, and all other forms of cold baths in which rubbing is desirable. In mixed applications of this sort it may be advantageous to employ a mitt for each hand. In general, however, the bare hand is better in these cases, as its warmth helps to secure the circulatory reaction which is one of the essential objects of the application. The use of the mitt somewhat intensifies the thermic effect of the bath.

Therapeutic Applications.— Cold friction may be locally 1211
applied over any part desired. When applied to the lower extremities, for example, the effect is revulsive or derivative. Cold water applied to the precordial region with friction influences the heart in a powerful manner. Cold friction applied to the back and scalp powerfully stimulates the cerebral functions.

Cold friction is indicated in all cases requiring tonic applications; hence it is invaluable in *neurasthenia*, and especially with very feeble neurasthenics who are either too weak to receive the douche or too exhausted to react to this powerful tonic procedure. Cold friction affords the best of all means for training patients to endure the contact of cold water with the surface. It has no equal as a measure for graduated hydriatic training.

This procedure may be advantageously employed in cases of *anemia*, *chlorosis*, in all forms of *wasting disease*, as *tuberculosis*, and in *convalescence* after fevers; in *cardiac dropsy*, as a means of stimulating the peripheral circulation; in *anasarca* from renal disease; in *chronic toxemia* accompanied by spasm of the peripheral vessels; in all cases of *cardiac insufficiency;* in *febrile conditions*, to reduce temperature, whenever cold in any form is indicated. It is a hydric measure of remarkable versatility, and may be employed in a vast variety of cases. There is no measure of greater value than cold friction in the treatment of *tuberculosis pulmonaris*. The application may be made twice daily with advantage, a temperature of 75° being used at first, and steadily lowered day by day until 35° can be readily endured. The "moist mitt" should be used. As it is the tonic effect which is especially desired, care should be observed that each surface treated is made to glow with vigorous reaction before proceeding to another part. This prevents pulmonary congestion.

Cold friction affords an excellent means of testing the ability of a patient to react. In *fevers*, it presents an excellent test for the state of the heart, and even affords a valuable means of prognosis. Great slowness to react, the parts remaining cold and pale, indicates excessive irritability of the vasomotor centers or nerves. This condition, which is commonly present in anemia, especially in grave cases, is often a cause of great difficulty in securing reaction. When present in acute fevers, vascular spasm is a positive indication of diminished heat elimination, and suggests at once the necessity of employing some means to increase the peripheral circulation, such as the short, hot-blanket pack, hot immersion for 3 to 4 minutes, fomentations to the spine, or some other heating process, to be followed by cold friction, and is a contraindication for prolonged cold baths. When the skin is very slowly reheated after an application of cold water, a mottled blue appearance remaining, the indication is great feebleness of the thermogenetic functions of the body, or diminished power of calorification. In fevers, this condition indicates impending collapse.

Cold friction must be mentioned also as a measure more or less indispensable in *typhoid fever* in *aged persons*, *children*, and *diabetics*, and in this disease when complicated by *ataxic* and *adynamic conditions;* in *dicrotic pulse*, *stupor*, *subnormal temperature*, *pregnancy*, *puerperal fever*, also in *chronic dysentery*, *malarial fever*, *coma* from any cause, *whooping-cough*, *yellow fever*, *plague*, *dengue*, *influenza*, *lithemia*, *leprosy*, *emaciation*, *scurvy*, *rickets*, *purpura*, *anorexia*, *hypopepsia*, *intestinal catarrh*, *chronic nephritis*, *hysteria*, *neurasthenia*, *Bell's palsy*, *migraine*, *chorea major*, *paralysis agitans*, and *morphia* and other drug habits. A *cyanotic skin* is always an indication for cold friction preceded or followed by heat, if the patient is very feeble.

When frequently repeated or prolonged hot applications are required, cold friction should be employed every two or three hours, or at least two or three times a day, *to maintain cardiac tone and general vital resistance.*

Contraindications.— There is scarcely any condition in 1212
which the cold friction mitt may not be employed. There are almost no contraindications except cutaneous lesions, in which the wet-towel friction should be substituted.

THE COLD TOWEL RUB.

This procedure consists in friction movements made upon 1213
a cold wet towel spread out upon the surface.

Requisites.— A towel for the head, several linen towels for the application; a sheet and a towel for drying; a pail of water at the temperature desired for the application, and a basin of water at a temperature ten degrees lower.

Method.—The patient should lie in a recumbent position with all his clothing removed, and wrapped in a Turkish sheet and a woolen blanket, a portion of the covering being laid aside so as to expose the portion to which the application is to be made. The head, face, and neck are first bathed with the colder water, in which one of the towels is also wet, and wrapped about the head. A linen towel is then wrung very dry out of the water prepared for the purpose in the pail. After being quickly shaken out, it is applied smoothly to the part to be treated; and with the hands applied in such a manner as to cover as large a portion of the towel as possible, they are rapidly moved from point to point with firm pressure, so as to bring each part of the towel successively in close contact with the skin. The rubbing should be continued until the towel is warm, when it may be removed; the dry towel is then placed upon or wrapped about the part, and it is rubbed until the skin is dry and *well reddened by reaction*. The corresponding part of the opposite side is then treated in like manner. If the patient is decidedly neurasthenic, special attention should be given to the back; while if the case is one of cardiac insufficiency, special attention should be given to the chest, arms, and legs.

The hands are rubbed upon the towel, but the towel is not rubbed upon the skin. Particular attention should be paid to this. The effect desired is not produced by mechanical irritation of the skin, but by the assistance rendered the circulation by the intermittent pressure upon the tissues. The hands are applied with long, rapid, alternating strokes, falling upon the surface with sufficient force to give a decided percussion effect. The friction movements may be alternated every few seconds with gentle percussion (**1227**). The whole surface of the towel should be gone over constantly, so as to avoid chilling by evaporation.

In order that the desired therapeutic effect may be obtained,

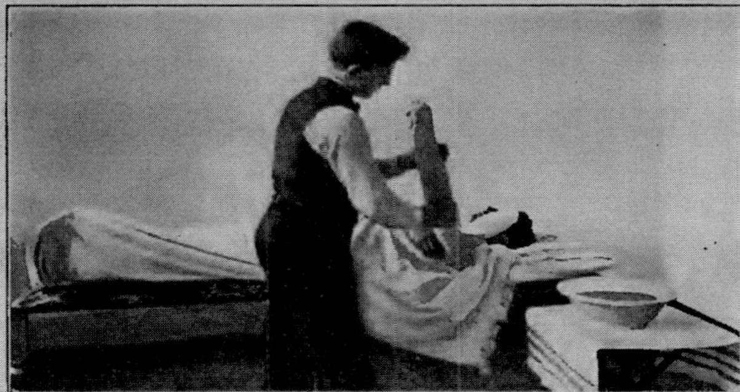

FIG. 99. COLD TOWEL RUB TO ARM (p. 649).

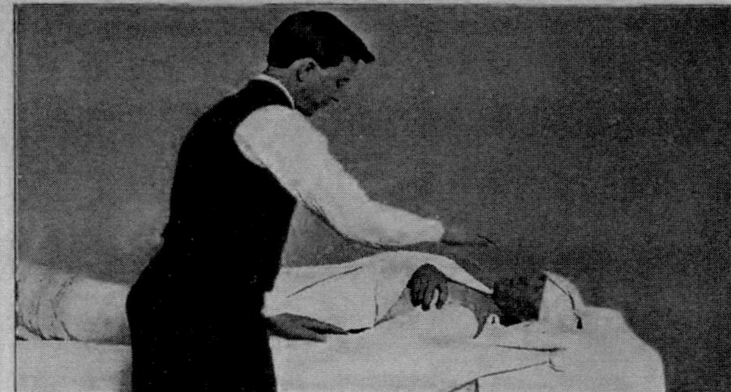

FIG. 100. COLD TOWEL RUB TO ARM — Patient Holding Towel (p. 649).

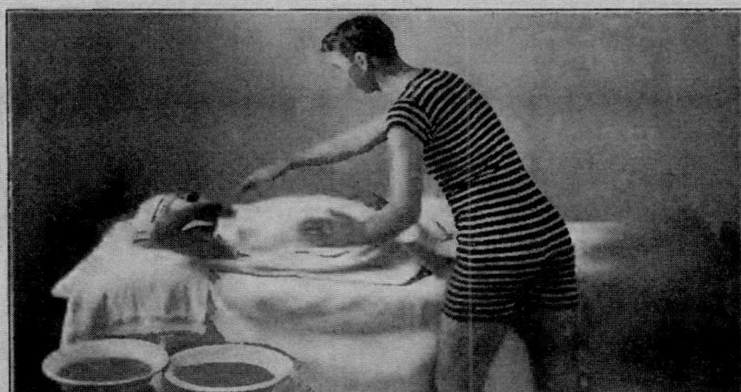

FIG. 101. COLD TOWEL RUB TO CHEST AND ABDOMEN (p. 649).

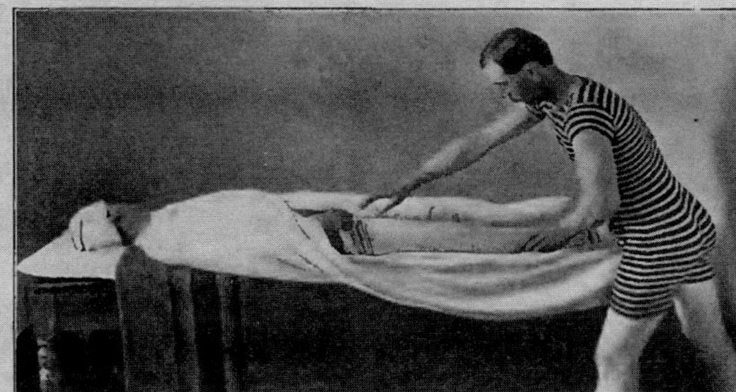

FIG 102. COLD TOWEL RUB TO LEG (p. 649).

the temperature of the water must be maintained at the initial temperature. This may be accomplished by employing a number of towels, so that no towel is used twice in the same application. A plan which the author prefers as more practical, however, is the following: Two pails or bowls of water are prepared, one of which is ten degrees lower than the temperature at which the application is to be made. The usual temperatures will be 60° and 50°. The face, neck, and head are cooled with the cooler water. After a towel has been applied to a surface and rubbed until warm, it is dropped into the cooler water, where it remains while the part is being dried and rubbed. In preparing the towel for a new application, it is gathered and squeezed, then dipped into the other pail (60°) and wrung out.

An excellent plan for institution work, where abundant facilities are supplied, is the following: Have ready several good-sized, rather heavy linen towels. Fold each one to half the length, wet in the cold water, twist, and leave in the water ready to wring out quickly when wanted. With the patient lying on his back, covered by a Turkish sheet, and the head cooled by one of the towels, uncover the chest, apply a well-wrung towel, rub well, then dry. Then uncover one arm, let the patient hold it up, and quickly wrapping a wet towel around it, let him catch the upper end with the hand of the arm under treatment (Fig. 99), holding the other end at the shoulder by his other hand while the attendant rubs vigorously, or the patient may hold the towel at the shoulder only, the arm lying by his side (Fig. 100). Then treat the other arm, and each leg. The patient holds one end of the towel for the leg, and both ends for the trunk (Figs. 101, 102). He then turns upon his face, and passing one hand over his shoulder and the other around back of the hip, he holds the towel spread out upon his back (Fig. 103); or the towel may be held at the upper end only (Fig. 104).

If the patient is too feeble to assist, the towel may be

kept in place by making the friction movements with the two hands simultaneously and from the center toward the ends or sides. It is far better, however, that at least one end of the towel should be held by the patient, so that the attendant may make long strokes with strong pressure, thus increasing the mechanical effect, which is an essential part of this procedure, especially when employed for the excellent tonic effects to be secured by it.

A towel is applied to the back of each leg, and lastly one to the feet, as follows: While the patient lies upon his face, the feet a few inches apart and the soles turned up, a towel is prepared and spread out under the feet, extending up above the ankles. The feet are separated, and the ends of the towel turned over and wrapped around each foot (Fig. 105). The soles are then percussed, and the ankles, instep, and toes rubbed until the towel is warm. Special care must be taken in drying the feet, to rub them until warm. The soles of the feet are important vasomotor areas, and have extended reflex relations; hence the importance of keeping the feet warm.

In drying, the dry towel should be applied and held in place in the manner described for the wet towel, or a corner of the Turkish sheet may be drawn over the part in such a way that long strokes may be made without displacing it (Fig. 106), or the patient may assist by holding one side (Fig. 107).

The amount of water in the towel may be regulated to suit each case. When refrigeration or antipyretic effects are required, the towel must be very wet, and its application renewed upon the same part several times in quick succession.

If the case is one of cardiac insufficiency, the treatment should begin with a limb, and end with the application of the towel over the chest. By this means, the small vessels are first dilated and stimulated to activity, thus lessening the work of the heart before the more powerful stimulating effect of the application to the chest is brought to bear upon it.

For very feeble patients, the temperature of the water employed at first may be as high as 70° to 75°, but it should

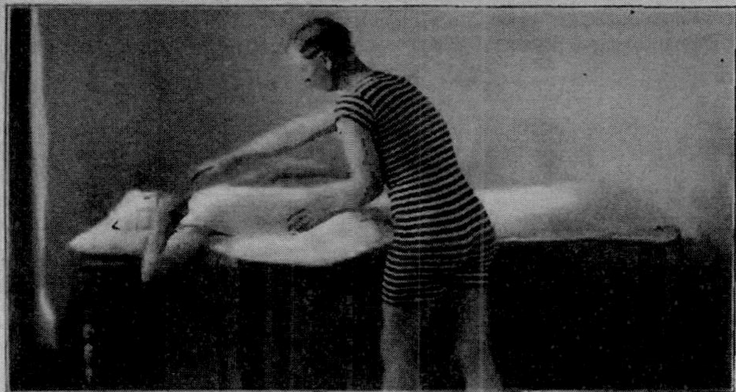

Fig. 103. COLD TOWEL RUB TO BACK — Patient Holding Towel in Place (p. 649).

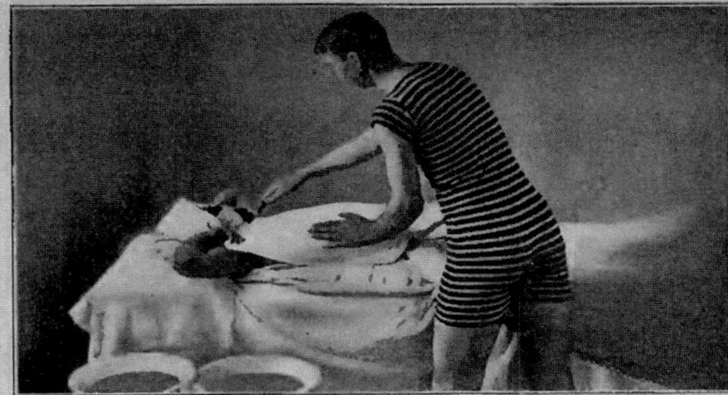

Fig. 104. COLD TOWEL RUB (p. 649).

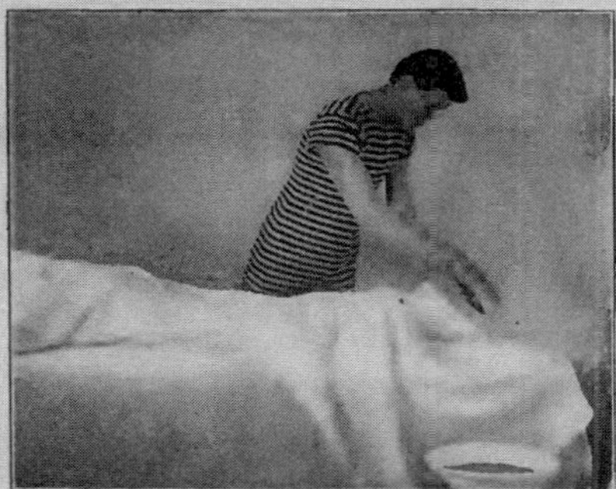

Fig. 105. Cold Towel Rub to Feet (p. 650).

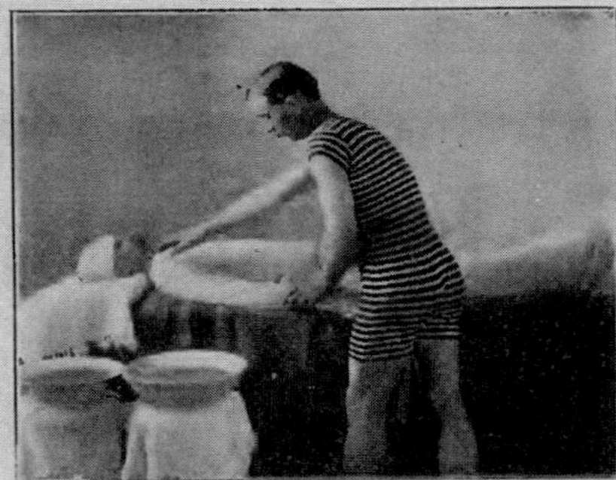

Fig. 106. Drying Patient after Cold Towel Rub (p. 650).

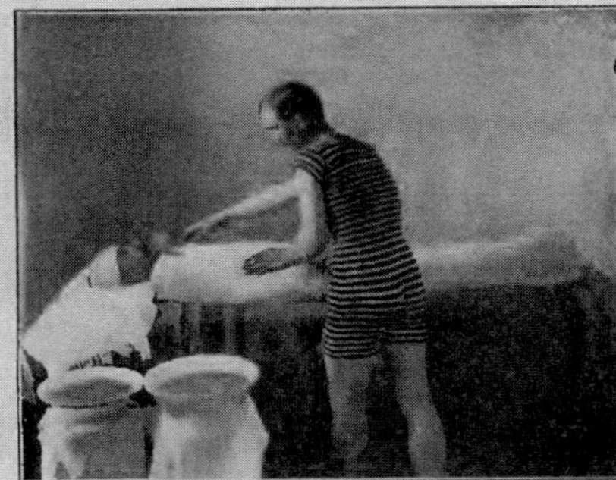

Fig. 107. Drying Patient after Cold Towel Rub (p. 650).

be lowered with each application until water at 55° or 60° may be used. Still better effects may be obtained at 50°.

The hot towel rub may be used when cold is positively contraindicated. As high a temperature as possible should be used (140° to 160°). Otherwise the method is the same.

Physiological Effects.—The physiological effects of the 1214
cold towel rub are precisely the same as those of the rubbing wet sheet, except that they are somewhat less pronounced. The nervous shock produced by the wet towel of a given temperature is very much less than that produced by the contact of the whole sheet with the surface of the body. At the same time, the reaction produced may be made just as complete as when the sheet is employed, and without producing any considerable degree of congestion of internal parts through retrostasis. As each part is successively treated, the cold application causes contraction of the vessels of the associated internal parts. As reaction occurs, the visceral vessels are dilated, and excited to increased activity. Thus vigorous fluxion is produced in one part after another until every internal organ has been awakened to new life and action, and all the bodily functions are quickened.

The fact that the inrush of blood and the succeeding reaction do not occur in all parts of the body at the same moment constitutes a most important distinction between the general rubbing sheet and the cold towel rub, the significance of which is great in the therapeutic applications of this procedure, since it renders the use of this measure possible and exceedingly useful in many cases in which the cold wet sheet as well as all other general cold applications must be interdicted, as in extreme cardiac weakness, acute renal congestion or inflammation, pulmonary or intestinal hemorrhage.

The intensity of the effect produced depends upon several factors, especially the following: —

1. The temperature of the water employed. Little effect is produced by water at a temperature above 60°, but a temperature of 70° to 75° may be used at the beginning in very

feeble patients with little power to react. The higher the temperature, the greater the amount of rubbing required to produce proper reaction.

2. The amount of water left in the towel when wrung out. The more water, the greater the thermic effect, because the greater the amount of heat abstracted from the skin. A very dry and very cold towel is very exciting, and if the rubbing is not excessive, may be even sedative and thermic.

3. The number of times the towel is applied in immediate succession.

1215 **Therapeutic Applications.**—Cold towel rubbing, being simply a diminished or partial wet sheet rubbing, may be employed in precisely the same cases in which cold sheet rubbing is employed, where patients can not endure the whole sheet,

The cold towel rub is of value in fevers not only as a means of improving the skin circulation, but by moistening the skin and thus encouraging evaporation of water, it promotes heat elimination, which is one of the most positive of all indications in fever. Weyrich has demonstrated that friction alone may increase evaporation over 50 per cent. The cold towel rub, then, is not only a direct antipyretic means in febrile conditions, but promotes in a high degree heat elimination through evaporation from the skin, amounting to more than 100 heat units per hour. The cold towel rubbing, as well as cold friction, affords a valuable means of preparing the patient in adynamic febrile cases to receive the cold bath, or the cooling pack.

The cold wet towel may often be used advantageously after a fomentation to the spine either as a local or as a general application; also after fomentations to the abdomen and other parts as a means of preventing too pronounced sedative or depressing effects from the hot application. When thus used, the towel should be wrung very dry out of very cold water. If applied after a fomentation, the first application should be made directly to the heated part. Cold wet-towel rubbing or cold friction at intervals of two or three hours is necessary to prevent depression of the heart and the central nervous system when prolonged hot applications are necessary, as in cases of acute nephritis.

This measure is of great service in the systematic treatment of chronic invalids, as a step in a progressive series of treatments increasing in vigor from wet-hand rubbing or cold friction to the shallow bath or the douche, and especially in the treatment of *anemia*, *chronic indigestion*, *neurasthenia*, and a long list of maladies requiring tonic measures, including *tuberculosis* of the *lungs*, *glands* (*scrofula*), *skin* (*lupus*), or *bones*, *chronic rheumatism* and *lithemia*, *diabetes*, *rickets*, *purpura*, *hemophilia*, *obesity*, *emaciation*, *dyspepsia*, *gastric ulcer*, and especially in cases of *cardiac weakness* either with or without organic or valvular lesion. In all these cases, great care must be taken to graduate the application, beginning with a very dry towel and lowering the temperature one degree each day till 40° is reached.

Contraindications.— In cases of asthma and cardiac affections attended by pronounced weakness of the heart or excessive compensation, the wet towel should not be applied to the chest. The chest should be rubbed with the moistened hand until good reaction is produced. Other contraindications are rare.

THE WET-SHEET RUB AND THE DRIPPING SHEET.

This procedure, perfected by Priessnitz, consists in a 1216
thorough rubbing of the body while enveloped in a wet sheet.

Requisites.— A linen sheet, a Turkish sheet, two towels, a tub containing hot water for the feet, a pail of water at 60° to 70°. Water at a higher or lower temperature may be employed when indicated.

Method.— The patient, being prepared, the head cooled in the usual way and protected with a cold wet towel, stands in the tub of hot water with the dry sheet wrapped about him.

The attendants prepare the wet sheet (Fig. 108), which should be wrung dry enough so it will not drip rapidly (Fig. 109).

When the sheet is ready, one assistant, holding one end of the linen sheet properly gathered in the right hand, and seizing the upper left-hand corner with his left hand, steps in front of the patient, while the other attendant withdraws the dry sheet and steps behind to assist. The patient holds up both arms, while the attendant in front places the upper left-hand corner of the sheet under his right arm (Fig. 110); the patient then lowers the right arm, holding the sheet in place, while the attendant passes the sheet quickly across the front of the body beneath the left arm, which is then also lowered. The sheet is then carried around the body by the assistance of the attendant who stands behind the patient, and pulls the bottom around. As the sheet is brought across the back of the patient, the attendant in front reaches over and seizes the upper edge of the sheet just above the point of the right shoulder, and pulls it first upward, then down upon the patient's chest (Fig. 111), while with his other hand he carries the sheet across the chest, covering the fold, and over the left shoulder, deftly tucking the corner under the edge of the sheet behind.

The attendant behind tucks the sheet between the patient's legs, which are then brought tightly together. The sheet is thus brought everywhere in close contact with the skin. As soon as the patient is thus enveloped,—an operation which should be completed in 5 to 8 seconds,—both attendants begin to rub vigorously, covering the whole surface as quickly as possible, one the legs and hips, the other the trunk and arms (Fig. 112). The rubbing should be continued for 1 to 3 minutes, or until the sheet is everywhere thoroughly warmed. The attendant should bear in mind that *the patient is not to be rubbed with the sheet, but over the sheet, with downward percussion strokes.* The bath does not depend for its effects upon irritation of the skin by the friction of the sheet, but upon the thermic stimulation and

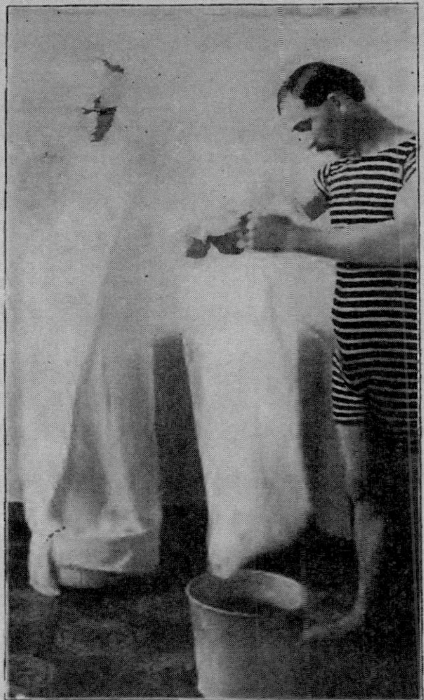

FIG. 108. WET-SHEET RUB — Sheet Ready for Wetting (p. 654).

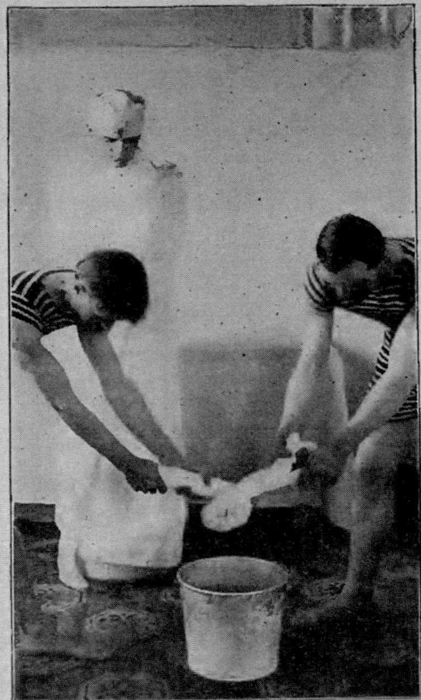

FIG. 109. WET-SHEET RUB — Wringing Sheet (p. 654).

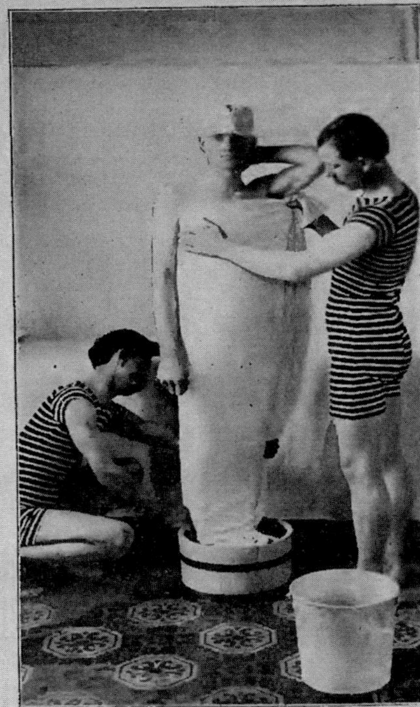

FIG. 110. WET-SHEET RUB — Applying Sheet (p. 654).

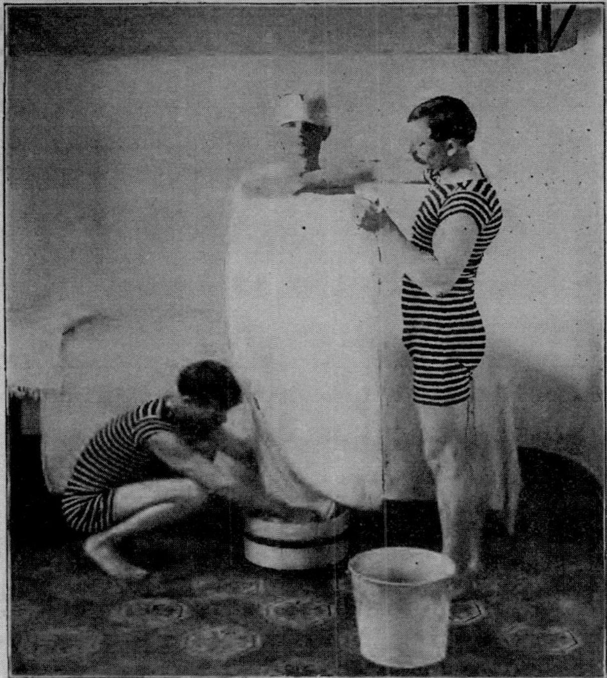

Fig. 111. THE WET-SHEET RUB. Applying the Sheet (Second Step).

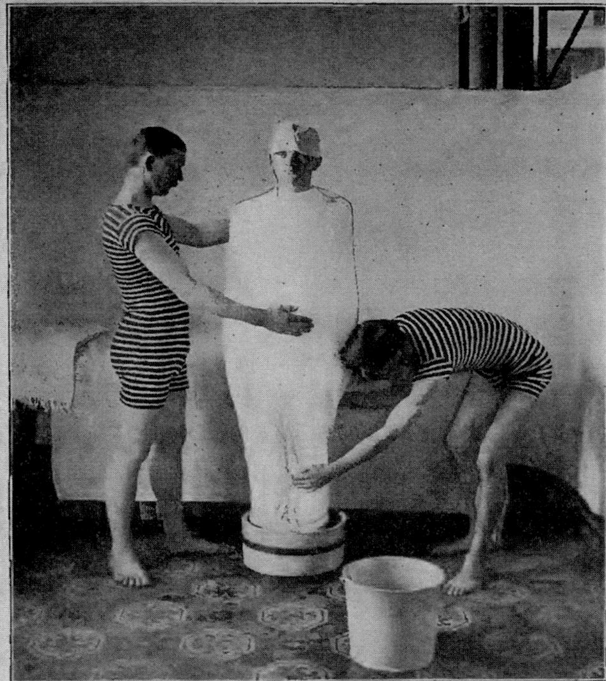

Fig. 112. WET-SHEET RUB (p. 654).

the assistance to the cutaneous circulation afforded by intermittent pressure upon the surface vessels. The rubbing movements are made with a sort of glancing percussion stroke from above downward. Percussion may be applied over the fleshy parts. Gentle patting may be applied to parts that are sensitive to rubbing. Care should be taken that the whole surface of the body is gone over many times and in rapid succession.

The rubbing must continue with vigor during the entire application. Very strong attendants are required, as a vigorous bath-man will usually find himself quite out of breath at the end of the procedure, if he has done his duty. When the sheet is well warmed, it is dropped, the Turkish sheet thrown about the patient, and the bath completed by vigorous rubbing over the Turkish sheet, followed by dry friction with the hand, with or without oil rubbing. Sometimes a Scotch douche follows the wet sheet before the drying.

The intensity of the bath may be readily varied in a number of different ways: (1) By the temperature of the water employed; (2) by the amount of water left in the sheet; (3) by using a thinner or thicker sheet; (4) by employing two or more wet sheets in succession, changing as soon as warm; (5) by the vigor of the friction movements applied; and (6) by the duration. This fact renders the rubbing wet sheet a most convenient measure for use outside of a regular hydriatic establishment, or where convenient appliances of various sorts are not at hand.

The longer the duration of the bath, the greater will be the thermic effect produced. Hence, when excitement of the nerve centers and tissue change is undesirable, the sheet should be wrung dry, the temperature of the bath should not be too low, the duration should be short, and the rubbing should be vigorous.

For very feeble patients the rubbing wet sheet may be applied in bed. Care should be taken to apply hot bags or hot fomentations to the feet during the application. For bedridden patients the sheet may be applied in much the same way as when the patient stands. The sheet being spread upon the bed over a blanket, the patient is placed upon it, and raises his arms above his head while one side of the sheet is passed across the body, the edge being tucked under the trunk and between the legs. The arms are then lowered, and the other half of the sheet is drawn across the body in such a way as to include both arms and to cover the shoulders, the free corner being tucked well under the shoulder, and care being taken to exclude the air. The patient is then vigorously rubbed from head to foot, the whole surface being gone over as rapidly as possible. If there is a tendency at the first to chill from too rapid evaporation, a warm blanket should be drawn across over the wet sheet, and the friction applied beneath it. The rubbing should continue until the whole surface of the body is well reddened and the sheet warmed, usually 1 to 3 minutes. The sheet should then be removed and the patient at once covered with a linen or Turkish sheet and a blanket, and dried beneath the blanket.

When it is necessary to avoid retrostasis in the use of the rubbing wet sheet, as in cases of cerebral hyperemia and marked visceral congestion, the patient should stand in very hot water (104° to 110°) during the application.

The rubbing wet sheet may be applied several times daily when necessary to procure the desired effect. When a saturated sheet is employed, it is sometimes necessary to apply vigorous percussion in addition to friction in order to secure proper circulatory reaction. In applying the cold rubbing sheet, care must be taken to see that the patient's skin is in a condition to receive a cold application with benefit. If the surface is cold, it must be warmed by a hot shower or some other heating bath. The wet-sheet rub should never be given when the skin is cold, or the patient chilly or apprehensive of a chill.

1217 **The Dripping Sheet.**—In giving the dripping sheet, which is a much more vigorous thermic application than the rubbing wet sheet, two or three pailfuls of water at different temperatures should be in readiness. The sheet is applied thoroughly saturated with water, and dripping. The patient is not rubbed, but vigorously spatted for 20 to 30 seconds. Then a half pailful of water at a little lower temperature than that in which the sheet was originally wet may be poured over each shoulder, and the spatting or percussion resumed. When evidences of reaction appear in returning warmth, another pailful of water at a still lower temperature may be poured over the patient if desired; but so vigorous an application is seldom indicated. The usual temperatures employed are 70° for the sheet, 65° for the first pail, 60° for the second pail. When higher temperatures are employed, it is difficult to get good reaction, since the exciting effect of cold is necessary to arouse the nerve centers to the requisite degree to produce the thermic and circulatory reaction which this procedure is intended to provoke.

By energetic percussion outside the sheet, the cutaneous circulation is maintained, and so the bath may be prolonged until the desired effect has been attained. Care must, however, be taken to terminate the application at once when the slightest symptoms of secondary chill appear; that is, when the patient begins to lose the sensation of glow and warmth which follow the first chill from the contact of the cold sheet, and is threatened with shivering, with goose-flesh and blueness of the skin. The full development of these symptoms should not be allowed to occur.

In cases in which it is unwise to allow the patient to stand erect, the application may be made thus: Place upon a bed a rubber sheet for protection. Spread upon this a linen sheet wet in water at 75°, and slightly wrung. Place the patient on the sheet, envelop him quickly as for a wet-sheet pack (**1179**); then let two attendants proceed to encourage circulatory reaction by moderate percussion and gentle rubbing of the whole surface, giving special attention to the extremities. As the sheet is warmed, cool by splashing over it water at

60° to 70°, continuing the spatting, and cooling by rewetting, until the patient begins to shiver. Then remove the wet sheet, wrap in a dry linen or Turkish sheet, cover with a woolen blanket, and after fifteen minutes take the rectal temperature. Renew when the temperature reaches 102° F.

In fever cases with extremely feeble heart, the hot reclining dripping sheet is sometimes useful as a preparation for the cold towel rub or cold friction. The sheet should be very hot, and should be applied quickly.

1218 **Physiological Effects.**—This procedure slows the pulse and energizes the heart, at the same time that respiration is increased, contrary to the usual physiological law. Plenninger noted a slowing of twenty beats a minute, while respiration increased five breaths per minute. Thermic reaction is usually less marked than in the immersion bath, circulatory reaction predominating; but thermic effects are obtainable at will in any degree of intensity. As the result of an ordinary application the rectal temperature falls two tenths to five tenths of a degree, while the axillary temperature is elevated. The very pronounced and lasting circulatory reaction produced, secures a vigorous cutaneous circulation and an increased rate of blood movement in the whole body. The effects of this procedure are intermediate between the douche and the wet-sheet pack; it is a sort of wet-sheet pack in the first stage, with mechanical effects added.

At the first moment, the application causes deep, gasping respiration, and sometimes slight shivering; but these sensations quickly give place to more prolonged and deeper respiratory movements, with slowed heart action and general feeling of warmth and glowing of the skin, as reaction begins. This procedure, combining, as it does, the mechanical effect of friction with the thermic effect of cold, produces at first a general contraction of the small vessels of the skin, very quickly followed by active dilatation.

During the first period of contraction there is dilatation of the vessels of the brain, lungs, and abdominal viscera, quickly followed by contraction when the blood returns to the skin with the reaction. Blood pressure is increased, as is also muscular capacity; there is improved assimilation of nitrogen, with increase of appetite and temporary lowering of temperature.

The most pronounced antipyretic effects, shown by lowering of temperature, are obtained by the use of a very wet sheet, a double sheet, repeated wetting of the sheet, by prolonged application, and by the use of the dripping sheet. By means of these several variations any degree of antipyretic effect may be produced. The most pronounced excitant effects are produced by a sheet wrung dry out of very cold water. The temperature ordinarily employed is 60°, but a lower temperature may be employed in robust patients, and a higher temperature (65° to 70°) with persons who are not accustomed to the use of cold water.

Therapeutic Applications.—A most important use for the 1219
cold dripping sheet is the lowering of temperature in cases in which the cold bath can not be readily employed. It may be used in such a manner as to secure all the good effects of the Brand bath without any of the inconveniences of that procedure. The author has employed this measure, with modifications, for more than twenty-five years in the treatment of continuous fevers, with excellent results.

Wet-sheet rubbing is a most excellent tonic procedure following the heating pack, the wet-sheet pack, the electric-light bath, and sweating procedures of all sorts. It has the advantage that it may be employed almost anywhere, as no apparatus is required; hence it is an especially valuable measure for use in the home. When tonic effects are desired, the sheet should be wrung very dry out of cold water (60°).

The fact that this procedure is capable of producing both thermic and mechanical effects of the most powerful character, and the readiness with which the intensity of the application may be modified, enables the physician to produce by this simple means alone nearly all the effects obtainable by hydric applications; hence the rubbing wet sheet may be properly designated as a pre-eminently useful hydriatic procedure. If the occasion requires strong derivative effects, with the minimum amount of metabolic change, as in the case of feeble, bloodless patients, with small heat-making capacity, very thin sheets wrung very dry out of water of low temperatures (50° to 60°) may be employed. The rubbing will be very vigorous, and the duration short (1 to 2 min.).

If, again, it is desired to produce decidedly alterative effects, through the production of strong tonic thermic reaction, a thicker or double sheet, wrung less dry, and renewed if quickly warmed, the application prolonged to 3 or 4 minutes, affords a means for securing any degree of effect which may be desired. The continued friction of the surface maintains the movement of blood in the skin, and thus prevents the shivering and other unpleasant symptoms arising from the internal congestion, which would otherwise require a speedy termination of the application before sufficient reduction of the temperature had been secured to call forth the requisite degree of heat production and accompanying tissue change.

Further, if it is desired to produce antiphlogistic effects, the dripping sheet prolonged to 10 or 15 minutes, or the rubbing wet sheet, if sufficiently long continued, is capable of producing any degree of refrigerant effect desirable. There are few other therapeutic measures, and certainly no medicinal agent known to man, capable of producing such versatile and desirable therapeutic effects.

The rubbing wet sheet is an excellent tonic measure for those unable to endure the douche. It is especially valuable as a derivative measure in cases of *cerebral congestion* and in *disorders* of the *liver*, *spleen*, *lungs*, and *digestive v s-cera*, in which congestion is a prominent symptom, as in *chronic gastritis*, *chronic bronchitis*, the chronically disordered *liver of dyspeptics*. It may also be used in some cases of chronic *congestion* of the *pelvic viscera* in which pain is not a prominent symptom.

The inactive skin of *dyspepsia*, *rheumatism*, *gout*, and *diabetes* may be excited to activity by this procedure. In cases of *anemia*, *chlorosis*, and *neurasthenia*, aged persons and feeble women, the wet-sheet rub affords an excellent tonic measure, which may be employed anywhere, and without apparatus. It is particularly valuable in relieving the passive hyperemia of so-called *chronic gastritis* or *gastric catarrh* and allied affections of the small and large intestines, known under the various names of *chronic enteritis*, *intestinal catarrh*, *pseudo-membranous colitis*, etc. It is applicable likewise to the *chronic splenic* and *hepatic congestions* which follow and accompany *malarial infections*. In *congestion* of the *spinal cord*, in *hypopepsia*, *apepsia*, *constipation*, *dilatation* of the *colon* and *stomach*, and most other functional disorders of the digestive organs, the powerful derivative effects of the rubbing wet sheet are indicated. The dripping sheet may be employed in all cases in which it is desirable to increase metabolic activity, as in cases of slowed nutrition (Bouchard). It is hence valuable in *obesity*, *chronic rheumatism*, *gout*, and *diabetes*. Under its influence, the dry, dingy, inactive, hidebound skin of the chronic dyspeptic and the arthritic becomes clear, transparent, supple, moist, and elastic after a daily application for a few weeks, especially when accompanied by the use of some suitable sweating procedure once or twice a week, as the electric-light or vapor bath, or the wet-sheet pack.

The wet-sheet rub affords an excellent remedy in *insomnia* due to *cerebral congestion* without special irritability of the cerebral cells. The effect of the application in stimulating circulatory reaction may be increased without thermic reaction by the addition of common salt to the water in the proportion of two pounds to the gallon (60°, 1 or 2 min.).

The rubbing wet sheet is especially indicated in insomnia when the skin of the sleepless patient is hot and dry. A temperature of 75° to 85° should be employed rather than a lower temperature, so that thermic reaction may be avoided.

When the skin surface is cool, the rubbing wet sheet produces undesirable effects in insomnia, increasing the wakefulness by exciting reflexes from the skin.

In cases of *cardiac insufficiency* due to valvular disease of the heart, the rubbing wet sheet renders valuable service as a means of stimulating the peripheral heart and fixing a considerable amount of blood in the skin. The dilated central heart is thus relieved, its action is slowed and energized, the whole circulation is improved, and the author has seen not a few cases permanently helped by this means when other measures had failed to afford more than temporary relief.

It may be applied twice daily in cases of *cardiac dropsy* if the patient has a fair degree of vigor. Generally it should be preceded by a short heating of the skin by means of the electric-light bath for 3 to 5 minutes, the vapor bath for 4 minutes, or a very short hot immersion bath (104° to 106°, 2 min.). Great care must be taken to avoid weakening the heart by overheating the patient. If necessary, an ice-bag may be employed over the heart during the heating process.

Gilles de la Tourette * has successfully employed the rubbing wet sheet to combat the febrile symptoms which occur in *exophthalmic goiter.*

This procedure furnishes also an excellent substitute for the spray or shower douche as a means of fixing the blood in the skin after a sweating pack, a vapor or an electric-light bath, or other heating processes, when a douche apparatus is not available. It may be advantageously used in cases of *myxedema,* and especially during the febrile exacerbations which frequently occur in this disease.

In the adaptation of the temperature of baths to different cases, it should be borne in mind that a low temperature is necessary for good effects with wet-sheet rubbing, on account of the quick reaction required. The body is exposed during the application to the cooling effects of evaporation, which to

---

* *Progrès Médical,* 1890, p. 101.

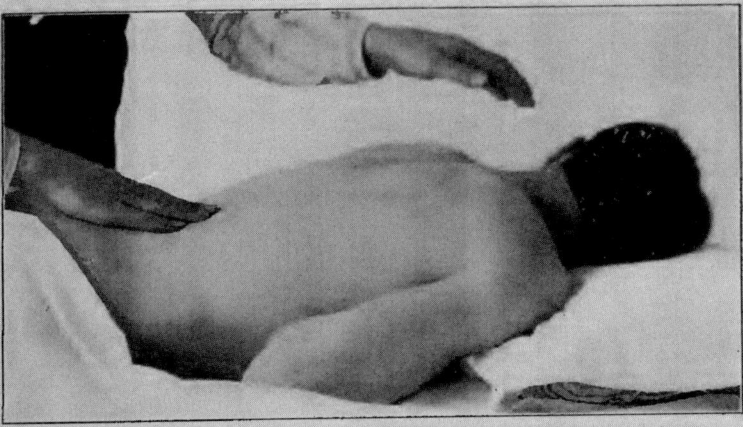

Fig. 113. FRICTION OF SPINE (p. 663)

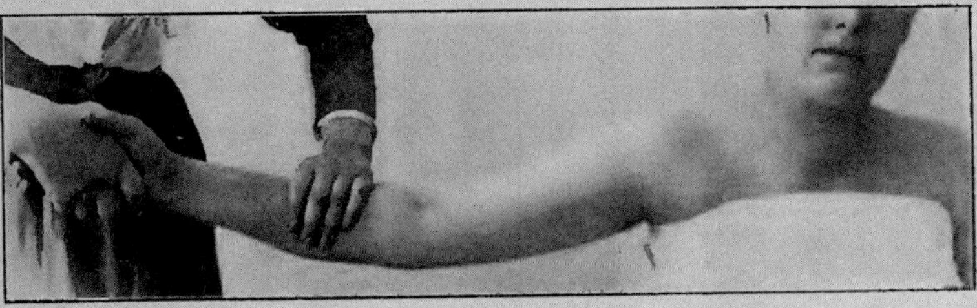

Fig. 114. CENTRIPETAL FRICTION (p. 664).

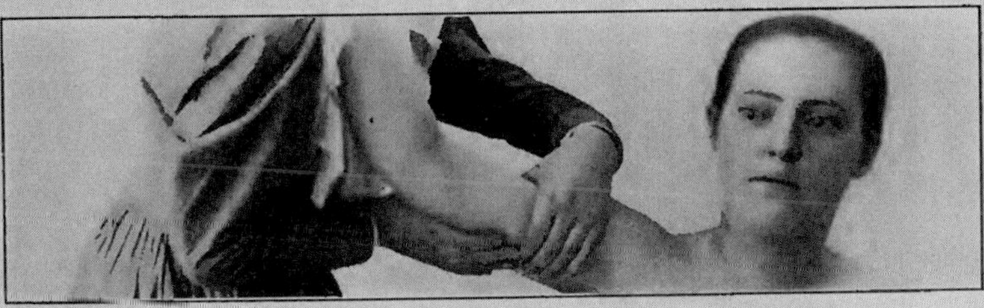

Fig. 115. CIRCULAR FRICTION (p. 664).

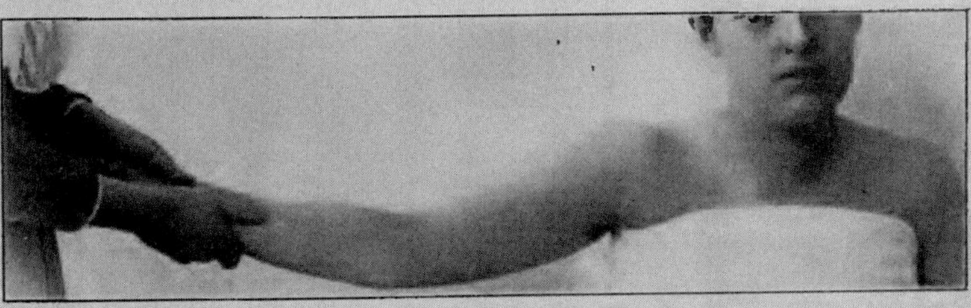

Fig. 116. SPIRAL FRICTION (p. 664).

a considerable degree interferes with reaction; hence the powerful influence of a low temperature, as well as the mechanical effects of friction and percussion, is necessary to secure the prompt return of blood to the surface after the primary contraction of the peripheral vessels occasioned by the first contact of the cold sheet with the skin. The best effects are obtained by temperatures between 50° and 60°.

Contraindications.—The principal contraindications for 1220
the rubbing wet sheet and dripping sheet are *cutaneous eruptions*, *extreme hyperesthesia* of the skin, *acute visceral inflammation*, *general neuritis*, severe *neuralgic affections* involving large nerve trunks, and such extreme feebleness of the circulation that proper reaction can not be secured. Persons who can not endure temperatures below 80° should not receive this bath, as reaction will be deficient. Other measures should be applied until reaction is improved, such as the cold wet-hand rub, cold mitten friction, and the cold towel rub.

DRY FRICTION.*

Massage is the natural accompaniment of hydrotherapy. 1221
The following procedures,—fulling, tapping, hacking, kneading, together with friction and joint movements,—encourage and assist in the development of the processes of accelerated tissue change and restorative metamorphosis which are set up by tonic hydriatic processes. Massage may be employed in such a way as to produce sedative as well as tonic and alterative effects of both a remote and a local nature, the same as hydriatic procedures.

Friction (Fig. 113) is simply one of the several valuable procedures of massage which may be advantageously employed in connection with hydriatic measures. It consists in systematic rubbing of the surface with the bare hand.

* For a full description of the forms and methods of massage, see the author's work, "The Art of Massage," Modern Medicine Publishing Company, Battle Creek, Mich.

Method.— In the ordinary employment of friction, as in drying a patient after a bath, the rubbing should be applied in both directions, as the effect desired is not only mechanically to assist the blood movement toward the heart, but to stimulate the cutaneous circulation.

In the systematic application of friction, the movements should, as a rule, follow the blood-vessels. This is especially true in friction of the extremities. We quote the following brief description of friction from the author's work on massage: —

"In this procedure the whole or a part of the hand is moved over the surface with a considerable degree of pressure, the pressure varying in different parts — heavy over thick, fleshy masses, light over bony surfaces and thin tissues. The pressure, however, should never be so great that the hand will not readily slip over the surface, nor sufficient to interfere with the movement of the blood in the arteries.

"The principal effect of friction is upon the superficial veins, the large venous trunks, and the lymph spaces and vessels. In the application of friction, the thumb only, or the whole or a greater part of the palmar surface of the hand, is brought in contact with the part operated upon. Five different forms of friction may be described, as follows: —

"*Centripetal friction* (Fig. 114), in which the movement is in the direction of the blood current in the veins, chiefly applicable to the extremities, the movement being from below upward, and from the hands and feet toward the body, the thumb or palmar surface of the hand being employed.

"*Centrifugal friction*, in which the movement is opposite to that of the blood current.

"*Circular friction* (Fig. 115), applicable to the extremities. The limb is grasped by both hands, which make an alternate wringing or twisting movement, beginning at the hand or foot and extending upward.

"*Spiral friction* (Fig. 116), a sort of combination of the preceding, executed with one hand, which progresses from the lower, or distal, to the upper, or proximal, end of the part with a sort of spiral movement.

"*Rotary friction* (Fig. 117), in which the hands are made to move over a broad surface in an elliptical, circular, or semicircular direction; especially applicable to such fleshy areas as the hip and that portion of the back lying above the spines of the scapulæ. In applying rotary friction, it is often necessary for one hand to support the tissues while the other hand is executing the movements.

"*Rate of Movement.*—The rate of the movement will necessarily vary according to the length of the strokes, and hence differs in different parts of the body. The rate may be from thrity to one hundred and eighty strokes per minute.

"*Direction of Movement.*—The direction of the movement in friction must necessarily vary more or less, according to the part operated upon. The general rule is to follow the large veins. Special care should be taken, in the treatment of the extremities, to follow the large venous trunks, making firm pressure directly over the large veins with the thumbs, passing from below upward.

"In the treatment of the forearm, the masseur will give special attention to the *radial* vein, which runs along the outer and anterior portion of the forearm; the anterior and posterior *ulnar*, which course along the anterior and posterior aspect of the inner border of the arm; and the *median*, which lies along the middle of the anterior surface of the forearm (Figs. 118 and 119).

"In the upper arm, special attention will be given to the *cephalic* along the outer side, and the *basilic* along the inner side, of the arm (Fig. 120).

"In applying friction to the leg, the thumb should at first be passed with firm pressure over the *long saphenous*, the course of which is from the instep along the anterior inner portion of the leg to the groin and the *short saphenous*, the course of which is from below the outer malleolus along the outer and posterior portion of the leg to the bend of the knee (Fig. 121).

"Centripetal friction is applied to the following parts in the direction designated: —

"*Head*, from before backward, and above downward.

"*Neck*, downward.

"*Back*, above shoulder-blades, circular; from shoulder-blades to sacrum, down; in the region of the loins, from the sides toward the spine.

"*Hips*, circular.

"*Chest*, from the sternum toward the axilla.

"*Abdomen*, upper part, from above downward and outward; lower part, from the median line downward and outward.

"*Arms and legs*, from below upward.

"*To promote absorption*, rub toward the heart (centripetal friction).

"*For sedative and derivative effects* upon the viscera and nerve centers, rub downward (centrifugal friction).

"Rubbing upward, or in the direction of the venous blood current, *increases the activity* of the circulation.

"Rubbing downward *decreases vascular activity.*

"In the application of friction, pressure should always be uniform for the part operated upon, and should be carefully graduated to meet each particular case.

"As a rule, some lubricant should be used,—fine vaseline, cocoanut oil, cacao-butter, or talcum powder.

"Friction is applicable to all parts of the body, but is especially useful to the limbs, head, and neck. It should always be used at the beginning of the application of massage, if the surface is cold.

"In the application of friction to large parts, both hands should be used either together or in alternation. In the treatment of a part which is small, it may be steadied by one hand while being treated by the other.

"*Mode of Applying Friction to Different Parts.*—A systematic order and method is essential in the application of friction to different parts of the body, which may be described for the chief divisions of the body as follows: —

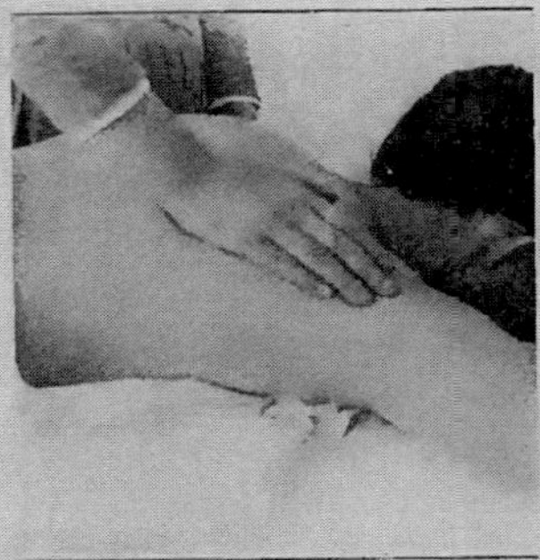

FIG. 117. ROTARY FRICTION (p. 665).

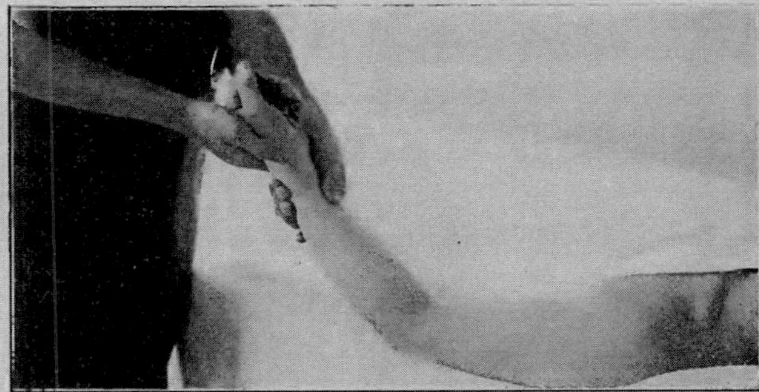

FIG. 118. FRICTION — Emptying Veins of Forearm (p. 665).

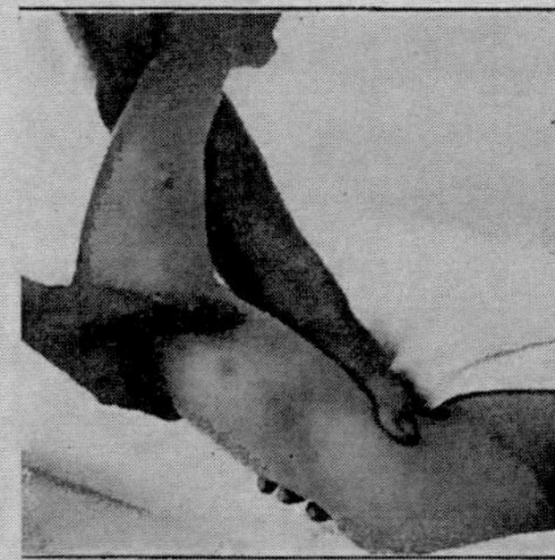

FIG. 120. FRICTION — Emptying Veins of Upper Arm (p. 665).

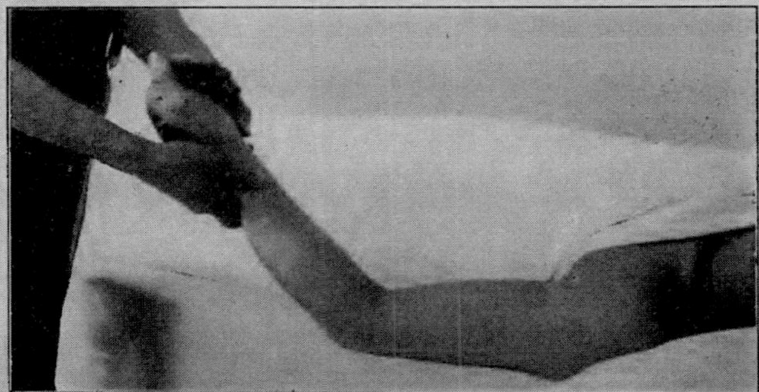

FIG. 119. FRICTION — Emptying Veins of Forearm (p. 665).

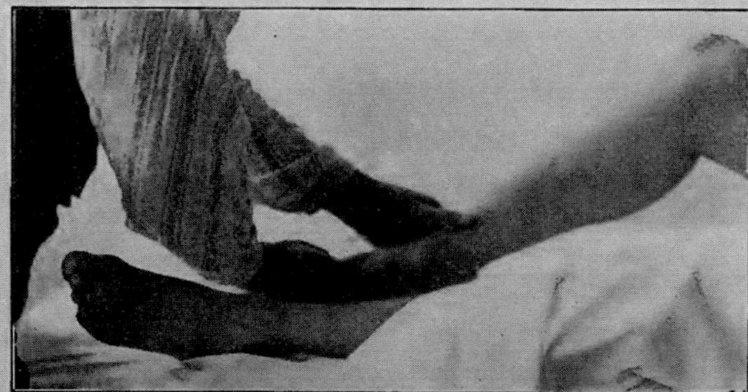

FIG. 121. FRICTION — Emptying Veins of Leg (p. 665).

"*The Hand.*—The patient's extended hand being allowed to rest in one hand of the operator, with the dorsal surface up, the masseur, holding the fingers of his other hand firmly extended, applies the tips of his fingers to the patient's hand in such a way that they will fall into the grooves between the adjacent fingers and metacarpal bones. The fingers are then pushed along in these grooves from the roots of the nails to the wrists. After repeating the movement several times on the back of the hand, the patient's hand is turned so that the palmar surface will be up, and the same movement repeated as before, with the modification that the fingers are carried a little farther up the wrist until the heel of the operator's hand rests in the hollow of the patient's hand, when slight rotary movement and firm pressure should be made, for the purpose of compressing firmly and emptying the numerous veins of the fleshy portion of the palm.

"The movements upon the back of the hand should be at the rate of sixty a minute; on the palmar surface a smaller number of movements will be executed per minute on account of the pause for one or two seconds in making rotary friction in the palm after each centripetal stroke.

"*The Forearm.*—With the arm of the patient half flexed, the masseur, facing the patient and operating with both hands, should make strokes from wrist to elbow, first with one hand upon one side, and then with the other hand upon the other side of the arm, in such a manner that each hand will include one half the circulation of the forearm, both thumbs resting upon the front of the arm. The operator may, if he prefers, stand with his back to the patient, making the strokes alternately with the two hands, as before.

"The masseur should keep constantly in mind the fact that firm pressure is to be made only with the ascending friction stroke. The hand is allowed to glide lightly over the surface in the descending or stroking movement, as a soothing measure, and not for the purpose of applying friction.

"In the treatment of very feeble persons, the patient may

be too much fatigued if the operator works with both hands at once, thus leaving him to support his own arm. In such case the patient's arm should be supported by the masseur, who will grasp the patient's hand with his own right hand, or the left hand with his left, applying spiral friction with the other hand upon the front side of the arm, then changing hands to operate upon the back surface of the arm.

"*The Arm.*— Work the arm in a manner similar to that described for the forearm.

"*The Shoulder.*— In applying friction to the shoulder, the masseur faces the side of the patient, operating with the two hands in alternation, following the surface of the joints, and always taking care to work centripetally; that is, toward the heart or toward the center of the body, and taking pains to follow the irregularities of the surface. The under as well as the upper side of the shoulder should receive attention.

"*The Foot.*— Begin with the hand, by friction with the ends of the fingers upon the dorsum of the foot, the operator standing in such a position as to face the sole of the foot. After finishing the dorsal surface, change the position so as to face the side of the foot, and make alternate transverse movements with the two hands on both sole and dorsum, working vigorously from toes to heel and instep. Lastly, extend the friction movements to the ankle, working with both hands, and following the grooves on each side of the tendon Achilles.

"*The Leg.*— With the leg half flexed upon the thigh, standing facing the patient, the masseur applies friction to the calf of the leg from ankle to knee, making eight or ten strokes, then turns his back to the patient, and operates upon the front of the leg by means of the thumbs working in alternation.

"*The Thigh.*— Standing with his back to the patient, the masseur grasps the leg in such a manner that the fingers fall behind and the thumbs in front, and makes very firm but rather slow strokes from knee to groin, not forgetting to give the knee due attention.

"*The Chest.*—The patient's arms should be separated a little from the sides, so as to straighten the outer portion of the pectoral muscles. The masseur, standing at one side, and facing the patient's feet, makes strokes from the insertion of the pectoral muscles at the humerus toward the median line, beginning at the upper border, just below the clavicle. The two sides may be operated upon simultaneously, or in succession, both hands being employed upon one side, one hand following the other in the movements. In progressing downward, the movements should be reversed below the pectorals, and the hands should be carried as far around the sides as convenient, care being taken to work toward the axilla above, and to follow the direction of the ribs and cartilages, until the whole surface has been covered, from the clavicle to the lower border of the last ribs

"*The Abdomen.*—Facing the patient, the masseur first makes long strokes from the upper to the lower portion of the abdomen, one hand following the other over the recti muscles, the two hands operating simultaneously over the lateral portions. After covering the whole surface six or eight times in this manner, strokes should be made more exactly in the direction of the veins, as follows: At the upper part of the abdomen, make strokes downward and outward, following the direction of the lower cartilages; for the middle portion, make strokes from the median line outward, reaching around as far as possible; for the lower portion, make the strokes downward and outward, in the direction of the hip joints.

"*The Neck.*—Facing the patient, place the hands one on each side of the head in such a manner that the little fingers will rest in the groove behind the lower jaw, the other fingers resting upon the mastoid processes and the inner border of the heels of the hands touching. Move the hands downward, and at the same time rotate them inward, so as to bring as large a portion of the palmar surface as possible in contact with the neck. At the lower border of the neck, move the hands outward toward the shoulders. After a few strokes, carry the hands a little farther back around the neck, so that as they move downward, the thumbs will rest one on each side of the larynx, thus compressing all the veins of the neck, both the superficial and the jugular, which lie deep. Finish with a few strokes applied to the back of the neck, starting at the occiput, and carrying the strokes downward and outward to the point of the shoulder.

"*The Face.*—Standing facing the patient, the operator places the palmar surfaces of his hands in contact, then applies them to the patient's face in such a manner that the little fingers touch the forehead at the median line. Separating the hands at the ulnar border, they are gradually spread out, as in opening a book, until the little fingers rest upon the temples, and the tips of the thumbs fall at the middle of the forehead.

"Fixing the thumbs at this point, the outer borders of the hands are moved downward by lateral flexion at the wrist until the forefingers fall at a level with the eyes. The whole hand is then moved downward in such a way that the nose is grasped and compressed between the thumbs while the palms of the hands and the fingers cover the cheeks. The movement is continued downward and finished by bringing the hands together below the chin. The object kept in view should be to bring as much of the hand as possible in contact with the face, and to touch every portion of its surface.

"*The Head.*—With the patient sitting or half reclining, and the masseur standing behind, the ends of the fingers and thumbs, with the fingers slightly flexed, are placed firmly in contact with the scalp, and a movement executed similar to that employed by a barber in shampooing. The mistake must not be made of applying the friction to the hair instead of the scalp. The movement begins at the vertex, gradually extending to the borders of the hairy scalp.

"*The Hip.*—In friction of the hip a very considerable amount of pressure is admissible, as the muscles and fleshy masses are very thick and firm. In applying friction to the hips, the masseur may face either the head or the feet of the patient.

"1. Make rotary friction upon the two sides simultaneously or in succession. In very fleshy persons it will be found necessary to support the tissues with one hand while operating with the other, on account of the great mobility of the muscular mass and the roughness of the skin, so frequently encountered in this region of the body.

"2. Apply centripetal friction, working from the great trochanter toward the crest of the ilium, and along the crest of the ilium from behind forward.

"*The Back.*—The patient lies upon his face, the masseur facing his head.

"1. A few light strokes are first applied from the occiput to the sacrum, along the center of the back, one hand following the other. The lateral surfaces are then covered by the two hands working simultaneously from above downward, and rotary friction is administered with greater pressure to the fleshy mass lying above the shoulder-blade. The two sides may be treated simultaneously or in succession, one hand being used to support the tissues. The latter method is usually necessary in very fleshy persons.

"2. From the shoulder-blades to the hips, lateral strokes are made, the masseur standing with his left side to the patient, facing his feet, the hands being placed as far around the sides as convenient, and simultaneously drawn toward the spine, the movement ending with the hands in contact. Great care should be taken to follow the ribs in the region of the thorax, which will give the movements a semicircular direction.

"3. Separating the index and middle fingers of the right hand, place one on either side of the spinous processes, and making firm pressure, move the hand downward from the occiput to the sacrum. The object should be to crowd the ends of the fingers as deeply into the tissues as possible on either side of the spinous processes, so as to influence the dorsal spinal veins. If necessary, the left hand may be used to increase the pressure.

"4. Finish the back by a few light strokes from above downward, using both hands simultaneously, covering as much surface as possible with the fingers in contact."

In the employment of friction in connection with hydrotherapy, the deliberate and elaborate methods above described are not always necessary or advisable. In cases in which the purpose is simply to encourage circulatory reaction and warm the skin, the whole surface should be gone over in a very vigorous manner, employing the larger movements as above indicated, while omitting the finer details, so that too much time shall not be lost, thus giving opportunity for chilling by evaporation. In many cases, however, it is advantageous to apply thorough and systematic friction after the patient has been well dried, not only as an aid to complete reaction, but as a means of supplementing the effects of the hydriatic application. In such cases, the methods described for different parts of the body may be followed out in detail.

When dry friction is quite disagreeable or produces marked irritation of the skin, the surface may be lubricated with talcum powder, fine vaseline, or cacao-butter.

If it is desirable to increase the stimulating effect of the friction to some degree, vinegar, or mustard water (a tablespoonful of ground mustard infused for ten minutes in a pint of hot water) may be employed, but these chemical stimulants are rarely needed.

1222 **Physiological Effects.**—The physiological effects of friction have been dwelt upon at length in an earlier chapter (**591**). Briefly summarized, these effects, as determined by Naumann* and Röhrig,† are as follows:—

1. Very light friction causes contraction of the surface

* Naumann, Prager, Viert, 1867.

† Röhrig, *Deutsche Klinik*, p. 254.

vessels, rise of blood pressure, and slight elevation of temperature.

2. Moderate friction causes, first, contraction of the blood vessels, with rise of blood pressure, then dilatation of the cutaneous vessels, with increase of blood movement and fall of temperature.

3. Very vigorous friction produces, almost from the very beginning, extreme dilatation of the small vessels, the stage of contraction being so brief as to be scarcely distinguishable; the pulse is slowed to a marked degree, also the respiratory movements. Heat elimination is so increased that the temperature is lowered to a very marked extent, one observer reporting a lowering amounting to 1.8° F. The amount of oxygen consumed as well as CO_2 is increased by friction, also the quantity of urea. When extremely violent friction is applied, albumin has been known to appear temporarily in the urine; in experiments upon animals the general temperature falls very decidedly, while both heart and respiration fail.

In hydrotherapy the effect usually sought is that of moderate friction; namely, preliminary contraction of the blood-vessels, followed by dilatation. By this means, the reaction which follows the cold application will be encouraged. The vigor of the application should be just sufficient to slightly encourage heat production without at the same time increasing heat elimination to such a degree as to cause an excessive loss of heat. In this regard, friction seems to operate in precisely the same manner as exercise. Too violent exercise after a cold bath, for example, causes an excessive loss of heat, and consequently, exhaustion. The same may be true of friction, whether the patient rubs himself or is rubbed by an attendant, if the application is too vigorous and long continued.

All the cutaneous functions are excited by friction. The skin becomes oily through stimulation of the sebaceous glands; and, according to Weyrich and Winternitz, perspiration may be increased more than 50 per cent. The temperature of the skin is elevated from two degrees upwards. Winternitz has shown that heat elimination may be increased more than 95 per cent. The powerful influence of friction in promoting heat elimination is readily shown by a simple observation based upon a method of determining the amount of heat elimination elsewhere pointed out (page 316). Increase by friction of the skin temperature of a patient with a warm skin, amounting to two degrees (95° to 97°), increased his heat elimination to the extent of 7 per cent.; while in the case of a patient with a cold skin warmed to the extent of ten degrees by friction (85° to 95°), the increase in heat elimination amounted to 66.6 per cent.

The mechanical effects of friction depend upon the direction in which it is applied.

1223 *Centripetal* friction, that is, dry friction movements made in the direction of the blood current in the veins, accelerates the movement of the blood toward the heart, and thus increases the vital activity in the part to which it is applied, the movements constituting a sort of pumping process by means of which the arterial as well as the venous circulation is accelerated. The lymph spaces and channels, as well as the blood-vessels, are emptied, and the lymph circulation is thus encouraged. The activity of the vital exchanges is increased, the tissues are rapidly freed from the waste matters produced in them, an increased amount of oxygen and of nutritive materials is brought to the part, and thus all the metabolic processes are encouraged.

1224 *Centrifugal* friction, in which the movements are made in a direction opposite to that of the venous blood current, retards the circulation, lessens vital activity, and hence produces a sedative effect.

In hydrotherapy the friction is for the most part applied either centripetally or in both directions.

1225 **Therapeutic Applications.**—Either moist or dry friction is employed in connection with nearly all hydrotherapeutic procedures. Dry friction naturally follows nearly every application of water. After cold baths, friction must always be employed for 3 to 5 minutes or longer. It may be moderate in intensity, so that the loss of heat shall not be so great as to induce secondary chill or vital exhaustion.

After a hot bath, vigorous friction movements are sometimes needed to encourage the effect of the bath by increasing cutaneous circulation and inducing perspiration. Care must be taken to protect the patient by warm covers. If the purpose of the hot bath is simply to produce a derivative effect, general perspiration being undesirable, care must be taken to avoid violent friction.

Light friction is applicable to cases in which the skin is congested and contraction of the blood-vessels desirable, such a condition as exists, for example, in the "feverishness" experienced in connection with a severe cold. This fact seems to have been discovered by the native masseurs of China, to whom the world is very largely indebted for the art of massage. A traveler in China informed the author that when at one time suffering from a severe cold, he employed a blind Chinese masseur, who immediately proceeded to administer very gentle centrifugal friction, and refused to employ centripetal movements, notwithstanding the request of the gentleman that he should do so, the latter supposing that the operator through ignorance was giving to his movements a wrong direction. Evidently the experience of the native manipulator had taught him that a hot, flushed skin should be stroked in a centrifugal rather than a centripetal direction. In the application of friction, either moist or dry, this principle must be kept in mind. If the tissues have been overexcited by excessive manipulation, if pain has been induced, or if excessive reaction has been occasioned by a Scotch douche, or the skin overexcited by a vapor, Russian, electric-light, hot immersion, or other heating process, an excellent antidote is offered in centrifugal friction applied in the form of gentle stroking.

A hot, flushed skin resulting from vasomotor disturbance

rather than a rise of temperature, is a condition not infrequently met in neurasthenics, and is often a distressing symptom in connection with the menopause. Centrifugal friction is indicated.

Friction is especially indicated in cases of *inactive, hide-bound skin*, when the skin is dingy, jaundiced, pale, cold, or insufficiently lubricated, the result of deficient activity of the oil glands.

Dry friction is excellent in *Bright's disease* and *diabetes*, either with, or independently of, appropriate water applications. It is also of great value in cases of very weak and feeble patients, in fever *convalescents*, in *consumptives* when in a nonfebrile state, in *asthmatic* persons suffering from *chronic bronchitis*, who often have a very strong antipathy to cold water, and are very sensitive to weather changes; also in *emaciation* and *dyspepsia*.

Dry friction may be advantageously employed as a means of lowering temperature in cases of *fever* in which the surface of the body is cold. The skin should be rubbed, preferably in a centripetal direction; that is, in the direction in which the venous blood flows; and the rubbing should be continued until the surface is warmed. The elevation of the surface temperature to the amount of ten or twelve degrees by rubbing may increase the rate of heat elimination 60 or 75 per cent. Lubrication of the surface with oil in connection with the rubbing enhances its effect, not only by facilitating the friction, but by increasing the loss of heat by radiation (**1232**).

In rubbing the patient, both in the bath and afterward, it is well to keep in mind the fact that rubbing is of special value at certain points. These points are as follows: First, the extremities; second, the back; third, the chest; fourth, the parts which are in immediate relation with external pain or internal congestion. For example, in cases of cerebral hyperemia, special attention must be given to rubbing the legs and arms. Again, in case of *pelvic* pain, the lower part of the back should be rubbed vigorously; for *ovarian* pain,

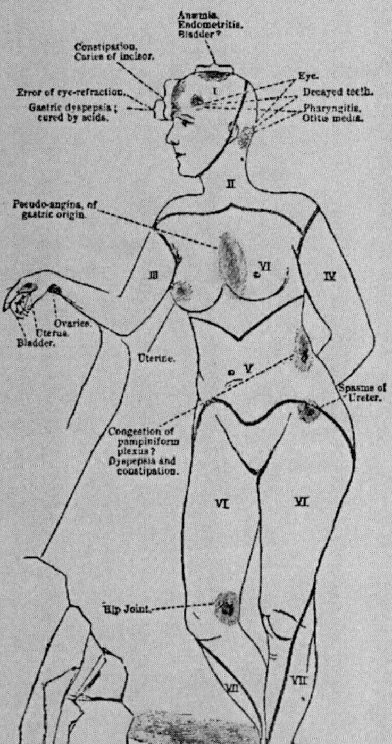

FIG. 122. Cutaneous Areas which are the Seat of Reflex Pain (p. 677). (Dana)

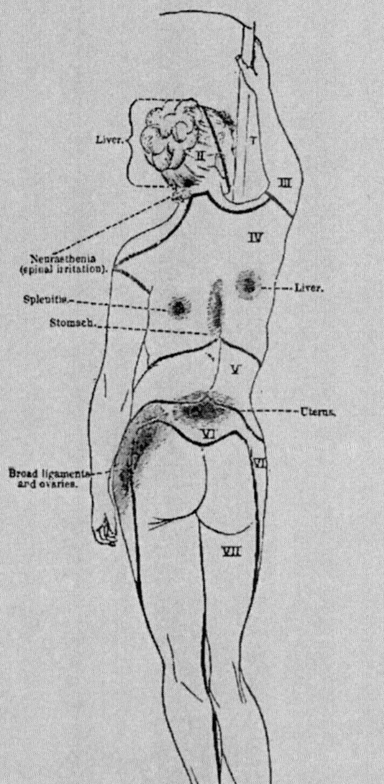

FIG. 123. Cutaneous Areas which are the seat of Reflex Pain (p. 677). (Dana)

the outer surface of the hips; for *gastric* pain, the dorsal region of the back; for *splenic* pain, under the left shoulder-blade; for *hepatic* pain, under the right shoulder-blade; in *neurasthenia*, the back of the neck, a common seat of pain, should receive especial attention; in *cerebral anemia* and in *uterine* disorders, the top of the head; in *constipation*, the abdominal surface; in *hypopepsia*, the epigastric region; and in *eye strain*, the supra-orbital and temporal regions; in certain *ovarian* disorders and some forms of *neurasthenia*, the hands and feet, especially the heels, wrists, and finger joints. These areas are shown in Figs. 122, 123, copied from Dana.*

A most valuable application of friction is in the treatment of *sprains*. At first, centrifugal friction — gentle downward stroking — should be applied. After the first forty-eight hours, centripetal friction may be used to increase the movement of blood through the part. The application should be made, not to the joint at first, but to the surfaces above the joint or between it and the heart, thus causing dilatation of both the arteries and the veins connected with the part. The blood channels being enlarged by this means, the movement of blood is accelerated and the healing process facilitated.

Contraindications and Precautions.— In some persons the 1226
skin is so sensitive that friction proves too exciting, giving rise to *insomnia*, *nervous irritability*, and general discomfort. Such persons are generally good subjects for the neutral bath and very gentle tonic measures.

Very light friction of the general surface hinders reaction by causing contraction of the blood-vessels. The effects on both the surface vessels and the heart are essentially the same as the first effect of a short, cold application. Hence, very light friction should be carefully avoided after a cold application, but may be employed with possible advantage after a hot application. On the other hand, energetic, but not violent, friction encourages the tonic reaction of cold, acting

* "A Clinical Study of Neuralgias."

in harmony with the vital movements of normal reaction, and hence naturally follows the cold bath.

Excessively severe or violent friction after a cold bath occasions depression of both heart action and respiration, and also gives rise to excessive loss of heat and too great activity of tissue change, producing various untoward effects, such as, (1) a secondary chill or succession of chills; (2) sweating and consequent depression, thus converting an application intended to secure a tonic effect into a reducing or sedative application; (3) nervous exhaustion and fatigue from excessive demands upon the reflex centers of the spine.

Care must be taken after cold applications of any sort, to avoid such vigorous friction as to induce perspiration.

It is especially necessary to avoid too vigorous rubbing after cold baths during the hot season, when the heated atmosphere encourages excessive reaction and perspiration. Gentle centrifugal friction may be properly and profitably employed as a means of combating excessive reaction, when this has been produced by a too cold bath, by too warm wrappings after a bath, by excessive exercise, or even by too prolonged or violent friction following the cold bath. If after tonic applications, perspiration appears, the effect of the bath has been spoiled, and the patient will be weakened instead of strengthened by it; hence it is easy to convert a tonic application into one of a very different character, thus producing most undesirable results, by neglecting properly to supervise the drying and rubbing of the patient after the bath.

On the other hand, care must be taken to avoid the opposite error. Very light, inefficient friction after a cold bath results in contraction of the blood-vessels, whereby reaction is hindered instead of encouraged; and the more prolonged an inefficient application of this sort, the more pronounced will be the ill effect produced.

It should be remembered that the effects of friction upon the heart closely resemble those resulting from irritation of

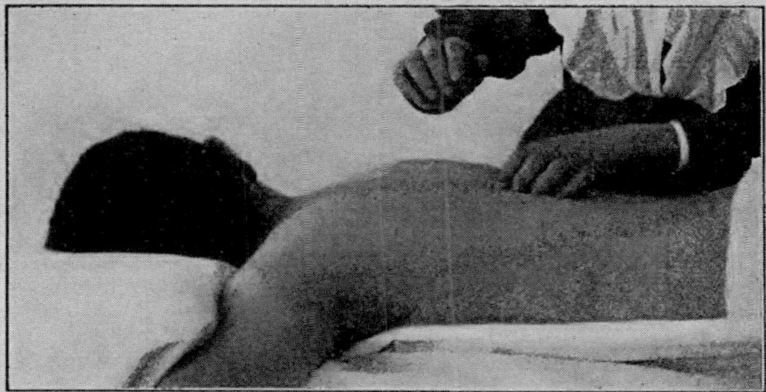

Fig. 124 (*a*). PERCUSSION — Tapping (p. 681).

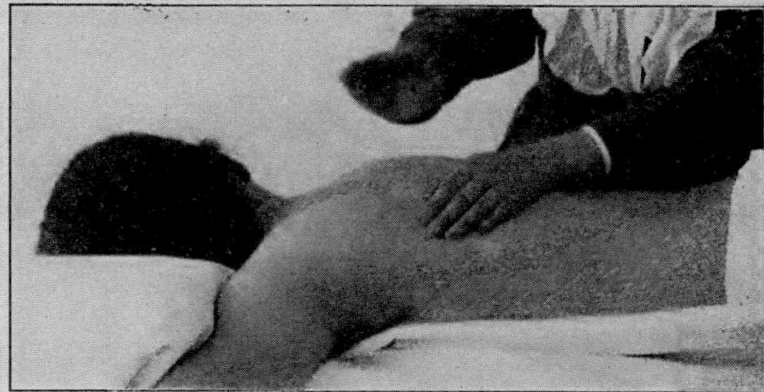

Fig. 124 (*b*). PERCUSSION — Clapping (p. 681).

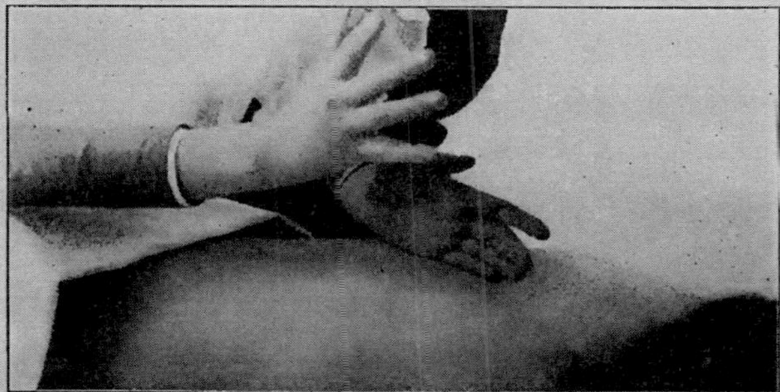

Fig. 124 (*c*). PERCUSSION — Hacking (p. 681).

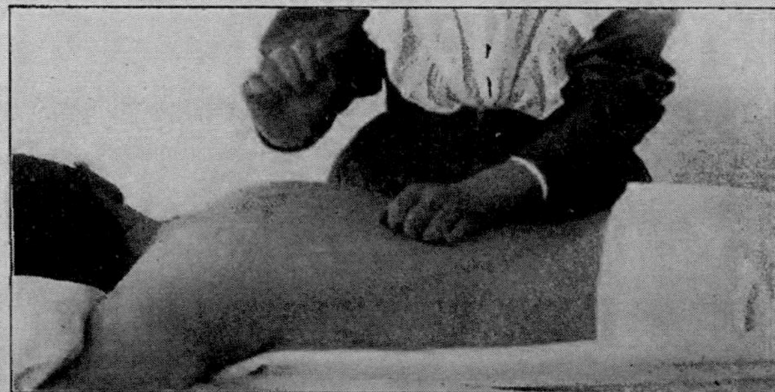

Fig. 124 (*d*). PERCUSSION — Beating (p. 681).

the pneumogastric. Slight irritation increases the heart's action, whereas violent irritation slows or depresses it.

Light rubbing or stroking should be employed only for the purpose of diminishing a tendency to excessive reaction. The stroking should then be centrifugal in direction, or from the center of the body outward.

If there is a tendency to excessive reaction, with a disposition to perspire, energetic rubbing should be avoided, and the patient should be dried by gentle patting over a towel, and the surface should be exposed now and then for a few seconds; or if considerably overheated, it may be cooled by a current of air set in motion by a fan or a towel. If the patient has a very sensitive skin which is irritated by rubbing with the dry hand, the hand may be moistened, or friction may be practiced with a wet napkin or a sponge, or talcum powder may be applied to the skin.

In rubbing the skin when slightly moist, it is very easy to produce abrasion by using too much force, as the hand often adheres quite tenaciously to the surface of the patient's body. This difficulty may best be remedied either by sprinkling a little talcum powder over the surface operated upon, after drying, or by using a little vaseline or cacao-butter.

During the friction, the attendant should take care that his own hand is thoroughly dry. If there is a tendency to perspiration of the palm of the hand, it should be dried with a towel, then well covered with talcum powder.

Friction can not be applied to an area of dry skin not lubricated more than six or eight minutes without producing irritation. It should be remembered that irritation of the skin may mean much more than simply a slight inconvenience —it may result in profound nervous disturbance, and may seriously interrupt a course of treatment which is very essential to the patient's welfare. In fever cases an abrasion may be the beginning of a bed-sore. Recent observations suggest the necessity of the same precaution in cases which have been subjected to examination by the X-ray.

There are cases in which light friction may be employed to very great advantage as an alternative with hydriatic procedures, when the patient's vital forces are too much reduced to allow of the daily employment of cold douches or similar applications. The author has not infrequently found it advantageous to suspend hydrotherapeutic measures for a short time almost altogether, substituting dry friction with the hand, a soft brush, or a linen, flannel, or Turkish cloth mitt.

In very sensitive patients, as certain neurasthenics, gentle patting over the sheet must take the place of friction as a means of drying the skin.

When patients are suffering from *rheumatic joints*, the parts should not be rubbed vigorously, but strong friction should be applied to each limb at a point just above the affected joint and in a centripetal direction. In cases of *acute inflammation* of any sort, the friction must be at first centrifugal, and on the distal side of the affected part.

Vigorous friction *after* the Brand bath is usually avoided, although a slight increase in temperature lowering might be effected thereby. There is a real gain in the omission, however, in the greater permanence of the temperature reduction.

Friction must be avoided altogether in cases of *eruptive disorders* of the skin, in *eruptive fevers*, also in cases of *erythema*, *dermalgia*, and *cutaneous hyperesthesias*. When the skin is hot, flushed, and dry, gentle friction may sometimes be employed, but as a rule, friction is to be avoided; also when perspiration is profuse. Gentle friction or stroking must be avoided when it is desirable to promote reaction; vigorous friction should be avoided when strong reaction is undesirable.

After a neutral bath, in which it is desirable to suppress both thermic and circulatory reaction, care should be taken to avoid friction as far as possible. The patient should be dried with gentle pressure with the hand outside the sheet, so as to bring it in close contact with the skin, the sheet being continually readjusted so as to bring new portions into contact with the moist surfaces. The same measures should be adopted after hot baths in which it is undesirable to further stimulate the cutaneous circulation, and after a short cold bath when there is a tendency to excessive reaction.

PERCUSSION.

Massage is the natural adjunct of hydrotherapy. It pro- 1227
duces both mechanical and reflex effects which result in the development of powerful circulatory reaction. The circulatory reaction produced by massage is very prompt, no delay being occasioned by contraction of the blood-vessels due to chilling of the patient, as when cold water is applied. Of the various procedures of massage, nearly all are efficient promotors of circulatory reaction; but aside from friction, the effects of which have already been described, percussion is the only form of manual manipulation which is systematically associated with ordinary hydric applications. In the massage douche, deep kneading in its various forms is also advantageously utilized, as elsewhere mentioned (1066).

Method.— "This procedure consists of blows administered by the hand in various ways and with varying degrees of force, the two hands being used in alternation [Fig. 124]. The movement is always from the wrist joint, which gives to the blow the quality of elasticity. The inexperienced operator holds the wrist rigid, and pummels the patient, much as a pugilist would do, thus producing disagreeable and painful effects; while a dexterous and experienced operator maintains a flexibility of the wrists which adds greatly to the good effects of the treatment.

"A stiff blow bruises the surface tissues without producing any beneficial effect upon the deeper structures, the force of the blow being expended upon the surface. An elastic blow, executed in the manner described, penetrates deeply without injuring the superficial structures. A skilled masseur gives springy blows, the movement being chiefly at the wrist joint. As a rule, the hand should strike the body transversely with relation to the muscles." *

Of the various forms of percussion, *spatting* and *clapping* are the only ones which are especially valuable in connection with hydrotherapy.

Spatting consists of percussion with the palmar surface of the extended fingers held rigid. This is the form in which percussion is most frequently employed. It is applicable to most parts of the body.

In clapping, the whole hand is employed, the palmar surface being so shaped as to entrap the air as it comes in contact with the skin, producing a sort of explosive effect and a loud sound. Clapping is used on fleshy parts where strong surface stimulation is desired.

1228 **Physiological Effects.** — The physiological effects of percussion are practically identical with the mechanical and reflex effects produced by friction (591). This procedure is a powerful excitant, acting not only upon the skin, but upon the tissues beneath. A short, light application produces spasm of the superficial vessels. It may be said that *light* percussion produces much the same effect as light friction; *moderate* percussion, the effect of moderate friction; and very *vigorous* and *prolonged* percussion, the effects of vigorous and prolonged friction (1222). Friction differs from percussion chiefly in the fact that by the movements made in friction, the blood is forced along the venous channels, thus mechanically aiding the circulation; while in percussion the mechanical effect is less, but the sensory impression is much stronger, and hence the reflex effects are more marked. Percussion and friction may be combined, as in the percussion friction stroke employed in the cold wet-towel rub and the wet-sheet rub.

1229 **Therapeutic Applications.** — Percussion, both spatting and clapping, may be usefully employed to intensify the effects of

* "The Art of Massage," Modern Medicine Pub. Co., Battle Creek, Mich.

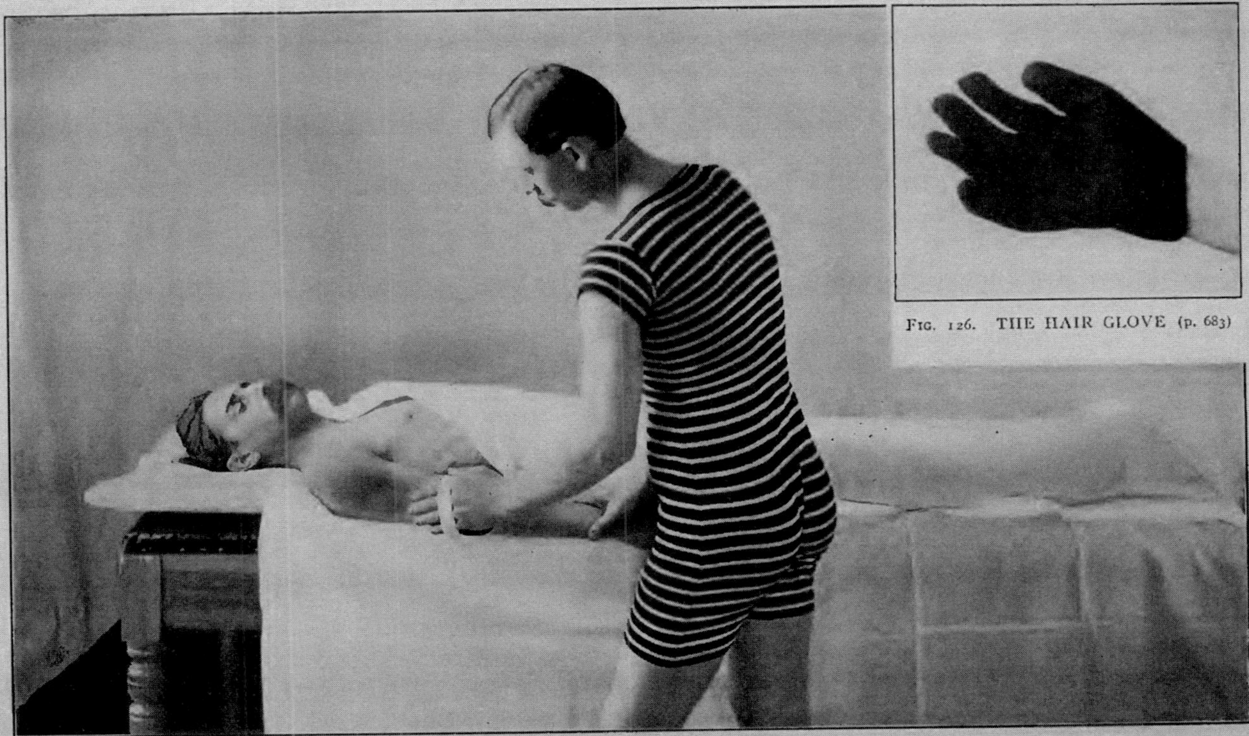

Fig. 126. THE HAIR GLOVE (p. 683)

Fig. 125. DRY SHAMPOO WITH FLESH BRUSH (p. 383).

friction in cases in which reaction does not promptly occur, or where the brief application of a more powerful stimulus than that induced by moderate friction is desirable, as in the wet rubbing sheet and the dripping sheet, and after a general cold application.

The suggestions made with reference to the therapeutic use of friction are also applicable to this procedure. It may be mentioned, in addition, that in *chronic sciatica* and *lumbago*, special attention should be given to these regions. In cases of *cirrhotic liver* or *spleen*, vigorous percussion is applied to the surface overlying these organs.

In *chronic constipation*, the effect of the cold douche to the abdomen may be intensified by vigorous percussion of this region. Percussion over the sacrum is an effective means of stimulating the genito-urinary organs in *atony* of these parts. In cases of *pleuritic adhesions*, *chronic pneumonia*, and *dropsy* of the *chest*, make percussion over the affected part.

Contraindications.— The contraindications are essentially **1230**
the same as for friction. Special care must be taken to avoid severe percussion in cases of *arteriosclerosis*, and when febrile conditions exist, with a hot, flushed skin.

DRY SHAMPOOING.

This consists of friction of the surface with the flesh-brush **1231**
(Fig. 125), the friction mitt (Fig. 97), or the hair glove (Fig. 126). The effects are identical with those described under the head of friction. The dry shampoo especially encourages circulatory reaction. The friction is applied with short and rapid to-and-fro strokes and little pressure ; hence the effects are largely reflex.

Therapeutic Applications.— Dry shampooing is sometimes useful in the treatment of patients who manifest great intolerance to hydric applications. It is especially adapted to persons with thick, tough, inactive skins. It may often be applied with advantage in alternation with hydric applications. It produces good circulatory reaction almost without thermic effect; hence is well adapted to persons who have little heat-making capacity, and who have habitually a cold skin. The author has made great use of this measure as an introductory application in the day's program, administered to the patient while still in bed before rising in the morning.

Rough treatment of the skin should always be avoided. Such an amount of friction, with the brush, the hair glove, or the hand, as gives rise to abrasion, eruption, or persistent redness of the skin, is harmful instead of helpful.

OIL RUBBING.

1232 This is one of the most ancient procedures used in connection with hydrotherapy. The old Romans always had themselves rubbed with oil after their baths. Oil rubbing is much practiced by the natives of savage countries, especially in tropical Africa.

Method.— The oil or unguent is applied by simple friction movements, generally centripetal in character, such as have already been described (**1223**).

The best effects are obtained when the application is made after a warm or tepid bath, as the epidermis then more readily absorbs the oil. The application of oil to the dry skin is generally disagreeable. Care should be taken to avoid the application of too much oil, and the surplus should be removed by gently wiping the surface with a soft towel at the end of the application. Care must be taken to avoid such vigorous friction as to induce perspiration.

Vegetable oils or fine vaseline should be employed, rather than animal oils of any sort. Cacao-butter is especially serviceable. Care should be taken that the oil used is not in the slightest degree rancid, and the patient should receive a thorough soap shampoo at least twice a week.

Physiological Effects.— The effects of oil rubbing are essentially the same as those of moderate friction, except

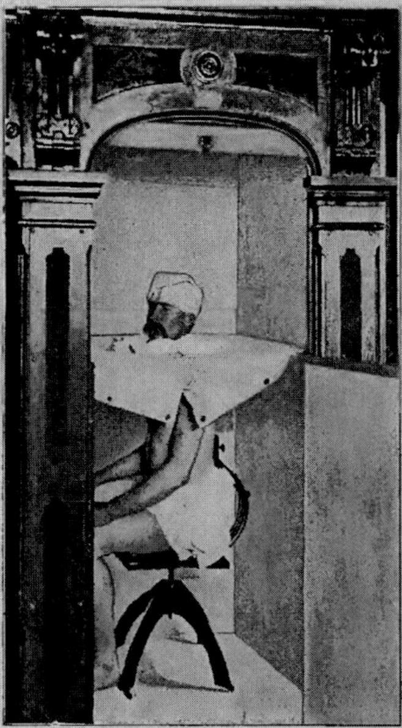

FIG. 127. HOT-AIR BATH (p. 687).

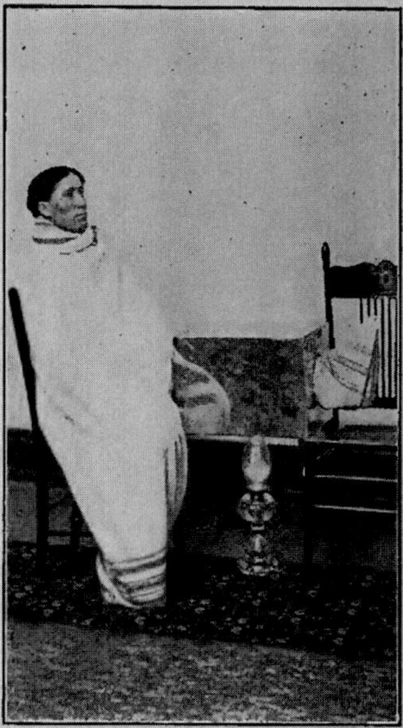

FIG. 129. LOCAL HOT-AIR BATH APPLIED TO KNEE JOINT (p. 692).

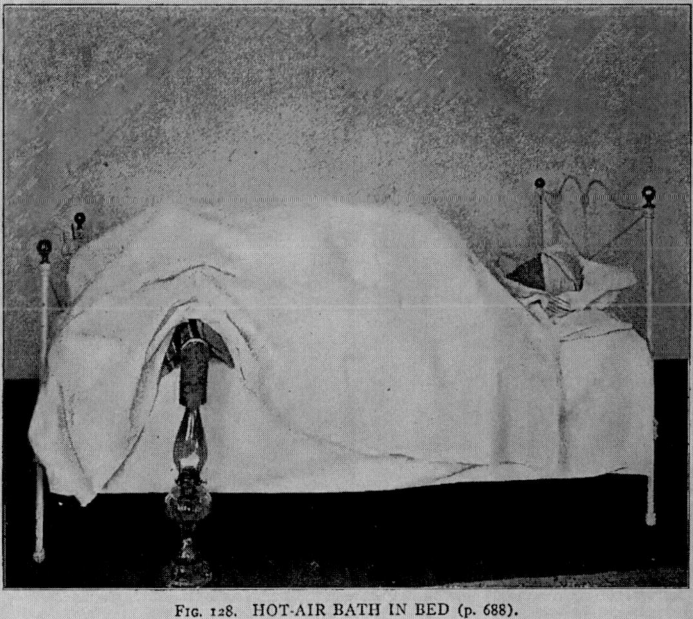

FIG. 128. HOT-AIR BATH IN BED (p. 688).

that it is a milder measure. The lubrication of the surface lessens the degree of reflex stimulation. The mechanical effects are the same as in ordinary friction. Oil rubbing may accordingly be practiced in cases where dry friction would be too exciting.

An important physiological effect which must be remembered in connection with oil rubbing is that the application of oil to the surface of the body to a marked degree lessens heat elimination by conduction while increasing radiation (Exp. 61). The natives of Samoa and other South Sea islands, who are great swimmers, and spend much of their time in the water, habitually smear themselves with oil before entering the water. On the other hand, heat radiation by the skin is very considerably increased by the application of oil. Peclet has shown (Schumann) that an oil surface radiates heat 50 per cent. more rapidly than a water surface. The amount of heat lost by radiation when the body is exposed is about twice that lost by conduction. The increase of heat loss by radiation thus overbalances the diminution of heat elimination by decreased conductivity.

The natives of Africa, when exposing their nude bodies to the direct rays of the tropical sun, habitually protect themselves by smearing the skin with melted fat of some sort. Smearing the skin with oil in cold weather affords protection only through the fact that the body is covered with clothing.

The popular supposition that the body may be nourished by the application of oil to the skin is an error. Probably very little, if any, of the oil applied to the skin enters the circulation; nevertheless, great care should be taken that the unguent used is not in the slightest degree rancid, for the poisonous fatty acids are apparently quite readily absorbed by the skin.

Therapeutic Applications.— Lubrication of the surface with oil facilitates the application of dry friction, and prevents the irritation likely to result from repeated and long-continued rubbing of a circumscribed area, as is often necessary in the treatment of joints for the removal of chronic exudates. Oil should also be applied to the surface as a protection for the skin against excessive masceration in cases in which the general or partial continuous bath is employed. Prolonged and vigorous friction of the feet and limbs with oil may be used with excellent effects for the relief of *cold feet*, a condition exceedingly common in *gastric neurasthenia*, and as a preparation of the feet for a cold pack if they are inclined to be cold.

Oil rubbing may be employed advantageously in most cases to which dry friction is applicable. It is a good plan to apply a little oil to the surface at least two or three times a week in most cases in which daily baths are administered, especially in cold weather. Oil or an unguent of some sort should always be applied after a shampoo in which soap has been used, as the removal of the natural oily covering of the skin increases heat elimination by conduction and the liability to take cold.

Patients who react poorly, and who are very susceptible to cold, should be rubbed with oil after each bath. Oil rubbing is especially needed in cases in which the skin is dry, through deficient activity of the oil glands of the skin. Great care, however, should be taken to avoid too vigorous rubbing in the application of the oil, as sweating from too strong reaction is very easily produced, to the disadvantage of the patient. In the treatment of infants and children, a marked and most favorable effect upon nutrition is produced by oil rubbing. Application of oil after cold baths encourages reaction. In most cases of *chronic dyspepsia* when accompanied by emaciation, in *diabetes*, and in most cases in which malnutrition with dryness of the skin is a prominent feature, oil rubbing is a valuable therapeutic resource.

Oil rubbing has been used in scarlet fever and other infectious fevers as a means of lowering the temperature, with some success.

THE HOT-AIR BATH.

This bath consists in exposure of the entire body, with 1233
the exception of the head (Fig. 127), to a superheated atmosphere.

Method.— The patient, undressed, is placed upon a stool in a suitably constructed cabinet inclosing the entire body with the exception of the head. The air of the cabinet is gradually heated to the desired degree by means of a steam coil, or a kerosene or gas stove; or the heating may be accomplished by means of alcohol or strong whisky burned in a cup or saucer placed in a basin of water. Burning alcohol or whisky does not, however, give an ideal hot-air bath, because of the large amount of watery vapor produced by the combustion of these substances. When an open flame of any kind is employed, great care should be taken to avoid burning the patient or setting fire to the cabinet.

The temperature employed is from 120° to 200°; a temperature of from 140° to 180° is usually sufficient to produce profuse perspiration.

Perspiration should be encouraged by making the patient drink a glass of water just before going into the bath, and if possible, one or two more during the bath.

The hot-air bath should nearly always be followed by a cold bath of some sort. This may be a wet-sheet rub, the shower or horizontal spray, the affusion, the full bath, or a sponge bath. In cases in which the bath has been employed for eliminative purposes, and has been continued for a half hour or more for the purpose of prolonging the sweating process, care must be taken not to make the cold application too abruptly. The cooling must be gradual, the initial temperature being a little below that of the body (about 98°), and somewhat rapidly but gradually lowered to 75° or 80°, at which point it may be continued for 30 to 60 seconds, or until the pulse becomes tranquil, the skin smooth and free from moisture, and the vascular excitement of the skin quieted.

The hot-air bath is not infrequently employed as a means

of heating the skin preliminary to a cold application of some sort. It may in this way precede a cold douche, a cold wet-sheet pack, a cold immersion, a cold sponge, or a wet-sheet rub. When used for this purpose, the bath should be continued just long enough to induce gentle perspiration. If continued longer, a sedative effect may be produced which will antagonize the tonic effect desired from the cold application which follows. As a means of inducing perspiration, the hot-air bath is inferior to no other measure except the electric-light bath.

Before the patient enters the cabinet, the hair of the scalp should be thoroughly wet and the face and neck well bathed with cold water. If there is a great tendency to cerebral congestion during the bath, a towel saturated with cold water or an ice collar may be placed about the neck.

If a regularly constructed cabinet is not available for a bath, an efficient hot-air bath may be administered by very simple means which can be improvised almost anywhere; for example, the patient may be placed in an ordinary cane-seated chair, the seat of which is covered with a moist napkin. Underneath the chair may be placed a kerosene oil stove or even an ordinary kerosene lamp, or alcohol or brandy may be burned in an open dish. Below the seat of the chair should be placed a sheet of metal, so that the patient will not be burned by the ascending current of superheated air. The hot air is retained about the patient by surrounding both the patient and the chair by a rubber blanket; or in the absence of this, several ordinary blankets, with newspapers placed between, may be substituted.

It is even possible to administer a hot-air bath in bed by building over the patient a sort of canopy by means of blankets spread upon hoops, as shown in the accompanying cut (Fig. 128). The hot air is conducted into the space about the patient by means of a metal pipe four or five inches in diameter, and connected with a kerosene stove or a large kerosene lamp. Care should be taken to protect the bed clothing from the hot pipe, by means of asbestos or other fire-proof material.

Care must be taken in administering the hot-air bath to avoid such sudden and excessive applications of heat to the skin as to cause dilatation of the surface blood-vessels before there has been time for the adjustment of the circulation of the viscera. Neglect of this precaution sometimes gives rise to vertigo and fainting. This danger may be obviated by the application of the cooling compress to the head, face, and neck of the patient. Excessive cold applications to the head and neck may, however, antagonize the effect of the bath by opposing the sweating process. The hot-air bath must not be employed too often, as it is a depleting or sedative measure, and if too frequently resorted to, may give rise to nervous exhaustion and debility.

The purpose of the cold application following the hot bath is to increase the tonus of the blood-vessels, to energize the nerve centers, and to change the condition of passive congestion of the skin to one of active vascular excitability.

In very susceptible persons, fainting sometimes occurs on the application of very cold water in the form of a shower, spray, or affusion, on emerging from a hot-air or other hot bath. The cause of this is the strong contraction of the blood-vessels of the brain the instant the cold water comes in contact with the skin. In persons liable to this inconvenience, the graduated shower or some other form of the graduated bath should be employed for cooling off.

In cases in which the hot-air bath is employed to induce sweating, the patient, after remaining for 15 or 20 minutes in the bath, may be removed and wrapped in warm blankets for half an hour or longer to continue the sweating. The sweating process may be encouraged by making the patient drink freely in the pack as well as in the hot-air bath. A quarter or half glass of water should be swallowed every five minutes.

1234 **Physiological Effects.**— The first effect of the hot-air bath is to heat the skin and the body. The heat is communicated to the skin by the dry, hot air, the temperature of the successive layers of the skin being elevated until finally the blood-vessels are reached and the temperature of the blood is raised to a sufficient degree to cause perspiration. The skin becomes red through the dilatation of the surface vessels, which are in a state of passive congestion. The temperature of the blood is generally elevated from two to five degrees according to the duration of the bath. When the bath is continued for some length of time, or for a short time at high temperature, respiration becomes very short, difficult, and thoracic. There is headache, and intense thirst, with nausea and vertigo. Quickening of the pulse and respiration nearly always occur in the hot-air bath. These symptoms usually disappear with dilatation of the surface vessels and the beginning of perspiration. They may be largely prevented by vigorous friction of the skin before the bath, and by raising the heat slowly until perspiration begins.

The temperature of the bath should usually be from about 130° to 160° F.; duration, 20 to 30 minutes. Local applications may continue for an hour or more at moderate temperatures.

The hot-air bath causes an elevation of the body temperature, and hence is not adapted for use in cases in which febrile action is present. This fact, however, gives it special value in the treatment of rheumatism, through the increased oxidation of proteid wastes (567).

1235 **Therapeutic Applications.**— The hot-air bath is seldom employed except in connection with other baths, though its effects may be either primarily or secondarily the object desired. The hot-air bath is one of the most convenient means of inducing perspiration. It is on this account quite liable to abuse. Perspiration is far less useful as an eliminative measure than is generally supposed, the perspiration usually containing but a small amount of toxic substances.

The chief value of the hot-air bath is perhaps as an exciting measure for the purpose of stimulating the skin during an application, and for some time after, if desired.

This bath is much employed in *rheumatism.* It is of service in the *toxemia* of chronic dyspepsia, biliousness, etc. It may be used in *obesity*, and with caution in certain cases of *Bright's disease.* It is useful in *cardiac dropsy*, but must be employed with great care and moderation to avoid depressing the heart. High temperatures must never be employed in cardiac cases, and the temperature must be very gradually raised. It must be wholly interdicted in cases of extreme *cardiac dilatation.*

The hot-air bath may be used to excellent advantage for revulsive effects in *sciatica*, *lumbago*, and other painful nervous affections involving large nerve trunks. In these cases the bath should be continued only long enough to heat the skin sufficiently to induce gentle perspiration, and should then be immediately followed by a very short cold general application with special attention to the part affected. For example, in sciatica a cold spray or douche would be employed over the course of the nerve in the affected limb, or a towel wrung out of cold water might be applied over the part, and the part vigorously rubbed for 30 to 60 seconds.

In making a cold application after a hot bath in rheumatism, an excessively low temperature must be avoided. Very cold applications in such cases have the effect to cause an immediate return of the pain and stiffness, which the hot bath usually relieves. A prolonged tepid spray may be safely employed in these cases, at a temperature of about 80° to 85°, the time, from 1 to 3 minutes, and followed by a gentle spray, shower, or a graduated immersion. Beginning at 95°, the temperature may be lowered to 80° within 2 minutes, with rubbing.

In extreme cases of *rheumatism* and *Bright's disease* in which cold applications can not be tolerated at all, the patient, on leaving the hot bath, should recline upon a cot, wrapped in a linen sheet, which should be partially opened now and then to admit of evaporation. After the first minute or two, a warm blanket may be thrown over him, which should be removed every five minutes for a few seconds, the covering being lessened as the patient gradually cools off. In the course of half an hour or an hour, when the pulse has become normal and the skin cool and smooth, the patient may be allowed to dress, but not before. Tepid sponging, fanning, etc., may also assist in the cooling.

Severe cold applications must likewise be avoided after a hot-air bath in Bright's disease, also in cases of weak heart. The sudden afflux of blood to the internal viscera may produce so intense a congestion of the kidneys as to damage these organs, and may so distend the right side of the heart as seriously to cripple its action.

1236 **Contraindications.**—The hot-air bath should be avoided in *eruptive skin disorders*, in cases of extreme *cardiac weakness*, in the *febrile condition*, in *diabetes* with emaciation, in *exophthalmic goiter*, in *arteriosclerosis*, and in advanced cases of *nephritis*.

In the employment of sweating processes of every kind, it must be constantly borne in mind that the natural effect of these applications is to produce inactivity of the bowels, as pointed out by Röhrig. The intestinal inactivity is of course caused by diminished secretion of moisture from the intestinal mucous membrane. The constipating tendency of the sweating processes may be largely overcome by copious water-drinking. Cold water is preferable to hot as a means of stimulating peristaltic activity. Cold water may be taken freely at proper hours (**1423**).

THE LOCAL HOT-AIR BATH.

1237 This measure consists in the application of superheated air to circumscribed portions of the body, as an arm, a limb, a knee-joint, etc. By means of a properly arranged chamber connected with a kerosene or gas lamp or other source of heat (Fig. 129), it is easily possible to bring to bear upon a

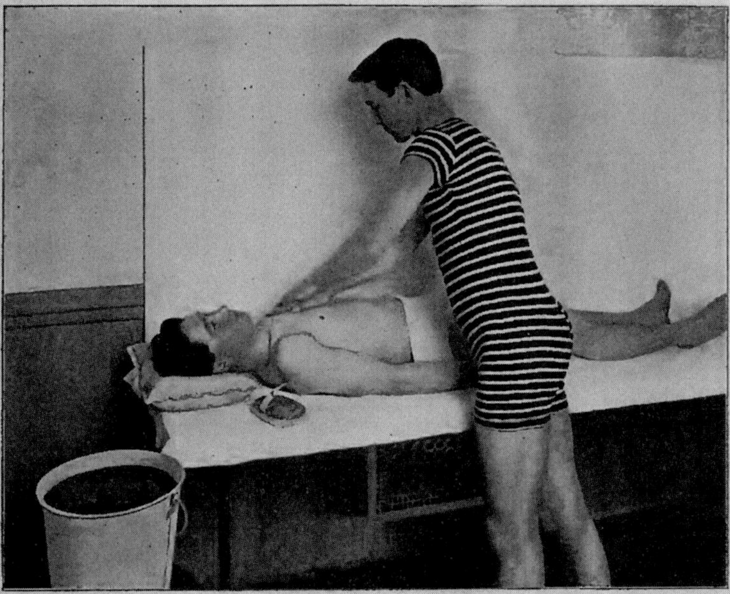

FIG. 130. TURKISH BATH — Shampooing (p. 695).

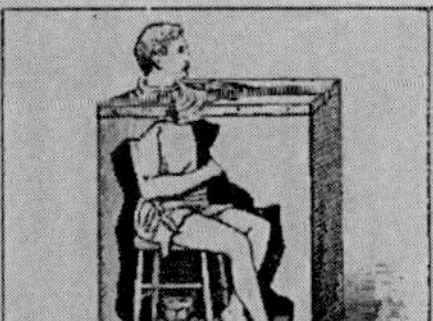

FIG. 131 (*a*). VAPOR BATH.

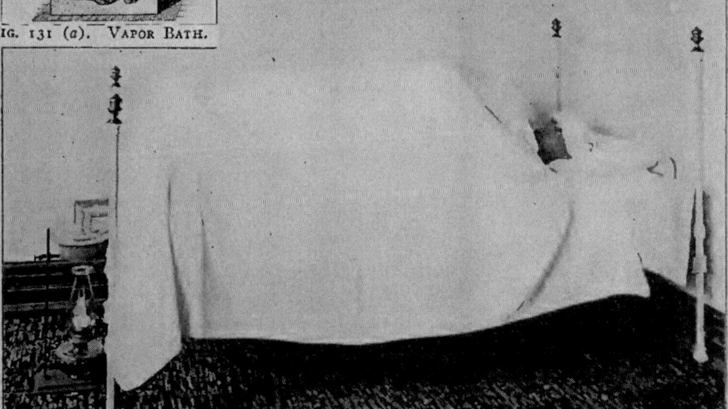

Fig. 131 (*b*). VAPOR BATH IN BED (p. 701).

circumscribed portion of the body a temperature of 300° to 400°.

The Japanese administer the local hot-air bath in a very simple manner. A properly constructed box is placed over a quantity of live coals until it is thoroughly heated. The limb to which the application is to be made is then placed in the box, and properly covered so as to retain the heat. As general perspiration is always induced when the application is prolonged, the patient should be undressed in preparation for the bath, and at its conclusion a short cold application should be made to the entire surface of the body as well as to the part treated. A cold mitten friction, a cold towel rub, or a wet sheet rub are the best measures for this purpose. Care should be taken to avoid chilling the patient. Immediate and thorough reaction should be promoted by careful drying and thorough rubbing.

Therapeutic Applications.—Remarkably excellent effects 1238
are certainly obtainable by the daily or frequent application of the localized hot-air bath, especially in cases of *rheumatic joints, chronic inflammation* of the joints with exudates, and allied affections. The duration of the application may be a few minutes to several hours, according to the intensity of the application, the sensations of the patient, and the nature of the case under treatment. In very chronic affections, prolonged applications are usually necessary. In more acute cases, short applications are preferable and sufficient.

When the limb is removed from the hot-air chamber, it may be wrapped in a large mass of cotton or wool, covered with oil or rubber cloth, then with flannel, to continue the effect of the bath. Before the dry pack is applied, a towel wrung very dry out of cold water may be wrapped about the part and vigorously rubbed for 10 or 15 seconds to secure a strong circulatory reaction whereby the blood will be fixed in the skin and the revulsive effect rendered more permanent. The localized hot-air bath is contraindicated in cases of acute inflammation, in general fever, and in cases in which the skin of the parts is diseased.

THE TURKISH BATH.

1239 This is a very old procedure, dating back to the time of the Romans. The author, with thousands of others, has explored in Rome and Naples the ruins of baths which were in active operation in the time of Nero; and while once wandering about the ancient places of Jerusalem, he one day accidentally stumbled upon an old Turkish bath which was built and used in the time of Herod, and after the lapse of nearly nineteen centuries is still in active operation. In this bath the air is heated by means of a huge brick furnace, the body of which is exposed in the room, the door for introducing fuel being outside the wall of the house. In a little grotto dug out of the limestone rock at one side, a man lay upon the floor perspiring, while an attendant, reclining by his side, supported himself upon his right elbow while leisurely kneading and shampooing the bather with his left hand.

The modern Turkish bath requires an establishment especially fitted up for its application, the essential features of which are: dressing-rooms, a warm room, or tepidarium (temperature 110° to 130°), a calidarium, or hot room (temperature 150° to 170°), a shampoo-room, a douche apparatus, a plunge bath, and a cooling-room.

The air of the rooms may be heated by steam coils, or so-called direct radiation, or by currents of hot air, or indirect radiation. The latter means is the most desirable, and is essential to good ventilation. Usually, Turkish bath rooms are provided only with steam-coils or pipes; and no provision being made for change of air, the atmosphere soon becomes so impure by emanations from the body that the good effects which otherwise might be secured by the bath are largely spoiled by the poisons inhaled.

Method.— The Turkish bath is similar to the hot-air bath, but differs in that it includes the whole body, and that it is accompanied by friction, kneading of the muscles, and shampooing. As practiced by the Turks at Constantinople and the Arabs at Cairo, the bath also includes joint movements of various sorts,—stretching, twisting, flexion, etc.

Before entering the bath, the patient should drink freely of either hot or cold water, as he prefers. A few minutes after entering the bath, another glass of water should be taken. Three or four glasses of water should be taken at intervals during the bath. During the first 10 or 15 minutes, the patient is frequently rubbed by the attendant for one or two minutes, to encourage dilatation of the surface vessels, and to induce perspiration. If perspiration is long delayed, apply a hot foot bath or a hot fomentation to the spine. If there is a disposition to cerebral congestion, the hair and the scalp may be moistened, and a cold towel may be placed about the head and neck. When the patient begins to perspire, he should enter the second apartment, the intense heat of which will give less discomfort after perspiration is well established than if entered at the beginning.

From the hot room the patient goes to the shampoo-room, where, lying upon a slab, he is first gone over from head to foot by the attendant with the hands dipped in water, the manipulations being calculated to remove as thoroughly as possible the layer of cuticle which has been loosened by the free perspiration. The first two manipulations are for the purpose of loosening the dead cuticle, the last removes it. These rubbings and strokings are continued until the skin is smooth and polished like marble. (Fig. 130.)

These movements are not easily described. They consist substantially of three sorts of manipulations:—

1. Simple firm pressure with the hand spread out and held firmly in contact with the skin with much pressure and with slight lateral movement.

2. Rapid to-and-fro movements, systematically applied to small areas in succession, as an arm, half the chest, the abdomen, etc.

3. Long stroking movements, applied after laving the part with water.

The next step is shampooing the patient with soap and water by the aid of a shampoo brush, a wad of horsehair or fiber, the hair mitt, or a mitt of Turkish cloth especially adapted to the purpose.

When the whole surface has thus been shampooed, the douche is administered. It is well to begin the douche with a warm shower, which should be heated to 104° to 106°. When the patient's skin has become well heated, and he feels a thirst for cold water, the hot water is suddenly turned off and the horizontal jet, spray, or multiple circle douche administered. After the shower, the patient enters the plunge bath for a few seconds if he desires. The temperature of the plunge should not be above 70°, and better effects are secured by a short plunge in water at 60°.

In the famous Hammam Turkish Bath in Paris, the author found the temperature of the water of the plunge to be 54°. A temperature even lower than this is sometimes employed, but is not to be recommended.

After the plunge, the patient is quickly dried, rubbed vigorously, then lies for 15 or 20 minutes, lightly covered, in the cooling-room. He should not leave the bathing apartments until the pulse has returned to the normal rate, and the skin is cool and perfectly dry.

1240 **Physiological Effects.**—The physiological effects of the Turkish bath are not very different from those of the hot-air bath. The body being completely surrounded with superheated air, so that the pulmonary mucous membrane as well as the cutaneous surface is exposed to its influence, somewhat more pronounced systemic effects are produced than by the hot-air bath, especially at the beginning of the application. Before perspiration begins, the heart is usually very much excited. The acceleration of the pulse is in direct proportion to the elevation of the temperature of the bath; the higher the temperature, the more rapid the pulse. With dilatation of the cutaneous vessels and beginning perspiration, the pulse is slowed, and blood tension lowered.

This interesting fact respecting the influence of the Turkish bath upon the circulation was well studied by E. Large.*

At a temperature of 150° to 180°, the respiration is purely thoracic, and more than doubled in frequency. The Turkish bath powerfully excites the sudoriparous glands. In his experience with this bath during the last twenty-five years, the author has often seen patients lose two pounds or more in a single bath of an hour's duration.

The amount of fluid which may escape through the skin under favorable conditions is very great, sometimes amounting, as in the case of a workman in hot weather, to as much as one fifth the body weight in twenty-four hours. Excessive activity of the skin is of course attended by an unusual movement of fluids toward the surface of the body. The amount of fluid poured into the alimentary canal is considerably reduced, and the result is constipation, the urine being also rendered scanty at the same time. It is thus evident that vigorous sweating must promote absorption from the alimentary canal. It is due to this fact that the sweating bath is such a powerful means of stimulating nutrition.

A lowering of blood pressure also occurs as the result of the diminished volume of blood. The rapid loss of fluid during profuse perspiration, amounting to three or four pounds per hour, emphasizes sufficiently the necessity for copious drinking in connection with sweating baths of every sort. The usual absence of perspiration during fever, also the absence of the normal odor of the perspiration during the febrile state, as observed by Bouchard, are interesting phenomena which indicate the importance of the skin as a heat-regulating organ, and as an avenue for the escape of toxic matters from the blood. The Turkish bath usually fails to excite perspiration in fever.

Therapeutic Applications.—The Turkish bath may be use- 1241
fully employed in the majority of chronic disorders. It is

* "Recherches Physiologiques sur les Bains de Vapeur Sèche" (Hamman Bains, Turcs).

an error, however, to suppose that the profuse sweating which may be induced by this bath is at all essential to good results in all classes of cases.

The therapeutic indications are essentially the same as those mentioned for the hot-air bath. The same suggestions and precautions are also applicable. It is especially important to investigate, by careful physical examination, the condition of every patient before submitting him to so vigorous a process as the Turkish bath. Like the hot-air bath, the Turkish bath may be used either as a sweating process or as a means of preparing the skin for cold applications of any sort (**1235**).

1242 **Contraindications.**—The Turkish bath should not be employed in cases of skin disease accompanied by eruptions, on account of the excessive congestion of the skin induced, whereby the eruptions are aggravated. The vapor and Russian baths are better in these cases. The Turkish bath must also be avoided in most cases of *organic disease* of the *heart*, in *Bright's disease* of the kidneys, in most *pulmonary affections*, in cases of *arteriosclerosis* in which the disease has reached an advanced stage, in cases in which a previous attack of *apoplexy* has recently occurred, in *diabetes* with emaciation, and in *febrile affections*.

Care must be taken to avoid the overuse of the Turkish bath. It is on the whole a very agreeable procedure, and may easily be employed to excess. Frequent long-continued exposure to the sedative influence of heat is debilitating. This effect of the bath is overcome, however, provided the application is not too prolonged or too frequent, by means of the cold shower or plunge with which the bath is completed.

THE RUSSIAN BATH.

1243 In this bath the patient lies upon a slab in a small room filled with steam, being rubbed at intervals by an attendant so as to promote the early appearance of perspiration. The temperature of the room is usually from 115° to 120°; 140°

is barely endurable, but can not be continued for any great length of time without danger. The length of the bath may be from 10 to 20 minutes. A cold shower bath is sometimes arranged in the apartment, so that the patient can, if he desires, expose himself to the alternate action of heat and cold by stepping under the shower bath for a few moments.

In Finland a Russian bath is produced by pouring water upon heated stones in a room provided for the purpose. This method is essentially the same as that used from the earliest times by the North American Indians.

The Russian bath, like the Turkish, is followed by a shampoo and a cold shower or plunge bath (**1239**). The same precautions should be observed at the conclusion of the bath respecting the cooling of the patient, as elsewhere indicated (**1233**).

Physiological Effects.— The effects of the Russian bath **1244**
are essentially the same as those of the hot-air bath (**1233**); but to the ordinary effects of other hot baths the Russian bath adds one disagreeable feature,— the interference with the respiratory process, because of the saturated condition of the atmosphere of the bath.

The elimination of CO_2 is diminished in the Russian bath, and perspiration is less active than in the Turkish or the hot-air bath at a temperature equally endurable.

One advantage possessed by the Russian bath over the Turkish or hot-air bath is that it is better tolerated by persons suffering from eruptions or cutaneous irritation of any sort.

Perhaps the most important characteristic of the Russian bath is the rapid and considerable rise of body temperature, due to the interference with heat elimination through the skin and lungs, as well as by the heat communicated. The body temperature rises higher and more rapidly in the Russian than in the hot-air or the Turkish bath. As a result, the oxidation of proteid elements is greatly increased, the condition being allied to that of fever. This increased oxidation of nitrogen gives to the Russian as well as the vapor bath and the sweating pack a special value in the treatment of chronic rheumatism and all forms of uric-acid poisoning and chronic toxemias, in which one of the chief indications is for increased oxidation and destruction of nitrogen-containing wastes and toxins. There is no bath which excels the Russian in this particular, except the electric-light bath, which rapidly heats the body, not by retention of body heat, but by the penetration of the rays of radiant energy into the depths of the tissues and powerfully excites metabolism.

1245 **Therapeutic Applications.**—These are essentially the same as those already mentioned in relation to the hot-air bath and the Turkish bath. The Russian bath is for some persons more agreeable than the Turkish or hot-air bath, because of the effect of the moist air upon the skin. Persons suffering from *acute bronchial catarrh* often experience very great temporary relief in the Russian bath. Its effect is likely to be transient, however; and unless extraordinary precautions are taken, the exposure ordinarily necessary after the bath is likely to result in an aggravation of the cold. The Russian bath whitens the skin by improving its circulation, relieves *rheumatic pain*, and may be advantageously employed in *diabetes* when there is no cardiac complication, in the *chronic toxemia* of *dyspepsia*, and in some *skin disorders* in which Turkish and water baths prove too irritating; it relieves pain in *sciatica*, and is generally useful in the *rheumatic diathesis*.

The Russian bath is not so well adapted to the treatment of cases of *obesity* as is the hot-air or the electric-light bath or the sweating pack. The reason for this is the tendency in obesity to overheating and systemic weakening in consequence of the exhaustion of the nerve centers.

Contraindications.—Extraordinary care must be exercised to avoid overheating the patient in this bath, as heat elimination is almost altogether suspended; and hence the bath must be avoided in *febrile cases*. The bath must also be interdicted in cases of *cardiac weakness*, in most cases of *advanced Bright's disease*, *pulmonary tuberculosis*, and in *arteriosclerosis*.

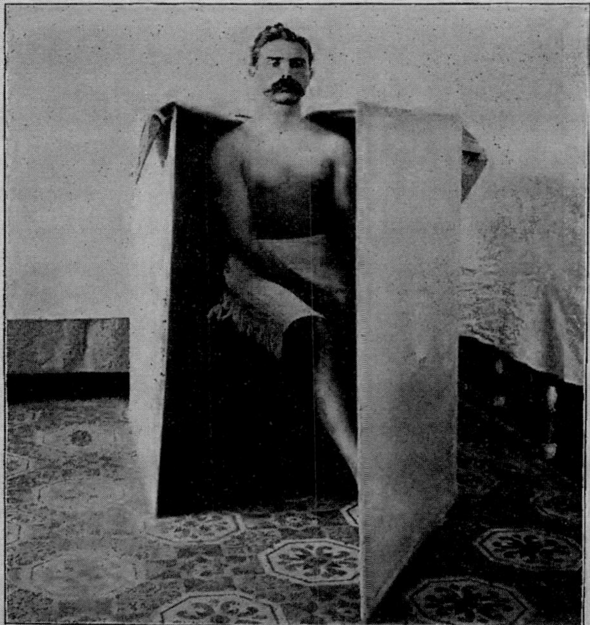

Fig. 132. PORTABLE VAPOR BATH (p. 702).

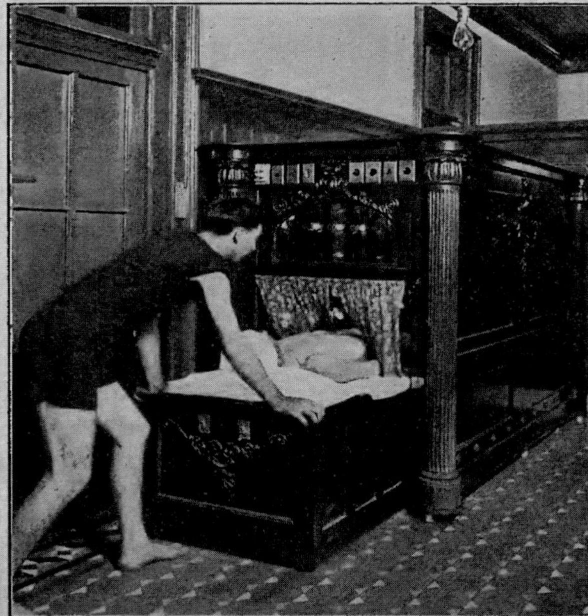

Fig. 134. HORIZONTAL ELECTRIC-LIGHT BATH (p. 708).

THE VAPOR BATH.

The vapor bath (Fig. 131) resembles the hot-air bath 1246
in the mode of administration. The same sort of cabinet may be used, and the emergency arrangements suggested for the hot-air bath are equally useful for the vapor bath (Figs. 127, 128). When the vapor bath is given in bed, however, an oil cloth must be placed under the patient to avoid wetting the mattress.

Among the different methods of giving a vapor bath may be mentioned the following:—

1. Water may be boiled in a flat-bottomed basin over an alcohol lamp or a small gas or kerosene stove. The basin should be wide, and the quantity of water small, so that it may boil quickly and vigorously.

2. A pail of boiling water may be placed in the cabinet beneath the chair on which the patient sits, and into this may be lowered one by one well-heated flat-irons, bricks, stones, or other mineral or metallic masses, a wire being attached to each so that the entrance into the water may be easily controlled. The mass should be gradually let down into the water, so that the steam may not be generated too rapidly.

3. A rubber tube attached to the spout of a teakettle with a tight-fitting cover is a useful method of conveying steam to the cabinet.

4. In the absence of a better arrangement, a vapor bath may be taken in an ordinary bath-tub supplied with hot and cold water, by the aid of the following simple arrangement devised by Winternitz: A board of a size sufficient to support the patient, and perforated with inch holes, is laid in the tub, and raised by proper supports three or four inches from the bottom. By means of a piece of ordinary garden hose three or four feet long, connected with the hot-water faucet, the hot water may be carried to the upper end of the tub beneath this board. By leaving out the plug, the hot water is thus allowed to run in and out of the tub; and as it passes the

whole length of the tub before escaping, it gives off a large quantity of steam, which, passing up through the openings in the board, surrounds the patient with warm vapor. The vapor is retained about the body of the patient by blankets placed over the top of the tub, and tucked around the neck in such a way as to protect the head from the warm vapor. The intensity of the heat may be regulated by controlling the flow of water. The inventor of this ingenious kind of vapor bath informed the author, when on a visit to his establishment at Kaltenleutgeben, near Vienna, that he had been able to administer a good vapor bath with two gallons of hot water.

Nothing could be simpler or cheaper unless it be the method adopted by the New Zealanders, who, as we have been informed by Mr. Maui Pomare, administer a vapor bath by the following unique but effective means: Several stones are laid upon a small heap of wood properly arranged; the wood being lighted, the stones are soon heated very hot. They are then covered with a thick bed of green leaves, upon which the patient lies down. The patient is covered with a blanket, which retains the moist vapor from the steaming leaves, and is thus made to perspire profusely. After the bath he is cooled by plunging into the sea.

An old French author describes a method of administering a vapor bath by placing an empty wine barrel from which one head had been removed over a fire until well heated, then reversing it and putting the patient inside, enveloping both the patient and the barrel in thick coverings to retain the heat and moisture.

The accompanying cut (Fig. 132) shows an extremely convenient portable cabinet which may be employed for either the vapor or the hot-air bath.

In certain cases it is desirable to administer a vapor bath with the patient reclining. This may be accomplished in several ways. A convenient arrangement devised by the author is shown in Fig. 131 (b).

Physiological Effects.— The pulse is greatly quickened, rising rapidly to 140 or 150 beats per minute. The heart is quickly tired out by the excitation of the hot bath, with the low vascular tension to which it gives rise, because its periods of rest are diminished. Beating at its ordinary rate, the heart has about forty seconds to rest out of each minute; but if its rate of beating is increased 25 to 50 per cent., its periods of rest are diminished proportionately. 1247

The pulse is much more profoundly affected in the vapor than in the hot-air bath. Sweating begins much sooner in the vapor than in the hot-air or Turkish bath, and less quickly than in the electric-light bath. It should be noted that the appearance of moisture upon the surface of the body is not necessarily an evidence of perspiration, as it may be the result of condensation of vapor upon the skin. Frey, in his interesting study of the hot-air and vapor baths,* calls attention to the interesting fact that while the respiration is quickened, the respiratory movements do not increase either in the hot-air or the vapor bath in proportion to the pulse. In the vapor bath, however, respiration is excited to a much greater degree than in the hot-air bath.

The absorption of oxygen is interfered with in the vapor bath for the reason that the respiration is not quickened in proportion to the increase in the pulse-rate. Oxidation is thus interfered with to some extent. When perspiration is induced by exercise, the breathing is quickened in proportion to the heart action, a larger amount of oxygen is taken into the system, and hence sweating resulting from exercise is less exhausting than that produced by the vapor bath or other sweating processes.

The effect of the vapor bath upon the body temperature is very profound, the rectal temperature rising in the course of 20 or 30 minutes sometimes to the extent of three or four degrees. The temperature of both the rectum and the axilla

* "Experimentelle Studien uber die Wirkung der heissen Luft und Dampfbäder," *Archiv für Psychiatrie*, Berlin, 1880, XI, 266–270.

rises much more quickly in the vapor bath than in the Turkish or dry hot-air bath (Exp. 62). The axillary temperature rises more rapidly and to a higher point than the rectal temperature. This is doubtless due (1) to the fact that vapor is a much better conductor of heat; and (2) to the further fact that cooling of the body by evaporation is suspended in the vapor bath as in the Russian bath, the hot immersion bath, and the wet-sheet pack.

In consequence of the elevation of temperature produced by the vapor bath, this procedure becomes a powerful factor in the oxidation of proteids, in common with all other hydriatic procedures which are accompanied by elevation of body temperature.

1248 **Therapeutic Applications.**—The vapor bath is indicated in the same class of cases as those for which the hot-air, Turkish, and Russian baths are recommended. It is especially useful as a means of heating the skin previously to a cold application of some sort (120° for 3 to 5 min.). For this purpose, however, it is inferior to the electric-light bath. Its only specific application is as a heating process in cases in which the skin is so irritable that the hot-air bath, the electric-light bath, and other similar processes are contraindicated. The contact of the moist vapor with the skin produces a soothing effect in these cases, provided an excessively high temperature is not employed. The vapor as well as the Russian bath has a further advantage in that it softens the epidermis, and facilitates the discharge of sebaceous matters and inspissated products from the perspiratory ducts, thus relieving a condition which one writer graphically describes as "constipation of the skin."

The physiological effects produced by the vapor bath, particularly its influence upon blood circulation and tissue activity, indicate it to be a powerful therapeutic procedure. The influence of the bath upon proteid oxidation especially adapts it to the treatment of those cases of retarded nutrition in which it is desirable to stimulate the oxidation of proteid

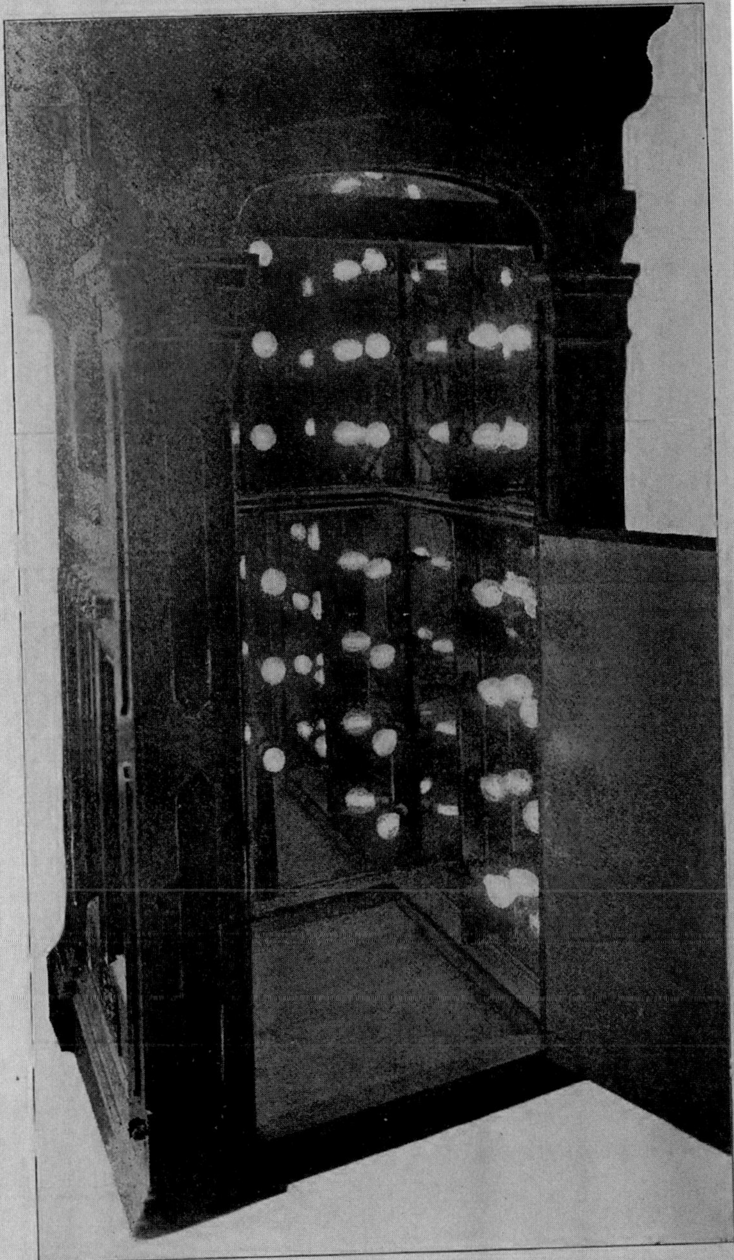

FIG. 133. ELECTRIC-LIGHT BATH (p. 707).

wastes, as in *rheumatism* or *gout*, and that very large class of chronic cases, including a large proportion of *neurasthenics*, in which the *uric acid diathesis* is the fundamental dyscrasia which forms the general background for the varied pathological pictures presented.

The vapor bath is a powerful eliminative measure. When employed for this purpose, its duration should be from 15 to 30 minutes. The prolonged vapor bath is indicated in *chronic rheumatism*, *jaundice*, *tertiary syphilis*, and whenever general spoliative effects are required, as in *obesity* with rheumatism.

The vapor bath is useful in all forms of *chronic toxemia*. It is especially well adapted to this class of cases, being exceeded in value by no procedure excepting the electric-light bath, which by its greater power to heat the tissues, stimulates still more actively the oxidation of the proteid substances of an excrementitious or toxic character, the presence of which gives rise to the exceedingly varied conditions so admirably described by Bouchard in his "Autointoxications."

Neuralgias, especially facial and spinal neuralgias, *sciatica*, *hemicrania*, *peripheral paralyses*, especially when due to syphilis, *paralyses* resulting from the exudates of gout or rheumatism, *functional disorders* of the *spinal cord*, *hysteria*, *hypochondria*, are all favorably influenced, often with remarkable rapidity, by the vapor bath. *Exudates* and *effusions*, whether of inflammatory origin or due to mechanical disturbance of the circulation, are absorbed under the powerful alterative and spoliative influence of the vapor bath; although for this purpose it is perhaps less effective than the hot-air or the electric-light bath. Paralysis resulting from *exudative meningitis* of the spine not infrequently yields rapidly to the influence of the vapor bath. This measure may also be appropriately applied in the treatment of *chronic nephritis* during an acute exacerbation, in *infectious jaundice*, in *acute alcoholic poisoning* in connection with the cold bath, in *tetany*, in *migraine* and *malarial neuralgia* (between at-

45

tacks), and as a heating procedure in connection with general cold applications, such as the douche, the half bath, and the wet-sheet rub, As a heating procedure (2 to 5 min.), it is very convenient, and is widely used in continental hydriatic establishments, although the electric-light bath is rapidly superseding it.

In the application of the vapor bath, it is important to remember that it is a very powerful measure. It is far more energetic than the hot-air bath, for moist air is a better medium of communicating heat to the body than is dry air.

Contraindications.—The contraindications for the vapor bath are the same as those for the hot-air and the electric-light bath as regards general conditions. The vapor bath is a more vigorous procedure than the hot-air bath, and hence better adapted to the strong and young than to old and feeble persons. Great caution must be employed in its use in advanced cases of cardiac or renal disease, in which it must be, as a rule, strictly prohibited. Exceptions to this rule are noted in the discussion of the hydriatic treatment of these affections.

THE LOCAL VAPOR BATH.

1249 While the chief use of the vapor bath is in general applications, it may be made to render valuable service in various partial applications as well. By suitable arrangements, the application may be confined to an arm, a leg, or any circumscribed portion of the body. When thus used, a much higher temperature may be employed than when the whole cutaneous surface is exposed.

Therapeutic Applications.—The powerful heating effect of the vapor bath renders it highly valuable as a means of relieving pain. It may be applied in nearly all conditions to which the fomentation is applicable. The fomentation itself is in fact little more than a crude form of vapor bath. As compared with the fomentation, the partial vapor bath has the advantage that it avoids mechanical contact with the affected part, and hence is better suited to cases in which there is extreme sensitiveness

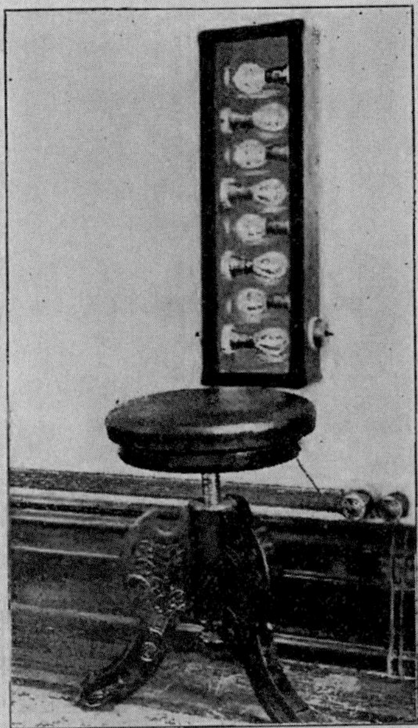

Fig. 135. Electric-Light Bath for Spine (p. 708).

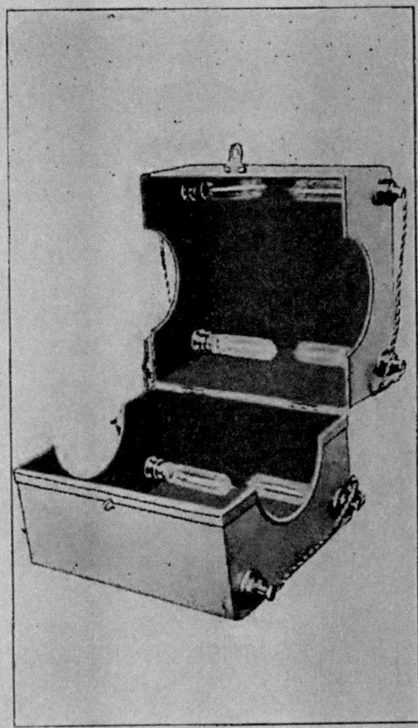

Fig. 138. Electric-Light Bath for Joint (p. 708).

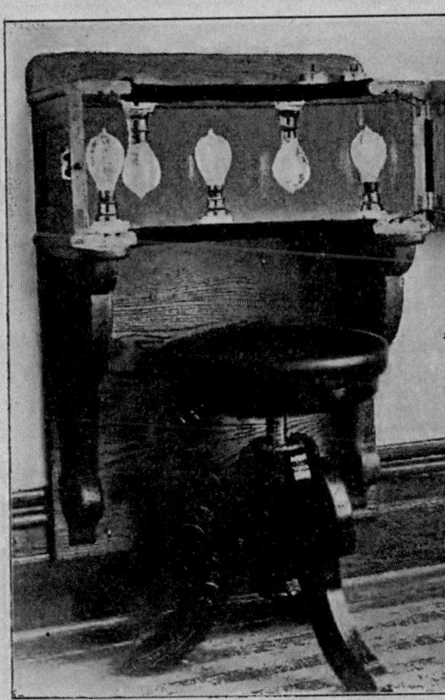

Fig. 136. Electric-Light Bath for Trunk (p. 708).

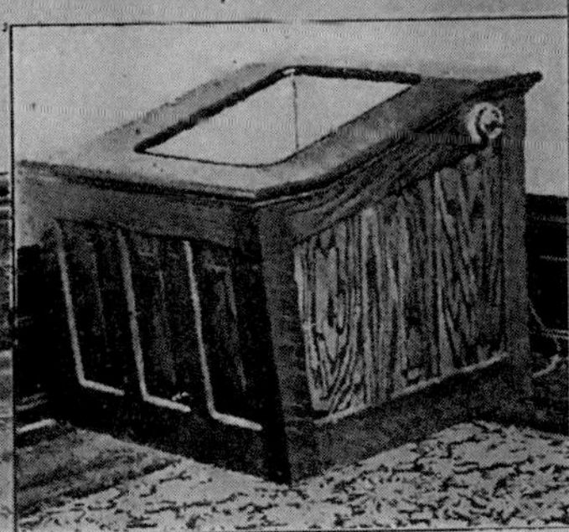

Fig. 137. Electric-Light Bath for Feet and Legs (p. 708).

of the skin, as in superficial inflammations and cutaneous hyperesthesias. Nearly twenty-five years ago the author learned from a patient who had long been a great sufferer from painful hemorrhoids and *rectal ulcer*, an application of the local vapor bath which is worth mentioning. This patient had made the discovery that by pouring into a pail a gallon or two of boiling water and sitting over it while evacuating the bowels and for a short time afterward, he was able to escape the terrible pain which he otherwise suffered.

By means of the *vapor douche* (**1102**), circumscribed vapor baths may be administered to any portion of the body, and at a temperature much higher than water in any other form can be applied.

THE ELECTRIC-LIGHT BATH.

In 1891 the author's attention was called by a colleague, **1250**
Dr. Kate Lindsay, to the convenience of the ordinary incandescent electric lamp wrapped in flannel as a means of applying heat in cases of pain. He had, some years previously, made extensive use of sunlight in the treatment of chronic invalids by a variety of means, especially the sun bath, modified by glass of various colors, and by means of large lenses which concentrated the rays of light upon painful points for the relief of hyperesthesia, particularly in the treatment of so-called spinal irritation. The observation above referred to, showing the electric light to be a convenient means of applying heat for local pain, led him to renew the study of the properties of light, and to begin experiments with various kinds of apparatus designed to make therapeutic applications of the electric light, which resulted in the development of the incandescent electric-light cabinet and various other devices for the general and local application of heat by means of the electric light. The first form of cabinet devised consisted of a compartment about eight feet in height (Fig. 133), upon the inside of which were placed between fifty and sixty incandescent lights, the spaces between the

rows of lights being filled with glass or metal mirrors to multiply the number of lights by reflection. The cabinet is so arranged that the whole body of the patient, sitting upright, can be exposed to the influence of the light, or the head may be excluded, as in the ordinary vapor bath. By means of switches and a proper grouping of the lamps in wiring, the number of lights in use can be instantly and perfectly controlled. As the heat effects of the bath are derived directly from the incandescent films by radiation, and do not at all depend upon the heating of confined air, the fullest provision is made for ventilation. It is not at all necessary that the air should be confined.

In another form of cabinet (Fig. 134), provided with sixty to ninety lamps, the patient lies in a horizontal position, the lights being placed on three sides. A suitable couch, provided with rollers, is pushed entirely within the cabinet, or only so far as to expose such portions of the body as it is desired to bring under the influence of radiant light and heat. By this plan, the influence of the light may be confined to the feet and legs, or any other portion of the body up to the neck. If preferable to do so, the attendant may protect by a sheet and a piece of mackintosh any portion of the body which it may be desirable to exclude from the action of the bath.

By means of other constructions, the effects of the incandescent light are localized for the spine (Fig. 135), the trunk, (Fig. 136), the legs (Fig. 137), and the joints (Fig. 138). These appliances are so quickly and easily managed that they constitute by far the most convenient and effective means of applying heat to the cutaneous surface. By the touch of a button the whole heating power of the apparatus may be brought to bear at once, or may be as quickly terminated. The intensity of the application may be regulated by a rheostat, or by the number and candle-power of the lamps employed.

Method.—There are two general forms of the electric-light bath; viz., the incandescent-light bath and the arc-light

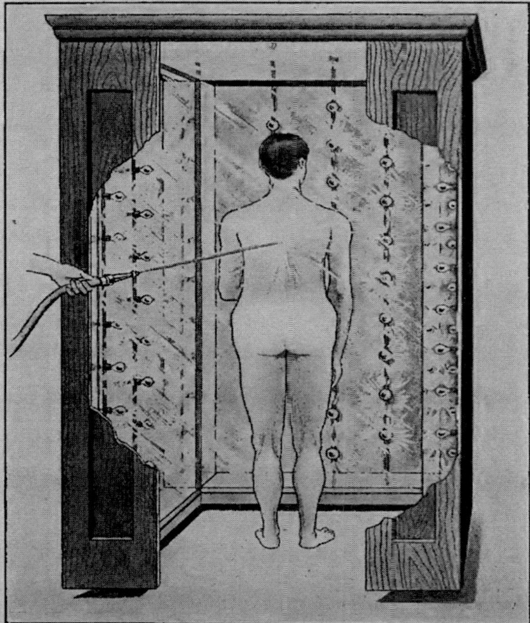

Fig. 139. ELECTRIC-LIGHT BATH AND COLD DOUCHE COMBINED (p. 709)

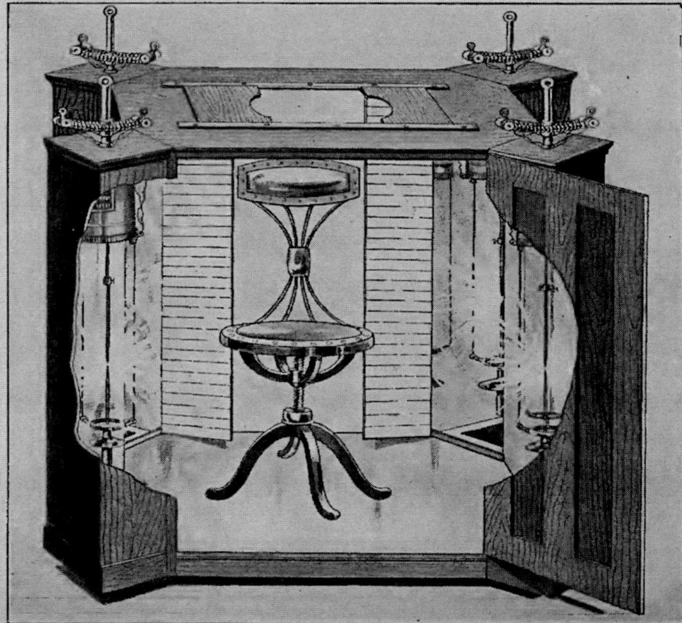

Fig. 140. AUTHOR'S ARC-LIGHT BATH (p. 711).

bath. Unless otherwise indicated, the term "electric-light bath" as used in this work refers to the incandescent electric-light bath, the several forms of which are shown in accompanying cuts. The author has also arranged cabinets in which the arc light and the incandescent light are combined.

The trunk electric-light bath has been found especially valuable in cases of disorders of the liver, kidneys, stomach, and bowels.

Employed in any of its localized forms, the application is usually followed by a cold trunk pack, cold friction, or a cold spray or douche to the surface which has been exposed to the heat.

The incandescent electric-light bath and the calorific or heating bath administered by means of the electric-arc bath may be regarded chiefly as heating procedures, and should be followed by cooling applications in precisely the same manner as the hot-air, Turkish, vapor bath, etc. The incandescent electric-light bath is superior to every other form of heating procedure in the quickness with which the skin may be heated when the object sought is simply a preparation for the cold bath. The time required may be not more than 3 to 5 minutes. When strongly derivative or eliminative effects are required, the application may be continued for 15 to 20 minutes. A longer application is likely to produce exhausting effects through overstimulation of the nervous system and excessive elevation of temperature.

For general revulsive effects, the author has devised a new form of bath, which combines the shower and douche with the electric-light bath. The cabinet is made in such form that the patient stands in an upright position (Fig. 139). After the skin has become thoroughly warmed by the heat from the lamps, a cold shower or horizontal jet douche of the desired temperature is applied, the lamps being protected from the cold water by an internal lining of plate glass. The revulsion thus produced is of the most powerful character, and may be repeated as many times as required. By repeating the cold application for 10 seconds at intervals of half a minute, this bath may be made very highly exciting and also tonic.

The sweating electric-light bath is usually followed by a shampoo and a cold douche, the finishing treatment being essentially the same as that for the Turkish and the Russian baths.

In cases in which the purpose is simply to excite the circulation of the skin, the daily shampoo is not required, as the heating process will be terminated when active perspiration begins. Feeble patients and persons not accustomed to cold water may be cooled by means of the wet-hand or wet-towel rub, by the cool friction mitt, or by affusion.

In the radiant-heat, or incandescent electric-light, bath the body may be subjected to the most intense heat desired without confining the patient, and without overheating the atmosphere surrounding him. This is due to the well-known fact that rays of heat pass through such transparent media as the air without heating them. This accounts for the intense cold experienced by balloonists and those who ascend high mountains, even in the tropics. As the woodchopper in the logging-camp roasts his back before a big log fire on a cold winter's evening, while the frost is taking sharp nips at his nose on the other side, so the patient in the incandescent electric-light bath, while perspiring freely, may be surrounded by air at the ordinary temperature.

If it is desired to heat the air of the bath, this may be accomplished by simply closing the cabinet, excluding the head. The glass globes of the lamps soon become heated, and in turn heat the air. The heating power of the globes depends upon the degree of vacuum. Winternitz has shown that the more air the bulb contains, the more the glass is heated. It thus appears that the incandescent electric-light bath may be so managed as to combine with the remarkable effects of radiant heat, all the effects of the ordinary hot-air bath, the value of which in promoting evaporation from the skin and thus encouraging perspiration, is certainly incontestible.

Local applications of the incandescent-light bath may be continued for half an hour or more, if desirable, as in the treatment of chronic inflammation of the knee-joint for resolvent effects, and in obstinate cases of sciatic neuralgia

Local applications to the spine are a most efficient means of exciting the spinal centers, and at the same time producing a powerful derivative effect. This is a most excellent measure in spinal neuralgia, in lumbago, and in reflex spinal pains arising from irritation of the sympathetic ganglia.

Application of the electric light to the joints is a more efficient method in old affections of these parts than any other known, and when combined with the heating compress and massage, accomplishes wonders in a class of cases most of which are generally looked upon as incurable. The heat and actinic rays penetrate the depths of the tissues, vitalizing and energizing the diseased and sluggish parts, and quickening the healing process.

A convenient appliance for a local application of the electric light may be easily improvised from an ordinary incandescent lamp by simply adding a conical tin shade of sufficient size to prevent contact of the lamp with the skin. If the heat is too intense, the skin may be protected by one or more thicknesses of white flannel cloth.

The Arc-Light Bath.—Experiments have shown that in 1251
the incandescent light bath only five per cent. of the electrical energy employed is thrown off as luminous rays; hence the great heating power of this bath.

In the arc light bath (Fig. 140), as stated elsewhere (599) in this work, we have other important factors. The electric arc light has been shown to contain actinic rays in even larger proportion than does the sunlight. In the arc-light cabinet which the author has had constructed, devices are introduced whereby the calorific, the actinic, or the combined rays of the electric arc may be brought to bear upon the patient. This cabinet consists of a quadrangular construction which permits the exclusion of the head of the patient. In each corner of the cabinet is placed a powerful arc light, so arranged that it may be moved up and down at will, thus bringing its rays to bear at any level. At each side of the opening through which the rays of each lamp are admitted, hangs a hinged door, one of red glass, the other of blue glass, so arranged that either screen may at will be brought before the lamp, thus excluding from the cabinet all rays except those which are desired. By means of a strong air current circulating through each lamp compartment, the accumulation of heat is prevented when desirable. The air of the cabinet is also constantly changed so that the patient may be subjected exclusively to the action of the radiant heat of the electric arc.

The author's experience with this form of bath is less extensive than with the incandescent form, but it has been sufficiently long to establish a reasonably fixed method for its employment. The calorific effects of the bath are secured by filtering the rays through red glass as described elsewhere (**596**), this being used when heating effects alone are desired. On the whole, the author's experience has shown the arc light to be less serviceable for this purpose than the incandescent light, as the light is less evenly distributed, and the method of obtaining heat much less economical. By means of the blue-glass screen the actinic rays are employed, with the exclusion of a large share of the luminous and calorific rays. The heating effects obtained with blue glass are very slight, but marked nervous and other vital phenomena may be elicited by a sufficiently long exposure, the experimental proof of which has been given elsewhere in this work (**599**).

The electric arc-light bath is only to a moderate extent a heating procedure, but the heat is sufficient to warm the skin thoroughly, so that tonic applications such as the cold douche may be employed directly after this bath.

1252 **Physiological Effects.**—In experiments conducted by the author, assisted by his colleagues, Drs. Paulson and Rand,

and Professor Gomberg of the University of Michigan, who superintended the chemical work, several very useful and interesting facts respecting the physiological effects of the electric-light bath have been demonstrated. It was ascertained, for example, that this bath is without doubt the most efficient and satisfactory of all modes of producing perspiration, as it stimulates the perspiratory glands and other structures of the skin in the most powerful manner. It causes the perspiration to appear in a remarkably short space of time, thus avoiding the exposure of the body to the exhausting effect of prolonged heat, as profuse perspiration generally appears in the electric-light bath in 3 to 5 minutes, even when the temperature of the air surrounding the patient is not above 85° F., while the dry pack not infrequently fails to produce vigorous activity of the skin within less than an hour and a half or two hours, a still longer time being sometimes required.

A fact which must be kept in mind in the employment of this powerful means of calorification, however, is that the body temperature, as indicated in the rectum, may rise to 103° or even higher in a prolonged electric-light bath.

It has also been ascertained that the lungs throw off, while exposed to the incandescent light, a decidedly larger proportion of carbonic acid gas than usual, showing increased oxidation. Hence the bath must not be excessively prolonged.*

The peculiar value of the electric-light bath is due to its efficiency as a source of radiant energy. In the Turkish bath, heat is communicated to the body chiefly by convection from heated air. Air, being a poor conductor, communicates heat to the body very slowly. Absorption of heat is further hindered by the skin, which is an excellent non-conductor, and by the rapid evaporation of moisture upon the skin, whereby it is cooled so rapidly that it is possible for a person to enter and remain for a considerable time in an atmosphere far above the boiling point. The heat of the electric light is in the form

* See paper, "The Incandescent Electric-Light or Radiant-Heat Bath," read before the Electro-Therapeutic Association at its fourth annual meeting, New York, Sept. 25–27, 1894.

of radiant energy. The electrical current of the incandescent electric-light bath develops light rays to the extent of only 5 to 8 per cent., while heat rays are developed to the extent of 92 per cent.*

This energy is not communicated to the body by convection. The skin, as well as the air, is to a large extent transparent to radiant heat, and the same is true of all the living tissues. This is evidenced by the gastrophone of Einhorn and other transilluminators. Through a speculum placed in the vagina with a suitably arranged electric light placed close to the abdomen, the author has seen the interior of the trunk illuminated and made to glow with a bright red light, the red color being due to reflection from the red corpuscles of the blood. Even the bones are translucent to light when in the living state. This is clearly shown by placing the hand between an electric light and the eye, with the fingers in close contact; if the hand is placed near enough to the light, the whole fingers will be seen illuminated, the bones as well as the soft parts. It may thus be said that heat from the electric light penetrates the body just as it would penetrate any other transparent or semi-transparent medium; while the heat of the Turkish, vapor, or Russian bath is communicated to the body by convection, and slowly works its way into the body by heating the successive layers of living tissue which, although, like glass, transparent to radiant energy, also possess to a greater or less degree the nonconducting quality of glass and allied substances.

Dr. Winternitz, professor of nervous diseases in the Royal University at Vienna, after having carefully reviewed the author's observations concerning the electric-light bath, and having himself made an extended study of the bath, states his conclusions in a recent work † as follows:—

"The electric-light bath presents an advantage over every other means of applying heat in the readiness with which the

* Kuhner, *Int. Klin. Rundschau*, Wein, 1894.

† Winternitz, "Fortschritte der Hydrotherapie."

dosage may be regulated as regards time and intensity. The instant the switch controlling the circuit is closed the whole force of the bath or that portion of it in use is brought to bear at once upon the body. The instant the circuit is opened the heat is wholly and absolutely withdrawn. By means of properly adjusted switches whereby the number of lamps in use may be controlled, the amount of heat applied may be exactly regulated.

"Another advantage of the electric-light bath is that it does not interfere with heat elimination. It in fact encourages heat elimination by encouraging free perspiration. Many other forms of hot applications, particularly hot water baths and sweating packs, cause retention of bodily heat. In the electric-light bath, the heat elimination and the excretion of effete matters which accompany vigorous perspiration proceed with increased activity at the same time the rays of radiant heat are penetrating the tissues, elevating the temperature of the blood, and quickening all the vital processes."

"The importance of this property of the electric-light bath is clearly shown by the interesting experiments of Conrad Klar.* This investigator showed by calorimetric experiment that with the body exposed in an atmosphere somewhat below the body temperature, heat elimination was during the first five minutes ten times the normal amount; while during the second five minutes the amount of heat eliminated was half as great. The diminished loss during the second five minutes was doubtless due to contraction of the blood-vessels of the skin. In the electric-light bath the cutaneous vessels are thoroughly relaxed, and this condition is maintained by the action of the rays of light falling upon the skin while the air about the patient is but little above the ordinary atmospheric temperature, a condition which in the highest degree favors heat elimination."

Professor Winternitz continues :—

"The electric-light bath is a new invention by Kellogg,

*Klar, *Wien. Klin. Woch.*, 1895, p. 180.

Battle Creek, Mich., U. S. A. It is undoubtedly true that radiant heat penetrates the tissues much better than conducted heat, and it is very probable also that the inner life of the cell is influenced by the radiant heat, either qualitatively or quantitatively, and to a higher degree. All the effects of the vapor bath can be produced by the electric-light bath. The loss of carbonic acid gas is considerably greater in the electric-light bath than in the vapor bath, and what is especially remarkable, perspiration occurs very quickly and at a very low temperature, and is very profuse. [Indications of perspiration are sometimes noticed at 28° R. (95° F.). The author has observed perspiration at 85° F., and Professor Winternitz stated to him personally (1899) that he had seen moisture appear upon the skin in a single instance at 65° F. The patient was a somewhat excitable neurasthenic, and very susceptible to the stimulus of radiant energy.]

"Ordinarily a much higher temperature is necessary before symptoms of sweating occur in the vapor bath. The time required to produce sweating in the electric-light bath is commonly 3½ minutes, whereas about 5 minutes are required in the vapor bath. Finally the quantity of perspiration is considerably greater in the electric-light bath. That the radiant heat is the main cause of this, and not the heated air, was evident from the observations made by us that the external part of the leg upon which the rays of light directly fell perspired very much more quickly and profusely than the internal part of the leg, which received only reflected rays. After 10 to 30 minutes the body temperature increased to 40° C. (104° F.), the pulse to 160, respiration to 42,—symptoms of the condition resembling fever. We have used the electric-light bath in ways analogous to the use of the vapor bath in a number of cases of sclerosis, rheumatism, and gout, and have been much gratified with the results. We have as yet made no further experiments. Kellogg reports very good results in sclerosis, arthritis, and many disorders of nutrition. Lehmann has been very successful in psoriasis. Since we

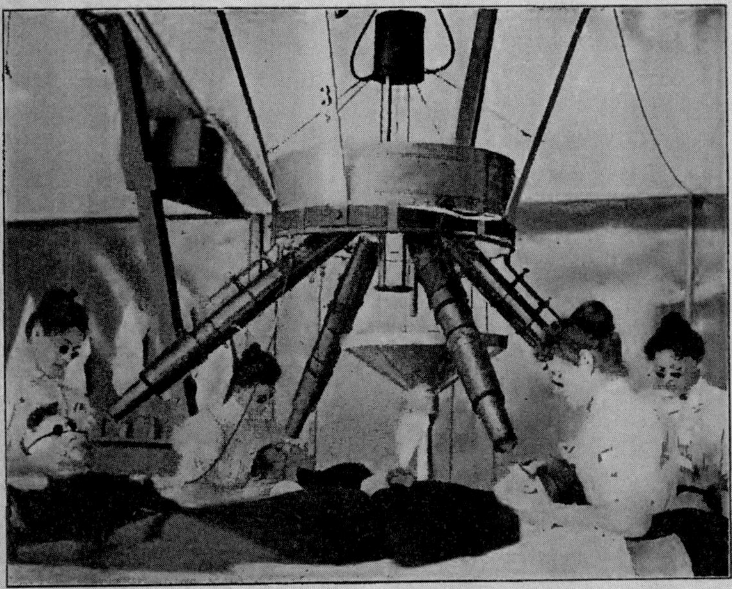

FIG. 141. FINSEN'S APPARATUS FOR PHOTOTHERAPY (p. 721).

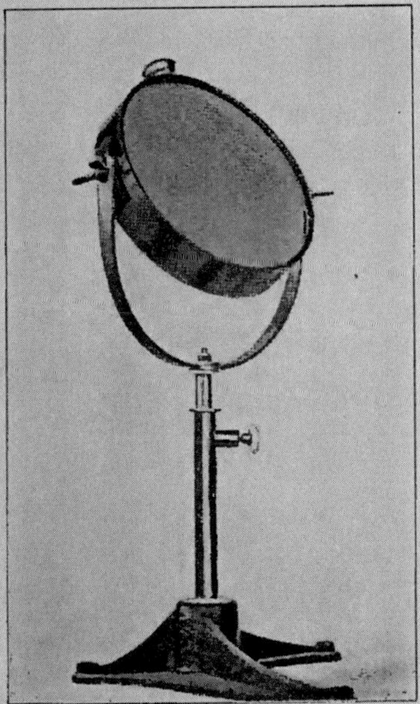

FIG. 142. LENS-BOTTLE FOR FILTERING OUT HEAT RAYS (p. 721).

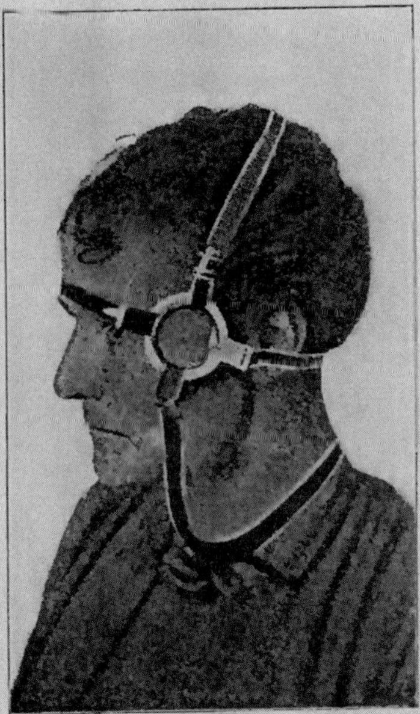

FIG. 143. COOLING COMPRESSOR (p. 721).

have in the electric-light bath a thermal method by which the degree of heat applied can be physiologically and exactly measured, and knowing the powerful influence of light upon the life of the cell and of the whole organism, we believe that this method will hold a prominent place among the forms of thermal applications, and that we shall be enabled by its use to influence a series of maladies more quickly, more effectively, and more satisfactorily than heretofore."

For a fuller discussion of the physiological effects of sunlight and of the electric light, see pages 168 to 180.

Therapeutic Applications.—The electric-light bath has 1253
proved, in the author's hands, of far greater value in the treatment of a large variety of maladies than any other means of applying heat except water, and admits of much more general employment than the ordinary Turkish, Russian, vapor, or hot-air baths. One reason of this is the convenience and rapidity with which the degree of heat may be graduated by turning on or off one or more groups of lamps, the amount of heat being thus rendered absolutely and instantly controllable, since the source of heat relied upon is the incandescent filaments of the lamps rather than a heated atmosphere. The instant the lamp is turned off, the heat which had previously been emitted is withdrawn from operation. If additional heat is required, the desired number of lamps may be turned on, and become instantly operative.

Another reason for the more universal utility of the incandescent-light bath is the fact that when properly applied, its effects are highly tonic in character. A short application of the bath at full force for a time just sufficient to induce powerful stimulation of the skin without provoking perspiration is a most effective means of cutaneous stimulation. The tonic effects of such an application may be still further intensified by instantly following the bath with a cold spray or other cold application, thus producing a revulsive effect of the most agreeable and effective character. The excessive heating of the skin prepares the way for the cold application, without at the same time so overheating and relaxing the blood-vessels as to render recovery of the tone of the cutaneous tissues so tardy as to involve the risk of exhausting the patient too greatly or exposing him to the liability of taking cold. In the experiments referred to, the amount of perspiration produced in the electric-light bath was found to be double that produced in the Turkish bath. The body temperature is also raised much more rapidly in the electric-light bath than in any other form of bath, because the rays of radiant energy pass through the skin and reach the interior of the body at once.

The electric-light bath is especially valuable in *cardiac disease* and in *diabetes*, in which prolonged sweating measures can not usually be employed without more or less risk. The penetrating nature of the heat of the electric-light bath stimulates oxidation of the residual tissues, and thus hastens the disappearance of redundant fat in *obesity*. In *dropsy*, associated with either cardiac or Bright's disease, in the *toxemia* of *chronic dyspepsia*, and in all conditions for which general and local applications of heat are applicable, the electric-light bath stands pre-eminent.

Chronic malarial cachexia, *syphilis*, *diabetes*, *obesity*, *neuritis*, *neuralgia*, *acute nephritis*, *migraine*, *neurasthenia*, *tetany*, *habit chorea*, and *hysteria* yield good results to the thermic impressions of the electric ray.

In *rheumatic* and *anemic* patients, and in all cases when the heat-making capacity is small, the electric-light bath serves an exceedingly useful purpose in preparing the skin for cold applications by storing up in it supplies of heat. And it serves a useful purpose in this way, not only in preparing the patient for tonic applications of water, but as a means of producing most excellent revulsive effects. For pure revulsive effects, only the circulatory reaction is desired, it being, in fact, necessary to suppress thermic reaction altogether. Hence the duration of cold applications which follow hot applications should be such as exactly to neutralize the heat

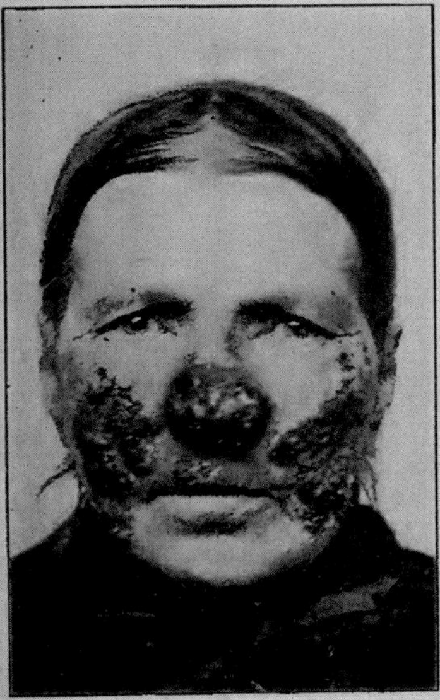

Fig. 144. A Case of Lupus before Treatment (p. 721). (Finsen)

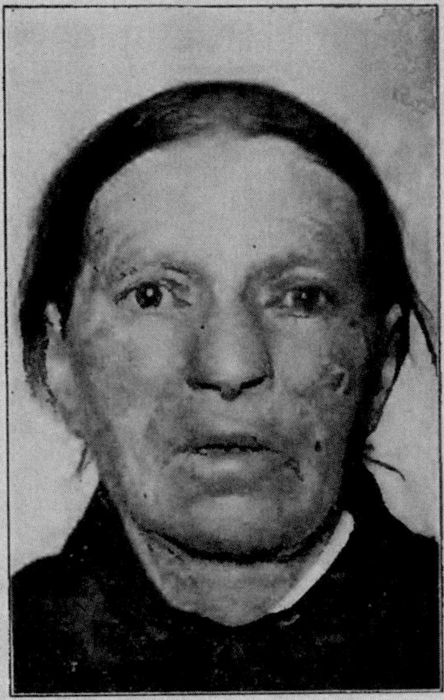

Fig. 145. A Case of Lupus after Treatment (p. 721). (Finsen)

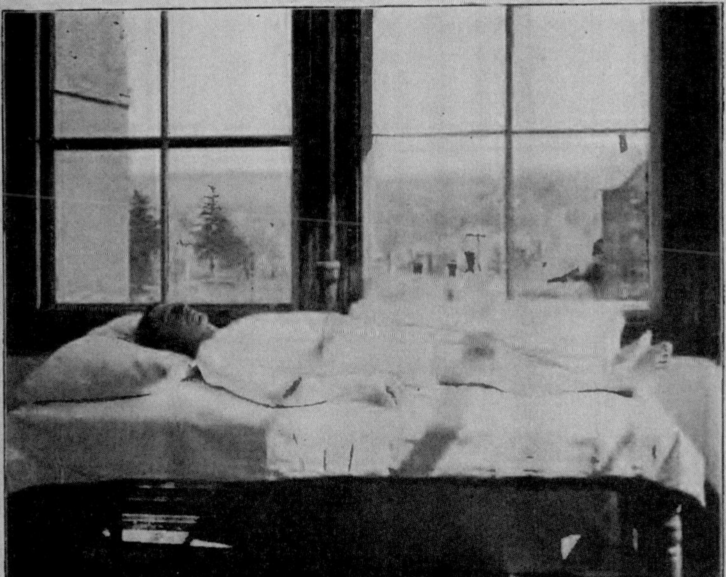

Fig. 146. SUN BATH (p. 722).

which has been absorbed by the skin in the previous hot application. The electric-light bath having the power to store up quickly a large amount of heat in the skin, it is consequently of special service in applications of this kind, which are the most effective means of relieving internal congestion, as well as the most powerful of all external agents for the relief of pain.

The electric-light bath is superior to all others in the treatment of *chronic rheumatism* and all maladies dependent upon the *uric acid diathesis*, owing to its ability to elevate body temperature while at the same time producing vigorous cutaneous activity. The elevated temperature stimulates the oxidation of proteid wastes, and augments vital combustion, while the increased skin activity carries off the waste products prepared for elimination.

Recent physiological experiments have shown that the elevated temperature in febrile conditions is one of the methods by which nature combats the causes of disease, or neutralizes some of the morbid conditions resulting from disease. The physiological effects of the electric-light bath may exercise in many cases a strongly curative influence by the elevation of the body temperature, thereby enabling it to produce antitoxins, or to render effective the curative efforts instituted by the *vis medicatrix naturæ* of the body.

As a *prophylactic*, this bath also possesses a high value, especially for persons who live a sedentary life, as teachers, doctors, lawyers, preachers, judges, and professional men generally, and to a still greater degree for the majority of women, as it is the best substitute for muscular activity in the open air.

The hygienic value of the sweating bath is certainly scarcely yet appreciated by the majority of civilized men and women. This can not be said of the Finns, however; for in Finland every house has connected with it a bath-house with conveniences for producing vigorous perspiration. Indeed, the author, while on a recent visit to Copenhagen, was told by an intelligent Finnish gentleman that it is the custom in his country for a young man anticipating matrimony to build as a foundation for his future home, first of all, a sweat-house. A vast multitude of city dwellers in civilized countries are suffering tortures from disease in various forms, and dying prematurely, because of the neglect of that important hygienic provision in the injunction of the Almighty to Adam, "By the sweat of thy brow shalt thou eat thy bread." Indeed, the neglect to sweat is one of the most prolific causes of disease in the conditions of civilized life. A modern writer has very sagaciously suggested that the chief difference between the savage and the civilized man is in the way he sweats. The savage sweats his brow in earning his bread, and taxes his brain but little; the civilized man earns his bread by the sweat of his brain, but seldom sweats his brow.

The electric-light bath, while not a complete substitute for the sweating produced by exercise, certainly comes nearer to being so than any other heating process; and when followed by some vigorous cold application, as the cold bath, possesses a hygienic value which can not be overestimated.

A local application of the electric light for 15 or 20 minutes, followed by an application of an ice compress or ice friction for 5 to 8 seconds, is almost a panacea for the pain of *sciatica* and for similar painful affections in which there is no inflammatory action.

The electric-light bath has been found superior to all other means for applying heat to circumscribed areas of the surface; and by the use of a number of simple appliances it is far more convenient in its application than the fomentation, hot bags, or any similar appliance (Figs. 135–138).

M. Below, who has for some time employed the electric-light bath constructed after the author's plan, reported in a paper read before the medical society of Berlin in 1898, a considerable number of cases in which the bath had been successfully used in the treatment of rheumatism, syphilis, and various other morbid conditions.

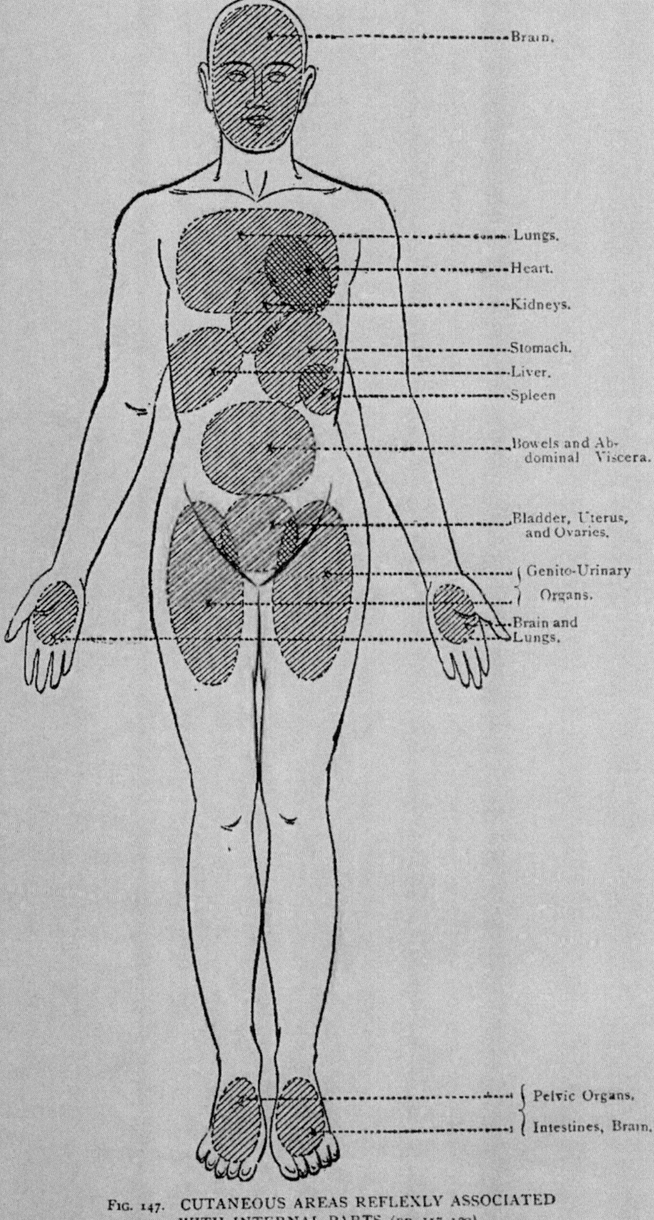

FIG. 147. CUTANEOUS AREAS REFLEXLY ASSOCIATED WITH INTERNAL PARTS (pp. 117-120).

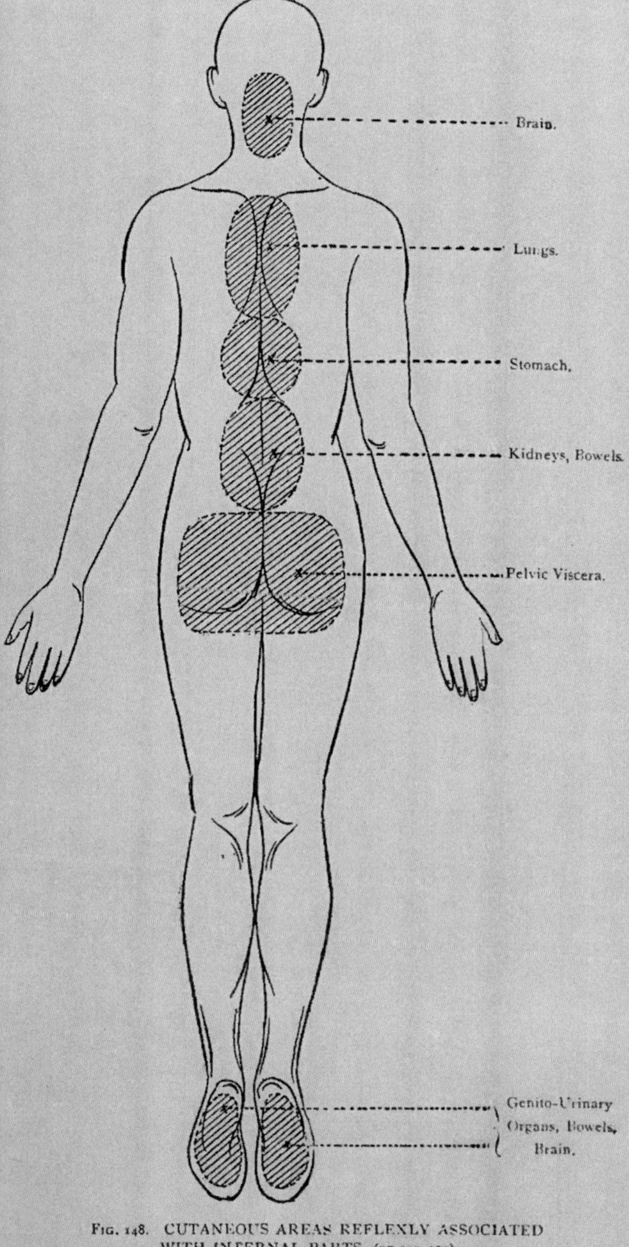

Fig. 148. CUTANEOUS AREAS REFLEXLY ASSOCIATED WITH INTERNAL PARTS (pp.117-120).

That the *electric arc light* acts powerfully upon the nervous system has been clearly proved by the experiments of Maklakow, Arloing, Paul Bert, and others. As yet, it is true, we are not fully acquainted with the exact measure of this influence; neither do we know precisely to what extent it may be utilized therapeutically; but knowing the fact, and having at hand the appliances necessary for exact observation, we are on the road to therapeutic discoveries which may prove to be not only interesting but of immense advantage to the human race.

That it is a true nerve tonic can not be doubted. It is daily in use in the treatment-rooms of the Battle Creek Sanitarium, and in the great hydriatic institution of Dr. Winternitz, at Kaltenleutgeben, near Vienna, and produces most excellent results, especially in the treatment of neurasthenics suffering from chronic toxemia.

Finsen, of Copenhagen, has shown that the actinic ray of the electric arc is capable of destroying the bacillus of tuberculosis in the skin under suitable conditions, and has utilized it in the successful treatment of hundreds of cases of lupus. On the occasion of a visit to the "Light Institute" at Copenhagen, an institution under the supervision of Professor Finsen, the author saw demonstrated most clearly the powerful therapeutic value of the actinic ray of the electric arc in the treatment of this disease (Figs. 141, 142, 143). There were numerous cases nearly cured, photographs of which, taken when they entered the institution, showed that the disease had already attained an advanced stage, while the history showed that these cases had proved wholly intractable to other methods of treatment. This is well shown by the accompanying illustrations (Figs. 144, 145). At the time of the author's visit, there were one hundred and twenty-five persons under treatment in the institute. A large number of these were personally seen, and the progress which had been made under the treatment was remarkable. The author is awaiting the opportunity to make a trial of this same method in the treatment of leprosy, believing that it may be found of value in dealing with this most obstinate malady, at least in the tubercular form of the disease.

THE SUN BATH, OR INSOLATION (Fig. 146).

1254 Sunlight is one of the most powerful of all hygienic and curative agents. As a hygienic measure it is of inestimable value in the destruction of dangerous microbes, the most of which are unable to resist the action of the direct rays of the sun for more than a few minutes. Sunlight is thus the most important of all disinfecting and sterilizing agencies. The value of sunlight in the maintenance of health is well shown in the dwarfed development or rapid deterioration of plants deprived of its stimulating influence. In caves, mines, and other places from which the light is excluded, plants, with the exception of the fungi, do not grow, or if they do, very quickly die, never attaining maturity. Animals also are dwarfed and sickly under these conditions.

It was long ago noticed that in hospitals a larger percentage of recoveries occurred on the sunny side than on the shady side of the ward. At least a part of the well-known good effects obtainable from an outdoor life or from systematic exercise out of doors must be attributed directly to the influence of the sun's rays.

In taking a sun bath, either the whole or a part of the body may be exposed to the direct influence of the solar rays, or some protection may be afforded by a covering of white cheese-cloth. The bath may be best taken in a room properly constructed for the purpose. The room should face the south (in the Northern hemisphere), and the windows should be sloping. The patient should lie on a cot placed before a window, the head being protected from the direct rays of the sun. The length of the exposure will depend upon the intensity of the sun's rays and the effects sought. If the light is very intense, or the patient very feeble, the duration of the bath should not be more than five minutes, if the whole body is exposed; while in less sensitive patients, or those accustomed to the sun bath, it may be continued from twenty minutes to half or three quarters of an hour.

Physiological Effects.—The sun's rays not only influence the skin, but pass through the skin into the body, exciting and stimulating every cell and tissue. The surface circulation is greatly accelerated, free perspiration occurs, the heart's action is increased, and the activity of all the vital functions is promoted. In many cases the patient experiences very pronounced sensations of languor or drowsiness during the bath, and not infrequently falls asleep. The effects of the sun bath are practically identical with those of the electric-light bath, which has been previously described.

The investigations of Finsen, of Copenhagen, Bert, and Maklakow, referred to elsewhere (597 to 599), have greatly broadened our knowledge regarding the physiological effects and therapeutic properties of light. Sunlight may be properly regarded as not only a source of radiant energy in the form of heat, but as a powerful tonic through its actinic rays. Its calorific, or heating, rays may be isolated by placing a red-glass screen between the sun and the patient, so that the actinic rays are filtered out. For tonic effects, the calorific rays may be separated by employing a blue-glass screen in like manner.

Therapeutic Applications.—The sun bath is useful in all 1255
cases of *mal-nutrition*, *anemia*, *inactivity* of the *skin*, *chronic dyspepsia*, most cases of *neurasthenia*, *indigestion*, *chlorosis*, *rheumatism*, *diabetes*, and *obesity*. The only class of cases in which the bath is positively contraindicated is that in which the patient has recently suffered from heat stroke, and is especially susceptible to the action of the direct rays of the sun.

The ancients made great use of the sun bath in the treatment of the sick. According to Plutarch, Diogenes, the renowned Athenian cynic, was in his old age accustomed to lie in the sunshine for the purpose of recruiting his energies, a custom which, according to Pliny, was common among old men in Greece. It is stated that Diogenes valued his sun bath so highly that when called upon by Alexander, who offered to render him any service in his power, he replied, "Only stand a little out of my sunshine."

According to Pliny, the sun bath was also in very common use among the Romans. Both the older and the younger Pliny were accustomed to spend an hour in exposure to the sun daily after dinner. Hippocrates prescribed the sun bath for chills. A noted French physician once said to some people who had brought their children to him for treatment: "Take these children to the country; feed them as well as you can; but above all, roast them — roast them in the sun."

Suggestions and Precautions.— It must be remembered that some people are so susceptible to the sun's rays that untoward effects resembling, or identical with, heat stroke, are very readily produced. On this account it is well to keep the patient under careful supervision during the bath, especially the first applications. If the sun's rays are very intense, a sheet should be thrown over the patient at the first application, to avoid the possibility of extreme effects. In all cases, the exposure of the head must be avoided. The actinic rays powerfully influence the brain. The author observed, as a common custom in Egypt, the protection of the head by a huge red shawl wound about it.

LOCAL OR PARTIAL HYDRIATIC MEASURES.

1256 A very great variety of local or partial hydriatic applications are in use, each experienced practitioner of hydrotherapy employing some measures which he has especially devised or modified to meet his own views or convenience, or in the adaptation of his resources to his needs. Thus, in the description of local or localized measures, the author will not attempt even to mention all possible applications, but only the leading and typical forms and their principal modifications. Several new measures, the outgrowth of the authors' personal experience, are presented, but only such as have borne the test of actual use and have proved their efficiency.

In a strict sense, all hydriatic applications are local or partial in character, since the most general measures, as a rain douche, an immersion or a vapor bath, act directly only upon the skin, thus immediately influencing only a small portion of the blood-vessels and nerves of the body. As fully shown elsewhere, however, an application to the entire cutaneous surface, though partial in an anatomical sense, becomes general through reflex action and reaction.

These general applications are often of service for securing purely local effects, as in the use of the hot bath in acute nephritis, which relieves the renal congestion by congesting the skin; the neutral bath to quiet the central nervous system; the wet-sheet rub to relieve cerebral congestion.

On the other hand, local or partial applications, while generally employed for purely local or localized effects, either at the seat of application or at some remote part by revulsive or derivative influence, likewise produce in many instances more or less decided general effects, as may be noted in the tonic influence of the running cold foot bath, the general sedative effects of prolonged cold applications to the head, the restorative and energizing effects of a cold douche to the spine, the excitant effects of very hot or very cold applications to almost any portion of the surface, even though the area be very limited.

The localized effects of partial applications depend upon a few well-established principles. These have been elsewhere briefly stated, but may be here recapitulated and extended :—

1. **Reflex Relations.**— Every portion of the cutaneous sur- 1257
face is in special reflex relation with some internal organ or vascular area. The most important of these reflex relationships are the following (Figs. 147, 148):—

(1) The skin of the scalp, face, and back of the neck is in reflex relation with the brain. The circulation of the scalp is also immediately connected with the brain through

the medium of the skull, the vessels of which anastomose with those of the scalp and those of the brain.

(2) The skin of the back is reflexly related to the centers of the spinal cord. This is also true of the entire skin surface of the trunk and limbs.

(3) The skin covering the neck is reflexly, through the spinal cord, related to the pharynx and the larynx.

(4) The upper dorsal region, the skin of the chest in front and behind, and the inner surface of the thighs, have special vasomotor reflex relation with the lungs.

(5) That portion of the chest wall overlying the heart (the precordia) is especially associated with the heart,— a fact often of priceless service.

(6) The skin covering the lower portion of the right chest is reflexly related to the liver.

(7) The skin surface of the lower left chest is associated with the spleen.

(8) The skin covering the lumbar region is reflexly associated with the uterus, ovaries, bladder, rectum, kidneys, and intestines.

(9) The skin covering the lower part of the sternum is especially associated with the kidneys.

(10) The dorsal spine is associated with the stomach, a fact which may often be made of great service in the suppression of nervous vomiting.

(11) The skin of the epigastrium has special relations with the stomach.

(12) The whole surface of the abdomen, and especially the umbilical region, is reflexly related to the intestines.

(13) The lower abdomen is associated with the uterus, bladder, colon, and rectum.

(14) The feet, and to a considerable extent the whole lower extremities, are associated with the brain, lungs, bladder, uterus, ovaries, and bowels.

(15) The skin covering the shoulders and upper portion of the back and the arms and hands is an area which is closely associated with both the cerebral and the pulmo-

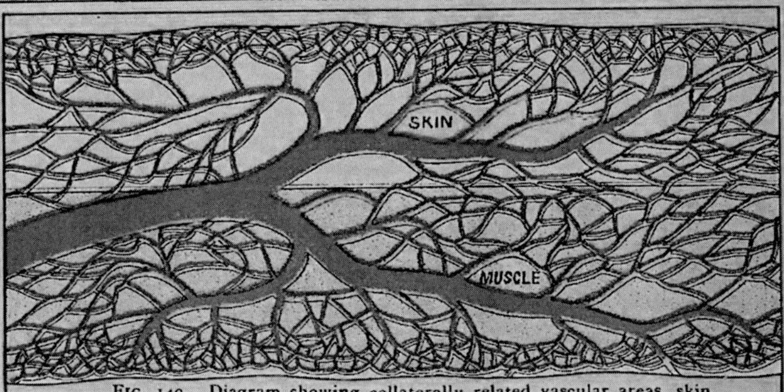

FIG. 149. Diagram showing collaterally related vascular areas, skin overlying muscle (p. 731).

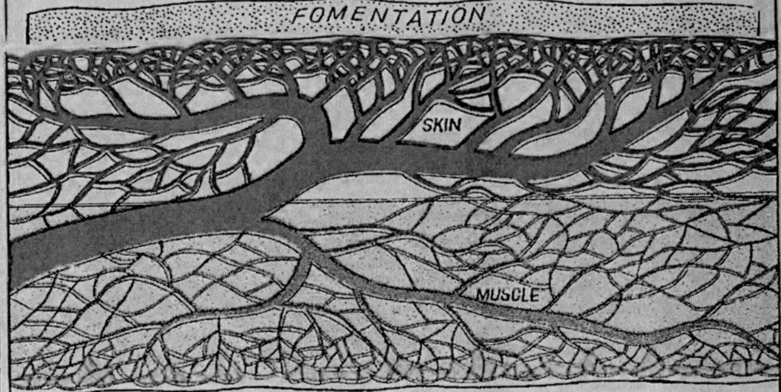

FIG. 150. Hyperemia of skin with collateral anemia of underlying muscle produced by a hot application (p. 731).

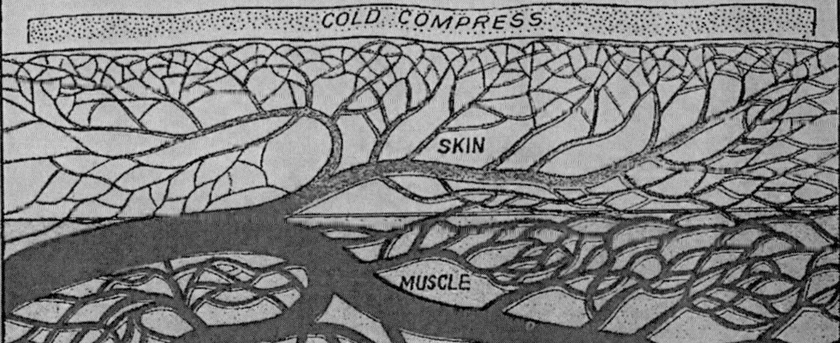

FIG. 151. Anemia of the skin with collateral hyperemia of the underlying muscle produced by a cold application (p. 731).

nary circulations, and may be employed in producing most useful therapeutic effects both by the reflex influence of cold applications and by the derivative effects induced by hot applications.

2. Internal Reaction.—The changes induced in internal 1258
parts by applications to the surface, especially by cold applications, may be not improperly termed *internal reaction.* (For full discussion of the phenomena of reaction, see paragraphs **429–481.**) These changes it is desirable sometimes to suppress or diminish, in other cases to encourage.

In general, it may be said that the more intense the external application, the more pronounced will be the internal reaction. The reaction of cold differs diametrically from the reaction following a hot application. The reaction following cold increases all kinds of vital work — heart and vessel work, brain and nerve work, gland work, respiratory work, tissue building, oxidation, poison destruction, poison elimination, heat production. Heat is followed by decrease of vital work.

It is often desirable to lessen the internal reaction to cold. This may be done in several ways, as follows: —

(1) By applying water of a *higher temperature*, thus lessening the external reaction.

(2) By means of the *Scotch douche* or other analogous measures. The greater the extremes of heat and cold, the greater the internal reaction. By raising the temperature of the cold application and lowering that of the hot application, thus lessening the difference between the two extremes, the intensity of the internal reaction may be diminished.

In the use of the alternate douche (**1044**), the greater the number of alternations, the greater the excitation induced.

Internal reaction may be diminished when alternate applications are employed, by *graduation* of the alternations,— increasing the difference between the extremes of heat and cold with each successive alternation, either by increasing the temperature of the hot application or lowering that of the cold application, or by changing both simultaneously.

(3) The *graduated bath*, either immersion or douche, lessens internal reaction and especially thermic reaction by the avoidance of an abrupt change of temperature. The zero of the temperature sense is gradually lowered by beginning the bath at a temperature near that of the body (98° to 100° F.), and gradually cooling to 90° during a period of from 30 to 60 seconds. The sensory impression made is thus greatly attenuated.

(4) By applying *before* the local application a general cold bath of some sort, the external and internal reactions may be generalized, and thus the local effect will be attenuated. The general application may be either a general douche or some form of nonpercutient application, as a wet-sheet pack (**1179**), a wet-sheet rub (**1216**), an affusion (**1103**), or general friction, either moist or dry.

(5) We may *precede* the local application by the general Scotch douche, the intensity of which may be graduated in any one of the several ways elsewhere pointed out (pp. 457, 459–461).

(6) We may *follow* the local application with a general douche or other cold application whereby general external and internal reaction may be produced.

1259 **3. Reflex Action.**—A cold application to the surface causes at first a brief contraction of the vessels in the internally related viscus as well as in the skin. This contraction is normally followed by reaction in both the skin and the internal parts. For the production of reflex effects the douche is the most powerful measure (**1070** to **1103**), but various other means may be employed, as the following:—

(1) Local cold affusion.

(2) Hot and cold affusion.

(3) Cold foot bath for 10 to 20 seconds, the water very cold and not more than one fourth of an inch deep.

(4) Alternate foot bath.

(5) Cold sponging.

(6) Cold compress.

(7) Ice rubbing.

(8) Fomentation followed by ice rubbing.

(9) Fomentation followed by an ice compress for a few seconds.

(10) Hot sponge bath followed by ice-water sponging.

(11) Vapor douche followed by cold affusion, ice rub, or ice compress.

The reflex effects resulting from localized hydriatic applications differ in both intensity and quality, according to the duration and temperature of the application.

4. **Fluxion.**—By the term *fluxion* is meant the movement 1260
of blood. There are four modifications of blood movement to be considered:—

(1) *Increasing the rate of movement* of blood through an organ.

(2) *Diminishing the rate of movement* of blood through a part.

(3) *Increasing the volume* of blood in a part containing too little blood (anemia).

(4) *Diminishing the volume* of blood in a part containing too much blood (congestion, or hyperemia).

In the preceding paragraphs the rationale of increased rate of blood movement resulting from reflex hydriatic applications (**1257**) has been explained, as has also the production of passive congestion for derivative effects (**1261**) It remains to consider more fully the rationale of the production of changes in the volume of blood by hydriatic means not acting reflexly.

When a cold application is made to the whole surface of the body, all the internal organs are thereby congested after the first momentary contraction of their vessels has passed away—by the mechanical displacement of blood from the skin inward, or *retrostasis*. During the first instant after the general cold application, while the internal vessels are contracted, the surplus blood, chased out of the systemic circulation, finds temporary refuge, so to speak, in the veins and the portal reservoir, from which, in the later moments, it is distributed among the internal organs. When the cold application is partial, however, this general retrostasis of blood does not occur except to a very limited extent, a very different readjustment of the blood distribution taking place. For example, if cold is applied to the lower part of the body, the blood-vessels, both external and internal, contract, and the blood is driven out of the lower extremities, pelvis, and lower abdomen. At the same time, the vessels of the head, chest, and arms are dilated, and the volume of blood in these parts is increased. The reverse is equally true. The umbilicus is the dividing line in this compensatory action. If cold is applied to one foot or hand, the effect is not, however, as might be supposed, to increase the volume of blood in the other hand or foot, but to decrease it, as shown by Brown-Sequard, through reflex action. A cold compress or a percussion douche over the spine does not produce general internal congestion to any marked degree, but causes contraction of the spinal vessels, which by reaction is followed by active congestion if the application is short and intense, and so produces a powerful tonic effect through exciting the spinal centers.

By means of hot applications, effects the opposite to those following cold are produced. The dilatation of the vessels of the legs following hot applications to these parts produces congestion of the vessels of the lower part of the body and anemia of the upper parts.

By the application of this principle, it is possible to combat either anemia or congestion of the brain, lungs, uterus, or other important vital parts. It should be said, however, that the principle is more often and more conveniently applicable to congestions and anemias of the upper parts of the body than to similar conditions of the lower parts, for the reason that intense congestion or anemia of the brain and lungs can not be induced with the same degree of safety with which we may congest the legs or lessen the blood supply of these parts.

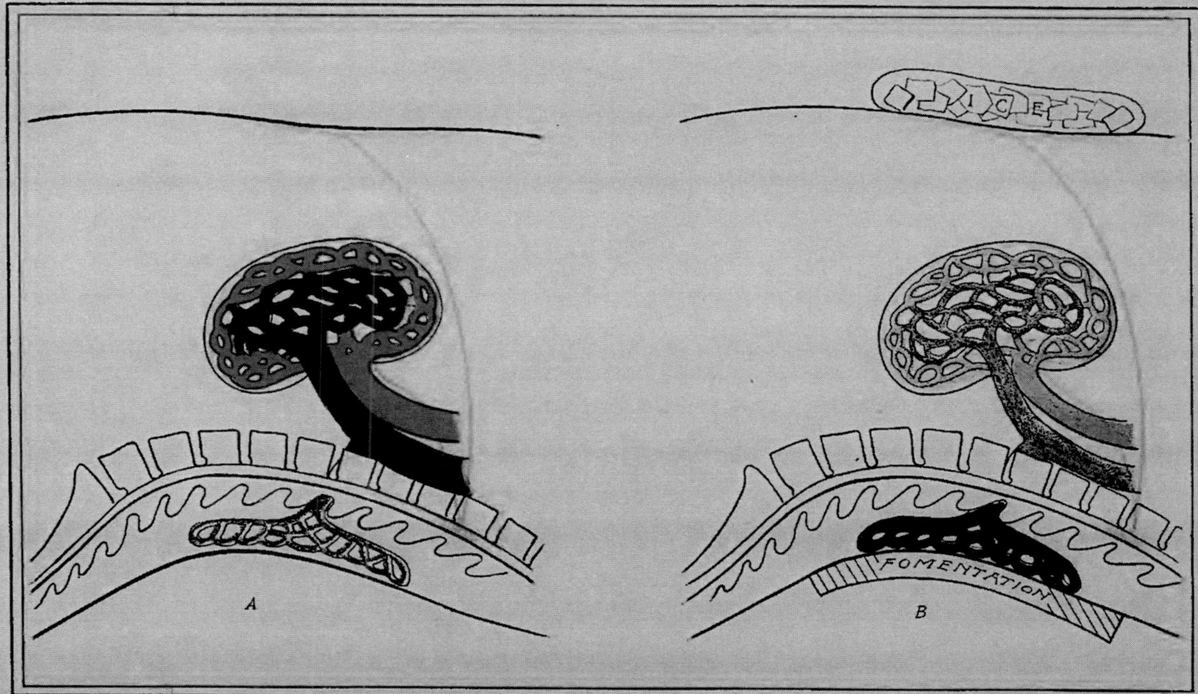

FIG 152. Co-operation of reflex and fluxion effects (*1361*). *A*. Renal congestion. *B*. Ice-bag to lower sternum with fomentation to loins — Congestion relieved (p. 732).

Collateral Anemia and Hyperemia.—Where all the parts 1261
concerned are supplied by a common arterial trunk, reciprocal changes in the volume of blood occur between the superficial and the deeper parts. This relation exists between any muscle, joint, or bone and the overlying cutaneous area. It also exists between the overlying skin and the following organs: The brain, the spinal cord, the eyes, the ears, the serous lining of the pleural and peritoneal cavities, the lungs, the kidneys, the uterus and ovaries in woman, the testicles and prostate in man. This relation between the skin and the uterus, ovaries, kidneys, bladder, and lungs is less intimate than between the muscles and joints; but clinical results as well as anatomical considerations indicate that such a relation really does exist, though more remote, and it is even possible to trace a very distinct and direct anatomical connection between the blood-vessels of the liver, stomach, intestines, spleen, and pancreas, and the contiguous superficial parts (**1270** to **1276**).

If, in illustration of this principle, we apply a cold compress over a fleshy part, as the front of the thigh, the result will be the production of pronounced anemia of the skin and a corresponding hyperemia of the underlying quadriceps extensor femoris muscle. If, on the other hand, a hot compress or fomentation be applied instead, the result will be the diversion of blood to the skin and the production of anemia of the muscle (Figs. 149, 150, 151).

It is by the application of this principle that we are able to combat inflammation, congestion, and pain in muscles and other deep parts which are directly connected with the skin through a common blood supply. By diverting blood into the skin by means of a fomentation or other hot application, the congested or inflamed muscle, nerve, or joint may be relieved.

In not a few instances, the collaterally related parts are not contiguous. The relation of the blood-vessels rather than the simple contiguity of the parts should be considered.

Many examples of this might be given. The cutaneous vessels of the arms are collaterally related with the brain circulation through the vertebral branches of the subclavian; with the lungs through the superior intercostals; the legs and hips with the head by diverting blood into the abdominal aorta and its branches; the legs with the pelvic viscera by diverting blood into the external branch of the iliac.

The most powerful effects possible are obtained by measures which combine the principle of induced hyperemia of collaterally related parts with that of reflex stimulation of the controlling vasomotor centers. Fortunately, the cutaneous areas which may be utilized for these respective purposes are often distinct, so that there is no anatomical obstacle in the way of their simultaneous employment. These relations are indicated in Figs. 152–155. Examples: The fomentation to the back of the chest with the cold compress to the front; a hot foot bath combined with a cold hypogastric compress.

Venous or passive hyperemia may likewise be induced as a means of draining collateral vascular areas. The means to be employed are the fomentation at a moderately high temperature (104° to 120°), and the protected heating compress applied without change until the desired effect has been obtained. Venous congestion is produced in connection with the arterial hyperemia resulting from a hot application. It may also be induced simultaneously with arterial hyperemia, by operating upon distinct areas (**1291**).

The portal system constitutes a most important arrangement for modifying the volume of blood in the systemic system. It is capable of holding all the blood in the body, and having no valves, there is easy fluxion in and out through the four gateways by which it communicates with the systemic veins (**1277**).

By means of induced collateral *arterial hyperemia* the arteries of a part are drained, the blood supply is lessened, and tension lowered. By induced *venous hyperemia* the veins of the part interested are drained, and the movement of blood through the part is accelerated by lessening resistance. An inflamed part does not need less blood, but less tension, and especially the rapid removal of toxins, CO_2, and disabled leucocytes, and an abundant and constant supply of fresh and pure serum, oxygen, and active leucocytes.

In active visceral congestion, as in the first stage of an inflammation, collateral arterial hyperemia is especially indicated. In passive congestion, collateral venous hyperemia is especially useful, but the best effects will be obtained by the simultaneous establishment of both conditions (**1291**).

Induced venous hyperemia may render most valuable service in many cases by association with cold compresses applied to another cutaneous area which is reflexly associated with the actively congested internal organ under consideration.

Cutaneous Areas which may be Utilized for Derivative 1262
Effects.—The anatomical arrangements whereby derivative effects in favor of various internal parts may be produced by hydriatic measures are scarcely less elaborate and interesting than those by which reflex effects upon both blood and nerve supply are secured. The following are only a few of the more important and clearly established collateral relationships whereby useful derivative effects in favor of important vital organs may be induced through the application of heat (**1286**) or combined heat and cold (**1290**), the skin surfaces named indicating the areas to which the application is to be made, and the blood-vessels the channels through which the fluxion takes place (heat produces hyperemia of the skin, and collateral anemia of the deep structures which are vascularly related thereto, while cold applications to the same surfaces induce anemia of the skin and hyperemia of the deep-lying parts) (Figs. 150, 151):—

The Brain.—The scalp, through the direct vascular connection between the cutaneous vessels and the vessels of the dura mater; the skin of the face, by diverting the blood into the cutaneous branches of the external carotid. This method is rarely practical, however, as the bones of the skull and face are so good conductors that the brain is quickly heated by a hot application, and thus the desired derivative effect is lost. The most practical method of lessening the blood supply of the brain is by means of alternate compresses or the reflex influence of cold applications. Hot applications must be brief.

Short hot applications to the back of the neck may divert blood from the cerebral branches of the vertebral arteries into the cervical, influencing especially the cerebellum.

Hot applications to the hands and arms may diminish cerebral congestion by diverting blood from the vertebral arteries, which are branches of the subclavian. If made very hot, favorable reflex effects will also be produced during the first moments of the application.

Warm applications about the neck, even warm wrappings, congest the brain by inducing dilatation of the carotid and vertebral arteries (cold produces the opposite effect [307]. Prolonged warm applications to the back of the neck congest the brain, as the vertebral arteries give off few cutaneous branches, so that their dilatation by prolonged warmth results in an increased supply of blood to the brain.

The direct connections between the venous sinuses of the brain and the cutaneous veins of the scalp afford opportunity for the relief of passive congestion of the brain by dilating the cutaneous veins, and thus enlarging the channels leading to the heart. The anatomical arrangements whereby the blood entering the cranium may be conveyed back to the heart through the cutaneous veins of the head are numerous and highly interesting. According to Woolsey,* the following relations exist:-

"(*a*) The *longitudinal sinus* communicates with the temporal veins through one or both parietal foramina when present, and, in the child, with the veins of the nose through the foramen cecum.

* "Text-book of Anatomy by American Authors." Gerrish.

"(*b*) The *lateral sinus* is connected with the occipital (or posterior auricular) vein through the mastoid foramen (the largest and most constant emissary), and sometimes with the vertebral vein through the posterior condylar foramen.

"(*c*) The *cavernous sinus* communicates with the pterygoid plexus through the foramen of Vesalius and the foramen ovale, as well as through the inferior ophthalmic vein; with the pharyngeal plexus through the foramen lacerum medium; and with the internal jugular vein by the carotid plexus through the carotid canal.

"(*d*) The *occipital sinus* communicates with the vertebral and extraspinal veins through the anterior condylar foramen.

"(*e*) A small vein occasionally passes to the *torcular* through a foramen in the occipital bone near the external occipital protuberance."

By hot or alternate hot and cold applications to the areas above indicated, any one of the principal sinuses of the brain may be drained into the veins of the adjacent skin. For example: —

1. To influence the *longitudinal sinus*, applications should be made to the parietal region, that is, the sides of the head.

2. The *lateral sinus* may be drained by applications to the back part of the head, especially the areas just behind the ears.

3. The *cavernous sinus* may be drained by applications over the ear, face, and side of the neck.

4. Blood may be diverted from the *occipital sinus* by applications to the back of the neck.

Applications made to the back of the neck influence especially the cerebellum, dilating the vertebral and the posterior jugular veins.

Applications to the side of the head and neck drain the brain through the internal jugular.

The Spine.—The skin of the back may be used to drain 1263

the spinal cord, through the dorsal branches of the aortic intercostals, which nourish the cord.

The dorsi-spinal veins, the superficial veins of the back, form a plexus which connects with the vertebral veins of the neck, with the intercostal in the dorsal region, the lumbar and sacral veins lower down. The dense plexuses formed by these veins in the skin and especially about the spinous processes, form a capacious reservoir into which the blood may be diverted from the venous plexuses which occupy the spinal canal (meningo-rachidian) with which they are connected by anastomosing branches passing through the intervertebral foramina and joining the vertebral, intercostal, lumbar, and sacral veins.

The veins of the spinal cord itself join the vertebral veins at the base of the skull. Applications intended to influence the blood supply of the vertebræ or structures connected with them should be applied the whole length of the spinal column. Applications directed toward the envelopes of the spinal cord should extend from the base of the brain to about the middle of the lumbar region. Applications intended to influence the spinal cord itself may cover the entire spinal area, but care must be taken to give particular attention to the extreme upper portion, including the lower and back part of the scalp.

1264 *The Eyeball.*—The skin of the eyelids and forehead drain the eyeball, by dilating the supra-orbital branch of the ophthalmic, a branch of the internal carotid.

1265 *The Middle Ear.*—The whole side of the head and face, diverting blood from the internal carotid and internal maxillary. If the hot compress extends below the jaw, the common carotid will be dilated. An ice-bag below the jaw with the fomentation increases its effect by contracting the carotid.

1266 *The Internal Ear.*—Receiving its blood supply from the vertebral artery, a branch of the subclavian, the internal ear is not influenced by heat over the ear, but may be relieved when congested by warm applications to the arms and cold

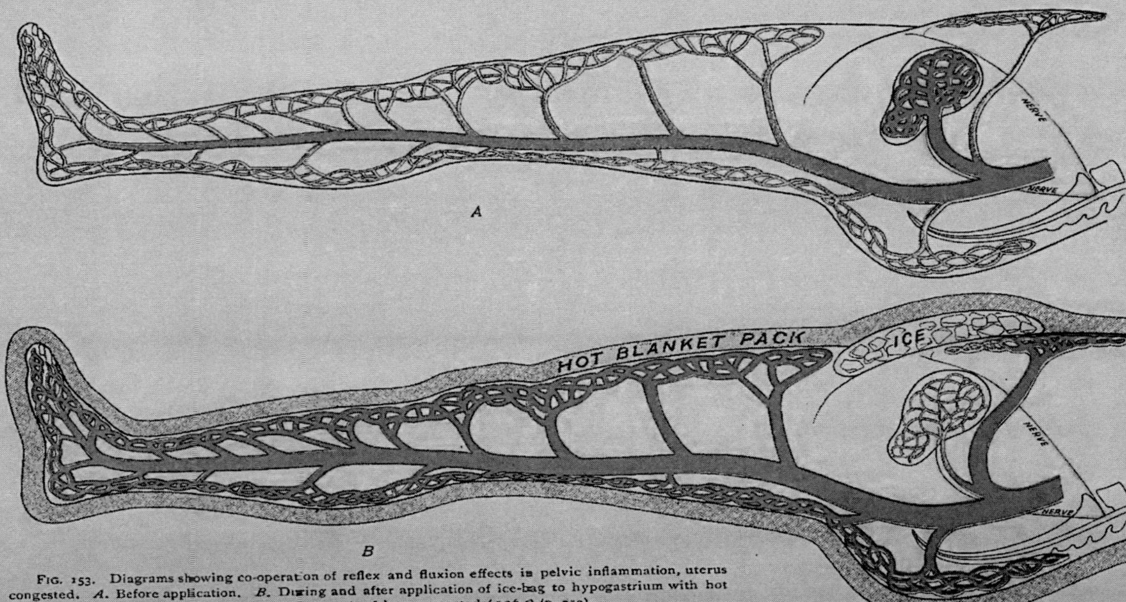

FIG. 153. Diagrams showing co-operation of reflex and fluxion effects in pelvic inflammation, uterus congested. *A.* Before application. *B.* During and after application of ice-bag to hypogastrium with hot hip and leg pack, uterine vessels contracted, vessels of legs congested (*1364*) (p. 752).

applications to the head and the back of the neck, thus diverting the blood into the arms from the vertebral arteries while at the same time contracting the vertebral arteries by a proximal cold compress or an ice-bag to the back of the neck.

The Nasal Cavity.— The face and sides of the head, 1267
diverting the blood from the internal carotid and the internal maxillary.

The Pharynx.— The whole face, diverting blood from the 1268
internal maxillary and the ascending pharyngeal.

The Larynx.— The skin of the neck overlying the larynx, 1269
and the arms, diverting the blood from the internal branches of the carotid and the subclavian into their external branches (the superior and inferior thyroids). The arms and back, and the sides of the upper chest may also be utilized. Chilling of the arms and shoulders should be avoided.

The Lungs.— The aim is to influence the bronchial arter- 1270
ies, the nutrient vessels of the lungs. The collaterally related cutaneous surfaces are: —

1. The anterior chest wall from the clavicle to the umbilicus, influencing especially the pleura (also the pericardium) through the cutaneous branches of the internal mammary.

2. The pleura of the posterior chest wall, through the cutaneous branches of the aortic intercostals.

3. The arms, through the diversion of blood from the superior intercostal, a branch of the subclavian, influencing especially the pleura of the upper part of the chest. Induced hyperemia of the arms also relieves congestion of the pleura of the anterior wall of the chest by diverting blood from the internal mammary, a branch of the subclavian.

4. A direct relation exists between the bronchial arteries and the skin of the right chest, through the fact that the right bronchial arteries arise from the aortic intercostals. The relation between the left bronchial arteries and the skin circulation is less direct; hence the importance of making applications to the whole chest in the hydriatic treatment of pneumonia, though one lung only may be affected. It is

especially important that the application should be made to the back of the chest.

It is interesting to recall the fact of the connection of the bronchial arteries with the pulmonary capillary plexus and veins, whereby arterial blood passing through the lungs may return at once to the left heart without entering the systemic venous system, and without visiting the right side of the heart, forming thus a sort of second pulmonary circuit, very small, but possibly very useful in many conditions for carrying on oxygenation of the blood independently of the pulmonary circulation proper.

5. Through the free anastomosis of the tracheal branches of the inferior thyroid and the bronchial arteries, the nutrient vessels of the lungs may be influenced by applications made to the front part of the neck. Cold applications made to this region will tend strongly to concentrate the blood in the lungs. By warm or alternate warm and cold applications the blood may be diverted from the lungs by facilitating the movement of blood through the collateral circulations, and passive congestion may be relieved.

6. The veins which return the blood from the nutritive arteries (bronchial) of the lungs empty on the right side into the azygos vein; on the left side either into the superior intercostal or the azygos vein. The intercostal veins are thus on both sides so connected with the bronchial veins that when dilated by hot or alternate applications the blood stream through the lungs may be accelerated, thus relieving passive congestion, a condition which constantly exists in pneumonia after the first stage, and in cardiac disease accompanied by dyspnea due to deficient compensation. Applications to be efficacious for this purpose must cover the whole thoracic cage, and especially the back and sides, as the intercostal vessels with which the bronchial arteries are associated are chiefly distributed to these portions of the chest. An appreciation of these anatomical relations is sufficient to impress the necessity for maintaining active circulation of the skin in pneu-

monia, and allowing opportunity for complete reaction to take place at short intervals when cold applications are made. If continuous cold applications are made to the front of the chest, care must be taken to maintain warmth, and to prevent collateral pulmonary congestion by applying heat behind.

The Kidneys.—The loins, through the renal branches of 1271
the lumbar arteries.

The Bladder, the Uterus and Adnexa, and the Prostate. 1272
—The sacrum, buttocks, perineum, external genitals, inner surface of thighs, groins, suprapubic region, through the sacral, gluteal, obturator, sciatic, inferior hemorrhoidal, superficial perineal, deep circumflex iliac, and deep epigastric arteries, derived from the internal iliac.

The Rectum.—The anal region and the perineum, through 1273
the inferior hemorrhoidal, superficial perineal, and other branches of the internal pudic.

The Stomach.—The arterial circulation of the stomach 1274
may be influenced through the free anastomosis of the gastric artery with the esophageal arteries, which in turn anastomose with the inferior thyroid, a branch of the subclavian. An arterial connection also exists between the vessels of the stomach and of the internal mammary, through the phrenic artery. The venous circulation of the stomach is connected with the skin through anastomosis of the gastric with the esophageal veins, which empty into the right azygos vein. The last-named vein also receives the intercostal veins, especially those draining the skin covering the sides and back of the chest. Applications intended to influence the arterial circulation of the stomach should be of such size as to cover the lower third of the sternum, the cartilages of the lower ribs, and the space between these structures and the umbilicus. When it is desired to influence the venous circulation, as in chronic gastritis, cardiac insufficiency, and hepatic cirrhosis, the applications are made to the back and sides of the chest.

The Liver and Spleen.—The arterial circulation of the 1275 liver and spleen may be influenced by the same measures described in relation to the stomach. The vessels of these organs are connected with the cutaneous circulation through the anastomosis of the phrenic arteries (right and left) with the internal mammary and the intercostals. Passive congestion of these organs is seldom of serious importance except when arising from disturbance of the portal circulation. Applications to relieve general portal congestion (1277) will relieve hepatic and splenic congestion, since such causes as tend to concentrate the blood in the portal circulation will influence in like manner the liver and spleen, together with the other abdominal viscera.

1276 *The Intestines.*—The intestines, especially the duodenum and the colon, have no vascular connection with the surface except through the renal circulation. Hot applications to the lumbar region by lowering the pressure in the lumbar veins may divert a portion of the blood from the left renal vein with which the veins from the duodenum and the transverse colon communicate. Similar applications over the front and lower portions of the chest exercise a like influence through the connection of the phrenic veins with the left renal vein on the one hand and the internal mammary on the other. Alternate applications may relieve the venous circulation of the duodenum and the colon through diversion of blood from the renal vein into the veins which accompany the branches of the renal artery distributed to the suprarenal capsule, the capsule of the kidney, and the overlying muscles.

1277 *The Portal Circulation.*—The portal veins contain no valves. This makes it possible for this appendage of the venous system to render the most valuable service as a blood reservoir, the capacity of which may be very easily and quickly varied, thus constituting a regulating or balancing mechanism whereby the delicate structures of the body are saved from injuries which they might otherwise suffer from sudden or excessive increase or diminution of the blood pressure. There is maintained a constant balance between the

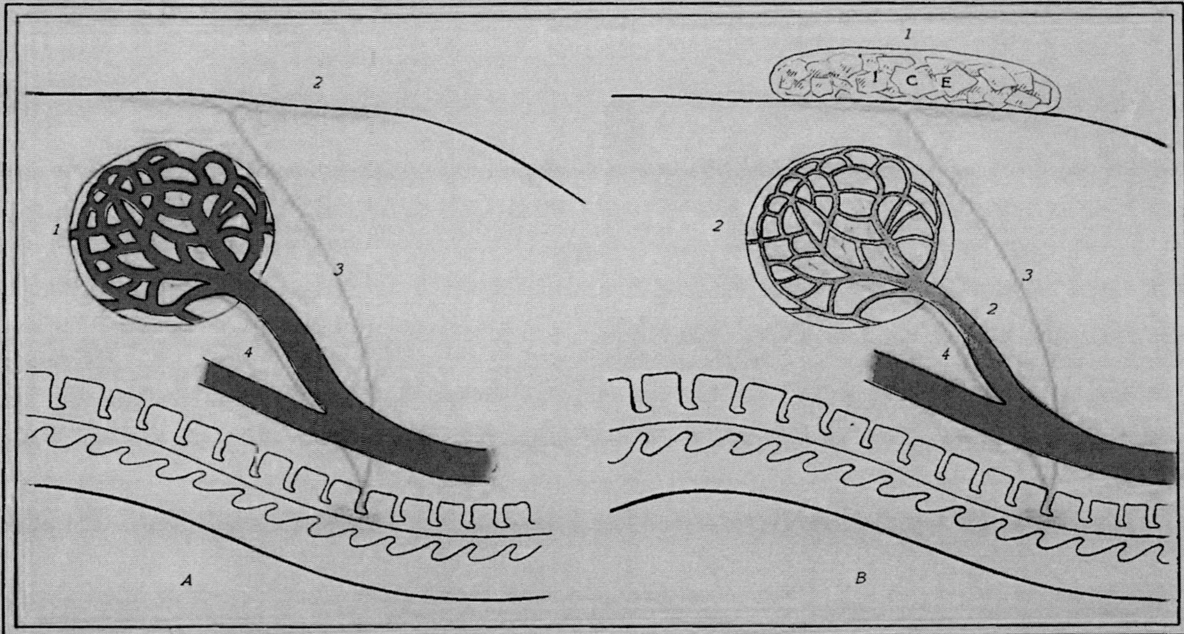

FIG. 154 *A*. Diagrammatic illustration of gastric congestion. 1. Arteries greatly dilated. 2. Cutaneous area reflexly related with the stomach. 3. Nerve trunk connecting this area with the spinal center connected with the stomach. 4. Sympathetic and vasomotor nerves which transmit to the stomach the sensory impulses received from the skin (p. 732).

FIG. 154 *B*. Diagrammatic illustration of the effect of cold applied to the cutaneous area reflexly connected with the stomach in case of gastric congestion or inflammation (*1319*). 1. Ice-bag. 2. Arteries contracted under the reflex influence of the cold application. 3. Nerve trunks by which the thermic impression made by the ice-bag is transmitted to the spine. 4. Vasomotor and sympathetic nerves which convey the impression to the gastric vessels securing their contraction and relieving congestion (p. 732).

intra-abdominal pressure and the general blood pressure. Even the volume of gases in the intestines and the tension of the abdominal muscles influence the blood pressure. The great splanchnic nerve is, through its control of the portal circulation, one of the most important factors in the blood-pressure-controlling mechanism of the body; it especially influences the cerebral circulation.

The study of the relations of the portal system to the 1278
general venous system and to the blood distribution of the skin, is exceedingly interesting, and of high practical value. The blood gathered up by the portal vein from the stomach, intestines, spleen, pancreas, and gall-bladder, in the main finds its way back into the general venous system only after it has passed through a second capillary network in the liver, from which it is gathered up, and conveyed to the ascending vena cava by the hepatic veins. There are, however, other channels well known to anatomists, of great practical value to the hydriatic practitioner. These are, as pointed out by Todd and Bowman * many years ago, as follows :—

1. The *hemorrhoidal plexus*, which communicates with the mesenteric veins on the one hand and the internal iliac on the other, thus furnishing an outlet for the blood of the portal circulation at its most dependent part,—an important safeguard against the development of diseased conditions of the hemorrhoidal veins.

2. *The esophageal veins*, which connect the gastric veins and the vena azygos minor.

3. A direct connection between the *left renal vein* and the veins of the duodenum and the colon.

4. A direct connection between the *phrenic vein* and the portal system at the surface of the liver (Kiernan).

According to Treves, the eminent English anatomist, the visceral vessels which anastomose with the parietal or cutaneous and muscular vessels are derived from the hepatic, renal, and suprarenal arteries, and also the vessels supplying the pancreas, cæcum, ascending and descending colon, and the duodenum. The connecting superficial vessels are derived

* "Physiological Anatomy," 1859.

from the phrenic, lumbar, ilio-lumbar, lower intercostal, epigastric, and circumflex iliac trunks. Schiff also has demonstrated an anastomosis between the portal veins and the epigastric veins at the umbilicus.

"In a case detailed by Professor Chiene (Journ. Anat. Phys., vol. 3) the cœliac axis and mesenteric vessels were plugged, but blood in sufficient amount to supply the viscera had reached the branches of these arteries through their parietal communications. The anastomosis gives an anatomical demonstration of the value of local blood-lettings and of counter-irritants in inflammatory affections of certain of the viscera, and also a scientific basis to the ancient practice of poulticing the loin and the iliac region in nephritis and in inflammation about the cæcum." (Surgical Applied Anatomy, Page 371.)

These interesting anatomical relations, when understood by the hydriatic physician, place at his disposal most powerful means of influencing the portal circulation. By warm or hot applications to the rectum the veins composing the hemorrhoidal plexus may be dilated, thus relieving any abnormal pressure in the portal circulation. By hot applications (5 to 15 min.) to the anal region, a hot pelvic pack or a hot sitz bath, followed by a short cold application (30 to 60 secs.), strong fluxion of the portal circulation may be produced, and passive congestion may be thus relieved.

Chronic portal congestion is best combated by the prolonged cool sitz (**1508**) and the wet girdle (**1347**). The temperature of the sitz should be 80° to 70°, the duration 15 to 30 minutes. The girdle should be protected by flannel only, and should be renewed every four hours, or just before it becomes dry, so that a tonic effect may be constantly maintained. These prolonged cold applications cause contraction of the external and internal branches of the iliac arteries, thus lessening the supply of blood to the iliac veins, and so lowering the pressure on the systemic side of the hemorrhoidal plexus, and increasing the outflow of blood from the portal veins. It is thus that the cool sitz affords relief in hemorrhoids, in catarrh of the rectum and colon, and in dysentery and diarrhea.

Cold applications either to the rectum itself or to the skin will temporarily produce the opposite effect; namely, interference with the movement of blood from the portal circulation into the systemic veins through the hemorrhoidal plexus. But if the application is short in duration, the reaction following may produce a result similar to that produced by warm or hot applications.

The effect of a prolonged hot application to the abdominal surface is quite different from that of a short application. The tone of the mesenteric vessels is constantly governed and modified by the reflexes sent in from the skin covering the abdomen. Cold causes contraction of the muscles of the intestinal walls as well as of the arteries, veins, and lymphatics, and even of the abdominal muscles; while heat produces the opposite effect. It is for this reason that we apply heat in colic and cold in tympanitis, acute inflammation, and hyperpepsia or hyperchlorhydria. A short hot application momentarily dilates the mesenteric vessels, but when it is removed, the subsequent cooling of the skin restores the normal tone. Thus passive portal congestion is relieved by short hot applications (5 to 10 min.), followed by cold (1 or 2 min.), through the energetic fluxion induced. For marked therapeutic effects the application must be renewed at intervals of two or three hours. The compresses may be alternated several times in succession at each application. When the application is prolonged, the mesenteric vessels lose their tone, and fill up with blood from the systemic circulation. It is thus that the prolonged (20 to 60 min.) warm sitz or the continuous heating abdominal compress or the wet girdle produces not only hyperemia of the skin, but also filling of the portal vessels. When this effect is desired, the compress or girdle must be protected by an impervious covering so as to secure the maximum amount of heating effect. When flannel alone is employed, the wet compress gradually dries by evaporation, through which means a cooling effect is produced just sufficient to maintain the tone of the mesenteric vessels, thus producing intense hyperemia of the skin with accelerated movement of blood, but without overfilling the portal veins.

The means by which the portal circulation may be influenced through the communicating vessels, have already been described. The hot trunk pack (15 to 20 min.), the sweating pack, the hot abdominal compress, the wet girdle covered with flannel only, the short hot sitz, and the Scotch douche to the spine and abdomen are the most effective means of draining the portal circulation through the cutaneous veins. A short cold application should always follow the hot application, to restore the tone of the visceral vessels.

1280 *The Upper Half of the Body.*— Induced hyperemia of the legs diverts blood from the brain, chest, and pelvis, and by induced hyperemia of the arms, shoulders, and chest, congestion of the pelvic viscera may be lessened.

The Rationale of Localized Measures.— In the following paragraphs (**1260** to **1291**) the practical application of the foregoing principles is illustrated by means of the compress.

1281 (1) Internal reaction, with dilatation of visceral vessels, occurs almost instantly after a *short cold* application, for the reason that the cause of the reflex vascular spasm (the cold application) being removed, the heat of the surrounding tissues (100° to 106°) quickly relaxes the parts. The rhythmical activity of the vessels of the part and the amplitude of their contractions are increased through the stimulation of the controlling ganglia. As a result, the supply of blood is increased, and with this arrive fresh and enlarged supplies of oxygen, leucocytes, and nutrient material. There is also a more thorough removal of CO_2 and other waste products, and hence an increase in the normal vital activities of the part, a higher grade of life, better tissue formation, and in time a restorative reconstruction in case the tissues of the organ concerned are in a morbid or diseased condition.

1282 (2) The effect of a *prolonged cold* application is to cause

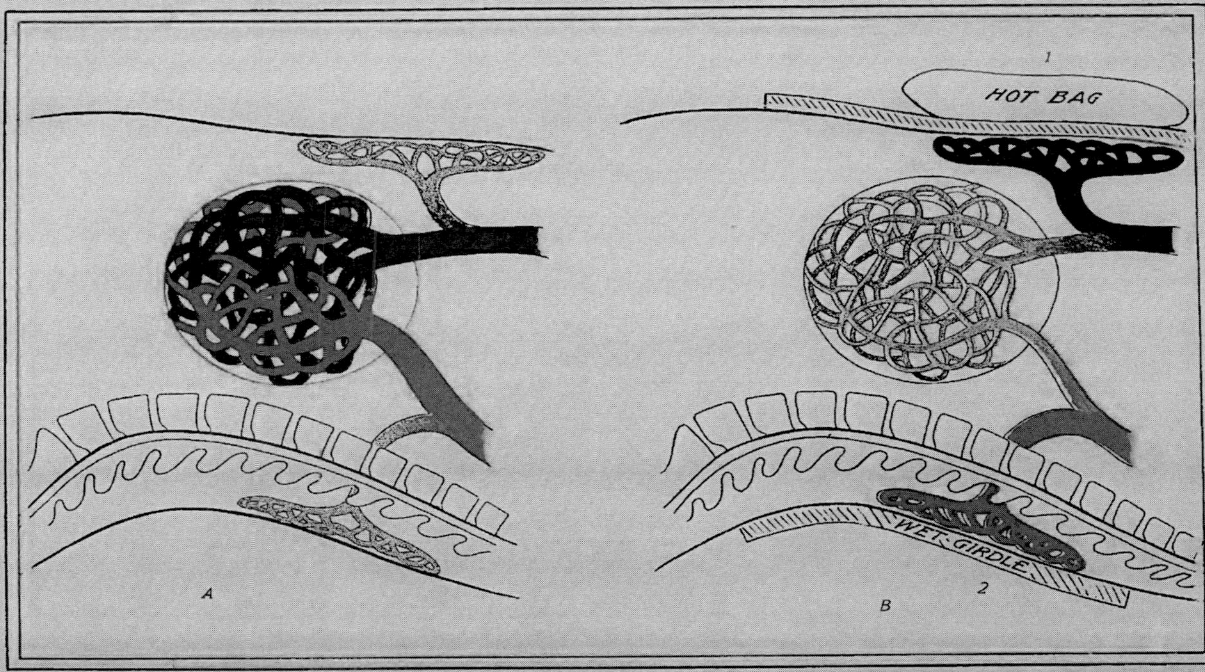

FIG. 155 *A*. Diagram representing visceral congestion (p. 732).

FIG. 155 *B*. Diagrammatic illustration of the effect of the hot and cold trunk pack (*1367*) in relieving visceral congestion. 1. The hot bag diverts blood from the stomach to the cutaneous veins by dilating the latter, while the wet girdle (2) at first causes constriction of the small arteries, later by reaction dilating both the arteries and the veins, thus relieving the visceral congestion (p. 732).

continuous contraction of the vessels of the internally related part so long as cutaneous sensibility is maintained; but when the application is so intense or prolonged as to destroy the sensibility of the skin, the reflex action ceases, and stimulation of the vasomotor centers no longer exists; hence, the vessels of the related internal vascular area relax. Thus a cold application, if too prolonged or too intense, may defeat its own purpose, producing an effect the very opposite to that intended. This interesting fact seems to be little known, or at least little regarded, if one may judge from the loose way in which instructions are given for the use of cold applications to the skin for relief of internal congestions and inflammations.

The reflex stimulation of cold may be maintained by removing the application for 3 to 5 minutes every 20 to 30 minutes, the parts being well rubbed with warm, dry flannel in the interim, or heat may be applied for 2 or 3 minutes.

The effect of a prolonged cold application, made in the manner suggested, is to lessen the blood supply of an internal viscus. This may sometimes be desirable, but is certainly far less often needed than is generally supposed. Injury does not result so much from the excess of blood in a part as from stagnation of blood. The blood is the chief healing agency in the body. It can not be too often reiterated—*it is the blood that heals.* Hence the aim should be to increase the supply of fresh blood to a part by encouraging the movement of blood through it, rather than to lessen the volume or the activity of the blood current.

While a cold application causes contraction of the vessels of the related viscus, the contraction of the cutaneous vessels may tend to fill the vessels of the part, if there exists collateral relation of the cutaneous and visceral vessels involved. The actual effect produced will depend upon the relative activity of the two forces. Care must be taken to arrange the compress in such a way as to avoid antagonistic effects of this sort. For example: In making cold applications to relieve cerebral congestion, the cold application should include the neck, so as to cause contraction of the main supplying trunks, thus preventing the collateral hyperemia of the brain, which may be induced by cold applications to the face alone.

In certain cases the effect of cold applications may be to increase internal congestion to such a degree as to make this the dominant effect, thus constituting a contraindication. A good illustration of this is seen in the case of the eye. A cold compress contracts the supraorbital artery, thus increasing the blood supply of the eyeball to which a collateral branch is distributed. For this reason the fomentation rather than the cold compress is indicated in inflammation of the eyeball. But the application must not be so prolonged as to heat the eyeball itself, thus dilating its vessels. In most cases inflammation of the lids is better relieved by short, very hot applications than by prolonged cold compresses. If cold compresses are used, they should be very small, not larger than the eye socket, and care should be taken that they do not extend above the brow.

1283 (3) The *proximal* cold compress controls local blood supply by contracting the supplying arterial trunk. This procedure is of special value in the treatment of congestion of the head, a cold compress, an ice-collar, or an ice-bag being applied to the neck. An ice-bag to the back of the neck contracts the vertebral arteries; cold applied to the sides or front contracts the carotids. The proximal compress is of greatest value when associated with heat applied derivatively, as in the treatment of cerebral congestion or inflammation, or inflammation of the pharynx, nasal cavity, or middle or internal ear (1327).

1284 (4) If the cold application is permitted to accumulate heat sufficiently to allow partial reaction to occur, being renewed only at intervals of 10 to 40 minutes, or when it has become warm, a still different effect is produced. At the first application of the cold, the blood-vessels are made to contract, thus forcing out of the diseased organ the accumulated and poison-laden blood. The lymph vessels share in the contraction, and likewise the muscular elements of the capsule and other structures. Thus the organ is well squeezed, so to speak, as one might compress a wet sponge in the hand. The germ-laden leucocytes are sent on their way to the spleen or other parts for repair or destruction, while a new supply of these most valiant and important body defenders is later brought into the part. As the compress warms up, internal as well as external reaction takes place, the vessels dilate, their rhythmical pumping is stimulated, and thus the introduction of a fresh and vital supply of blood is effected. By this means, leucocytosis is encouraged, and the supply of fresh leucocytes is constantly renewed, just as a wise general continually brings against the enemy fresh relays of soldiers, retiring those who are worn out by the combat, in order to maintain a vigorous fight.

From the foregoing it will be seen that the *frequently renewed heating compress* has characteristic properties which commend it for use in specific inflammations of deeply seated parts, as in pneumonia, typhoid fever, hepatitis, gastritis, pelvic and other internal inflammations.

It may be further remarked in relation to this form of partial application, that *by permitting sufficient reaction to maintain an active cutaneous circulation, an excellent derivative effect is produced*, the value of which is often overlooked.

(5) By *alternate hot and cold* applications to a limited 1285
cutaneous area, a most active fluxion of blood through an associated internal part may be produced; and this effect may be many times repeated, by reason of the constant renewal of the sensibility of the skin surface by hot applications, thus maintaining a high degree of reflex activity. The frequent change from heat to cold (every 15 secs.) powerfully excites the nerve centers in charge of the parts, and thus the nerve supply; hence, this form of application is contraindicated by pain or acute inflammation.

Each application of cold causes instant contraction of

the associated visceral vessels; each application of heat instantly restores the normal temperature of the skin, and terminates the reflex effect of the cold. Thus the organ is alternately emptied and filled, much as a sponge may be squeezed and filled, and this may be accomplished almost as rapidly as the compresses can be applied, and may be continued indefinitely,—a veritable pumping process by which blood may be passed through any internal organ, a genuine vasomotor gymnastics, applicable to a multitude of acute and chronic conditions.

On the other hand, an application so capable of exciting both vascular and nervous activity is especially adapted to cases of passive congestion, chronic exudates, and atonic and indolent states, such as malarial enlargement of the liver and spleen, rheumatic joints, serous and fibrinous exudates in the chest, muscles, or joints.

1286 (6) *Very hot* applications produce internal vascular effects somewhat similar to those of cold applications; but the contraction is briefer in duration, and occurs only when the application is sufficiently hot to cause pain, and to induce contraction of the cutaneous vessels. The contraction of the cutaneous vessels quickly gives way to dilatation, especially of the veins, because of the direct influence of the heat upon the sympathetic ganglia of the small vessels; but the stimulation of the vasomotor centers continues as long as the temperature of the application is sufficiently high to excite pain, and thus the influence upon the reflexly related parts may be much more prolonged. It must be remembered, moreover, that the application of heat to large surfaces, or over the heart, has the effect to excite the action of the heart, which is usually undesirable. The arterial trunks are also dilated, an effect often desirable and indicated, but which must sometimes be avoided. Hot applications for purely local effects should be not larger than necessary, and the duration must be carefully regulated.

1287 (7) A *warm* or *neutral* compress is soothing in its effects.

This fact is due to the shutting off from the internal related viscus of all external stimuli. It is by these stimuli, chiefly thermic in character, that the vascular tone and functional activity of internal parts is maintained. These vital conditions are, at least in very great measure, dependent upon the fusillade of sensory impressions constantly playing upon the spinal and cerebral centers. When these impressions become too intense, or the nerve centers abnormally sensitive, the phenomena of irritation appear — pain, spasm, hyperesthesia, etc. Neutral applications protect the skin against external irritants. This explains the soothing effect of the poultice. It must be remembered, however, that a warm compress, when applied across an arterial trunk, has the effect to dilate the vessel, and thus to increase the volume of blood flowing into the parts supplied by it. Hence the fulness in the head and the discomfort resulting from too warm clothing of the neck.

(8) *Moderately hot* applications generally produce con- **1288**
gestion of the associated vascular areas. It is in this way that a warm hip or foot bath encourages the menstrual flow, and the heating abdominal compress fills the portal circulation with blood, and thus relieves the brain. The fomentation (**1328**) and the heating compress (**1344**) are the most important partial measures for accumulating or concentrating blood in parts in which such an effect is desirable either to combat a local anemia or to produce a derivative effect in favor of some remote or associated part, though many other procedures are of great service in special cases.

(9) By means of the *prolonged heating compress* it is pos- **1289**
sible permanently to increase the volume of blood in a part, thus lessening the volume of blood in some collaterally related area. For example, the prolonged heating abdominal compress not only distends the cutaneous vessels, but also the portal circulation, thus drawing away from the brain or lungs a considerable amount of blood, and relieving an existing congestion, either active or passive. (*a*) When the effect desired is increased volume of blood in a given part, for the

purpose of producing anemia in some proximate or remote part, the wet towel should be protected not only by flannel, but also by rubber cloth or other impervious material. The purpose is to retain as much heat as possible, so as to secure the fullest dilatation of the cutaneous vessels. (*b*) When it is desired to increase the movement of blood in a reflexly related part, while at the same time combating stagnation or passive congestion, a compress covered only with flannel should be employed, so that by the limited but constant evaporation taking place, there may be maintained an *active* congestion of the skin and related parts, with derivative effect, and at the same time a vigorous fluxion in the reflexly related viscus, and a stimulation or energizing of the nerve supply of the part, and of all those vital activities whereby disease processes are opposed and the integrity of the body conserved.

1290 (10) *The hot and cold compress* (**1356**) produces remarkable effects by combining derivative and reflex effects. For example, (*a*) a fomentation to the upper back diverts blood from the bronchial vessels, while cold simultaneously applied to the front of the chest contracts the same vessels by reflex influence, thus intensifying the effect (**1270**); (*b*) Cold over the sternum with a fomentation over the lumbar region relieves congestion of the kidneys in the same way, by diverting blood into the cutaneous branches of the lumbar arteries while contracting the renal vessels (**1271**); (*c*) The pelvic circulation is controlled by a cold bag over the hypogastrium in conjunction with a hot pelvic pack (**1272**); (*d*) To relieve congestion of the liver, stomach, spleen, or pancreas, the application may be reversed, the heat being applied to the anterior surface and the cold application behind; or if pain is not present, the compress may be applied to the whole trunk, thus acting derivatively upon the whole portal system, while an ice-bag is placed over the stomach to contract the gastric vessels, and thus combat congestion, which is likely to be the cause of the pain; or for distension of the stomach with gas, a frequent accompaniment of hyperpepsia or hyperchlorhydria, which depends upon the escape of gas from the blood rather than upon fermentation (**1275**); (*e*) The intestines are most strongly influenced by the cold compress to the umbilical region combined with the fomentation over the lumbar region.

(11) The *hot and cold* pack (**1365**) consists in a hot bag or 1291
coil combined with a heating compress or partial pack. The action differs from that of the hot and cold compress in that the principal action is a remarkable derivative effect through drainage of the arteries of the affected part by the passive hyperemia induced by the heating compress, while at the same time blood is diverted from the veins by the dilatation of the collaterally related vessels by means of the hot bag.

The hot and cold pack very strongly influences both the arteries and the veins. It is, perhaps, our most powerful derivative procedure, its effects being almost wholly derivative in character, while the hot and cold compress concerns chiefly the arteries, which it influences both reflexly and derivatively.

Special Indications and Precautions Respecting Localized 1292
Applications.—Great care must always be employed in the application of douches or affusions to the head. (1) A short cold application excites the brain, and may be used in melancholia and cerebral anemia, and in sunstroke with pallor. The prolonged cold douche to the head is one of the most powerful of all depressing agencies. Unless very short, the depression may be too great; hence the cold affusion is better.

(2) Hot and warm as well as cold applications to the head must be managed with great care, and should be at first employed in a tentative manner, carefully noting effects.

(3) A cold or very hot douche to the back of the neck stimulates the respiratory centers. If too cold or too prolonged, suffocation or arrest of the heart may result. The very hot or very cold compress, alternate compresses, or

sponging are milder measures which produce similar effects, and are in general to be preferred.

(4) A short tepid douche to the head or a tepid affusion will allay excitement. It may be usefully employed in insomnia, maniacal excitement, and cerebral irritation. The temperature should be from 80° to 92° for 3 to 5 minutes; a slightly higher temperature causes congestion. Affusion is to be preferred to the douche. In the application of water to the head, percussion should always be avoided.

(5) Hot affusions to the head are useful in syncope and collapse, and in cases of migraine with low arterial tension, but should be employed with great precaution. In cases of cerebral anemia, alternate applications may be employed instead of the short cold douche, or hot or cold compresses may be applied. In syncope, especially when the condition is prolonged, hot or alternate hot and cold compresses or affusions should be applied to the head and face.

(6) Long cold applications to the head are usually exceedingly depressing, but may be used in fever, in cerebral congestion, and in sunstroke with congestion of the skin.

(7) The affusion, the ice-compress, and the evaporating compress are usually more convenient for application to the head than the douche, and safer, because less likely to be overdone.

(8) Hot applications must not be indefinitely continued. By degrees the beneficial effect often disappears. The vessels of the deeper-lying parts fill up from the anastomosing vessels and from heating of the deeper parts of the vessels, and consequent dilatation of the vessels, so that the advantage at first gained is after a time lost, and thus the derivative or revulsive influence of the heat in dilating the surface vessels is effaced. To renew the effect, however, it is only necessary to make a short cold application, withdrawing the heat for the purpose. The cold application must be very intense (40° to 60°), and the duration must be brief (10 to 60 secs.), just long enough to contract the sur-

face vessels, sending the blood on into the veins, and thus making room for another diversion of blood from the deep parts through the application of heat. The cold application also serves a most useful purpose in causing reflex contraction of the vessels of the deeper parts, thus aiding in the production of the desired anemia, which is increased and maintained by the succeeding hot application.

(9) As a corollary from the above principles, it appears that, in general, partial cold applications should rarely be absolutely continuous, but should either be allowed to accumulate heat sufficiently to permit slight reaction, or should be interrupted by a short hot application at intervals, or by brisk rubbing of the skin. Continuous cold is indicated only in cases of superficial inflammation at the very onset of the morbid process, and then must not be so intense as to suspend tissue activity, which condition is indicated by numbness of the parts when induced by cold.

(10) Hot applications likewise, when long applied, must be interrupted at intervals of 15 to 30 minutes by a very short cold application.

THE COLD FOOT BATH (Fig. 156).

The *cold* foot bath (45° to 55°, 1 to 5 min.) though less 1293
useful than the hot foot bath, is of great service in producing reflex, revulsive, and other effects. The sole of the foot is one of the most important vasomotor areas in the body, having very direct connection with the nerve centers which control the circulation of the pelvic and abdominal viscera.

The brain circulation may also be influenced by stimulation of the rich vasomotor nerve supply of the plantar region, a fact of practical interest in cases of cerebral congestion.

Method.—The water at proper temperature should be placed in a small tub adapted to the purpose, to a depth of three or four inches. The feet, previously warmed, are immersed in the tub for 1 to 5 minutes. Friction should be applied to the feet continuously during the bath, either by the hands of the attendant or by the patient's rubbing one foot against the other in alternation.

Physiological Effects.—Among the most interesting effects of the cold foot bath are the vasomotor and other reflex effects set up in the pelvic viscera, causing contraction of the vessels and muscles of the uterus (in women) and the organs connected with it. The blood-vessels of the brain, the stomach, the liver, the bladder, and the intestines, are made to contract at the same time. Intestinal peristalsis and contraction of the bladder are also excited. To obtain the most pronounced effects, the temperature must be very low (45° to 50°). The duration will vary with the effect desired.

1294 **Therapeutic Applications.**—The revulsive effects of the cold foot bath are very decided, and continue for a long time —much longer than those obtained from a hot foot bath or similar applications. As a derivative and revulsive application, the *short* cold foot bath is useful in *cerebral congestion* and *uterine hemorrhage*. For these purposes, however, the application must be very short (20 to 60 secs.), as it is the primary effect alone that is desirable. In cases in which the feet are constantly cold, and in persistent sweating of the feet, the rubbing cold foot bath is a most useful measure, making the feet glow with circulatory reaction (50° to 60°, 1 to 3 min.). It must be repeated daily.

The prolonged cool foot bath (60° to 70°) may sometimes be employed as an antiphlogistic measure in cases of injury to the feet, such as *sprains*, *strains*, *inflamed bunions*, and similar conditions. The feet must be well warmed before the application is made, by walking, running, rubbing, or by heat.

Contraindications.—The cold foot bath must generally be avoided in cases of *cystitis*, *pelvic cellulitis*, *salpingitis*, and in all forms of pelvic and abdominal congestion and inflammation, as *peritonitis*, *prostatitis*, *proctitis*, and in *hepatic*, *uterine*, *renal*, and *intestinal congestions*. In these cases the very hot foot or leg bath should be employed (115° to 125°).

THE SHALLOW FOOT BATH.

The shallow foot bath is a variety of the cold foot bath in which the amount of water employed is small, barely sufficient to cover the toes. After being held in the bath for one-half minute, one foot is taken out and rubbed for half a minute and returned, then the other is treated in like manner, this being continued until the whole surface is well reddened with strong circulatory reaction. Lastly the feet are wiped dry and thoroughly rubbed with the dry hand. The soles are vigorously percussed. The water should be very cold, or at a temperature of 45° to 55°. The shallow foot bath gives rise to powerful reflex effects upon the pelvic viscera, causing contraction of the vessels, and thus relieving uterine congestion. The intestines and even the brain are also influenced. 1295

Therapeutic Applications.—The shallow foot bath produces powerful reaction effects to the feet, and is thus of great service in chronic cases of *cold* and *sweating feet.* Its applications are the same as those of the ordinary cold foot bath, only differing in being somewhat more intense.

THE RUNNING OR FLOWING FOOT BATH.

This bath is a modification of the shallow foot bath, in which, through the constant change of water by means of suitable arrangements, the initial temperature is maintained. Water from a natural source, at as low a temperature as can be obtained, is commonly employed. The outlet should be so placed that the water can not accumulate to a depth greater than one-half inch. Circulatory reaction is promoted by the movement of the water in contact with the feet, and constant alternate rubbing of the feet one upon the other. The purpose of the flow of water is to maintain a uniform and low temperature, while at the same time reaction is promoted by the incomplete submergence of the feet and constant friction. The sole of one foot is rubbed against the dorsum of the other for 10 to 15 seconds, then the feet 1296 are reversed; and thus each foot is treated. The bath is prolonged until the toes are reddened by reaction.

The running foot bath may be conveniently taken in the full bath tub, by allowing cold water to run with the outlet partially or fully open.

Therapeutic Applications.—This bath is indicated in all cases in which the ordinary cold foot bath may be used (**1294**), and is more effective. It is a powerful derivative measure, and a highly valuable remedy in cases of ***habitually cold feet*** from vasomotor spasm of the extremities. The remedial effect in these cases is obtained not alone by means of the very decided hyperemia induced in the vessels of the feet and legs, but by reflex influence upon the sympathetic centers, especially the lumbar ganglia. Incidentally, ***cerebral congestion*** is relieved both by reflex spasm of the meningeal vessels during the bath, and by the diversion of blood to the lower extremities through the reaction following.

This bath is of special value in the management of ***neurasthenics*** suffering from cold extremities and cerebral congestion, producing an excellent general tonic effect.

In cases of ***insomnia*** due to cold feet, it is well to precede the application by a hot foot bath (110° to 115°, 2 to 5 min.).

When the hands as well as the feet are cold, a rubbing cold hand bath may be taken at the same time with the foot bath, rubbing the hands together in very cold water.

Contraindications.—The flowing foot bath should be avoided in ***catarrh*** of the ***bladder***, ***irritable rectum*** and ***bladder***, and other forms of ***pelvic inflammation***. It is also contraindicated in ***ovarian neuralgia***, ***neuralgia*** of the ***bladder***, ***sciatica***, and ***rheumatic affections*** of the ***toes*** and ***ankles***.

THE HOT FOOT BATH.

1297 The requisites are a suitable receptacle for the feet, and a supply of very hot water, with cold water for tempering.

Method.—The temperature required for positive effects is 104° to 122°. The bath should begin at a temperature

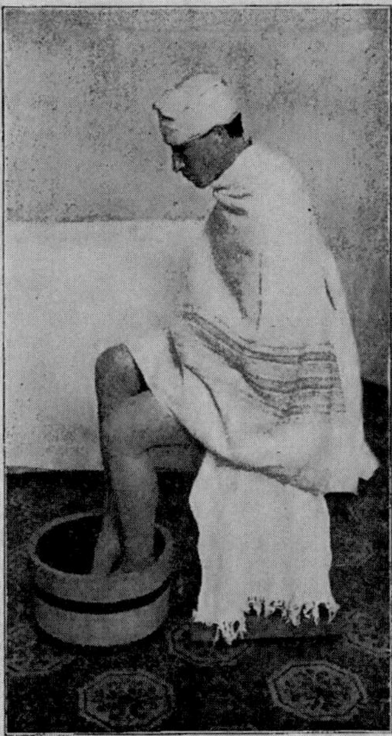

FIG. 156. COLD FOOT BATH (p. 753).

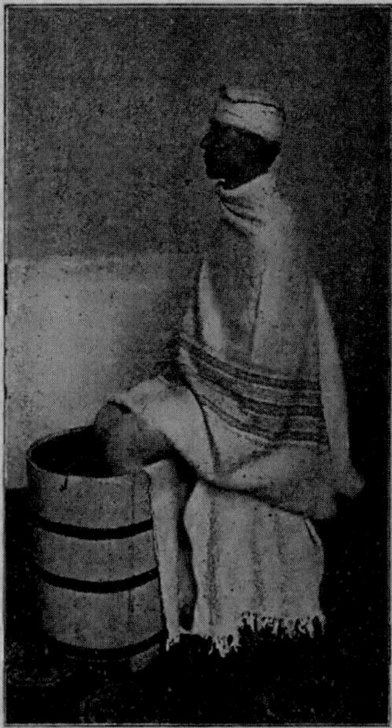

FIG. 157. LEG BATH (p. 758).

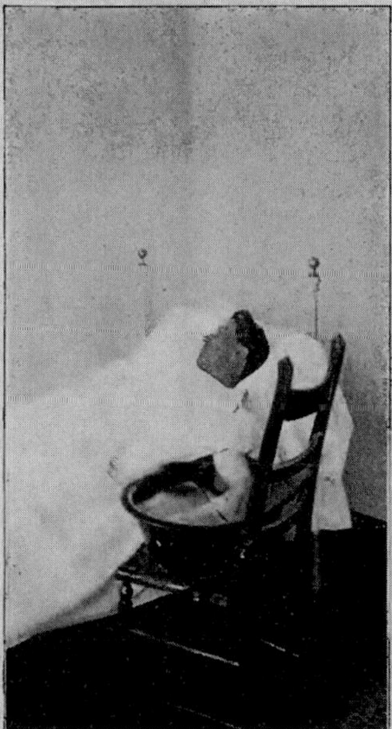

FIG. 158. ARM BATH (p. 759).

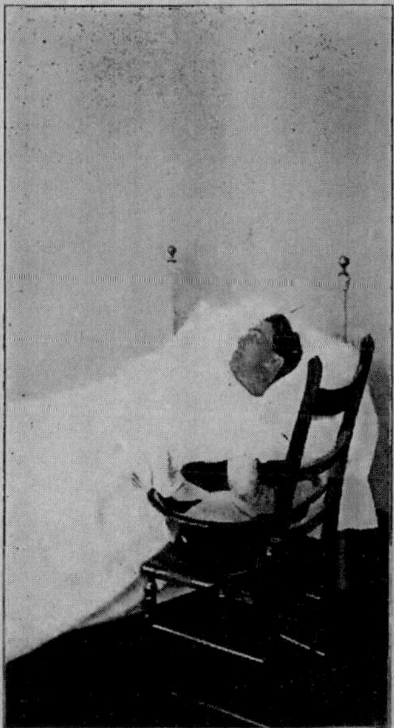

FIG. 159. ELBOW BATH (p. 759).

of 102° to 104°, and should be gradually increased until by the end of two or three minutes a maximum temperature of 115° to 122° is reached. The duration may be from 5 minutes to half an hour. The feet should be completely immersed in the water; the effect may be intensified by increasing the depth of the water.

After the very hot foot bath, the feet should receive a dash of cold water,—affusion, jet, or spray,—to produce the true revulsive effect by suddenly cooling the skin and encouraging tonic circulatory reaction.

Physiological Effects.— Bergesio has shown that the hot foot bath produces in a diminutive way precisely the same effects as the general hot bath. At first the pulse is slowed and the brain congested, but after three or four minutes the pulse rate is increased, and the brain becomes anemic, this condition persisting for some time after the bath is terminated. Shokovsky showed that the foot bath at 108° to 115° for 20 minutes caused elevation of the temperature in the external auditory canal amounting to one degree Fahrenheit. The rectal temperature at the same time *fell to the same extent.* Arterial tension was increased 8 mm.*

Therapeutic Applications.— This bath is more commonly used, perhaps, than any other, as a derivative measure. At a temperature of 103° to 110° the hot foot bath is an exceedingly useful means of balancing the circulation, by the dilatation of the blood-vessels of the legs relieving congestion of the brain and other organs in the upper half of the body.

Very hot (115° to 125°) as well as cold applications to the feet stimulate the involuntary muscles of the uterus, intestines, bladder, and other pelvic and abdominal viscera. Heat may be used at first in cases in which cold is not well tolerated. The dilatation of the blood-vessels produced in the feet by this application extends to the upper parts of the limbs, and even to the vessels of the pelvic viscera. This is shown by the vigorous pulsation of the femoral artery after

*Wratsch, *Lyon Médical*, 1883, page 541.

a hot foot bath. By vaginal examination it may be readily noted that the pulsation of the pelvic vessels is greatly increased in vigor, indicating a heightened vascular activity. By this means the uterus and ovaries receive an increased supply of blood, which renders the foot bath a useful measure for restoring the function of menstruation when suspended.

The very hot foot bath is exceedingly useful in cases of *sprain* of the ankle joint. *Anesthesia* of the plantar region and *neuralgia* of the foot and gout are relieved by the very hot foot bath. The application should be made two or three times a day, and continued for 20 to 30 minutes each time.

The hot foot bath is also of very great service as a means of relieving or preventing a cold resulting from accidental chilling of the feet, if applied soon after exposure.

The prolonged warm or hot foot bath (98° to 106°) dilates the vessels of the feet, and produces collateral anemia of the pelvic viscera. A short, very hot foot bath (110° to 120°, 5 min.) produces the same effect. The hot foot bath (104° to 110°) accompanies the cold sitz.

THE ALTERNATE FOOT BATH.

1298 In the employment of the alternate foot bath, the feet are placed in hot water for 2 or 3 minutes, then in cold water for 20 seconds to 1 minute. They are then returned to the hot water for 2 minutes, then replaced in the cold water, this operation being repeated a number of times. The alternate foot bath is a more highly excitant measure than the cold foot bath. It is especially useful in *chilblains*, in *local asphyxia*, in habitual *coldness* of the feet, and for *sweating* feet.

THE LEG BATH.

1299 This bath (Fig. 157) is essentially the same as the foot bath, with the exception that a deeper tub is used, with a larger amount of water. Any desired temperature may be employed.

The leg bath is a powerful derivative measure, and may be used in cases which do not readily yield to the employment of the foot bath. It is especially serviceable in the treatment of *insomnia*, *pulmonary congestion*, *dysmenorrhea*, *suppression* of *menstruation*, *hyperpepsia*, *ovarian congestion*, and *pelvic pain* from other causes. In all the above-mentioned conditions the warm or very hot leg bath is employed. Low temperatures are rarely called for with this procedure.

The contraindications for the cold leg bath are the same as for the cold foot bath.

THE ARM BATH.

Immersion of the arm in water (Fig. 158) is frequently **1300**
a useful measure, especially in surgical cases. In cases of *felons*, *sprains*, and various other injuries to hands and arms, antiphlogistic effects may be obtained in this way. *Chronic ulcers* and some forms of *chronic skin disease*, and especially *burns* of the arms, may be successfully treated by prolonged immersion. The temperature in cases in which deeply seated inflammatory conditions are present should be 92° to 97°, or neutral. A cold bath under such conditions will be followed by reaction with increase of congestion and pain. A long hot bath will cause local elevation of temperature and increased fulness of vessels, and will likewise increase the local pain and intensify the morbid process. A *neutral* temperature, preferably as near 92° as possible, especially if prolonged for several hours, lessens pain, lowers local temperature, diminishes congestion, and thus favors resolution. A short hot arm bath relieves pain by producing hyperemia of the skin and collateral anemia of deep inflamed parts. Superficial pains or inflammations require neutral applications.

The Elbow Bath (Fig. 159) is a modification of the arm **1301**
bath which is best suited to the treatment of inflammatory affections of the hand. Immersion of the elbow in cold water lowers the temperature of the hand more efficiently than does cold immersion of the hand itself. This interest-

ing fact, first discovered by Priessnitz, is dependent upon the principle that an application of cold across the trunk of an artery contracts the artery and all its distal branches (Exp. 63). The same results may be obtained by a cold compress about the arm.

THE HAND BATH.

1302 Immersion of the hands in very cold water exercises a powerful influence — much greater than might be expected — upon the cerebral and pulmonary vessels. Vasilieff showed (1885) that immersion of the hands in cold water for a sufficient length of time is capable of slowing the pulse and the respiration, lowering the temperature in the external auditory canal, lessening the pressure in the cerebral arteries, and narrowing the veins of the retina. The hot hand bath produces opposite phenomena. These observations explain the effect of the cold hand bath in controlling epistaxis. Holding a block of ice in the hand is an excellent means of checking nosebleed, and in the author's hands has proved of service in pulmonary hemorrhage, checking the bleeding very quickly even when other measures seemed to be unsuccessful.

Brown-Sequard and others demonstrated long ago the powerful reflex influence of immersion of the hands in hot or cold water, observing that the immersion of one hand in cold water caused a lowering of temperature in the other hand, while placing one hand in hot water produced an elevation of temperature in the other hand.*

THE PARTIAL CONTINUOUS BATH.

1303 This bath, first introduced by Langenbeck,† consists in the continuous immersion of a limb in water at a neutral temperature. Langenbeck resorted to its use as a method of treating surgical wounds, and reported many hundreds of cases dressed by this method. The results claimed

* *Archives de Physiologie*, v. 3, pp. 497–502.

† *Deutsche Klinik*, 1855, No. 39, pp. 409–419.

by him were as follows: (1) Lessening of pain from the wound; (2) lessening of fever; (3) lessened secretion or suppuration; (4) accelerated healing process. Many leading German and French surgeons adopted this method of dealing with surgical wounds; and had it not been for the wonderful discovery of Lister, the partial immersion bath might have remained for a long time the most successful method of dressing surgical wounds. Figures 160 and 161 show the ingenious devices of Langenbeck for the practical and convenient employment of this bath. Duplicates of these were used by Dr. Frank Hamilton in his practice in Bellevue Hospital. Dr. Hamilton certainly deserves credit for his earnest advocacy of the immersion treatment of wounds at a time when amputation was the almost inevitable result in cases of badly contused injuries of the limbs. While the author was a student under Dr. Hamilton in Bellevue Hospital in 1874, numerous grave cases were successfully treated by this method in the hospital wards.

The author had the pleasure of listening to a heated discussion upon the utility of the method, which occurred at the Academy of Medicine in the winter of 1874–75, Dr. Hamilton defending the immersion treatment, while Dr. James Wood and others as vigorously denounced what they chose to denominate the "maceration method." The antiseptic treatment of wounds and injuries has since rendered this method of comparatively little value, but circumstances still occasionally arise in which it may be utilized to advantage, as in the treatment of senile gangrene, severe burns, painful or lacerated wounds, and in the absence of antiseptic dressings.

THE SITZ BATH.

The sitz bath (Fig. 162) is one of the oldest and most 1304
serviceable of hydriatic procedures.

Method.—The tub may be of metal, porcelain, or wood. It is usually of such form and size that the patient may be comfortably seated in it by leaving the feet outside and flexing the limbs, the feet being placed in a separate and smaller tub during the application. The flexion of the limbs in a sitz bath is, however, to some degree objectionable, as it interferes somewhat with the circulation; and on this account the author is much inclined to exchange the sitz bath for the half-bath (**1174**) in dealing with a large class of cases. The temperature of the sitz bath may be cold, cool, neutral, tepid, hot, or very hot. There are also the rubbing sitz, the flowing sitz, and the revulsive sitz.

The sitz bath may be made to serve the purpose of a general bath by rubbing the body during the bath with the hands or with a towel wet in water of the same temperature.

THE COLD SITZ BATH.

1305 In this procedure, either still or running water may be employed, according to the effect desired.

The temperature of the cold sitz bath is 55° to 65°. A lower temperature is seldom required. The time should be 1 to 15 minutes. The duration of the cool or the tepid sitz may be considerably longer (70° to 80°, 10 to 15 min., with rubbing; 88° to 92°, one-half hour to several hours).

In a cold sitz bath the patient should always be rubbed sufficiently to prevent chilling, and care should be taken that the feet are kept warm, either by the hot foot bath or by hot bags, or flannels wrung out of hot water and placed about the feet and legs. The limbs should be so adjusted that there will be no pressure upon the popliteal space, as this will interrupt the circulation in the feet, and interfere with the results of the bath. If necessary, the foot bath may be elevated a little, or the edge of the sitz bath may be covered with a thickly folded flannel to prevent compression of the vessels.

In the *flowing sitz* bath, cold water is admitted to the tub at such a rate that the temperature may be maintained at the initial point, the surplus water being allowed to flow out through an opening properly placed.

The bath may be administered two or three times a day with advantage in some cases, but the practice of using the bath five or six times a day, which prevails at some hydropathic establishments, is not to be recommended.

Physiological Effects.—In the sitz bath an impression is 1306
made upon the cutaneous areas which are reflexly connected with the viscera of the pelvis and also those of the lower part of the abdomen; namely, the lumbar region, the hypogastric region, the outer and inner surfaces of the thighs, the perineum, and the external genitals. The physiological effects depend, as in other baths, upon the temperature, the duration, and sometimes the mechanical effects combined with the thermic impressions.

The cold sitz bath produces a profound effect upon all the bodily functions. The general effects are those which pertain to the application of cold water, such as lessened activity of the skin, goose-flesh, contraction of the cutaneous vessels, slowing of the pulse, increased arterial tension, lowering of the temperature of the parts immersed, and if the bath is short, a powerful reaction in the parts brought in contact with the water and reflexly related parts.

A short cold sitz (30 secs. to 2 min.) produces active dilatation of the vessels of the lower abdomen, increasing the movement of blood through these parts. The thermic reaction produced, heightens the nutritive processes in the parts concerned, and excites contraction of the muscular structures of the viscera, thus influencing the bladder, pelvic organs, and the structures involved in the acts of defecation and urination, together with the various musculo-ligamentous structures which support the abdominal and pelvic viscera. During the first moments of the bath, the cold sitz produces increased activity of the heart and a temporary rise of the blood pressure.

Therapeutic Applications.—Short applications (70° to 1307
50°, 5 to 8 min.) produce tonic effects. Prolonged applications may be sedative. The bath is most frequently employed for fluxion effects upon the pelvic viscera. The cool sitz bath is derivative when continued for 15 to 20 minutes, or long

enough to cause very decided dilatation of the surface vessels. The special advantage of the bath depends upon the persistence of this dilatation, which fixes a large quantity of blood in the skin. Contraction of the internal vessels produced at the same time by the irritation of cold, aids in establishing a condition of relative anemia in the internal parts.

The cold sitz may be advantageously applied in cases of *jaundice* after the hot enema or in alternation with the sweating process. It stimulates the outflow of bile by strongly increasing the tension of the portal circulation.

The cold sitz bath is an excellent derivative measure for patients who are moderately vigorous, and who suffer from *congestion* of the *brain*, or from *hepatic* or *splenic congestions* or *chronic enlargement* from *malarial poisoning*, or other chronic conditions of like character. This measure is especially useful in atonic and paretic conditions of the genito-urinary organs, and in the *nocturnal urinary incontinence* of young children. In *chronic uterine affections* accompanied by a relaxed condition of the vessels, ligaments, and muscles, this measure is invaluable (70° to 80°, 10 to 15 min.). It is equally valuable in *chronic congestion* of the *prostate*, *gleet*, in the atonic forms of *seminal weakness*, and in *constipation* and *atony* of the *bladder* in both sexes.

Contraindications.—The cold sitz must not be prescribed in cases of acute inflammation of the pelvic or abdominal viscera, in painful affections of the bladder or genital organs, in sciatica, nor in cases of acute pulmonary congestion.

THE PROLONGED COLD SITZ BATH.

1308 The sitz bath at 60° to 70° for 15 to 40 minutes causes prolonged contraction of the vessels of the pelvic and abdominal viscera, thus making it a most effectual measure in combating chronic congestions or so-called chronic inflammations. A hot foot bath must be given simultaneously.

In many cases a temperature of 75° to 80° (usually about 75°) is preferable to a lower temperature, especially for

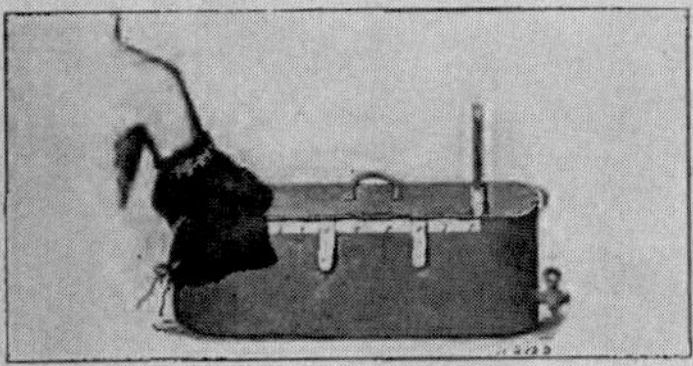

FIG. 160. PARTIAL CONTINUOUS BATH (p. 761). (Langenbeck)

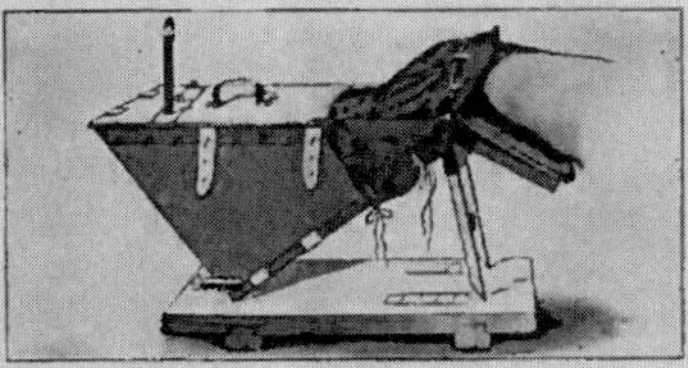

FIG. 161. PARTIAL CONTINUOUS BATH (p. 761). (Langenbeck)

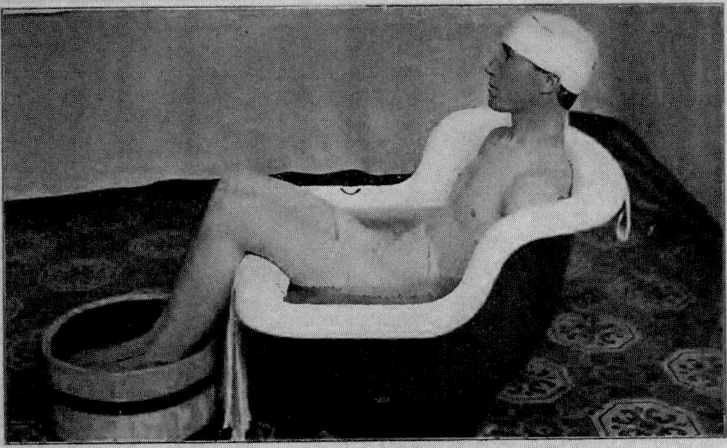

FIG. 162. SITZ BATH (p. 762).

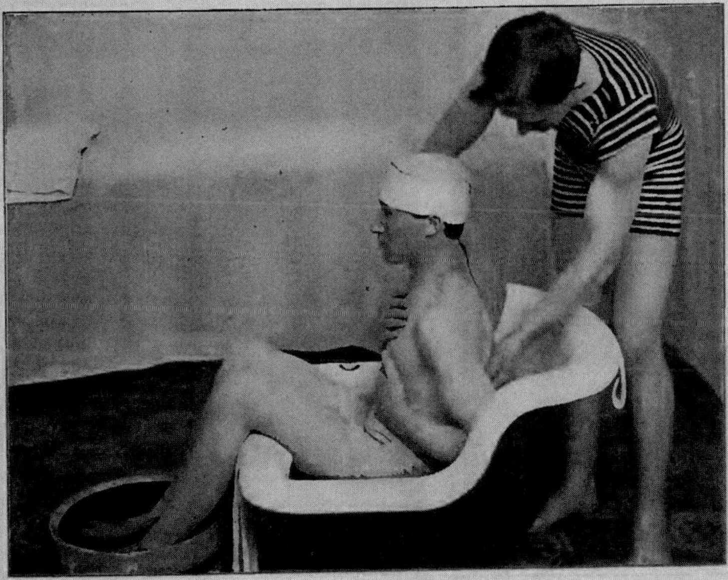

FIG. 163. COLD RUBBING SITZ (p. 763).

patients who have not been accustomed to cold water, and in whom a lower temperature produces pain or other unfavorable excitation, due to the intense internal reaction. The bath may be continued in cases of passive pelvic congestion for 30 to 40 minutes with excellent effects. In some cases it is desirable to begin the bath at a temperature of 85° to 90°, lowering it, after the first few minutes, to 75°. The duration of the bath should ordinarily be 15 to 20 minutes. For chronic congestion, a bath at 65° to 75° affords most satisfactory results. The cold must always be accompanied by the hot foot bath (104° to 110°).

Physiological Effects.— The prolonged cold sitz causes very pronounced effects upon the pelvic circulation. The contraction of the cutaneous branches of the internal iliac tends to produce hyperemia of the pelvic viscera, while the reflex effect is to contract the pelvic vessels. If the parts are rubbed so as to maintain strong surface circulation, the balance of effect will be to decongest the pelvic viscera. Without friction, the internal parts will be congested. This may be obviated by the simultaneous hot foot bath, which drains the iliac vessels through the femoral artery, while the reflex from the skin contracts the visceral vessels, affording a most beautiful example of the advantage of simultaneous hot and cold applications. The temperature of the foot bath should not exceed 110°. A higher temperature may dilate the pelvic vessels.

Therapeutic Applications.— The prolonged cool sitz affords excellent results in *chronic menorrhagia* when not due to vegetations of the endometrium. It should be used in connection with other measures of treatment. A Russian observer finds the prolonged cold sitz following the hot vaginal douche the most effective means of relieving *pelvic congestion.* Winternitz recommends the prolonged cold sitz after the wet-sheet rub as the most effective of all measures for the relief of *chronic diarrhea.* Both these observations the author is able to confirm by many clinical examples.

The cold sitz bath is also indicated in *hemorrhage of the bladder*, *intestines*, *uterus*, *urethra*, and *rectum*, in *hemorrhoids*, *chronic inflammation of the prostate*, *chronic metritis*, *circum-uterine inflammation*, and in most chronic inflammations of the pelvic viscera when pain is not a prominent symptom. The hot foot bath should be administered simultaneously. The pelvic vessels are thus drained of blood while they are at the same time reflexly contracted.

The *revulsive* sitz is a very short cold sitz, simply a dip into cold water for a few seconds, following a very hot sitz (115° to 120°), of 3 to 8 minutes' duration. It is a most powerful sedative measure in painful affections of the pelvic viscera. It may be very advantageously employed in cases of *ovarian* or *uterine neuralgia*, *enteralgia*, and in *painful affections* of the *bladder*, *rectum*, and *prostate*.

The cold sitz, accompanied by rubbing of the whole surface with cold water, is a powerful means of stimulating cerebral activity. Winternitz has shown by plethysmographic observations that the cold sitz increases the volume of the arm. This is accomplished through the contraction of the mesenteric vessels, which, with the spleen, constitute a sort of flexible reservoir into which the blood may escape from other portions of the body, and from which, by various means, it may be driven back again into the general circulation. The cold enema and the cold abdominal douche are the only other measures capable of acting in so direct a manner as the cold sitz upon this great reservoir of the blood. An eminent London preacher, Mr. Joseph Parker, has a small bath-room fitted up in the rear of his pulpit, in which he habitually takes a cold sitz just before appearing before his audience. He testifies that the effect of this application upon his cerebral activities is most remarkable, and asserts that if he can have his cold sitz bath, he feels able to command any audience that can be gathered before him.

Contraindications.— On account of the considerable increase of blood pressure at the beginning of the bath, the cold sitz is always contraindicated in cases in which suddenly increased arterial pressure is likely to prove detrimental. On this account it must be avoided in most affections of the heart. It is also contraindicated in all acute inflammations involving the viscera of the abdomen or pelvis, as in *cystitis*, *prostatitis*, *metritis*, *ovaritis*, *enteritis*, *colitis*, *appendicitis*, *peritonitis*, *salpingitis*, and so-called *cellulitis;* in affections of the bladder, uterus, and intestines attended by *muscular spasm;* in *vaginismus;* in *enteralgia*, *lumbo-abdominal neuralgia*, *neuralgia* of the *ovaries*, *bladder*, *testicles;* in *coccygodynia* and *sciatica;* and in most *painful affections* of the *genito-urinary organs*. The cold bath in any form must be avoided in *spermatorrhea* accompanied by hyperesthesia of the prostatic urethra, or frequent losses; the cold sitz is especially harmful. In many cases in which the cold bath is contraindicated, a sitz bath at 85°, gradually cooled to 75°, may, however, be employed with benefit. The length of the bath when employed in this manner should be 15 to 20 minutes.

THE COLD RUBBING SITZ BATH (Fig. 163).

The patient's head having been properly cooled and pro- 1309
tected by a wet towel, he steps into the hot foot bath, and then seats himself in the sitz bath. The attendant at once begins a vigorous rubbing of the hips, back, and thighs. The rubbing should continue during the entire bath, the patient rubbing the abdomen and thighs while the attendant rubs his back and sides (duration 3 to 4 min., temperature 65° to 55°). Friction mitts may be employed to facilitate reaction in persons very susceptible to cold and who do not react well. At the end of the bath it is well to administer the Scotch douche to the hips and legs. When this is not available, a douche at a temperature ten degrees below that of the bath may be applied over the hips and feet (20 secs.).

Physiological Effects.— The effect of this bath is to produce decided thermic and mechanical impressions upon the reflex areas associated with the viscera of the pelvis and lower abdomen. A most powerful and lasting circulatory reaction is produced in the surface vessels, which depletes the circulation of the associated internal areas by collateral influence, producing a strong revulsive effect.

Therapeutic Applications.—The cold rubbing sitz is a powerfully tonic measure, influencing especially the genito-urinary organs, and is applicable to all atonic conditions. It is one of the best of all measures for the relief of *constipation*, and of *atony* of the *bladder* accompanied by incontinence or retention of the urine, when pain and active inflammation are not present. It is an excellent procedure in cases of *subinvolution* of the *uterus* and *adnexa* in women, and *enteroptosis* in both sexes, especially when the abdominal muscles are greatly relaxed; in *nocturnal enuresis* of children; in *impotence* in men, *sterility* in women; and in cases of *uterine* and *ovarian displacement*, in conjuction with other appropriate measures of treatment.

This measure may be used with advantage in certain cases of *insomnia*, being repeated two or three times during the night if necessary. Usually two or three hours of good sleep will be obtained after each application. It is also valuable in *constipation* with *apepsia* or *hypopepsia*, and in *dilatation* of the *stomach* and *colon*. It may be employed in *delayed labor*, cold water being poured upon the spine while the patient is in the bath.

In certain cases in which the rubbing sitz is indicated, so great intolerance to cold water exists that the patient must be very carefully trained for some time before a vigorous application can be made; in such cases the bath may be given at 80° to 85°, being lowered one or two degrees daily until a really effective cold bath may be administered. When the higher temperatures are employed, the duration of the bath may be prolonged with advantage to 6 or 8 minutes.

1310 **Contraindications.**— This bath is not admissible in cases of *acute inflammation* and *congestion*, and in *painful* or *spas-*

modic affections of the *pelvic* and *abdominal viscera*, as *neuralgia* of the *ovaries* or *testicles*, *tenesmus* of the *bladder* or *rectum*, and *vaginismus*. It may be added, however, that the cold rubbing sitz is of high value in cases of *ovarian neuralgia* and other painful non-inflammatory affections of the pelvis, if made of short duration (one-half minute to a minute), and preceded by a hot pelvic pack or a hot sitz bath for 10 or 15 minutes. When employed in this way, it serves to fix in the skin, so to speak, the blood which has been brought to it by the preceding hot application, and thus intensifies and prolongs the analgesic effect.

THE VERY HOT SITZ BATH.

Temperature, 106° to 120°; duration, 3 to 10 minutes. **1311**
It is well to begin with a temperature of 100°, rapidly adding hot water until the maximum temperature is reached. A hot foot bath is taken with it (110° to 120°).

Physiological Effects.— The general effects are essentially the same as those of the hot immersion bath (**1126**). The cutaneous branches of the external iliac are widely dilated, diverting blood from the internal viscera. The hot foot bath, by dilating the branches of the external iliac, still further drains the portal circulation. At temperatures above 110°, especially if the bath is continued beyond three or four minutes, the effect is to excite the pelvic circulation, and to concentrate the blood in this portion of the body.

Therapeutic Applications.—The hot sitz is of great service in restoring the menstrual function when suspended as the result of general chill or other cause. The shallow, very hot sitz is an excellent measure in relieving the pain of inflamed *hemorrhoids*. It is likewise of great value in *vaginismus*, *spasm* of the neck of the bladder, *anal tenesmus*, in *uterine colic*, in *nephritic colic*, in *sciatica*, *lumbo-abdominal neuralgia*, *neuralgia* of the *ovaries*, *testicles*, and *bladder*, and in all painful affections of a non-inflammatory character, involving the viscera of the pelvis and lower abdomen. The hot sitz

49

bath is a most powerful analgesic measure. For the best effects, it should be followed by a short cold application.

In cases in which this bath is employed for the relief of acute visceral congestion, great care must be exercised to cool the surface of the body gradually, so as to restore the tone of the vessels without producing a general and sudden contraction of the surface vessels, whereby the good effects of the bath may be immediately destroyed (affusion or spray, 80°, 5 min.; or 40°, 5 to 10 secs.). The slightest chilly sensation following the bath will be accompanied by a return of the unpleasant symptoms which have been removed by the application.

1311½ A most useful form of the sitz bath is what the author has termed the *revulsive sitz*. The bath begins at 100° F., the temperature being rapidly raised to 115° or 120°. The patient remains in the bath 3 to 8 minutes, the head being carefully protected by a cold compress upon the head or about the neck. As the patient rises from the bath, a pailful of cold water is dashed upon the hips, so as to produce a tonic reaction, and fix in the skin the blood with which it has been well filled by the hot bath. There is no better analgesic measure than this for the various *neuralgias* and *hyperesthesias* of the genito-urinary organs to which women, and occasionally also men, suffer most persistently, and often without any substantial relief.

THE NEUTRAL SITZ BATH.

1312 The character of this bath is essentially the same as that of the neutral full bath. It is simply a circumscribed neutral bath. The temperature is 92° to 97°; the duration may be from 15 minutes to an hour or two.

Physiological Effects.—The effects are those of a limited neutral bath. No decided thermic or circulatory reaction is produced by it, and as a consequence it exercises a pronounced calmative effect upon the viscera of the pelvis and lower abdomen.

Therapeutic Applications.— The neutral sitz bath is an exceedingly useful means of relieving *nervous irritability* and *congestion* of the *pelvic viscera*. It is of great service in the treatment of *painful* and *inflammatory affections* of the genito-urinary organs in both men and women, in *pruritis* of the vulva and anus, in *strangulated hemorrhoids*, *frequent urination* from irritability of the bladder, *spermatorrhea* arising from excessive irritability of the genito-urinary center, —frequent losses,—*neuralgia* of the *spermatic cord* and *testicles*, and in cases of *enteroptosis* accompanied by extreme hyperesthesia of the lumbar ganglia of the abdominal sympathetic, also in *chronic backache* from rectal and uterine disorders or *enteroptosis*, and *coccygodynia*.

The neutral sitz bath is highly antiphlogistic in character, and may be employed in subacute and even acute inflammatory conditions, such as *acute catarrh* of the *bladder* and *urethra*, and in subacute inflammations of the *uterus*, *ovaries*, and *tubes*. This bath is especially useful as a means of relief in *neuralgia* of the *Fallopian tubes* or of the *testicles*, in *vaginismus*, *pruritis* of the *anus* and *vulva*, *vesical* and *rectal tenesmus*, *hyperesthesia* of the *lumbo-aortic plexus*, and in *hyperesthesias* of the *genito-urinary organs*. It is indicated as a sedative means in *erotomania* in both sexes, in *priapism*, and in cases of *spermatorrhea* accompanied by a marked hyperesthesia of the urethra and ejaculatory ducts, and in all cases of pelvic disease in which cold applications are inadmissible on account of pain or the inflammatory conditions which may be present.

THE COMPRESS.

This is simply the application of water at any temperature 1313
by means of a cloth, a sponge, spongiopyline, or other suitable medium. More than a century ago Benjamin Rush used a compress of clay with excellent results. The ordinary old-fashioned poultice is a compress, but inconvenient and uncleanly. For ordinary purposes, a linen cloth of two to

four thicknesses and of proper size, or cheese-cloth doubled four to eight thicknesses, renders the best service. If the compress is to be greatly prolonged, a rubber bag filled with water at the proper temperature, or a rubber coil through which water at a suitable temperature is continually passed, may be applied over the compress so as to maintain the desired temperature. In addition to the compress, there may be needed a piece of flannel for covering, also in some cases, oilcloth, mackintosh, or rubber cloth, and a Turkish sheet and towel for drying the parts at the conclusion of the treatment.

Compresses may be classified according to their temperature, as: (1) *very cold* (55° or less); (2) *cool* or *cooling* (60 to 70°); (3) *warm* or *neutral* (92° to 98°); (4) *hot* (102° to 110°); (5) *very hot* (110° to 160°); (6) *alternate* (very hot and very cold in alternation); (7) *revulsive* (short cold following prolonged very hot); (8) *hot and cold* (simultaneous); (9) *hot and cold pack;* (10) *heating* or *stimulating* (applied cold, more or less protected, and prolonged until warmed by the body heat); (11) the *proximal compress;* (12) the *irrigating compress.*

These several forms of the compress produce effects so characteristic as to demand particular consideration of each as a special procedure.

THE VERY COLD COMPRESS.

1314 This application may consist of folded cloths saturated with ice-water, and changed every 4 or 5 minutes, or the low temperature may be maintained by bits of ice placed between the folds of the compress. Other methods consist in the use of the ice cap (Fig. 164), the rubber or aluminum *coil* (Fig. 165), or a specially constructed rubber sac (Fig. 166), through which a stream of water at a low temperature is made to flow continuously, a rubber bag filled with broken ice (Fig. 167), or a rubber sack containing a cooling mixture.

When ice or very cold water can not be obtained, as in many tropical countries, a very satisfactory substitute may

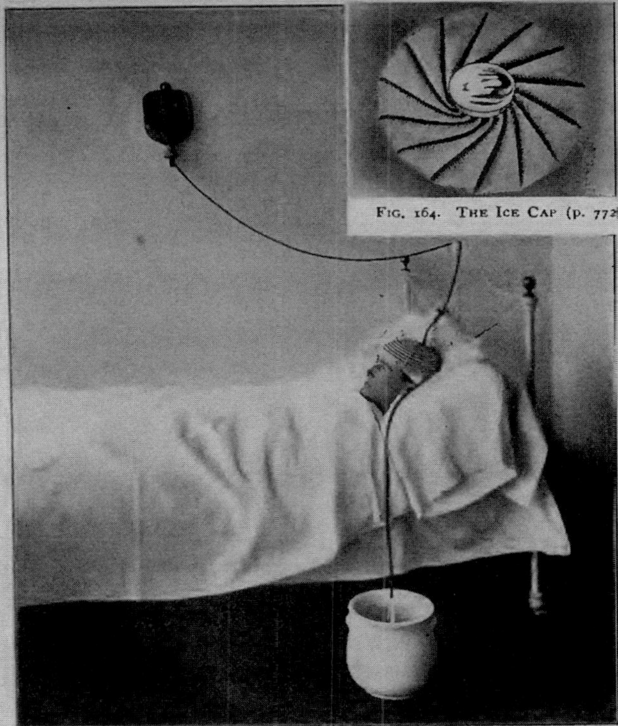

Fig. 164. The Ice Cap (p. 772).

Fig. 165. ALUMINUM COOLING COIL TO THE HEAD (p. 772).

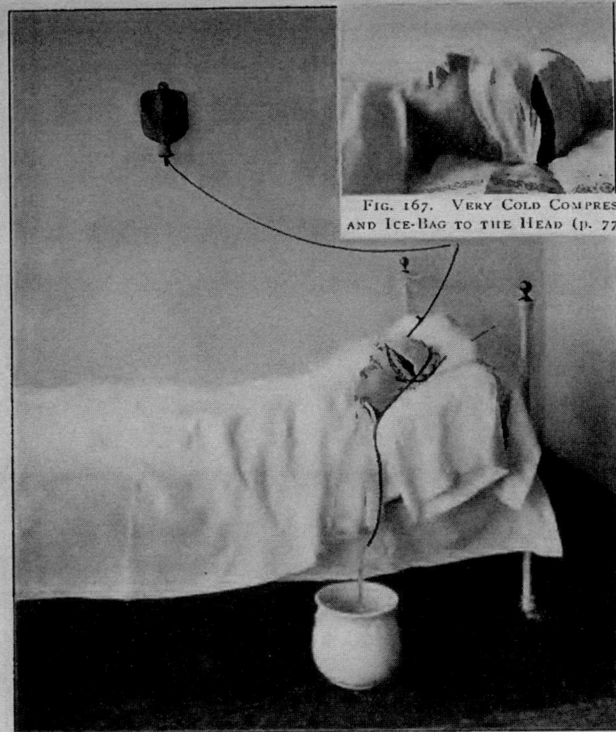

Fig. 167. Very Cold Compress and Ice-Bag to the Head (p. 772).

Fig. 166. IRRIGATING BAG TO THE HEAD (p. 772).

be found in ammonium nitrate. This chemical substance has the property of absorbing an enormous amount of heat in passing from the solid to the liquid state. By adding to a quart of water eight ounces of nitrate of ammonium, a temperature of 41° was secured, the initial temperature of the water being 70°, and the temperature of the room in which the experiment was made being 70° F.

A very intense degree of cold may be obtained by means of carbonic acid gas condensed in the form of snow, known as the "CO_2 compress." For this purpose a flannel bag is used, filled with absorbent cotton. A short pipe leading from the reservoir containing the liquid carbonic acid gas is passed into the middle of the bag, and the liquid gas is then allowed to escape. The rapid evaporation quickly fills the bag with a white snowy mass which has a temperature of —80° F. When the bag is filled, it may be slipped inside a sack made of thin mackintosh.

The cold of the carbonic acid gas compress is exceedingly intense and penetrating. In certain cases the author believes this compress has advantages which are not possessed by any other application or any other mode of utilizing cold. In application, the skin should be protected by flannel placed between it and the bag. This precaution is also necessary in most cases in the use of the ice-bag.

Schultze has shown* by numerous experiments that the deep tissues may be cooled by applications of ice to the cutaneous surface, contrary to the conclusions drawn by some other observers. According to his observations, the temperature of the tissues half a centimeter (one fifth of an inch) below the surface was found to have fallen 18° F.; at a depth of two centimeters (four fifths of an inch), the lowering of temperature was 3.6° F.; and at a depth of seven centimeters, nearly three inches, there was still a lowering of temperature amounting to nearly one-half degree. A ther-

* Joffroy, "These d' Aggregation," Paris, 1878, p. 176.

mometer applied to the internal surface of the chest in a case of thoracentesis showed a diminution of temperature of nearly 7° F. A clinical thermometer placed against the inner surface of the cheek while ice was pressed against the outer surface showed a diminution of more than fourteen degrees in temperature. A thermometer placed in the vagina indicated a fall of nearly one and one-half degrees, as the result of an application to the hypogastrium of a large bladder filled with ice (Exp. 64, 65, 66, 67).

1315 **Physiological Effects.**—These depend upon the length of the application and the part to which it is applied. A *short, very cold* compress has the effect to produce a primary contraction, followed by dilatation of the surface vessels and of the visceral vascular area in reflex relation therewith. By means of such an application, it is possible to influence the circulation in an internal viscus, to awaken vital activity, to relieve passive congestion, to encourage leucocytosis, and to increase vital resistance, as in pneumonia. The ice-water compress produces more powerful cooling effects than ice or the ice-bag, as the skin is more easily wet.

Prolonged very cold applications cause spasm of the surface vessels, together with contraction of the vessels of the reflexly related internal part, and hyperemia of collaterally related vessels.

Continuous very cold applications lower vital action, and may even suspend all vital activity in the parts cooled. The surface becomes blue from excessive absorption of oxygen from the slowed blood stream in the veins. The nerve ends are benumbed, and reflex activity between the surface and the corresponding internal area is interrupted. This effect is sometimes very useful, and may be employed to abolish reflex activity when indicated; but more frequently this effect is undesirable and contraindicated, and must be prevented by frequent removal of the cold compress, and restoration of the parts by warm rubbing or allowing an interval for reaction.

Continuous cold causes contraction of the arteries of the cooled parts; hence the value of the continuous ice-bag or poultice in the proximal compress, as in the ice-collar.

Prolonged cold applications (an ice-bag for 15 to 30 min.) over the heart slow the pulse and raise blood pressure. Continuous cold applications depress the activity of the heart.

Very cold applications made to such extremely vascular parts as the head may lower the temperature of the entire body, when carried to the extent of producing shivering.

Intense cold to the head becomes decidedly painful when prolonged. Continuous cold to the head operates somewhat differently than applications to any other portion of the body. The vascularity of the scalp is so great that the circulation is not suspended even when ice is employed. The bones of the skull are thin; and being, like other bones, good conductors, the continuous cold application to the head is capable of lowering the temperature of the brain, and by depression of the cerebral thermic centers heat production is diminished, and thus general vital activity is lessened.

A short cold application to the head (1 to 5 min.) excites cerebral activity through the reaction which follows. But by rewetting the cold application every three or four minutes, a renewed contraction of the vessels is induced at each contact of the cold water, and thus the vessels are made to contract more vigorously, and the effect of the application is more intense than if continuous, as by an ice-bag or ice-compress.

Intense cold applications, especially when made to the head, become very painful when prolonged. Such a degree of cold is unnecessary to secure the therapeutic effect desired.

Therapeutic Applications.—The *very cold* compress ren- 1316
ders valuable service in many cases, but its usefulness is small compared with that of the cool or cooling compress, which will be mentioned later. It may be usefully employed in the suppression of *local inflammation* in *joints*, *inflamed wounds*, and other conditions in which powerful sedative

effects are required. Applied to the head, it lowers the temperature in *fever*, relieves *delirium* in febrile conditions, may control excitement in *acute mania*, and renders invaluable service in *meningitis*, used in connection with the warm bath.

The ice-bag over the stomach for a half hour before meals is exceedingly useful in *anorexia*. Ice-cold applications are also of service in certain cases of *neuralgia*. Ice compresses may be applied for the relief of *inflamed hemorrhoids*. An ice-bag laid across the trunk of an artery is more effective in reducing the blood supply of the part in which the artery is distributed than an application made directly to the part itself; and an application made to the axilla, the bend of the elbow, the groin, or the bend of the knee, will control inflammation in the distal portion of the limb more effectively than a cold application to a hand or foot. The ice collar or very cold compress about the neck is a powerful means of relieving *cerebral congestion*. An ice compress over the heart lowers the general temperature by cooling the blood, while it energizes the heart. It must be removed for five minutes at intervals of 20 to 30 minutes, so as to allow reaction, thus maintaining the sensibility of the skin upon which its energizing effect upon the heart depends; or the skin may be rubbed or heat applied for one minute every 15 or 20 minutes.

A cold compress to the face and the upper spine causes contraction of the vessels of the nasal mucous membrane, and will thus control nosebleed. This measure is also useful in cases of acute and subacute *nasal catarrh*. Prolonged cold applications to the back of the neck and the face constrict the vessels of the brain, and so relieve *cerebral congestion*.

Cold compresses to the inner portion of the thighs, the perineum, the vagina, and the lumbar region cause contraction of the vessels of the uterus, and are useful in *uterine hemorrhage*, *intestinal* and *vesical hemorrhage*, *bleeding hemorrhoids*, etc. Ice-bags to the spine aid in lowering the general temperature in *fever*.

A cold compress to the thighs, perineum, and hypogastrium in conjunction with a very hot fomentation (10 min.) over the lumbar region, is a valuable means of arresting hemorrhage from the kidney when the bleeding is from small vessels and not due to malignant disease. The cold compress contracts the renal vessels, while the fomentation to the loins diverts blood from the renal circulation into the collateral vessels.

The cephalic, spinal, and cardiac compresses act in special ways in lowering temperature. The head compress lowers the temperature of the blood in the brain, and lessens the activity of the cerebral centers. The cardiac compress lowers the temperature of the blood as it passes through the heart and lungs. The spinal compress causes dilatation of the vessels of the lower extremities, and thus exercises a refrigerative effect, extending over a much larger surface than that to which it is directly applied.

Dieulafoy recommends the application of ice-bags to the whole length of the vertebral column in *ataxic* cases of *typhoid fever*. The author has made use of this measure in many cases of typhoid fever, with excellent results. In some instances, however, the alternate hot and cold spray is more effective. This measure combats the tendency to meningitis and other lesions of the cord. Care must be taken to avoid injuring the vitality of the skin.

The ice compress may be applied directly to a wound as a means of checking *bleeding*, but the compress must be large; instead of covering the wound only, it must extend over the whole part, or the greater portion of it. The circulation of a wounded part must not, however, be restricted to such a degree as to interfere with its nutrition. Hence the cold must be withdrawn as soon as possible. Pure blood is the great healing power in the body, the source of life and energy, in health and disease alike. In case of wounds of the hand or foot, the cold proximal compress may render inestimable service.

Nosebleed may be checked by the application of cloths wrung out of ice-water to the face or to the upper part of the spine.

An ice-bag applied over the stomach or to the spine opposite will often check *vomiting*, and will relieve the excruciating pain of *cancer* of the *stomach* or *chronic ulcer*.

An ice-bag or ice compress renders great service in cases of *inflamed* and *prolapsed hemorrhoids*, and affords marked relief to the pain which accompanies *ulcer* and *cancer* of the *rectum*. The pain of *orchitis* is relieved by the cold compress, the parts being supported meanwhile. It must be remembered, however, that in such cases the parts may be easily damaged by a too intense or prolonged application, the tissues being sometimes so chilled that sloughing occurs. It is only necessary to employ ordinary care and discretion, however, to prevent this. The cold applications should be continued until the parts are no longer sensitive to pressure.

The pain of toothache from *alveolar inflammation* is often more readily relieved by a cold application to the side of the neck just below the jaw, than from a hot application to the cheek. The two applications may be used simultaneously.

Dr. Chapman pointed out many years ago that the ice-bag or intense prolonged cold applications made to the back produce a sedative influence upon the spinal cord, and also upon the vasomotor sympathetic nerve centers. Dr. Chapman's idea was that this effect is to be attributed to the benumbing effect of cold resulting in lessened activity of the centers brought under its influence. According to him, an ice-bag applied to the lower portion of the spine, will dilate the vessels of the lower extremities, and increase the blood supply of the pelvic viscera. While not prepared to support all of Dr. Chapman's claims, the author has noted a number of cases in which the application of the ice-bag to the lower portion of the spine has produced a very marked effect upon the circulation of the lower extremities. A young lady, a bed-ridden invalid, who had for years suffered from cold feet and legs, noted that her limbs became warm and filled with blood within ten or fifteen minutes after the application of the ice-bag to the lower spine. The patient was first to call attention to this effect of the ice-bag as a curious and interesting circumstance. Many similar cases might be cited. When used for this purpose, the cold application should be continuous and prolonged.

Applications of ice across the neck, just above the sternum, influence the pneumogastric nerve, and will often relieve spasm of the bronchioles in *asthma* within a few minutes. Care must be used to avoid contact of cold water or ice with the chest, and heat may be used to the back of the chest.

The *ice collar* is a valuable measure in the treatment of diphtheria, the application being exchanged at intervals of 15 to 20 minutes for a very hot short fomentation. The effect of this procedure is to diminish the blood supply to the inflamed parts by its influence upon the carotid, the peripheral branches of which are made to contract by the application of cold over their trunks. A beneficial influence is also exerted by the reflex effect of the cold application upon the vessels of the affected region; and thus in two ways the blood supply of the part is diminished, and the inflammatory process controlled to a corresponding extent. In cases in which the inflammatory action is extremely intense, and after the first onset of the disease, the cooling or even the heating compress should be employed instead of the cold compress.

Applications of ice to the mucous membrane of the nose and lips have been shown by Drs. Beer and Forges, of Vienna, to be efficient in restoring respiration in cases of *asphyxia* from opium, chloroform, or other narcotics. The cold application excites the respiratory center.

By a mixture of two parts of finely pounded ice with one part of common salt, a very intense degree of cold may be produced, sufficient to quickly freeze the parts to which the mixture is applied when necessary for surgical purposes.

1317 **Contraindications and Precautions.**—If ice is used, one thickness of flannel should be placed between the ice and the skin.

In cases in which ice must be used for a long time, it is wise to withdraw the application for a few minutes at intervals of half an hour, and to make an application of very hot water from 1 to 3 minutes, as a precaution against too great depression of the vitality of the parts, or the parts may be rubbed until warm and red.

The very cold and the cold or cooling compress must be avoided in all cases in which the collateral hyperemia produced by it may do injury. This collateral effect must always be borne in mind. Examples: *Inflammation* of *muscles* and *joints;* deeply seated *abscesses* vascularly connected with the cutaneous surface; *parietal pleurisy* or *peritonitis; inflammation* of the structures of the *eyeball.*

It must also be remembered that the same reflex impulse which excites the vasoconstrictor nerves, causing vascular spasm in a deeply seated part, likewise excites all the other nerves of the part, and so may intensify pain when present. Hence the cold compress is contraindicated in most cases in which pain is a prominent symptom. The revulsive compress (1341) or the fomentation followed by the neutral or heating compress, is to be preferred in these cases.

Sometimes, however, the cold compress may be employed by combining with it a hot application, thus realizing its good effects while antidoting by means of heat its untoward effects. Examples: A hot foot bath with an ice-bag over an inflamed ovary or tube; an ice-bag to the epigastrium in gastritis, with a fomentation to the back; a fomentation to the ear and cheek in otitis media, with an ice-bag over the carotid.

THE COLD OR COOLING COMPRESS.

1318 Hippocrates was familiar with the cooling compress, employing it in the treatment of fevers by having linen cloths dipped in cold water and applied to the hottest parts, while the patient was at the same time given cold water to drink.

The temperature to be employed is 55° to 70°. For sedative effects, the compress may be changed every 5 or 10 minutes. The higher temperature may be employed when thin compresses are used, as the evaporation taking place from the surface will keep the temperature down so that reaction and dilatation of the vessels will not quickly occur, but renewal must be more frequent. The lower temperature named is greatly preferable, because of the decided effects upon the arterial trunks. After the first onset, the cold compress, changed every 20 to 30 minutes, is most useful. For the principles which govern the mode of application of the cold compress, see paragraphs **1256** to **1292**.

The compress should always cover an area larger than the part to be influenced. The recommendation of a leading physician, published in a well-known medical journal, that thin cloths four inches square be laid over the region of the appendix as a means of combating appendicitis, is a veritable travesty of hydrotherapy. The smallest viscera of the trunk requires a compress at least one foot square.

Physiological Effects.—The cooling compress has been **1319**
very carefully studied by Winternitz and Baginsky.* It is a powerfully revulsive measure, and one of the most valuable of all means of controlling, through the cutaneous circulation, the circulation of the viscera. When the cold compress is applied to the skin, causing contraction of the surface vessels, with dilatation of the deeper-lying vessels which are supplied by the same artery, the blood-vessels of the reflexly associated viscera are, through reflex influence, maintained in a state of contraction so long as the application is so managed as to avoid reaction, or so great lowering of the skin temperature as to destroy sensation, and thus abolish reflex action. When the skin becomes numb under the influence of a cold compress, the vessels of the associated vascular area dilate

* Baginsky, "Lehrbuch der Kinder Krankheiten," 1896, p. 292.

through loss of the influence of the skin reflexes, while the blood is diverted from the collateral surface vessels into the deep vessels. This is a most undesirable effect, against which the nurse or physician who makes use of cold applications must be constantly on his guard. Neglect of this precaution is responsible for failure to obtain good effects in multitudes of cases.

Sometimes the cold compress produces a tendency to general chilliness. This must be prevented by a simultaneous hot application to some surface where hyperemia of the skin will be advantageous, as to the feet or the back. If the feet are cold, the hot foot bath or hot leg pack is always indicated as an adjunct of the cold compress to the head, abdomen, or pelvis.

A prolonged cold proximal compress, that is, a cold application, as an ice-bag, placed over an arterial trunk, causes contraction of the artery and all its distal branches. A warm or hot application produces the opposite effect. This principle is especially important in relation to compresses applied to the neck, axilla, bend of elbow, groins, or popliteal space.

The effectiveness of the cool or cooling compress depends upon the continued maintenance of a moderately cool temperature, with frequent renewals, whereby continuous stimulation of the vasoconstrictors is maintained.

It must not be forgotten that the action of the cool compress involves more than its direct influence upon the nerve centers. It sets up and maintains a regular play of reflex nervous impulses between the skin and the related internal parts, through the medium of the nerve centers. When the area involved is general, the whole nervous system is excited to a most pronounced degree. This play of nervous activity is a dominant factor in the revulsive effect produced by the cold application. Through it there is produced an increase of vital work in the parts interested,—local metabolism, secretion, excretion, heat production, etc.

The most important effect of the cool compress in many

cases is the fluxion produced by it in deep parts. Fluxion is without doubt one of the most powerful hydriatic resources which we possess. The correct management of this therapeutic force is the most severe test to which an individual's knowledge of hydriatic principles and procedures can be brought (1260-1291).

Cool compresses may be employed in such a manner as to influence the circulation and the functions of the liver, spleen, stomach, kidneys, intestines, lungs, brain, pelvic viscera — in fact, all the internal structures of the body.

When used as an antithermic or antipyretic measure, the compress should cover at least one fourth of the skin area (page 316). The size of the compress may be estimated from the weight of the patient by a simple calculation based upon the proportion $180 : W :: 87 : x^{1}$, in which W represents the weight of the patient, and x the skin area. Dividing the result by four, the required size of a cooling compress for use in reducing temperature will be: for a person weighing 180 lbs., 5 sq. ft.; 120 lbs., 4 sq. ft.; 60 lbs., 2½ sq. ft.; for a child weighing 30 lbs., 1½ sq. ft., or 12 x 18 inches.

In Dr. Thompson's experiments upon dogs, published in 1320
1892, it was found impossible to lower the rectal temperature by applications to the sacrum or abdomen. In these experiments an incision was made in the abdominal wall, the bulb of a thermometer was introduced, and an ice-cold application made to the surface. The thermometer indicated no change of the temperature of the inner surface of the abdominal wall so long as the animal remained alive, though cold applications to the head produced a very decidedly cooling effect upon the brain.

The experiments of Schultze give somewhat different results, showing actual reduction of temperature from cold applications to the abdomen (1314). Nevertheless, it is doubtless true that the chief effects of the cold abdominal compress in cases of visceral inflammation, unless large enough to cover one fourth of the body surface, are obtained through its influence upon the circulation and innervation of the diseased structures by reflex action through the vasomotor centers.

The temperature of a deeply seated part is dependent upon its functional activity, and the rate of blood movement through it. The slower the movement of blood, the higher will be the temperature. Hence passive congestion favors local elevation of temperature. The active fluxion of blood through a viscus, which may be induced by the cold or cooling compress, may thus lower the temperature of the most deeply seated organs, and exercise a decided antiphlogistic influence without actually lowering the temperature of the intervening parts.

It is by this reflex influence that we are able to control inflammations in the lungs, spinal cord, stomach, liver, intestines, uterus, ovaries, and other deeply seated organs.

1321 **Therapeutic Applications.**— The cool compress may be employed in such a manner as to render invaluable service in all forms of *localized inflammatory processes*, whether superficial or deep. In superficial inflammations the compress produces vasoconstriction, and thus sedative effects are brought about as soon as the application is made. In case of visceral inflammation, the beneficial results obtained are through reflex action, the application being made to the surface which is in reflex relation with the inflamed part (Figs. 168, 169).

The compress is exceedingly useful in *typhoid fever*. It should be covered with flannel only, not with oilcloth, so that there may be little retention of heat, and so as to encourage fluxion in the mesenteric vessels and leucocytosis rather than retention of blood in the portal vessels. The object of the abdominal compress in typhoid is to encourage leucocytosis and vital resistance in the diseased structures, rather than to reduce the temperature.

Care must be taken that the application never be made in such a way as to cause numbness or even lowered sensibility of the skin, as it depends for its effects upon the main-

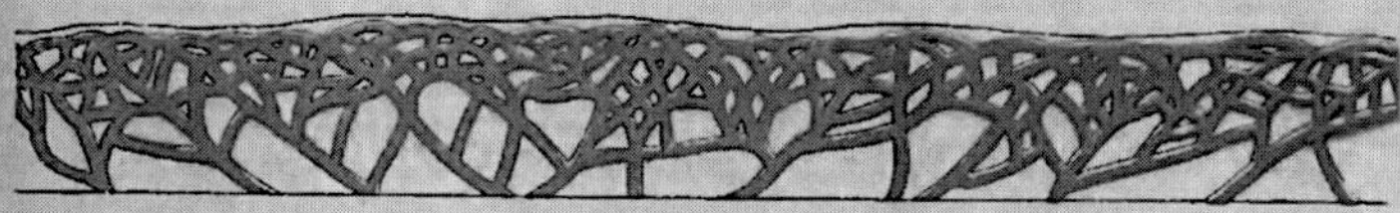

A. Congested skin.

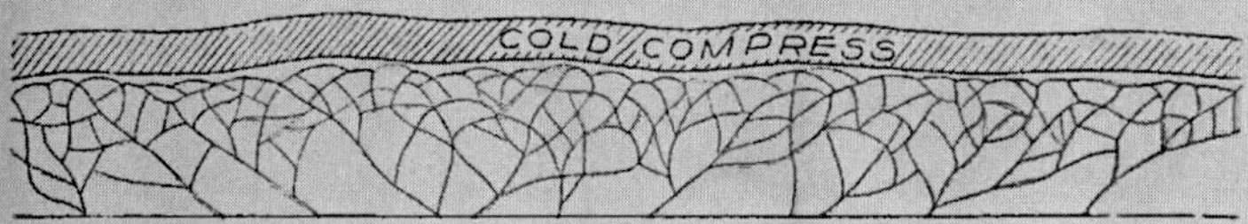

B. Cutaneous vessels contracted by cold compress.

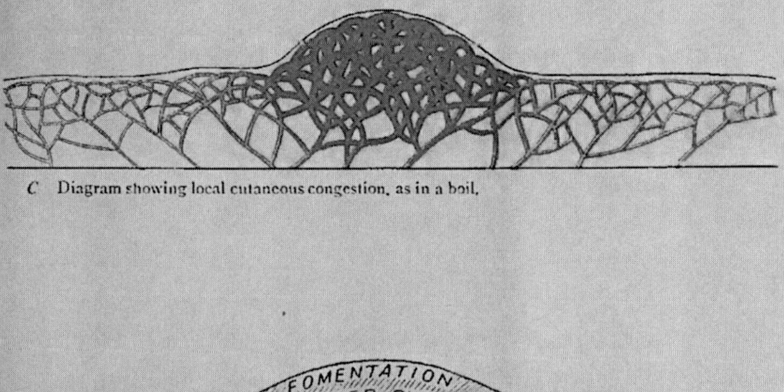

C. Diagram showing local cutaneous congestion, as in a boil.

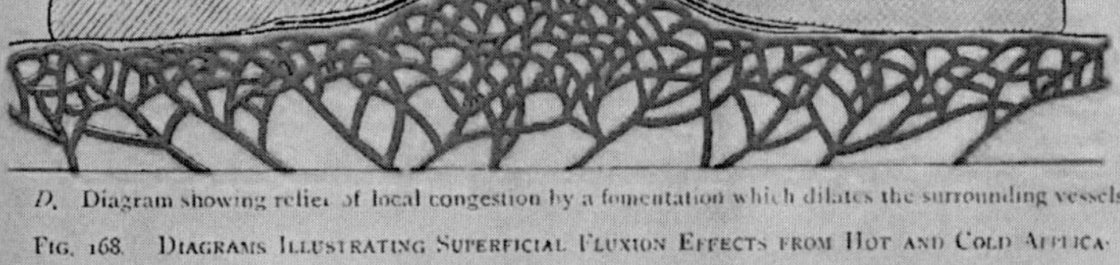

D. Diagram showing relief of local congestion by a fomentation which dilates the surrounding vessels

FIG. 168. DIAGRAMS ILLUSTRATING SUPERFICIAL FLUXION EFFECTS FROM HOT AND COLD APPLICATIONS (p. 784.)

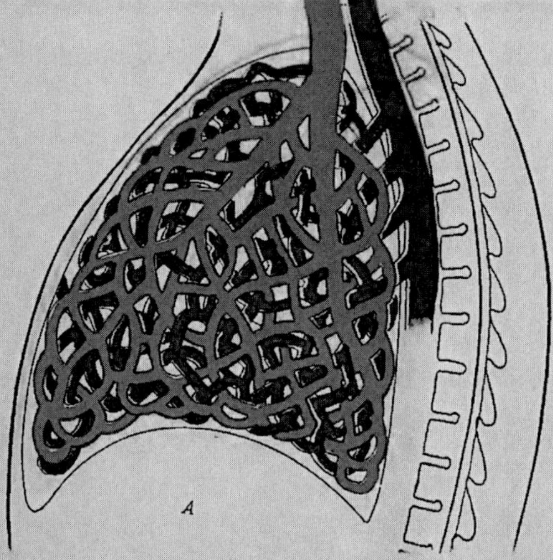

Fig. 169. Diagrams showing: *A*, Pulmonary congestion. *B*, Beneficial effects of cold chest compress. (P. 784.)

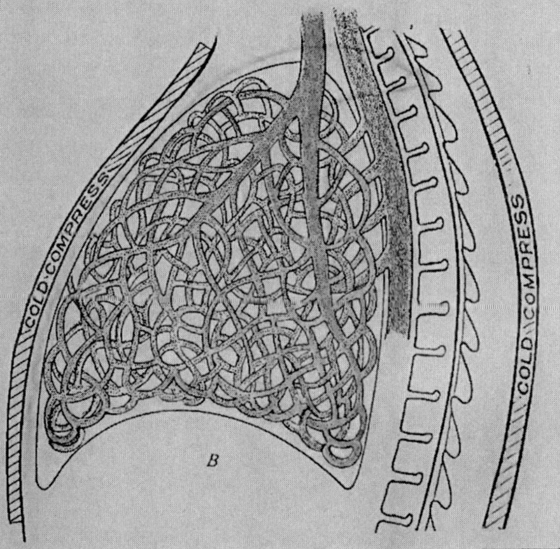

tenance of reflex activity between the skin and the viscera.

The cold compress is of greatest service in *pneumonia.* It must be applied to the whole front chest and the affected side, and changed as soon as well warmed (**1284**).

The cool compress is highly useful as an application in cases of *cardiac insufficiency,* either in fevers or as the result of disease of the heart. It is applicable in nearly all cases except those in which there is degeneration of the cardiac muscle; in *myocarditis* it is valuable, notwithstanding the affection of the muscle, for the reason that it controls, to such a remarkable degree, inflammatory processes. In cases of *erysipelas,* except when affecting the face or scalp, a cool or cold application is more serviceable than the ice compress as an antiphlogistic application.

In *dermatitis,* the cool compress is exceedingly valuable. In *inflammation of the external portions of the eye,* the cooling compress is more effective than ice-cold applications, but it is effective only when the inflammation is confined to the eyelid itself. When the eyeball is the seat of the inflammatory process, the fomentation or the revulsive compress applied over and above the eye, is the proper measure. The application should be made to the eyelid and cheek only, not extending above the eyebrow (**1262**).

Cold applications for superficial inflammations should be made as long as the parts have a bright red appearance, but a mottled blue appearance of the skin is always an indication for the application of heat, as it shows excessive contraction of the small arteries and slowed movement of blood. Such a case requires the hot compress every two hours (10 min.) with the heating compress between applications.

When renewed every 5 to 8 minutes, the effect of the cooling compress is to maintain contraction of the cutaneous vessels and simultaneous contraction of the vessels of the reflexly associated visceral vascular area. When the compress is left in place long enough for reaction to be established (15 to 30 min.), the effect is somewhat different. The reflexly associated visceral vessels are dilated, as well as those of the skin. When the application is renewed, the freshly cooled compress causes contraction of the cutaneous vessels and renewed contraction of the visceral vessels. This effect, frequently repeated, serves to maintain a vigorous circulation through the affected organ, and thus combats in the most decided manner the tendency to stagnation or passive hyperemia which is always present in visceral inflammation. This measure is consequently a most efficient means of combating *hypostatic congestion* of the lungs in surgical cases and prolonged helplessness from any cause, in resisting the action of specific bacteria in *typhoid fever*, and also renders most valuable service in the early stages of *pneumonia*. When the febrile activity is very great, the compress may be renewed as often as every 5 to 10 minutes. Later, when the activity of the inflammatory process is somewhat lessened, as shown by the slower heating of the compress, it may be left in place for an hour. The skin must be well rubbed at each renewal. In all deep-seated visceral inflammations, the same principles hold good.

The abdominal compress, frequently renewed, maintains active contraction of the mesenteric vessels. The cooling may be made continuous by ice-bags, but a more moderate temperature is, on the whole, better. This compress should be employed as a routine measure in typhoid fever, and may sometimes become the chief reliance, as in cases of intestinal hemorrhage and other conditions contraindicating the general cold bath. The cold abdominal compress was used successfully in fevers by Le Drau, of France, in 1731.

Often the patient's feelings are a good guide as to whether heat or cold should be applied. The organic intuitions of the body are marvelously correct guides in the application of rational and physiological measures. It is a common thing to hear a patient say, when a correct hydriatric prescription is made, "That will do me good, I am sure." And it does. Nature is a wise teacher and a watchful nurse.

Mays, of Philadelphia, has for several years advocated the ice-bag to the chest in pneumonia, and the results he reports * are certainly much superior to those obtained by other methods in common use. For more than twenty years the author has employed the cold compress or ice compress in the early stages of pneumonia, exchanging it every three hours for a fomentation, during the early stages of the disease, and applying the cooling compress as soon as the crisis was passed and the period of resolution begun. 1322

The prolonged application of the cold compress to the cutaneous surface produces contraction, not only of the blood-vessels of the skin, but also those of the deeper tissues underlying the area to which the application is made. This effect is reached, however, only after long application. The first effect of an application over a muscle, for example, is to cause collateral hyperemia of the muscle simultaneously with the cutaneous anemia produced.

The cold compress or ice-bag over the heart for half an hour twice a day is of great value in cases of palpitation and cardiac insufficiency. The continuous application of the ice-bag is equally serviceable in cases of cardiac irritability (**1383**). Winternitz very strongly urges the value of this procedure as a substitute for digitalis, to which it is infinitely superior. Its use is indicated by the appearance of dicrotism in typhoid fever or in depression of the heart from shock.

Contraindications.— The precautions and contraindications relating to the cooling compress are the same as have elsewhere been indicated for the very cold or ice compress (**1317**). It needs only to be added that the compress at a temperature of 60° to 70° is generally useful, while a lower temperature is often injurious.

THE COOLING COIL.

A refrigerating method much employed in Germany is the 1323
cooling coil (Fig. 170), consisting of a flat coil of rubber

* Transactions of the Philadelphia County Medical Society, 1895, p. 302.

tubing through which cold water is passed. The coil is placed over a thin wet compress. The author has devised a rubber sack (**1336**) so constructed that its walls can not become too widely separated, and provided with an inlet and outlet on opposite sides. The sack is put in place, and connected by two pieces of rubber tubing with a fountain placed at a proper level and a receiving vessel placed on the floor. By regulating the temperature of the water in the fountain and the rate of the flow, any desired heating or cooling effect may be obtained. When ice-water is used, the same water may be employed continuously, it being only necessary to dip the water back from the lower into the higher vessel as the latter is emptied and the former filled.

Therapeutic Applications.— The cooling coil is especially useful only in those exceptional cases in which continuous cold is desirable, as in *meningeal inflammation*, as a precordial application in *fever* with very high temperature and bounding pulse, and as a proximal application (**1327**) in cases of wounds of the extremities.

THE EVAPORATING COMPRESS (Fig. 171).

1324 This consists of a thin compress or other absorbent material kept moistened with water and cooled by evaporation. In the evaporation of a pound of water about 1,000 heat units are rendered latent; that is, the evaporation of a pound of water absorbs as much heat as would be required to raise 1,000 pounds of water 1° in temperature. The rate at which the water evaporates from a compress of this sort depends upon the heat of the part, the temperature of the surrounding air, and the amount of air brought in contact with it. A compress twelve inches square, covering an area of 144 square inches, may remove from the body under favorable circumstances 150 heat units in an hour; but in order that the evaporating compress may accomplish its work, it must be in direct contact with the skin, must be kept constantly moist, and must not be protected. The moistened hair

Fig. 171. EVAPORATING CEPHALIC COMPRESS (p. 788).

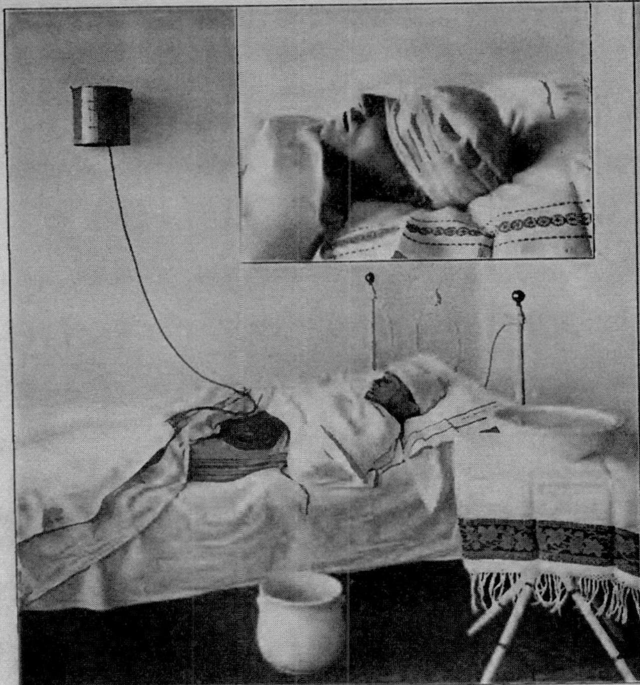

Fig. 170. ALUMINUM COOLING COIL (p. 787).

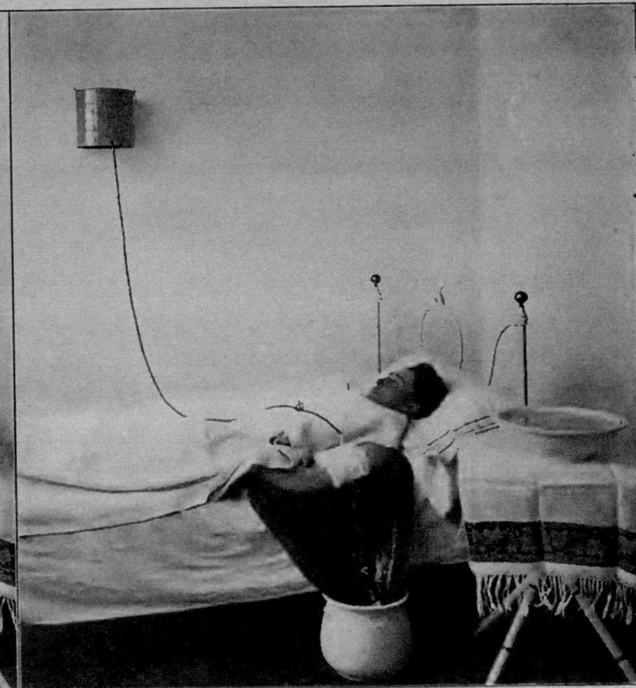

Fig. 172. IRRIGATING COMPRESS (p. 789).

serves very well the purpose of an evaporating compress to the head, but the hair must be kept wet. A moist compress laid upon the surface of the dry hair is practically without effect in cooling the head.

Therapeutic Applications.— The evaporating compress is 1325
of great value in fevers as a means of cooling the head. Benjamin Rush employed clay poultices as a cooling measure in the latter part of the last century. The evaporating compress is a most excellent means of maintaining a moderate degree of cold in cases of *erythema*, and in various conditions of *irritation* of the *skin* in which an intense inflammatory process is not present, so that more vigorous cooling measures are not indicated. The wet head-cap is a very useful measure in cases of *acute cerebral congestion*, and not infrequently proves a sovereign remedy for the *insomnia* which so often accompanies this condition. The evaporating head compress is contraindicated in rheumatics because of the tendency to cause rheumatic pains of the scalp.

THE IRRIGATING COMPRESS.

In this procedure a compress consisting of several thick- 1326
nesses of cheese-cloth or soft muslin, or a mass of absorbent cotton, having first been saturated with cold water (60°), is laid upon the part to be treated. It is kept moist by an arrangement whereby cool or cold water is made to trickle slowly upon the compress, thus keeping it saturated, and constantly changing the water which it contains, so that as fast as the water in contact with the skin becomes warm, it is displaced by that of a lower temperature. The parts treated should be so disposed as to be inclined somewhat, that the water which enters the compress at the upper end may run away at the lower end. By means of a surgical cushion or oilcloth the water may be collected as it runs away in a vessel at the side of the bed or couch. A convenient arrangement for conducting the cold water from the container to the limb is a simple siphon, as shown in Fig. 172. The tube should

be so constricted by tying a string about it or by other means that the water will flow at just the proper rate to maintain the temperature desired. If a fountain with a stopcock is employed, the flow of water may be regulated by the cock.

The *physiological effects* and the *therapeutic applications* of this procedure are the same as with the ordinary cold compress, the only difference being that by the method of irrigation the temperature of the application may be maintained at a certain point as long as desirable, and thus reaction may be easily suppressed. Irrigation is especially applicable in cases of *wounds*, *burns*, *bruises*, and other injuries in which the dressing can not be readily removed without irritating the injured surface.

Suggestions and Precautions.—It should be remembered that when a very low temperature is employed, the parts may be so devitalized by the long-continued application of cold as to be injured. Consequently a fomentation should be employed for 5 to 10 minutes once in two or three hours, to maintain proper activity of the circulation.

THE PROXIMAL COMPRESS (Fig. 173).

1327 This procedure differs from other compresses in that the application is made, not to the part which it is desired to influence, but at a point near the part and between it and the heart. It is not always convenient to apply a wet cloth to the part to be cooled. This is especially true in the case of wounds, which must be antiseptically treated, it being quite impossible to maintain asepsis with the use of the water dressing in the case of an open wound. This treatment of open wounds won great success half a century ago, before antiseptic treatment was understood, but the present method of dry antisepsis is so much superior, that this method is not to be considered in comparison with it. In many cases, however, great advantage may be gained in the relief of pain and the control of inflammation by the antiphlogistic effects of the cooling compress applied in the manner suggested. The principle on which this compress rests has a sound experimental basis. The application of cold to the trunk of an artery has been shown to cause contraction of the artery and of its distal branches (Winternitz). The clinical advantage of the application of cold in this way was well understood before the physiological explanation was experimentally discovered. Priessnitz employed the cold elbow bath for the control of inflammatory processes of the hand, and recognized the same principle in the treatment of wounds and inflammations in other parts of the body. The proximal compress may be usefully applied either by means of a cooling compress, frequently changed, at a temperature of 60° to 70°, or by means of the cooling coil or sack, or a bag filled with ice or ice-water, and protected by one or two thicknesses of flannel (Exp. 68).

The following are the most useful applications of the cold proximal compress: —

To the knee and the calf of the leg as an antiphlogistic measure for the foot.

To the whole thigh or an ice-bag to the popliteal space to influence the portion of the leg below the knee.

An ice-bag in the groin to influence the whole leg.

The cold compress around the elbow joint as an antiphlogistic measure to the hand.

An application to the whole upper arm as a measure to influence the forearm.

An ice-bag to the axilla as an antiphlogistic measure for the whole arm.

An ice-bag at the bend of the elbow as a means of lowering the temperature of the hand.

An ice collar about the neck to control congestion of the brain. This is also a most effective measure in laryngeal inflammation, and may be used in meningitis.

THE FOMENTATION (Fig. 174).

This is an application of a hot compress, usually a thick 1328
folded flannel cloth, applied a number of times in succes-

sion at a high temperature. It is essentially a local vapor bath. There is no such thing as a "cold fomentation."

Requisites.— The material for a fomentation may be a piece of an ordinary woolen bed blanket, spongiopiline, a large flat sponge, or a thick woolen cloth of any sort, or, in the absence of anything better, a thick mass of cotton cloth, as cheese-cloth, towels, etc.

The flannel cloth should be large enough so that when folded to four thicknesses, it will well cover the part to which the application is to be made. Fomentations are generally made to cover too small an area. If the affected part involves an area the size of the hand, the fomentation should cover a territory three or four times as large, as the good effect depends much upon the size of the surface to which the application is made. A pain confined to a point not larger than a finger-tip, if acute and persistent, may require for its relief an application covering one or two square feet.

In addition to the flannel used for the fomentation, a much larger dry flannel or blanket and a piece of mackintosh should be at hand to cover the moist cloth, so as to retain the heat. Two or three large towels are also needed. A supply of water at boiling heat should be ready for use. If the fomentation must be given at some distance from the source of supply, a pailful of hot water may be made to retain its heat for some little time by covering and wrapping it well with a woolen blanket or a piece of carpeting.

Method.— The proper application of a fomentation consists of the following steps: (1) Preparation of the patient; (2) wringing the flannel out of hot water; (3) renewal of the application one or more times; (4) finishing treatment. These several steps are executed as follows: —

1. The patient should lie on a bed or couch, with the part to be treated thoroughly exposed. A little vaseline or cacao butter should be first rubbed over the surface to be treated, especially when the treatment is to be given daily. The patient's clothing, and the bed-clothing should be so arranged

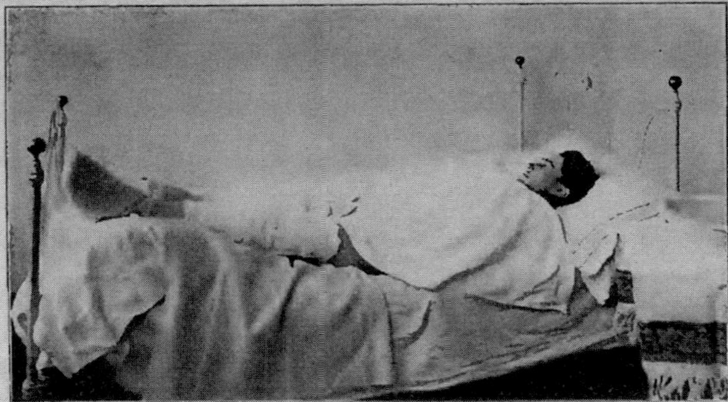

FIG. 173. PROXIMAL COMPRESS (p. 790).

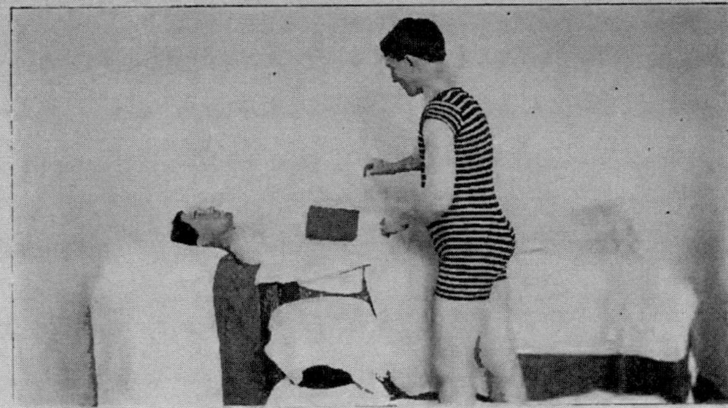

FIG. 174. FOMENTATION TO CHEST (p. 791).

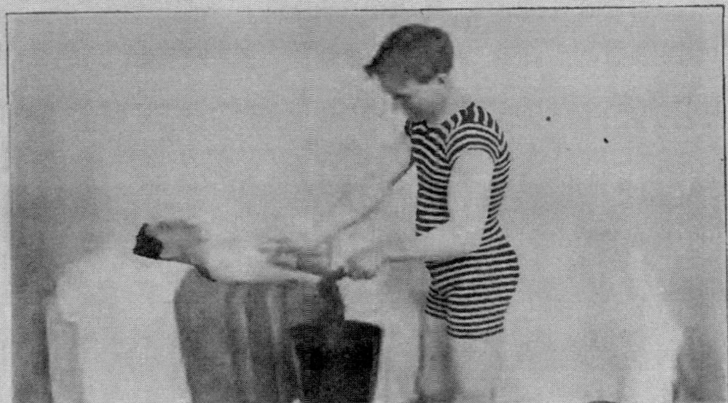

FIG. 175. WRINGING FOMENTATION CLOTH IN A TOWEL (p. 793).

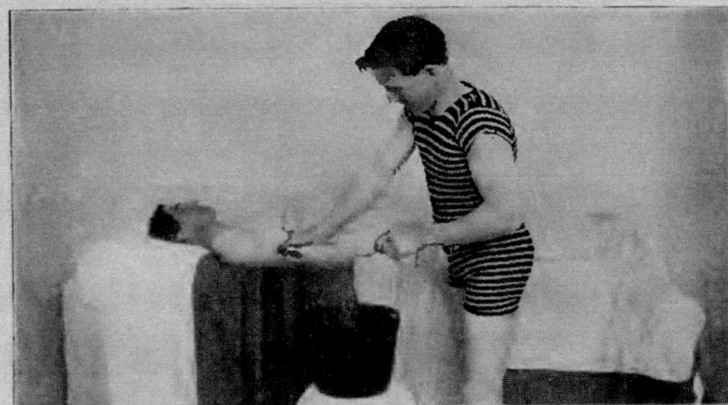

FIG. 176. WRINGING FOMENTATION CLOTH (p. 793).

that it will not be wet, as otherwise he may take cold after the treatment. Care must be taken that the extremities are warm; and if there is cerebral congestion, a cold cephalic compress (**1371**) should first be applied.

2. Unless too large, the fomentation cloth is placed in a strong towel, the towel being folded around it so as to leave the ends free; the attendant then grasps the towel by the ends, dips the whole in the hot water until completely saturated and heated to the temperature of the water, then wrings it over the pail by twisting the ends of the towel and stretching lengthwise (Fig. 175). A convenient method is partially to unfold the cloth, dip one end into the water, and fold together again in such a way that the dry portion will be on the outside. Then, by wringing, the dry part will become saturated by the absorption of water from the wet portion. By using an extra large fomentation cloth, the central portion only may be wet, leaving the ends dry to be grasped by the hands for twisting and wringing (Fig. 176).

The intensity of the application and the length of time the fomentation will retain its heat will depend upon the amount of water left in the cloth, as well as the temperature of the water. When very hot water is used, the cloths must be wrung very dry, otherwise there will be danger of blistering the patient. Another precaution which it is well to observe is to place a dry flannel next the skin, so that the heat of the fomentation may reach the skin gradually. More water may be left in the fomentation and a higher temperature may be employed when the skin is thus protected. When so intense a heat is not needed, but rather a poultice effect is desired, very soft flannel may be used and a considerable amount of water should be left in the cloth, but for this effect the temperature should not be so high as to make the application painful at first contact.

3. Ordinarily, when a mass of flannel of considerable thickness is used, the fomentation will require renewal at the end of about five minutes. When very intense heat

is required, or a thin compress is used, the renewal must be made at more frequent intervals. In other cases, a sufficient amount of warmth may be retained to last for eight to ten minutes. If desirable or convenient, a rubber bag, a bottle filled with hot water, or some other heated object, may be applied between the moist cloth and the dry covering to maintain the heat.

When the fomentation cloth is removed for renewal, the dry wrappings should be quickly replaced and the cloth wrung out of hot water and replaced as quickly as possible, so that the surface will not become chilled by evaporation, and the effect of the fomentation be thus neutralized. An excellent plan, when continuous heat is required, is to have a second cloth wrung out and ready for instant application when renewal is necessary.

4. The duration of the fomentation must depend upon various conditions, most of all upon the patient's own sensations, especially when it is applied for the relief of pain.

The beneficial effects of the fomentation should be still apparent several hours after the application. If the symptoms return after having been relieved, the application may be renewed. Occasionally, continuous application for several hours is necessary, especially in cases in which acute pain is present. So long as the pain or other urgent symptom is relieved by the application, and returns when it is removed, the application may be continued. Every half hour, however, the hot compress should be replaced by a well-wrung cold wet towel for 1 or 2 minutes.

In concluding the treatment, a cold application should always be made. This usually consists of a towel wrung very dry out of cold water—the colder the water, the better. This should be applied quickly over the whole surface which has been reddened by the fomentation, and should be retained in place for 30 to 60 seconds. It should then be removed and the part rubbed slightly, and immediately covered with dry flannel. In cases in which pain is not present, no harm could result from a more thorough cooling of the part, but it is only necessary to remove from the skin the heat which has been introduced by the fomentation. By this plan, circulatory reaction is produced and a thorough revulsive effect is secured, without producing thermic reaction, which is undesirable when either pain or acute inflammation is present. In the last class of cases it is often desirable to follow the fomentation by a cooling (**1318**) or heating (**1344**) compress, as in pneumonia, pleurisy, and erysipelas, and sometimes in acute arthritis.

Fomentations may be improvised in a great variety of ways, as the author has often had occasion to learn by personal experience. When stopping at a Western hotel some years ago, he was suddenly aroused in the middle of the night by a loud outcry, and being called to the bedside of the patient, found a young woman suffering from a distressing pain in the head. She was almost beside herself with pain, and writhed in agony as every fresh paroxysm came on. No hot water being obtainable without considerable delay, the following plan was adopted: A towel was folded and wet, then laid upon the bottom of a large dipper placed bottom upward. The inverted dipper was then held over a kerosene lamp, as close as possible to the top of the chimney without producing smoke. In two or three minutes the compress was steaming hot, and by the time the first one was cooled, another was ready for instant application. The patient experienced almost immediate relief, and in ten or fifteen minutes she was sleeping comfortably, and in the morning seemed in usual health.

In an emergency a flannel cloth or a cloth of any sort may be wrung out of cold water and wrapped around a stove-pipe or laid upon the top of a stove, or held against its side for a few seconds until heated. To prevent soiling by contact with the stove, the cloth may be placed between the folds of a newspaper; the newspaper, being moistened, will not burn.

1329 **Physiological Effects.**—The fomentation is a powerful excitant measure, stimulating tissue activity, increasing metabolism or tissue change, quickening the circulation and general nutritive processes, and encouraging absorption and repair. The excitation of the sensory, vasomotor, and sympathetic nerves produces highly important functional effects.

Fomentations, like other forms of hot applications, have not only a primary or direct *excitant* effect, but also a secondary *sedative* effect.

When applied at a sufficiently high temperature, the fomentation produces a temporary blanching of the parts from the contraction of the small vessels, which is quickly followed by relaxation or paralysis of the constrictors. When long continued at a high temperature, the vasomotor paralysis produced and the turgidity of the cutaneous structures is very pronounced, and continues for a considerable time, as shown by the dusky redness. The dilatation of the surface vessels produced by the hot application is passive in character, while cold produces active dilatation. The relaxing effect seems to influence the veins somewhat more than the arteries, thus showing the blood stream, which, with the increased rate of hemoglobin reduction (Henocque), accounts for the dusky color produced.

When applied to a cutaneous area reflexly associated with some internal part, the vessels of the latter are through reflex influence relaxed simultaneously with those of the surface. When the fomentation is thus employed to concentrate blood in any internal part, its size should be limited to that of the reflexly associated area; otherwise the derivative effect of the application may counterbalance and nullify its reflex effect.

Very hot applications lessen the sensibility of the cutaneous nerves. When applied to a reflex area, an anodyne effect is produced in deeply seated, painful parts through the thermic nerves.

The parts brought under the influence of the high temperature are, for the time being, excited to increased action.

Very soon after the application is withdrawn, however, an atonic thermic reaction occurs, as the result of which all kinds of vital activity are lowered. An examination of the blood of the part to which the fomentation has been applied for a short time shows a notable diminution in the proportion of the hemoglobin and red cells and an increase of white cells to two or three times the normal. Hot applications encourage migration of the white cells and thus leucocytosis. The actual number of blood cells in the part is, however, greatly increased because of the increased volume.

When the blood-vessels of the skin over a deeply seated part are widely dilated and filled with blood as the result of a hot application, a collateral anemia exists in the vascularly associated areas; that is, deep parts supplied by the same arterial trunk.

The effect upon the deep structures underlying the surface to which the fomentation is applied, and supplied by the same artery, is exactly the opposite of that resulting from a cold application. The dilatation of the cutaneous vessels causes contraction of the vessels in the deeper structures. It is in this way that fomentations relieve pain when applied to the skin overlying a deep part which is the seat of an inflammatory process. This explanation also applies to applications to the abdominal surface for the relief of visceral inflammations, since there is a connection between the venous circulation of the abdomen and that of the cutaneous covering of the abdomen. This fact becomes very apparent in cases of hepatic cirrhosis, by the enormous enlargement of certain cutaneous veins (1277–1279).

Through this means, heat becomes a valuable antiphlogistic measure, notwithstanding the fact that inflammatory processes are attended by an increase of heat. It is more than probable that the increase of heat accompanying inflammatory action is not simply an incidental result from the morbid process present, but is one of the methods adopted by nature for the cure of inflammatory processes or the mitigation of their evil effects. This may explain the wonderful benefit derived from the use of heat in a large number of local inflammatory processes. Recent experiments go to support the idea that elevation of the temperature of an inflamed part may sometimes serve as a valuable aid to the natural processes of defense, stimulating vital activity, and encouraging the development or the efficiency of those subtle elements by which nature renders the tissues inhospitable to the microscopic parasites upon which inflammation almost always depends.

The fomentation is one of the most efficient means of producing dilatation of the surface vessels of a circumscribed part, and thus producing local hyperemia and collateral anemia. Derivative effects are also produced by dilatation of the veins of the part to which the application is made, thus diverting the blood from the veins of some associated part. It is in this way that the portal circulation is relieved, when it is the seat of passive congestion, by large abdominal fomentations or a hot trunk pack.

1330 **Therapeutic Applications.**—Local revulsive, derivative, analgesic, and excitant effects follow the use of the fomentation. The fomentation is always indicated when it is necessary to reduce a swelling, stimulate the absorption of an effusion or an exudate, excite tissue change, increase local blood supply, promote leucocytosis, and awaken functional activity. For these purposes it is best used in alternation with the heating compress. Remote antiphlogistic and hemostatic effects are induced by derivative applications. The abdominal fomentation is indicated when the abdominal muscles are contracted. This remote effect is exceedingly valuable in cases of visceral congestion and inflammation; hence the efficacy of the fomentation in relieving both pain and congestion in *inflammation of the liver, acute* and *chronic gastritis, splenic congestion* and *enlargement, acute* and *chronic intestinal catarrh, peritonitis, ovaritis, metritis,* and *inflammatory* *affections* of the muscles and nerves, in all of which cases the application is made directly over the affected part.

The most valuable therapeutic action of the fomentation, to which its remarkable pain-relieving properties are due, is based upon its power to produce prompt and most pronounced revulsion. There is no means by which such certain, immediate, and such intense and efficient, revulsive effects may be produced, as through the dilatation of the cutaneous vessels under the influence of moist heat.

The methods by which hot applications may be best employed for the relief of congestion and inflammation of the brain, the lungs, the liver, and other internal organs, have been pointed out in preceding paragraphs (**1260–1292**).

In case of *acute inflammation* involving the surface structures, the fomentation may be usefully employed for a short period (5 or 10 min.) at intervals of two or three hours, cool applications being employed in the interim. By this means the analgesic and sedative effects of the hot applications are obtained.

Hot applications are perhaps most frequently employed **1331**
for their analgesic, or pain-relieving, effects, for which they certainly afford a most efficient resource. The analgesic effects of heat are obtained chiefly through its revulsive effects, which have been previously explained (**667–678**). For the best results, the application must be made at a very high temperature, the compress being hot enough to cause slight pain when first brought in contact with the skin. Its actual temperature should be from 140° to 160°. There will be little or no danger of burning the patient, provided the compress has been wrung as dry as possible, and the skin has been carefully covered with vaseline, and protected by a single thickness of flannel. When these precautions are observed, the hot water does not come in actual contact with the skin, but only the highly heated air or vapor, the fomentation thus becoming really a local vapor bath.

As an analgesic, the fomentation generally gives magic

relief. The fomentation may be applied in nearly all conditions in which pain is present, whether of functional or organic origin. Its powerful derivative effects often afford temporary relief even in maladies which are incurable. There is no more effective means than the fomentation for the relief of pain from *strain* or *sprain* of joints and muscles, and other injuries in which the skin is unbroken. It may also render very valuable service in the relief of pain and relaxation of tense tissues in cases of *dislocation* and *fracture* of *bones*, thereby greatly facilitating the adjustment of the displaced parts. The author has made it a practice for more than twenty years to administer a fomentation just before applying the dressing in a fresh fracture, unless the patient presented himself immediately after the injury. The effect is greatly to mitigate the patient's suffering, as well as to prevent subsequent swelling, and thus facilitate healing. The fomentation should be applied after the bones have been restored to position; or if the parts are so swollen and sensitive as to make it difficult to manipulate them, fomentations may be applied for 20 to 30 minutes before any attempt is made to readjust the bones to their normal position. Heat relaxes, or rather causes expansion of, the white fibrous tissue of the joint ligaments. By the use of the fomentation in this manner, the administration of an anesthetic may often be avoided.

For the relief of *chronic pains*, the pain from *gall-stones*, *renal calculi*, *hepatic pain*, *infectious jaundice*, and for *neuralgias* and other painful affections of the joints, the fomentation is of immense service, if applied thoroughly. In the painful conditions often present in *hyperpepsia*, a fomentation applied half an hour after meals, or when the pain begins, affords great relief. The applications should be very hot, but not very long continued, as continuous heat over the abdomen after meals is an exciting measure.

1332 A very short fomentation over the heart is useful in *collapse* under *anesthesia*, in *opium poisoning*, and in cases of heart failure due to other causes. The application should be followed by a cold compress or an ice-bag, which should be left in place for half an hour, when the hot application may be renewed for a few minutes if necessary.

For diseases of the *eyeball*, very hot applications to the eye, avoiding the cheek, but extending over the brow, afford great relief, and greatly facilitate recovery (**1264**).

The fomentation may be applied to the whole head for the relief of *headache* due to *anemia* of the brain, a condition generally found present in neurasthenia, and indicated by a sense of weight or pressure, while the face is pale and the pulse feeble.

The pain of *toothache*, *migraine*, and *earache* is greatly mitigated, if not wholly relieved, by fomentations. Care must be taken to confine the application to the face. If the hot compress extends to the neck below the jaw, the congestion will be increased by dilating the common carotid. It is for this reason that cold applications often relieve a painful affection of the jaw more readily than heat, by causing reflex contraction of the deeper vessels. In such a case still better effects will be obtained by applying the ice-bag or cold compress lower down or below the jaw, so as to contract the large vessels of the neck simultaneously with the fomentation to the face or the side of the head. The very best effects are obtainable by revulsive applications (**673, 1041, 1341**).

In cases of *hyperesthesia* of the solar plexus and the umbilical ganglia of the abdominal sympathetic, the fomentation not only relieves the local distress, but also a great number of reflex symptoms which have their origin in sympathetic nerve disorders, such as *cold hands* and *feet*, *giddiness*, *pain* in the loins, between the *shoulder-blades*, in the *back*, of the *neck*, and various other *reflex neuralgias*, *paresthesias*, and *vasomotor disturbances*.

Farquharson recommends fomentations to the anal region in *incontinence* of urine when of spinal origin, and especially when due to a sort of chorea of the lumbar cord.

Fomentations to the throat are of great value in *inflammatory affections* of the *larynx*, *fauces*, and *tonsils*, through the strong revulsion which they produce, diverting the blood away from the internal parts to the skin. The application should be continued for 15 to 20 minutes; then the cooling compress (**1318**) should be applied for an hour or two, when the fomentation should be renewed. Hot compresses are applicable in *croup*, both true and false, but especially in false croup, in which they always afford relief. In *true croup*, it aids, to some degree at least, in the loosening of the obstructing membrane; and in *false croup*, the fomentation causes relaxation of the contracted air passages by relieving the irritation which gives rise to the disease. After the fomentation, the heating compress should be applied.

The fomentation is exceedingly useful in combination with cool or cold compresses in many cases, as for example, to the throat in *diphtheria* and *tonsillitis*, and to the chest in *pneumonia* and *pleurisy*. The application should be applied for 5 to 10 minutes at a temperature as high as can be borne.

In *ulcerations* and *inflammations* of the *cornea*, in *pannus*, *iritis*, and in affections of the deeper parts of the eyeball, hot applications render great service. The application should not be continued for more than 15 to 20 minutes at a time, however, and should be followed by very short cold applications lasting for 10 to 15 seconds, after which the parts should be covered with warm cotton or flannel to prevent cooling by evaporation, or a neutral compress (96° to 98°) may be applied. The neutral compress must be changed every 10 to 15 minutes to prevent elevation of temperature through accumulation of heat, whereby the stimulating effects of the poultice will be produced; it should also be covered with dry flannel or oilcloth to prevent cooling by evaporation. The compresses should be applied over the eye and the forehead just above, rather than to the cheek.

Fomentations to the *spine* may be applied in fever as a means of stimulating the spinal centers, especially the sweat centers, and warming the surface, thus increasing heat elimination.

Fomentations over the *abdomen* relieve the *painful tympanitis* of typhoid fever; and in peritonitis and inflammatory processes of the *pelvis* they not only relieve the pain, but lessen the inflammatory process by bringing the blood to the surface, and contracting the distended vessels of the affected internal part. The atonic reaction which follows hot applications also aids in combating the inflammation.

In the case of *pelvic* and *abdominal inflammations*, a hot hip pack or hot trunk pack is, however, generally much more serviceable than the simple application of a fomentation, since a larger surface is rendered hyperemic, thus diverting more blood from the abdominal or pelvic viscera.

In all forms of *gastric pain* the fomentation is an invaluable remedy. It must cover the area from the fourth rib to the umbilicus, and between the two axillary lines.

The cold compress to the epigastrium in combination with the dorsal fomentation produces most happy effects, acting reflexly to contract the gastric vessels while the fomentation drains them by dilating the intercostal veins (1362).

In the early stages of *erysipelas*, and also of *meningitis* of the brain and cord, the fomentation is of great service. It relieves pain in both classes of cases. In *meningitis* it likewise acts as a derivative and an antiphlogistic through the atonic reaction induced. The application of heat should not be continued more than 3 to 5 minutes, and should be followed by a continuous cold application.

Very hot applications (135° to 160°) are exceedingly serv- 1333
iceable in cases of swollen internal *hemorrhoids* or prolapsed rectum, with large external hemorrhoids. The water should be applied as hot as can possibly be borne, by means of a soft cheese-cloth or sponge. The application should be continued for 15 or 20 minutes, when the hemorrhoids, if internal, should be gently pressed up into the bowel, to avoid strangulation by contraction of the sphincter muscle, and a cold compress

should be applied. If the bowel, or hemorrhoids, can not be reduced, the hot applications should be renewed for 10 to 15 minutes every hour, the cold compress being continued during the intervals.

The fomentation should be employed on the same plan in *orchitis*, *acute inflammation* or *congestion* of the *ovaries*, *uterus*, and *kidneys*, and in *prostatitis*, *proctitis*, and *vaginitis* when accompanied by much pain. In *inflammation* of the *bladder* the cold compress must be omitted, the parts being simply kept warm.

The hot fomentation to the perineum is indicated in *inflammation* of the *prostate*.

Hot applications over the hypogastrium, thighs, and the vulva and perineum are likewise indicated in *inflammations* and other painful affections of the *uterus* and *ovaries*.

Intercostal neuralgia, *pleurodynia*, *lumbago*, *sciatica*, and other pains of similar character may generally be made to vanish as if by magic under the potent influence of the fomentation vigorously applied. *Hemicrania*, being an acute toxemia, in most cases, at least, is more obstinate, but is often greatly relieved.

In *neuralgia* and *acute articular rheumatism*, in which the application of cold as a finishing measure may cause a return of the pain, the parts may be allowed to cool gradually, by leaving the last fomentation cloth in place for 15 or 20 minutes, or until it has become nearly of the temperature of the skin. It should then be removed, the part dried and gently rubbed, then covered with a warm dry soft flannel folded to several thicknesses.

The accompanying cuts (Figs. 149, 150) show at a glance the areas over which hot applications should be made for relief of the most common localized painful affections and for combating congestions in the internal viscera by means of derivative measures. Further details respecting the methods of controlling the visceral circulations have been given elsewhere (**1260–1291**).

In *pneumonia, pleurisy*, and *acute bronchitis*, the fomentation is an invaluable remedy. In the acute stage of the disease, fomentations should be employed only for short periods, the cool compress or the ice-bag being applied in the interval, changing every 20 minutes for the fomentation.

In pneumonia, cold or cool compresses should be applied immediately after the removal of the fomentation, which should be renewed at intervals of one, two, or three hours.

In *pulmonary congestion* from any cause, fomentations to the chest often render important service, relieving pain and diverting the blood from internal to external parts, thus lessening the congestion of the diseased lung. In making the application, the region of the heart should be avoided if possible. The application should be made to the whole chest or to the back and sides especially **(1270)**.

A fomentation to the back of the chest accompanied by a cold compress to the front (the hot and cold compress **(1356)**, is perhaps the best of all means of combating passive pulmonary congestion. By means of the fomentation the bronchial vessels are drained into the skin, while the cold compress stimulates contraction of these vessels by reflex action.

In cases of *hemorrhage* of the *lungs* a very hot fomentation may be applied to the upper part of the spine and back of the neck in connection with the cold chest compress. The application should be very short (3 to 5 min.), and should be repeated every 15 minutes.

In the application of heat for derivative effects upon a lung, an ovary, or other viscus, the temperature should be high enough to cause a painful sensation of excessive heat, or as high as possible without actually injuring the skin. Thus the reflex effect of sharp irritation of the cutaneous nerves will be obtained, with contraction of the vessels of the part which it is designed to influence, and the collateral anemia which it is desirable to establish by diversion of blood to the skin, will be aided by excitation of the vasomotor centers.

Very hot fomentations should be applied in the early stage of *boils*, not only for the relief of pain, but to stimulate the vital activities whereby the disease may be aborted. Fomentations promote suppuration in fully developed boils, or "bring them to a head," as the laity say, but it is exceedingly questionable whether under any circumstances the suppurating process should be encouraged. If pus is present, it should be reached as quickly as possible by means of the surgeon's knife, and antiseptic treatment should be applied at once. Fomentations are, however, exceedingly valuable in these cases, notwithstanding the wrong theory of their use; for if applied early enough, suppuration may be averted by the stimulation of the vital activities of the tissues, and the increased fluxion of healthy blood through the infected parts. During the painful stage, when pus is forming, very short hot applications afford relief by producing strong revulsion, distributing the blood to surrounding parts. The common practice of applying hot poultices to boils is uncleanly and inconvenient, and has no advantages over moist heat derived from fomentations with soft and easily moistened fabrics, as the hot cotton poultice.

The moist heat of a fomentation, properly managed, affords more relief than any other measure in cases of *rheumatic pains* in either muscles or joints. The fomentation should be applied all about the joint, and should also cover the limb for several inches above and below the joint, if possible. These applications may all be made several times daily. During the day it is best to follow the fomentations with dry coverings to protect the joints, and at evening the application, made just before the patient retires for the night, may be followed advantageously by the heating compress. The latter should be made of soft, very thin-material,—four to six thicknesses of cheese-cloth, — and covered with oiled muslin or some other water-proof material, then with a thick layer of wool or cotton, and several layers of woolen bandage outside of all.

Very hot applications made to the upper part of the neck

or back of the head, also the top of the head and the face, constitute one of the most efficient means of relieving *cerebral congestion.* This measure is especially useful in that form of congestion or hyperemia of the brain due to overwork. *The temperature should be 135° to 140°, or high enough to induce slight pain at the beginning of the application. A lower temperature than this has the effect to produce slight congestion in a normal brain, or to increase the congestion when the blood-vessels are overdistended.* The compresses should be light, and should be renewed every two or three minutes. Two compresses are required for applications of this sort, so that when one is removed, a freshly heated one may be applied instantly, allowing no time between for cooling of the surface by evaporation. The sensation of weight and pressure at the back of the head, of which anemic neurasthenics often complain, and which commonly results from excessive mental work, loss of sleep, and other exhausting influences, generally yields promptly to these applications.

Light, very hot fomentations are exceedingly useful in nearly all forms of nervous headache, whether occipital or frontal. The compresses should not be large or heavy, and should be frequently changed.

In cases of low-pressure headache (anemia of the brain) relief is best obtained by the heating compress to the head and by moderately warm applications around the neck, whereby the blood supply of the brain is increased.

In cases of great *loss of blood,* fatal syncope may be prevented by making moderately hot applications to the head, and so encouraging the circulation of blood in the brain. The application should be made especially to the neck and the top of the head. Hot applications made to the face alone, or to the sides of the head or the occiput, might temporarily decrease the volume of blood in the brain. Very hot applications may also momentarily increase the anemia.

For *indigestion, colic, suppression of urine, constipation* accompanied by abdominal pain and tenderness, *torpid liver,* and *dysmenorrhea*, the very hot fomentation is a remedy of great value, and may be used with brilliant results. The efficiency of this measure in relieving *sick-headache* is unrivaled, the applications being made to the spine, head, neck, or stomach.

When employed to relieve suppression of the urine from *congestion* of the *kidneys* or in *acute nephritis*, the fomentation should cover the whole central and lower part of the back, extending well around to the sides. The application should be as hot as the patient can bear, for 10 minutes, and should then be followed by cold friction for 1 minute, the parts being afterward well protected by dry flannel. The procedure may be repeated every 30 minutes. If the patient has good power to react, the heating compress may be applied instead of cold friction, and may be left in place until the following application of heat.

In *hysteria*, very hot fomentations may with great advantage be applied over the hysterogenous zones when pain is present.

Dr. Noir, a French physician, a few years ago pointed out the fact that very hot applications are of great value in the treatment of *herpes circinatus*, the applications being made daily, at a temperature of 122°. When the disease affects the scalp, bichloride of mercury should be added to the water employed for the fomentation, in the proportion of one part to two thousand. It is well in some cases of this kind to make the bichloride application continuous by means of layers of gauze saturated with the solution and covered with oiled muslin.

Very hot water (140° F.) is wonderfully successful in the treatment of *acne* of the *face*. For many years the author has made use of hot applications to the face in the form of the hot spray or small hot fomentations, or hot water applied by means of a soft sponge, in cases of this sort. The temperature required is about 140°. The greatest inconvenience in the use of this remedy for acne is the fact that the effect of the hot water can not be confined to the diseased parts. In order to avoid this objection, the author has had made a simple device for applying moist heat to acne, which he finds very convenient. It consists simply of a conical, hollow copper cone (Fig. 177), furnished with a handle. The cylinder is closed with a small cork, and the point covered with a small mass of moist cotton. Being filled with boiling water, and the cork placed so as to prevent spilling, it is ready for use. The cotton-covered tip is moistened, then applied to each pimple or blotch, and held there for one or two seconds, or as long as the heat can be endured. By this simple device, the applications can be made in rapid succession, and to the diseased structures alone. The application should be renewed at least twice a day, each pimple being touched from four to six times at each sitting.

Fomentations have been successfully used for the relief of *irreducible hernia*.

The fomentation to the spine or abdomen may be used as a heating measure preparatory to a general cold procedure. Used in connection with cold wet friction, it aids in lowering the temperature in febrile conditions accompanied by diminished heat elimination.

It is impossible to enumerate all the morbid conditions in which the fomentation is found useful. We might mention, further, the following: *Hysteria*, *hysterical anorexia*, *leptomeningitis*, *spinal irritation*, *acute chorea*, *chorea major*, *general tic*, *paralysis agitans*, *tetany*, *occupation neuroses*, *angioneurotic edema*, *scleroderma*, *muscular contraction*, *alcoholism*, *delirium tremens*, *morphinism*, *cocainism*, *lead poisoning*, *heat stroke*, *dermalgia;* over the liver and spleen in *malarial fever;* as a means of relieving *abdominal pain* occurring during *gestation;* as an application to the abdominal surface in *parturition;* as a *spinal*, *cardiac*, or *cephalic application* in *collapse* or *shock;* in *retinitis*, *keratitis*, *chronic granular conjunctivitis*, *typhus*, *typhoid fever*, *the plague*, *smallpox*, *scarlet fever*, *influenza*, *chronic dysentery*, *miliary fever, febricula, locomotor ataxia, diabetes, chronic gastritis, tuberculosis* of the *lymph glands, Weil's disease, lithemia, increased peristalsis, gastric ulcer, cholera morbus, cholera infantum, Asiatic cholera, appendicitis, torticollis, ascending paralysis, Bell's palsy, Meniere's disease, paralysis* of the *circumflex nerve, myelitis, anterior poliomyelitis.*

The thorough application of the fomentation two or three times a day for a week or two preceding an abdominal operation, in cases in which chronic or subacute peritonitis is present, aids much in preparing the patient for safe transit through the perils of the operation. The operation should not be delayed, however, when urgently indicated.

The hot compress has many uses in connection with other procedures, particularly the cold compress in producing analgesic, revulsive, and derivative effects.

1334 **Contraindications and Precautions.**—1. The fomentation has been greatly abused. When this procedure gives rise to profuse and weakening general perspiration, it should be discontinued, and hot sponging substituted. The temperature of the water in hot sponging may be some degrees higher than that used for the fomentation, for the reason that a smaller area of the skin is involved in the treatment at a given moment.

2. It is generally wise to follow the fomentation by a very brief application (4 to 30 sec.) of cold by means of a compress wrung very dry out of cold water.

3. Great care must be exercised in the use of the fomentation to avoid damage to the skin in cases of paralysis or diminished sensibility.

4. When used for the relief of neuralgic pain, as sciatica, toothache, and nervous headache, and also when employed for the purpose of producing remote vasomotor effects, as for the relief of congestion of the liver, in hyperesthesia of the lumbar ganglia of the abdominal sympathetic, in cases of chronic gastritis, pelvic inflammation, and in similar conditions, the heat of the fomentation should be as great as can

be borne without injury to the skin, and sufficient to produce slight pain when the application is first made.

5. As the fomentation usually produces more or less perspiration, care should be taken to protect the patient after the removal of the fomentation, and in most cases a tepid or cool shower, towel, or sponge bath is advisable. When for any reason a cold application can not be made, the patient should be wiped dry with a soft towel, and covered sufficiently to prevent chilling; but the covering should not be so warm as to induce continued perspiration.

6. In cases in which the fomentation is applied for the relief of an acute inflammatory condition in which the part affected is so situated that the application comes in immediate contact with it, it must be very brief (not more than 5 to 10 minutes) repeated at intervals of two or three hours, cold compresses being applied during the interval. In case the inflammatory affection is situated in an internal viscus, the application may be continued for half an hour, or even for a longer period, provided there is not at the same time a considerable general elevation of temperature. The reason for this will be apparent when it is considered that heat is directly stimulating; and while heat may be briefly applied directly to the inflamed parts, as a means of relieving pain, a long-continued application might result in stimulating the inflammatory process. When the inflamed part is more deep-seated, however, the heat of the fomentation does not reach the diseased part, but its blood-vessels are made to contract through the influence of the heat upon the vasomotor nerves, and through the induced collateral hyperemia.

7. In some painful affections, especially when the skin is in a state of hyperesthesia, the application of intense heat aggravates the pain as well as other symptoms. In such cases more moderate heat — neutral or even cold or heating compresses — should be employed.

8. It should be remembered that if a fomentation is left in contact with the part long enough to allow the temperature

to fall very considerably, an effect the very opposite from that desired may be induced.

9. Vaseline should be freely applied to the skin before the fomentation, when the latter is employed daily.

10. The fomentation must be avoided, or, if employed at all, only with great care and for short periods (5 to 10 minutes), when the abdominal walls are relaxed and the intestines distended with gas, since the natural effect of heat is to increase these conditions.

THE HOT-WATER BAG (Fig. 178).

1335 Heat, either with or without accompanying moisture, may be applied by a variety of other methods, as by means of a rubber bag filled with hot water. The exact effect of the fomentation may be secured by wrapping a hot bag with a moist flannel cloth. Hot bricks, bottles filled with hot water, and other heated objects may be used in a similar manner when it is desirable to employ heat for a considerable time.

Dr. Chapman recommended the use of a hot bag to the spine, the effect being, he claimed, to stimulate the sympathetic nerve centers, and thus diminish the size of the small vessels throughout the body. He insisted that the temperature of the application to the spine should not be higher than 120°. I have for twenty years made use of the spinal hot bag, and had constructed for the purpose a rubber bag somewhat broader and longer than that of Chapman. The application is made not to the spine, but to the back, and hence should cover a sufficiently broad area to bring under the influence of heat a considerable portion of the cutaneous branches of the posterior spinal nerves. The results to be obtained are due, not to the action of heat upon the nerve centers, but to reflex and fluxion effects.

THE SYPHON HOT-WATER BAG.

1336 The syphon bag (Fig. 179) devised by the author some twenty-two years ago is a convenient method for applying

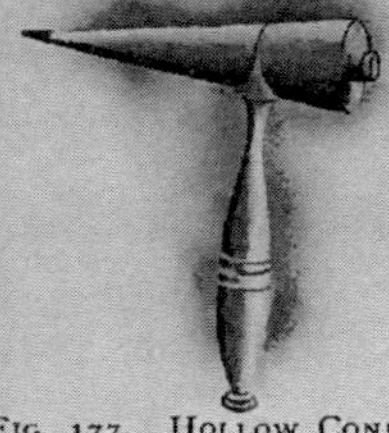

Fig. 177. Hollow Cone for Acne (p. 809).

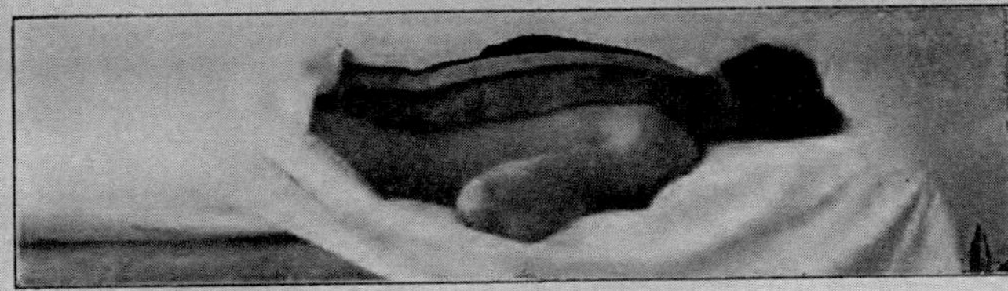

Fig. 178. HOT-WATER BAG (p. 812).

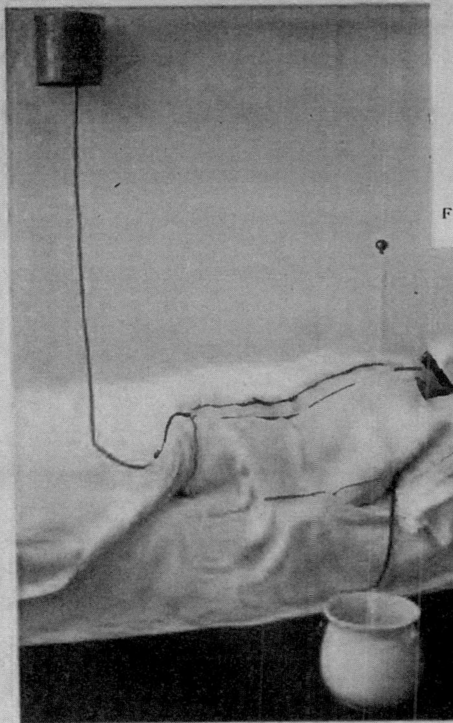

Fig. 179. APPLICATION OF SIPHON BAG TO SPINE (p. 812).

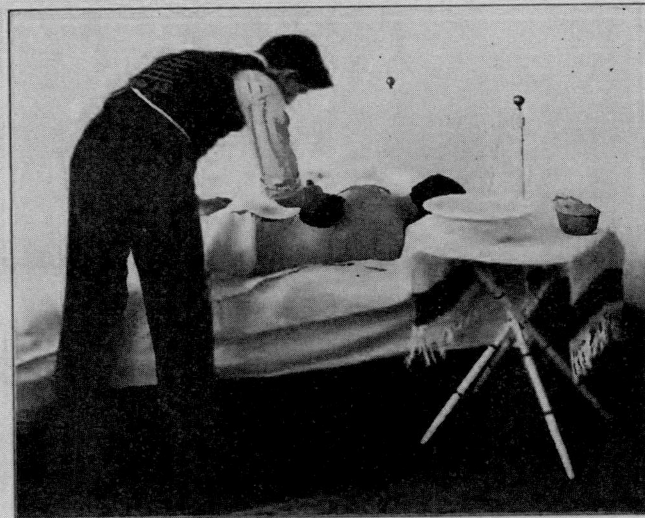

Fig. 180. (*a*) ALTERNATE APPLICATIONS TO SPINE (p. 822).

either heat or cold continuously. It is used in precisely the same manner as the cooling or heating coil (**1323**). The device consists of a bag, the sides of which are connected to prevent excessive bulging, and with an opening at either end. A tube connected with one end of the bag communicates with a fountain, either in the ordinary manner or on the syphon principle. Another tube connects the opposite end of the bag with a receptacle at the bedside. The flow of water is easily regulated by means of a proper stopcock, or simply by tying a string about the outlet tube. By means of a series of bags properly constructed for fitting different parts of the body, either heat or cold may be continuously applied in a most effective manner, and the temperature may be perfectly regulated. The author has had prepared bags of different shapes, which are adapted to use for different parts of the body. He prefers the bag to the coil for the reason that the amount of non-conducting material between the water and the patient is less. The bag also fits the surface more smoothly and completely than does the coil, and is more uniformly heated.

THE THERMOPHORE.

This is a rubber bag containing a quantity of a chemical **1337**
compound which acquires the property, after being heated for a definite time, of giving off heat at quite a uniform rate for several hours,—from two or three to ten hours, according to the conditions. Wrapped with a moist flannel, the thermophore makes an excellent continuous fomentation. Without the moist covering, it constitutes a most convenient and serviceable means of applying dry heat for any desired therapeutic purpose. In preparation for use the bag is immersed in boiling water for some minutes, until the contents are liquefied.

The thermophore is especially indicated in cases in which continuous and long-continued heat is necessary.

THE MUSTARD FOMENTATION.

1338 This measure consists of an ordinary fomentation in which mustard is added to the water employed in the proportion of a tablespoonful of ground mustard to the quart of water. It is not necessary to prepare a large quantity of water. One quart of boiling water into which a tablespoonful of mustard has been thoroughly stirred, and steeped for a few minutes, should be poured upon the fomentation cloths placed in a basin or pail.

The effect is that of the fomentation intensified by the addition of the chemical irritation of the mustard.

The mustard fomentation is especially applicable to cases in which a very quick and strong revulsive effect is desired, as for the relief of severe pain, or to secure strong derivative effects. Care must, however, be taken to avoid excessive irritation or blistering of the skin.

THE NEUTRAL COMPRESS.

1339 This is a compress at 92° to 97°, its temperature being so nearly that of the skin that neither thermic nor circulatory reaction is produced. Its effects are simply those of a poultice. The sensibility of the cutaneous nerves is lessened by the imbibition of moisture, as in the neutral bath. The surface covered by the compress is protected from external irritants of all sorts. A quieting effect is thus exerted upon that portion of the interior of the body which is in reflex relation with the cutaneous surface treated.

Therapeutic Applications.—The neutral compress is by no means so useful as the cool or the cold compress, but nevertheless renders extremely valuable service in special cases. It is useful as an application to the spine in *locomotor ataxia*, especially as a means of relieving *lightning pains*. When applied to the spine for this purpose, it should cover the whole lower half of the back. It may be usefully applied over the abdomen in cases of *hyperesthesia* of the skin due to an irritable condition of the abdominal sympathetic centers. It may *replace the poultice* in all cases in which this old-fashioned measure might be profitably employed. It should be remarked, however, that the use of a poultice or any substitute for it as a means of encouraging suppuration is not in harmony with the principles of modern rational medicine. The retention of the body heat encourages the growth of the pathogenic microbes, causing the diseases together with the toxins.

The neutral compress may be usefully employed as a soothing application for *painful wounds*, and in *dermatitis*, when the acute stage of the inflammatory process is past. The addition of an antiseptic of some sort in very small proportions is often useful in preventing the development of micro-organisms, which is favored by the compress.

The heating compress applied after a fomentation is useful in relieving the excrutiating articular pain of *acute rheumatism*. As the compress is rather lightly covered, and with flannel only, the neutral rather than the stimulating effect is obtained. The same measure renders valuable service in cases of *sprain*, joint injury from *dislocation*, *chronic inflammation* of the joints, and even in cases of *tuberculosis* of the joint.

The neutral compress sometimes proves more serviceable in relieving the pain of *neuralgia* in certain cases than either hot or cold applications. The temperature should be about 95°, or as near that of the body as possible. It operates simply by excluding irritation, preventing contact with the air, and filling the tissues with water, whereby the nervous sensibility is diminished. It is especially indicated in cases of neuralgia affecting nerves very near the surface, as in *dermalgia* and the neuralgia following *herpes zoster*. It sometimes proves successful also in most obstinate cases of hyperesthesia of the skin in which other measures have failed.

The heating chest pack and the moist abdominal girdle, also the general pack, owe certain of their effects to the properties which are characteristic of them in common with the neutral pack. It is largely through its nerve-quieting influence as a general neutral compress that the wet-sheet pack renders such signal aid in combating insomnia. The author could easily cite many scores of cases of insomnia which have been promptly relieved by this simple means. The neutral abdominal compress acts with equal efficiency in relieving hyperesthesia of the "abdominal brain," the solar plexus, and the lumbar ganglia of the sympathetic.

THE ALTERNATE COMPRESS.

1340 This measure consists in the application of very hot and very cold compresses in alternation.

Method.—The procedure is simply a succession of compresses renewed every half minute,—every other compress consisting of a fomentation, and the alternate a compress wrung quite dry out of cold or very cold water. The duration of each application respectively may be timed so as to meet any special condition. For example, the hot compress may be given a duration twice that of the cold compress, or the reverse. As a rule, the duration of the hot application should be equal to or greater than that of the cold. The procedure must always begin with a hot application and end with a cold one.

Physiological Effects.—The effects of alternate or successive applications of heat and cold to some extent combine the effects of both the cold and the hot compress. The sedative effects of both applications are, however, absent, as only the first effects are developed. The general effect of the application is exciting or stimulating. The hot application, with which the procedure begins, widely dilates the cutaneous vessels, and especially the veins. The cold application causes, first, contraction, then with the reaction which immediately follows, active dilatation of all the vessels of the skin, with an increased movement of the blood. When the hot and cold applications are of equal length, or when the cold application exceeds the hot in intensity, a decided thermic reaction occurs, with marked stimulation of the metabolic processes. The application is thus both revulsive and exciting to a high degree.

The internal vascular spasm occasioned in reflexly related internal organs by the cold application is quickly terminated by the hot application which follows in alternation at regular intervals during this procedure. After the ordinary cold compress the internal vascular contraction gradually disappears as the skin returns to its natural temperature; but when the skin is suddenly heated by the fomentation, the irritating effects of the cold application are abolished at once, and the blood-vessels of the part are dilated, thus encouraging the general movement of blood.

There is probably no other procedure which is capable of so intensely and rapidly exciting the movement of the blood in superficial parts and in deeper parts associated with them, either in sharing the blood supply, as in the case of an underlying muscle, or through reflex nerve connections (**1259**), as when applied to a cutaneous area having vasomotor relations with the liver or some other viscus.

Therapeutic Applications.—The alternate compress may be advantageously employed to combat the tendency to suppuration in cases of *localized suppuration* when beginning blueness of the parts shows stasis of the blood and the establishment of a condition of the circulation favorable to the suppurative process. By these alternate applications better effects may be obtained than from the application of either heat or cold alone. Continuous cold lowers the vitality of a part, and thus lessens the ability of the tissues to combat the microbes present, and lessens the supply of oxygen, by slowing the movement of the blood. Hot applications excite the the tissues to increased activity which is increased by the thermic reaction following the short cold application. Heat applied to the skin widens the surface vessels, and narrows the vessels of the deeper structures; while cold produces the very opposite effect. Thus by the alternate application of heat and cold the vessels of the deeper parts, in which suppuration is threatened, may be kept in such constant movement, contracting and dilating, that the cell-paralyzing ptomains will be washed out, the stagnant blood will be moved on, and a new supply of fresh, active leucocytes will be brought into the part. This effect of the alternate procedure in some cases renders it superior as an analgesic measure to either the cold or the hot compress alone, through the relief of *venous stasis*.

The alternate compress is superior to most other measures for combating the tendency to *bed-sores*, which are so likely to appear in typhoid fever, tuberculosis, and other wasting disorders. The alternate compress may be usefully employed as an application to *paralyzed limbs*, and to parts affected by *chilblains*, also as a means of stimulating absorption in *dropsy* of the abdomen, dropsy of the chest, and in *chronic pleurisy* and *pneumonia*, in which the parts damaged by the acute inflammatory process have not been wholly restored. Alternate hot and cold applications made to the spine powerfully impress the whole central nervous system, and form a most effective means of arousing a patient from the lethargy of *opium poisoning*, profound *alcohol intoxication*, or poisoning by any other narcotic drug. The author recalls very vividly a case of opium poisoning to which he was called in consultation some twenty-five years ago, in which a patient's pulse was reduced to less than twenty, and respiration to four per minute. Thoroughgoing hot and cold applications to the spine quickly brought the pulse to a nearly normal count, the respiration became twelve per minute within five minutes, and the change in the entire aspect of the case was so marvelous as to seem little short of a miracle to the by-standers, who had never before witnessed the powerful stimulating effects of thermic applications properly managed.

THE REVULSIVE COMPRESS.

1341 The revulsive compress differs from the alternating compress in its mode of application only in the different timing of the heat and cold. In the alternating compress the applications are of equal time, or at least the hot application does not exceed the cold. In the revulsive compress the hot application is applied for several minutes, while the time of the cold application is only a few seconds. Usually the hot application, or fomentation, remains in place for 4 or 5 minutes, or at least until its maximum heating effect is reached. It is then withdrawn, and a cold compress is instantly applied and allowed to remain in place for 20 to 40 seconds, or just a sufficient length of time to absorb from the skin the heat communicated to it by the fomentation.

Physiological Effects.—The purpose of this mode of procedure is to secure a strong circulatory reaction without thermic reaction. The vascular dilatation resulting from heat is transient in character. Within a short time after the heat is withdrawn and the skin exposed to the air, the blood-vessels are made to contract by the cooling resulting from the evaporation and contact with the air at the ordinary atmospheric temperature. The circulatory reaction following a cold application is, however, much more lasting in character, and is also more thoroughgoing, since it is an active rather than simply a passive or paralytic dilatation of the blood-vessels, and influences the arteries to fully as great an extent as the veins. By a short cold application following a hot application, the atonic reaction is converted into the tonic reaction of cold, the state of the blood-vessels being thus very materially changed, and active fluxion of the blood in the skin is thereby maintained for a considerable length of time (667).

The alternate compress produces both circulatory and thermic reaction. In the revulsive compress the procedure is so managed that the thermic reaction is wholly suppressed. This gives to it superior power as an analgesic measure, in which respect it is, in fact, superior to all other hydriatic processes. This end is attained by superheating the skin before the cold application, then making a cold application of just sufficient intensity and duration to absorb the surplus heat without reducing the skin temperature below the normal point. Under these conditions, thermic reaction can not possibly occur; hence metabolic activity is not increased, neither do systemic or local disturbances occur, and a purely revulsive, non-excitant, and analgesic effect is obtained.

Therapeutic Applications.— The revulsive compress is especially applicable to all forms of *neuralgia* and painful affections of every description. In some cases relief may best be obtained by very hot applications, in others by cold applications, and in still others by alternate applications; but in quite a large proportion of cases in which pain is present, applications of a character which produce thermic reaction increase the pain by exciting the affected nerves. This is especially true of cases in which inflammation is present. For this class of cases the revulsive compress is indispensable.

This compress is also a powerful decongestant and derivative. It is of value in cases of *visceral congestion*, especially in such painful conditions as *gastric congestion*, *gastritis*, *enteralgia*, *acute sciatica*, *neuritis*, *painful affections* of the *eye*, and *spinal irritation*. It often affords immediate relief from the excruciating pain of *toothache*. It is applicable also in cases of *gastric crises*, and other painful conditions accompanying *locomotor ataxia*.

ALTERNATE APPLICATIONS TO THE SPINE.

1342 The importance of this special procedure will amply justify its separate consideration as a special measure for securing other than purely local results. In addition to hot, cold, and neutral applications, there may be made to the spine a number of alternate applications in the form of either the Scotch douche, the alternate douche, or the revulsive douche, all of which are useful under special circumstances. There are other non-percutient applications capable of producing similar effects, which may also be employed.

Alternate applications so managed as to produce the effects of the Scotch, the revulsive, or the alternate douche, minus the percutient or mechanical effects, may be conveniently made by the use of two bags, one filled with very hot water, the other with cold water; by the fomentation and the cold or ice compress in alternation; by alternate hot and cold sponging; and by the hot and cold pour. The method of applying these several measures to the spine is not different from that pursued with other regions of the body, but may be briefly described by way of general illustration. The hot and cold water bags, hot and cold compresses, hot and cold sponging, are all best applied with the patient lying down upon the face, or upon the side and inclined toward the face. The hot and cold pour must be applied with the patient sitting upon a stool, leaning slightly forward, with the arms folded in front. The hot and cold water bags are the most convenient means for prolonged applications. The hot and cold compress, or the fomentation followed by the cold compress, or rubbing the spine with a piece of ice covered with two or three thicknesses of cheese-cloth, are more vigorous measures which may be employed when it is desired to secure results by a short intense application.

Alternate sponging is a less vigorous application than the alternate compress, and is most frequently employed when calmative effects are desired, through the tonic influence of this application upon the spinal centers. The alternate pour may be used in cases in which the alternate douche is not readily available.

In the use of the hot and cold water bags, the hot bag may remain in position for 10 to 15 minutes, the cold bag 30 seconds to 2 minutes. In the employment of the alternate compress, the fomentation is first applied for 10 or 15 minutes, then a very cold compress for half a minute. A thin compress wrung very dry out of ice-water is best for the purpose when the object sought is the relief of the pain which accompanies so-called spinal irritation. If exciting effects are desired, the hot and cold applications should be of about equal length; viz., 15 to 20 seconds each.

Alternate sponging is a measure which may be continued for as long a time as is found agreeable to the patient, and may be repeated as often as indicated. The hot sponging is best done with a very soft sponge attached to a handle (Fig. 180). The sponge should be of good size, and great care should be taken to press out the hot water sufficiently to avoid risk of blistering the spine. A sponge wet in cold water may be used in alternation with the hot sponge, or a piece of ice wrapped in thin muslin, or a couple of thicknesses of cheese-cloth wet in cold water may be quickly rubbed up and down the spine for 3 to 10 seconds after the hot sponging has been continued for a few seconds.

In the employment of the hot and cold pour, care must be taken to adapt the application carefully to each individual case. A somewhat prolonged (5 to 8 min.) hot pour to the spine, followed by a cold pour for 15 to 20 seconds, is a most excellent means of relieving congestion of the cord. The pour may be very conveniently administered with the patient sitting over the edge of a full bath-tub, or upon a low stool in a bath-tub, the feet being placed in hot water for derivative effects, and to protect them from contact with the cold water. When exciting effects are desirable, the duration of the heat and the cold should be about 15 seconds each. Powerful exciting effects may be produced by this means.

Therapeutic Applications.—The alternate process is of great value in *neurasthenia;* especially in very feeble cases, a remarkable reviving effect is at once experienced by the patient during the application, and for some time afterward.

Alternate compresses or sponging to the spine afford one of the most efficient means of arousing the patient from *opium* or *alcohol narcosis*. It is equally indicated in *Prussic acid poisoning*, and in cases in which there is a depressed condition of the *spinal* centers, as in *syncope*, *asphyxia* from coal-gas or carbonic acid gas poisoning, or *drowning*. The application should be continued not only until the patient shows evidences of returning consciousness, but for some time

Fig. 180. (b) ALTERNATE APPLICATIONS TO THE HEAD (p. 823.)

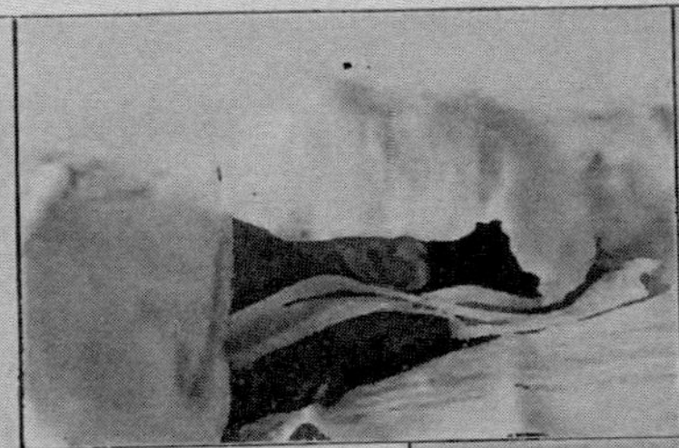

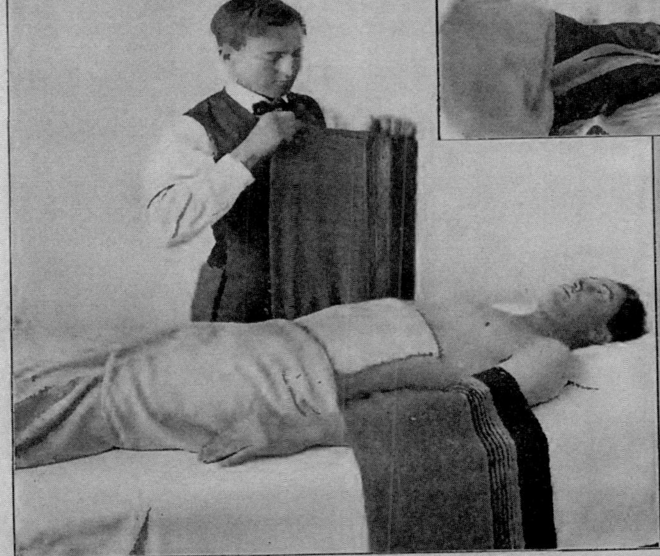

Fig. 181. ABDOMINAL HEATING COMPRESS— Unprotected (p. 824).

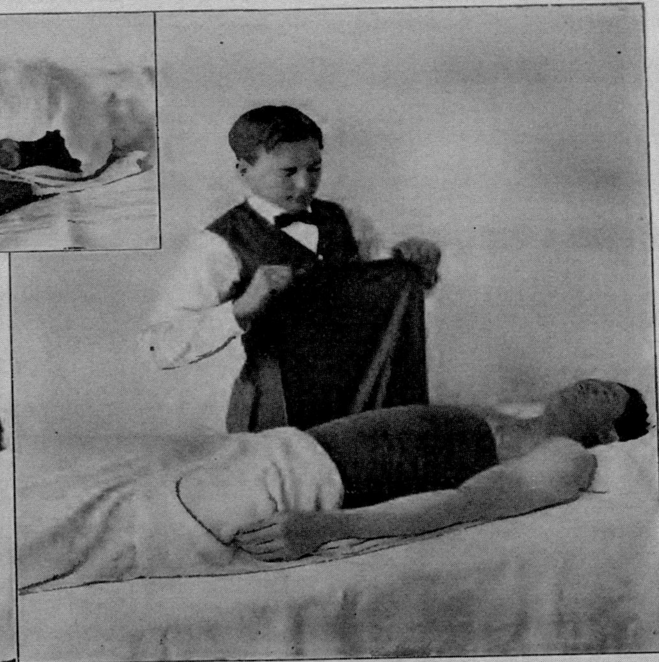

Fig. 182. ABDOMINAL HEATING COMPRESS— Protected with Mackintosh (p. 825).

after, to maintain the necessary degree of nervous and vital activity. The author has more than once employed this measure with success in threatened *collapse* under *chloroform*, and to combat grave symptoms arising from the injection of cocaine, years ago, when the anesthetic properties of this drug were first known and its toxic properties not so well understood as now. Alternate applications to the spine may be systematically employed in *general paresis*, *acute ascending paralysis*, *pachymeningitis*, and *muscular atrophy*. It is frequently serviceable in *chronic anemia*, *toxemia* from gastrointestinal disorders, and general systemic depression in various acute and chronic affections.

ALTERNATE APPLICATIONS TO THE HEAD.

In some cases of violent headache, especially the con- 1343
gestive form, most excellent results are obtained by alternating hot and cold compresses, or hot and cold sponging of the upper portion of the spine. The application should begin at the occiput, and extend to a point midway between the shoulders.

Very hot sponging (160°), followed by the application of an ice-bag, is one of the most efficient means of relieving cerebral congestion. In severe cases an ice compress may be applied over the top of the head and the face, the hair being well moistened, at the same time that the hot sponging is being applied at the back of the neck.

Another alternate measure which the author has found serviceable in relieving cerebral congestion and headache is the application of steam to the face by means of a metal mask constructed for the purpose, alternating with a cold blast. The face is exposed to the action of steam for 2 or 3 minutes, then for about half a minute to a strong blast of cold air from a fan. Thus the face is cooled not only by contact with the cold air, but by the rapid evaporation taking place from the moist surface (Fig. 237).

THE HEATING COMPRESS OR LOCAL PACK (Fig. 181).

1344 This most valuable hydriatic procedure consists in a thick moist linen compress well covered with flannel, with or without an outer covering of impervious material.

The heating compress may be applied to any part of the body. Its most useful applications are to the trunk, the chest, the neck, the spine, and the joints.

Method.— The principle upon which the effects of the heating compress depend is the production of reaction by a primary cold application, and the accumulation of heat by protecting the cold compress in such a manner as to prevent, wholly or in part, the escape of heat by means of radiation or evaporation.

The degree of protection may be regulated by the number of thicknesses of flannel applied as a covering, or if complete protection is desired, by the application of an oilcloth, rubber cloth, or some other impervious material. Oiled paper may be used in an emergency, in the absence of anything better. In all cases it is necessary to cover closely the edges of the compress so as to prevent the formation of air currents at any part, as such currents produce cooling by evaporation. Even though the area thus cooled may be very small, the refrigerant effect produced may be sufficient to greatly disturb or even wholly destroy the legitimate effect of the compress.

The degree of protection will be regulated by a number of conditions; as,—

1. If the patient's temperature is elevated and the skin hot, one or two thicknesses of flannel sheeting or one thickness of flannel blanket will suffice, as the purpose is simply to limit evaporation so as to prevent too rapid cooling. When the surface is cool or cold, even though the temperature may be elevated, several thicknesses of flannel (three or four) may be employed. The covering should be sufficient to insure slight warming of the compress, but not enough to prevent drying by evaporation.

2. When the purpose is to control a deep-seated inflammation by producing fluxion of the parts, the compress being changed once in 30 or 40 minutes for this purpose, the compress should be covered with flannel, so as to cause prompt reaction.

3. When it is desired to produce the effect of a poultice by the fullest possible accumulation of heat and consequent dilatation of the surface vessels, the compress should always be protected, not only by several layers of flannel, but also by some impervious covering, as thin mackintosh, or rubber cloth, or oilcloth; or in the absence of some convenient, impervious material, ordinary newspapers may be employed. The efficiency of paper may be increased by saturating it with oil, wax, or paraffin. This is the *protected heating compress proper* (Fig. 182).

The rate at which the heat accumulates in the heating compress depends, of course, primarily upon the degree of protection; but many other factors are involved, as the temperature of the water employed, the amount of water left in the compress, the reactive powers of the patient, and the condition of the cutaneous circulation in the surfaces to which the application is made.

Other things being equal, very cold water produces a quicker and more vigorous reaction than water of a higher temperature. The more water the compress contains, the longer the time required to heat it, hence the longer the delay in the establishment of the reaction. If the protection is but partial, evaporation may take place at such a rate as to prevent accumulation of heat, the heat being dissipated by the evaporation as rapidly as it is generated. If the compress dries rapidly, this fact is evidence that rapid evaporation is taking place; and of course the heating of the compress will be much less than when it is protected by an impervious covering.

Physiological Effects.—The effects of the heating com- 1345
press are like those of the wet-sheet pack, somewhat mixed

or varied. At the beginning and for some minutes after the cold wet cloth is brought in contact with the skin, there exists strong contraction of the vessels, and by reflex action the same condition is produced in the related internal area. When reaction takes place, however, heat begins to accumulate, and dilatation of the vessels occurs, which increases with the accumulation of heat,—a characteristic which gives to the procedure its name. This dilatation is at first an active or tonic dilatation, in which there is an increased movement of blood to the skin; but later, when the temperature has risen above the normal temperature of the skin, the vessels lose their tone and become relaxed. This is especially true when an impervious covering is employed, so that the highest degree of heating effect is produced. The degree of this paralytic dilatation of the blood-vessels and the congestion will, of course, depend upon the exact mode in which the bandage is applied, and the degree of the protection. A series of experiments made by Winternitz and Strasser, which the author has repeatedly verified, shows that heating takes place at quite a different rate, the maximum temperature being reached at very different periods, according to the mode of applying the bandage and the degree of protection afforded (Exp. 69, 70).

When lightly covered, the heating compress slowly cools by evaporation, producing an active fluxion in the associated viscera; and by the improved circulation and nutrition, the normal conditions are restored, and the passive congestion is overcome. With each reapplication there is contraction of the arterial walls, which empties the blood-vessels, and dislodges the leucocytes which may be adhering to the vessel walls, thus antagonizing inflammation and chronic congestion. As the compress warms up, the vessels gradually dilate again, and the blood moves with increased velocity.

The degree of reaction also depends very much upon the condition of the patient. Bloodless, very feeble patients sometimes react very slowly, and in a particular case the effect

Fig. 184. HOT AND COLD HEAD COMPRESS (p. 843).

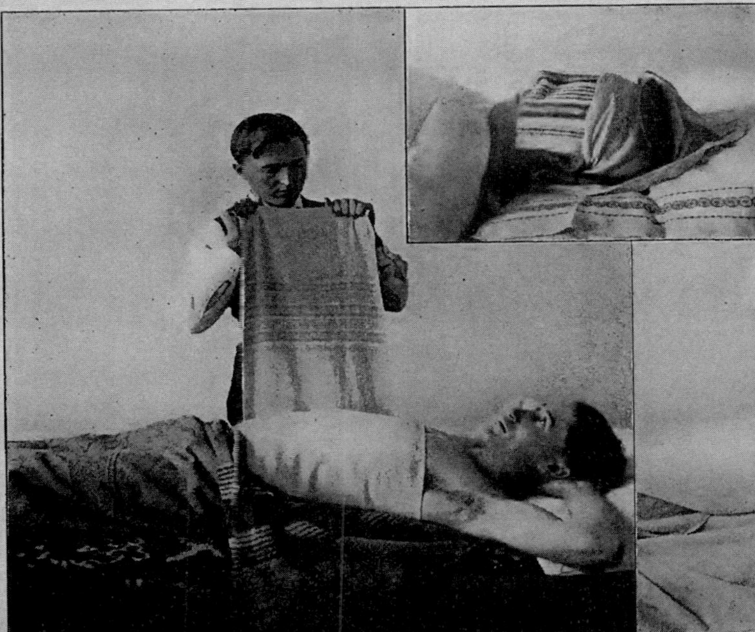

Fig. 183. WET GIRDLE (p. 829).

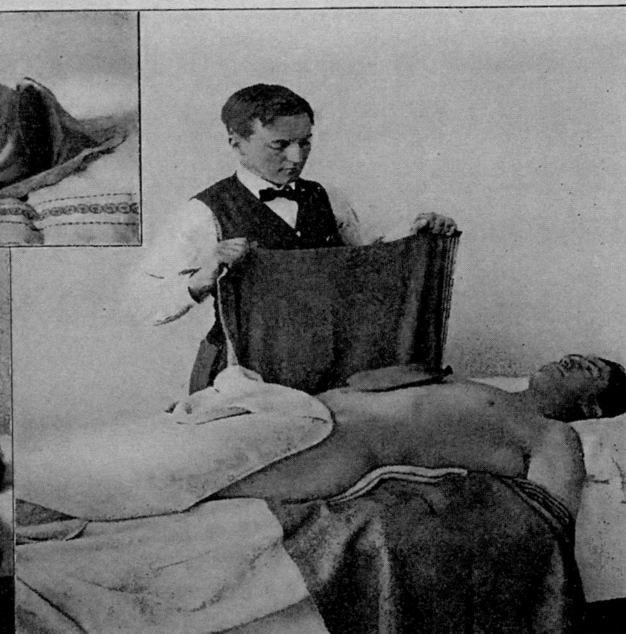

Fig. 185. HOT AND COLD RENAL COMPRESS (p. 846).

of a well-protected compress may not be greater than that of a partially protected compress with another person. This fact must be constantly considered in giving directions respecting the application of the heating compress.

In persons in whom reaction takes place very slowly after the application of the compress, so that uncomfortable chilliness and other disagreeable symptoms are experienced, the surface with which the bandage is to come in contact should be vigorously rubbed with the dry hand until red, or with the hand or a friction mitt dipped in water at a temperature ten or fifteen degrees below the temperature of the bandage.

The colder the water, the drier should be the compress. The smaller the compress, the sooner will reaction occur. During the warming-up period, before superheating begins, the effect of the heating compress is highly tonic, exciting all the functions of the skin and the internal parts connected with the area treated. During the period of superheating, or that in which the temperature rises above the normal temperature of the skin, the peculiar excitation characteristic of heat is produced, including analgesic effects upon the skin and associated parts, and also developing atonic thermic reaction, and producing powerful derivative or revulsive effects.

If it is desired to emphasize the tonic effect of the application, it is only necessary to lower the temperature and make the covering relatively less, so that excessive heating may not occur.

If the effects of heat are desired, with the strongest possible revulsive effects, the moist bandage should be very warmly covered with blanket flannel, and the impervious protection carefully applied. It may be well to remark that when the greatest heat accumulation is secured by the impervious covering, the skin is most strongly stimulated, and the most powerful derivative effects are induced; but when the impervious covering is omitted, vascular activity and tone being maintained in the skin, a strong tonic effect is exerted upon the viscera, and most powerful fluxion effects occur.

These facts should be borne carefully in mind in the therapeutic application of the heating compress, especially in its use in the form of the abdominal compress or the wet girdle.

1346 **Therapeutic Applications.**—This measure is indicated in *insomnia, indigestion, constipation, bronchial catarrh, laryngitis, articular rheumatism*, and a great variety of other conditions. Whenever there is need for increased movement of blood, absorption of *exudates* or *effusions*, quickened functional activity, or to relieve *swelling* from venous stasis, the heating compress may be advantageously used. The protected heating compress proper should be used in cases of *old joint trouble*, in which the leading object sought is to promote absorption of exudates; in cases of *chronic bronchial catarrh;* to relieve cough in *tuberculosis* and spasm of the bronchioles in *asthma;* for the abdominal compress and the leg compress when strongly derivative effects in favor of the cerebral circulation are desired; to the head for the relief of *acute coryza, headache, vertigo*, or *insomnia* due to anemia; to the spine for spinal irritation (1355).

Impervious protection should also be used for the gastric or abdominal heating compress in cases of *hypopepsia*, in *hyperesthesia* of the abdominal sympathetic, and in cases in which patients chill easily, and whose circulation and heat-making powers are so sluggish that the compress does not become sufficiently heated to accomplish the result desired unless evaporation is wholly prevented.

One of the most practical and effective applications of this compress is in the treatment of chronic rheumatism for the relief of pain and to restore lost joint motion. Hot fomentations applied night and morning, followed by the heating compress to be worn during the succeeding twelve hours, constitutes a good method in the treatment of *rheumatic joints*.

A very important use for this procedure is in the treatment of *pneumonia*. The compress should be large enough to cover the whole chest, and should be renewed as soon as well warmed, so as to encourage energetic fluxion in the lungs, the importance of which has been pointed out elsewhere.

The heating compress likewise finds useful employment as an application to the trunk in *acute* and *chronic peritonitis* (frequently renewed, in the acute form), *amyloid infiltration* of the *liver*, *amyloid kidney*, *acute ascending paralysis*, *congestion* of the *spleen*, *ascites*, *infectious jaundice*, *icterus neonatorum*, *appendicitis*, *enteralgia*, *intestinal catarrh*, *gastric ulcer*, *hyperorexia*, *Addison's disease*, *chronic migraine;* to the spine in *locomotor ataxia* and *occupation neuroses*, *spinal neuralgia*, *hyperpepsia*, and as a local measure in *muscular rheumatism*, *chronic appendicitis*, *chronic ovaritis* and *salpingitis;* to the scalp in *anemic insomnia;* and as a derivative measure in *acute coryza*.

Precautions.—Few measures of treatment are capable of producing more disastrous results than the heating compress when improperly used, and especially when so applied that prompt reaction does not occur. The slow but prolonged chilling produced by the evaporation resulting from the loosely applied or imperfectly protected heating compress, when not indicated as a therapeutic measure, is certain to result in visceral congestion and aggravation of the condition for which it is applied, with rheumatic pains and numerous other inconveniences, both general and local. The effects, in fact, are precisely the opposite of those desired. There is no other hydriatic measure the success of which depends more wholly upon exact technique; and few which yield more gratifying results when properly applied.

THE WET GIRDLE (Fig. 183).

This application is practically the same as the half-pack, 1347
except that it covers a more limited area. The region to which it is applied is bounded by the nipple line above and the hip joints below. The application is addressed especially to that portion of the skin having most immediate reflex relation with the abdominal viscera.

This measure has been exceedingly popular in Germany for at least a hundred years, and possibly a much longer time, under the name of "Neptune's girdle."

Requisites.—A linen bandage usually eight or nine inches wide and about three yards in length, or sufficiently long to pass three times around the body; a flannel bandage three or four inches wider; and a water-proof covering of oiled silk or other impervious material.

Method.—The application is to be made in accordance with the principles already pointed out in relation to the heating compress (1344). The girdle may be wide enough to reach from the axillæ to the hips, when it is termed the *trunk pack*. In some cases also it is better to reduce the size of the bandage at the start, covering only the abdominal surface instead of passing the bandage around the whole trunk. The impervious covering may be applied or omitted as indicated.

1348 **Physiological Effects.**—The wet girdle certainly produces a powerful effect upon the vasomotor centers, and through them upon the abdominal viscera. It is without question one of the most effective and well-known means for combating visceral irritation and congestion. The slight chilliness which is at first produced disappears more quickly than when a larger surface of the body is involved, as in the wet-sheet pack. The patient soon experiences a pleasant, cool sensation, and a sense of well-being, with relief of any sensation of heaviness of the epigastrium or of the head, vertigo, and other unpleasant symptoms which may have previously existed. Later, perspiration may appear. General perspiration is less likely to occur than when the wet-sheet pack is employed. If the covering is properly adjusted, the pack may be continued for several hours without inducing perspiration or other than a simple prolonged tonic reaction with powerful derivative and calmative effects upon the internal viscera. The wet girdle acts powerfully upon the sympathetic, the moist warmth which follows the first chill soothing and relieving the visceral irritation. That there is a most intimate relation between the viscera and the structures of the abdominal wall is clearly shown by the strong contraction of the abdominal muscles frequently occurring in connection with visceral irritation. In these cases, extreme hyperesthesia is often present in both the right and the left ganglia, and in the sub-umbilical sympathetic ganglia, or the so-called lumbar ganglia of the sympathetic and the lumbo-aortic plexus. The application of cool water to the abdominal walls stimulates contraction of the bladder, uterus, and bowels,— another evidence of the intimate nervous relation between the skin and the muscles of the abdomen and the viscera contained within its cavity. The wet girdle may be so managed as to be practically a prolonged neutral bath; or it may be made a powerfully derivative procedure, according to the degree of protection provided.

Elsewhere full explanation has been made of the influence of induced cutaneous hyperemia upon the portal circulation, and both the arterial and the venous circulation of the stomach, liver, lungs, and other viscera (1271 to 1277).

Therapeutic Applications.— The moist abdominal bandage 1349
is one of the most valuable of what might be termed the minor hydrotherapeutic measures. Its use is applicable to all cases in which there is evidence of visceral irritation or hyperesthesia of the abdominal sympathetic ganglia, a condition which is almost universally present in *chronic dyspepsia*, *constipation*, *gastric* and *intestinal catarrh*, *hepatic congestion* and other disorders of the liver which result from chronic gastric disorders, and in many *chronic pelvic disorders*. It is almost a panacea in cases of *chronic backache*, also in heaviness across the abdomen, when the seat of the discomfort is not located in the pelvis.

The therapeutic effect of the wet girdle differs somewhat, according to the exact point at which it is applied. Over the lower portion of the abdomen the chief effect is concentrated upon the bowels, allaying irritation, increasing secretion, and thus tending to promote normal activity and to relieve *chronic constipation.* Applied around the upper portion of the abdomen, the bandage is useful as a means of promoting healthful activity of the stomach and liver. Its effect is powerfully revulsive. It stimulates the vasomotor centers, and hence relieves *congestion* of the *liver*, *kidneys*, and other abdominal viscera. It is also of much service in ordinary *dyspepsia* with *dilatation* and *prolapse* of the *stomach*.

There is no more serviceable measure in the treatment of chronic indigestion in all its forms. In *hyperpepsia*, it should be applied very cold, wrung very dry, covered just sufficiently to secure good reaction, superheating being avoided by omitting the impervious covering. This is also true in each of the conditions above mentioned.

In *hypopepsia*, the bandage should be wrung out of water at a temperature of 60° to 70°, very dry, and should be well covered with flannel, the impervious covering being also applied when necessary to secure good reaction, as it is desirable to secure the most powerful revulsive effects possible, and also the atonic thermic effect of heat.

For *flatulence* of the stomach or intestines, a cold, well-wrung bandage with a moderate amount of flannel covering should be employed. *Dilatation* of the *colon*, *enteroptosis*, lack of normal sensibility in the lower bowel, are best treated by the bandage wrung very dry out of very cold water, and lightly covered with flannel. The bandage should be renewed just before it becomes dry, or every three to four hours.

A well-protected heating compress may be advantageously employed in cases of *hyperesthesia* of the *lumbar ganglia*, general *sensitiveness* of the *abdominal sympathetic*, *enteralgia*, *chronic peritonitis*, painful conditions resulting from peritonitis, recurring *appendicitis*, or inflammation of the cecum when the case is for any reason not suitable for operation.

The moist abdominal bandage, either with or without the impervious covering, is a most excellent means for combating *insomnia*. The reaction should be strongly pronounced, so as to divert the largest possible amount of blood into the skin of the trunk as well as into the portal circulation, which is alone capable of holding all the blood in the body. As this system is associated with the venous vessels of the abdominal wall, it is possible by means of the heating compress to divert a large portion of the blood into this portion of the circulatory system, thus causing contraction of the cerebral vessels and an accumulation of lymph beneath the dura mater, whereby conditions favorable for sleep are secured (Schüller).

For the relief of insomnia the wet bandage or girdle should be applied at bedtime, and may be renewed to advantage at least once during the night, as the bandage must be kept moist in order to be effective. The patient is apt to be nervously irritated when the bandage becomes perfectly dry. It is also highly important that reaction should take place promptly, as otherwise prolonged chilliness may result, and the patient become so nervous and disturbed that the hypnotic effect of the application is wholly lost.

The wet girdle, when properly managed, is a more valuable hypnotic in combating insomnia than any or all medicinal drugs.

The wet girdle may be advantageously employed in nearly all forms of *visceral irritation*. Care should be taken, however, to avoid impervious covering. In *hyperpepsia* especially, this is necessary, and the bandage should be changed every three or four hours. In *hypopepsia* the impervious covering should be applied, especially in cases in which there is marked evidence of congestion, as in *chronic gastritis*, and in congestion of the mucous membrane arising from *cardiac insufficiency* or *cirrhosis* of the *liver*. The wet girdle is of value in disorders of the menopause, serving to lessen morbid sympathetic reflexes and vasomotor disturbances. In the preparation of patients for abdominal operation the wet girdle without impervious covering is of service. The bandage should be covered with flannel only, and should be changed every four to six hours, the purpose being to increase the movement of blood through the viscera, and thus prepare them for the ordeal which the patient must undergo. This measure is also of great advantage in *gestation*. It may be used with benefit during the entire period, and especially during the later months.

1350 **Precautions and Contraindications.**— 1. It should be remembered that the wet girdle is serviceable only when moist. When it becomes dry, it should be removed, and a dry flannel put in its place, after rubbing the parts with the hand dipped in cold water; or it should be renewed.

2. With the majority of persons it is sufficient to wear the girdle at night only. In cases of enteroptosis in which patients suffer from backache and abdominal pain when on their feet, the moist girdle may, however, often be advantageously worn during the day, and should be supplemented by an abdominal supporter.

3. When worn night and day, the wet girdle frequently gives rise to an eczematous, or, in some cases, herpetic eruption of the skin; sometimes boils make their appearance in the region covered by the bandage. These morbid processes are in no way desirable, and care should be taken to prevent them. The old notion that effete matters are eliminated through purulent discharges was long ago exploded. Neither is any special benefit to be derived from the irritation produced by an eruption or any other morbid process. The resources of hydrotherapy enable us to stimulate the skin to the highest degree, and a healthy skin is more ready to respond to physiological stimuli than is a diseased skin.

The eruption occurs as the result of wearing the moist abdominal bandage only when it is not kept scrupulously clean. It should be boiled daily, or rinsed in a ten-per-cent. solution of chloride of lime, or a ten-per-cent. solution of sulphate of zinc, or a one-to-one-thousand bichloride of mercury solution. If cleansed daily by any of these methods, the troublesome eruption which sometimes follows the prolonged use of the bandage may be readily prevented. There is no advantage whatever in this eruption, but on the contrary, a positive disadvantage. There are always present upon the skin pus-producing germs, the development of which is encouraged by the continuous warmth and moisture secured by the bandage. The accumulation of perspiration in the bandage furnishes a culture medium for the development of these germs, and thus encourages the infection to which the eruption is due. The surface treated should be daily washed with hot water and yellow soap, and a little vaseline should be applied.

4. Chronic invalids sometimes become addicted to the wet girdle. They rely upon it to such an extent that they may be said to be quite dependent upon it. This is quite undesirable. As a means of preventing irritation and other inconveniences arising from the constant employment of the girdle, it is wise to omit the application either during the day or night, as may be most advantageous and convenient; or if for any reason it must be worn continuously night and day, it should be left off for a day at least once a week, a dry flannel bandage being worn in its place.

5. As the protected heating compress, when applied to the trunk, accumulates blood in the portal system, it is obviously unwise to make use of this measure in conditions involving chronic disease of the liver or spleen, and in *inflammatory affections* of the *stomach* and *bowels*, in *ulcer* of the *stomach*, in *varicose* conditions of the *gastric veins*, in *hemorrhoids*, *intestinal catarrh*, *bleeding fibroid* of the uterus, and in acute pelvic inflammations or congestions. In these cases the wet girdle covered with flannel only may be used with great advantage.

THE ABDOMINAL HEATING COMPRESS.

This is a procedure similar to the wet girdle, but more 1351
limited in extent, being applied only to the anterior portion of the trunk, from the pubis to a point an inch or two above the epigastrium, and extending to the loins on either side.

Method. — The same materials are needed as for the wet girdle. A compress of proper size, consisting of six or eight thicknesses of soft cheese-cloth, fits the skin better than one consisting of coarse toweling. The compress wrung out of cold water is applied to the front of the trunk between the sternum and the pubis, and a dry bandage placed over it in such a manner as to hold it in place. The woolen and water-proof coverings are then added.

Physiological Effects. — The effects of the abdominal heating compress are essentially the same as those of the wet girdle (**1347**), but somewhat less pronounced. This application acts especially upon the sympathetic centers and the viscera.

Therapeutic Applications. — This procedure is extremely useful in minor cases of *visceral irritation* or *congestion*, indicated by sensitiveness in the region of the liver, spleen, or bowels, *hyperesthesia* of the *lumbâr ganglia* of the abdominal sympathetic, *constipation*, *flatulence*, *gastric* and *intestinal catarrh*, *insomnia*, and other nervous affections arising from irritation of the abdominal sympathetic. The abdominal heating compress may be used as a milder or introductory procedure in all cases in which the wet girdle is indicated.

1352 **Precautions and Contraindications.**— In the use of the wet girdle or the abdominal compress for the relief of insomnia, it must be remembered that the brain is relieved at the expense of congesting the portal circulation. The portal system is a reservoir capable of containing all the blood in the body. When the heating compress is applied in such a way as to accumulate the largest possible amount of heat, as when covered very thick with flannel or protected by oilcloth, mackintosh, or other impervious material, both the cutaneous and the visceral vasoconstrictors are relaxed, thus diverting into these parts an enormous amount of blood, and relieving the cerebral vessels by a sort of internal blood-letting.

If kept moist, and not too warmly covered, the walking

powers are improved; but when excessively covered, it becomes exciting and weakening, and when worn at night, may cause dreams, fidgets, and insomnia, by reflexly producing cerebral congestion. This is a point worthy of the most careful consideration in the use of the procedure.

This intense portal congestion is wholly harmless in conditions of health, for it is evidently a part of the function of the portal system and the distensible and elastic viscera connected with it, especially the spleen, to serve the body in this fashion as a sort of overflow reservoir, whereby the regulation of the circulation may be effected under conditions which without this aid would baffle the efforts of the other regulators of the blood supply. But what is true in normal conditions by no means always holds good in conditions of disease. When the portal system is the seat of pathological states involving changes in the vessel walls, as in the *varicose condition of the veins of the stomach* and intestines which often accompanies *hepatic sclerosis;* in the *acute congestions* of the spleen and liver which are present in chronic malarial infection, typhoid and other continued fevers; in acute congestions of the liver due to infection from the alimentary canal, as in *catarrhal* or *infectious jaundice;* in *chronic gastritis* and *gastro-intestinal catarrh;* in *abdominal dropsy;* and in *constipation* due to atony and dilatation of the colon,—in these and kindred states, any procedure whereby the portal congestion already present is increased can not be otherwise than damaging in a high degree; and hence in these conditions the portal reservoir can not safely be utilized as a means of diverting blood from the cerebral circulation. In such cases the desired end may be accomplished by other means almost, if not quite, as effective. The cutaneous envelope of the body, while a less capacious reservoir than the portal system, is, nevertheless, capable of holding fully one half of all the blood of the body, and, fortunately, can not be easily filled to a really dangerous degree. By means of the heating pack (**1186**), the wet-sheet rub, cold friction, or even the shallow bath and the Scotch douche, the skin may be readily congested to such a degree as to render the cerebral vessels anemic while the lymph spaces are filled, thus securing the conditions necessary for sleep and repair of the cerebral energies.

A *varicose* condition of the abdominal veins should always be taken as an indication that the protected abdominal girdle should not be employed. This condition is easily discovered, when present, by making the patient stand up. The varicose vessels will then be seen just above the pubes running outward, nearly parallel with the groin. Other veins may be seen near the epigastrium.

It should be remarked that in these cases the abdominal girdle is not altogether interdicted, but only when imperviously covered so as to cause superheating of the skin and consequent paralysis of the vasoconstrictors; the flannel-covered compress may often be advantageously used, as in dropsy of the abdomen.

The abdominal compress has a decidedly laxative effect. The cold abdominal compress, renewed every hour or two, is a most efficacious remedy in diarrhea and intestinal flatulence.

When necessary to employ the abdominal compress in cases of menorrhagia, the bandage should be confined to the region of the umbilicus, to avoid congesting the pelvic viscera.

To obtain the best tonic effects, the compress should be renewed every two or three hours.

In feeble persons, the measure may begin with a small folded napkin applied over the epigastrium.

THE DRY ABDOMINAL BANDAGE.

1353 This measure consists in a broad flannel bandage of sufficient length to extend two or three times around the body. In cold weather, it should be applied whenever the moist abdominal bandage is omitted. If the moist bandage is worn during the night, the dry bandage should be applied in the morning, and worn during the day, after cool sponging and rubbing of the parts on removal of the moist bandage.

The dry abdominal bandage is valuable, first, as a means of supporting the viscera when enteroptosis exists, although for this purpose it is not very effective as an abdominal supporter, as it constricts the trunk to some degree, and does not elevate the viscera to the extent desirable in most cases.

The warmth afforded by the abdominal bandage is exceedingly helpful in many cases in which the digestive functions are feeble and the sympathetic ganglia irritable. Indigestion and other disorders may be greatly mitigated by a dry flannel bandage applied about the abdomen.

THE HEAD PACK.

A cheese-cloth compress wet in very cold water is applied 1354
to the head after the hair and scalp have been thoroughly wet with cold water. A rubber cap like a lady's bathing cap is then placed over all, and the retention of heat soon warms the compress and develops the usual effects of such an application. Where there is a heavy growth of hair, simply wetting and covering it with the rubber cap is sufficient to develop the full effects of the stimulating compress.

On rising in the morning, the scalp should be well drenched with cold water, then rubbed dry, and protected by a cap during the day to prevent taking cold. This is an excellent measure for promptly relieving an acute "cold in the head."

The use of the stimulating head cap is indicated in *chronic headache*, when due to *anemia;* in *chronic neuralgia* and *rheumatic affections* of the *head;* in *chronic nasal catarrh* with *diminished secretion*, and in *acute coryza*. The stimulating compress may be preceded by a very short hot application for the relief of *headache*—to the face when due to nasal catarrh, to the top of the head when due to anemia. It is also useful in *baldness* due to failing nutrition of the scalp.

THE SPINAL PACK.

While less frequently employed than many other forms of 1355
the heating compress, the spinal pack is sufficiently useful as a hydriatic procedure to be worthy of brief description.

Requisites.—The requisites are: an ordinary towel, a piece of woolen blanket sufficiently large to cover the entire back when folded four thicknesses; if special protection is required, a piece of mackintosh a little larger than the folded flannel, and a roller cheese-cloth bandage one foot wide, three thicknesses, and four yards long.

Method.—The towel is folded lengthwise and wrung dry from water at 60°, and applied the whole length of the spine from the cervical region to the coccyx, after first rubbing the skin surface with the hand dipped in water at 50° until reddened. The flannel is laid over the towel, over this the mackintosh, and the cheese-cloth bandage is then applied in such a manner as to hold the pack in snug contact with the skin.

Therapeutic Applications.—The spinal pack produces, first, strong fluxion in the spinal vessels; later, hyperemia of the skin, whereby the spinal cord is drained. If impervious protection is employed, the superheating of the skin finally produces accumulation of blood in the spinal vessels. This procedure may therefore be employed either to combat *anemia* or *hyperemia* of the *cord*, according as it is more or less protected. Partial protection (**1344**) maintains active fluxion in the spinal vessels, and thus combats passive congestion. The prolonged protected spinal pack, by congesting the spinal vessels, antagonizes *chronic degenerations* of the *cord*. It is very useful in some cases of *insomnia*.

The neutral pack, applied at 80°, covered with two thicknesses of flannel only, without mackintosh, is a calmative procedure of great value in *spinal irritation* with *hyperesthesia* of the *spine*, and in conditions in which *irritability* of the *spinal centers* exists, as in *locomotor ataxia* and other degenerations at certain stages.

THE HOT AND COLD COMPRESS.

1356 This procedure consists in the simultaneous and continuous applications of a hot and a cold compress to separate skin surfaces collaterally related to a single internal part

This unique procedure is not applicable to all parts of the body, but may be applied under appropriate conditions to the head, chest, spine, abdomen, pelvis, and legs. The hot and cold compress is a combined application of peculiar interest and value, since it can be relied upon to accomplish, under certain conditions, results which can be attained in no other way, and sometimes affords relief in cases of great suffering and imminent peril.

Method.—The adjustment of the hot and the cold compresses respectively varies for different parts of the body and the different viscera, the circulation of which it is desired to influence. The management of the cold and hot compress should be the same as previously indicated for continuous applications; that is, the nervous sensibility of the cutaneous surface to which the cold application is made must be kept alive by rubbing the parts with a dry warm flannel for one minute each time the compress is changed. The compress should be renewed every 10 or 15 minutes, or as soon as its temperature begins to approach that of the body. The hot application likewise should be exchanged every 15 or 20 minutes for a cold application of 30 seconds to 1 minute, so as to empty the veins, restore the tone of the vessels, and prevent too great accumulation of heat in the deeper parts.

The duration of the hot and cold compress may be from 15 minutes to one or two hours, or even longer. A good rule is to continue the application until the effect desired is produced, unless decided indications for its interruption appear.

In the employment of the hot and cold compress it must be borne constantly in mind that the application should be made in such a way that the blood-vessels of the congested organ in the interest of which the application is made will be caused to contract by the cold compress, the veins or the arteries of the part being at the same time drained into another collaterally related cutaneous area by means of the hot application, in accordance with principles explained elsewhere (1290).

To secure the best effects, the compresses should be

adjusted with special relation to internal parts, as explained for each special form of this procedure.

1357 **Physiological Effects.**—The hot and cold compress is a hydriatic measure of great power. It is perhaps the most effective means of controlling the movement of the blood in internal parts. It acts both reflexly and derivatively. A cold application applied to one cutaneous surface causes contraction of the vessels of the associated internal organ through stimulation of its controlling vasomotor centers, while the hot compress applied to another cutaneous surface, the vessels of which are collaterally related to those of the part, drain off a portion of blood into the dilated cutaneous veins and arteries. The partial reaction following the first impression made by the cold compress and the frequent renewal of the cold application facilitates the movement of blood through the affected part, thus insuring a constant supply of oxygen, fresh nutrient material, the removal of wastes, and the influx of leucocytes, while at the same time the hot application combats stasis by drawing the blood into collateral venous and arterial channels, at the same time facilitating the rate of movement of the blood through the arteries of the parts by lowering the pressure in the veins. By this combination of effects the distension of blood-vessels and stasis of blood is prevented, while the movement of blood is accelerated, thus restoring the normal status of the circulation and greatly facilitating the healing processes. How this may be accomplished in the interest of any particular internal viscus may be clearly seen by a careful study of paragraphs **1262–1291.**

Therapeutic Applications.—The conditions under which the hot and cold compress attains its special successes are those in which ordinary hot or cold applications, if they afford any relief at all, secure no more than partial amelioration of the urgent symptom present, the beneficial effects which might be obtained through the revulsion produced by cold being antidoted by the thermic effects produced by the application;

while, on the other hand, hot applications prove too exciting, depressing the heart when long continued, or causing other untoward effects. By a combination of the two, however, in these cases the evil effects resulting from each are antidoted, while the good effects of each are intensified.

The following forms of the hot and cold compress have been tested and found practical and useful:—

The Hot and Cold Head Compress.— Place an ice-bag to the 1358
back of the neck and the ice compress to the vertex (Fig. 184). Apply very hot compresses to the face and ears. The hot compresses should not extend below the level of the jaw, thus avoiding the heating of the large vessels of the neck. The ice-bag causes contraction of the vertebral arteries; the cold compress to the vertex causes reflex contraction of the meningeal and cerebral vessels, and cools the brain; while the fomentation to the face and ears dilates the external branches of the carotid artery, thus establishing collateral anemia of the brain. The fomentation also dilates some of the venous channels by which the cerebral sinuses are drained (**1262**).

A reverse method may sometimes be used advantageously in applications to the head, as follows:—

A rubber bag filled with hot water and covered with a moist flannel, or a fomentation, is applied to the upper and back part of the neck, while a soft cheese-cloth compress wrung out of cool or very cold water is applied to the face and the top of the head.

The effect of the compress in relieving cerebral congestion is greatly increased by the application of the ice compress or ice-bag to the front of the neck, whereby the blood supply of the brain is lessened by contraction of the carotid arteries.

The combination of heat and cold to the head in this manner renders it possible to make applications of heat to the head for a much longer time than could otherwise be tolerated, the cold antidoting any ill effect which might be produced by the heat, while encouraging the good effects of the application.

The author has made use of this application for many years as a means of relieving certain forms of *neurasthenic headache.* It is exceedingly useful also in so-called *nervous headache* accompanied by marked congestion of the brain.

This procedure is especially useful in *passive congestion* of the brain, and serves a useful purpose as an adjunct procedure in the treatment of *insomnia* when due to cerebral hyperemia. It should be avoided, however, in cases of insomnia due to excessive excitability of the cerebral cells, and is of course contraindicated in insomnia due to anemia.

1359 **The Hot and Cold Lung Compress.**—A thick and very hot fomentation is applied over the back, reaching from the middle of the neck to the lumbar region, and extending to the axillary line on each side. The cold compress should cover the top of the lungs, the lower half of the neck in front, and the whole anterior surface of the chest to the level of the lowest ribs. The fomentation diverts the blood from the bronchial arteries by dilating the cutaneous branches of the intercostals, while the cold compress contracts the bronchial arteries through reflex stimulation of the vasomotor ceniers controlling them. The effects of the application may be intensified by hot applications to the arms and legs applied simultaneously, especially hot packs, which produce decided derivative effects.

This procedure is exceedingly useful in the early stages of *pneumonia*, in *broncho-pneumonia*, in *pulmonary hemorrhage, acute pulmonary congestion*, and the congestion resulting from the use of ether in anesthesia. Its use in the last-named condition is especially important when much mucus is present, and when cyanosis, or blueness of the skin, indicates stasis from cardiac weakness or interference with oxygenation. It has for some time been the author's custom to apply a heating chest pack immediately after removing the patient from the operating table when the foregoing symptoms were present. More recently the plan of applying the hot and cold lung compress in cases in which an anesthetic is administered has been tested. When ether is employed, the application extends to the whole chest surface, as above described; when chloroform is used, a hot bag is placed to the back and an ice-bag or a cold compress over the heart. The compress should be at least as large as the surface covered by the patient's two hands placed side by side. The cold compress should be removed for a few seconds every ten minutes, and the surface rubbed with a dry, warm flannel till red, so as to maintain the cutaneous reflexes upon which this compress depends for its efficiency as a cardiac stimulant.

The author has made use of the hot and cold chest pack for fifteen years or more, and believes it to be one of the most valuable of all means for combating pulmonary congestion. The circulation of the lungs is controlled by the vasomotor centers located at the upper portion of the dorsal region, and the purpose of the hot application is to stimulate the activity of these centers; while the cold application to the anterior portion of the chest causes first a contraction, and later active dilatation and fluxion of the vessels of the lungs, thus combating passive hyperemia and inflammation.

This is an excellent means of relieving acute congestion of the lung in pulmonary hemorrhages, and combating the hypostatic congestions which occur in fevers of a low type. The application may be continued for half an hour or more, and should be repeated two or three times a day.

This measure is of very great value for removing the pulmonary congestion which follows ether anesthesia, and thus combats the tendency to bronchial pneumonia, which is often a greater risk in old subjects than the operation itself.

A special form of the hot and cold compress is of particu- 1360
lar service in asthma. An ice compress is applied to the back of the neck and head while a fomentation is applied to the whole front part of the chest, extending from the clavicles to the umbilicus. The back may be included. The cold application lessens the blood supply of the medulla, and so dimin-

ishes the excitability of the respiratory centers, while the fomentation relaxes the spasm of the bronchioles.

1361 **The Hot and Cold Renal Compress** (Fig. 185).—The hot application covers the back from the middle dorsal region to the coccyx. The cold application should consist of an ice-bag or a cold compress covering the lower third of the sternum. The connection of the portal circulation with the renal vein makes it undesirable that any of its outlets should be closed or its tension raised by reflex impressions from the general abdominal surface. The fomentation diverts the blood from the branches of the lumbar artery which are distributed to the capsule of the kidney and leads off a portion of the blood from the renal vein into the anastomosing muscular branches, while the cold application causes reflex contraction of the blood-vessels of the kidney and increases its activity (1098). (See Fig. 152.)

This measure is of special service in cases of acute congestion of the kidney, especially in connection with acute febrile diseases, as scarlet fever, typhoid fever, smallpox, and diphtheria. It should be used in connection with the hot blanket pack or other general hot applications in the intervals as a means of continuing the effect of the general hot application. Care must be taken that the patient does not become chilled by the cold application.

1362 **The Hot and Cold Gastro-Hepatic Compress.**—This compress influences not only the stomach and liver, but also the spleen and the pancreas through the intimate association of the circulation of these organs. The application is almost exactly the reverse of that of the renal compress. The fomentation is applied anteriorly from the fourth rib to the umbilicus, extending to the axillary line on each side, while a cold bag at least eighteen inches long is applied to the dorsal and lumbar spine. Through the dilatation of the branches of the internal mammary arteries and associated veins, the blood is drawn off from the stomach, liver, spleen, and pancreas while the reflex stimulation of the controlling vasomotor centers contracts the vessels of the arterial circulation.

The Hot and Cold Intestinal Compress.—The cold compress is applied over the whole abdominal surface, extending from the xyphoid cartilage to the pubes. The fomentation is simultaneously applied to the lumbar region and the left side, as it is desirable to divert the blood from the left kidney both by establishing collateral hyperemia of the overlying structures, and also by diverting the venous blood from the kidney into the anastomosing muscular channels. 1363

This procedure is of special value in chronic duodenitis and colitis.

The Hot and Cold Pelvic Compress.—The cold compress is applied to the hypogastrium in combination with a fomentation across the lower part of the back. The fomentation may also profitably become a hip pack, or a hot leg and hip pack. When the inflammation is confined to one side, an ice-bag instead of the cold compress may be placed over the affected part. The ice-bag may be used in combination with the hot pelvic pack (Fig. 153.). 1364

This measure is especially valuable in the treatment of *acute inflammations* of the *uterus*, *tubes*, *ovaries*, and *bladder*, in *appendicitis* and *pelvic peritonitis*. In cases of *inflammation* of the *prostate*, in *proctitis*, and *cystitis*, the ice-bag may be applied to the perineum in connection with the hip pack, or with the hip pack and the hot leg pack or foot bath applied simultaneously.

THE HOT AND COLD HEATING COMPRESS OR PACK.

This procedure differs from the hot and cold compress in the same way in which the ordinary heating compress differs from the cold compress. In the hot and cold compress the hot application is made continuous, or practically so, by the frequent renewal of the compress. In the hot and cold heating compress or pack the cold application is not renewed, but allowed to accumulate heat through reaction. The area covered by the cold application in this procedure is usually much greater than in the hot and cold compress. The duration is usually from one to two hours. 1365

This procedure is especially applicable to the chest, the abdomen, and the pelvic region.

Physiological Effects.—The hot and cold pack is, next to the hot and cold compress, perhaps the most powerful of all known means of controlling the movement of blood through the viscera of the chest and abdomen. The heating pack depends for its special features upon the anatomical fact that the collateral relation between the arteries and the veins with internal parts does not closely coincide as regards the location of the related vessels in the skin, thus making possible the simultaneous application of two procedures differing in method, but each assisting the other.

The explanation of the effects of the hot and cold compress (**1356**) applies only in part to the hot and cold heating compress or pack. In the former, the action of the cold application is continuous or nearly so, while in the heating process the stimulant effect of the cold soon disappears, giving place, under the influence of the powerful reaction, to extreme dilatation and great activity of the cutaneous vessels. As the heat accumulates, venous stasis is developed, producing powerful derivative effects upon the associated venous trunks, and thus by lessening the pressure in the veins, hastens the movement of blood through the arteries of the congested part. At the same time, the hot compress, being applied to a cutaneous area, the arteries of which are collaterally related to those of the deeper structures which it is designed to influence, produce powerful collateral anemia of the vessels of the congested organ. Several very powerful therapeutic factors are thus brought to bear simultaneously upon the diseased part as follows:—

1. By the application of the cold compress the vessels of the part are made to contract, thus forcing the stagnating blood onward into the veins.

2. As the heating compress warms and the cutaneous veins become filled with blood, the veins of the congested viscus are emptied, thus draining the tissues of the toxins which have accumulated in them.

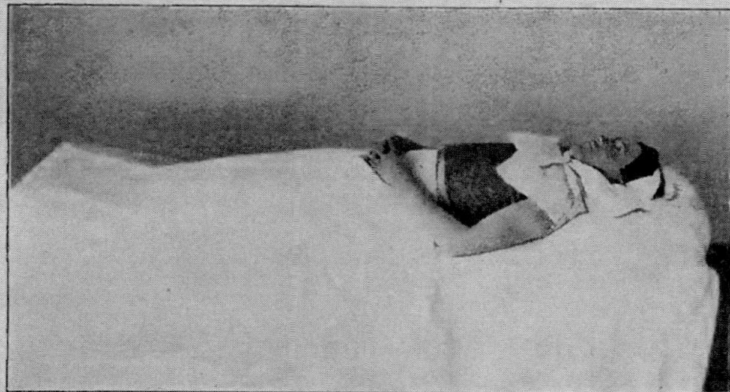

Fig. 186. HOT AND COLD CHEST PACK (p. 849).

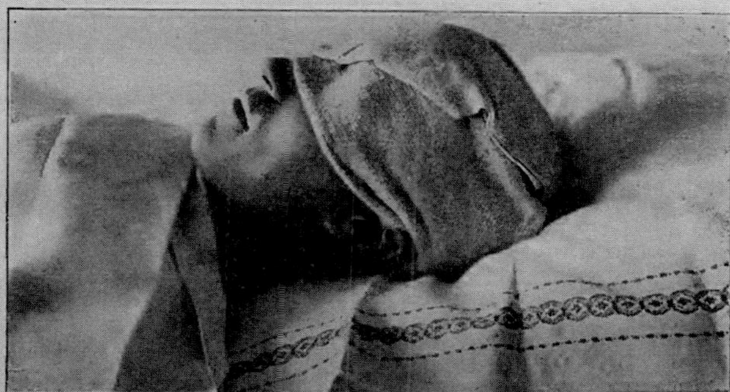

Fig. 188. COLD CEPHALIC COMPRESS (p. 853).

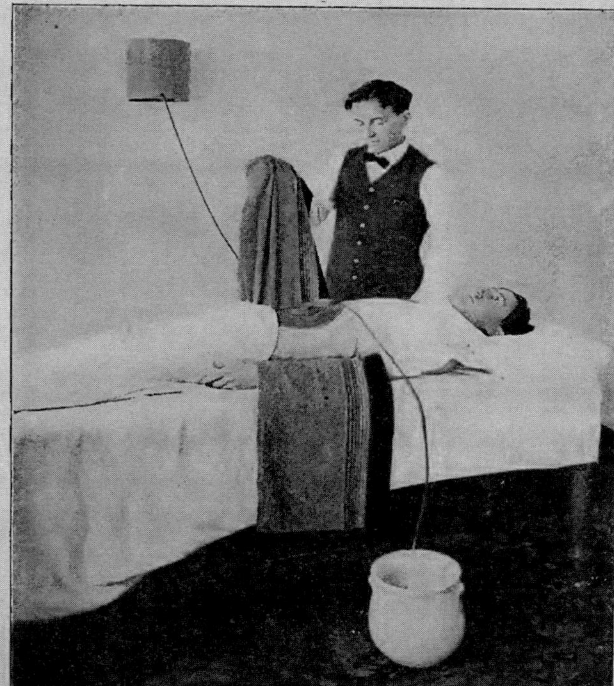

Fig. 187. HOT AND COLD ABDOMINAL OR TRUNK PACK (p. 849).

3. By lowering the pressure in the veins, the arterial circulation through the affected part is facilitated, thus encouraging the nutrition and functional activity of the cells which are engaged in combating living germs, or which are seeking to repair damages which may have originated in any way.

4. The hot application diverts the blood into the cutaneous branches of the collateral arteries or into anastomosing vessels, thus preventing undue accumulation of blood and consequent embarrassment of the affected tissues. The anatomical relationships through which these results are attained have been described elsewhere (**1262–1278**).

The Hot and Cold Chest Pack.—The chest pack is applied in the ordinary way. The form known as the square chest pack (**1374**) is preferable. After the wet pack has been adjusted and before the woolen wrapping is arranged, a spine bag filled with water as hot as can be borne safely (140° to 160°) is applied between the shoulders, reaching from the lower cervical to the lumbar region. The woolen wrapping is then brought snugly in place, and fastened in such a manner as completely to cover the back, leaving no openings about the neck. As an extra precaution it is a good plan to adjust a flannel about the neck in the manner shown in Fig. 186. 1366

The Hot and Cold Abdominal Pack (Fig. 187).—In this procedure the moist bandage is placed around the trunk at the level of the umbilicus in the usual manner for the *umschlag*, or wet girdle (**1347**). A rubber or aluminum coil is placed upon a wet towel just over the epigastrium. The blankets are then tucked snugly about the patient, and a stream of hot water is kept flowing through the coil continuously during the application, at a temperature as high as the patient can bear. The author has made use of this application ever since it was first suggested by Professor Winternitz, using instead of a coil, however, a rubber bag filled with very hot water, a thermophore, or a syphon sack. 1367

The first information printed in this country in relation

to this valuable hydriatic measure was an article contributed by Professor Winternitz, by request of the author, to his journal, *Modern Medicine.**

If necessary to continue the application for a considerable length of time, the hot water bag may be refilled once or twice. In general, however, it is better to remove the hot bag or coil at the end of the first 30 minutes, thus avoiding overheating.

The hot and cold abdominal pack has rendered most valuable service in a great number of cases; and so positive and satisfactory have been its results in the hands of the author that in his estimation it stands almost unrivaled as a hydriatic procedure in the certainty with which it produces the effects expected from it. This measure has proved especially successful in both *sensory* and *motor disturbances* of the *stomach*, especially in cases in which the patients complain of *pain* soon after eating, *flatulence*, *eructations* and *regurgitations* of *food* and *vomiting* of *bile*.

In one case in which a lady had suffered four months from regurgitation of bile into the stomach, being reduced to a very low state, the reflux of bile was at once controlled by the application of this pack. It was applied half an hour before each of the two daily meals given the patient, and was retained two hours, so that the process of digestion was begun under the influence of the pack. During the first few weeks of the treatment the difficulty returned occasionally when the compress was omitted, but after a few months, the patient was able to dispense with the pack, and was not only entirely relieved of the distressing symptom, but had gained twenty-five pounds in flesh, and was restored to health. In another case a man had been for years afflicted in the same manner, having frequent attacks, lasting for several weeks, during which time vomiting occurred within a few minutes after each meal. The patient was brought to the Battle Creek Sanitarium in an extremely feeble condition. The hot

---

**Modern Medicine*, Vol. I, page 50.

and cold abdominal compress, however, controlled the vomiting in a few days, and the patient's stomach was soon trained to the digestion of a reasonable amount of wholesome and simple food. Scores of similar cases might be related.

Hyperesthesia of the lumbar ganglia of the abdominal sympathetic and of the solar plexus, when extreme in degree, also requires the application of this powerful analgesic procedure. By its daily application for a few weeks, cases in which the ganglia are so sensitive that even very slight pressure excites almost excruciating pain, and in which as a result the abdominal viscera are subject to painful affections of various sorts, may often be made completely comfortable, other constitutional measures being of course employed at the same time. In nervous asthma and disturbances due to disorders of the abdominal sympathetic, this measure renders invaluable service, as may also be noted in the majority of cases of *nervous headache*, or *migraine*, which is likewise a sympathetic nerve disorder. Obstinate vomiting, nausea, including the nausea and *vomiting* of *pregnancy*, yield to this procedure with most satisfactory readiness in nearly all cases.

The hot and cold trunk pack has been found of great service in cases of *hyperpepsia* and in *hypopepsia* attended by *gastric irritation*.

The Hot and Cold Lumbar Pack.—This application is 1368
made the same as for the hot and cold abdominal pack, except that the hot bag or coil is applied over the lumbar region. A large square bag is used for this purpose. This application is of special service as a means of combating portal or renal congestion. Care must be taken to apply the heat over the left kidney, as there is a direct communication between the left renal vein and the portal system.

The Hot and Cold Spinal Pack.—A half sheet, one thick- 1369
ness, wrung out of very cold water, is placed about the trunk in the usual manner for the trunk pack. The patient then rolls to one side, and a long rubber bag half filled with

hot water is placed in such a position that when he returns to the dorsal position, the bag will lie in contact with the center of the back its whole length. The blankets are then drawn around the patient in the usual manner.

This procedure is especially valuable in cases of spinal irritation which are aggravated by cold applications, and in which there is general passive congestion of the viscera of the chest and abdomen,—conditions present in a large proportion of cases of chronic dyspepsia, especially in women. In these cases there is generally an exceeding tenderness of the lumbar ganglia, of the intercostal nerves, and of the whole dorsal region. Hot applications to the spine usually afford temporary relief, but are exhausting and weakening when long continued or often repeated. Much better results are obtained by the application of heat and cold as described.

1370 **The Hot and Cold Pelvic Pack.**—This measure is applied in the same manner as the ordinary cold pelvic pack (**1390**), with the exception that a rubber bag filled with hot water or a coil is placed over the lower abdomen next the wet sheet. The effect of this application is to afford relief in congestions of the pelvic viscera, in which it is as useful as is the hot and cold abdominal pack (**1367**), in congestions of the abdominal viscera.

Method.—The mode of application is precisely the same as that of the ordinary pelvic pack (**1390**), except that a hot water bag or coil is slipped in between the folds of the blanket with one thickness intervening, and so placed as to fall over the uterus and bladder.

Therapeutic Applications.—The hot and cold pelvic pack is indicated in hyperesthesias of the uterus, ovaries, and bladder, in *acute congestion* of any of the *pelvic viscera*, accompanied by *pain* or *muscular spasm*, as *tenesmus* of the *bladder* or *rectum*, and *vaginismus*. Painful *ovarian congestion*, *congestion* and *hyperesthesia* of the *uterus*, *vesical irritation*, *ovarian irritation*,—these and other like conditions indicate the employment of this useful measure, and are generally very readily relieved by it. *Sexual erethism, irregular* and *painful menstruation*, and the heaviness and indescribable but distressing symptoms with which so many invalid women suffer, yield to this remarkably efficient measure.

SPECIAL FORMS OF COMPRESS.

In addition to the various forms of compress which have been described in the foregoing pages, there are several special compresses worthy of description because of their great practical utility, and concerning which there are various practical points which need to be understood, especially in relation to the technique of their application. These are the *cephalic compress*, the *chest pack*, the *throat compress*, the *neck compress*, the *joint compress*, the *cotton poultice*, the *hip pack*, the *pelvic pack*, the *leg pack*, the *foot pack*, and the *hot* and *cold compress*.

The *roller compress* consists of a long strip of cheese-cloth folded to three thicknesses, and of proper width. Thus prepared, the bandage is rolled up. When wanted for use, it is immersed, wrung out quickly, and applied as soon as possible, so that its temperature may not be modified by contact with the air of the room. A number of such bandages of different widths should always be in readiness for use.

THE CEPHALIC COMPRESS (Fig. 188).

The application is usually made to either the top or the 1371
back of the head. When applied to the back of the head, the upper part of the neck is usually included in the application. The application may be made to the top of the head and the face, to the face and the neck, or to the entire head, —scalp, face, and neck.

In the application of the cold cephalic compress it is necessary to bear in mind the fact that a cold application to the face may have the effect to produce collateral hyperemia of the brain, by contracting the external branches of the carotid artery (1282, 1262). A napkin moistened with ice-water and laid upon the forehead may do more harm than good, by contracting the supraorbital branch of the internal carotid, and thus diverting more blood into its internal branches in the cerebrum. This effect may be readily antagonized by a cold application about the neck, which will contract the carotids and the vertebral arteries and all their branches, and thus aid the reflex action from the face and scalp in lessening the volume of blood in the brain.

These contrary and undesirable effects of cold applications are most likely to occur in conditions in which the vascular tension is low and fluctuating. They may give rise to local or circumscribed cyanosis from vascular spasm, and simultaneous collateral congestion.

In making cold applications for the relief of cerebral congestion, special care should be given to the eyes. The compress should always cover them, and should be well pressed down upon them, so as to utilize the powerful reflex relations which exist between the eye and the brain through the sympathetic.

The same principle governs applications to the hands and feet for relief of inflammatory conditions involving deep structures. An ice-bag over the trunk of the supplying artery (axilla, bend of elbow, groin, popliteal space) will lessen the local congestion, as well as or even better than an application to the whole arm or leg; while an application to the part alone might produce collateral internal congestion.

Physiological Effects.—The effects of the application of cold to the head have already been considered (**1315**). It may be mentioned further that the head compress is less exciting and more sedative than the cephalic douche. Applied continuously, or frequently renewed, the prolonged cold head compress is highly sedative, lessening the cerebral blood supply, and diminishing the activity of the brain. In active congestion, a continuous *very cold* application is best; in passive congestion, it is better to secure vasomotor exercise and fluxion of the brain by means of the repeated impressions obtained by frequent renewals of the cold compress, allowing

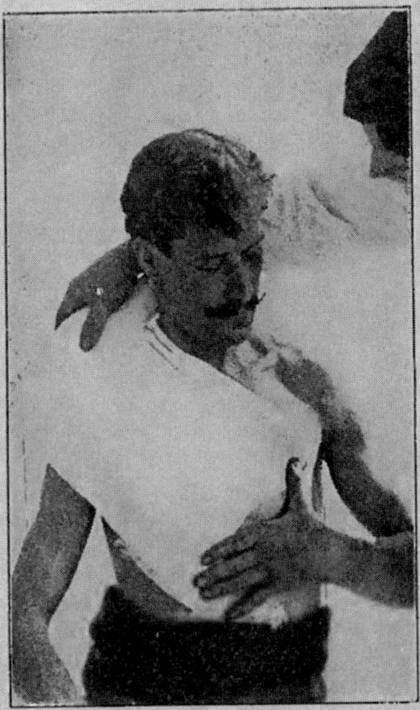

FIG. 189. ROLLER CHEST PACK — First Step (p. 858).

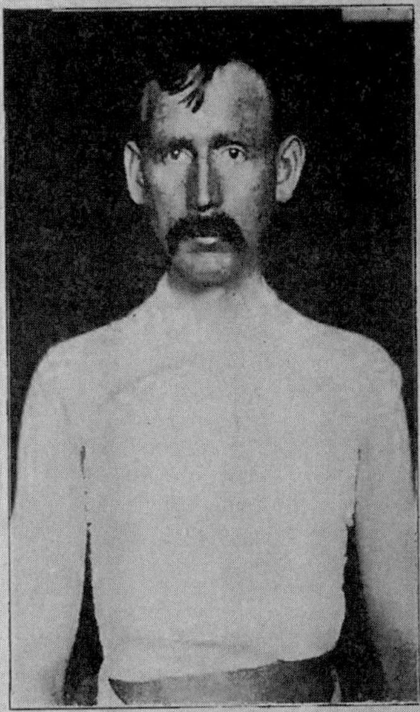

FIG. 190. ROLLER CHEST PACK — Second Step (p. 858).

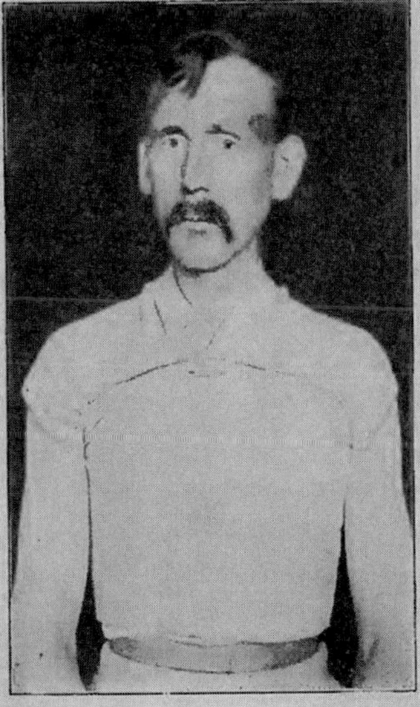

FIG. 191. ROLLER CHEST PACK — Complete (p. 858).

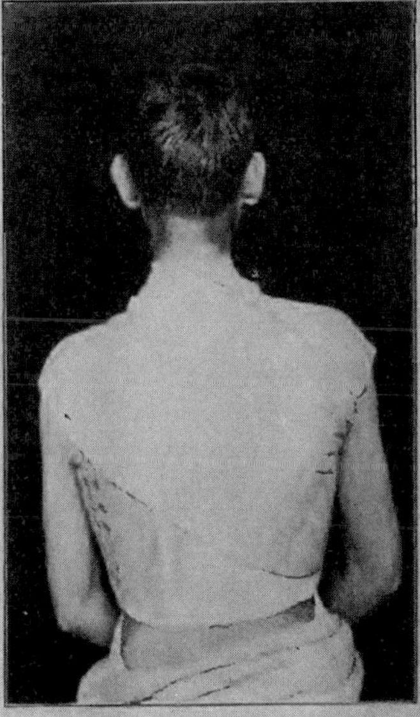

FIG. 192. ROLLER CHEST PACK — Complete (p. 858).

only time for the beginning of reaction effects or slight warming of the compress.

The *short cold* compress increases the cerebral blood supply by reflex reaction effect.

The *hot* or *warm* cephalic compress, or fomentation to the head, congests the cerebral vessels when long applied.

A *short hot* application acts by revulsion to diminish the blood supply of the deeper parts.

Therapeutic Applications.— All forms of *cerebral congestion*, *insomnia* from *cerebral hyperemia*, the *delirium of infectious fevers*, and *congestive headache*, require the cold head compress.

The *hot* head compress, or fomentation to the head, excites cerebral activity, and is of great service in *anemia* in *syncope*, *shock*, and in *collapse* from any cause when associated with cerebral anemia.

The *short cold* compress, followed by drying and rubbing of the scalp, may be used in the same conditions. The hot compress is to be preferred when pain is present, because of its powerful revulsive and analgesic effects.

Continuous cooling of the head may be secured by wetting the hair and allowing the head to remain uncovered. This mode of cooling, however, as also the use of the evaporating compress, is likely to give rise to rheumatic pains of the scalp, because of the long-continued action of a degree of cold sufficient to chill by slow abstraction of heat, but not vigorous enough to induce reaction. The pain is doubtless due to disturbance of the blood supply of the nerve trunks.

The ice-bag applied to the back of the head is a valuable measure in *spermatorrhea* accompanied by frequent losses. The application should be prolonged. It should be applied before going to bed at night, being so adjusted as to rest against the base of the skull while the patient is asleep. In *vaginismus*, and in *masturbation* in women due to sexual erethism, the ice-bag may be applied with advantage to the upper cervical region for twenty minutes several times a day.

In *anemic headache*, the ice-bag may be applied to the upper part of the neck for 1 to 3 minutes. The reaction following increases the supply of blood to the brain. In *nervous asthma*, prolonged applications of the ice-bag to the back of the head will be found advantageous (1360). For very rapid beating of the heart, apply the ice-bag for 10 to 20 minutes to the back of the head or to the neck. A precordial compress should be applied at the same time.

THE COLD SPINAL COMPRESS.

1372 Cold may be applied to the spine by means of the cold wet compress, or by long rubber bags filled with ice, ice-water, or some cooling mixture. The application may be made to the entire spinal column, or to a particular region, as may be desired. Those portions of the spine which it is most commonly designed to influence are the cervical, central, upper dorsal, middle dorsal, and lumbar regions.

In all cases in which the very cold spinal compress is employed for reflex effects, the compress should be removed every 15 or 20 minutes, and the surface rubbed with warm, dry flannel for half a minute, or until reddened. The surface should never become blue or numb. The frequently renewed cold compress (60°, changed every 15 to 30 minutes) produces powerful fluxion of the spinal cord, and is a useful means of improving the nutrition of the cord, and combating degenerative processes.

Therapeutic Applications.—By means of ice-bags or ice poultices, or cloths wrung out of ice-water and renewed every 3 or 4 minutes, most powerful and useful antiphlogistic effects may be obtained in *meningeal inflammation* of the *spine.* The same measure is useful in *apoplexy* of the spine, in cases of *fever* with very high temperature when spinal complication is feared. Localized cold applications to the cervical region are useful in *congestion* of the *brain*, *paroxysms* of *dyspnea* in nervous asthma, and *irritation* of the *cerebellum;* to the upper dorsal region for *pulmonary hemorrhage;* to the lower dorsal region in *nervous vomiting;* to the lumbar region in *uterine* and *renal hemorrhage;* to the whole spine in certain cases of *hysteria*, and in connection with the cephalic compress in the *epileptic state;* to the lower dorsal and the upper lumbar regions in cases of extreme *irritability* of the *genito-urinary centers.*

Cold applications of all sorts to the spine are *contraindicated* in most cases of so-called *spinal irritation*, and in cases of *locomotor ataxia* in which lightning pains or gastric crises are present.

THE CHEST PACK.

This procedure does not differ essentially from packs to 1373
other regions, except that it is confined to the chest. It is commonly applied to the entire chest, both front and back, extending from the neck to the level of the floating cartilages.

Method.—The chest pack may be conveniently applied by means of a sort of jacket fitted to the patient, or better still, by means of a bandage made of one or two thicknesses of linen, or four to six thicknesses of cheese-cloth. The bandage should be eight to ten inches in width, six to eight feet in length, and should be loosely rolled up, dipped into water at the proper temperature, and wrung out without unrolling. The bandage is applied in a sort of "figure 8" fashion, which may be described as follows: The nurse taking the roll of bandage in her right hand, and seizing the end of the bandage with her left, stations herself in front of the patient, who is sitting or standing with the clothing removed to the waist. The end of the bandage is placed against the right side of the chest, and held in place by the patient's hand; or, the application may begin under the patient's right arm, which is pressed against the bandage to hold it in position. The bandage is then carried obliquely across the chest and over the left shoulder; then, passing obliquely downward across the back, it is carried forward under the right arm and then horizontally across the chest in front, under the left arm obliquely upward to the right shoulder, over which the end of the bandage is drawn and tucked under the transverse fold crossing the chest. The transverse portion of the bandage is then pulled up toward each shoulder, and fastened as snugly as possible by means of safety-pins. The wet bandage should be made to fit the patient tightly everywhere (Figs. 189–192).

A flannel bandage of the same width and a little greater length is applied over the moist bandage in precisely the same manner, care being taken to cover the wet bandage completely, and to make it fit snugly at every point so as wholly to exclude the air. The flannel bandage may be long enough to extend several times about the chest so as to protect the wet bandage as thoroughly as necessary. A bandage of mackintosh cut as in the square pack (Fig. 193) may be placed next the wet bandage when needed.

1374 **The Square Chest Pack.**—This is one of the most convenient and perhaps on the whole the most satisfactory of all the several forms of the chest pack (Figs. 193–197).

Requisites.—A rectangular linen bandage of the proper length, and a woolen bandage of the same shape but larger. The length of the linen bandage should be one and one-half times the circumference of the patient's chest over the largest part, and the width should be sufficient to reach from the top of the shoulder to the lowest rib; the woolen bandage should be two inches wider and the same length. The thickness of the linen bandage depends upon the effect desired: a single thickness of heavy linen toweling is sufficient; if linen sheeting is employed, two thicknesses will generally be required, or four thicknesses of cheese-cloth. The woolen bandage should be of blanket stuff, heavy, soft, and at least two thicknesses. Starting at a point one third the distance from the upper edge of the linen bandage, a slit is torn one third its length; a similar slit is torn at the other end. The woolen bandage is prepared in the same way; also a mackintosh if needed.

Method.— The woolen blanket is spread out on a smooth surface. The linen bandage is now wrung dry out of water

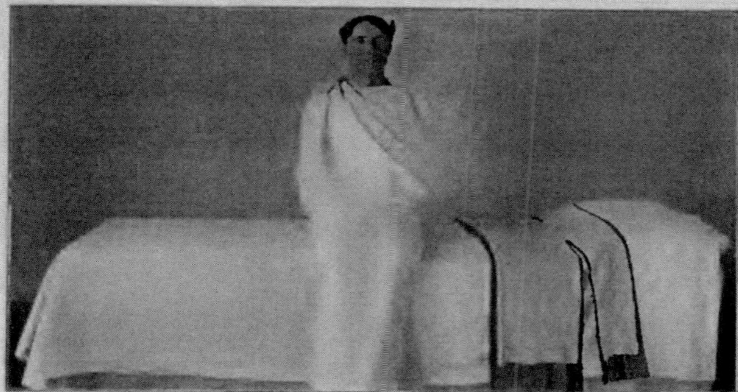

Fig. 193. SQUARE CHEST PACK — First Step (p. 858).

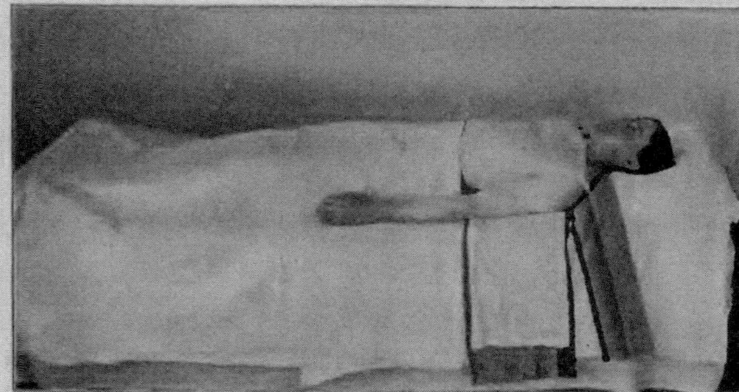

Fig. 194. SQUARE CHEST PACK — Second Step (p. 858).

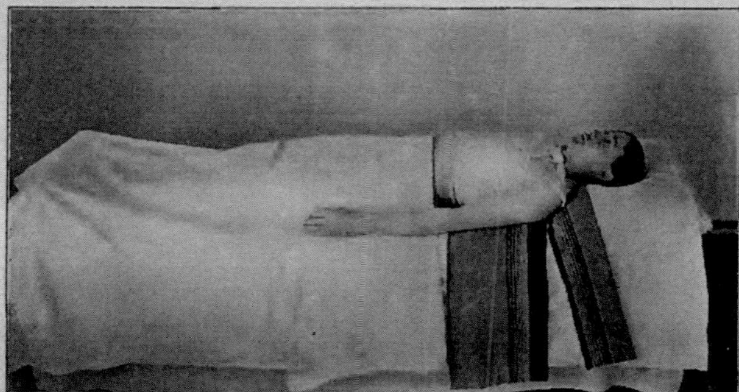

Fig. 195. SQUARE CHEST PACK — Third Step (p. 858).

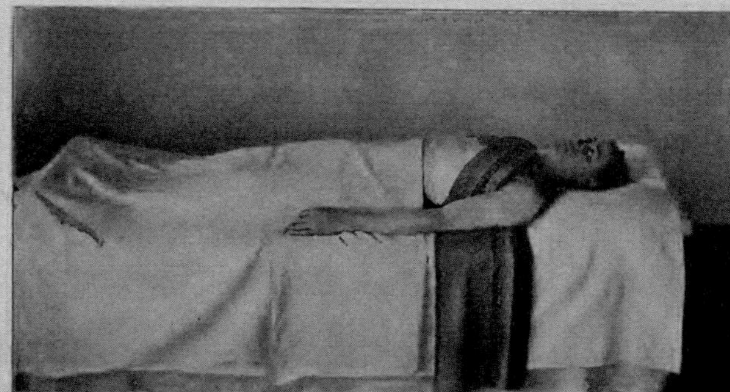

Fig. 196. SQUARE CHEST PACK — Fourth Step (p. 858).

at 60°, and spread out upon the woolen blanket (Fig. 193). The patient having been previously prepared, he sits or is held up for a few seconds while the bandages are spread out on the bed beneath him in such a position that the end of each slit falls exactly at the top of the axilla on each side. When the patient lies down, the upper edge of the woolen bandage should just reach the hair.

The upper tail of the bandage on one side is now drawn across the shoulder toward the opposite side, and the surplus folded back (Fig. 194). The corresponding part of the bandage on the opposite side is adjusted likewise. The rest of the bandage is then adjusted, one side and then the other being drawn over, as shown in Fig. 195. In cases of pharyngitis in connection with acute catarrh of the lungs, the edges of the two shoulder pieces may be brought together close up under the chin, thus making a throat compress. The flannel bandage is now brought across in like manner, care being taken to cover thoroughly all portions of the moist bandage so as to prevent cooling by evaporation. This bandage has the advantage that it is simple, can be very easily and quickly applied, and completely envelops the chest.

The Triangular Chest Pack.—This is a very convenient 1375
form of bandage for use in cases of acute inflammatory processes in the lungs, as pleurisy, pneumonia, bronchitis, tubercular disease, and in patients too feeble to sit up, as in some typhoid cases.

Requisites.—One thick woolen blanket, one linen sheet folded twice lengthwise, one woolen sheet folded cornerwise, a triangular linen or cheese-cloth bandage of three thicknesses, with base four to six feet, height of triangle, three feet.

Method.—Spread the woolen blanket on the bed. Lay the linen sheet folded lengthwise across the bed at such a point that the upper edge will fall an inch above the level of the axilla when the patient lies down. Lay the triangular woolen bandage across the bed with the apex down and the base at such a point as to be level with the occiput when the patient lies down. Now, wet the triangular linen bandage in the following manner: Fold it by placing the two equal angles of the triangle together, grasping the bandage with the left hand at the middle of the base. Continue folding in like manner until three or four inches wide, then turn the lower end upward, still retaining the hold with the left hand. Dip the whole in water, wring out dry so as not to drip, still retaining hold with the left hand as at the beginning. After the bandage is wrung dry, shake with the left hand until it is completely unfolded. Spread out with the apex down, the base upward, falling parallel with the base of the triangular woolen bandage and one inch below it (Fig. 198). Now let the patient lie down in such a position that the occiput will fall just below the upper edge of the bandage. Next let the attendant lay hold of one lateral angle of the wet bandage, and draw over the shoulders, then the other, covering each shoulder well, and carrying the tips of the bandage across the chest and under the side opposite, leaving the arms out. The woolen triangle is then adjusted in similar fashion, and lastly the folded sheet is brought around the chest, first one end and then the other, binding all together (Fig. 199). When necessary to renew the compress, it may be easily withdrawn after opening the woolen wrappings.

1376 **The Towel Chest Pack.**—This is the simplest and one of the best of all the various forms of the chest compress or pack. It differs from the preceding only in having two large towels used in place of the linen triangle. These are wrung out very dry, and then applied one over each shoulder and across the chest in front and behind, care being taken to cover the whole surface of the chest (Fig. 200). The outer wrappings are then closed about the chest as in the triangular pack. The wet towels must be wrung as dry as possible.

In applying the chest pack in either form described, it is of the utmost importance that the application be made accurately. If the compress is applied in such a way that evaporation takes place, the parts will be chilled, producing an effect the very opposite to that desired. On the other hand, overheating with too much covering, or by impervious covering, is equally harmful in cases in which it is desired to maintain vascular tone rather than to produce strong hyperemia for derivative effects.

The temperature should be 60° or less, except for very feeble patients who are not accustomed to cold, in which case it may be 70° to 75°, for the first application. If from previous experience it is known that the patient is not able to warm the bandage rapidly, the hand should be dipped in water at 50°, and this should be applied to the chest and neck with vigorous rubbing, followed by drying and rubbing with a warm flannel just before the bandage is applied. This insures good reaction.

The Half Chest Compress.— In certain cases it may some- 1377
times be best to confine the application of the cold compress to one half of the chest. The following simple device answers the purpose admirably, covering the top as well as the sides of the chest, a precaution which should not be forgotten in the treatment of chest affections:—

A broad towel about two feet in length is split down the middle one third its length. It is then wet and wrung out in the usual way, and applied in such a manner that the arm occupies the slit, while one of the two legs passes in front of the shoulder, falling over the top, while the other covers the back of the shoulder (Fig. 201). The flannel covering is then applied in the usual way, and lastly a flannel bandage of square or triangular form, as most convenient.

Another method employs a wide towel of the ordinary length. After being wet and wrung out, it is laid across the shoulder. The upper corners of the towel are carried across the chest, one in front, the other behind, and made to overlap close under the axilla, well covering the side (Fig. 202). The application of the flannel bandage secures the towel in position. The towel may be doubled if necessary, and if long enough, or two towels may be used. If necessary, a safety-pin may be applied at the top of the shoulder in such a way as to attach the towel to the flannel to prevent its slipping down over the shoulder.

The hot and cold chest pack (**1366**) and the hot and cold lung compress (**1359**) have been fully described elsewhere. They are important modifications of the chest compress which are of special value in the morbid conditions in which they are particularly indicated. The special directions for the use of the chest compress in pneumonia and other pulmonary maladies are given elsewhere.

1378 **Physiological Effects.**—There is no therapeutic agent the use of which rests upon a more thoroughly sound and rational basis than does the employment of the compress in pulmonary affections, especially in pneumonia.

The experiments made by Winternitz and Schlikoff showed that the temperature of the cavity of the chest is diminished within ten minutes after the application of the cooling thoracic compress. The blood-vessels of the chest are made to contract instantly when contact with the cold compress is made. The tidal air is increased more than one third in volume (Exp. 71).

1379 **Therapeutic Applications.**—The chest pack acts powerfully upon the pulmonary mucous membrane. It is of great value in *pulmonary congestion*, and has also been used with considerable success in *pulmonary tuberculosis*. In this disease it controls the *cough*, lowers the temperature, lessens the *night sweats*, and facilitates the healing process by aiding leucocytosis. In *bronchial catarrh* it is of very great service, relieving the congestion by bringing the blood to the surface, thus relieving the cough and the *expectoration*.

In spasmodic asthma the application of the chest pack sometimes brings on a paroxysm of difficult breathing. This tendency may be largely obviated by the application of fomentations to the chest just before the application of the cold compress. The chest pack is a very valuable measure in all cases of *chronic bronchitis*, *chronic pneumonia*, and *chronic pleurisy*, in connection with fomentations, which should in these cases precede the application of the pack, and especially in that very common affliction known as a cold on the lungs. The fomentations should be very hot and of short duration — 5 to 8 minutes.

The cooling chest compress is applicable in all cases of *congestion* and *inflammation* of the *lungs* and in *pulmonary hemorrhage*. Its employment is especially important at the beginning of pulmonary inflammation. In cases of hemorrhage, very cold compresses should be applied and frequently renewed. Special attention should be given to the surface above the clavicle. The effect of the compress may be intensified by applying ice-bags to the apices of the chest over the cold compress.

A cold compress over the whole chest or over the cardiac region alone is valuable in cases of over-action of the heart, cardiac irritability, or threatened cardiac failure. The effect secured by this application is often very remarkable and almost immediate.

The heating chest compress has great therapeutic value in the treatment of tuberculosis and in chronic bronchial catarrh. When employed for this purpose, the compress should be covered with thin mackintosh or gutta-percha tissue if the patient is feeble and reaction defective. When febrile action is marked, flannel covering only should be used.

The heating chest compress is very useful in cases of chronic pleurisy accompanied by affusion. The pack should be removed once in three or four hours for the application of the revulsive compress, consisting of a fomentation for 4 or 5 minutes, followed by a cold compress for 15 to 20 seconds, the alternation being repeated three or four times.

In cases of chronic bronchitis, the compress should be covered with mackintosh, and should be changed as often as once in every four hours. If allowed to remain too long, so that it becomes superheated, palpitation of the heart and faintness are likely to occur.

When considerable fever is present, as indicated by a temperature of 101° to 102°, the compress should be wet in cool water, or water at a temperature of 60° to 70°, and wrung lightly, so that it may contain, when applied, as much water as possible without dripping. While the fever lasts, this chest compress should be worn night and day. It should be covered lightly, with flannel only, in the summer-time. In the winter-time, if the temperature of the sleeping-room falls below the ordinary living-room temperature, and the patient's powers of reaction are deficient, the impervious covering may be applied. When the cough and the fever are both troublesome, the compress may be worn both night and day.

Precautions.— 1. Every precaution must be taken to avoid chilling the patient. If the towel is too wet, a feeble patient may not be able to warm it up, and may chill.

2. Especial care must be taken to make the dry flannel bandage extend an inch beyond the wet towel above and below, in order to prevent the air from getting under the bandage.

3. When the chest pack is applied at night, the chest must be bathed with cold water and vigorously rubbed on arising in the morning, and a thick flannel wrapping must take the place of the pack, to be worn during the day.

THE HOT CHEST PACK.

1380 This differs from the ordinary chest pack chiefly in that the wet bandage is of flannel, doubled, and is wrung out of hot water. The square form of pack is preferable (**1374**).

The hot chest pack stimulates the circulation of the surface of the chest, thus withdrawing the blood from the bronchial arteries into the intercostals. The pleura is drained into the cutaneous branches of the internal mammary.

The hot chest pack relieves the *pain* of *pleurisy* and *pneumonia*, *cardialgia*, and *spasm* of the *bronchioles* in nervous asthma.

It should not be forgotten that in applying heat to the chest the heart, as well as the lungs, is profoundly affected;

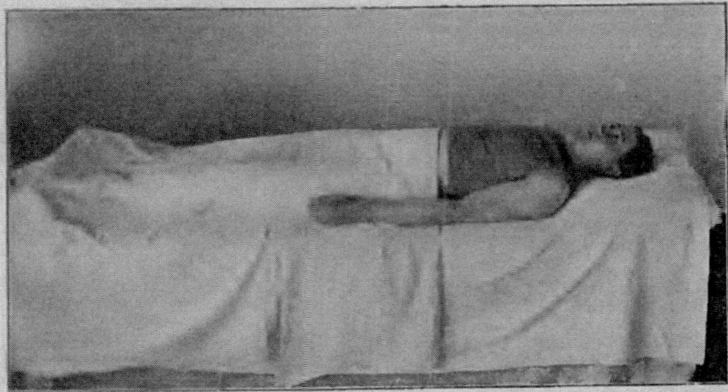

Fig. 197. SQUARE CHEST PACK — Complete (p. 858).

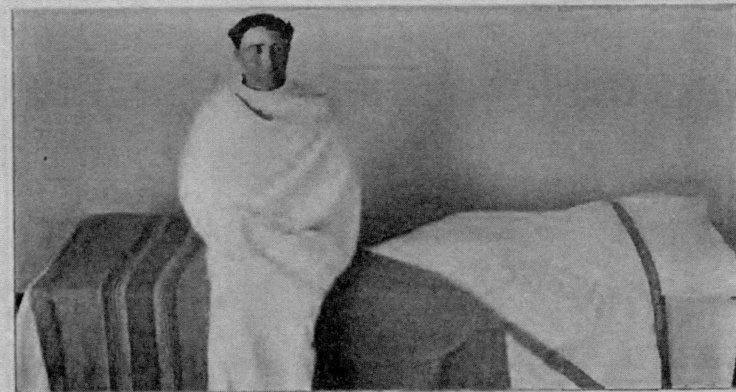

Fig. 198. TRIANGULAR CHEST PACK — Ready for Application (p. 858).

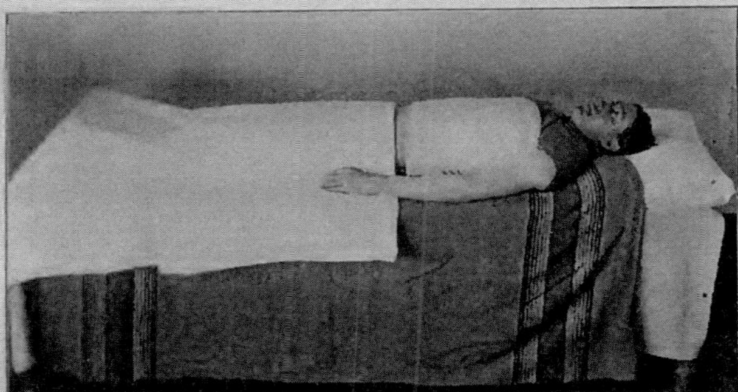

Fig. 199. TRIANGULAR CHEST PACK — Complete (p. 860).

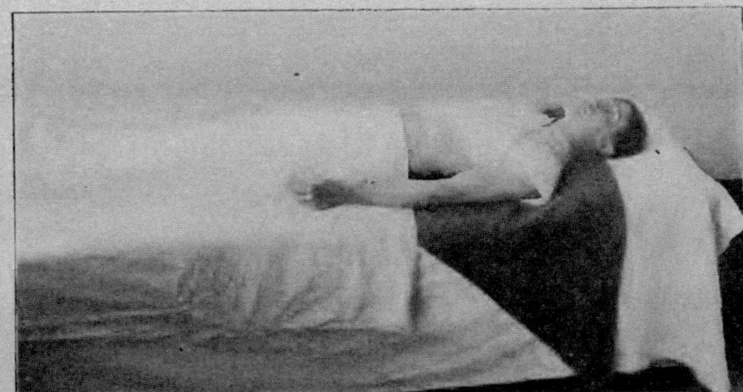

Fig. 200. TOWEL CHEST PACK (p. 860).

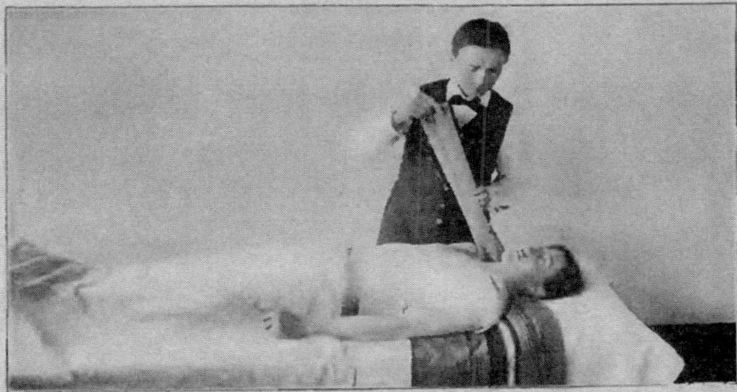

Fig. 201. HALF CHEST COMPRESS (p. 861).

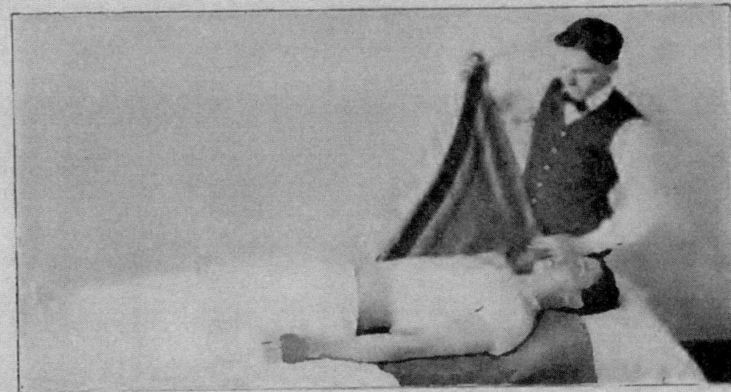

Fig. 202. HALF CHEST COMPRESS — Applied (p. 861).

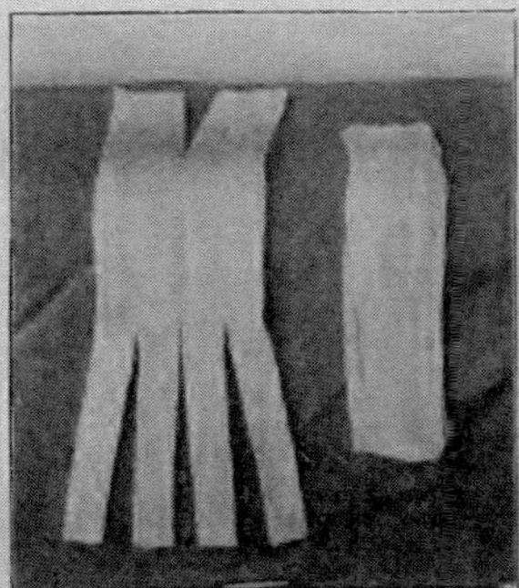

Fig. 203. Compresses for Throat (p. 865).

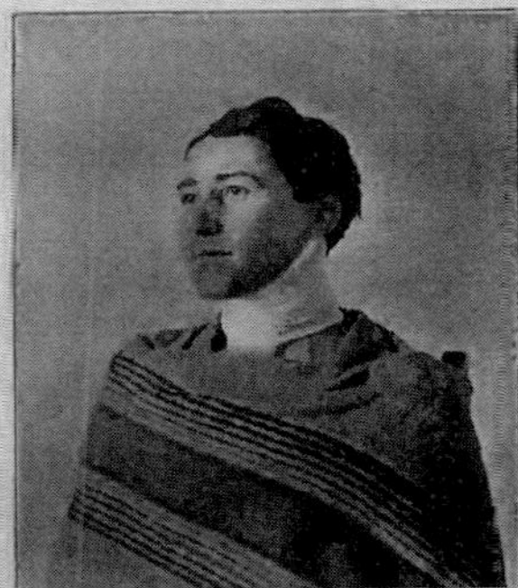

Fig. 204. Throat Compress — First Step (p. 865).

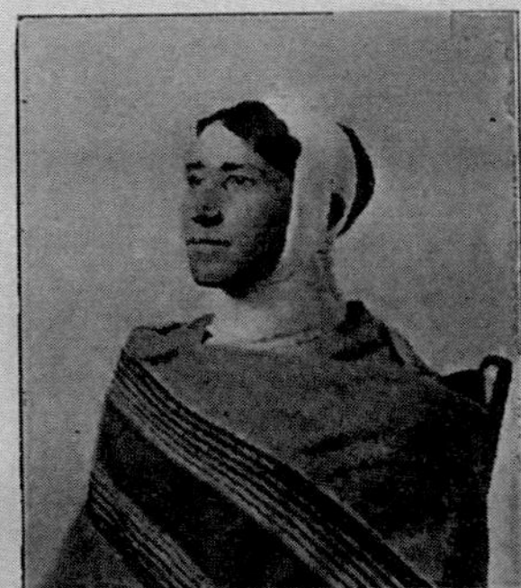

Fig. 205. Throat Compress — Second Step (p. 865).

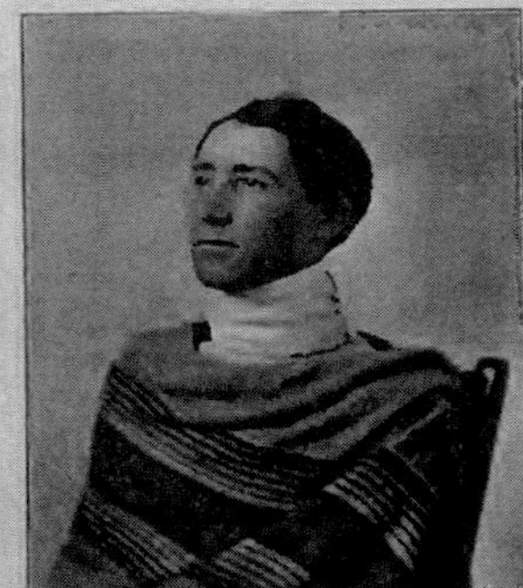

Fig. 206. Neck Compress (p. 865).

hence care must be taken to avoid this application in cases in which there is grave organic disease of the heart, especially when cardiac weakness is marked.

THE THROAT COMPRESS.

In this compress it is desirable to bring under the influ- 1381
ence of the application the skin covering the lower jaw from the chin backward, the sides of the face from the angle of the jaw to the ear, and the sides and back of the neck. The compress wound about the neck is of very little use for the ordinary sore throat in which the fauces and perhaps the tonsils are involved.

The compress is prepared as follows: For the wet compress, fold a piece of cheese-cloth to four or six thicknesses, four inches in width, and length sufficient to reach one and one-half times around the neck. For the flannel covering, provide a piece of soft blanket flannel eight inches wide and long enough to reach around the head and beneath the chin and overlap an inch. Fold the flannel crosswise, and split it down the middle to within an inch of this fold. Open, and split again each of the two legs of one end. Apply first the wet bandage from behind, crossing the ends under the chin and folding up against the sides of the neck, covering also the back of the cheek to the ear. Now apply the flannel bandage as shown in Figs. 203, 204, 205. If protection is required, apply a strip of mackintosh next the wet cloth.

This is a very excellent application for the relief of chronic sore throat. It may be applied at bedtime and removed in the morning. On removal rub the throat with very cold water.

The throat compress in acute inflammation should be covered with flannel only. If mackintosh is used, apply flannel outside to prevent too rapid radiation.

The hot compress for sore throat is applied across the jaws behind the chin and to the sides of the face. The dry ends may be fastened above the head, and a cold compress applied about the neck at the same time.

THE NECK COMPRESS (Fig. 206).

1382 This consists simply of a linen cloth wrung out of water at the right temperature and wound about the neck, covered with flannel or flannel and oilcloth.

For acute laryngitis the bandage should be wet in water at 60° to 70°, wrung moderately dry, and covered with flannel only. It should be changed just before the bandage becomes dry. In cases of chronic laryngitis the bandage should be wrung out of very cold water, and covered with flannel and mackintosh. On removing the bandage in the morning, the parts should be thoroughly rubbed with cold water, and should be protected by the dry bandage during the day.

Physiological Effects.—Through the reflex effects to be obtained by the application of this bandage to the skin over the larynx, and through its influence upon the sympathetic centers of the neck, the procedure is capable of exerting a very decided influence upon the mucous membrane of the larynx and the various organs concerned in speech, promoting activity of the mucous membrane, and relieving congestion and irritation of the larynx and the pharynx, which are often the cause of chronic cough.

It must be remembered, also, that warm applications to the throat enlarge the great arterial trunks conveying blood to the head, and hence may produce cerebral congestion. For this reason, throat wrappings should not be unnecessarily warm. The compress should generally be covered with flannel only, and *should not be left in place after it becomes dry.*

Therapeutic Applications.—The heating throat compress is useful in *colds*, *acute inflammation* of the *larynx* and *pharynx*, in *whooping-cough*, *diphtheria*, *croup*, *clergyman's sore throat*, and in all cases in which a derivative effect is indicated in this region of the body.

Sore throat, *catarrh* of the *larynx*, and so-called "cold in the head" are promptly relieved by the heating compress, if applied immediately after the cold has been contracted. The compress should be wrung out of cold water; and if applied for sore throat, should be lightly covered with flannel, and changed every four hours; if for *chronic catarrh* of the *larynx*, it should be covered with impervious material, so as to secure vigorous revulsive effects. General treatment is also required.

The continuous warm compress to the throat may sometimes render useful service in cases of marked *cerebral anemia*, as also in *pernicious anemia*.

When used for antiphlogistic effects, a simple compress of six or eight thicknesses of cheese-cloth is required. This is freshly wrung out of cold water every four or five minutes. It should never be allowed to become heated, it being necessary to suppress reaction completely and contract the deep vessels, in order that the antiphlogistic effect desired may be produced.

Duval* reports a case of very severe *torticollis* cured by the heating compress in connection with general cold ablutions. The compress was renewed every two hours, and remained in place until profuse sweating was occasioned.

THE PRECORDIAL OR CARDIAC COMPRESS.

The application consists of a compress applied to the por- 1383
tion of the chest wall over the heart. This comprises the space bounded by the second rib above, the right border of the sternum, a line falling one-half inch to the right of the nipple, and the sixth rib below. The compress should be large enough to cover this space and to extend at least two inches outside it. Ordinarily, the best effects are produced by employing water at a temperature of about 60°. The compress should be wrung moderately dry, and should be very lightly covered. It is desirable that cooling by slow evaporation should be encouraged, and should continue for some time. The heating compress, when applied over the heart, may produce a depressing effect. The compress should be changed as soon as it becomes decidedly warm, or before.

* "Ann. de Cher et d'Orthod.," 1896, IX, 73, 76.

Ordinarily the cooling compress will need to be changed every 15 to 20 minutes. The ice-bag may be used in place of the cold compress, and has even been used continuously with excellent results to control high temperature. A single thickness of flannel should protect the skin.

Physiological Effects.—The effect of the precordial compress is first to increase the activity of the heart. The heart makes stronger, more vigorous and frequent contractions than before the application; within a few minutes, however, the rate of the heart-beat will become slower; and within half an hour, when the application has been rightly adapted to the case, the pulse-rate will be considerably slowed, arterial tension increased, and the first sound of the heart considerably accentuated, the upstroke in the sphygmographic tracing being much quicker and longer, indicating a larger movement of the heart (Fig. 207, A and B). (Exp. 72).

Experiments made with the heart separated from the body have shown that cold water dropped upon the heart slows its action, while hot water quickens it. That the opposite effects are produced by the application of hot and cold water to the skin is due to the fact that the impression made upon the heart by cutaneous applications is reflex. When the heart is directly cooled by an ice-bag long applied, the uniform effect is slowing of its action.

The effect of cold upon the heart has been quite fully discussed elsewhere in this work, and need not be further dwelt upon here (**514**).

1384 **Therapeutic Applications.**—Frequent application of cold over the heart is indicated in the feeble heart of *low fevers*, especially when *cardiac failure* is threatened, in the early stage of the disease. Very cold or continuous cold applications should not be made when there is evidence of cardiac degeneration resulting from neglect of proper treatment of the case during the first week or two after the beginning of the attack. If continuous applications are employed, the compress or ice-bag should be removed every half hour. and the

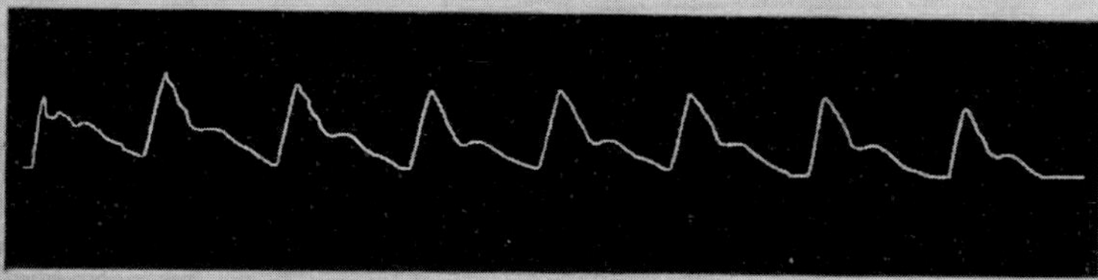

(*a*). Before Application (Tension Low).

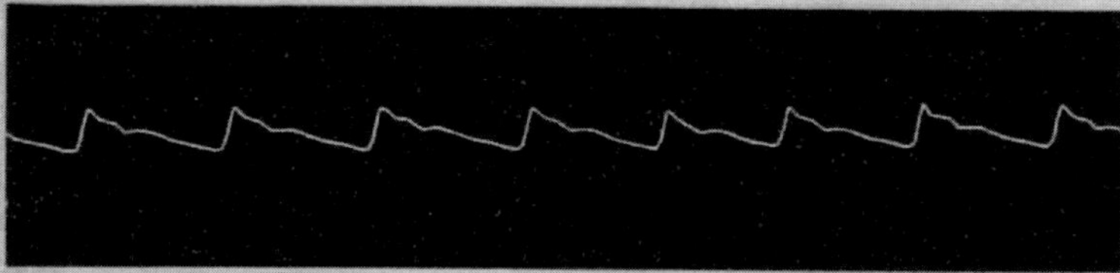

( ). After Application (Tension High).

FIG. 207. SPHYGMOGRAPHIC TRACINGS SHOWING THE EFFECTS OF THE COLD CARDIAC COMPRESS IN RAISING THE BLOOD PRESSURE (p. 868).

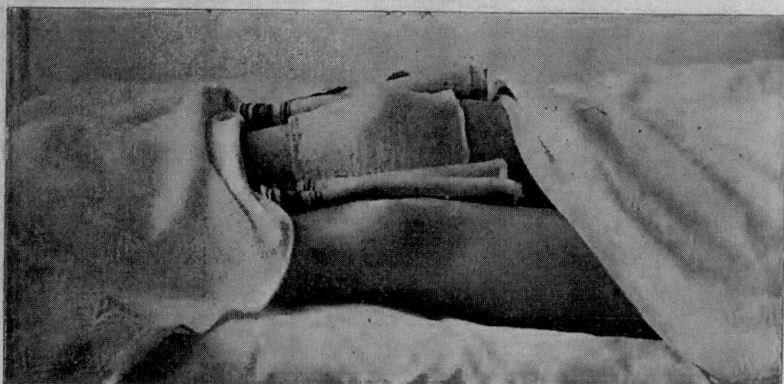

FIG. 208. JOINT COMPRESS (p. 872).

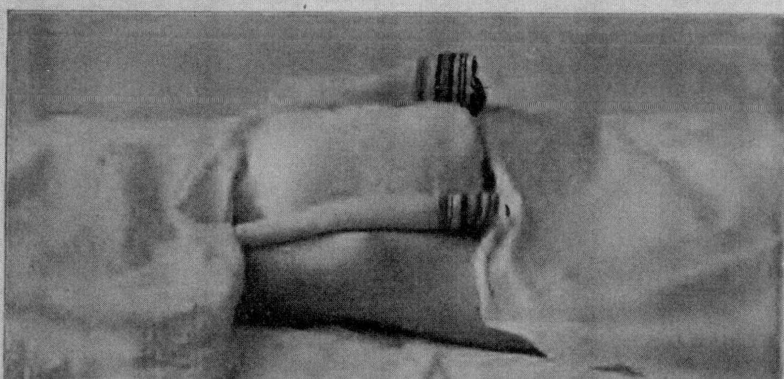

FIG. 209. COTTON POULTICE (p. 872).

skin surface to which the application is made should be rubbed vigorously, or sponged with hot water. In many cases of cardiac weakness, especially in *chronic cardiac insufficiency, bradycardia, tachycardia*, and other functional disorders of the heart, the cool or cold compress may be applied three times a day (15 to 30 minutes). This measure is also valuable in cases of overaction and irritability due to valvular disease of the heart in which there is no degeneration of the heart muscle.

In the acute form of *endocarditis*, and in *myocarditis*, the cool compress should be applied continuously. Each time the compress in changed the moistened surface should be rubbed with the warm hand until red through reaction. In *chronic endocarditis*, the cold compress should be applied for half an hour three times a day. The effects of the precordial compress are greatly augmented by general cold friction and other general procedures.

The cold compress is indicated in most cases in which the prevailing practice calls for alcohol, digitalis, or strychnia. All the good effects which it is possible to obtain from these drugs may be secured by the precordial compress, combined with other hydriatic measures, thus avoiding the undesirable effects of the drugs. Alcohol lowers the blood pressure instead of raising it, and adds to the toxic elements in the blood, lessening vital resistance, and also weakening the heart. Digitalis and strychnia, while they seem to strengthen the heart, at the same time increase its work, and add to the toxins already present in the body another powerful poison. The precordial compress is valuable in cases of aortic insufficiency with dilatation, or beginning degeneration of the vessels, also in endocarditis, whether acute or chronic.

A very useful application for the cold precordial compress is during *chloroform anesthesia*. It is the author's invariable custom to employ a cold compress for this purpose whenever the administration of chloroform is necessary. An ice-bag is used, which is applied, not directly to the skin, but over one thickness of thin flannel. Every ten minutes the ice-bag is removed, and the parts rubbed with dry flannel until warm and reddened. A failure of the parts to react or the appearance of an areolar cyanosis (a mottled bluish appearance) constitutes a warning sign of excessively depressed nerve centers, so that the application becomes a guide to the physician administering the anesthetic. Its most important use, however, is to support cardiac activity by maintaining powerful reflex stimulation of the cardiac centers. It is the author's opinion that few deaths from chloroform would ever occur if this measure were uniformly resorted to. The ice-bag should not be applied at the beginning of the anesthesia, except in cases of extreme cardiac weakness. The proper time for the application is after the first or irritant effects of the anesthetic have disappeared, and the secondary effects have become pronounced. This will usually be within five to six minutes after the beginning of the administration.

The same measure is also of value in *ether anesthesia*, but it is well in the latter case to employ a cheesecloth compress rather than the ice-bag, and to extend the application to the whole anterior surface of the chest. The compress should be applied at 60°, and changed every 15 or 20 minutes. The square compress wrapping may be advantageously used in these cases. If the anesthesia be prolonged, the pack may be changed once in 10 to 15 minutes and the precordial region vigorously rubbed with the hand dipped in ice-water for 20 seconds. This procedure may be employed in connection with anesthesia with very little inconvenience, and enormously lessens the risk of death from heart failure in chloroform poisoning or from acute pulmonary congestion or bronchopneumonia after ether administration.

1385 *Indications for the Application of the Cold Cardiac Compress.*—According to Winternitz, the indications for this measure are the same as for digitalis:—

"1. The application of cold over the heart diminishes its temperature, and is therefore useful in inflammation of the heart and pericardium.

"2. The temperature of the blood is by this means reduced, and hence this measure may be usefully employed in fever in connection with other antithermal measures. If antithermal drugs are employed, cold applications should be applied over the heart, for the reason that antipyrin acts injuriously upon the heart, and lessens the tone of the vessels, thus leading to collapse; whereas the cold precordial compress has the opposite effect.

"3. In all conditions of cardiac weakness, no matter from what cause, cold applications over the heart may be employed.

"4. When the blood pressure is low, the application of cold is especially useful; hence this measure may be employed in all serious disturbances of the heart, as in adynamic fevers and in functional disorders of the heart.

"5. By aiding the pulmonary circulation, cold applications over the heart are useful in a congested condition of the lungs, in bronchial hemorrhages, and bronchial catarrh resulting from stasis in the pulmonary vessels."

A moderately hot compress may be applied over the heart in the weakness of that organ which occurs in hysteria with anemia (110° for 10 min.).*

Contraindications.—The cold precordial compress is to be 1386
avoided in the *fatty degeneration* of the *heart* muscle which occurs in the advanced stages of cardiac disease, and in *diabetes* and *nephritis*. In *emphysema*, when the disease is well advanced, the beneficial effects of cold applications upon the heart are diminished, because of the condition of the lungs. One of the most important, but not sufficiently appreciated, effects of hydric applications consists in the modification of the elasticity and tonus of both the vessel walls and the tissues. As a loss of tonus and elasticity in the vessels produces stasis, hyperemia, and predisposes to inflammation, the restoration of the tonus of the vessels and tissues removes the disease of the vessels thus caused.

---

* Thermes. *Ann. Soc. Hydrol. Med.*, Paris, 1879-80, XXV, 224-295.

It has been clearly demonstrated that diminished tone of the vessels and tissues produces a positive and decided diminution of cardiac energy, and that the restoration of the vessel tone will, to a marked degree, remove the derangements which may be produced by organic ailments of the heart. From a hydriatic standpoint, the loss of vessel tone is a symptom the removal of which is of the highest importance to restore normal conditions of the circulation.

THE JOINT COMPRESS (Fig. 208).

1387 This consists simply of a bandage wet in water of the proper temperature, wound around the joint, and covered with flannel, cotton, and oiled muslin, or some other impervious material. In cases of acute joint disease with pain and swelling, a moderately wet compress should be applied, at a temperature of 60° to 70°, and flannel or cotton-wool protection should be used. In *chronic joint affections* accompanied by stiffness, *exudates*, etc., the compress should be wrung dry, out of very cold water, and should be very thoroughly protected by means of several coverings of flannel or a thick mass of cotton and oiled muslin or mackintosh outside of all. In the acute form of the disease, the compress should be changed often enough so that it will not become dry. In chronic cases, the compress may be worn at night only, in ordinary cases. In the morning the joint is rubbed first with the hand dipped in cold water, then with oil, and protected by several thicknesses of flannel bandage, properly adjusted, to be worn during the day.

THE COTTON POULTICE (Fig. 209).

1388 This consists simply in the application to a part of a mass of dry cotton covered with mackintosh or other impervious material. The cotton is soon moistened by the retained perspiration, and thus the effect of a poultice is obtained, but in a much more cleanly and convenient manner. The cotton poultice is especially valuable in *chronic joint affections.*

THE HIP PACK (Fig. 210).

This application is confined to the skin area extending 1389
from the umbilicus to the middle of the thighs.

The materials needed are the same as for the half-pack (1196), and the method is the same. For the cold pack a folded linen sheet is used; for the hot pack, a folded woolen blanket.

The cold hip pack has a pronounced effect upon the pelvic viscera, just as the trunk pack affects profoundly the abdominal viscera. Judiciously used, it has a powerful tonic and alterative effect upon the organs of the pelvis.

The *cold* pack should be avoided in cases in which severe neuralgic pain is present, in *acute inflammation* of the appendages, *chronic uterine* or *ovarian pain*, and *menstruation*.

The *hot* hip pack is a highly stimulating procedure, and one of the most excellent means of relieving, temporarily at least, *menstrual pains*, whether of uterine or ovarian origin, by the powerful revulsion produced. If the menstrual flow is increased by the application, this tendency may be counteracted by the hot vaginal douche applied immediately before or afterward, the patient remaining in bed.

Not infrequently the good effect of a hot hip pack is lost by exposure of the body to chill directly afterward. It should be remembered that, like all other very hot applications, it usually gives rise to general sweating, and hence may readily expose the patient to chill with all the resulting consequences, if proper precautions are not adopted.

Some form of the cooling bath, as cold friction (1209), the wet-hand rub, or cool towel rub, should be employed directly after the hot hip pack, and care should be taken to secure gradual cooling off.

THE PELVIC PACK (Figs. 211, 212, 213).

Spread a woolen blanket on the couch as for the wet-sheet 1390
pack. Fold a woolen sheet once lengthwise, place transversely across the couch in such a way that when the patient lies

down upon it, the sacrum will fall in the center of the sheet each way. Fold another woolen sheet cornerwise, and lay across the table with the apex pointing down and the base at such a point that when the patient lies down, the upper edge of the blanket will fall a couple of inches above the umbilicus and a little below the sheet folded lengthwise. Now wring out a cotton sheet cut or folded cornerwise in the shape of a triangle a little smaller than the woolen triangle, and place upon the couch with the apex down and the base an inch below that of the woolen triangle.

The patient should now lie down upon the couch face upward, and in such a position that the upper border of the wet sheet will fall at about the level of the umbilicus. The legs are drawn up and the knees widely spread, and the feet placed one on each side of the apex of the triangular wet sheet. The apex of the wet sheet is drawn upward until it fits the perineum tightly, the apex lying upon the sternum, the sides being spread out over the abdomen as much as possible. The legs are now extended, and the lateral triangles of the wet sheet are brought over one by one and wrapped about the thighs in such a way that the skin of the abdomen, hips, thighs, and perineum is everywhere covered by one thickness of sheet. The apex of the triangle is now turned down over the abdomen so that the fold will come at the level of the umbilicus.

The woolen sheet is adjusted in just the same way, only the lateral angles are carried over and tucked under the opposite thigh. Now draw over the ends of the folded sheet, and tuck under the sides, drawing as snugly as possible, so the patient will warm up very quickly. Last of all, wrap the patient in the large woolen blanket first spread upon the couch. The remainder of the procedure is now the same as for the general wet-sheet pack.

Three stages may be recognized:—

1. The *tonic* stage,—from the beginning of the pack until the patient feels warm and comfortable. The effect upon the pelvic viscera is to excite vascular and nervous activity.

2. The *neutral* stage,—while the patient is reacting until the normal temperature of the skin is reached. When the temperature of the skin begins to rise, the neutral stage ends. This stage is quieting, calmative.

3. The *heating* stage commences when the temperature of the skin begins to rise, and continues to the point when perspiration begins. This stage is *derivative*.

4. The *sweating* stage begins at the end of the heating stage, and lasts as long as the patient continues to perspire, which may be two or three hours. This stage is exciting. It is rarely used with the pelvic pack.

In cases in which reaction is poor, a hot sitz may be administered for 4 or 5 minutes just before the pack, or a hot hip pack for 6 to 8 minutes, or a fomentation over the hypogastrium. This pack is generally used for tonic effects and as a training for the cool sitz bath. The application is continued from 20 to 30 minutes, or until the patient feels comfortable.

In the *hot and cold* pelvic pack when used to relieve chronic pain, ovarian irritation, etc., for which it is a most excellent measure, the procedure is precisely the same, except that a bag filled with hot water is slipped between the blankets over the lower abdomen in such a way that one thickness of flannel will intervene between it and the wet sheet. The temperature of the bag should be as high as the patient can bear. The thermophore is preferable to the hot water bag, as the heat is more evenly distributed, and lasts longer. The duration of the pack varies from 20 minutes to two hours, according to the indications.

In applying the *hot pelvic pack*, the procedure differs somewhat from the preceding. The several coverings are arranged exactly as in the wet-sheet pelvic pack, except that the triangular linen sheet is folded so as to be about two feet greater in width, and is not wet. The triangular woolen sheet is wrung as dry as possible out of water at 160°, and laid over the triangular sheet. The patient, his head having been previously protected by cooling and the application of a cold towel, lies down upon the couch, and is enveloped as previously described, the dry triangular sheet being adjusted so as to maintain close contact with the body at every point. Then the side angles are brought up and tucked in; the apex is firmly drawn up between the legs and securely fastened. The cotton sheet is then adjusted in like manner, and a folded woolen blanket drawn about the hips.

1391 **Physiological Effects.**— The pelvic pack is intended especially to influence the pelvic viscera, the bladder, the lower colon, the rectum, the testes and prostate in men, and the ovaries and uterus in women. Applied in the manner indicated, it acts upon those surfaces which are in most intimate reflex relation with the viscera of the pelvis; namely, the cutaneous surfaces of the lumbar region, the lower abdomen, the inner surface of the thighs, and especially the cutaneous covering of the external genitals. If the sheet is simply wrapped about the hips, instead of being drawn up between the legs in the manner described, the genital surfaces and the inner surfaces of the thighs are not reached, and hence these most important reflex areas are not brought under the influence of the procedure.

The effects of this procedure upon the pelvic viscera depend upon the exact mode of application, the temperature of the water employed, the length of the application, and the special conditions or susceptibility of the patient, as is the case with other hydric procedures. If the wet sheet is wrung very dry out of very cold water, and the application continued only until reaction is well established, the effect is to encourage the circulation of the pelvic viscera and to energize all the other functions. Such an application is in brief an excellent physiological tonic for the pelvic viscera. If an application given in the manner described is continued for an hour or two, or until the skin is strongly excited, a powerful revulsive effect is exercised upon the viscera of the pelvis. This is one of the most effective means of decon-

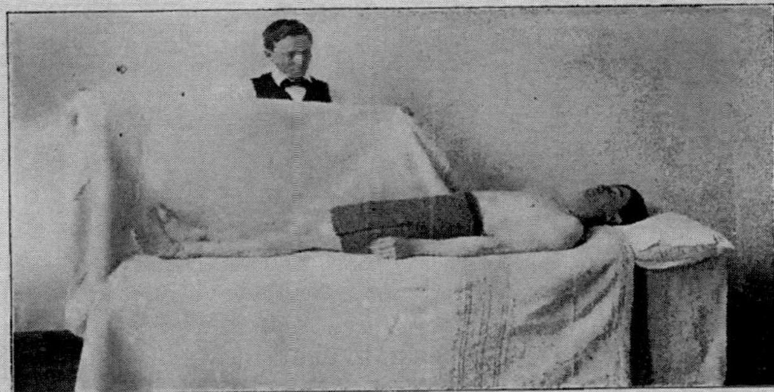

FIG. 210. HIP PACK (p. 873).

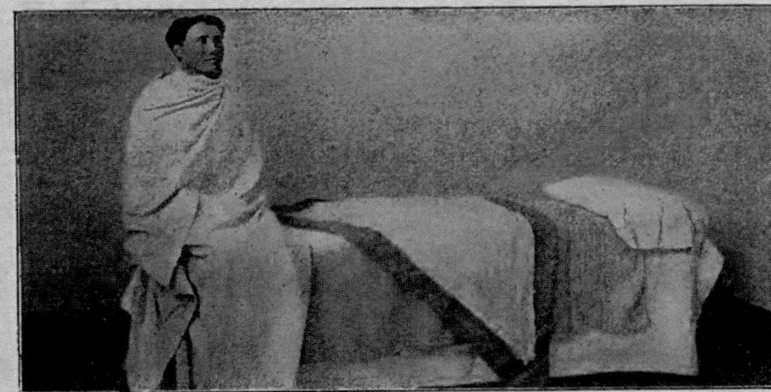

FIG. 211. PELVIC PACK — First Step (p. 873).

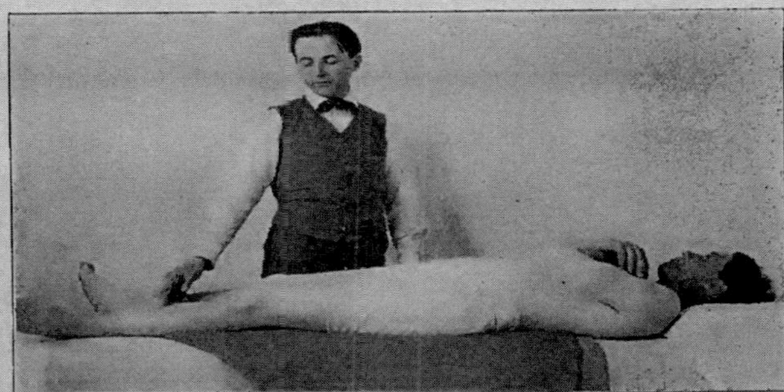

FIG. 212. PELVIC PACK — Second Step (p. 873).

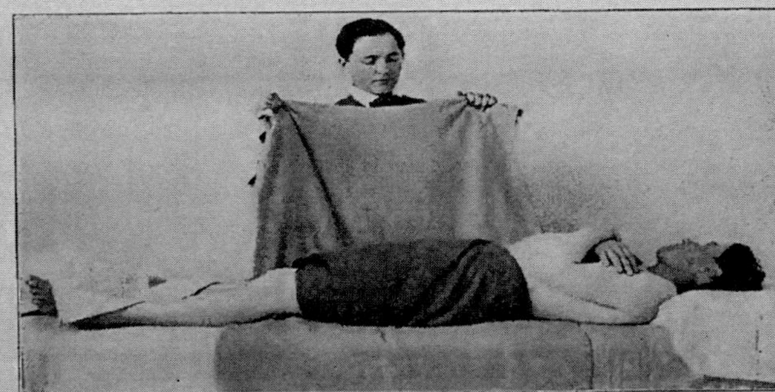

FIG. 213. PELVIC PACK — Third Step (p. 873).

gesting these organs. The application of the pelvic pack at a temperature of 60° to 70°, the application being renewed every 20 to 30 minutes, exercises a powerful influence upon the pelvic blood-vessels. By its continued excitant effect upon the vaso-constrictors, permanent contraction is produced in the small vessels of the pelvic circulation. If the wet sheet is slightly wrung out of very cold water, the effect is to produce powerful constriction of all the pelvic vessels.

The hot pelvic pack exercises a powerful revulsive effect upon the pelvic viscera. If continued for some time, pronounced excitant effects are produced through the stimulation of the sympathetic nerves in relation with these parts. Very pronounced and permanent derivative effects may be produced by the hot pelvic pack, followed by a prolonged cold pack applied to the same surface.

Therapeutic Applications.—Of the four principal methods 1392
of applying the pelvic pack, each has its special therapeutic indication. The *short cold* pack, with the wet sheet wrung very dry, is tonic in its effects, and is of the greatest value in most cases of *chronic pelvic disease* in which neither active inflammation nor acute congestion is present, and in which pain is not a prominent symptom. It is indicated under the same conditions as the rubbing sitz, but is a less vigorous procedure, and may be employed with very feeble patients who have poor powers of reaction or who are too fatigued to react properly to the rubbing sitz. It is a hydriatic procedure of great service in cases of *uterine* and *ovarian prolapse* due to a relaxed condition of the muscles and ligaments connected with the pelvic viscera, in *amenorrhea*, *irregularities* of *menstruation*, *chronic inactivity* of the *lower bowel*, *backache*, *enteroptosis*, *sexual weakness*, and *impotence*.

The cold-sheet pelvic pack, prolonged until cutaneous excitation is produced, or as it may be termed, the *heating* pelvic pack, may render special service in cases of *chronic passive congestion* of the pelvic viscera, as *chronic colitis*, *chronic metritis*, *chronic ovarian congestion*, *amenorrhea* resulting from arrested development, *excessive involution* after childbirth. It should be followed by a short cold application, as the cold douche, cold friction, affusion, or cold rubbing sitz for 20 to 30 seconds, at a temperature of 70° to 75°. The length of the application and the temperature must of course be suited to the particular case in hand.

The *repeated* pelvic pack, employing water at 60° to 70°, with a quite wet sheet, changed every 30 to 40 minutes, is a measure of great efficiency in cases of acute *congestion* or *inflammation* of the *pelvic viscera*. The blood-vessels of the viscera are not only contracted, thus preventing stasis and an increase of the inflammatory process, but the vital activities are excited and maintained by stimulating impulses continually received from the surface; and thus the disease process is antagonized and brought to an early and successful issue. This measure is of great value in *non-suppurating inflammations* of the *ovaries* and *tubes*, *pelvic peritonitis*, *acute metritis*, *vaginitis*, *proctitis*, *dysentery*, *prostatitis*, *urethritis*, and *orchitis*. By the application of water at a moderate temperature to the entire cutaneous surface reflexly associated with the pelvic circulation, much more pronounced effects may be obtained than by water at a lower temperature applied to a smaller surface. These cool and moderately cold applications are also much more effective than extreme cold in relieving visceral congestion. Their efficiency is greatly increased by a hot leg pack given at the same time.

When an acute inflammation or congestion is accompanied by pain, a *hot* pelvic pack or fomentation may be substituted every hour or two for the cold application; but the duration of the hot pack should not be more than 15 to 20 minutes, and the temperature should be as hot as can be endured.

The *very cold* pelvic pack sometimes renders valuable service in cases of *uterine hemorrhage*. The author has been able by this means to control at once uterine hemorrhages which had resisted all other measures for weeks. A hot application must be made to the feet simultaneously.

The *hot* pelvic pack is most useful as an analgesic measure in all *painful affections* of the *pelvis*. It renders the highest service in cases of *dysmenorrhea, ovarian neuralgia,* and all neuralgiac affections of the pelvic viscera, also in *enteralgia, sciatica,* and *coccygodynia.*

The *hot and cold* pelvic pack (1370) may render special service in cases in which the combined influence of heat and cold is desirable. The procedure may consist of a hot pelvic pack with an ice-bag over the inflamed part, or a cold pelvic pack with a hot bag over the part interested.

Contraindications and Precautions.—The pelvic pack, to be of real service, must be carefully adapted to the condition in hand. For example, prolonged cold applications must not be made in cases in which pain is a prominent symptom, as the almost certain result will be a great increase of the pain. The very cold pack should also be avoided in inflammatory conditions, because of the resulting reaction and the collateral hyperemia induced. Long-continued hot applications also tend to increase inflammatory action in salpingitis, peritonitis, and other similar conditions. In such cases the hot pack may be used only at intervals of three to four hours, the cooling pelvic pack being employed in the interim.

Care should be taken in the employment of the cool or cold pelvic pack that general chilliness is not induced, or the proper effect of the application will be negatived. Likewise, in applications of the hot pelvic pack profuse perspiration is to be avoided.

THE LEG PACK (Fig. 214).

Either one or both legs may be included in this procedure. 1393

Requisites.—The same materials are needed as for the trunk pack, though the wrappings may be smaller.

Method.—In the application of a leg pack, each leg should be wrapped in the wet sheet separately and closely (Fig. 214). The legs may be rubbed outside the wrappings, if necessary, to encourage the circulation. The temperature should be

60° for the cold pack, and as hot as can be borne for the hot pack. A linen sheet is used for the former, a blanket for the latter.

Physiological Effects.—The leg pack is a powerful derivative measure. Applications made to the legs affect to a marked degree the circulation in the head, throat, chest, and pelvis.

Therapeutic Applications.—The leg pack may be used to excellent advantage as a derivative measure in quite a large class of cases, as in *cerebral congestion*, *pulmonary congestion*, *coldness* of the *feet* and *legs*, resulting from irritation of the sympathetic nerves and spasm of the blood-vessels of the lower extremities. The cold leg pack is of special value in cases of *paralysis* in which the skin is cold, purplish, and inactive. The application should be preceded by a hot leg bath. The *hot* leg pack is exceedingly useful in cases of *neuralgia* of the legs, in *hemiplegia*, and *paraplegia* with defective circulation, as shown by a purplish tint of the skin. It is also a very useful measure in cases of *chronic rheumatism* confined to the knee and ankle joints, and as a derivative measure.

THE FOOT PACK (Fig. 215).

1394 This resembles the leg pack, but differs from it in that the feet and ankles only are involved.

The patient lies upon a cot while each foot is separately wrapped in a towel wrung out of cold water, and a blanket carefully folded about the feet and legs to the height of the knees. The entire body is then wrapped in another blanket, so as to suppress any disposition to chilliness.

Therapeutic Applications.—The foot pack is of great value as a means of relieving *cold* or *sweating feet*, and for *insomnia*. The pack should be applied at night, and allowed to remain in place for a few hours, or overnight. On its removal, the feet should be carefully sponged with cold water, and afterward dried and rubbed.

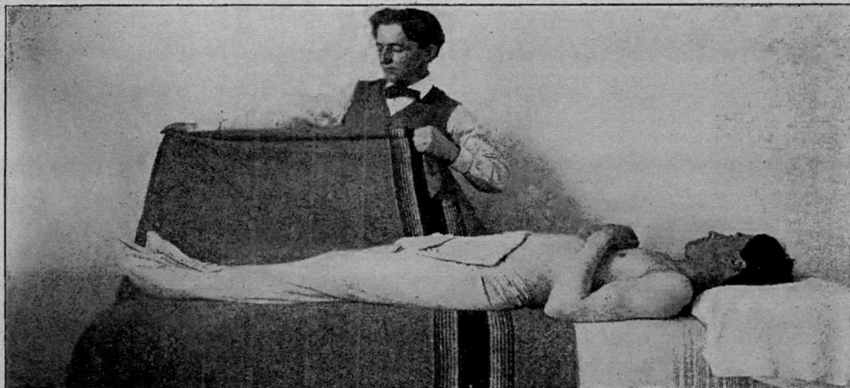

FIG. 214. LEG PACK (p. 879).

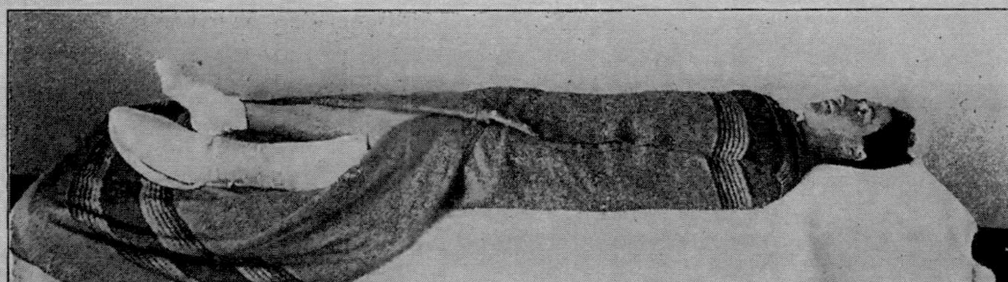

FIG. 215. FOOT PACK (p. 880).

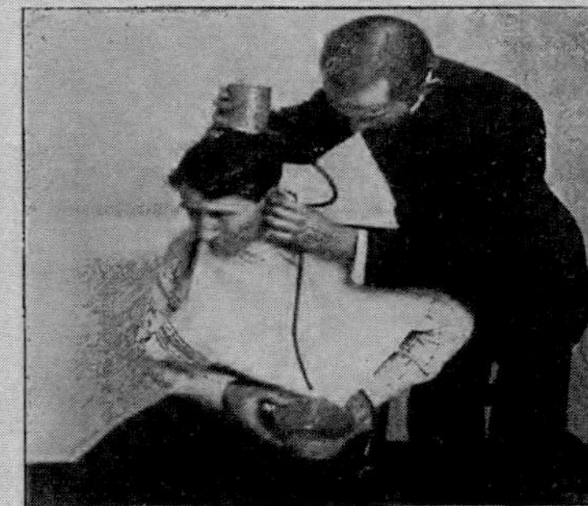

FIG. 216. IRRIGATION OF EAR (p. 881).

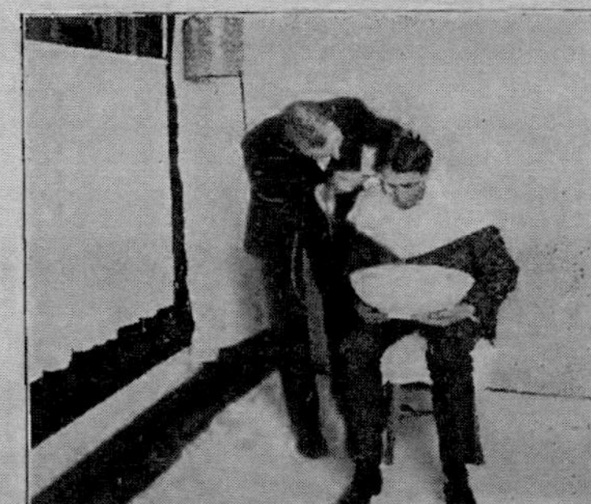

FIG. 217. IRRIGATION OF EYE (p. 883).

THE PERINEAL COMPRESS.

For rectal, bladder, or genito-urinary affections requiring 1395
antiphlogistic treatment, the cold compress may be applied in such a manner as to cover the perineum and the external genitals, extending over the bladder in front and the anus and nates behind. The temperature of the water employed should be about 60° to 70° F. The compress should be changed every 20 to 40 minutes. It should be lightly covered.

Therapeutic Applications.—This measure is especially valuable in cases of *rectal irritation*, *leucorrhea* of the *rectum*, *acute inflammation* of the *prostate*, *chronic gleet*, *vaginal leucorrhea*, and *uterine* and *ovarian congestion*. Fomentations may be applied to the region when required for revulsive effects, or to relieve pain or tenesmus in the rectum, bladder, urethra, or uterus. A hot perineal compress combined with a heating pelvic pack (**1390**) is a most efficient analgesic and antiphlogistic procedure.

IRRIGATION.

Irrigation differs from the douche in the fact that the element of mechanical excitation is entirely eliminated through the application of water without pressure. Irrigation is applied to both the skin and the mucous membrane. The application is made by means of a reservoir or fountain placed a few inches above the surface to be irrigated, the water being allowed to flow through a small rubber tube, and the stream regulated to the amount desired by compression of the tube or regulating the height of the reservoir. Either hot or cold water may be applied by this as well as by other means, or alternate applications may be made.

The principal applications of this procedure are to the ear, eye, nose, throat, stomach, rectum, bladder, vagina, and uterus.

IRRIGATION OF THE EAR.

Fig. 216 shows an excellent method of applying the 1396
irrigation to the ear by means of a glass or hard-rubber de-

vice. The water passes into the ear and out through a tube, thus enabling the patient to receive the treatment in any position, as the instrument exactly fits into the outer extremity of the external canal of the ear. The temperature may be from 100° to 130°, according to the effect desired. The fountain should be on a level with the top of the head. Force should never be employed, for the reason that perforation of the ear often exists, and serious injury might result from the introduction of the water into the middle ear with any considerable degree of force. The head should be inclined toward the side under treatment.

The canal of the ear should afterward be carefully dried and covered with a napkin or with the warm hand for a few minutes. In cold weather the ear should not be exposed out of doors for at least an hour after the application of a warm ear douche, and even then it is well to protect the canal by a little cotton placed in the outer extremity.

This measure affords great relief in the pain of acute *otitis media* and earache due to other causes. In chronic suppurative disease of the ear, this measure is indispensable as a means of cleansing and disinfection.

NASAL IRRIGATION.

1397 Nasal irrigation may be administered by means of an ordinary good fountain syringe, a properly constructed tube being passed into one nostril, and the water allowed to flow into one and out the other, the head being held forward to permit of this taking place. This measure of treatment was formerly considered indispensable as a means of cleansing the nasal cavity in catarrh, but is now seldom used, and might well be entirely discarded, as it is a fruitful source of acute and chronic disease of the ear. The nasal cavity can be much better cleansed by means of antiseptic volatile oils, or by cleansing solutions introduced into the nose by means of vaporizers or atomizers.

The very hot nasal irrigation (104° to 105° F.) is useful

for checking hemorrhage from the nose. A saline solution, one or two drams to the quart, is best for the purpose.

POST-NASAL IRRIGATION.

The post-nasal douche or irrigation is administered by 1398
means of a curved tube passed into the post-nasal space by introducing it behind the uvula, and throwing a stream of water forward toward the anterior nares. The irritation produced in the region of the Eustachian tubes is frequently a source of serious inconvenience, and it is probable that more harm than good results from the use of this measure in chronic nasal catarrh.

This measure, which was once very generally employed, is now rapidly becoming obsolete.

IRRIGATION OF THE EYE (Fig. 217).

This application should be made with very little pressure. 1399
The reservoir should be placed not more than six inches above the head. With the eyes closed, the water is allowed to fall upon the outer surface of the lids and the forehead above the brow. The hot eye douche is very valuable in cases of chronic inflammation of the mucous lining of the eyelids.

Hot irrigation of the eye has been proved to be more useful as a means of relieving even acute inflammatory troubles of the eye than cold applications. The beneficial effects are the result of powerful revulsion, producing hyperemia of the skin with collateral anemia of the inflamed mucous membrane.

IRRIGATION OF THE THROAT.

This is perhaps the proper term to be applied to the appli- 1400
cation commonly known as "gargling." A large sip of water is taken into the mouth and passed to the back of the throat and held there by closure of both the esophagus and the epiglottis. Air is then forced upward through the epiglottis, thus producing a violent agitation of the liquid, and so bringing it in contact with all the structures of the post-nasal

region. The application of very hot water by this means may be recommended in cases of *chronic pharyngitis* with tickling of the mucous membrane and dryness of the throat, *irritation*, *hacking cough*, and *rawness*, giving rise to frequent clearing of the throat or a *tickling cough*.

IRRIGATION OF THE STOMACH, OR GASTRIC LAVAGE (Figs. 218, 219, 220).

1401 This procedure does for the stomach precisely what the enema or the coloclyster does for the colon. By its aid the stomach may be washed out, hot or cold applications may be made to it, and cleansing and medicated solutions may be applied to the gastric membrane.

Method.— In the use of the stomach-tube, several points require special attention: First, the tube should be of the most approved pattern, of medium size, very soft and flexible, and perfectly smooth. It should not be forced into the stomach, as in the use of the old-fashioned stomach-pump, but should be simply swallowed as one would swallow food or drink. One end of the tube being passed into the mouth and well back into the throat, the patient makes movements of swallowing, while the attendant gently urges the tube along into the stomach. Water at about the temperature of the body is poured in either with or without the addition of common salt and soda in the proportion of a teaspoonful of each to a quart of water.

A powder consisting of three parts of bicarbonate of soda, one part of sodium sulphide, and one part of chloride of sodium may be advantageously used in cleansing the stomach. Use one teaspoonful of this powder to each pint of water. After a pint or so of water has been poured into the stomach, the outer end of the tube is lowered, and by coughing or similar movements the contents of the stomach are forced through the tube into some proper receptacle. The operation should be repeated until the water is clear.

In withdrawing the tube it should be pinched tightly be-

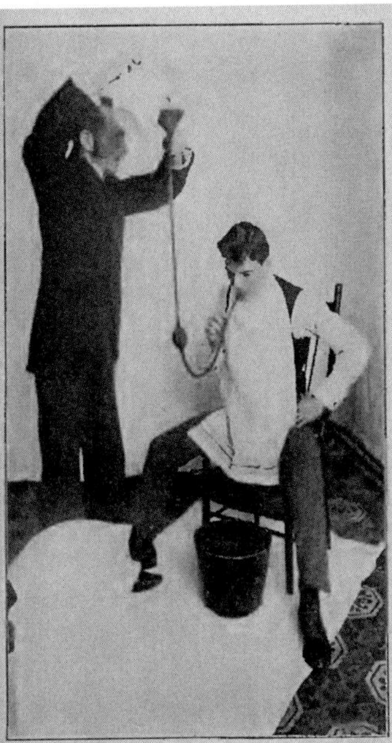

FIG. 218. GASTRIC LAVAGE (p. 884).

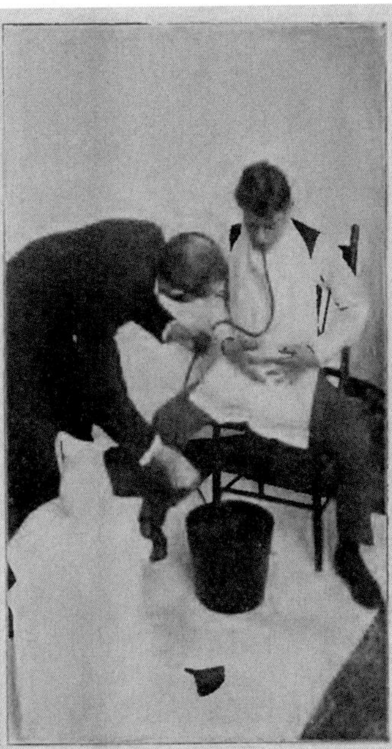

FIG. 219. GASTRIC LAVAGE — Emptying the Stomach (p. 884).

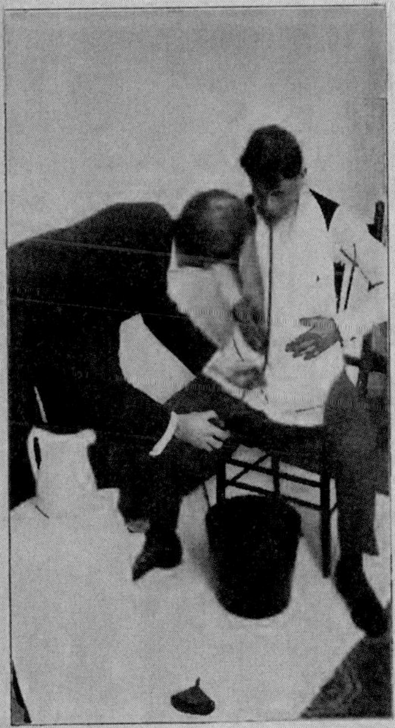

FIG. 220. GASTRIC LAVAGE — Withdrawing Tube (p. 884).

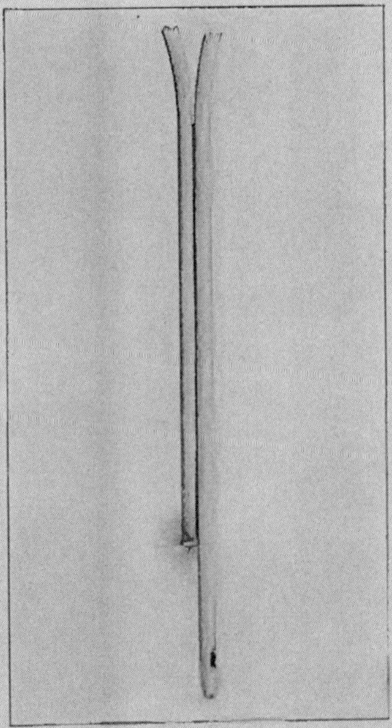

FIG. 221. GASTRIC IRRIGATOR (p. 886).

tween the thumb and finger just in front of the teeth, so that it is completely closed, before beginning the withdrawal. It should then be drawn out quickly. The object of this is to prevent the entrance into the larynx of the fluid or portions of food which the tube may contain. Such an accident has sometimes resulted in serious dyspnea and even syncope.

When lavage is employed in cases of catarrh of the stomach, or for removing decomposing contents, the cleansing solution of which the formula has been given above, or some similar preparation, should be employed. It should be remembered, however, that washing the stomach is not in itself a radically curative measure. The stomach is simply cleansed for the time being of mucus or decomposing food or of noxious substances which may have been swallowed. It is not directly curative except through the fact that removal of the products of disease from the stomach greatly aids the natural curative process by which the organ may be brought back to its normal healthy state.

The application of very hot water to the mucous membrane of the stomach in cases of hyperpepsia and gastrorrhea may be made by means of the ordinary stomach-tube or by the use of a return-flow tube. The maximum temperature of the water employed for this purpose should be 140°, the application being begun with the water at 110°, and the temperature rapidly increased to the desired degree. The temperature must be regulated somewhat by the patient's sensations. Two or three pints of water may be passed through the stomach in this way with advantage. Care must be taken to employ the tube very gently.

The cardiac excitation resulting from very hot irrigation may be readily controlled by an ice-bag over the the heart (1383).

Rosenbaum maintains that great benefit is derived from the application to the inside of the stomach of a spray consisting of many streams of water applied with considerable pressure, at a temperature of 95° to 110°. This measure he finds especially beneficial in so-called *nervous dyspepsia* and *gastritis*. Dr. Türck, of Chicago, Ill., has made large use of this measure in gastric disorders, and places a high value upon it. A return flow tube is employed for the purpose (Fig. 221).

In cases of *hypopepsia* and *apepsia* the tonic circulatory reaction and excitation which follow cold applications may be advantageously induced by the aid of the stomach-tube. The depressing effect of severe cold, however, when applied to such large surfaces as the gastric membrane, suggested to the author the advisability of employing alternate applications instead. The variations of temperature should not be so great as those employed upon the skin, because of the active sympathetic reflexes connected with the stomach.

At the beginning of the treatment, the temperature of the hot water should be 105°, that of the cold, 80°. The temperature of the hot water may be gradually raised, and that of the cold water lowered, one or two degrees at a time, until a temperature of 115° for the hot and 70° for the cold is secured. The application must be made with the greatest care, and should be discontinued at once on the appearance of any untoward symptoms. By means of this application, powerful stimulation of the stomach and its glands may be induced, resulting in the return of the patient's appetite, an increase in the amount of hydrochloric acid secreted, and a radical change for the better in every way, in many cases which have resisted ordinary measures of treatment.

The hot water should be introduced first, the quantity being about a pint. This should be retained from 20 to 30 seconds, and then passed out, and an equal quantity of cold water introduced. At first only one alternation should be made; but later, after the patient has become accustomed to the treatment, the number of alternations may be increased to five changes. Patients to whom the lavage is administered should also receive the alternate douche or cold epigastric douche daily.

When necessary to employ lavage for infants, a small-sized tube, as a No. 8 Nelaton catheter, is employed. The child is held in an upright position by the nurse, while the tube is introduced. A large glass funnel or fountain should be in readiness, with two or three pints of water at 100°, containing one-half teaspoonful each of salt and bicarbonate of soda to the quart. The rubber tube should be connected with the catheter, and the tube completely filled with the liquid to avoid introducing air.

After introducing from four to eight ounces, according to the size of the child, the tube is disconnected, and the liquid allowed to escape. The greater portion generally passes out around the tube, as the catheter is so small that it will not allow free exit for the hard and undigested curds of cow's milk which are often found present in these cases. The catheter should be held firmly in place, drawn to one side during vomiting, but kept in the stomach if possible.

Lavage for young children is perfectly safe, and is by no means so difficult as might be supposed. The younger the child, the more easily the maneuver is executed. The tube passes without difficulty, and the whole operation is over in a short time, to the great relief of all concerned. Clinical evidence is overwhelming that gastric dilatation and the retention of undigested food in the stomach, giving rise to the development of microbes and of ptomains resulting from their growth, is one of the chief causes of the gastric disorders of children which prevail so extensively in the summer-time. The use of unmodified cow's milk is without doubt chiefly responsible for the intestinal disorders of children, and these maladies will continue rife among them until a more natural and appropriate diet can be generally provided for young human beings.

Therapeutic Applications.—Gastric lavage is absolutely 1402
necessary as a means of cleansing the stomach in cases of *obstruction of the pylorus* from any cause, when the closure is complete or nearly so. In such cases it must be employed

systematically daily, or in some instances even twice a day. In *chronic dilatation* of the stomach, in which organic changes have taken place in the walls of the stomach, resulting in the formation of pouches or an extreme degree of motor insufficiency, the habitual use of the stomach-tube is sometimes required, although it is not always necessary that lavage should be administered daily. Complete emptying and cleansing of the stomach every other day or three times a week is generally sufficient to maintain a comfortable degree of asepsis.

In cases of *gastric catarrh* in which large quantities of mucus are present, the stomach-tube must be used; but it should be dispensed with as soon as possible. In cases of *hypopepsia*, in which there is little or no irritation of the mucous membrane, the use of the stomach-tube once or twice a week for a short time sometimes affords useful stimulation of both the muscular and the secreting structures. Occasionally the use of the tube may be advantageously resorted to in *gastric ulcer*, though generally it is contra-indicated in this condition.

In *persistent vomiting*, especially when the vomited matters have a green color, or consist of bile, and even in fecal vomiting, gastric lavage not infrequently produces the most happy results.

The therapeutic indications for gastric lavage are, in the author's opinion, by no means so numerous as is generally supposed. It was at one time the author's custom, after making a bacteriological examination of the stomach fluid and finding many germs present in it, to order systematic washing of the stomach twice or thrice weekly; in occasional cases, lavage was applied daily. But more careful study of the subject, and larger clinical experience in the adaptation of dietetic remedies to these cases, has convinced him that lavage is necessary only in a very small proportion of cases, even when the stomach is thoroughly infected. A fruit diet will starve out all the microbes that can grow in the stomach, with the exception of yeasts and molds, and even these disappear when a simple, rational dietary is adhered to for a reasonable length of time. Many persons have injured themselves greatly by the too frequent use of the stomach-tube. Even in gastric catarrh a properly adjusted dietary will accomplish all that can be done by means of lavage, and much more, except in cases in which large quantities of tough, tenacious mucus have accumulated in the stomach, and require removal as a foreign body, or when the stomach is enormously dilated from atony or pyloric obstruction. This measure is of immense utility in cases in which it is required, but it may be easily abused.

A very useful application of lavage is to abort a threatened attack of migraine. Repetition is sometimes necessary.

The introduction of two or three ounces of ice-water after a cleansing lavage is useful in increasing motility in cases of atony or motor insufficiency. This measure should not be employed when hyperpepsia or gastric catarrh is present. In *chronic gastritis*, water at a temperature of 105° to 120° should be employed in washing the stomach.

Gastric irrigation is recommended by Turck as a cardiac stimulant. It is certainly a powerful means of exciting the heart, but the inconvenience of its use leads the author to recommend as preferable the precordial compress (1383), the effects of which are decidedly marked, rendering it a most efficient remedy in cases of cardiac failure.

Lavage of the stomach may be successfully employed as a preliminary remedy in cases of *intestinal obstruction* in a large proportion of cases. The author has been able to relieve what seemed to be hopeless cases by this means. It may be said that, as a rule, whenever *fecal vomiting* occurs, gastric lavage may be properly administered, as the powerful peristaltic movement thus set up not infrequently restores the normal relations of the disturbed parts, and so relieves the obstruction.

Contraindications.—The habitual use of the stomach-tube is highly detrimental to the stomach, and should be prohibited except when made absolutely necessary by organic disease. The habit many patients have of passing a stomach-tube and emptying the stomach whenever they feel a slight inconvenience in the gastric region or experience headache or other slightly unpleasant symptoms, is a most detrimental practice. In recent years, since the use of the stomach-tube has become so very common, the author has found himself under the necessity of prohibiting its use as frequently as he has been called upon to recommend its employment.

The use of the stomach-tube should be carefully avoided in cases of *ulceration* accompanied by *hemorrhage*, and in cases of *cirrhosis* of the *liver* in which there is reason to suspect an accompanying varicose condition of the gastric veins. In *hemorrhagic tubercular* cases, in *aneurism* of the aorta within the chest, in advanced cases of *arteriosclerosis*, and in cases in which *cerebral apoplexy* has occurred, the use of the stomach-tube must be either wholly interdicted, or undertaken with most extraordinary precaution.

THE WATER EMETIC.

1403 Copious drinking of water at a temperature of 95° to 100° is an excellent means of provoking emesis. A single glassful will not generally produce the effect desired, but three or four glasses are almost sure to do so. If any medicinal agent is employed, as mustard or other substance by means of which emesis may be provoked, a copious draught of water at the temperature named should be employed at the same time. If the desired effect is not produced after three or four glasses have been swallowed, another glassful to which a teaspoonful of common salt has been added, should be taken.

The emetic is by no means a certain means of emptying the stomach; even though there may be considerable quantities of liquid removed from the stomach by vomiting, it is impossible to say that there is not a considerable quantity still left; and in any case it is evident that the stomach can not be thoroughly cleansed by this method. The stomach-tube is in every way preferable to the emetic, the use of which is necessary only in cases in which the stomach-tube can not be safely employed, or when the patient's fear of the stomach-tube is so great that its use is quite impossible. It is sometimes useful to suggest to an apprehensive patient contemplating the use of the stomach-tube with great horror and distress, that it is not necessary to swallow the whole tube, but only the tip end of it. As a rule, it is only the nervous fear of the patient which makes the use of the stomach-tube at all painful or even seriously inconvenient.

IRRIGATION OF THE COLON.—THE ENEMA.

This very useful procedure consists of the introduction of 1404
a quantity of water into the colon. The author employs the enema in three forms: First, the *simple* enema, the method of using which is well known; second, the *graduated* enema, a method devised by him a few years ago for the purpose of enabling persons who had become accustomed to the daily use of the enema to dispense with this very inconvenient procedure; third, the *coloclyster*, termed by the French "enteroclyster," which consists in an enema taken in the right Sims's position or the knee-chest position, a long rectal tube being employed.

In the simple enema the water is commonly employed at about the temperature of the body, or 98°. Better results are obtained by employing water at 70° F. The water is introduced by the aid of a syringe of some sort. Various excellent forms of syringes have been devised, of which the accompanying cuts illustrate the most useful and typical forms (Figs. 222, 223; 224).

The temperature must also be adapted to the use for which the measure is employed. If for mere mechanical effects, a temperature near that of the body is proper. It is generally better to introduce the water gradually, so that the bowels may not be stimulated to contraction, causing the fluid introduced to be discharged before a sufficient quantity has been received.

While the water is being introduced, the patient lies upon his back, with the hips slightly elevated. If a strong desire is experienced to expel prematurely the liquid introduced, the difficulty may be overcome by asking the patient to resist the expulsive impulse strongly, if necessary by compressing the anus with a napkin for a short time, until the peristaltic movement has ceased.

In the employment of the enema only such an amount of water as is necessary should be used. Many persons have been damaged by distending the colon so as to compel it to receive three or four quarts of water at once, as advised by a well-known empiric of New York City. On the very day of this writing the author has been called upon by a patient who was seriously damaged by following the advice of the charlatan referred to. The colon had evidently been stretched and dilated to such an extent that it had never returned to its normal condition, although considerable progress had been made in overcoming the obstinate intestinal inactivity caused by the habitual mechanical emptying of the colon.

In the application of the enema great care must be taken to avoid the introduction of air into the bowels, as this may be a source of severe colic pain. It is also important that the quantity of water employed should be only sufficient to accomplish the purpose sought.

The enema may be usefully employed in the cases of feeble patients as a preparation for surgical operations. In such a case, the bowels should be first washed out, then two or three pints of water at 100° should be slowly introduced into the rectum, the purpose being to increase the volume of the blood by absorption.

The warm enema (98° to 100°) may be usefully employed as a means of introducing water into the system in cases in which for any reason the patient can not swallow liquids without injury, as after operations upon the stomach, in cases of *persistent vomiting* requiring complete gastric rest, in *hemorrhage* from the *stomach*, in *typhoid fever* with *gastric dila-*

tation, and similar cases. Absorption takes place from the intestine much more rapidly than from the stomach.

The enema is certainly most useful as a means of temporarily relieving chronic intestinal inactivity; but great care must be taken to avoid creating dependence upon it. However, it is far better to be a slave to the enema than to "after-dinner pills."

A small cold enema is usually preferable to a large warm one. A pint of cold water may be introduced into the rectum at night or before or after breakfast to be retained.

The warm enema soon loses its efficiency because of its relaxing effect upon the intestines. The tone of the muscular walls is gradually lessened from day to day, until the bowel may become enormously stretched. Large quantities of water should never be used, as they overstretch the bowel and produce atony. Three or four pints is the limit for a daily application. The colon will hold a considerable quantity more than this, but should not be stretched to its full capacity under the relaxing influence of the warm water. The introduction of cold water into the small intestine is entirely free from this objection. Half a pint or a pint of cold water may be employed daily without injury, for the reason that the cold water energizes the muscles and nerves of the intestine. In the ordinary use of the enema, the temperature should be (80° to 70°).

In cases of extreme atony of the colon the enema sometimes fails to produce evacuation, the water being in large part retained, in these cases contraction of the colon may be induced by applying a cold wet towel to the abdomen, lower back and perineum while the patient is at stool or by massage of the colon or by a small enema of very cold water.

Not the least valuable service rendered by this simple procedure is the post-operative management of cases of abdominal surgery. It is the author's custom to administer an enema immediately after the operation in all cases in which adhesions have been broken up, for the purpose of "placing" the intestines, as a precaution against obstruction. The value of this procedure, in combination with other measures, pertaining chiefly to regimen and care, is attested by the fact that in dealing with more than seven hundred cases of abdominal surgery, nearly all ovariotomies or hysterectomies, the author has never once been compelled to reopen the abdomen to relieve obstruction, and has been able to record a mortality rate of less than three per cent, and a series of one hundred and sixty-five successive operations for the removal of uterine or ovarian tumors and diseased appendages, without a single death.

1405 **The Cold Enema.**—The enema is recognized as one of the most valuable means of reducing the temperature in febrile conditions, and not simply as an antithermic, but as a measure which aids in the removal of the causes of the abnormal temperature by exciting renal and cutaneous activity.

The cold enema was employed by the De Hahns in Germany in 1737 in the treatment of fevers. The same measure was also used by Dr. Benjamin Rush in the treatment of yellow fever in Philadelphia in 1794 with "good effects."

The enema renders invaluable service in typhoid fever, not only as a means of reducing the temperature, but of encouraging the action of the liver and kidneys, and especially in cleansing the alimentary canal. For twenty-five years it has been the custom of the author to begin the treatment of every case of typhoid fever with copious enemas.

A simple illustration will show the efficiency of the enema as a means of lowering the temperature: Suppose, for example, the quantity of water introduced to be five pounds (pints), and the temperature 70°, the patient's temperature 105°, and his weight 150 pounds. If on the withdrawal of the water, its temperature is found to be increased to 85°, there will have been absorbed by the water 75 pound Fahrenheit heat units ($5 \times 15 = 75$). This would be an equivalent of one half a heat unit to each pound of the body weight, or .5° fall in temperature for the whole body. In other words, if there had been, in the meantime, no increase of heat production, the temperature of the body would be lowered .5°.

A very convenient method of administering the cooling enema is to supplement the ordinary tube of a fountain syringe by a shorter piece of tubing, two or three feet in length, connected to it in such a way that it can easily be disconnected. The short piece of tubing should be somewhat larger than the ordinary size, so that it will not be easily obstructed. After being slowly introduced, the water should be retained for 5, 10, or 15 minutes, if possible. Then by disconnecting the short tube, and without removing the rectal tube, the water may be allowed to escape into a suitable vessel, and another portion of cool or tepid water may be immediately introduced.

In a fever case under the author's care a number of years ago, the cold enema was employed in this manner continuously for two or three hours, with the result that the temperature of the patient, which was between 105° and 106°, and had proved refractory to every other measure, was reduced to 102° and was thereafter readily controlled by the repetition of the same procedure.

The lower the temperature of the water employed, the greater will be the effect. Ordinarily it is not necessary to employ water at a temperature lower than 70°, and excellent effects may be obtained by means of the enema at 80°, provided a large quantity is introduced and the measure repeated a number of times in immediate succession. To prevent premature expulsive efforts, it is well to begin at a temperature near that of the body, gradually but quite rapidly lowering it by adding cold water in sufficient quantity to produce the temperature desired. Suppose, for example, that it is desired to administer an enema of four pints of water and to obtain the effect of water at 70°; the enema is started with a pint of water at a temperature of 100°, and three pints rapidly added at a temperature of 60°.

Stolz, in experiments to determine the antithermic effect of the cold enema in cases of *typhoid fever*, found that by the administration, at intervals of 5 to 10 minutes, of the enema at a temperature of 46°, the pulse was slowed twenty to thirty beats, and the temperature as taken in the mouth was lowered 3.6°.

The cold enema has rendered great service in the treatment of jaundice, as first shown by Krull.* The author prefers the enema at 105° to 110°, followed by the cold enema (60°).

The cold enema is most effectual as a means of relieving *constipation* through its tonic effects upon the structures of the rectum and mucous membrane.

1406 **The Hot Enema.**—The hot enema, or hot irrigation of the colon, is a useful means of combating an inflammatory condition of the pelvic viscera. Hot water introduced into the rectum and colon is brought nearer to the ovaries and other pelvic viscera than is possible in any other way. For this purpose it may be administered three or four times a day, or if necessary once every three or four hours. The temperature should be 110° to 120°.

Reclus prefers very hot rectal irrigation (130°) to vaginal irrigation or injection, in *congestions* of the *pelvic viscera.* It is of great value in the treatment of *prostatic inflammation,* causing disappearance of the swelling and pain and difficulty in micturition, often in a few hours, and in the majority of cases securing a complete cure of acute prostatitis in three to four days.

The hot enema is one of the most valuable of all hydriatic measures for combating *threatened collapse* in typhoid fever as well as in cholera and other conditions in which the vital failure is due to toxemia. The hot enema may even be used in cases of typhoid complicated by intestinal hemorrhage, and with marked benefit, when there is reason to believe that

---

* Krull, *Berliner Klin. Woch.*, 1877.

the patient is suffering in consequence of absorption of toxins resulting from the decomposition of retained blood clots. An immediate change in the aspect of cases of this sort is often apparent after freeing the colon of the fetid clots with a simple hot enema. The application should not be made while the hemorrhage is in progress, as the increase in arterial tension would involve serious risk. But a day or two later the bowel may be washed out without apprehension. The coloclyster, or copious enema, is the most rational method of establishing intestinal asepsis, at least when combined with an aseptic dietary of farinaceous gruels, fruit juices, and systematic water drinking.

The hot enema (104° to 115°) may be used with great benefit for its relaxing effect upon involuntary muscular tissue, in cases of *hepatic* or *biliary colic.* It is found equally useful in quieting excessive *uterine pains* during *parturition*, and in combating *irregular contractions* of the uterus.

The large hot enema has for many years been employed by Cantani and Wonte in the treatment of colic and infantile diarrhea. These sagacious observers also recommend its use in intestinal occlusion and *pseudo-membranous* colitis.

The hot enema is one of the most helpful of all measures in surgical shock and other forms of *collapse.* It may be safely used in all cases of shock in which the skin is pale and the pulse weak. The temperature should be from 110° to 120°. It should be followed by cold friction.

THE COLOCLYSTER, OR ENTEROCLYSTER.

The purpose of this mode of applying the enema is to fill 1407
the entire colon, or at least to introduce the largest quantity of water possible without overdistending the colon. In the ordinary enema it is difficult to introduce more than a pint and a half to three pints of water; but by placing the patient in the right Sims's or knee-chest position (Fig. 225), the amount of liquid may be increased to four or even five or six pints, and in some cases even more, without inconvenience to

the patient. In the right Sims's position the water is passed upward through the sigmoid flexure, and then runs along the descending colon, and on reaching the transverse colon, follows down toward the ascending colon, in which it accumulates until the colon is gradually filled. In the knee-chest position the action of gravity is still more helpful in completely filling the colon. This filling of the colon is necessary in cases in which fecal accumulations are present in the cecum; in catarrh of the cecum, a condition often mistaken for appendicitis, and which is doubtless the precursor of appendicitis in the great majority of cases; also in cases in which the cecum is infested with threadworms; and in cases of pseudo-membranous colitis.

Physiological Effects.—The physiological effects of irrigation of the intestine have been carefully studied by Krull, Stadelmann, and Kemp. Krull held the cold enema to be a powerful hepatic stimulant, but Stadelmann concluded from his researches that its action is mechanical only, aiding the liver by removing from the intestine large quantities of decomposing stuffs, with swarming microbes and the ptomains and toxins produced by them. This result seems rather surprising when one considers the powerful influence upon the mesenteric circulation, of cold water introduced into the intestine. Very powerful fluxion of the liver must be excited by this measure, and the reaction following must certainly be attended by decided increase in the activity of the portal circulation.

The introduction of very hot water into the colon increases blood pressure, improves and accelerates the heart action, and produces a marked effect upon renal secretion. A temperature of 110° to 120° has been found much more effective in increasing renal secretion than a lower temperature. The author has often noted in cases of patients to whom the enema has been administered, the passage within a very short time of a large quantity of clear urine. This was observed and pointed out by the empirical hydropaths more than fifty years ago.

Cold water produces a movement of fluid toward the intestine by the reaction which follows the application. This fact renders the cold enema of value in the treatment of constipation due to excessive dryness of the fecal matters. When used for relief of an *acute inflammation*, as in *dysentery*, the application must be moderate, prolonged, and continuous.

The hot enema, on the other hand, stimulates absorption from the alimentary canal, and raises the blood pressure by filling the blood-vessels and by reflex stimulation of the heart.

For most pronounced effects upon the heart and kidneys, the temperature should be 110° to 120°. The author is confident that he has saved the lives of a number of persons suffering from renal suppression by the repeated employment of this simple measure during periods varying from one to three or four hours. He has used the hot enema for this purpose for more than twenty years. The effects obtained are much more prompt and in every way more satisfactory than those obtained from jaborandi or any other diuretic drug.

The ordinary hot enema at 100° to 104° produces little effect upon blood pressure, but has a marked diuretic effect.

Cerebral congestion may result from the use of the warm water enema, as shown by the experiments of Schüller.*

According to M. Von Genersch † it is possible by the employment of the coloclyster to introduce a liquid into the small intestine, through which it may be rejected by the mouth.

Therapeutic Applications.—The coloclyster affords marvel- 1408
ous relief in a class of patients, unfortunately by no means small in number, who, suffering from *atony* and *dilatation* of the *colon*, are always carrying about with them an enormous accumulation of fecal matters. The patients are variously classified as *neurasthenics*, *hypochondriacs*, *simple dyspep-*

* *Arch. für Klin. Med.*, 1874.

† Von Genersch, *Progrès Médical*, 1893, p. 162.

tics, etc., and are treated for ***biliousness, insomnia, exhaustion***, and a multitude of ailments, all of which conditions are the simple result of *chronic autointoxication*, and are promptly relieved by a cleansing bath administered to the large intestine. The quantities of fecal matter removed in these cases is sometimes enormous; and not infrequently quantities of old putrefying fecal masses, semi-hardened by long retention, make their appearance after a free coloclyster has been thoroughly administered every day for a week or more, showing that a single irrigation of the colon, no matter how thoroughgoing, is not sufficient to establish the fact of its thorough cleansing. In this class of cases the coloclyster should be administered daily for two or three weeks if need be, or as long as the patient complains of gaseous distention of the bowels and fetid flatulence.

After the discharge of the warm water, the temperature of which should be 92° to 95°, a pint of water at 60° to 70° should be introduced and retained if possible, as a tonic bath for the colon. Care should be taken to avoid distending the colon with an excessive quantity of water at once. The amount need never exceed two quarts, and the quantity should be reduced from day to day after the colon has been thoroughly cleansed, until only a pint or a half pint of cold water is employed. Cold water stimulates and tones the bowel, whereas hot water is relaxing. The cold coloclyster may be used indefinitely without producing constipation, if the quantity of water employed is small. It acts as a sort of gymnastic trainer for the bowel, strengthening its muscular structures, and increasing the activity and energy of its controlling nerves and nerve centers.

The author's attention was early called to the observations of Krull, already referred to, and he has for more than twenty years made use of the enema in cases of *jaundice*, whether suspected to be due to *gall-stones*, or clearly due to infection of the liver and *catarrh* of the *bile ducts* in so-called "*infectious jaundice.*" The results have been almost uniformly excellent. Patients rarely fail to show marked improvement within a few days, and complete recovery has been secured in all cases of infectious jaundice. Careful regulation of the diet and other measures have been employed at the same time, but the coloclyster has been regarded as a measure of primary importance. The temperature for the clyster should be 90° to 100°, the purpose being to flush the portal circulation while at the same time cleansing the alimentary canal. A much larger quantity of water can be introduced by this method than when a lower temperature is employed, and may be retained for a much longer time. A small cold enema (70°, one pint) should be injected as soon as the warm water is discharged, to counteract the depressing and relaxing effect.

The coloclyster by means of the Sims's position is an exceedingly useful measure in fevers. By placing the patient in this position a much larger quantity of water may be introduced, and in certain cases this method is one of the most effective of all means of lowering the temperature.

That many cases of intestinal obstruction may be relieved by the coloclyster properly administered has been abundantly proved by Lesage, von Genersch, and others. Four to six quarts of fluid are often employed. The patient should take the knee-chest, or right Sims's position, or may be inverted, and the water should be introduced with a long rectal tube. The temperature should be 104°, and care should be taken to introduce the liquid slowly, the fountain being placed at an elevation of eight to twelve feet.

THE GRADUATED ENEMA.

This form of intestinal irrigation is administered in the 1409
same way as the ordinary enema or the coloclyster, and differs from it only in the fact that each day the amount of water is diminished and the temperature lowered. A very good plan to adopt is as follows: Beginning with three pints of water at a temperature about that of the body, the amount

of warm water introduced each day is diminished by half a pint, one-fourth pint of cold water being added, making the total amount of the fluid one-fourth pint less each day. At the end of the twelfth day the enema will consist of four ounces of cold water. In the majority of cases the decrease in temperature will compensate in stimulating effect for the diminished quantity; so that the bowel is thus brought to a more natural state, and weaned from the necessity of distension with warm water in order to provoke an evacuative movement. The graduated enema is exceedingly useful as a means of overcoming the enema habit.

RECTAL LAVAGE OR IRRIGATION.

1410 The author a number of years ago devised a hard-rubber instrument for this purpose, which has proved very convenient (Fig. 226). Numerous other forms of irrigators have been devised for the same purpose.

The temperature of the water used should be 100° to 125°, beginning with the lower temperature at first, and gradually increasing as tolerance is established. A normal saline solution, about a dram and a half to the quart, is more serviceable when the purpose is to relieve local irritation. When a cleansing effect is desired, as in catarrh of the bowels, a mixture consisting of equal parts of carbonate of soda and common salt (one dram and a half to the quart) may be used.

Hot irrigation of the rectum or the small hot enema frequently repeated is very useful in cases of *inflammation* of the *prostate*. Hot irrigation is also valuable as a means of relieving *leucorrhea*, *catarrh* of the *rectum*, *rectal irritation*, *spasm* of the *sphincter*, and *rectal ulcer*.

Cold rectal irrigation is useful as a means of allaying acute inflammation (60° to 40°, 5 to 10 min.). Repeat hourly. Fig. 227 shows an instrument for dry cooling.

Alternate irrigation (60°, 15 secs.; 110° to 120°, 15 secs., repeating) may be usefully employed in cases of constipation due to loss of normal nerve sensibility. Employed daily, or twice daily, at night and after breakfast.

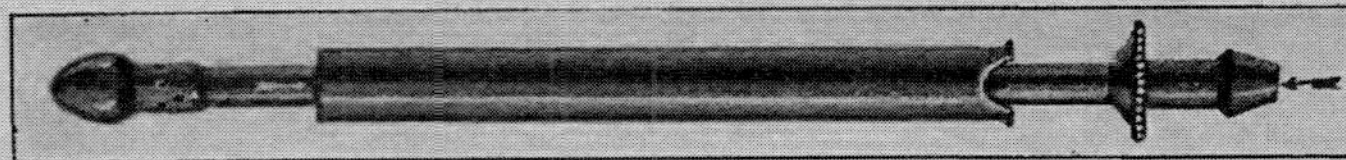

FIG. 226. RECTAL IRRIGATOR (p. 902). (Kellogg)

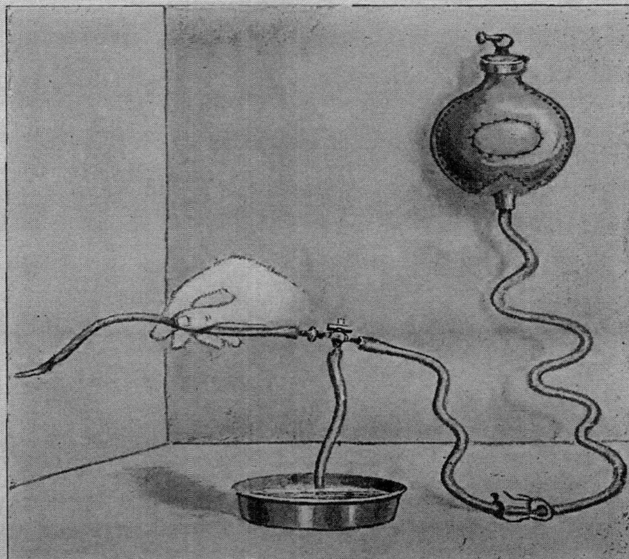

FIG. 228. INSTRUMENT FOR BLADDER IRRIGATION (p. 903).

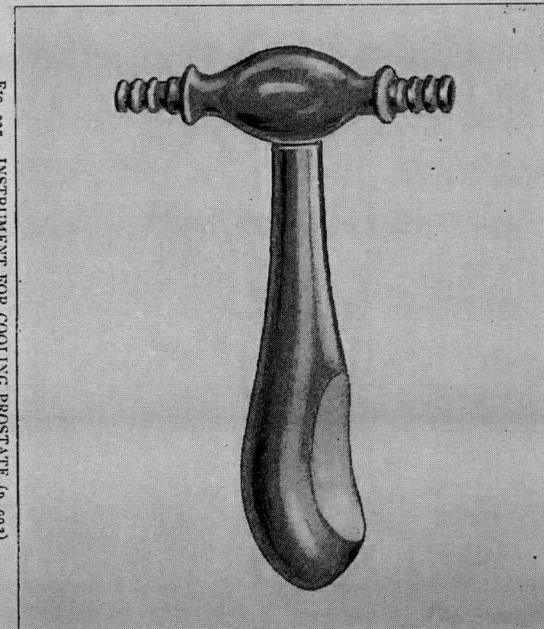

FIG. 227. INSTRUMENT FOR COOLING PROSTATE (p. 902).

IRRIGATION OF THE BLADDER.

The instruments required for this procedure are a fountain 1411
syringe (Fig. 228) or a funnel with three or four feet of rubber tubing attached, and a smooth, soft-rubber catheter. Special forms of catheter are necessary in some cases of prostatic disease. The connection of the syringe with the catheter should be made by means of a "Y" connection piece to one arm of which a piece of tubing two or three feet in length is attached for the purpose of conveying the water into some proper receptacle. The patient should lie upon a couch or treatment table with the clothing conveniently adjusted. The fountain should be placed a foot and a half or two feet above the couch Both the supply and the waste tubes of the instrument should be furnished with convenient stop-cocks, so that the flow of water may be easily and perfectly controlled.

Great care should be taken in introducing the catheter to preserve strict asepsis. Not only should the catheter be thoroughly aseptic, but the genitals, and the hands of the physician or nurse, must be as carefully prepared as for a surgical operation. When these precautions are taken, the so-called "catheter-fever" will very rarely occur. The temperature of the water employed should be, for ordinary cleansing purposes, 100°. Water containing chloride of sodium, in the proportion of one and one-half drams to the quart, is less irritating than fresh water. The water should be boiled after the salt is added, so as to make sure that it is thoroughly sterile.

The bladder should first be emptied, then the water should be introduced in small quantities, from one to three ounces at a time. It should flow in with little force, and should be allowed to pass out immediately; but the bladder should not be pressed upon to hasten the discharge of the fluid, and a new quantity of fluid should be introduced before the bladder is completely emptied, so as to avoid the irritation produced by strong contraction of the bladder upon itself.

By the same apparatus employed in vesical irrigation, certain useful mechanical effects may be brought to bear upon the bladder. In cases in which the organ has become abnormally contracted, so that the patient is continually annoyed by distressing demands for micturition, the normal capacity of the organ may be restored by gradual distention by means of the hydrostatic pressure of the water column connected with the fountain. To accomplish this, the outflow tube is closed, the fountain is placed about one foot above the patient, and the bladder is allowed to fill as full as possible with this amount of pressure; then the fountain is slowly raised until the patient experiences a very strong desire to empty the bladder. The inflow is now shut off, the outlet opened, and the bladder allowed to empty itself; after a rest of three or four minutes, the operation is repeated. The bladder should thus be filled and emptied three to six times at each treatment, and the treatment should be repeated daily. The temperature of the water employed should be 104° to 106°.

We are indebted to Daggett, of Buffalo, for a method of irrigating either the bladder or the urethra, or both, which is exceedingly practical, and is superior to the hydrophore. A cut of the instrument employed is shown in Fig. 229. The irrigator is connected with a fountain syringe containing a solution of salt in the proportion of a dram to a quart, at a temperature of 115°. The instrument is introduced into the meatus far enough so that it can be grasped and held in place. The tube is then connected with the inlet, the end of the finger being held over the outlet. The fountain is placed two or three feet above the patient's head, so as to give moderate pressure. As the urethra is gradually distended, the fluid finds its way backward, and finally enters the bladder if permitted to do so. When the bladder is filled, it is only necessary to pinch the tube connecting the irrigator with the fountain, and allow the water to escape. By repeating the operation several times, the bladder may be thoroughly cleansed, and without running the risk of injury, catheter fever, etc., which is so likely to occur even when great care is practiced, in the daily passage of an instrument into the bladder. Of course there are cases in which this simple device will not answer the purpose on account of obstruction at the bladder outlet; but it is practical in a very large proportion of cases, even in cases of enlarged prostate, and can be used by the patient himself after proper instruction.

Physiological Effects.—The mucous membrane of the bladder is exceedingly sensitive to temperatures either above or below the average temperature of the interior of the body. The healthy bladder expels with great force water at a temperature of 77°, even when the quantity is not more than two or three ounces (Mellez), and at a temperature of 41° so small a quantity as one or two drams will cause prompt and vigorous contraction. Very hot water likewise produces powerful contractions of the bladder.

Therapeutic Applications.—The bladder douche at a temperature near that of the body is a highly valuable measure in the treatment of vesical catarrh or chronic cystitis. This measure is in fact indispensable in dealing with that form of bladder catarrh which is met with in old men suffering from enlarged prostate, and who have lost the power to empty the bladder without mechanical assistance. In such cases it may be employed daily, twice a day, or every other day, as may be indicated by the conditions present. When mucus is formed rapidly and in làrge quantities, when the bladder is infected and decomposition takes place to such an extent that the urine is ammoniacal when withdrawn from the bladder, the irrigation should be sufficiently often to prevent accumulation of mucus and advanced decomposition.

In inoperable cases of calculus of the bladder, vesical irrigation renders valuable service as a palliative measure, the patient's suffering being greatly mitigated by its use. Irrigation is indicated in most cases of *atony* of the *bladder* and in cases of *paralysis* of the organ associated with *paraplegia*, *locomotor ataxia*, and other affections of the nervous system. Vesical irrigation is usually required whenever the urine is ammoniacal, and when it is turbid when passed; when pus or blood is present; and when minute calculi, so-called gravel, are sometimes passed. In certain cases of *atony* in which there is no irritation, and in which no evidences of vesical catarrh are present, the powerful stimulus of cold water may be carefully tried. The first injection should consist of one or two ounces of water at 80°. If this produces no unpleasant effect, the temperature may be gradually lowered to 60°. Hot applications may likewise be employed with advantage in these cases, but the temperature should not exceed 115° to 120°. Alternate hot and cold irrigation of the bladder is the most powerful means of stimulating its muscular structures. The extreme temperatures should at first not exceed 110° and 85°, and the highest and lowest temperatures should be gradually approached.

In *hemorrhage* from the *bladder*, very hot irrigation (118° to 122°) may be employed. An ice-bag may be applied over the bladder at the same time, and a hot foot bath or a hot blanket pack to each leg separately may be employed with advantage.

Contraindications.—Irrigation of the bladder must generally be avoided in *acute cystitis* until after the extreme sensitiveness of the mucous membrane has to some degree subsided. Irrigation can generally be undertaken if special care is employed within two or three days after the onset of the disease. Most relief will be obtained in the early stages of cystitis by external applications, such as the hot pelvic or hip and leg pack or the very hot sitz (110° to 120°) for 5 or 10 minutes, followed by a very gentle affusion at 80°.

Special care must be taken to avoid the baneful effect of cold in cases of either *acute* or *chronic cystitis*. Chilling of the patient during the treatment may produce an acute exacerbation of the inflammation, and greatly aggravate all the symptoms. To counteract any tendency in this direction, it

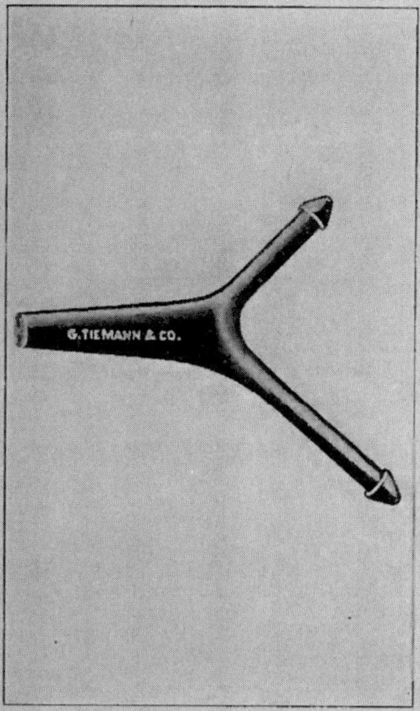

FIG. 229. IRRIGATOR FOR URETHRA AND BLADDER (p. 904).

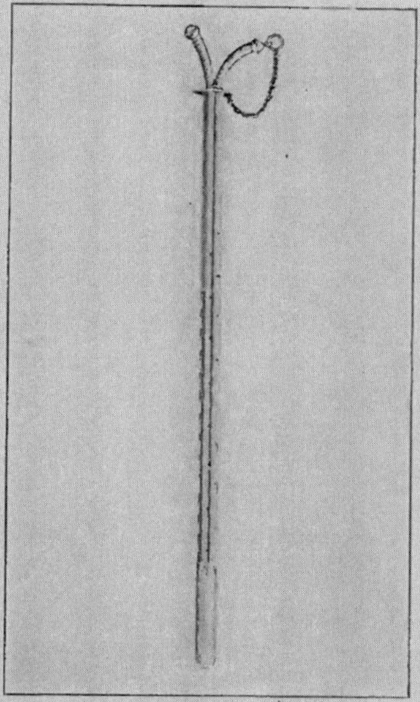

FIG. 230. URETHRAL IRRIGATOR, YDROPHORE OF SCHUTZ (p. 907).

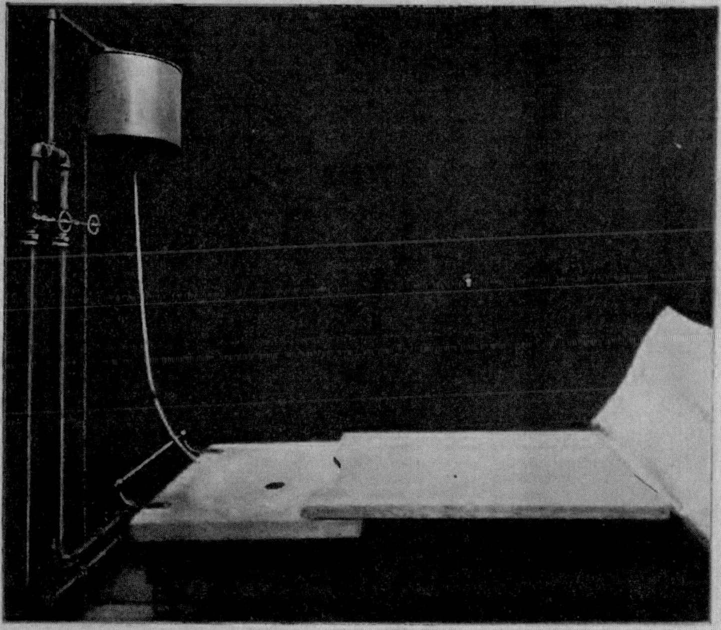

FIG. 231. MARBLE-COVERED COUCH FOR VAGINAL IRRIGATION (p. 909).

is well to administer a hot or warm sitz bath immediately after irrigation of the bladder, in cases in which the patient is able to sit erect. Special care must be taken to keep the feet warm during the application, and there should be as little exposure as possible. The limbs should be wrapped in flannel blankets, and the patient should on no account be allowed to feel the slightest sensation of chilliness.

Irrigation of the bladder must be avoided in cases of *acute urethritis*, in consequence of the danger of conveying the infection backward into the bladder and other of the deep passages.

IRRIGATION OF THE URETHRA.

Numerous instruments are employed for the application of 1412
liquids to the urethra. One of the best of these is the hydrophore of Shutz (Fig. 230), which consists of a fluted tube, with small openings in the sides. As this instrument is introduced, the water flows backward toward the meatus, cleansing the canal as the tube advances, thus preventing the conveyance of infection to the deeper parts of the urethra. The instrument should be introduced until it passes beyond the sensitive area, but should be checked at this point. Daggett's instrument (Fig. 229) may also be used. When it is desired to treat the urethra exclusively, as in gonorrhea, for example, the urethra should be shut off from the bladder by pressure upon the perineum with the finger. It is sometimes important to distend the urethra, so as to spread out the folds of the mucous membrane, and thus secure complete cleansing of the surfaces. To accomplish this, it is only necessary to compress the parts at the meatus about the catheter with sufficient firmness to prevent the escape of liquid, while also compressing the urethra at the perineum.

Ordinarily, the temperature of the water employed for irrigating the urethra should be about 100°. Curtis reported many years ago (1833) remarkable results in the treatment of *chronic urethritis* by very hot water. He employed simply a fountain syringe, consisting of a tin pail with a rubber tube attached, and a No. 8 English catheter. An alcohol lamp was adjusted under the pail, so as gradually to elevate the temperature of the water during treatment. The temperature was allowed to rise very slowly, by which means a tolerance was established to such a remarkable degree that a temperature of more than 180° was sometimes employed. This was probably the temperature in the fountain, the temperature of the water actually in contact with the mucous membrane naturally becoming considerably lowered by cooling while passing through the tube. The catheter was introduced into the urethra to within about an inch of the prostate, and the fountain hung high enough to give sufficient force to the stream to carry it backward through the urethra, but not into the bladder. Curtis claimed for his method that it cut short the disease very promptly; that it gave almost immediate relief from pain and swelling; and that it was equally successful in acute and chronic cases. The author has found the very hot urethral douche a very effective procedure.

The employment of hot urethral irrigation (110° to 130°) in gonorrhea secures the early absorption of exudates, and thus prevents deformity, cicatrization, and stricture. This is also the best remedy for *chordee*. The quantity of water employed should usually be several quarts, or until the pain is relieved. A short hot sitz bath (110° to 118° for 5 or 10 min.) is a valuable measure to be used in combination with hot urethral irrigation. In chronic cases, with exudates, employ alternate hot and cold irrigation.

VAGINAL IRRIGATION.

1413 This procedure, more commonly but incorrectly termed the vaginal douche, consists of the injection into the vaginal canal, with little or no pressure, of a stream of water, either hot, cold, or of intermediate temperature. This procedure has rendered immense service in the treatment of uterine, ovarian, and other pelvic disorders in women, but a lack of understanding its physiological effects and therapeutic application at various temperatures has resulted in numerous failures and disappointments.

Following the example of Peasley and Emmett, who were among the first to champion the vaginal douche as a therapeutic measure in gynecological practice in this country, most American practitioners make habitual use of vaginal irrigation at as high a temperature as the patient can comfortably bear, or from 105° to 122° F. Fortunately, vaginal irrigation at this temperature is applicable to a large proportion of cases; but other temperatures, higher or lower, may often be employed to much better advantage. The application is best made with a fountain syringe, which consists of a reservoir containing water placed at a height of two to three feet above the patient. By means of a rubber tube of suitable size (the size ordinarily employed is too small) and a glass or hard rubber vaginal nozzle, the water is conducted to the vaginal canal. The patient lies upon her back with the hips elevated, a proper receptacle being arranged to catch the water as it flows out from the vagina.

Fig. 231 shows a douche table devised by the author, which has borne the test of many years' use. The top consists of a marble slab, hollowed somewhat to fit the form of the body, and provided with an opening and channels to conduct the water rapidly away. The arrangements for asepsis are perfect, and the patient's clothing never becomes wet or soiled.

In introducing the vaginal tube, care should be taken to direct it backward behind the cervix uteri, to the very farthest limit of the *cul de sac*, so as to avoid any possible danger of forcing the water into the uterine cavity. As the water enters from the fountain, it flows about the neck of the uterus, and circulates through the vagina, bringing every part of it under the thermic influence of the application, thus affecting not only the mucous membrane with which the water comes in actual contact, but through reflex influence the circulation of all the pelvic viscera.

1414 Many years ago Max Runge made an exhaustive study of the effects of vaginal irrigation upon the circulation and muscular excitability of the uterus, applying a gentle stream of water at different temperatures to the exposed uterus in living rabbits. As a result of these interesting studies, he found that the application of water at 41° F. produced at first strong tetanic contractions, lasting for a full minute, which were followed by rhythmical contractions and relaxations, continuing for some time. When the cold application was continued for 10 to 15 minutes, the contractions slowly ceased, the pale color of the uterus induced by the primary contraction of the uterus under the influence of the cold, giving rise to a pronounced red colorization, showing active movement of blood through the organ. After the close of the experiment, the parts returned to their normal state at the end of a half hour. That the cessation of the contraction was not due to the exhaustion of the uterine muscle, was shown by the fact that subsequent applications of heat or electricity gave rise to violent contractions.

Applications of hot water at a temperature of 122° produced, on the other hand, rhythmical contractions of the uterus, but less vigorous than after applications of cold, and without any tendency to tetanic contraction, as after the cold application. When the hot application was continued for 10 minutes, the contractions finally ceased, leaving the uterus as before, and of a bluish color, but incapable of contracting, as shown by applications of cold, electricity, strychnia, and other excitants. No effect whatever was produced, showing that the uterine muscle was, temporarily at least, completely paralyzed. After the lapse of half an hour the uterus acquired its normal condition. Further investigation showed that the passively congested and paralytic state of the uterus, as described, was produced only by temperatures above 104° or very hot applications.

It is interesting to note the similarity, with marked differences, however, between the applications of heat and cold to the uterus. Stronger and more prolonged contractions were produced by the cold than by the heat. Muscular excitability was not diminished, but was palpably increased by the cold application, whereas in ten minutes it was completely obliterated by the hot irrigation.

From these facts it will readily appear that both hot and cold applications may be employed for relieving hemorrhage due to uterine congestion, but that the cold application is a more powerful hemostatic agent than heat. Hot applications, on the other hand, possess remarkable power to lessen and even completely to annul uterine excitability and contractility of the uterine muscle, which is decidedly increased by cold irrigation. But the tendency of cold irrigation to produce painful uterine contraction and to provoke an exacerbation of neuralgic and other pains to which the pelvic viscera are so particularly subject, accounts for the almost universal preference for hot irrigation in the treatment of pelvic disorders of women. The author has found not a few cases in which temperatures above 104° were badly tolerated, a fact which was doubtless due to the paralytic congestion produced by high temperatures. The douche at 90° is found highly useful in relieving pelvic congestions, which are extremely productive of discomfort. The author has never found it expedient to employ as low a temperature as 41°, but vaginal irrigation at 75° to 80° has often produced excellent antiphlogistic results in cases in which hot irrigation could not be tolerated.

Hot irrigation is indicated when the effect desired is to relieve pain, to promote the absorption of exudates, and to stimulate vascular activity in cases of salpingitis or so-called cellulitis; also in cases of chronic metritis, ovaritis, and so-called endometritis.

Very hot irrigation, as shown by Emmett and proved by the experience of nearly every other gynecologist, is of high value as a means of checking hemorrhage. For this purpose the application must be made at as high a temperature as can be borne, a temperature of 125° to 130° being desirable.

If hot irrigation fails, employ cold, boiled water (65° to 55°). If cold irrigation produces pain, employ simultaneously a hot sitz bath or hot hip or leg pack. Hot irrigation is sometimes better tolerated in connection with the cool or tepid sitz bath (75° to 85°). Rub the surface well to promote reaction.

In relation to vaginal irrigation during pregnancy, it may be remarked that careful vaginal irrigation, even at a temperature of 115° to 118°, may be made at any time during gestation before labor has begun, without the slightest danger of producing uterine contractions or any tendency to miscarriage. After the beginning of labor, however, very hot irrigation produces prompt dilatation of the cervix.

The ordinary effects of vaginal irrigation will be increased by employing an intermittent jet obtained by attaching an ordinary bulb syringe to the fountain douche apparatus. Alternate irrigation is sometimes useful in relaxed conditions and in promoting absorption of exudates when pain and congestion are not present. Two fountains with tube attachments may be employed, one containing cold (60° to 80°), the other hot (104° to 120°), water; or two fountains may be joined to a single tube by a suitable connection.

The percussion vaginal douche is an effective means of cleansing irrigation, and also powerfully stimulates the pelvic circulation. It is administered by means of a modification of the ordinary fountain douche in which the fountain is closed and the air pumped in by a rubber compressor bulb, a small amount of air being mingled with the water so that there is an alternate discharge of water and air expelled with considerable force.

1415 **Intra-Uterine Irrigation.**—The application of water to the interior of the uterus requires a special instrument for the purpose, so constructed as to allow a ready outflow of the liquid introduced, known as a double current or irrigating sound. In uterine irrigation only distilled or well-boiled water should be employed. If no other medicament is used, it is

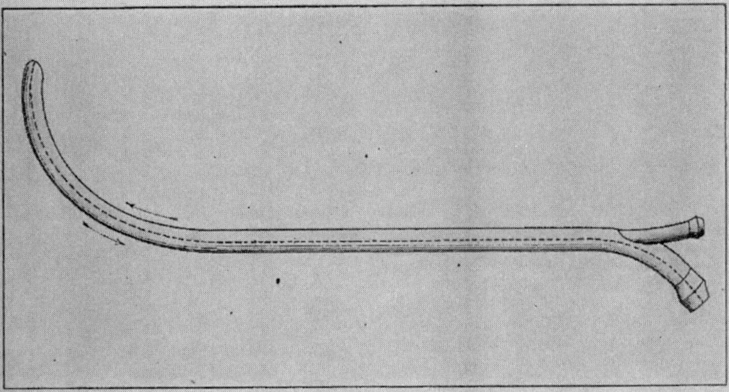

FIG. 232. PSYCHROPHORE (p. 913). (Winternitz)

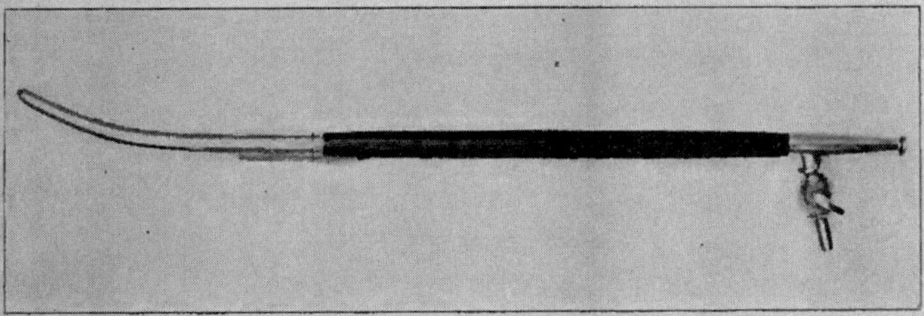

FIG. 233. HOLLOW SOUND FOR MAKING THERMIC APPLICATIONS TO UTERUS (p. 914). (Kellogg)

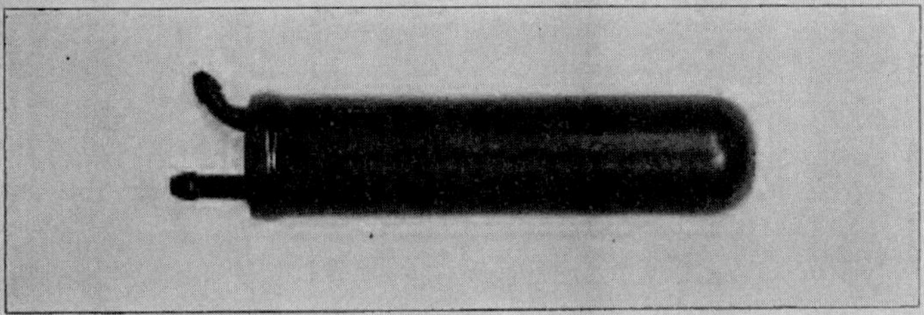

FIG. 234. HOLLOW CYLINDER FOR MAKING THERMIC APPLICATIONS TO VAGINA (p. 914). (Kellogg)

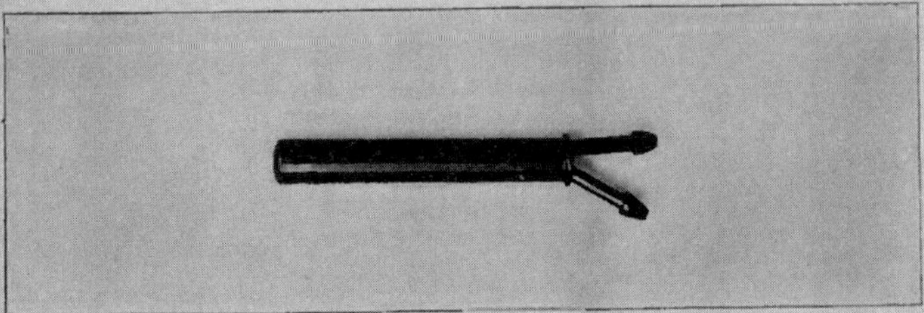

FIG. 235. HOLLOW CYLINDER FOR MAKING THERMIC APPLICATIONS TO RECTUM (p. 914). (Kellogg)

well to add to the water common salt, one gram to 100, or 10 grams to the gallon. The application should be made with all antiseptic precautions after curettement or other operations upon the interior of the uterus, and in obstetrical cases in which blood clots or membranes are retained, from which the patient is liable to infection through absorption of septic matter from the uterine cavity.

MEANS OF MAKING HOT, COLD, AND ALTERNATE APPLICATIONS TO THE MUCOUS PASSAGES.

Fig. 232 illustrates an instrument devised by Professor 1416
Winternitz, known as the *psychrophore*, and intended for making applications to the urethra when hot or cold applications are desirable. The author has found this measure serviceable in the treatment of certain cases of extreme hyperesthesia of the urethra. Both prolonged cold applications and short hot applications may be used with success. In some of these cases alternate hot and cold applications are most effective. This is especially true in cases in which the tone of the parts is lowered or passive congestion exists.

Alternate cool or tepid and very cold applications may sometimes be made with advantage, the warm at 78° to 80° for 5 minutes, then an application at 50° to 57° for 5 minutes.

The bladder should be emptied just before the use of the psychrophore, and should not be emptied again for a couple of hours after the treatment.

The psychrophore likewise renders valuable service in the curative treatment of *nocturnal enuresis*.

The author a number of years ago devised a series of hollow applicators shown in the accompanying cuts (Figs. 233–235), which have proved very successful for the several purposes for which they were designed. By means of a hollow uterine sound (Fig. 233) either hot, cold, or alternate applications may be made to the interior of the uterus with great convenience. By compressing the outflow tube, the rate at which the water passes through the instrument may be regulated, and by the same means also the temperature. If the water at the outlet is made to fall upon a thermometer, the temperature of the water may be observed at every moment, and may be made to rise or fall by adjustment of the gauge. The author has frequently made applications to the body of the uterus at 160° with excellent effect, although this temperature is somewhat painful. A temperature of 140° is usually sufficiently high to accomplish the desired results. The instrument also proves useful in cases of subinvolution, vegetations, catarrh of the cervix, and flexion or relaxed uterine walls and arrested development.

1417 In Fig. 234 is shown a hard-rubber instrument which has been found very useful as a means of applying heat to the pelvic viscera through the vagina, in cases in which the bed-pan or douche apparatus can not be used without injurious disturbance to the patient. The instrument is simply introduced into the vagina, and a current of hot water passed through it. The patient may lie in any position, and thus is in nowise inconvenienced by the application; the relief experienced from this procedure is often very remarkable. The effect of moist heat is easily obtainable by simply covering the instrument with a mass of absorbent cotton and saturating with water.

1418 Fig. 235 shows an instrument constructed on the same plan as the preceding, but smaller in size, and designed for *thermic applications to the rectum.* Either hot or cold applications or alternate hot and cold applications may be made as desired. This measure is of great value in the treatment of rectal irritation, and constipation due to lack of tone in the structures of the rectum, as well as in cases of enlarged or irritable prostate, etc. Short cold applications or alternate hot and cold applications are employed in cases in which excitant effects are desired, as in relaxed conditions in which there is loss of muscular tone, in hemorrhoids, and in some cases of chronic ulcer requiring stimulation. The extremes of heat and cold should in such cases be made as great as possible, or as great as the patient will bear. Very hot applications are useful in cases of *internal hemorrhoids*, *rectal catarrh*, *rectal ulcer* and *fissure*, *enlarged prostate*, and *spasm* of the *sphincter*.

The analogous instrument for the vagina the author has used with great satisfaction in relieving the pain which is often most distressingly persistent after a *laparotomy* involving the pelvic viscera. The instrument may be applied with water at any temperature desired. Most excellent analgesic effects may be obtained with cold water in *local inflammatory processes*.

Arzberger, to whom the credit of having first employed instruments of this sort is ascribed, employs a temperature of 70° to 60°. The temperature at first may be higher (80° to 85°), and may be gradually lowered. Numerous modifications of these instruments, possessing varying degrees of merit, have been constructed by various instrument-makers.

STEAM INHALATION.

The inhalation of air saturated with moisture and warmed 1410
by mixture with steam, improperly called steam inhalation, is a very old-fashioned but an extremely valuable remedy for both acute and chronic inflammations of the air-passages. The so-called "croup-kettle," though a crude affair, has been the means of saving many lives, and alleviating the sufferings of hundreds of little ones. When it is desirable that the patient should breathe the vapor continually, very effective means may be conveniently arranged by aid of the portable oil-stoves and gas-stoves now in use. The stove should be placed by the bedside of the patient, with a teakettle, or in the absence of anything better, a basin in which water may be continuously and vigorously boiled. By means of a yard of wire mosquito netting, rolled into the proper shape, and covered with oil-cloth, rubber cloth, or newspapers, it is possible to construct a cone whereby the vapor may be brought to the face of the patient lying close to the edge of the bed; or

for a small sum a tinner may be employed to make a more convenient and durable arrangement for conducting the steam from the boiler to the patient. It is not necessary nor desirable that all air should be excluded except that which comes through the apparatus. It is only important that the patient should breathe the air as moist and at as high a temperature as possible.

In cases of *croup* and *diphtheria*, the moist, hot inhalation aids greatly in maintaining the resistance of the tissues, and facilitates the separation of the false membranes. It must be remembered, however, that complete saturation of the air with moisture seriously interferes with the absorption of oxygen by the lungs; so that if marked cyanosis is present, the inhaling apparatus must be removed, or the inhalation of pure oxygen gas may be employed in connection with it.

1420 By far the most important use for steam inhalation is in the treatment of *acute* or *chronic catarrhal affections* of the nose and throat. The simplest form of inhaler consists simply of a tin cup with a loosely fitting cover, through which a tube passes, by which the patient is enabled to draw from the interior of the cup, warm sautrated air, which finds its way in about the edge of the cover. More than twenty years ago the author devised a convenient inhaler which is illustrated in the accompanying cut (Fig. 236). This construction permits the addition of some medicament to the water when desirable, and provides an extra water compartment outside the inhaling cup, by which the heat of the latter is retained for a long time. In *acute inflammations* of the *pharynx*, the *post-nasal region*, the *larynx*, and even in *acute bronchitis*, the faithful employment of the steam inhaler aids greatly in securing early recovery. The inhaler should be used many times a day in order to secure the best results. Ten or fifteen minutes in each hour is the usual prescription. In acute conditions, in which the parts are very sensitive and painful, the temperature of the inhalation should be moderate. The effect of the application should be soothing. In chronic conditions, especially when there is thickening of the mucous membrane and hypertrophy of the glandular structures, as in cases of large or *elongated uvula*, *enlarged tonsils*, *follicular hypertrophy* of the *tonsils*, or *adenoids*, the temperature of the inhalation should be as high as can be borne. A tolerance for heat is quite readily established by the mucous membrane, so that after a few minutes a higher temperature can be employed than at first. It is not necessary to change the temperature of the water on this account, however. At the beginning of the inhalation the patient makes short, quick drafts through the inhaler; then, as tolerance is established, he draws longer and deeper breaths, especially if the bronchial mucous membrane is involved. It is easily possible to manage the inhalation so as to confine the effect almost wholly to the naso-pharynx.

The effect of the hot vapor upon the mucous membrane is precisely that of circumscribed applications of heat to the cutaneous surface. The tissues are excited to increased activity, the movement of blood through congested parts is encouraged, and the improved circulation aids the reparative processes, assists the absorption of exudates, and promotes the resistance of the tissues against invasion by parasitic microbes, to which the chronicity of catarrhal affections of the naso-pharynx is chiefly due.

Another method of administering steam inhalation, de- 1421
vised by the author, has been shown by experience, to be possessed of so much merit that it is entitled to brief mention here. It consists of the inhalation of steam from a receptacle to which it is conducted by a pipe communicating with a powerful generator or with the steam-heating system of the building. The receptacle is of such shape that the entire head in front of the ears may be pushed into it, thus exposing the skin of the face to contact with hot steam, at the same time that the heated moist air is drawn in through the nose or the nose and mouth. By this means the entire mucous surfaces and a large part of the cutaneous surface, associated

directly and reflexly with the diseased parts, are brought under the influence of the hot application. Thus while the vasomotor stimulating influence of the heat is acting upon the mucous membrane of the nose and throat, this direct action is greatly assisted by the strong hyperemia of the skin produced, and consequent draining of collaterally associated vessels of the mucous membrane. Patients experience from this treatment a degree of immediate relief such as is afforded by no other measure with which the author is acquainted. Obstructed nostrils are opened up, viscid and inspissated masses of secretion are loosened and discharged, pain and pressure are removed, hoarseness is relieved, and the patient recognizes so thoroughly the benefit received that it is not necessary to urge him to persevere in the employment of the measure until permanent results can be obtained. The treatment should be administered three times a day, 15 minutes each time. At the conclusion of the treatment, a towel wet in ice-water is applied to the face for half a minute. The latter procedure restores tone to the relaxed cutaneous vessels, while at the same time securing continued activity and a lasting hyperemia, thus prolonging the effect of the treatment.

In cases in which there is great loss of tone of the vessels of the naso-pharynx, exposures to the hot steam may be alternated with ice-water applications, the steam being employed one minute and the ice compress 15 seconds. The alternations should be repeated ten or twelve times.

In the apparatus shown in the accompanying cut (Fig. 237), devised by the author, a strong draft of cold air is produced by the aid of an electric fan. The patient controls the fan with a button, and exposes his face alternately to the action of the hot steam and the cold air. By this means a powerful alterative effect is brought to bear upon the naso-pharyngeal membrane with most excellent results. The treatment is, of course, associated with the inhalation of antiseptic vapors and the application of antiseptic sprays to the affected membranes, for the purpose of maintaining an aseptic condition until the parts have become sufficiently restored to resist successfully the attacks of their microbic enemies.

Adopting the suggestion of Brown-Sequard, the author has also utilized the cold draft as a means of training sensitive patients in such a way as to establish immunity against slight exposures to cold air or drafts, allowing the breeze from the electric fan to fall upon the back of the neck or other sensitive parts, while they are at the same time submitted to a vigorous rubbing to encourage their ability to react. As the training advances, the application of the breeze is made longer and stronger, while the force of the rubbing is diminished until the skin becomes capable of taking care of itself without either protection or the mechanical aid of rubbing. This condition being one which must be reached by every person who desires to become free from catarrhal affections, any system of treatment which does not accomplish it, or which confines itself to the treatment of the diseased mucous surfaces, will certainly fall short of the object sought.

The whole skin must be made so healthy and vigorous that it will be proof against the circulatory disturbances which give rise to colds. A relaxed skin which is bathed in perspiration by slight exercise renders the person very liable to colds. By cold bathing the skin becomes accustomed to contracting its blood-vessels firmly, so that the loss of heat which gives rise to chill and the accompanying internal congestion, does not occur. This condition can be secured only by long training by means of daily cold applications.

THE STEAM JET.

The steam or vapor jet is so called only by the license of 1422
common usage, as steam proper can not be brought in contact with the living tissues without destructive effects, although a Russian physician (Snegirjow) a few years ago called attention to the value of this agent at 212° for controlling hemorrhage, and Pincus Kiliani, who continued the experiments and observations, has clearly shown that steam has powerful

styptic properties, and that it might be used advantageously in operations upon the liver, kidneys, lungs, and other parenchymatous organs. Bleeding from quite large arteries is readily controlled by it. Under the influence of the steam jet, the parts shrivel, and acquire a cooked appearance. This action of steam does not, however, appear to interfere with immediate union of the cut surfaces to which the application has been made. The steam jet has also been advantageously used in morbid conditions of the uterus, accompanied by bleeding, especially in malignant disorders.

The steam jet is applied by means of an ordinary steam generator such as was formerly used for surgical operations by Lister's spray method. The steam is conducted to the part to which the application is to be made by rubber tubing, as short as possible without inconvenience, provided at the end with a suitable holder. The author has devised a special nozzle for applying the steam jet, which prevents the ejection of the water of condensation which, having a greater specific gravity than steam, is likely to fall where not desired. The nozzle is so arranged as to combine handle and nozzle in one piece, and provides for the safe disposal of the water of condensation (Fig. 238). The value of the steam jet for the purpose suggested has yet to be determined by the test of further clinical experience. It may prove to be an exceedingly useful measure in certain classes of surgical cases.

WATER DRINKING.

1423 Water drinking as a therapeutic measure is of very ancient origin. Hippocrates prescribed it as a remedy in fevers, and the drinking of cold water has been practiced among the Egyptians from the most ancient time in the treatment of fevers. Cold water drinking was used by Hahn in the treatment of fevers in Germany in the first half of the eighteenth century, fully sixty years before Priessnitz prescribed the internal use of water in such prodigious quantities at Graefenberg.

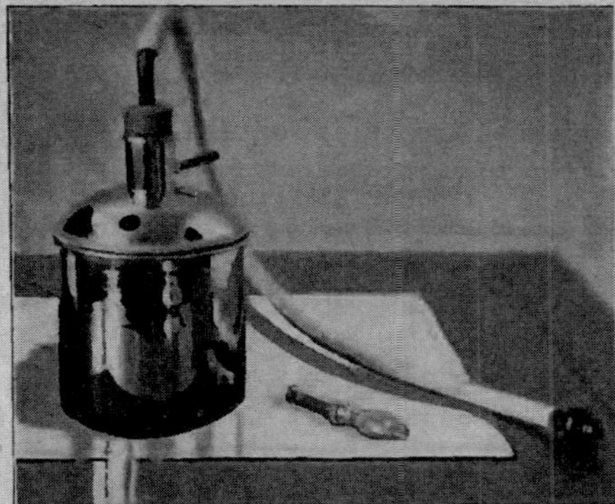

Fig. 236. STEAM INHALER (p. 916).

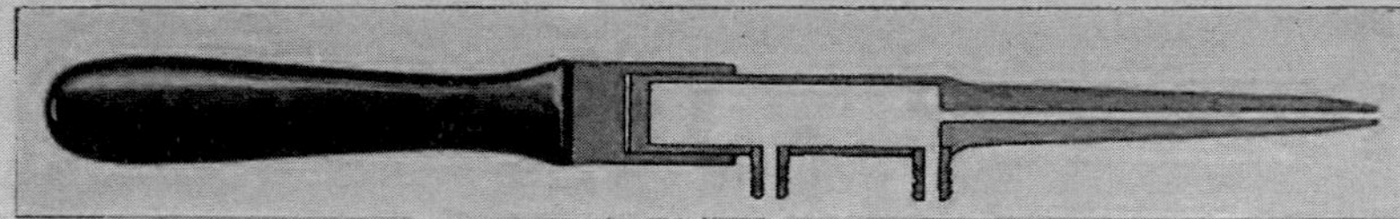

Fig. 238. STEAM-JET AND NOZZLE FOR HEMOSTASIS — Diagram (p. 920). (Kellogg)

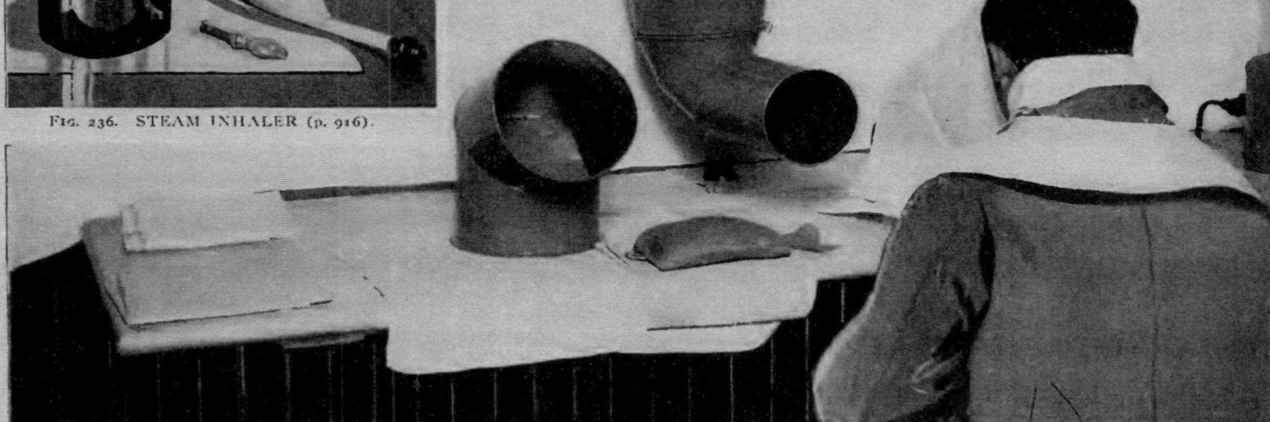

Fig. 237. STEAM FACE BATH ALTERNATING WITH COLD BLAST (p. 918).

Todano, an Italian contemporary of Hahn, made his fever patients drink five pints of ice water every three hours. The patient was placed in a hammock without covering, and the treatment was continued until perspiration occurred. If he became comatose, ice was placed over the heart. This extraordinarily vigorous refrigerative treatment must have sometimes produced most undesirable results, and it is these excesses in the use of an efficient and valuable remedy which are doubtless to a great degree responsible for the slowness with which the merit of water drinking as a systematic procedure has acquired recognition and appreciation.

Sir John Chardin, a French traveler in Persia, relates how that in May, 1674, he was treated by a native Persian physician for a very grave intermittent or "fever of Bender." One of the most important measures to which he was subjected was the drinking of large quantities of water cooled with snow.

Currie also recommended water drinking in the treatment of fever, as follows: "While the different modes of applying water to the surface are employed, it ought also to be poured into the stomach in large quantities when the patient's heat will permit it, and the presence of nausea and vomiting are no objection to this practice."

The importance of water to the vital economy must be recognized when we remember that the living organisms which compose the human body, as well as those of all other animals, are submerged in water.

Bernard, the great French physiologist, sagaciously remarked concerning the aquatic life of man, "Life exists only in a liquid medium. It is only by certain artifices of construction that the organisms of man as those of other animals, can live in the air; but all the active cells upon which their functions depend, live, without exception, like the infusoria, in an interior liquid medium." *

---

* "Études Physiologiques sur Quelques Poisons Américains." Cl. Bernard, Paris, 1864.

Water drinking is an internal bath; it dilutes the fluids of the body in which the cells and fibers are bathed; it purifies the body by diluting the medium in which it lives. By the free use of water the movement of the mass of liquid in which the living elements of the human body perform their work is quickened, and the stream of life runs clear and pure. It has been shown that water is absorbed from the stomach very slowly. This takes place chiefly in the intestine. Absorption is stimulated, however, by the presence of CO_2. Distilled water charged with CO_2 is the best of all drinks as a beverage for use in connection with hydrotherapy. It is soothing to the stomach, and is rapidly absorbed; hence more readily quenches thirst. The presence of mineral salts of any kind lessens the rate of absorption.

1424 Schultz has shown that copious water drinking increases the proportion of water in the blood nearly six percent; but Böcker has shown that this increase lasts only a short time, not more than fifteen to twenty minutes. Half an hour later the blood is thicker than before, and contains a smaller proportion of water than when water has been wholly withheld for twenty-four hours. Another effect upon the blood noted by Böcker was that blood clots formed after copious water drinking contain a smaller number of damaged corpuscles, which indicate their incapacity to absorb oxygen by not turning red when exposed to the air,—an evidence of the great value of water drinking as a means of improving the quality of the blood through bettering its constituents as well as by elimination of waste matters through assisting their solution.

To the great thinning of the blood which follows copious water drinking is due the remarkably increased activity of the kidneys, skin, and bowels which it produces. Examination of the urine shows not only that the quantity is increased by water drinking, but that the urea and other solid constituents are also increased. Fleming,* in experiments for the purpose of determining the physiological effects of the Turkish

* "Physiology of the Turkish Bath," Glasgow.

bath, showed that the perspiration produced in profuse sweating after copious water drinking contains a larger per cent of the chloride of sodium than does the urine. An increase in the amount of urea and other nitrogenous principles (1.55 per cent) was also noted.

Baron Liebig showed long ago (and his observations have been many times confirmed) that water drinking powerfully influences metabolism, increasing both assimilation and disintegration, but especially the former.

Water is the medium by which nutritive material is conveyed to the tissues and waste matters conveyed out of the body. Thus it is evident that by increasing the amount of water introduced into the body, the movement of the vital fluids, the blood and lymph, may be accelerated almost at will. By the increase in the volume of blood, the blood pressure is raised, the heart movements become more energetic, and the functions of the glands and other forms of activity are increased. This is true of the secreting glands as well as of the kidneys and other excreting glandular organs. Increased movement of blood through the lungs secures greater absorption of oxygen by which the various metabolic and catabolic processes are facilitated; retrograde metamorphosis is more completely accomplished; uric acid, urates, oxalates, and other products of imperfect oxidation are diminished or made to disappear entirely; in short, the patient lives a more highly vitalized and functionally active life.

Therapeutic Applications.—The effect upon the blood of 1425
copious water drinking suggests it as a valuable measure in cases of ***dropsy***, whether general or local in character, especially the latter. The increase in the specific gravity of the blood due to the rapid withdrawal of water by the kidneys and the skin, even to the extent of impoverishing the blood, prepares the way for the absorption of the dropsical fluid; and by a repetition of this measure from day to day most remarkable therapeutic results may sometimes be obtained. Distilled water charged with carbonic acid gas should be em-

ployed, without the addition of sugar or any substance, unless it be fruit-juices of some sort. The dose should be from one to two pints, and should be taken preferably before breakfast or an hour or so before dinner. The author well remembers a case with which he became acquainted while in Bellevue Hospital nearly twenty-five years ago, under the late Dr. Austin Flint. A patient under treatment for general dropsy from organic disease of the heart, which had proved so refractory to all measures which had been employed, including diuretics of all sorts, was finally given up as a hopeless one, and the patient was permitted to drink copiously of water, which had previously been denied or allowed only in very stinted quantities. She drank in the course of the day two or three quarts of water. As a result, profuse diuresis occurred, the dropsy disappeared, and the patient made, for the time being at least, a very good recovery, and was soon able to leave the hospital.

Profiting by this experience, the author has made use of this measure in many cases of dropsy with most-gratifying results, and has never found it necessary to require dropsical patients to refrain from drinking water freely. It should be taken *in large quantity and rapidly*. When practiced for the purpose of carrying off the dropsical effusion, the water drinking should be confined to two periods daily, morning and evening, no fluid whatever being taken between these hours.

When it is desired to increase the volume of the blood and to introduce permanently a larger proportion of water, the water drinking should be managed in quite a different manner. A small quantity should be taken at frequent intervals, and the amount in the course of a day may sum up to several pints; but the quantity taken at any one time should not exceed four to six ounces. This quantity may be taken every hour or hour and a half with advantage.

When the amount of water supplied to the body is insufficient, the condition of the body becomes in some degree comparable to that of a stagnant pool; while an abundant supply of liquid so encourages its activities that it may not inaptly be compared to the flowing mountain stream.

Cold Water Drinking.—Priessnitz required his patients to 1426
drink large quantities of water, many patients taking as high as twenty to forty glasses a day. It is curious to note that at the time when this empiric was requiring his patients to swallow such prodigious quantities of water, he had a rival, an old schoolmate, by the name of Schrott, living in a little village four miles from Graefenberg, who required his patients to abstain wholly from water for five to eight days at a time.

Water is not a mere mechanical conveyor of poisons out and of foods in; it is a powerful vital stimulant, a divinely appointed agent which the *vis medicatrix naturæ* can use in her healing work. Dietl, the famous pupil of a world-renowned master, Rokitansky, writing so long ago as 1845, uttered the following wise and philosophical words, which every physician who undertakes to rely upon the virtues of water and other physiological agents in dealing with human maladies should accept as a confession of faith:—

"Nature alone can cure; this is the highest law of practical medicine, and the one to which we must adhere. . . . Nature creates and maintains; she must therefore be able to cure."

The deluging practice of Priessnitz is still recommended by the German water-cure empirics and by some scientific hydrotherapists, but cases are certainly very rare in which such quantities of cold water can be swallowed with advantage. As a measure of treatment, water drinking may be practiced to the extent of six or eight or even ten glasses a day with advantage, when required, but not infrequently three or four glasses are sufficient, and there are cases in which it is more important to interdict the use of liquids by the stomach than to commend their use. In such cases water may be introduced by the enema in small quantity, to be retained.

Cold water drinking is especially indicated in all the

cachexias and diatheses. In rheumatism it is useful as a means of diluting the blood so that it can dissolve and carry out of the body a larger amount of uric acid and allied substances; and as a means for encouraging activity of the skin and kidneys, it is always useful in this disease.

In *obesity*, water drinking is essential as a means of dissolving and carrying out of the body the large amount of broken-down material which results from the increase in tissue destruction set up by exercise, hot and cold baths, and other means employed to reduce weight. To forbid the free use of water in obesity is a grave error.

In *diabetes* the free use of water is not injurious, but advantageous. The blood contains an excess of sugar. All the sugar that is not oxidized must be removed from the body by the kidneys and skin, chiefly by the former. The specific gravity of the urine in these cases is always high, indicating a similarly high specific gravity of the blood. It is evident, then, that water is needed in cases of this sort for the purpose of maintaining a proper degree of fluidity of the blood and for facilitating the removal of the unused sugar, the presence of which interferes more or less seriously with the various vital functions. While the free use of water in diabetes will of course have the effect to increase the quantity of urine daily discharged, the amount of sugar, which is a matter of most serious importance in this disease, is not increased. Indeed, the amount of sugar has appeared to be somewhat decreased, doubtless as the result of the increased oxidation which takes place within the body under the influence of free water drinking.

In *fevers* water drinking is essential as a means of aiding the kidneys and the skin in the elimination of the toxins to which the rise of temperature is due, in aiding the liver in its work of destroying the fever poisons, oxidizing leucomains, and promoting the reduction of temperature by securing an increased evaporation from the skin.

Winternitz and numerous other observers have shown that

when water is taken in sufficient quantities, the temperature of the body may be lowered by the absorption of heat from the water. Suppose, for example, a patient having a temperature of 102° should swallow three pints of water at 60°. In acquiring the temperature of the body the water swallowed will absorb 126 heat units. In the case of a patient weighing 120 pounds this would induce a fall of temperature of more than 1°, provided, of course, that the heat production and heat elimination continued at a uniform rate.

A general fall in the temperature of the body of .4° C., sometimes more, was observed after drinking water at a temperature of 60° to 65°. Water taken at a lower temperature and in larger quantity has been shown by Winternitz to be capable of reducing the pulse twenty beats and the temperature .8° C. (1.4° F.). The temperature of the urine was found to be .7° C. (1.3° F.) below the normal.

Winternitz, by means of a thermometer introduced into the stomach itself, made interesting observations upon the effect of water drinking upon the local temperature. A half hour after drinking a pint of cold water the temperature of the stomach was found to be .6° C. (1.08° F.) below its normal temperature. The rectal temperature was found to be still lower, sinking gradually from the time the water was taken for nearly half an hour, when the maximum reduction of more than 1° C. (1.8° F.) was found. The axillary temperature at first rose slightly, then fell, the temperature remaining below normal for more than an hour. The pulse was decreased ten beats. This curious fact was noted,—that the temperature reduction was greater in the rectum than in the stomach. On reversing the experiment and introducing the water into the rectum, it was found that the temperature in the stomach was reduced more than was that of the rectum, falling to .9° below the normal.

A decided fall of the surface temperature at the epigastrium may be observed after cold water drinking, as well as general reduction of temperature, indicated by thermometers placed in the axilla and rectum (Exp. 73). This fact was first observed by my assistants, Drs. Otis and Edwards, while conducting a series of observations (1898) to determine the effect on temperature reduction of water taken at different temperatures.

In cases of *chronic inactivity* of the *skin*, cold water drinking is an exceedingly valuable measure, but it must be employed with discretion, as inactivity of the skin usually means an inactive mucous membrane, so that liquids are absorbed with difficulty. In cases of chronic dilatation of the stomach, water drinking, while indicated as a means of relieving the general condition, may be inadmissible on account of the state of the stomach. In these cases water may be introduced by enema.

Copious water drinking is one of the most effective means of relieving a common cold, by aiding in the elimination of tissue poisons, the accumulation of which gives rise to the difficulty known as "a cold."

One or two glasses of cold water taken half an hour or an hour before breakfast prove in many cases an almost perfect panacea for *chronic inactivity* of the *bowels*. Hundreds of patients have been cured by the use of this simple remedy alone. At a meeting of the New York Academy of Medicine attended by the author more than twenty years ago, a leading physician of New York City stated that he had successfully treated more than one hundred cases of constipation by this simple means.

Chronic biliousness, which is nothing more or less than *chronic toxemia* resulting from the putrefaction of animal food substances in the alimentary canal, requires the free use of water. Eight or ten glasses a day would be none too much in cases of this sort.

In cases of *gall-stones* and *infectious jaundice*, water drinking is certainly indicated. The amount taken should be ten or twelve glasses a day, if possible, so that the liver will be thoroughly flushed and the bile so diluted that it will be able to dissolve and remove any concretions which may be present. In *cirrhosis* of the *liver* arising from either indigestion or alcohol, water drinking is essential as a means of aiding the liver and the kidneys to perform the work required of them in the removal of a large quantity of alimentary poisons in addition to the toxins naturally produced within the body by the physiological processes of tissue change.

In the treatment of the opium, alcohol, tobacco, and other drug habits, water drinking renders important service by hastening the elimination of the drug and in aiding liver work and general oxidation.

The *temperature* of the water drunk should ordinarily be about 70° F. In special cases water at 60° and even 50° may be employed. Very cold water is indicated only in fevers, in constipation, and in small quantities in hypopepsia.

The *quantity of water* taken must depend on the effect 1427
desired. In fevers, a good rule is to take a glass of water every hour. In hypopepsia, one third or one half a glassful of cold water may be taken half an hour before eating. For inactivity of the bowels, one or two glasses of cold water should be taken on retiring at night, and as much more on arising in the morning. A thirst for water is almost always an indication that it may be taken with advantage, no matter whether such use is in harmony with the established canons of hygiene or not. It is safer to trust to the natural instincts than to pin one's faith to a theory. Almost the only decided contraindication is in connection with meals when free water drinking prevents proper insalivation of the food.

The Best Water.—The purest water is universally the 1428
best. Whatever beneficial effects are obtained from water drinking must be attributed to the water itself, and not to any ingredients which it contains. Mineral waters are simply diluted drugs. The ingredients may be obtained at any drug-store, and if diluted to the same extent as that in which they are found in the so-called natural waters, the effects obtained from their use would be the same. Medical experience has

shown that the best of the so-called mineral waters are those which contain the least mineral ingredients. The very best water is distilled water which has been well aërated. Water obtained from natural sources is generally more or less contaminated, that from lakes, streams, and rivers being necessarily defiled by the fish and other creatures which live in natural bodies of water, and by surface drainage, which, after every rain, washes out quantities of filth.

Water obtained from public supplies should always be boiled; indeed, this precaution is a wise one under nearly all circumstances.

Hard water should always be boiled for a long time to eliminate, so far as possible, the lime which it contains; but even when boiled it is by no means free from this injurious ingredient. The larger the amount of saline ingredients, the more slowly the water is absorbed. The presence of acids encourages absorption. Carbonated distilled water and diluted fruit juices without sugar are the best drinks.

HOT WATER DRINKING.

1429 Hot water drinking has of late years been enormously overdone. In the United States, and doubtless in other countries, many persons have been injured by deluging their stomachs with quantities of hot water several times daily. The author has met a number of patients who were taking three or four glasses at once in this way at a temperature which would seem positively incredible. In one instance a gentleman was found sipping a glass of water at a temperature of 160°. The free use of hot water has been largely encouraged by physicians who recommend an exclusive meat dietary, experience having taught them that the free use of meat must be accompanied by copious water drinking as a means of ridding the system of the ptomains, toxins, and various other poisonous substances which are always to be found in the body of a dead animal. Water drinking in these cases is doubtless a means of saving the patient's life

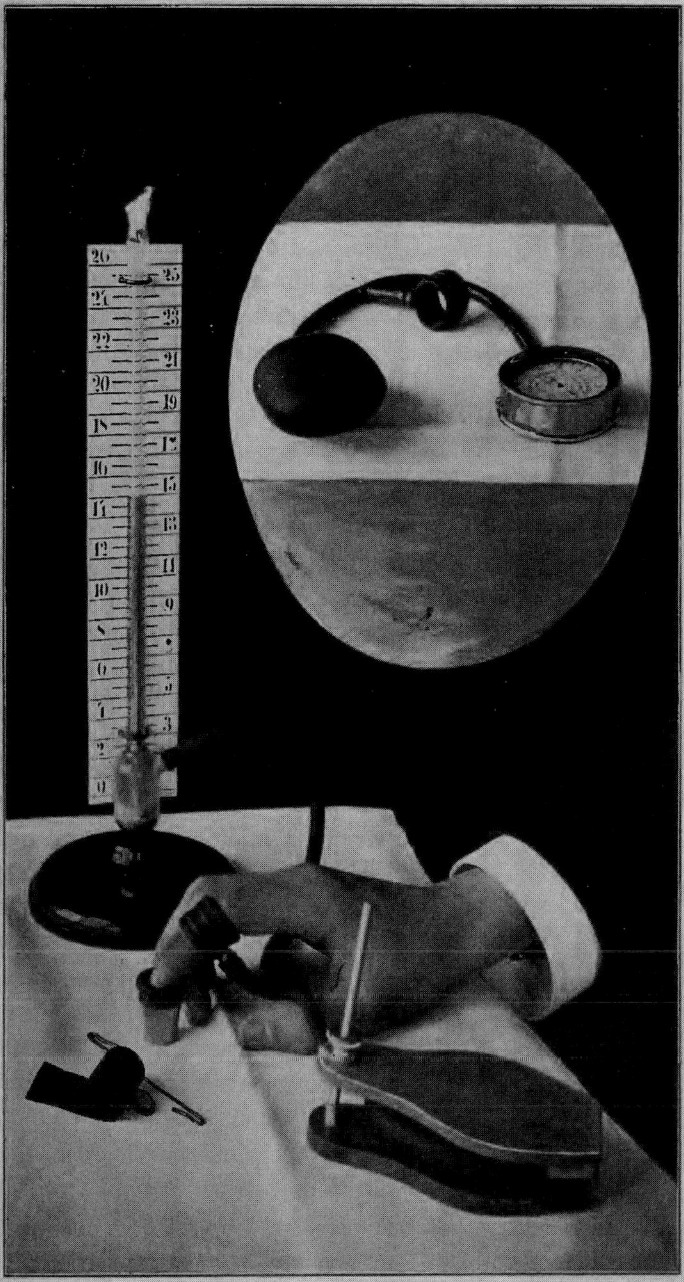

FIG. 240. GÆRTNER'S TONOMETER.

FIG. 239 GÆRTNER'S TONOMETER (p. 931).

under conditions which would otherwise lead to speedy exhaustion of the defenses of the body, and thus precipitate some acute and perhaps fatal malady, as Bright's disease, organic changes in the liver, arteriosclerosis, etc.

The fact that hot water has proved serviceable in some cases has led to its excessive use by a large number of persons who have suffered serious consequences from the practice. The general effect of hot water drinking is to debilitate the digestive system, while cold water acts as a tonic. Heat and cold, when brought in contact with the mucous membranes, produce effects entirely analogous to those resulting from their application to the skin. When heat is applied, the result is first a stimulation, quickly followed by a tonic reaction lasting for a considerable length of time. In this condition the blood-vessels of the stomach are contracted, the circulation is less active, and the activity of the peptic glands, if not entirely suspended, is greatly diminished, so that the quantity of hydrochloric acid produced is smaller than under ordinary conditions. When cold is applied, the opposite effect is produced. The blood-vessels are first contracted, but later, tonic reaction occurs, the movement of blood in the vessels is accelerated, the glands become more active, and the functions of the stomach are quickened.

From these facts it is apparent that hot water drinking is a measure likely to prove of great service in *hyperpepsia*, and likewise in gastrorrhea, as in these conditions there is an excessive production of hydrochloric acid. In order to be beneficial in cases of this sort, the water swallowed must be very hot, the temperature being 130° to 140°; and should be swallowed rapidly, so that it may be cooled as little as possible before coming in contact with the stomach.

The tonometer of Gærtner, an instrument by means of which the level pressure may be quickly and exactly determined, may be advantageously employed in connection with water-drinking. The two forms of this instrument are shown in Figs. 239 and 240.

Hot water drinking is very useful in *gastralgia*, especially when accompanied by vomiting. Slowly sipping hot water will sometimes relieve vomiting not only in gastralgia, but in other conditions. Hot water drinking also affords relief in the colic pains frequently the result of the habitual use of milk from a neglected nursing-bottle or some similar cause. It is an invaluable remedy in chronic gastritis, or gastric catarrh.

In cases of *hypopepsia* and *apepsia*, a few ounces of cold water should be rapidly swallowed half or three quarters of an hour before the meal, the purpose being to produce a vigorous reaction in the mucous membrane of the stomach. The result is an improved appetite and increased digestive power.

1430 *When Free Water Drinking Should Be Avoided.*—In *extreme dilatation* of the *stomach*, water drinking must be avoided for the reason that a dilated stomach does not readily absorb, and from lack of muscular tone it can not readily relieve itself of its contents by transferring the water to the small intestine. Very little absorption takes place in the stomach, the intestine being the great absorbent organ of the body. Thus when water is swallowed freely in cases of this sort, the stomach is simply filled up, and the thirst is not relieved until the stomach is completely filled, so that it runs over into the small intestine.

The effect of this overburdening of the stomach with liquids which are not readily disposed of, is to increase the dilatation or prolapsus of the already disabled organ.

In colic, cold water drinking should be entirely avoided, though hot water often affords relief if taken in ample quantity. At the same time that the hot water is taken into the stomach, the hot enema should be employed.

Dr. Lawson Tait laid down a law that liquids of all sorts should be avoided for two days after an *abdominal section.* His idea was that by withholding liquids in this way, the intestine would be compelled to absorb the stagnant fluids from the abdominal cavity. This method is quite a hardship to patients who are subjected to it, many suffering more from thirst than from the pain of the operation. It is certain, however, that as Mr. Tait has pointed out, patients do better under this regimen. The withholding of fluid from the stomach is certainly a useful means of combating the nausea and vomiting which so commonly follow operations of this kind, and the author is inclined to think that this latter is the most important advantage obtained by withholding fluids in cases of this sort. No harm has seemed to result from the use of the tepid enema as a means of affording the necessary amount of liquid.

Drinking very freely of cold water must be strictly avoided when a person is both fatigued and sweating profusely. It is generally better not to drink freely of cold water when perspiring freely, even though one may not be seriously fatigued; as when the body is actively perspiring, the elimination of heat is very great, several times the normal amount, and the additional loss of heat occasioned by the cold water is sometimes sufficient to produce a chill, with internal congestion and serious results. If very cold water be taken when a person is perspiring freely, it should be in very small amount, and should be very slowly sipped.

Feeble patients should avoid the free drinking of cold water except when walking, when just setting out for a vigorous walk in the open air, or when about to engage in some other exercise. Water drinking is also entirely safe just before and during a hot bath. Avoiding the free use of water at meals is a very important hygienic rule. The cold water interferes with the digestion of starch, delays peptic digestion, and is the cause of many other mischiefs.

ELECTRICITY AS A COMPLEMENT TO HYDROTHERAPY IN THE TREATMENT OF CHRONIC DISEASE.

1431 The efforts of some enthusiasts to find in electricity a panacea for all human ailments, and the subsequent failure of this agent to accomplish in the hands of others all that was claimed for it, has been a fruitful cause of prejudice against its use as a substitute for the empirical, irrational, and artificial methods which have come down to us as a legacy from the infantile days of our beneficent art, or which were engrafted upon it during the ages when all the arts and sciences were stifled by the universal prevalence of superstition and intellectual darkness,— methods which still cling to us like the barnacles upon the bottom of an ocean steamer, and hinder our advancement toward the goal of all scientific progress in medicine; viz., the attainment of a system of dealing with the sick in which every measure employed and every application shall have for its basis a thoroughly rational and physiological foundation. No medical practice can properly claim to be strictly rational which is not at the same time physiological. Those measures which accomplish so-called therapeutic results by means of toxic effects are pathological rather than physiological agents; and with the onward march of laboratory research, clinical observation, and physiological and pathological knowledge, they must in time be wholly eliminated from our therapeutic armamentarium.

The author has for more than twenty-five years given special and earnest study to the practical application of physiological agents of all sorts in the treatment of disease. Water, gymnastics, massage, manual and mechanical exercise, heat, sunlight, diet, and other agents, as well as electricity in its various forms, have all been carefully studied and utilized in the treatment of the various forms of acute and chronic disorders. Relying upon none of the agents as a cure-all, the effort has been made so to combine them all as to secure for each the greatest possible efficiency, utilizing each one for those things to which it is best adapted, and applying two or more in succession or simultaneously in such a way as to enable the effects of each one to supplement or complement the effects of each other one. Special attention has been given to the utilization of water and electricity, for the reason that these two agents have been the object of more exact scientific study and research than any others employed in physiological therapeutics.

The chronic invalid rarely has a fair chance unless he can have brought to bear upon his case simultaneously all the various physiological agents which are indicated. To undertake to cure a chronic dyspeptic by diet alone, by water alone, or by electricity or exercise alone, or by any other single agent, is very much like trying to raise a great building with one jack-screw. All the lifting agencies possible must be set at work to get these chronic sufferers out of their pathological ruts.

It requires but a very superficial study of the subject to show the remarkable similarity between the methods of hydrotherapy and electricity in effecting results. The most important results of each are attained through their influence upon the nervous system, as the therapeutic effects of both agents are based upon their physiological effects.

The researches of Schüller, Vinaj, Winternitz, and others have shown that prolonged moderately cold applications to the surface produce prolonged contraction and decongestion of internal vascular areas reflexly connected with the cutaneous area acted upon. Local cold applications in this respect differ from general cold applications, which cause dilatation of the visceral and cerebral vessels through contraction of the surface vessels.

Warm applications, that is, a temperature of 92° to 98°, on the other hand, cause immediate contraction of the vessels of the interior of the body, corresponding with dilatation of the cutaneous vessels.

Every portion of the cutaneous surface is reflexly associated with some internal vascular area, the conditions of which may be controlled by the application to the associated cutaneous area of thermic or other agents capable of producing vascular changes; for example, any agent which causes contraction of the cutaneous vessels will cause a corresponding action of the associated visceral vascular area, this being also true respecting vasodilatation.

From clinical observations and from the study of practical electrotherapy in connection with hydriatry or rational hydrotherapy, the author is fully convinced that many of the effects of percutaneous applications of electricity are produced by the same means through which most hydriatic effects are obtained; viz., through nervous impressions propagated from the skin to the spinal cord through the sensory nerves, and sent out from the spine as motor influences, then carried outward by the non-medullated vasoconstricting fibers of the sympathetic and the medullated inhibitory fibers which pass directly from the vasomotor centers of the cord to their distribution in the vessels. In other words, the condition of anelectrotonus and catelectrotonus, as the case may be, established in the cutaneous vessels, is propagated through a reflex arc to the associated internal vascular area. It seems to the author that this view alone affords a rational explanation of the influence of percutaneous applications of galvanism upon the internal organs.

1432 A galvanic current of twenty to forty milliamperes applied, the anode electrode over the hypogastric region, the cathode over the lumbar region, produces decided effects in relieving uterine and ovarian congestion. Yet the location of these organs is such as to bring them practically at the neutral point between the two poles, and hence outside the sphere of influence of either the cathode or the anode. It is true that by increasing the strength of the current, the neutral point may be moved nearer to the cathode; while decreasing the current moves the neutral point nearer the anode, thus bringing in either case a larger area under the influence of the opposite pole. Knowing this fact, and taking advantage of it, we may bring under the influence of either pole desired, structures not too far removed from the surface; but in the case of organs located approximately in the center of the body or far beneath the surface, as the uterus, the ovaries, the abdominal viscera in general, and the spinal cord, it is evident that we are powerless to produce in them an electrotonic condition of any considerable degree of intensity.

In the case of the pelvic organs, and likewise with the **1433**
stomach, we are able to produce either anelectrotonus or catelectrotonus, as we may desire, by means of suitable electrodes; but in the case of the spinal cord, the sympathetic ganglia, and most of the abdominal viscera, and indeed, nearly all the deep-seated structures of the body, we are unable to produce electrotonic states, for the reason that the action of electrical currents, when applied to the body, is practically confined to the immediate vicinity of the electrodes. As the current leaves the electrodes, it spreads out, utilizing the whole body as a conductor instead of passing from one electrode to the other, as might be supposed by one not familiar with the laws of electrophysics.

These and other considerations show us that in explaining the effects of percutaneous applications of electricity we must keep in mind the interesting anatomical and physiological relationships which form the basis of a large share of the applications of water in rational hydrotherapy.

The researches of Brown-Sequard, Charcot, Winternitz, **1434**
Beni-Barde, Fleury, and other hydriatrists, have established a distinct reflex relationship between the principal internal organs and particular cutaneous areas, as elsewhere designated (**372–382**).

In general, the skin overlying an internal organ is reflexly associated with it. This is the reason why percutaneous applications of electricity made over an organ usually affect it, and not altogether because the electrical current is passed through the organ.

1435 For nearly twenty years, the author has made use of this principle in the application of electricity, especially in the treatment of genito-urinary diseases, and has seen excellent results from the application. For example, in applications intended to influence the genital glands and associated organs,—the uterus, ovaries, and tubes in women, and the testicles and prostate in men,—it has been found distinctly advantageous to make applications to the inner surface of the thighs and perineum, as well as to the epigastric and lumbar regions. The anatomical relations of the nerve supply of these regions suggested the method before the reflex relationships between cutaneous and visceral vascular areas was so thoroughly understood as at present. The author has also for many years utilized anodic applications of the galvanic current to the face as a means of relieving coryza, and has often seen a patient relieved of headache, presumably congestive in character, by applications of the galvanic current to the abdominal and cervical sympathetic.

It requires but a cursory review of the physiological effects of water and electricity to note the remarkable parallelism between the effects of hydriatic applications and those of electricity. With equal readiness it may be seen how, by simultaneous or successive use of electricity and water, if applied with scientific precision, these two potent agents may render mutual aid in a great variety of conditions.

1436 Special note may be made of the following points:—

Water moistens the skin, and thus increases electrical conductivity.

Hot applications cause immediate dilatation of the blood-vessels, increasing the vascularity of the skin, and thus also increasing its electrical conductivity; while cold water causes first a contraction of the small vessels, lessening the blood supply of the skin, and diminishing its conductivity for both heat and electricity. In the reaction which follows, however, the amount of blood in the skin is greatly increased, thereby lessening its resistance.

Both very cold and very hot applications to the skin diminish the sensibility of the nerves, and thereby lessen their susceptibility to electrical effects. Anemia of the skin, on the other hand, increases sensibility, while saturation of the skin with moisture diminishes irritability and nerve sensibility. Steiner has shown that temperatures below 59° and above 77° lessen the velocity with which nerve impulses are conducted, while Hermann has shown that the application of cold diminishes notably the phenomena of electrotonus.

Heat, being relaxing, produces effects analogous to the cathode; while cold, produces contraction or anodal effects.

Neutral applications are likewise sedative, thus resembling the anode in their effects. Short cold applications, because of the reactionary excitation produced, give rise to effects resembling the cathodic influence of the galvanic current or the excitation of the faradic; while the atonic reaction which follows prolonged hot application results in sedative effects similar to those of the anode.

Granting the truth of those statements respecting the mode of action of percutaneous applications of electricity upon the visceral circulation, it needs no lengthy argument to show the great advantage of combining electrical and hydriatic applications in a great variety of morbid conditions.

According to the author's personal experience, two general 1437
rules may be established for applications of this sort: *First*, increased movement of blood and accelerated functional activity of an internal organ may be induced by short, vigorous, cold applications in combination with cathodic applications of galvanism. The electrical application may be either simultaneous or may immediately follow the cold application. Bipolar, faradic, or sinusoidal currents may also be applied

with advantage, but the effect is less distinct than that of the galvanic current. The electrical application should, in general, be as strong as the patient can bear without pain.

Secondly, congestion and undue functional activity of an internal organ may be diminished by a prolonged, moderately cold application (60° to 70° continuing from thirty minutes to several hours), combined with the simultaneous anodic application of the galvanic current of moderate strength.

By the application of these principles, results which appear really marvelous to one not familiar with applications of this sort, may be obtained in cases of congestion of the brain, lungs, liver, uterus, ovaries, likewise in atonic conditions of the stomach and bowels, and in amenorrhea and hypopepsia.

1438 In applications for the relief of pain, in which electricity so often renders most valuable service, the association of heat with the electrical application is an exceedingly valuable measure. When the pain is neuralgic in character, the strong application of the sinusoidal or faradic current, combined with a fomentation at a temperature high enough to produce slight pain when first applied, continued for 15 or 20 minutes, gives very positive and gratifying results. The current should be as strong as the patient will bear. When the pain is due to congestion or inflammation, an anodic application of the galvanic current should be employed instead of an induction current. The application should be prolonged, and not so strong as to produce decided sensation.

1439 Anodal galvanic applications may likewise be associated with cold as an analgesic measure. In cases of cardiac insufficiency in which the application of electricity may be thought to be a necessary or useful measure, advantage may be gained by the application, two or three times daily, of a cold compress for 40 to 60 minutes, over the anterior surface of the chest. Slowing of the pulse and an increase in arterial tension, as indicated by a sphygmographic tracing, indicate at once the therapeutic power of this simple application.

In cases of atony of the bladder, and inactivity of the 1440
bowels due to dilatation of the colon, the cold douche to the feet and over the lumbar, umbilical, and hypogastric regions, in combination with faradic and sinusoidal applications to the rectum and abdominal walls, achieve prompt success in many most obstinate cases which have failed to yield to other measures. Cold douches applied to the parts named may also be used to advantage in combination with the galvanic current applied percutaneously to the abdominal and lumbar surfaces. The strength of the current should be 60 to 80 milliamperes.

In cases of apepsia and hypopepsia, in which hydrochloric 1441
acid is absent or greatly deficient in quantity, most excellent results may be obtained by the application of the cathodic galvanic or the sinusoidal current applied to the epigastrium in combination with the ice-bag, for half an hour before each meal. Painful congestion is relieved by very hot fomentations half an hour after a meal in combination with a faradic or sinusoidal current of moderate strength.

Very short, very hot applications over the liver (130° to 1442
140°, for 5 to 8 min.), combined with a prolonged anodic galvanic application, act powerfully in relieving hepatic congestion.

Very hot fomentations over the lumbar regions, combined 1443
with an anodic galvanic application to the same parts and to the lower third of the sternum, are indicated in renal congestion.

The hemostatic effects obtainable by hydriatric applica- 1444
tions in connection with the galvanic current have been proved of invaluable service in hemorrhage due to ovarian congestion, intra-uterine vegetations, and intra-uterine and submucous and interstitial fibroids of the uterus. In cases in which persistent hemorrhage follows the employment of electrolysis, the cold pelvic pack and the hot vaginal douche in many cases render continuation of the treatment possible when otherwise its interruption would be necessary.

1445 In amenorrhea, the effects of cathodic, faradic, or sinusoidal applications to the uterus are greatly increased by short cold applications to the lumbar regions, the inner surface of the thighs, and the feet.

1446 In applications of electricity to paralyzed and paretic muscles, the effects of the electrical application may be greatly increased by the previous application of cold water in the form of the ordinary cold douche, the percussion douche, the Scotch douche or cold friction, or the heating compress. The marked increase of muscular irritability produced by hydriatric applications of this sort increases the susceptibility of the muscle to the influence of the electrical current, whether the galvanic, faradic, or sinusoidal current be employed.

1447 For relief of pain in neuralgic joints, hot applications followed by the sinusoidal or galvanic current, are a most useful measure in cases in which joints are not painful nor stiffened or thickened by inflammatory products. The alternate hot and cold douche and other exciting hydriatric measures may with much advantage be employed in connection with cataphoresis. The author has found this combination exceedingly useful in treating many cases of this sort.

1448 In chronic congestion of the pelvic and abdominal viscera, the good effects obtained from local electrical applications, either internal or percutaneous, may be continued and intensified by the use of the heating compress, consisting of a towel wrung dry out of very cold water, placed over the parts and covered with several thicknesses of flannel sufficient to maintain the heat produced by reaction, but not an excessive accumulation.

1449 Faradic, sinusoidal, and cathodic galvanic applications may be employed in connection with the revulsive douche and other revulsive applications in all cases in which pain is not a marked feature, but in which the purpose is to produce strong circulatory reaction. When pain is present, the faradic or sinusoidal current should not be employed; the galvanic current should be used instead of the cathode.

The form of revulsive applications referred to consists of a prolonged hot application followed by an exceedingly short cold application. The respective times of the applications may be hot, 5 to 15 minutes, cold, 15 to 30 seconds, if compresses are employed; or 3 to 5 minutes for the hot douche, followed by a cold douche of 4 to 10 seconds.

For general hypnotic effects, applicable to nearly all cases 1450
of insomnia, a neutral bath — that is, a bath at a temperature of 92° to 96° for 30 to 40 minutes, or a douche with little pressure at the same temperature, with a duration of 1 to 5 minutes — succeeds in securing sound sleep without the use of hypnotic drugs of any sort, especially when combined with the static insulation and breeze to the head and spine, or a galvanic application to the inferior cervical sympathetic and solar plexus, the anode being placed at the neck.

The neutral full bath, combined with the galvanic, faradic, 1451
or sinusoidal current, is perhaps the most powerful of all hypnotic measures. The author has employed this bath with success for nearly twenty-five years; and it has rendered valuable service not only in relieving insomnia, but in helping patients through the trying time which immediately follows the withdrawal of opium, cocaine, and other drugs, in the treatment of various forms of drug addiction.

The faradic, sinusoidal, static, and high frequency currents 1452
are all tonic in character, stimulating metabolism, arousing the nerve centers; and directly exciting the brain and all portions of the central nervous system. Short applications of cold water, especially when accompanied by strong me-mechanical effects, as in the cold douche, constitute the most powerful of all known tonics. By combination of the cold douche with the faradic and sinusoidal electrical currents, the tonic effects of each measure are intensified. The electrical application should be made soon after the douche, when reaction is well established, the nerve and muscle tone elevated, and the nervous reflexes in full swing.

1453 The refrigerant effects of the cold bath may be greatly increased by the simultaneous application of a slowly alternating sinusoidal current in such a manner as to secure vigorous contraction of the large muscular masses. Three sets of electrodes should be employed: one for the arms, another for the legs, and another for the back and the abdomen. The contractions should be at the rate of four to six per minute. The temperature should be 78° to 75°. The duration of the bath should be 10 to 15 minutes. The patient should be rubbed during the bath so as to maintain an active cutaneous circulation.

1454 The analgesic effects of water may be most advantageously employed in connection with the electrolytic treatment of uterine fibroids for the relief of the pelvic pains which are not infrequently awakened when currents of large quantity are employed. It has always been the author's custom to administer a very hot vaginal douche just before and just after the electrical treatment. A very hot sitz, 115° to 120°, for 3 to 5 minutes, followed immediately by a dash of cold water over the hips, prevents pain and hemorrhage.

1455 In applications for the relief of headache due to cerebral congestion, in which the cold applications do not produce favorable results, applications of galvanism may be made to the head in the usual manner in connection with very hot applications to the cervical region. Excellent and almost immediate results may thus be frequently obtained in cases which are rebellious to other measures.

1456 Dana, in his masterly work, "The Clinical Study of Neuralgias," fixes the location of a considerable number of areas which are the seat of transferred pain in neuralgias, and which have by clinical observation been definitely associated with internal pathological conditions.

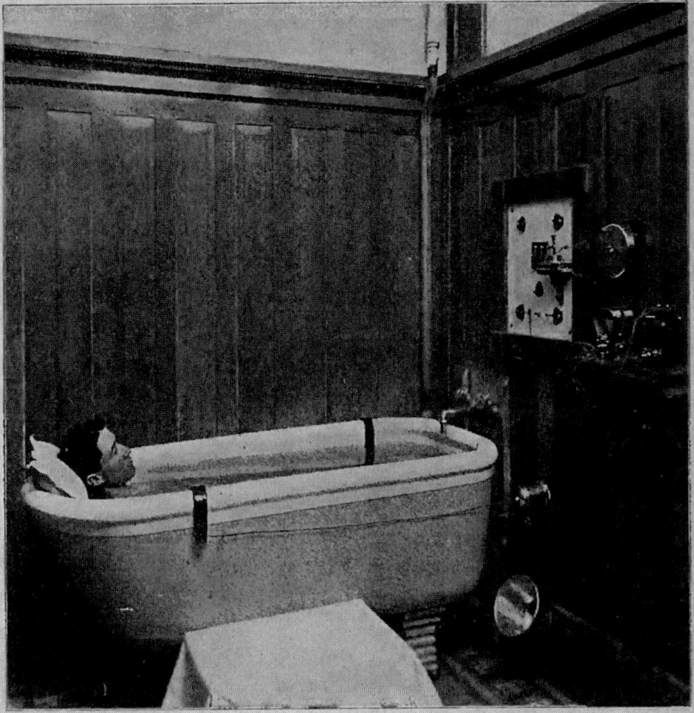

FIG. 241. ELECTROHYDRIC BATH (p. 946).

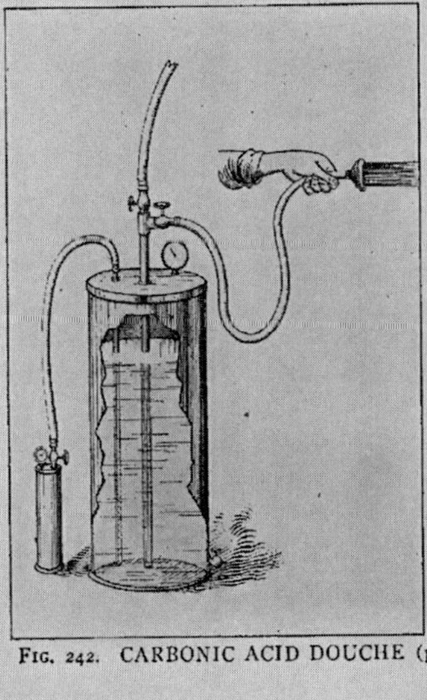

FIG. 242. CARBONIC ACID DOUCHE (p. 937).

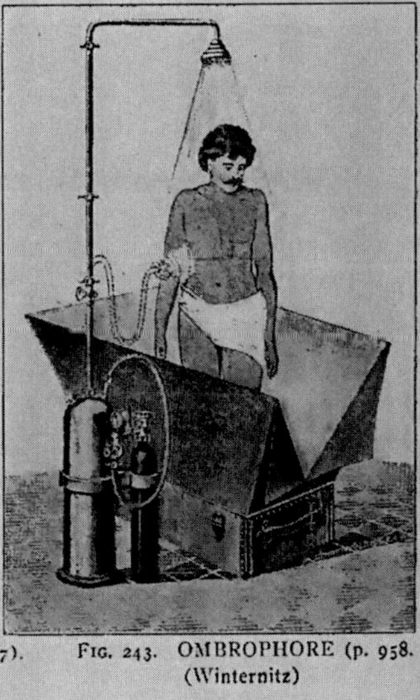

FIG. 243. OMBROPHORE (p. 958.)
(Winternitz)

By the combined application of fomentations, revulsive compresses, or other analgesic hydriatic procedures with the sinusoidal, faradic, or static electrical currents, most excellent results may be obtained, such as could not be looked for by other means than by the combination of water and electricity,— the two most powerful known agencies in influencing the nervous system. These several areas as located by Dana may be enumerated as follows:—

1. Vertex (anemia, endometritis, bladder).
2. Frontal region (constipation, hypopepsia, error of eye refraction, caries of incisors).
3. Occiptal region (pharyngitis, diseases of the ear and teeth).
4. Sternal region (gastric irritability, hypopepsia).
5. Mammary region (uterine disease).
6. Dorsal area below right shoulder-blade (liver).
7. Dorsal area below left shoulder-blade (spleen).
8. Central dorsal region of the spine (gastric disease).
9. Wrists (ovaries).
10. Thumbs (uterus).
11. Fingers (bladder).
12. Area between crest of the ilium and ribs (dyspepsia and constipation).
13. Sacral region (uterus).
14. Outer surfaces of hips (broad ligaments and ovaries).
15. Groins (spasm of ureter).
16. Inner aspect of knee-joint (the hip-joint).
17. Heels (neurasthenia, disease of the ovaries, rheumatic diathesis).

The location of these areas may be clearly seen by reference to Figs. 122, 123, for which the author is indebted to Dana's work previously mentioned.

THE ELECTRO-HYDRIC, OR ELECTRIC-THERMAL, BATH.

This bath is simply a water bath with the addition of 1457
electricity. The author employs the faradic, galvanic, or

sinusoidal electrical currents in this way. The electricity is communicated to the patient in a porcelain tub by means of a stationary head plate and sliding metallic electrodes on either side (Fig. 241). The electrical apparatus may be placed at the head of the tub or in any other convenient place within easy reach of the operator. The temperature of the bath depends upon the effects desired. The temperature most commonly employed is from 92° to 98°.

When tonic effects are desired, the faradic current is generally found preferable. The temperature of the bath may be from 92° to 95°, for 5 to 6 minutes, and at the last end cooled to 80°, the patient being rubbed in the meantime to prevent chilling. The strength of the current should be such as to produce distinct tingling in the various parts of the body to which it is directed, but not sufficiently strong to cause contraction of the muscles.

When sedative effects are desired, the temperature of the bath should be 92° to 97° (ordinarily about 95°), and the galvanic or sinusoidal current should be employed. The bath should be continued for 12 to 15 minutes. The direction of the current should be from head to foot; that is, the positive pole should be connected with the head of the bath, the negative with the foot.

The neutral electro-hydric bath is an excellent application for the relief of insomnia. It is, in fact, adapted to all classes of cases in which the nervous system is abnormally irritable. The sinusoidal current is especially useful in cases in which neuralgic pains are a prominent feature of the nervous irritability.

In administering the electro-thermal bath the current should be entirely turned off before the patient enters the bath, and then turned on very gradually until the current is just sufficient to produce decided sensations of tingling and prickling. Great care should be taken to avoid giving the patient a shock of any kind by the sudden interruption of the current. This is of special importance in the case of the galvanic bath. If the bath is supplied with electricity from a street-current of high tension, as a 500-volt or 1,000-volt current, great care must be taken to avoid the possibility of a sudden afflux of current, which might be in the highest degree dangerous to life. On this account, it is better to supply the galvanic bath with a current from a cell battery of such size that the total amount furnished by it will not be capable of producing more than temporary inconvenience.

Electro-Vapor Bath.— This bath consists of a cabinet 1458
arranged as for an ordinary vapor bath. In addition, stationary electrodes are placed upon the foot rest, the seat, and the back rest, and several movable electrodes are provided suitable for application to the abdomen, or chest, or to be held in the hand. These electrodes are connected with a switch board placed upon the outside of the cabinet. An ordinary faradic battery is connected with the switch board in such a way that the current may be directed through the body in various directions by connecting the different electrodes through the switch board.

It is possible that certain therapeutic advantages may be gained by the combination of electricity with the vapor bath. The skin when moistened by vapor is certainly rendered a better conductor, and the entrance of the electric current into the body is thus facilitated. The tonic influence of electricity will, to a certain extent, counteract the sedative and depressant effects of the heat of the bath, and thus, the patient may possibly be enabled to endure a longer application when prolonged sweating is required for eliminative purposes. It can not be clearly shown, however, that equally good effects may not be obtained by the application of electricity after the bath; and it is probable that the tonic effects obtained from the electrical current are so much less intense than those derived from the cold application which should always follow the vapor bath, that the advantages gained by the combination of electricity with this procedure are hardly worth considering.

1459 **Thermo-Electric Bath.**— In this bath, an application of electricity is combined with a hot-air bath (1233). The physiological effects are essentially the same as have been elsewhere indicated in the description of the hot-air bath (1234). The mechanical arrangements are essentially the same as those described above for the electro-vapor bath; the only difference is that provision is made for heating the air without adding moisture to it. The cabinet may be so arranged that it may be used for either the vapor or the thermo-electric bath. The remarks made above respecting the therapeutic value of the electro-vapor bath apply equally to this procedure, and need not be repeated.

1460 **Electro-Chemical Bath.**— This bath is simply an electro-hydric bath in which a solution of some chemical substance is employed instead of plain water. Various compounds have been used for this purpose. The addition of chloride of sodium increases the conductivity of the water, and is a measure which may be usefully employed to increase the intensity of the bath when the electrical current is too feeble to obtain the effects desired. For this purpose two to ten pounds of salt may be added to the water of the bath.

The bath may be rendered alkaline, if desired, by the addition of sal soda in quantity of two to four pounds. This combination is thought by some to be especially desirable in cases of rheumatism in which the perspiration is strongly acid. If the bath is administered at a temperature of 90° or less, it is possible that there may be some slight absorption of alkali into the system; but the amount thus taken in is, as has been experimentally shown, exceedingly minute, and scarcely worth considering.

Certain observers claim special tonic effects from the employment of an acid solution, the water of the bath being acidulated by the addition of an ounce or two of sulphuric acid. It is doubtful whether any special advantage is gained by this means.

In cases of cardiac and renal disease in which the effervescent bath is indicated, an electrical current may sometimes be advantageously added, thus enhancing the tonic effects of the bath, and rendering it possible to repeat it at more frequent intervals and to prolong the duration of the application, thus producing a more intense degree of cutaneous stimulation, the special object aimed at in the employment of this procedure.

Some attempts have been made to combine applications of static electricity with hydriatic procedures, but without very appreciable results. It is possible that this current might be substituted for that obtained from the induction coil, but it is doubtful whether any material advantage would be gained thereby. Possibly future experimentation may develop something of interest in this direction. The writer has long made use of the static current obtained from a very powerful influence machine in connection, but not in combination, with hydriatic procedures, and has found it a valuable aid, especially as a hypnotic, particularly in cases of insomnia and as an analgesic in cases of chronic articular rheumatism and neuralgia of the joints.

MASSAGE WITH HYDROTHERAPY.

In addition to the remarks made elsewhere (1221-1230), 1461
there remain to be discussed a few points in relation to the combined use of massage and hydriatic measures. The value of massage as a measure associated with hydriatic procedures depends chiefly upon the following characteristic physiological effects: —

1. Increase of circulatory activity.

2. Stimulation of all the functions of the skin and promotion of reaction.

3. The promotion of nutritive changes in the muscles.

Massage may be advantageously associated with hydriatic procedures not only as an accompaniment of the hydriatic process entering into the technique of the application but it may be employed either as a preparatory or a supplementary measure.

All the procedures of massage may be associated with hydrotherapy. Friction, percussion, and deep massage are especially of service.

Friction.— Friction, as elsewhere explained (**1225**), is almost universally employed as an essential means of promoting reaction after general cold baths. It has other uses of almost equal importance, of which the following may serve simply as illustrative examples:—

1. Friction of the skin at intervals of 15 to 30 minutes in connection with the cold compress, to prevent benumbing of the skin and obliteration of the reflexes upon which the efficiency of the compress depends. This measure is especially of use in connection with the cold precordial compress (**1383**), the cold chest compress in pneumonia (**1374**), ice-bag to the back of the neck (**1314**), the ice-cap (**1314**), and the spinal ice-bag (**619, 670**). Friction should be avoided when the purpose of the cold application is to allay superficial inflammation. The hot fomentation (**1328**) should be employed instead of friction in cases in which deep-seated pain exists, which is aggravated by the friction, and in cases in which the superficial parts are tender. The friction should be applied with sufficient vigor and duration to redden and warm the parts.

2. Friction may often be employed advantageously before an application to accelerate the surface circulation, and prepare the parts to react quickly after a cold application is made. This method is of special value in connection with the wet girdle (**1347**), the abdominal compress (**1351**), and the chest pack (**1373**). It may also be usefully employed as a general measure before cold applications when there is a tendency to gooseflesh or the patient complains of slight chilliness, or when reaction is difficult, especially when the application of heat as a preparation for the cold procedure can not be conveniently utilized.

3. Vigorous friction may be advantageously used after either hot or cold localized applications which are employed for derivative effects, such as the cold running bath (**1296**), the standing shallow (**1174**), Scotch douche to the feet and legs (**1037**), and the revulsive compress (**1341**). It is only contraindicated in connection with these measures when pain or cutaneous hyperesthesias or eruptions are present.

Percussion may be employed in the same manner as friction and for the same purposes, either by itself or in connection with friction, but is a less useful procedure, its specific effects being less frequently indicated.

1. Percussion is especially indicated in cases in which very powerful circulatory reaction is required, and in which pain is not a marked symptom and the superficial parts not at all sensitive. When percussion is employed, it should be continued until the surface is well reddened. The special purpose of percussion is to produce a very intense and prolonged circulatory reaction.

2. Percussion as well as friction may be employed after the Scotch douche (**1037**) to the legs for relief of asthma or cerebral, pulmonary, or spinal congestion. It may likewise follow the leg pack (**1393**) or the leg bath (**1299**).

3. Percussion as well as vigorous friction must be avoided in cases in which inflammation is present, as in peritonitis and all acute inflammation of the pulmonary or abdominal cavities, in pelvic inflammations, and in most cutaneous eruptions and hyperesthesias of the skin.

General Massage.—General massage, including massaging of the muscles, so-called petrissage, or deep massage, may be administered with special advantage after general cold applications for the reason that the application of cold to the skin produces a marked effect upon the muscles, rendering them susceptible to the circulatory and nervous impressions made by the manipulations of massage.

1. The application of massage after the cold bath is especially useful after prolonged cold procedures such as are

appropriately employed in obesity and fat diabetics, as the plunge (**1108**), the shallow (**1174**), the prolonged cold douche (**1010**), and the dripping sheet (**1216**). Massage following the cold bath is indispensable in cases of obesity in which the patient is too weak to secure good reaction by vigorous exercise after the cold bath.

2. Very vigorous massage may be applied with advantage after the cold bath in cases of rheumatism, especially in cases in which the patient is so crippled that vigorous or prolonged exercise is impossible, either on account of general weakness or of a crippled condition of the limbs.

3. Gentle massage may be administered with very great advantage after moderate general cold applications in Bright's disease. These measures are not applicable to cases of advanced Bright's disease, but are especially useful in cases in which the patient has been gradually trained to the employment of cold water at a moderate temperature. Massage should not be employed in cases in which active inflammation is present as shown by elevation of temperature.

General and thorough massage may be advantageously employed to promote sweating in connection with the Turkish or the Russian bath, or the hot immersion bath. It is especially indicated in cases in which the skin is dry and inactive so that perspiration begins with great difficulty. It should be employed during the first fifteen minutes of the Turkish bath and the first two or three minutes of the Russian bath. It may be discontinued as soon as perspiration begins.

5. Massage may sometimes be administered with special advantage in connection with the hot immersion bath, the bath having the effect to relax the tissues and to lessen their sensibility. In this way, manipulation for the purpose of reducing joint dislocations may be made to succeed. Taxis for returning the prolapsed bowel into the abdominal cavity in case of hernia often succeeds with the patient in a hot bath after most persistent efforts of other means have failed.

Abdominal massage for replacement of prolapsed viscera

is, in some cases, only possible when the patient lies in a warm immersion bath because of the abnormal rigidity of the abdominal muscles. The hot immersion bath also facilitates manipulation of the abdominal and pelvic viscera in certain cases, thus rendering valuable aid in diagnosis.

6. Massage may by employed with great advantage after various localized applications, as the cold abdominal douche (1081), the cold plantar douche (1083), cold muscle douche (1101), in cases of degeneration of the muscles from neuritis, spinal cord disease, or other disorders of the central nervous system. These combined procedures are indicated in a general way in all cases of localized paralysis.

7. General massage may sometimes be employed after the general hot bath as a means of promoting vigorous perspiration, especially in cases of chronic rheumatism. This measure is also useful for the removal of exudates such as are found about joints after the subsidence of acute inflammatory processes; in the muscular shortening and rigidity which follow muscular rheumatism; in cases of sciatica after the employment of the Scotch douche (1037), and in cases of old, badly united fractures in which pain is a prominent symptom.

MISCELLANEOUS BATHS.

Hydrotherapy, strictly speaking, relates solely to the employment of water-baths applied in such a way as to produce thermic impressions by communicating heat to the body, or abstracting heat from it. It may not be out of place, however, to make brief mention of a few special forms of baths in which other substances are employed, either alone or in connection with water.

1462 **Emollient Baths.**—In certain forms of cutaneous irritation great relief is afforded by the employment of an emollient bath, which consists of an ordinary full or immersion bath at a temperature of 93° to 96° to which some emollient substance has been added. Either one of the following may be employed, the quantity of each substance named being calculated for 30 gallons of water; 4 to 6 pounds of bran previously softened by soaking for fifteen minutes in a sufficient quantity of water to completely saturate and cover the bran; or, 1 pound of corn-starch previously made into a thin smooth paste, with 1 or 2 gallons of water; or, 1 to 2 pounds of isinglass dissolved in 1 gallon of water. Of the above, corn-starch or gelatin are to be preferred.

1463 **Alkaline Baths.**—The fame of many mineral springs, as Vichy, Ems, and various American mineral spring resorts is wholly due to the agreeable effects of the alkaline ingredients of the water upon the skin. All the beneficial effects of these waters may be obtained by adding to the water of an ordinary full-bath, carbonate of soda or potash in proportion of 4 to 12 ounces of the carbonate to 30 gallons of water. The water should have a neutral temperature,—92° to 96°. This bath is useful in many forms of skin diseases and also as a means of relieving the intense itching of jaundice and urticaria.

Alkaline solutions may be employed in various partial applications, particularly the hot sponge bath for relief of urticaria, and the evaporating compress in certain forms of eczema. Carbonate of soda or potash should be employed in proportion of ½ ounce to the quart of water.

Saline Baths.— The typical saline bath is the sea-water 1464
bath. The water of the sea contains in solution from ¼ to ⅓ pound of solids to the gallon of water. The principal ingredients are common salt, magnesium chloride, and magnesium sulphate. These substances have a decided stimulating effect upon the skin and thus encourage reaction. This enables the patient to tolerate the bath at a temperature two or three degrees lower than when fresh water is employed, thus increasing both the tonic and the derivative effects of the bath. For an artificial sea-water bath employ 8 pounds of sea-salt, for 30 gallons of water, or the following mixture: Chloride of sodium, or common salt, 7 pounds; magnesium chloride 1 pound; magnesium sulphate ½ pound; water, 30 gallons. Practically identical effects may be obtained by the employment of ordinary salt in the proportion of 5 to 8 pounds of salt to 30 gallons of water. Cutaneous stimulation will be increased by the addition of half a pound to 1 pound of chloride of calcium (do not make the mistake of employing the substance commonly known as chloride of lime, the proper chemical name for which is calcium hypochlorite). The stimulating effects of various partial applications may be increased by the addition of common salt, in the proportion of 4 ounces to the quart of water. This solution may be used in place of common fresh water in connection with cold friction (**1201, 1209, 1213, 1216**).

The Pine-Needle Bath.— To an ordinary full-bath add pine- 1465
needle extract. The amount required is small, but should be sufficient to cause reddening of the skin of the whole body. The temperature of the bath should be adapted to the patient's condition. The temperature may be somewhat lower than when ordinary water is employed. This bath produces powerful cutaneous stimulation. It is useful in chronic renal and cardiac disease, at a temperature of 92° to 94° and may be used in the place of effervescing baths.

1466 **The Mustard Bath.**—Add to the water of an ordinary full bath 2 ounces of freshly ground mustard which has previously been steeped for ten minutes in a quart of hot water. The mustard should be thoroughly stirred into the bath before the patient enters it; the effect is much the same as that of the pine-needle bath.

For a hot *mustard sponge,* add to the water employed ground mustard in proportion of 1 ounce to the quart and proceed as in an ordinary hot sponge bath,

For a hot *mustard fomentation,* wring a towel or a cheese-cloth compress out of hot water to which ground mustard has been added in proportion of ½ ounce to the quart. Spread this upon the part to which the application is to be made, then apply the fomentation over it.

Alcohol Sponge Bath.—To 3 parts of water at the tem-
1467 perature desired, add 1 part of proof spirit. The alcohol sponge is useful in relieving the night-sweats of phthisis. The efficiency of the evaporating sponge bath as a cooling measure is also increased by the addition of alcohol to the water. Vinegar may be employed in the place of alcohol, and in the same proportions.

The Sulphur Bath.—In certain forms of skin disease the
1468 sulphur bath is sometimes employed, although the writer has never found it necessary to resort to it. It may be easily administered by simply burning a small quantity of sulphur in connection with the hot-air or vapor bath. One-half ounce of sulphur may be burned in an iron basin placed over an alcohol flame in the hot-air or vapor bath cabinet. Great care must be taken to protect the patient from the sulphur fumes by tightly closing all the openings in the cabinet. Special care must be exercised during the removal of the patient from the bath. An excellent plan is to connect the bath with a ventilating shaft, so that by suitable arrangements the sulphur fumes may be removed before the cabinet is opened.

1469 **The Carbon Dioxide Bath.**—The carbon dioxide bath has for many years been used in some parts of Continental Europe in two forms: simply immersing the body in an atmosphere of carbon dioxide gas, the head being of course excluded, and in the form of the carbon dioxide gas douche. The effect of these procedures has been said to be a marked stimulation of the skin. The writer, however, feels exceedingly doubtful whether the application of pure carbon dioxide gas in this manner is capable of producing any very decided physiological effect. It seems more probable that whatever effect may have been observed, was due rather to the systemic disturbance induced by the incidental inhalation of the gas during the administration of the treatment. The gas, carbon dioxide, (CO_2) is an inert substance; but when this gas is concentrated in water, it is capable of producing decided effects if brought in intimate contact with either the cutaneous or the mucous surfaces.*

Observation of the effects of the effervescent bath (1139) led the writer to devise a method for a carbon dioxide bath. This bath consists simply in the application of water artificially impregnated with carbon dioxide. The saturation of the water with the gas is effected by means of the apparatus ordinarily employed for charging so-called "carbonated" or "aërated" drinks and mineral waters (see Fig. 242). The water thus charged may be used for immersion baths, the full bath, the foot bath, or other partial immersions, or in the form of the general or localized douche. This bath is of the greatest service in the form of the douche. It must be administered at a low temperature in order to secure its characteristic effects. At a high temperature, the gas is rapidly dissipated. The stimulating effects of the bath encourage reaction, and thus permit the employment of a lower temperature than when ordinary water is used; by this means both circulatory and thermic reaction are encouraged to an unusual degree. When the jet douche alone is employed, any desired degree of pressure may be obtained by opening the valve and connecting

* Verrier, Précis d'Hydrothérapie Scientifique.

with it a cylinder containing liquid carbon dioxide gas. For localizing this douche, an ordinary siphon bottle with a connecting rubber tube and nozzle may be utilized in the absence of any better apparatus.

Professors Winternitz and Gaertner, of Vienna, have recently devised an apparatus for administering a cold shower bath, which they have named the "Ombrophor" (Fig. 243). This apparatus, which through the courtesy of Prof. Winternitz the writer has been permitted to add to his collection of hydriatic devices, consists essentially of the following parts: First, the water cylinder, with which is connected a small cylinder containing liquid carbon dioxide. With the water cylinder connect pipes, valves, and nozzles suitable for a shower and a spray bath. By means of an ingenious valve either the spray or the shower may be employed separately or together as may be desired. While the application is being made, the patient stands in a metal-lined box which also serves as a case in which to pack the instrument for transportation when desired. The whole apparatus is exceedingly ingenious, practical, and convenient. In their description of the apparatus the inventors do not mention that they expect to derive any special effects from the carbon dioxide gas in connection with the apparatus, but by taking pains to agitate the water cylinder after admitting the gas, or by filling the cylinder with water and bringing the gas in contact with it some hours in advance of the bath, the water may be well impregnated with carbon dioxide gas, and the apparatus may thus become an efficient means of administering the carbon dioxide bath.

The carbon dioxide bath is especially indicated in cases in which it is desired to obtain good circulatory reaction with as little thermic or mechanical irritation as possible. It is most advantageous in connection with the short cold douche. It is valuable as a remedy for insomnia when due to cerebral hyperemia, and when there is no considerable irritability of the cerebral cell. It may likewise be used with advantage in chronic cardiac and renal cases, but in cases of this sort its use must be managed with a high degree of discretion, and it must be employed only when a proper preparation of the patient has been made, so that injury may not be done by the induction of too powerful retrostasis.

The Air Bath.—The effect of cold air when brought in 1470
contact with the surface of the body is essentially the same as that of cold water, though less intense. The powerful tonic effects of cold air are well illustrated by the refreshing influence of a current of air when one is greatly oppressed by heat. The fan, so much in vogue with ladies of all countries, owes its existence and popularity to this fact. The remarkably refreshing effect of a gentle breeze on a hot day, even though the temperature of the air may remain the same, is another common illustration of the physiological influence of air when applied to the surface of the body.

Air, as well as water, may be applied to the body in either a quiescent or an active state; that is, the body may be simply surrounded by air of a given temperature,—what might be called an immersion air bath corresponding to the full or immersion water bath; or the surface of the body may be exposed to a current of air having any desired temperature and rate of movement, which I have named the fan bath or air douche. Benjamin Franklin was one of the first to call attention to the value of the air bath, and it was the custom of this great philosopher to administer such a bath to himself just before retiring at night by removing his clothing, and walking about in his apartment. He declared that he derived great benefit from thus exposing the surface of the body to contact with the air.

There can be no doubt that the constant protection of the body from air and light by clothing, which is rendered necessary by the artificial customs and conditions imposed by civilization, in no small degree interferes with the normal functions of the skin by overheating this organ, retaining noxious secretions in contact with it, and depriving it of the normal stimulating effect of the actinic rays of the sun and the important gymnastic exercise of the vasomotor nerves and centers and the contractile tissues of the small vessels and capillaries resulting from the never-ceasing storm of thermic impressions made upon the unprotected skin by contact with the ever-changing atmosphere.

The writer has for more than twenty-five years made use of the air bath in connection with various hydriatic procedures in the systematic treatment of chronic invalids, and has employed it in various forms, the principal of which may be briefly described as follows: —

1. The Outdoor Bath.—This bath is best administered by means of the outdoor gymnasium: A high-walled enclosure provided with dressing rooms and all necessary conveniences for out-of-door exercise at all seasons of the year. An outdoor gymnasium arranged under the writer's direction, consists of the following: A wide walking or running track extending around the outside of the enclosure, just 1-10 of a mile in length; a swimming tank 75 feet long, 30 feet in width, 4 feet in depth at one end and 8 feet at the other, with an arrangement for an abundant supply of water so as to keep the contents of the tank always fresh and clear and at the proper temperature (from 65° to 70°); a supply of wood-saws, axes, and plenty of material in the shape of logs of different sizes, from 3 inches to 3 feet in diameter, a large pile of fine white beach sand for those who wish to indulge in the sand bath, swinging rings, horizontal ladders, a May-pole, appliances for lawn-tennis, pitching quoits, and various gymnastic games (Figs. 244, 245).

On entering the outdoor gymnasium the patient removes all his ordinary clothing, and dons a thin bathing-suit or a pair of trunks; shoes, stockings, and hat are discarded, for he desires to bring himself as nearly as possible into a state of simple savagery, and to throw off all the unwholesome restraints of conventionalism. A pair of sandals may be worn if desired, but it is better to expose the soles of the feet to

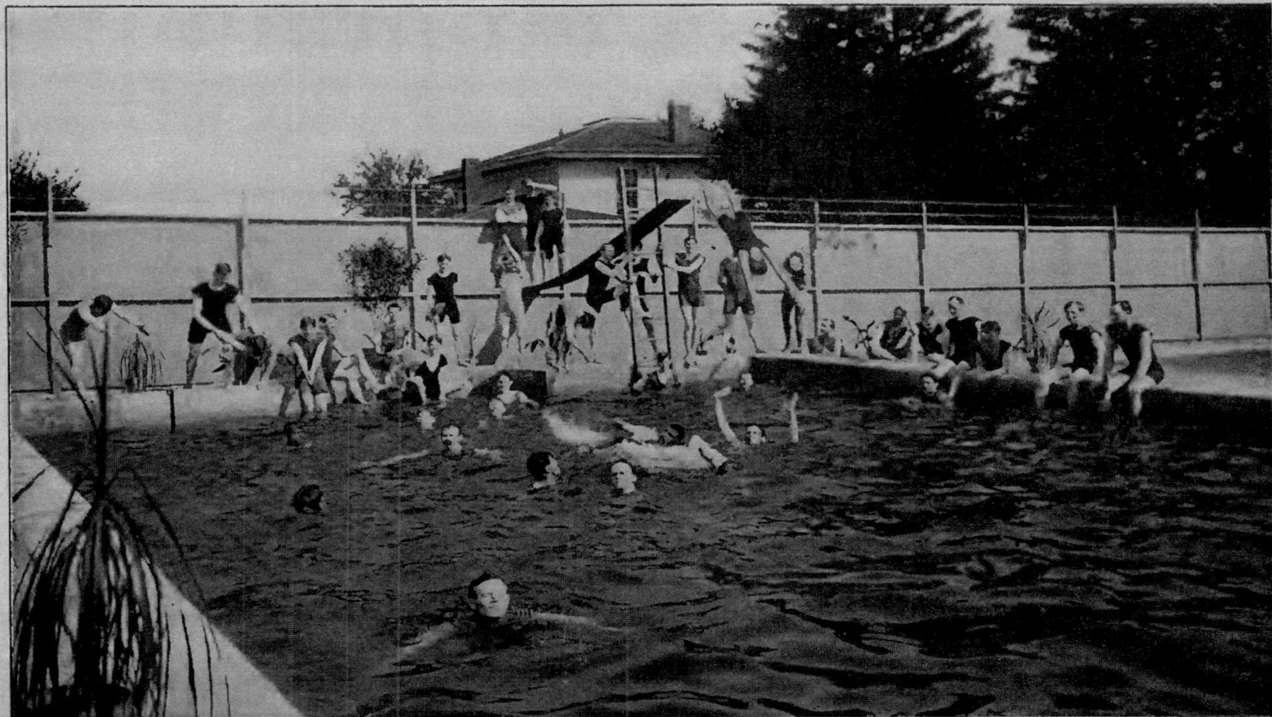

FIG. 244. OUTDOOR GYMNASIUM — Swimming Bath (p. 960).

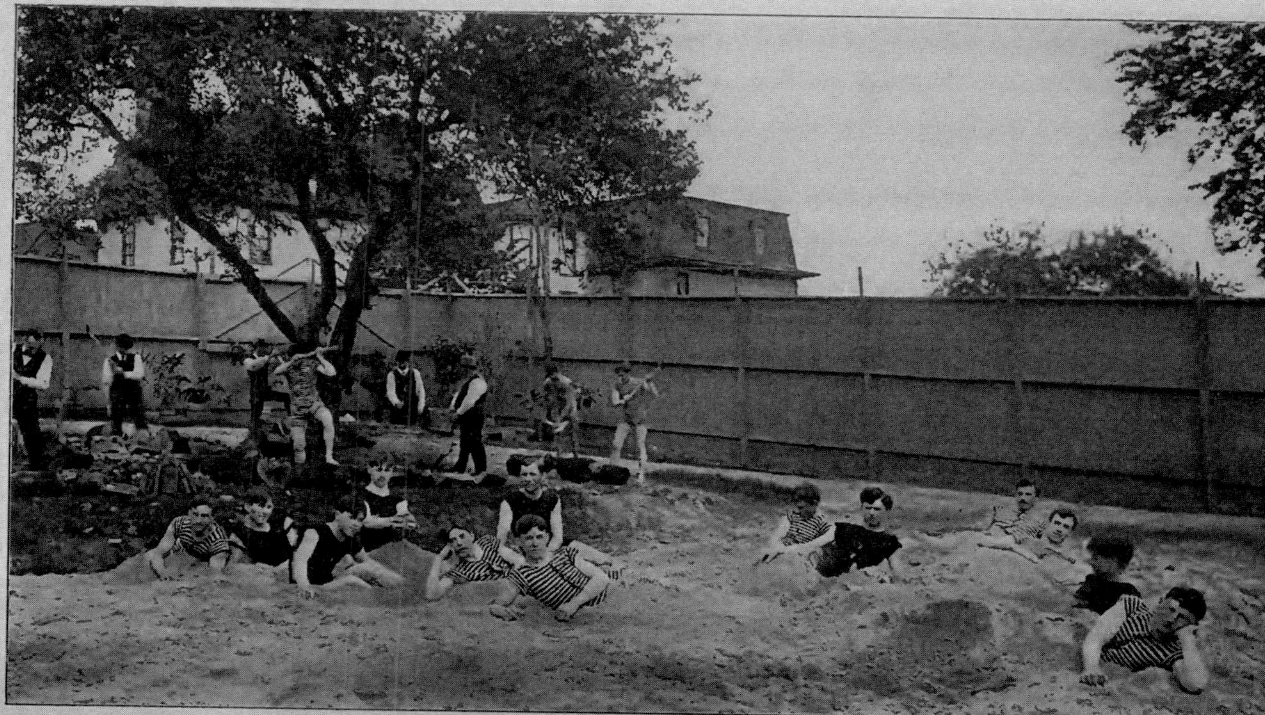

Fig. 245. OUTDOOR GYMNASIUM.—Wood Chopping (p. 960).

contact with the earth and the grass. He imagines himself a boy again, frolicking in the freedom of unrestrained activity,—he walks, runs, leaps, rolls about on the grass, buries himself in the sand, chops or saws wood, laughs, shouts, whistles, and fairly runs wild with exhilaration as he feels the impulses of new life and vigor thrilling through his nerves and bounding in his veins, and finally plunges into the pool for a swim, which cools and tones the skin. As he returns again to the prison house of conventional clothing in which civilized human beings are compelled to live, he wishes heartily that civilization and nature had not drifted so far apart.

The outdoor gymnasium is a marvelously potent means for developing the restorative and healing powers of the body, and is the natural complement of the various thermic procedures of the hydriatic method. No sanitarium can be considered as scientifically complete without a well-equipped outdoor gymnasium.

More or less of the benefits of the outdoor gymnasium may be obtained by such out-of-door exercises as cycling, horseback riding, walking, boating, surf-bathing, swimming, mountain-climbing, golfing, and various other out-of-door sports, to which may well be added horticulture, floriculture, and light gardening. The outdoor gymnasium has the advantage, however, that it may be employed at all seasons of the year, that the exercises may be accurately regulated and under the constant supervision of a competent director, and that the seclusion of the gymnasium affords opportunity for a more thorough exposure of the body to the influence of light and air than ordinary out-of-door exercise.

For feebler patients, carriage riding provides a partial sort of air bath, which may be advantageously utilized while strength for more vigorous exercise or a more considerable degree of exposure is being accumulated. Very feeble patients may be allowed to lie out on the verandas or in sheltered places on cots or reclining chairs. This measure the writer has employed extensively for more than a score of years, and with most excellent results. The patient is as lightly covered as is consistent with comfort, and the wraps should consist of white woolen blankets in cold weather, and white fabrics at all seasons, so that as much light as possible may penetrate to the skin. The writer's general instruction to his patients is to spend as much time as possible in the open air. Simply lying in the cool fresh air promotes appetite and normal metabolism and greatly adds to the beneficial effects derived from other therapeutic measures.

2. **The Sand Bath.**—The sand pile, with which every outdoor gymnasium should be provided, affords an excellent opportunity for the sand bath. Under the influence of the summer sun the sand becomes intensely heated and when heaped about the body is a most effective means of calorification. The head should be protected as in the hot water bath by a cold napkin, and should be shielded from the direct rays of the sun. Perspiration is quickly induced. By regulating the duration of the bath any desired eliminative effect may be obtained. The bath is followed by a cold shower or a plunge into the swimming pool. This bath is especially serviceable in cases of chronic rheumatism and inactive skin, which is so commonly associated with dyspepsia, diabetes and in certain forms of autointoxication.

Local applications of the sand bath may be made at any season of the year by heating the sand in an oven and heaping it about the part.

3. **The Indoor Air Bath.**—This bath may be administered in different ways: The patient may simply remove his clothing, and walk about the room, or sit, or lie, as his strength or inclination may indicate. The best effects are obtained by active exercise with the clothing wholly removed, rubbing and chafing the surface with the hands, and executing free-hand gymnastics or resistive movements. Feeble patients may be assisted by an attendant. Chilling is prevented even when the temperature of the air is quite low, by vigorous rubbing of the surface and the employment of active and passive move-

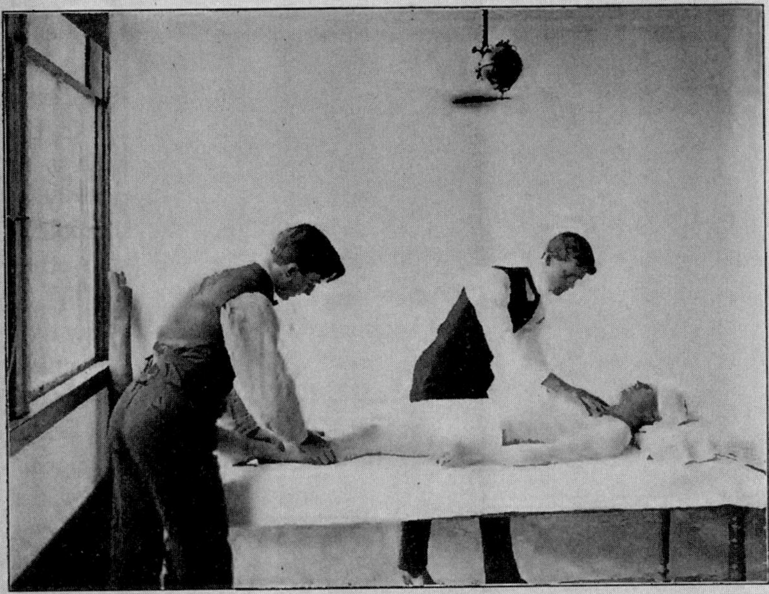

FIG. 246. AIR BATH (p. 963).

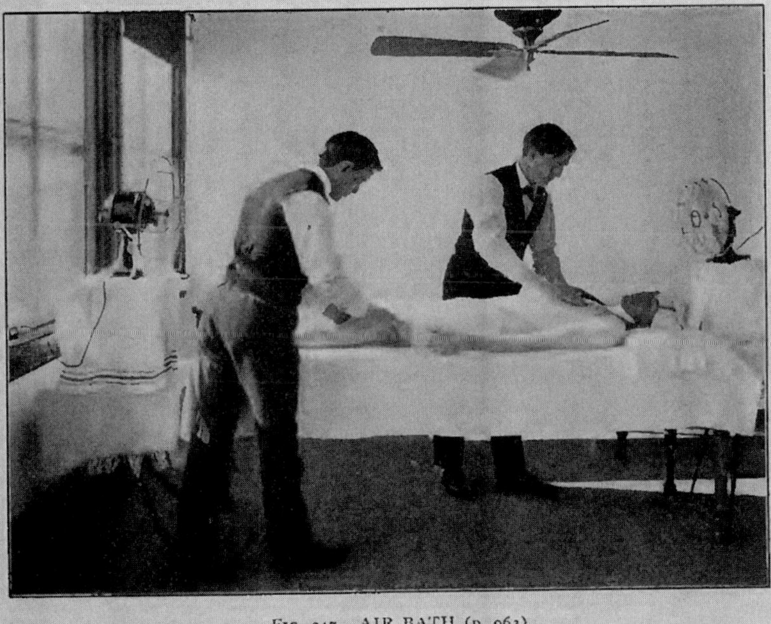

FIG. 247. AIR BATH (p. 963).

ments. Systematic massage may be administered advantageously in many cases. The temperature of the air should be as cool as it can be secured without artificial means during the summer, spring, and autumn months. During the winter months the temperature may range from 50° to 60°. A lower temperature may be tolerated for a short time, but for very feeble patients it is not advisable when the whole surface of the body is exposed. A much lower temperature may be employed, however, by affording the body the protection of a white woolen blanket, exposing only the head and a single arm or leg or some other circumscribed portion of the body where friction is being applied to maintain an active cutaneous circulation. For best effects, the indoor air bath should be combined with the sun bath.

4. **The Air Douche or Fan Bath.**—This bath consists of exposure of the whole body, or a circumscribed portion of the surface, to the influence of a current of air set in motion by an electric or blast fan. The writer first made use of this method in the year 1883, when he had constructed for the purpose an apparatus by means of which air artificially heated or cooled, might be applied to any desired portion of the body. The bath may be employed as a general tonic measure or as an antipyretic procedure. Cold air only is utilized for this bath. The hot fan-bath has a very limited range of usefulness.

When employed for general tonic effects, the patient is exposed to a strong blast of cold air while being at the same time vigorously rubbed by two attendants, so that strong cutaneous circulation is constantly maintained. By this means powerful thermic impressions may be made upon the skin without wetting it. Very satisfactory effects may be obtained by the employment of ceiling fans or any of the several forms of movable electric fans, which may now be readily obtained (Figs. 246 and 247).

For the most intense effects, as when it is desired to reduce the temperature of the body, the surface may be moistened by sprinkling or by covering it with a wet sheet.

Part Four.

HYDRIATIC PRESCRIPTION MAKING.

A CLEAR conception of the nature of disease is the first essential in the building of a hydriatic prescription and in searching for therapeutic indications. To say that disease is disharmony, a morbid state, a perverted vital activity, is merely to say that when a man is sick, he is not well. In a condition of health the body is not only in a state of ease and comfort, but possesses the ability to maintain itself in such a state. This faculty which the body possesses of maintaining a physiological equilibrium, of resisting the encroachments of microbes and other enemies, is termed vital resistance. This most important factor is always to be taken into consideration in formulating a rational prescription.

The diseased body heals itself by precisely the same processes by which it maintains itself in health. Napoleon recognized this fact when once he protested against the polypharmacy of his day, exclaiming, "Life is a fortress. Why throw obstacles in the way of its defense? Its own means are superior to all the apparatus of your laboratories."* To say that the thoroughly well man never falls sick, is not a paradox. The morbid manifestations or pathological states which are commonly known as disease, either acute or chronic, result not only from the recognized immediate or exciting cause, but from a lessening of the natural resistance to disease, or the innate ability to keep well. For example, typhoid fever, as Bouchard has shown, chooses for its victims persons whose stomachs have lost the power to destroy the typhoid bacillus which thus finds entrance to the intestines, and finding there a favorable habitat, rapidly grows and produces the series of morbid processes which constitutes the

*Emerson's Essays.

clinical picture of typhoid fever. Cholera germs, likewise, are unable to develop in the healthy alimentary canal, but only obtain a permanent footing in the body when the stomach has been weakened by indigestion or subacute gastritis. The tubercle bacillus is not able to establish itself in the thoroughly healthy organism, but thrives in the body which is rendered a favorable soil for this parasitic organism by errors in diet, neglect of exercise, and other unhygienic habits.

The rational treatment of disease requires first of all the removal of causes. The second step is to stimulate and regulate the normal physiological activities. This is the essential particular in which rational medicine differs from empiricism and the artificial method, the evils of which were so well pointed out by Dr. Jacob Bigelow, of Boston, half a century ago. When the body is in a disordered state, it is evident that it is far better to restore the physiological equilibrium by removal of the disturbing element or by encouraging those physiological activities which constitute the normal defenses of the body, than simply to antidote or neutralize one disorder or disturbance by creating a counter-disorder, or in other words, as suggested by the famous Baron Liebig, to undertake to cure one disease by producing another. There are of course conditions under which such measures may be commendable, but only as a last resort for relief of pressing symptoms which do not yield to other measures, or in cases recognized as incurable, and in which only palliation can be expected.

The Natural Defenses of the Organism.—The natural meth- 1471
ods by which the body resists disease must be clearly understood. First of all is the blood, of which Holy Writ declares, "The blood is the life." The nerve supply of a part may be destroyed,—a limb, for example, may have lost entirely both sensation and power of motion, yet its life is maintained through the fact that the living blood is still circulating through its vessels. Cut off the blood supply, and even though no other injury be done to the limb, death will

speedily occur. The blood is not only the source of life, but is the great healing agent of the body.

In disease, the blood carries oxygen directly to the part in which the life-battle is being fought, whereby the cells engaged in the conflict are stimulated and sustained while the accumulated poisons are burned, or are carried away by the serum with which the tissues are bathed. Through the control of the general blood movement and of the local blood supply, hydrotherapy is capable of influencing almost every morbid process.

One of the most remarkable and useful methods by which the body defends itself against morbid processes is that known as phagocytosis, in which the white corpuscles of the blood destroy or remove from the circulation disease-producing microbes of various sorts which may find entrance.

The destruction of germs is also carried on in the body by other cells than the white corpuscles of the blood. The spleen doubtless possesses the power of attenuating parasitic organisms, even though they may not be entirely killed. The lymph glands wage a fierce and often successful battle against the encroachments of microbes of various sorts. It is this fact which gives rise to the rapid enlargement of the lymphatic glands in the vicinity of an infected part. The same enlargement and increase of activity of the glands and other structures usually takes place after removal of the spleen. Various cells lining the nasal cavity and the alimentary canal are able to destroy microbes of many sorts, and thus to protect the body from disease.

The destruction of poisons by the liver, by the thyroid gland, the suprarenal capsules, and doubtless by other structures, is a most important and admirable method of automatic defense, which is of the highest value in both health and disease; but in certain forms of disease, especially in acute infectious fevers, it is indispensable to the saving of life.

As pointed out by Charrin, the alkalinity of the blood plays a most important part in the defense of the organism, both in ordinary health and disease. A lowering of the alkalinity of the blood diminishes the activity of the leucocytes, lessens the energy of the normal reflexes, diminishes the promptness and energy of those manifold reactions upon which so many of the life processes depend. The alkalinity is lowered in various diseases, especially in fever, in rheumatism, gout, diabetes, and in many cases of indigestion. This lessening of the alkalinity is always accompanied by lowered vital resistance. This is well shown in the frequency with which skin diseases, gangrene, cataract, and various other affections due to lowered resistance occur in diabetes. Milch cows are not infrequently subject to diabetes, and when in this condition, suffer more than usual from phlegmon.

The thyroid and perhaps other glands not only destroy poisons, but act as general regulators of nutrition through the internal secretions formed. These secretions produce various physiological effects, as vaso-dilatation and stimulation of the spinal cord.

The kidneys aid in the defense by eliminating poisons, especially those resulting from the oxidation of proteids. The suprarenal capsules are active in destroying certain poisons. The liver purifies the blood by removing the alkaline wastes, and forming urea from uric acid and other more highly toxic substances.

The skin plays a very important part in defending the body, not only in acting as a non-conductor and a regulator of the bodily temperature, but by opposing the entrance of germs, and by maintaining the various interesting reflex activities whereby the internal machinery of the organism is kept in motion.

General Indications.—The general indications for the employment of hydriatic procedures which are encountered in the management of different acute and chronic maladies, may be enumerated as follows:—

Activities to be Encouraged.

1. General vital resistance.
   a. Destruction of toxins.
   b. Elimination of toxins.
   c. Destruction and elimination of bacteria.
2. Oxidation.
3. The functions of the automatic and reflex centers.
4. General and local metabolic processes, blood formation, glandular activity, etc.
5. Cardiac activity and general blood movement and local blood supply.
6. Heat production.
7. Heat elimination.

Activities and conditions to be diminished, combated, or mitigated.

1. Nervous irritability.
2. Bacterial growth.
3. Blood movement and volume.
4. Exaggerated metabolism.
5. Heat production.
6. Heat elimination.

In addition to the above indications which are drawn chiefly from a study of the etiology and pathology of disease, we may find through a study of the clinical history, course, complications, and termination of various chronic and acute diseases, a great number of special indications for the employment of both palliative and curative measures. Many of these have already been indicated in the section on "Therapeutic Effects," to which section the reader is referred to avoid unnecessary repetition here.

To deal exhaustively with each one of these several indica tions would require an extensive volume. We will undertake to present in the briefest manner possible only the most useful facts in relation to the use of hydriatic measures in meeting these several important indications.

1472 **Procedures for Increasing Vital Resistance.**—Vital resistance, as Charrin has suggested, is a property of the individual cells. To increase the vital resistance, the energy and activity of the cell must be increased. Hydrotherapy affords a most excellent means of accomplishing this in the application of cold water to the cutaneous surface. It is generally conceded that the increase of vital resistance is one of the greatest advantages presented by the Brand bath (**1150**) in the treatment of typhoid fever and other infectious diseases. The Brand bath is not applicable, however, to all cases in which it is necessary to increase vital resistance. Fortunately, there are numerous procedures whereby vital resistance may be increased which differ sufficiently in form and intensity to make possible the most complete adaptation of the therapeutic means to the requirements of every case. The most useful of these procedures are elsewhere named in the order of their intensity (**1625**).

There are various partial or mixed procedures of greater or less value as a means of increasing the vital resistance through their exciting or tonic effects, of which the following may be especially mentioned: The wet-sheet pack (**1179**), the wet girdle (**1347**), the chest pack (**1373**), the rubbing sitz (**1309**), alternate sponging of the spine (**1342**), the alternate spinal compress (**1340**), cold water drinking (**1426**), the small cold enema (**1405**).

Any of these tonic procedures may be preceded by a short hot application as a preparation for the cold procedure, but the hot application must be very brief and the cold application must be prolonged sufficiently to produce the dominant effect. It must be remembered, however, that cold is primarily a depressing agent, and hence applications intended to increase the vital resistance must be very brief, and must be promptly followed by reaction. The lower the temperature, if the duration is short, the more highly tonic the effect of the application (**632**). Nearly every case of chronic disease requires cold applications of some sort twice a day, even if nothing more intense than the cold mitten friction (**1209**). In cases of fever, cold applications, such as the cold mitten friction (**1209**), or the cold towel rubbing (**1213**), should be applied every three or four hours, unless a cold bath of some other sort, such as the wet sheet pack (**1179**) or the Brand bath (**1150**), has been administered.

The principal ways in which the body resists the encroachments of disease are, (*a*) destruction of toxins, (*b*) elimination of toxins, (*c*) destruction and elimination of bacteria.

1473 *a. Procedures Which Encourage Destruction of Toxins.*— All procedures which encourage vital resistance, at the same time encourage the destruction of toxins by stimulating the toxin-destroying cells of the thyroid gland, the liver, the spleen, the lymphatics, and other tissues. The efficiency of these organs is also increased by the increased rate of blood movement which always follows tonic cold applications. The hepatic douche (**1096**) and the splenic douche (**1097**) increase the activity of the two largest glands in the body, while the general cold douche (**1010**) powerfully stimulates all the bodily activities by which destruction of toxins is promoted.

1474 *b. Procedures To Encourage the Elimination of Toxins.*— In observations made upon rabbits some seven or eight years ago, the writer demonstrated that the perspiration of the ordinary healthy man contains toxic substances in such quantity that from 100 to 120 c.c. of the liquid collected from the surface of a sweating man, is, when injected intravenously, capable of killing a rabbit weighing one kilogram. It has been shown that in epileptics the toxicity may be enormously increased. In one case of this disease, 20 c.c. of the sweat thrown off during a paroxysm was found to be sufficient to kill a rabbit weighing one kilogram. Bouchard has also shown that certain poisons are thrown off by the skin. Hence eliminative baths (**642-659**), especially the electric-light bath (**1250**), the sweating wet sheet pack (**1179**), and the vapor bath (**1246**), are valuable means for encouraging the elimination of toxins resulting from bacterial action or perverted metabolic processes. The kidneys, liver, and bowels are the most important outlets for toxic substances. The liver disposes of alkaline wastes, the kidneys remove urea, also uric acid and other products of deficient oxidation, while a variety of poisons find their way out through the intestines.

c. Water can not be employed in such a way as to act 1475
directly as a germicide; but by increasing the alkalinity of the blood, and especially by increasing leucocytosis and the activity of the lymphatic glands and other organs capable of destroying bacteria, the encroachments of these enemies of life may be successfully opposed.

The observations of Metchnikoff and others have shown clearly the importance of leucocytosis as a means of combating bacterial infection. By the regulation of the local blood movement and volume, leucocytosis may be encouraged to almost any desired degree. Winternitz, Thayer, Thermes, and numerous others have shown the enormous influence of the general cold bath in producing general leucocytosis (**383**). By means of the heating compress (**1344**) frequently renewed, and the alternate compress (**1340**), local leucocytosis may be encouraged to a marvelous extent, and most admirable results in utilizing the natural defenses of the body may be secured. This fact has been demonstrated in multitudes of cases in the management of pneumonia, typhoid fever, and other maladies in which the pathological process is circumscribed and due to micro-organisms.

The most effective procedures for encouraging leucocytosis are the heating compress or pack (**1344**), the alternate compress (**1340**), the Scotch douche (**1037**), and the alternate douche **1044**). The elimination of bacteria by the skin and kidneys is encouraged by sweating baths (**1239-1250**), copious water drinking (**1423**), and especially by the vapor bath (**1246**), the sweating pack (**1191**), and the prolonged neutral bath (**1130**), each followed by the cold mitten friction (**1209**), the cold towel rub (**1213**), or some other cold procedure.

Procedures Which Increase Oxidation.—Strasser and others 1476
have shown that the application of the cold bath increases the absorption of oxygen and the elimination of CO_2 (**402**),

and it is evident that general oxidation is thereby increased throughout the body. By the employment of hot baths in such a way as to elevate the body temperature, the oxidation of proteid substances is increased (567). We are thus in possession of means by which either the oxidation of carbon — in other words, the burning up of sugar or fat — or the oxidation of nitrogen, and the more perfect combustion and elimination, through conversion into urea, of uric acid, creatin, creatinin, and other proteid wastes, may be effected at will.

Cold applications for the purpose of increasing oxidation should be general in character, or at least should be sufficiently extensive to lower the body temperature a few tenths of a degree, in order to develop the reaction necessary to increase heat production, and consequently consumption of the carbonaceous elements. More prolonged baths, such as the dripping sheet (1217), rubbing shallow (1174), cold immersion (1114), plunge (1108), and the cooling pack (1189), are the measures most effective for stimulating oxidation of fat and carbohydrates.

The hot immersion bath (1126), the heating pack (1197), the dry pack (1192), the vapor (1246), hot air (1233), and Turkish baths (1239), sun bath (1254), and especially the electric-light bath (1250), are the most efficient means of stimulating nitrogen oxidation. By means of these measures the body temperature may be elevated a few tenths of a degree, or even three or four degrees, according to the duration of the bath. These general hot applications should always be followed, as has been elsewhere pointed out (644), by a very short general cold application, to counteract the depressing effects of the hot bath, and to restore the tone of the skin.

1477 **Procedures Which Excite the Central Ganglia.**— In adynamic fevers, in many neurasthenic states, in cardiac failure, hypopepsia, renal insufficiency, and various visceral congestions, general or localized excitation of the central ganliag is clearly indicated. This may be admirably accomplished by various hydriatic procedures, especially by very cold, very hot, or alternate hot and cold applications. The alternate general douche (**1044**), percussion or alternate spinal douche (**1342**), alternate spinal sponging (**1342**), alternate spinal compresses (**1340**), alternate immersion (**1113**), with all the various forms of cold (**1318**), alternate (**1340**), and hot and cold localized compresses (**1356**), are most efficient means of exciting the central ganglia.

Measures Which Encourage General and Local Metabolic Processes.— In most forms of chronic diseases, there is either primarily or secondarily a grave disturbance of the general nutrition, arising from failure of the tissues to maintain normal metabolism. The failure may be either general, as in some forms of autointoxication, or local, as in hypopepsia. In both classes of cases, hydrotherapy furnishes efficient and potent measures which may be relied upon to awaken the sluggish organs to normal activity, provided the integrity of their tissues has not been too extensively damaged. This may be accomplished by the same measures which have been mentioned above as capable of increasing vital resistance, and stimulating the central ganglia. Tissues to which applications may be directly made are most quickly excited by hot applications; as, for example, when it is desired to produce cutaneous activity, the results may be most quickly secured by a general hot bath of some sort. The best and most permanent effects are produced, however, by somewhat prolonged hot applications followed by a brief cold application. The most effective means of stimulating visceral activity is by applying to the related skin area a short cold douche (**1070**) with strong pressure, the alternate douche (**1044**), the alternate (**1340**) or the heating compress (**1344**). These measures also increase blood formation and glandular activity, as elsewhere shown (**383-388, 390-399**). 1478

That general cold applications to the cutaneous surface promote to a high degree the processes of blood formation, is well shown by the efficiency of the cold bath in combating the most inveterate forms of anemia, even when all other measures have failed. It is certainly safe to say that there is no known remedy of such great value in promoting blood formation as short general cold baths. The lower the temperature, the better, but the application must be very short. The cold mitten friction (1209) and the cold towel rub (1213) applied two or three times daily are especially valuable for this purpose. For patients who have been trained up to its use, the cold douche (1010) is most effective of all.

1479 **Procedures Which Increase General Blood Movement and Local Blood Supply.**— By the regulation of the general movement of the blood, all the nutritive processes of the body may be influenced. Since the blood is the great healing agent of the body, measures whereby the movement of the blood throughout the body may be encouraged or controlled are of the greatest importance in dealing with both acute and chronic diseases of almost every sort. Cold applications to the surface excite the heart, increase the blood pressure, and increase the movement of the blood and lymph throughout the body. All tonic measures may be used for this purpose. The cold precordial compress (1383) serves a like purpose, and may be employed in many cases when general cold applications may be inadmissible, and also when hot applications are required for some other purpose, thus antagonizing the depressing effect of heat. The cold mitten friction (1209) and the cold towel rub (1213) are especially useful in reenforcing the energy of the heart and encouraging the circulation in almost all cases in which these indications are present, whether in cases of fever, cardiac or renal diseases, or in cases of neurasthenia with general feebleness, and in chronic tuberculosis and other wasting disorders.

General hot applications at first stimulate the heart and increase blood pressure, but later lower the blood pressure (1025), diminish the energy of the heart, and lessen the rate of the movement of the vital fluids. Hot applications are seldom required for this purpose, though the neutral bath (1130) is sometimes useful in quieting excessive activity. It is important to bear this fact in mind whenever it is thought necessary to employ hot baths in cases in which there is pronounced cardiac weakness, so that excessive or prolonged general hot applications may be avoided. Being thus forewarned, it is also possible to guard against cardiac failure by the application of the cold precordial compress (1183) during the hot application. This is very often necessary in the administration of the vapor bath (1246), the electric-light bath (1250), and especially the Russian (1243) and hot immersion baths (1126), in cases of cardiac disease.

Cold applications first quicken and then slow the action of the heart, raise the blood pressure, and increase the movement of the blood and the lymph through their proper channels in all parts of the body (298–316, 1256–1292).

Measures Which Increase Heat Production.—That cold 1480
applications to the skin promote heat production has long been recognized as a thoroughly established fact (290). The processes of thermogenesis, or heat production, are brought into play through the impression of cold upon the thermic nerves of the skin. The more intense and prolonged this impression, the greater the effect in increasing heat production. The most intense effects are produced by prolonging the application until the temperature of the body has been slightly lowered. If the application of cold is greatly prolonged or is repeated at short intervals, the thermogenetic reaction fails, and the depressant effects of cold appear (417).

Measures Which Increase the Elimination of Heat.— 1481
Increased heat elimination is indicated in nearly all cases of fever, as it has been shown by Winternitz (1164), that in febrile disorders the elevation of temperature is due less to increased heat production than to decreased heat elimination. The measures most essential are such as will maintain active cutaneous circulation, while at the same time cooling the skin. This may be accomplished by vigorous

rubbing in a cold immersion bath,— the so-called Brand bath (**1150**), — by the rubbing wet sheet (**1216**), the wet-sheet pack (**1179**), very short hot applications followed by short cold applications to the surface, the cold friction bath (**1209**), the cold towel rub (**1213**), cold water drinking (**1426**), cold enema (**1405**), cold applications to the spine (**1372**). In certain cases the hot-blanket pack (**1197**), the hot evaporating sheet (**726**), and various other measures, may be usefully employed (**744, 745**).

1482 **Measures Which Relieve Pain and Nervous Irritability.**— Nervous irritability and pain may be most successfully combated by hydriatic applications, which are not only successfully directed to the removal of the cause, but also act efficiently in palliation. The measures most useful for this purpose have been discussed elsewhere. See **693, 644.** Also **1130, 1031, 1318, 1351, 1355, 1344, 1328.** The general neutral bath (**1130**) and the neutral douche (**1031**) are marvelously efficient in relieving nervous irritability, and inducing sleep, not only in chronic forms of insomnia, but the neutral bath or pack in the delirium and vigil of acute fevers. The moist abdominal bandage (**1351**), cool head-cap (**1371**), and in certain cases the heating spinal compress (**1355**) are equally useful. The hot fomentation (**1328**) and the heating compress (**1344**) are as useful in relieving localized pain and diminishing local irritability, whether cutaneous or visceral, as are cold applications in arousing activity in sluggish parts. The cold compress (**1318**) and the ice compress (**1314**) are likewise useful in relieving pain in superficial parts to which these applications may be made directly.

1483 **Measures Which Combat Bacterial Development.**— The development of invading bacteria in cases of infection may be delayed by prolonged applications of cold, when it is possible to make the application directly to the parts involved. When deeper parts are affected, the growth of parasites may be combated by increasing the alkalinity of the blood by means of general cold applications (**388**), and by

the application of measures which have already been described as favoring local leucocytosis, such as the frequently renewed heating compress (1344), and the alternate compress (1340). These measures, by increasing the movement of the blood through the affected parts, bring constantly into contact with the growing bacteria fresh supplies of alexins and antitoxins, whereby their growth is discouraged, while at the same time the white cells are actively engaged in capturing 1484
and destroying the parasites.

Means of Controlling Blood Movement and Volume.— Stasis of the blood and lymph encourages morbid processes by favoring the development and the accumulation of waste and toxic substances in the tissues, thus leading to perverted metabolism or unhealthy tissue formation, and by weakening the resistance of the cells, which become asphyxiated by the accumulation of CO_2 and poisoned by their own excretions, so that they are unfitted for combat with the invading parasites.

The same measures which have been described as encouraging leucocytosis may be successfully employed in combating stasis of the blood in inflamed or congested parts. Derivative measures (682), the cold compress (1318) over the affected viscus, Scotch douche (1037), and revulsive measures 1485
(680) of all sorts are indicated. See also 1256 to 1292.

Measures Which Lessen Heat Production.— Heat production, which must be discouraged in febrile states, is best inhibited by short hot applications to the surface, and by prolonged or frequently repeated cold applications. The short hot immersion bath (1126), the hot-blanket pack (1197), fomentations to the spine (1328), the hot evaporating sheet (726), and the short hot immersion (1126) are the best means of applying heat for this purpose. The graduated bath (1120), the prolonged tepid bath (1123), (88°), and the cooling pack (1189) are the best cold applications for diminishing heat production (744).

Measures Which Lessen Heat Elimination.— It is seldom 1486

necessary to discourage heat elimination, except in cases of syncope, in which the dry pack (**1192**), the hot-blanket pack (**1197**), the hot enema (**1406**), and hot water drinking (**1429**) are efficient means of preventing excessive heat loss, and an aid to nature in accomplishing the end which it is sought to gain, by contraction of the peripheral vessels. When hot applications are made, great care must be taken to avoid exposing the patient during the changing of the application or after it has been removed. It is wise to alternate the hot application by a short cold application, with friction, vigorous cold wet-hand rubbing (**1213**), and cold mitten
1487 friction (**1209**). See **752.**

General Metabolic Activity Is Diminished, first of all, by maintaining absolute rest in bed. The neutral bath (**1130**) is an efficient measure for the same purpose. In cases of hypopepsia, intestinal, uterine, and vesical catarrh, overexcitation of the secreting glands may be lessened by withdrawing the blood from the part by various derivative measures (**667-682, 1286-1291**).

1488 **Hydriatic Incompatibilities.**—Wise discretion must be used in the combination of procedures, lest one measure shall undo the therapeutic work accomplished by another. The combination of hydriatic processes in such a manner as to enable one procedure to intensify or to prolong the effect of another is perhaps the best test of a physician's experience and skill. The following meager suggestions barely touch the surface of the subject.

1. Tonic procedures must be carefully avoided when a sedative effect is desired, such as cold and neutral baths or other measures. The tonic application may be accidental. The contact with pure cold air after a neutral bath, or of the feet with a cold floor, may destroy the sedative effect of the bath altogether.

2. Sedative measures must be as carefully suppressed when tonic procedures are employed for their specific effects. When a hot bath precedes a cold bath, if too prolonged, or

if the cold application is too short, or if the patient is exposed to an overheated atmosphere after the bath, the tonic effect will be lost.

3. In the use of antipyretic measures, the procedures must be so managed that heat production will not be increased so much as to more than counterbalance the increase in heat elimination; hence, short cold or cool applications may be injurious. Cool sponging often raises the temperature by increasing heat production.

THE ADAPTATION OF HYDRIATIC PRESCRIPTIONS TO INDIVIDUAL DISEASES.

In the study of individual diseases with reference to the making of a hydriatic prescription, we must first of all consider in each case what are all the therapeutic indications present or likely to be present in the case in hand. The information sought will be found by carefully studying, first, the etiology of the disease; second, its pathology; and third, its clinical history, including the clinical course, complications and possible terminations and sequelæ.

TYPHOID FEVER.

The hydriatic treatment of typhoid fever may be taken as a 1489
type and model for the treatment of all acute infectious fevers, although each presents special indications to which attention will be called.

Etiological Indications.

1. **Prevent Further Introduction of the Bacillus.**— Boil the drinking water, or administer only distilled or other water known to be free from micro-organisms.

2. **Suppress the Growth in the Intestine of the Specific Bacillus and Putrefactive Organisms.**— Withhold all solid food, and food rich in nitrogen. Especially avoid meat extracts, broths. Give fruit juices and fruit purées, and dextrinized or predigested cereals, as zwieback, granola, granut, syrupy malt extracts.

Pathological Indications.

3. **Combat the Local Morbid Process in the Intestine.**— (*a*) Pay thorough attention to indications especially as regards

a dietary which will not furnish a favorable nutrient media for the growth of the bacillus. Administer a coloclyster (**1404**) at 75° to 80° twice daily, placing the patient in the right Simm's position so as to insure a complete evacuation of the entire colon.

(*b*) Avoid irritating foods and drugs, especially purgation, mercurials, and salines.

(*c*) Increase the local resistance by the cold abdominal compress (**1318**) changed every ten to twenty minutes, rubbing the surface until red whenever the compress is changed. The compress should be employed through the entire course of the disease. It should never be allowed to remain sufficiently long to produce heat accumulation.

(*d*) Relieve local congestion and pain by applying fomentations (**1328**) to the abdominal surface, or the hot trunk pack (**1197**) for ten minutes every three hours, and by taking care to maintain the activity of the cutaneous circulation by frequent rubbings and proper covering in connection with the cold compress. See that the hands and feet are kept warm, if necessary by hot hand (**1302**). or foot baths (**1297**), or by warm wrappings and hot-water bottles.

4. **Increase and Sustain General Vital Resistance.**— Employ the cooling pack (**1189**), the graduated bath (**1120**), the prolonged neutral bath (**1130**), the Brand bath (**1150**), the cold enema, (**1405**), and other rational antipyretic measures. See **711** to **745.** The cold mitten friction (**1209**), cold towel rub (**1213**), or cold wet-sheet rubbing (**1216**) in bed should be employed systematically three or four times daily for general tonic effect.

Water drinking (**1423**), to the amount of 4 to 8 pints daily, half a glass an hour, counting liquid food. Water may be administered by enema (**1404**) when not readily swallowed.

5. **Energize the Heart and Blood-Vessels and Facilitate General Blood Movement.**— The cold bath, especially when accompanied by friction, increases the energy of the heart and the activity of the peripheral vessels. The cold mitten friction (**1209**), the cold towel rub (**1123**), and the Brand bath (**1150**), are most effective. Cold friction should be applied whenever the surface is blanched and cold or cyanotic. When the spasm of the blood-vessels is pronounced or the circulation feeble, precede the cold application with a short hot application, hot affusion (**1103**), large hot fomentations (**1328**), or hot sponging (**1204**). Apply

the cold precordial compress (1383) and the ice-bag (1314) over the. heart for fifteen minutes at intervals of two to four hours.

6. **Prevent Wasting of the Muscles and the Tissues.**— Complete mental and physical rest. See also 4.

Clinical Indications.

The clinical symptoms of this disease are wonderfully mitigated by the application of those measures which are required to meet the etiological indications as presented before. There are various palliative measures, however, which may be employed for the relief of special symptoms, and as means of preventing various complications and sequelæ, and which may be employed with great advantage. Special indications also arise from variations in the type of the disease, in mixed infections, etc. The indications presented by the leading symptoms of the disease are as follows: —

7. **Headache.**— Cold compress (40° to 60°) to the head (1371) and face. Wet the hair thoroughly, and renew the compress before warmed. If the pain is very severe, apply the ice-bag or ice compress to the head (1315), and ice-collar (1316) or ice compress to the neck (1314); the hot and cold cephalic compress (1358) for ten minutes, the cold compress during the interval. Sponge forehead and neck with very hot water. Shampoo scalp with fingers dipped in cold water.

8. **Pain in the Neck.**— Fomentations (1328) applied for 3 minutes followed by the heating compress (1344), changed every 15 minutes. Repeat the fomentation hourly.

9. **Nose-Bleed.**— Ice to the back of the neck (1314); very hot compress to the face (1286); ice to the hands (1302); hot foot bath (1297); very hot nasal douche (1397). Compression of soft parts of nose against bone.

10. **Cough.**— Fomentation to the chest (1328) for 5 minutes. Heating compress (1344), changed every 2 hours or hourly, when temperature is above 102°. Continue so long as bronchial catarrh exists.

11. **Foul Tongue and Sordes.**— Cleanse the mouth with dilute peroxide of hydrogen or hydrozone, 1 to 6, four times daily. Mois-

ten the mouth frequently with cinnamon water. Keep the tongue moist by a mass of cotton placed between the teeth moistened frequently with cinnamon water, made by adding ten drops of cinnamon essence to half a glass of boiled water.

12. **Constipation.**—Copious coloclyster (**1407**) at 75°, twice daily, followed by enema, one pint at 70°; oil enema.

13. **Diarrhea.**—Copious coloclyster (**1407**) at 95° after every evacuation of the bowels; hot enema (105°) (**1406**), two or three pints followed by cold (70°) one pint. Cold abdominal compress (**1318**) at 60°, changing every half-hour; hot leg pack (**1393**), if extremities are cold. An exclusive diet of fruit juices for a day or two.

14. **Tympanites.**—Very hot fomentation (**1328**) for 5 minutes, followed by cold compress (**1318**), changing every 15 minutes. Coloclyster (**1407**) at 75° to empty colon. Yellow soap may be added to the water, if necessary. This symptom is rarely troublesome under hydriatic treatment.

15. **Fever.**—Cooling pack (**1189**); graduated bath (**1120**); prolonged tepid bath (**1123**) 88°; Brand Bath (**1150**); cold towel rub (**1213**); cold mitten friction (**1209**); large cold compress (**1318**); cooling enema (**1405**); cooling bath when temperature rises about 101.5°. See **703–765**.

a. **High Temperature with Hot Dry Skin.**—Cooling pack (**1189**); graduated bath (**1120**); Brand bath (**1150**); prolonged tepid bath (**1123**). See **744**.

b. **High Temperature with Cold Skin.**—Hot-blanket pack (**1197**), 5 to 10 minutes, followed by cooling pack (**1189**); hot full bath (**1126**) 3 minutes, followed by graduated bath (**1120**); fomentation to spine (**1328**) or hot enema (**1406**), followed by cold mitten friction (**1209**). See **745**.

16. **Insomnia.**— Prolonged neutral bath (**1130**) at 92°–95°, neutral wet sheet pack (**1182**); cold compress to head (**1371**); hot foot (**1297**) or leg pack (**1393**) when legs are cold.

17. **Delirium.**—Ice-cap (**1323**); ice-collar (**1316**); alternate sponging (**1206**) or compress to upper spine (**1340**); prolonged tepid bath (**1123**), 88°, 1 to 4 hours; cooling pack (**1189**), three to five changes, last application prolonged to heating stage; hot foot (**1297**) and hand bath (**1302**), if extremities are cold; cooling enema (**1405**) every 3 hours.

18. **Coma.**—Cold towel rub (**1213**); cold mitten friction (**1209**); prolonged neutral bath (**1130**); wet-sheet pack (**1179**); alternate spinal compress (**1340**); cooling enema (**1405**) every 3 to 4 hours; alternate spinal compress (**1342**).

Complications are due to special localized manifestations of the disease, chiefly either to secondary infection of the bacillus itself or to intense local action of the toxins.

19. **Gastric Irritation.**—Large fomentations over the stomach or around the body (**1328**), for 20 minutes. Repeat every 3 hours. Cold compress (**1318**) at 60°, renewing every 15 minutes, during the interval; hot and cold gastric compress (**1362**); ice-bag to epigastrium (**1316**); ice pills, feed by nutritive enemas.

20. **Intestinal Ulcerations.**—Fomentation over the abdomen (**1328**), 5 minutes every 2 hours, followed by cold compress (**1318**) at 60°, changing as soon as warmed; hot foot bath (**1297**) or leg pack (**1393**).

21. **Intestinal Hemorrhage.**—Withhold food till hemorrhage ceases. Extreme quiet for 2 to 3 days, ice-bag over abdomen (**1314**), hot foot bath (**1297**) or hot leg pack (**1393**). Rectal irrigation with ice-water (**1410**). After 2 days, a cleansing enema to remove decomposing clots (**1404**), 75°.

22. **Inflammation of Bile Ducts.**—Large fomentation (**1328**) over the right side for 15 minutes every 3 hours followed by cold compress (**1318**) at 60°, changing every 15 minutes during the interval. Water drinking (**1423**); an exclusive diet of fruit juices and fruit purées for 3 or 4 days; cooling enema (**1405**) repeated every 3 hours.

23. **Appendicitis.**—Fomentation (**1328**) for 20 minutes over right iliac region every 2 hours. Cold compress (**1318**) at 60°, renewed every 10 minutes during the intervals. Hot foot bath (**1297**) or leg pack (**1393**) with the fomentation.

24. **Laryngitis.**—Fomentation (**1328**) to the throat for 10 minutes every 2 hours. Cold compress (**1318**) renewed every 15 minutes during the interval. Steam inhalation (**1419**).

25. **Bronchitis, Broncho-Pneumonia, Lobar Pneumonia.**—Fomentation to the chest (**1328**) for 10 minutes every 2 or 3 hours, followed by cool chest compress (**1321**) renewing, every 15 to 30 minutes during the intervals. See **1570, 1571, 1498**, taking into consideration the patient's condition.

26. **Pulmonary Congestion.**—Alternate compresses (**1340**) to the chest for 15 minutes, renewed every 3 hours; heating chest pack (**1374**) during the interval, at 60°, changing once an hour. Rub the chest well at each change. Hot foot bath (**1297**) or leg pack (**1393**).

27. **Cardiac Failure.**—Cold mitten friction (**1209**) whenever the skin is cold or cyanotic. Avoid the Brand bath and extreme general cold baths. Lower temperature by cold mitten friction (**1209**), graduated bath (**1120**), prolonged tepid bath (**1123**); ice-bag over heart (**620, 1314**) for 15 minutes at intervals of 2 hours. (Avoid in endocarditis.) Hot fomentations (**1328**) over the heart for ½ minute followed by cold compress for 10 minutes when cold alone is not sufficiently stimulating.

28. **Endocarditis—Pericarditis.**—Hot fomentation (**1328**) for 30 seconds followed by ice-bag (**620, 1314**) to be taken off and parts rubbed till red every 15 minutes. Repeat the fomentation hourly, if necessary to relieve pain.

29. **Myocarditis.**—Fomentation (**1328**) 30 seconds, followed by compress (**1314**) at 60°, 15 minutes. Repeat hourly or every 2 hours. General cold friction (**1209**). Avoid the cold immersion bath and general cold applications.

30. **Arteritis and Phlebitis.**—Fomentation (**1328**) for 15 minutes every 2 hours. After each fomentation apply a heating compress (**1344**) or a dry cotton poultice (**1388**) to remain until the next fomentation. Complete rest of the affected parts.

31. **Mania.**—Neutral wet-sheet pack (**1182**); prolonged neutral bath (**1130**), 92° to 95°; cold to the head and neck.

32. **Meningitis.**—Hot-blanket pack (**1197**); ice-cap (**1323**); ice-collar (**1315**); ice-bag to spine (**1372**); hot immersion bath (**1126**), 103°, 2 to 5 minutes, followed by wet-sheet pack (**1179**) with ice-bag (**1323**) to head and ice compress (**1314**) to neck during bath. The wet-sheet pack should be prolonged in the heating stage (**1183**). Prolonged neutral bath (**1130**). Copious enema or coloclyster once or twice a day (**1407**).

33. **Apoplexy.**—Cold compress (**1314**) to the head and neck; hot leg pack (**1393**) for 30 minutes every 2 hours; dry pack to legs (**1192**) during intervals; brief application of cold friction (**1209**); catheterization of bladder (**1411**).

34. **Hysteria.**—Hot-blanket pack (**1197**) followed by neutral wet-sheet pack (**1182**); ice to head (**1314**) and spine (**1372**); cooling enema (**1405**).

35. **Neuritis.**—For general neuritis, prolonged neutral bath (**1130**) 1 to 3 hours, twice daily. Water drinking (**1424**), copious cooling enema (**1405**), hot-blanket pack (**1197**), 15 minutes, followed by heating pack (**1183**). For local neuritis, fomentation every 2 hours, with heating compress during interval, or revulsive compress for 5 to 10 minutes every hour or two.

36. **Multiple Sclerosis.**—Fomentation to the spine (**1328**) every 3 hours; followed by heating spinal compress (**1344**) renewing every 30 minutes during the intervals; prolonged neutral bath (**1130**); cold friction (**1209**); warm enemas (**1406**); cooling enema (**1405**) at 75° three times daily.

37. **Contractures.**—Fomentations to spine (**1328**) and affected parts followed by heating compress (**1344**).

38. **Periostitis.**—Fomentation (**1328**) to the affected part for 20 minutes repeated every 3 hours; continuous heating compress (**1344**) during interval.

39. **Arthritis.**—Fomentation (**1328**) for 15 minutes every 3 hours; heating compress (**1344**) during interval, changing hourly or more often when the local temperature is high.

40. **Abscess of the Muscles.**—Fomentation (**1328**) for 10 minutes every 2 hours followed by continuous heating compress (**1344**) at 60° during the interval. Prevent general septicemia by prolonged neutral baths, copious water drinking, large enemas twice daily, and early opening and antiseptic treatment.

41. **Suppurating Kidney.**—Fomentation for 10 minutes over the kidney, repeating every 2 hours; continuous heating compress (**1344**) during interval; revulsive compress every 3 hours (**1341**); irrigation of bladder (**1411**).

42. **Orchitis.**—Fomentation (**1328**) for 20 minutes every 2 hours followed by the cooling compress (**1318**) extending over the hypogastrium and inside the thighs; hot pelvic pack (**1390**) for 15 minutes every 3 hours; hot foot bath (**1297**); ice-bag (**1372**); take care to maintain vigorous surface circulation.

43. **Ovaritis.**—Hot and cold pelvic compress (**1364**); ice-bag

over ovary, removing for 5 minutes every half-hour, with hot leg pack (**1393**); keep the extremities warm.

44. **Pelvic Hematocele.**—Hot pack to the hips (**1389**) and legs (**1393** and **1197**), 10 to 20 minutes; repeat every 2 to 3 hours; ice-bag over tumor during intervals. After first 24 hours, revulsive compress (**1341**) three times daily; hot rectal (**1410**) or vaginal irrigation (**1413**) twice daily; fomentation (**1328**); hot enema (**1406**).

45. **Acute Nephritis, Albumin in Urine.**—Hot-blanket pack (**1197**) continued, if possible, to vigorous perspiration; repeat (**1314**) every hour. Ice-bag over heart during pack. Hot full-bath (**1126**) 103° to 105° for 6 minutes, followed by neutral bath (**1130**) 92° to 94° for 1 to 2 hours; fomentation to back (**1328**) for 20 minutes every 2 hours; heating compress (**1344**) applied at 60° during intervals; enema (**1404**) at 92° three times daily; small ice-bag (**1314**) over lower third of sternum, remove for 5 minutes every half-hour; copious water drinking (**1423**).

46. **Scanty Urine.**—Enema (**1405**) at 80° every 4 hours; copious water drinking (**1423**) from 1 to 2 pints every 4 hours, employing carbonated distilled water if possible; may add fruit juices, but avoid cane sugar, which causes tympanitis; small cold compress (**1318**) or ice-bag (**1314**) over sternum; fomentation (**1328**) over the loins for 15 minutes every 3 hours, well-protected heating compress during intervals.

During Convalescence.

47. **Subnormal Temperature.**—Fomentation to the spine (**1328**) accompanied by cold mitten friction (**1209**); dry pack (**1192**). Hot enema (**1406**); hot water drinking (**1429**); warm flannels and hot water bottles.

48. **Cardiac Weakness.**—Cold (60°) precordial compress (**1383**), 15 minutes, 3 times daily; cold mitten friction (**1209**) or cold towel rub (**1213**) twice daily.

49. **Palpitation of Heart.**—Cold precordial compress (**1383**) or ice-bag (**1314**) over heart; may be relieved by the use of the stomach-tube (**1401**), if due to retained, undigested food stuffs; enema (**1404**) if bowels distended.

50. **Lack of Appetite, Hypopepsia.**—Fomentation (**1328**) over the stomach for 5 minutes followed by ice-bag (**1314**) half an

hour before eating; wet girdle (1347) worn at night; cold mitten friction (1209) or cold towel rub (1213) twice daily.

51. **Anemia.**—Graduated tonic treatment (1625), twice daily. Out-of-door life; nitrogenous diet.

52. **General Weakness.**—Alternate spinal sponging (1342) or compresses (1340) twice daily, followed by cold mitten friction (1209) or cold towel rub (1213) twice a day; massage (1221, 1461); manual Swedish movements.

Complications.

53. **Boils, Phlegmons, and Bed-Sores.**—Scrupulous cleanliness of the skin; hot soap bath twice daily; dependent parts, the axilla, groins, nares should be smeared with laundry soap, which should be allowed to remain for 10 minutes; apply alternate compress (1340) to parts subjected to pressure for 15 minutes twice daily; the parts should be carefully masséed (1221, 1461), taking care to avoid abrading the surface; pimples should be dressed antiseptically. Hot fomentation (1328); neutral compress (1339); ice-bag or ice compress (1314).

54. **Ataxo-Adynamic State.**—Hot full-bath (1126) for 5 minutes followed by cold affusion (1103) for 3 minutes at 75° to 73°; the affusion should be followed by vigorous rubbing. Hot full-bath (1126) 104° to 105° followed by cold affusion (1103), 75° to shoulders, head, and spine, the patient being held in sitting position during the affusion. The affusion should begin with two pails, increasing in number to 6, adding one at each application if effects are satisfactory. Ice-bag (1314) over heart 10 minutes every 2 hours. Prolonged neutral bath (1130), 92° to 95°, rubbing gently if inclined to chill; gradually lower temperature to 88°; continue for several hours. A general cold friction (1209); ice-bag to the spine; fomentations to the spine (1328), or hot-blanket pack (1197) followed by cold friction (1209).

55. **Typhoid in Infants.**—Graduated bath (1120); prolonged neutral bath (1130); cooling pack (1189); continuous abdominal compress (1351); cooling enema (1405). Avoid Brand bath.

56. **Typhoid in Aged Persons.**—Graduated bath (1120); prolonged neutral bath (1130); cooling pack (1189); cooling enema (1405); cold friction (1209) over heart and chest every 3 hours, heating compress (1344) between. Special attention

should be given to the administration of water by the mouth and by enema (**1404**). Avoid Brand bath.

57. **Typhoid with Puerperal Fever.**—The prolonged neutral compress (**1339**); graduated bath (**1120**), avoiding temperatures lower than 80°. Cooling pack (**1189**); hot-blanket pack (**1197**), followed by cold towel rub (**1213**) or cold mitten friction (**1209**); hot pelvic pack (**1390**); hot enemas (**1406**); hot uterine irrigation (**1415**); hot vaginal irrigation (**1413**); cold precordial compress (**1383**) or ice-bag (**1314**) over heart; fomentation (**1328**) over abdomen 5 to 10 minutes every 2 to 3 hours; heating compress (**1344**) applied at 60°, renewing every 20 minutes during the intervals.

58. **Typhoid with Pregnancy.**—Prolonged neutral or tepid bath (**1130**); cool enemas (**1405**); cold towel rubs (**1213**); cold friction (**1209**). Wet-sheet pack (**1179**); abdominal compress (**1318**). Avoid Brand bath.

59. **Typhoid with Erysipelas.**—The same measures as in ordinary typhoid, adding ice-cold compress (**1314**) to inflamed surfaces, changing every 15 minutes; fomentation (**1328**) for 5 minutes every 2 hours; after 24 hours, cooling compress (**1318**) to the inflamed parts, changing every 20 minutes. As inflammation diminishes prolong the intervals (**1344**).

60. **Typhoid with Diabetes.**—Prolonged tepid bath (**1123**); cooling enema (**1405**); fomentation to spine and abdomen (**1328**) followed by neutral pack (**1182**); cold mitten friction (**1209**); cold towel rub(**1213**).

61. **Typhoid with Obesity.**—Cooling pack (**1189**); cold mitten friction (**1209**); cold towel rub (**1213**); revulsive compress (**1341**) to the chest twice daily; cooling enema (**1405**); lightly covered chest compress (**1377**) changed every 2 hours.

62. **Typhoid with Influenza.**—Hot foot bath (**1297**) followed by heating pack (**1183**) continued to sweating (**1187**) if possible; hot leg packs (**1393**); prolonged neutral baths (**1130, 1182**). Short hot immersion bath (**1126**), with cold to the head, followed by prolonged neutral bath (**1130**). Cold compress to head. See also indication 28.

63. **Typhoid with Tuberculosis.**—Neutral bath; cold towel rub (**1213**); chest compress (**1344**) changed every 2 hours. Avoid Brand Bath.

64. **Typho-Malarial Fever.**—Short hot immersion bath (**1126**) or hot-blanket pack (**1197**) followed by short cold pail douche (**1103**), spray (**1055**), shower (**1047**), or percussion douche (**1035**) followed by dry pack (**1192**) just before chill begins. During the chill the douche may be administered best as pail pour (**1103**), patient sitting in tub; when temperature is high, cooling pack (**1189**), cooling enema (**1405**), cold abdominal compress (**1318**). Treatment the same as for ordinary typhoid.

65. **Contraindications.**—The following measures are to be avoided: prolonged hot applications, short cold applications, vigorous friction; and in cases complicated with myocarditis, hemorrhage, and perforation, avoid the Brand bath, affusion, and all disturbing procedures. The same measures are to be avoided also in cases complicated with nephritis, pelvic hematocele, meningitis, appendicitis, pneumonia, bronchial pneumonia, multiple neuritis, spinal meningitis, arthritis, and ovaritis, diabetes, obesity, or tuberculosis, in infants and aged persons.

General Method.—Antipyretic measures should begin at the earliest possible moment without waiting to make the diagnosis absolutely certain. Vigorous measures at the outset will shorten the duration of the disease, greatly diminish its intensity, lessen the danger of a fatal issue, and abbreviate the period of convalescence. If the patient is first seen after the temperature has reached a high point (103° or 104°), most vigorous hydriatic measures should be employed at once to bring the fever under control if possible. As the disease advances, milder measures, such as the neutral bath (**1130**), the graduated bath (**1120**), the rubbing wet sheet in bed (**1216**), and repeated wet towel rubbing (**1213**) are the measures indicated. During the first few days of the fever (3 to 7 days) the diet may consist exclusively or nearly so, of natural fruit juices,—unsweetened grape-juice is best; later, gruels prepared from heat-dextrinized cereals (**1630**) or malted preparations (**1631**) should be employed in addition.

By a careful study of the above paragraphs it will be noted how many different indications are met by a single simple hydriatic procedure, as for example, the abdominal cooling compress.

MALARIAL FEVER—REMITTENT. INTERMITTENT.

1490 ***Etiological Indications.***

1. **To Suppress Infection.**—Boil drinking water, and if necessary and possible remove to a salubrious locality. Avoid mosquito bites.

Pathological Indications.

2. **Increase General Resistance.**—Tonic hydriatic applications, especially the wet-sheet pack (1179); cold mitten friction (1209); cold towel rubbing (1213); wet-sheet rub (1216); half-bath (1174); cold douche (1010); cool coloclyster daily (1407); copious water drinking (1423). The vigor of the applications must be suited to the patient's condition (1625). Repeat two to three times daily during remission or between the paroxysms.

3. **Increase General Leucocytosis as a Means of Destroying the Parasites.**—The hot bath followed by vigorous cold applications,—hot-blanket pack (1197) followed by cold towel rub (1209); vapor bath (1246) or electric-light bath (1250) followed by cold douche (1010) or wet-sheet rub (1216); hot-blanket pack (1197) followed by cold douche (1010) or shallow bath (1174); sweating bath (832, 1191) followed by wet-sheet rubbing (1216).

4. **Combat Hepatic and Splenic Enlargement.**—Fomentations (1328) or the revulsive compress (1341) over the liver and spleen three times daily, followed by the heating compress (1344) be worn during the intervals.

5. **Interrupt Malarial Paroxysm or Periodicity.**—The hot bath (1126) followed by a short very cold douche or affusion (1103), with vigorous rubbing followed by dry pack. (1192). Apply an hour before the chill and repeat in half an hour. Approach of chill is indicated by rise of temperature.

6. **Combat Anemia, Changes in the Blood and Organic Changes and Degenerations of the Liver, Spleen, and Other Viscera.**—Copious water drinking (1424) to eliminate the poisons; cold applications as indicated for increasing vital resistance; hot baths followed by cold douches or affusions (1103); sweating pack (1191) followed by wet-sheet rub (1216); enema, 70°,

(1404) or coloclyster (1407) twice a day; careful feeding; easily digestible foods, especially well-dextrinized cereals and fruits.

Clinical Indications.

7. The indications for the treatment of continued malarial fever are almost identical with those for the treatment of typhoid. The typhoid state is not infrequently present. The abdominal compress (1351) is as useful in combating lesions of the liver and spleen in the remittent or continued forms of malarial infection as in typhoid.

In the intermittent form special attention is given to suppression of the chill and less to the employment of antifebrile measures.

8. **Fever.**—The temperature rises higher than in typhoid. The cooling pack (1189) is especially indicated. The cooling enema (1405), graduated bath (1120), rubbing wet sheet in bed (1216), cold towel rubbing (1213), and cool sponging (1204) are indicated. Water drinking (1424). In intermittent fever care must be taken to avoid precipitating a chill by cold applications, which should not be made until all tendency to rigor has disappeared.

9. **Chill.**—The prevention of the paroxysm, or interruption of the periodicity of the disease is of the highest importance in intermittent malarial fever. The best measures are the sweating pack (1191), or the very hot immersion (1126) or shower bath (1054), 3 to 5 minutes, followed by a very cold douche or affusion (1103), and this followed by vigorous rubbing (920), and the dry sweating pack (1192). When the chill occurs, give the patient hot water to drink, wrap in warm blankets, place bags filled with hot water, or heated bricks, to the sides and loins. Avoid hydriatic applications of all sorts. Moistening of the skin causes chill by evaporation.

10. **Sweating.**—Wipe with a soft cloth, taking care to avoid too much exposure of the body. If the sweating is greatly prolonged, sponge the surface with very hot (1204) water. Make no cold applications while the patient is sweating.

11. **During Interval.**—If intermittent, on well day administer a sweating bath followed by cold wet-sheet rub (1216) and other vigorous tonic measures. A fomentation (1328) should

be applied over stomach and liver, morning and night. The wet girdle (**1347**), without impervious covering, should be worn constantly and changed just before becoming dry, or three or four times daily.

12. **Mixed Infections: Typho-Malarial Fever, Malarial Dysentery, and So-called Malarial Pneumonia.**— Should be treated especially with reference to the primary or most prominent disorder. See Dysentery (**1530**), Pneumonia (**1498**), Typhoid (**1489**).

13. **Hematuria.**— Continuous rest in bed; hot-blanket pack (**1197**) for 30 to 40 minutes, followed by cold mitten friction (**1209**), twice or more times daily, administered so as to avoid chilling. The skin must be well reddened and very active cutaneous circulation maintained. Ice-bag (**1314**) over sternum during interval; withdraw ice-bag for 5 minutes every half-hour to allow reaction to occur. Fomentation (**1328**) to back for 15 minutes every 2 hours followed by well-protected heating compress (**1344**) Between fomentations (**1328**), maintain vigorous surface circulation by hot-water bags, etc.

14. **Syncope.**— Hot-blanket pack (**1197**) for 15 minutes, followed by very cold and vigorous friction (**1209**), and wrapping in warm, dry blankets. Hot fomentation over heart 1 minute followed by cold friction to the chest 2 or 3 minutes, repeated every hour or more if necessary. Hot water drinking (**1429**); hot enema (**1406**). Induce sweating if possible by fomentation to spine and over liver (**1328**). After a few minutes follow by general cold friction (**1209**).

15. **Convulsions.**— Heat to back (**1335**) with ice to head (**1314**), or hot immersion bath (**1126**) with ice cap (**1323**); copious water drinking (**1424**) and hot enema (**1406**). After the bath, wrap the patient in dry blankets.

16. **Malarial Enlargement of Liver and Spleen.**— Alternate compress (**1340**) or alternate douche (**1044**), over liver and spleen; wet girdle (**1347**) to be changed every 4 hours.

17. **Malarial Cachexia.**— Electric-light bath (**1250**), vapor bath (**1246**), hot-blanket pack (**1197**), or sweating wet-sheet pack (**1187**), followed by tonic cold applications suited to the patient's condition, once daily, as cold mitten friction (**1209**) or towel rubbing (**1213**), wet-sheet rub (**1216**), half bath (**1174**) or douche (**1010**) once or twice daily; fomentation

(**1328**) over the liver twice a day with heating compress (**1344**) during the interval; water drinking (**1424**); an aseptic dietary.

18. **Complications.**—These are for the most part similar to those of typhoid fever and require the same treatment.

General Method.—In cases of intermittent malarial fever the first object to be gained is the interruption of the paroxysm. If the patient's system is greatly deteriorated and his blood corpuscles greatly diminished in number, either by the long continuance of the malarial disease, or some pre-existing malady, the vital resistance may be in nearly all cases sufficiently developed by means of simple hydriatic procedures, carefully administered as above described, to interrupt the paroxysm without the administration of a medicinal agent of any sort. If, however, after one or two thoroughgoing attempts to interrupt the paroxysm by hydriatic means, success is not attained, antiperiodic doses of quinia (5 to 15 grains) may be administered. The drug should be given within the six hours just preceding the expected paroxysm. The hydriatic measures recommended for interrupting the paroxysms should also be employed, and between the paroxysms strongly tonic measures should be steadily kept up to fortify the patient against a new attack. These measures should be continued for several weeks after the interruption of the paroxysm. The use of large doses or many-times repeated doses of quinine is never necessary in the treatment of intermittent fever when the resources of hydrotherapy are effectively brought into operation.

In chronic malarial infection, which is often refractory to quinine, hydrotherapy is marvelously successful. See "Malarial Cachexia" (17).

Remittent malarial fever can not be so readily brought to a quick termination as the intermittent form of the disease. The general method is the same as in typhoid fever. When the temperature is high, administer vigorous antipyretic measures, especially the cooling pack (**1189**); during the remission apply fomentations (**1328**) over the liver, cold towel rubbings (**1213**) every two or three hours, and thus build up the patient's resistance. In cases which have resisted antiperiodic doses of quinine, arsenic, and other drugs, a few days' application of hydriatic measures rarely fails to effect a radical change for the better. If hydroherapy alone proves insufficient, one or two small antiperiodic doses of quinine may be administered with the happiest results.

SCARLET FEVER.

1491 ***Pathological Indications.***

1. **Encourage General Resistance.**—Hot-blanket pack (**1197**), 3 to 8 minutes followed by cooling wet-sheet pack (**1189**). (The cold sheet should be well heated before removing.) Or, the hot pack (**1183**) may be followed by cold towel rub (**1213**), wet-sheet rub (**1216**) in bed, or tepid affusion (**1103**), 85° to 80°, the patient sitting in a bath tub. Cold mitten friction must be avoided.

2. **Eliminate Poisons.**—Copious water drinking (**1423**), two to six glasses in 24 hours. Carbonated water, fruit juice, fruit purées, etc.

Clinical Indications.

3. **Fever.**—Cooling pack (**1189**), hot-blanket pack (**1197**), followed by cold towel rub (**1213**) or wet-sheet rub (**1216**), graduated bath (**1120**), copious water drinking (**1423**), cooling enema (**1405**).

4. **Delayed Eruption.**—Wet-sheet pack (**1183**) prolonged to heating stage.

5. **Diarrhea.**—Enema (**1405**), 75° to 80° after each movement. Fomentation (**1328**) for 15 minutes over the abdomen every two hours, followed by heating compress (**1344**), changed every half-hour. If the general surface is cold, the hot full-bath (**1126**) for five minutes, followed by short cold towel rubbing (**1213**).

6. **Vomiting.**—Hot and cold trunk pack (**1367**), ice-bag (**1314**) over the stomach or spine opposite, lavage (**1401**) if vomiting is persistent.

7. **Convulsions.**—Hot-blanket pack (**1197**) for 10 minutes, followed by cold wet-sheet pack (**1179**) with ice to head (**1314**). Hot bath (**1126**) for 5 minutes followed by neutral bath (**1130**) 92° to 95°. Water drinking (**1423**); large enema (**1404**).

8. **Pharyngitis.**—Fomentation (**1328**) to throat 10 minutes every hour with ice compress (**1314**) during interval. Steam inhalation (**1419**) 5 to 10 minutes every half-hour. Gargle throat with very hot water hourly. Throat compress (**1381**) at 60°, changed every 15 minutes; protected heating compress (**1344**)

changed once in 3 hours. Spray throat with weak solution of peroxide of hydrogen or hydrozone every hour.

9. **Delirium with Insomnia and Nervous Agitation or Chorea.**—Ice bag (1323) to head, hot fomentations (1328) to spine, followed by prolonged wet-sheet pack (1179).

10. **Desquamation.**—Neutral (92° to 95°) alkaline bath daily (1112, 1463), 15 minutes to 1 hour.

11. **Nephritis, or Suppression of Urine.**—Hot-blanket pack (1197) for 20 to 30 minutes followed by heating compress (1344) to the loins. Copious water drinking (1423); enema (1405) 80° to 90°, twice daily.

12. **Pleurisy.**—Fomentation to the chest (1328) for 15 minutes every 2 hours with heating compress (1344) during the interval. Tight muslin bandage about chest if pain is intense.

13. **Rheumatism.**—Sweating pack (1191); copious water drinking (1424); fomentation (1328) to joints every 3 hours with heating compress (1344) during interval.

14. **Pericarditis, or Endocarditis.**—Ice-bag (1314) or cold compress (1314) over heart to be removed for 5 minutes every 15 to 20 minutes.

15. **Enteritis.**—Hot trunk pack (1197), with hot foot bath (1297) or hot leg pack (1393) for 20 minutes, followed by cold abdominal compress (1318) at 60°, to be changed every 30 minutes. Enema (1404) after each stool, at 95°.

16. **Pneumonia.**—Fomentation (1328) for 15 minutes every 2 or 3 hours, cold compress (1344) at 60° during interval, changing every 10 to 20 minutes. Hot hip and leg pack (1393) once or twice daily to relieve congestion. Keep skin warm and active. Hot-blanket pack (1197) if patient is chilly, followed by heating wet-sheet pack (1183).

17. **Enlarged Spleen or Liver.**—Fomentation (1328) over part for 10 to 20 minutes twice daily. Follow by ice-water compress, to be changed every 2 hours during interval.

18. **Contraindications.**—Avoid short cold baths, prolonged hot baths, and all other measures which diminish heat elimination or increase heat production.

General Method.—At the beginning encourage eruption by hot-water drinking (1429), very hot baths (1126), heating pack (1183).

After eruption is fully developed, cooling pack (**1189**), graduated bath (**1120**), cool enema (**1405**), and other antipyretic measures. Copious water drinking (**1426**) is especially important.

Give attention to throat, to prevent infection of the ears. Steam inhalation (**1419**); irrigation (**1400**); heating compress (**1344**).

If albumin appears, the blood must be kept in the skin by hot packs (**1197**) and warm wrappings; and the cold applications must be "partial," such as wet-hand rub (**1201**), cold mitten friction (**1209**), cold towel rub (**1213**).

Prolonged chilling of the skin must be carefully avoided.

MEASLES.

1492 ***Pathological Indications.***

1. **Maintain General Resistance.**—Wet-sheet pack (**1179**); graduated bath (**1120**).

2. **Prevent Pulmonary Complications.**—Fomentation to chest (**1328**) twice a day, chest pack (**1373**) during interval.

Clinical Indications.

3. **Naso-Pharyngeal Irritation.**—Apply light very hot compresses (**1286**) to the face. Inhale steam (**1419**) and vapors of aromatic oils and balsams. Fomentation (**1328**) to the throat every 2 hours, heating compress (**1344**) during the interval, changing every 15 minutes at first, less frequently later.

4. **Headache.** See **1554**, 11–15; **1562**.

5. **Delayed Eruption.**—Hot-blanket pack (**1197**) 10 minutes followed by heating wet-sheet pack (**1183**).

6. **Inflammation of Middle Ear.**—Ice to throat of same side (**1314**); fomentation (**1328**) over ear.

7. **Nephritis.** See **1537**.

8. **Hemorrhagic Form.**—Hot-blanket pack (**1197**) or short hot immersion bath (**1126**) followed by heating wet-sheet pack (**1183**). Repeat every 3 or 4 hours. Prolonged neutral (**1130**) bath at 95° to 93°.

9. **Bronchial Catarrh.**—Fomentation to chest (**1328**), cold towel rub (**1213**), or cold mitten friction (**1209**) twice daily. Moist chest pack (**1373**) night and day.

10. **Lobar Pneumonia — Broncho-Pneumonia.**— Fomentation (**1328**) for pain and irritable cough, repeated every 2 or

3 hours; cold compress (1344) during interval, at 60°, changing every 15 to 30 minutes; hot hip and leg pack (1197) if the local inflammation is severe. See Pneumonia (1498).

11. **Cough.**—See 1570, 4-7.

12. **Nosebleed.**—See 1496, 4.

13. **Inflammation of the Eye or Eyelids.**—See 1602.

ERYSIPELAS.

Pathological Indications. 1493

1. **General.**—Cold mitten friction (1209) or towel rub (1213) every 3 hours.

2. **Combat Local Inflammation and Extension of the Disease.**—Cold compress (1318) during the early stage of the disease, renewing before it becomes warm, later, less frequently. Avoid ice-bags or ice compresses, which involve risk of sloughing; Fomentations (1328) for 2 to 5 minutes every 2 hours. Ice-collar (1316), when the skin of the head or face is affected.

Clinical Indications.

3. **Fever.**—Graduated bath (1120); prolonged neutral bath (1130); cooling enema (1405); cooling wet-sheet pack (1179).

4. **Recurring Chills.**—Dry pack (1192); hot water drinking. (1429).

5. **Vomiting.**—Ice-bag (1314) over stomach; hot and cold trunk pack (1367).

6. **Pericarditis, Endocarditis.**—See 1576. Fomentation (1328) over heart 30 seconds, followed by precordial compress (1383) at 60°; change every half-hour.

7. **Myocarditis.**—See 1489, 29; 1576, 5.

8. **Arthritis.**—See 1499; 1489, 39.

9. **Albuminuria, Acute Nephritis.**—See 1537.

10. **Delirium.**—See 1489, 17.

General Method.—During the early stage of the disease, while the surface is bright red and the inflammation extending, apply cooling measures, changing every few minutes (3 to 5), as often as warm. Prevent extreme depression by a fomentation (1238), not too hot, every hour or two. When the parts become a dull red color, or the rapid extension is checked, employ the heating compress (1344), changing at intervals of 15 to 30 minutes, prolonging the interval as the fever and inflammation subside.

SMALLPOX.

1494 ***Pathological Indications.***

1. **General.**—Spare, aseptic diet (**1626**); water drinking (**1423**). See Scarlet Fever (**1491**, 1).

Clinical Indications.

2. **Lumbar Pain.**—Fomentation (**1328**) or hot trunk pack (**1197**) every three hours; heating pack (**1183**) during interval, change every 30 to 40 minutes.

3. **Nausea and Vomiting.**—Ice-bag (**1314**) over stomach, hot and cold trunk pack (**1367**).

4. **Constipation.**—Cold enema (**1405**) daily; coloclyster (**1407**) 70° daily.

5. **Diarrhea.**—Enema (**1404**) at 95° after each movement; fomentation (**1328**) to abdomen; cold compress (**1318**) to be changed every hour.

6. **Delayed Eruption.**—Hot-blanket pack (**1197**) or hot bath (**1126**) followed by sweating wet-sheet pack (**1183**).

7. **Fever.**—Graduated bath (**1120**); prolonged tepid bath (**1123**); cooling wet-sheet pack (**1189**); cool enema (**1405**), with simultaneous fomentation (**1328**) to back if necessary to prevent chill; large cooling compress.

8. **Stage of Suppuration.**—Prolonged or continuous neutral bath (**1130**).

9. **Tumefaction of Face.**—Hot compress (**1286**) to face for 5 minutes every hour; cold compress (**1318**) during interval, at 60°, renewed every 20 minutes.

10. **Pitting.**—Cooling compress, using red cloth, covering face completely. Red curtains to windows.

11. **Headache and Delirium.**—Ice-cap (**1323**), ice-collar (**1316**). Hot and cold cephalic compress (**1358**).

12. **Broncho-Pneumonia.**—See **1576**, 5.

13. **Endocarditis.**—See **1573**.

14. **Laryngitis.**—See **1568**.

15. **Nephritis.**—See **1537**.

16. **Inflammation of Eye.**—**1602**.

17. **Contraindications.**—After the eruption appears, avoid the wet-hand rub, cold mitten friction, and all friction baths.

General Method.—Keep the temperature down, and maintain activity of the skin by prolonged neutral (**1130**) and tepid baths (**1123**); aid elimination by copious water drinking (**1423**); prevent visceral complications by continuous cold to the head (**1323**) and the frequently changed abdominal compress (**1318**). In confluent cases, general septicemia is prevented by prolonged immersion baths (**1136**).

CEREBROSPINAL MENINGITIS.

Pathological Indications. **1495**

1. **General.**—Careful cold mitten friction two to four times daily.

2. **Combat Congestion of the Brain and Cord.**—Ice-cap (**1323**); ice-collar (**1316**); cooling coil to the head (**1323**); ice-bag to the spine (**1372**). General derivative treatment; hot hip (**1389**) and leg packs (**1393**); hot-blanket pack (**1197**); hot immersion bath (**1126**) 102°. The head should be protected by the ice-cap (**1323**), cooling coil, or the ice-collar (**1316**) during all hot applications. Fomentation to the spine every 2 hours. Spinal ice-bag during intervals. Vigorous cutaneous circulation must be maintained.

3. **Prevent Bronchitis.**—Fomentation (**1328**) to the chest twice daily; well-protected heating compress (**1374**) during interval. Keep shoulders dry and well protected while in bed. In cold bath, see that water covers shoulders. The chest compress must cover the shoulders.

Clinical Indications.

4. **Headache.**—Fomentation (**1328**) to the back of the neck; ice compress (**1314**) to head and neck; hot and cold head compress (**1358**).

5. **Pain in Back and Legs.**—Fomentation (**1328**) to back; hot hip pack (**1389**). Repeat every 4 hours or more often. Heating compress (**1344**) or ice-bag (**1314**) during interval.

6. **Vomiting.**—Ice-bag (**1314**) over stomach; hot and cold trunk pack (**1367**).

7. **Diarrhea.**—Enema (**1404**) at 95° after each movement. During interval cold abdominal compress (**1318**) at 60°, renewed every fifteen minutes with fomentations to the abdomen 15 minutes every two hours (**1328**).

8. **Muscular Rigidity.**—Hot-blanket pack (**1197**); hot immersion bath (**1126**); hot fomentation (**1328**), followed by well-protected heating compress (**1344**).

9. **Hyperesthesia.**—Neutral bath (**1130**), 94° to 96°.

10. **Delirium or Mania.**—Prolonged wet-sheet pack (**1179**); ice-cap (**1323**) and ice-collar (**1316**).

11. **Muscular Spasm.**—Hot immersion (**1126**) 102° for 15 to 30 minutes, with ice-cap (**1323**) and ice-collar (**1316**). Prolonged neutral bath (**1130**). Heating spinal compress (**1355**).

12. **Contraindications.**—Cold immersion bath, Brand bath, and other general cold procedures.

General Method.—The object to be sought by treatment is to relieve congestion of the brain and spinal cord by diverting as much blood as possible into the skin, hence the skin must be kept constantly warm. General cold procedures such as the cold immersion bath and the cooling pack must be avoided. Undue excitement of the brain and cord during hot applications is prevented by protecting these parts by ice compresses (**1314**) and the application of an ice-bag (**1314**) over the heart. Partial cold applications, as cold mitten friction (**1209**), should be administered several times daily to maintain vital resistance, care being taken to maintain surface warmth by the application of heat to the spine and legs (**1328, 1393**) or other parts during the treatment, so as to avoid retrostasis.

MUMPS.

1496 ***Pathological Indications.***

1. **General.**—Cold mitten friction (**1209**) or cold towel rub (**1213**) two to four times a day. Neutral bath one hour daily (**1130**); copious water drinking (**1423**).

2. **To Combat Local Inflammation.**—Hot-blanket pack (**1197**) followed by heating or sweating wet-sheet pack (**1187**), continued 1 to 2 hours. Repeat the application twice a day. Fomentation (**1328**) over the affected parts every 2 hours for 15 minutes, followed by heating compress (**1344**) at 60°, to be changed every 10 minutes or as soon as warm; ice-bag over swollen glands until active inflammation is subdued. Remove ice every half hour and apply fomentation for 5 minutes.

Clinical Indications.

3. **Headache.**—Cool compress (**1314**).

4. **Nose-Bleed.**—Ice (**1314**) to back of neck; hot compress (**1286**) over face; ice to hands; elevate hands to vertical position; if necessary, hot foot bath (**1297**), or hot leg pack (**1393**); very hot nasal douche (**1397**).

5. **Diarrhea.**—Enema (**1404**) at 95° after each movement. Abdominal compress (**1318**) at 60°, renewed every 15 to 30 minutes. If pain is present, abdominal fomentation (**1328**) for 15 minutes or until relieved, every 2 hours; large hot soap enema to empty colon if due to fecal accumulation.

6. **Vomiting.**—Ice (**1314**) over stomach or spine opposite, or hot and cold gastric compress (**1362**); ice pills; sipping very hot water.

7. **Earache.**—Ice bag (**1314**) to neck of the same side, fomentation (**1328**) over ear; hot ear douche (**1396**) if necessary. Protect the ear with warm cotton to prevent chilling by evaporation after treatment.

8. **Convulsions.**—Hot blanket pack (**1197**) or hot immersion (105° to 108°) (**1126**) with cold to head.

9. **Inflammation of the Mammæ.**—Fomentation (**1328**) over the breast for 15 minutes every 3 hours. During interval, heating compress (**1344**) at 60° renewed every 15 to 30 minutes. Hot pack (**1197**) to arm of the same side. Hot hip (**1389**) and leg pack (**1393**) for derivative effect if pain is severe.

10. **Inflammation of Testicle.**—Ice compress (**1314**) covering entire genitals and inner surfaces of thighs with simultaneous hot hip (**1389**) and leg pack (**1393**) for 30 minutes. Repeat every 4 hours. During interval, heating compress (**1344**) at 60° in place of ice compress, renewed every 15 minutes.

DIPHTHERIA AND TONSILITIS.

Pathological Indications. 1497

1. **Increase and Maintain Vital Resistance.**—Hot fomentation (**1328**) to the spine or short hot bath (**1126**), followed by cold mitten friction (**1209**) or cold towel rub (**1213**) two to three times a day.

To Combat Local Inflammation.—Fomentation (1328) to throat every 2 hours for 15 minutes; ice compress (1314) to throat during interval. If inflammation becomes intense, and suppuration or sloughing is threatened, the heating compress (1344) at 60°, changing every hour. Steam inhalation (1419); antiseptic lotions to throat; hot-water gargle.

2. **Combat General Toxemia and Resulting Degenerations and Localized Inflammations.**—Copious enemas (1404) twice daily. Copious water drinking (1423), three to six pints daily. The free use of fruit juices. Hot fomentations (1328) to the spine or short hot bath (1126), followed by cold mitten friction (1209) or cold towel rub (1213) two to three times a day.

3. **To Combat Local Inflammation.**—Hot-blanket pack (1197) followed by sweating wet-sheet pack (1183); repeat every 3 or 4 hours if necessary. Fomentation (1328) to throat every 2 to 3 hours for 15 minutes; ice compress (1314) to throat during interval; ice pills; if inflammation becomes intense and sloughing is threatened, the heating compress (1344) at 60°, changing every hour. Steam inhalation (1419); antiseptic lotions.

Clinical Indications.

4. **Fever.**—Hot-blanket pack (1197) followed by wet-sheet pack (1179); prolonged neutral bath (1130) when rectal temperature rises above 101°; fomentation (1328) followed by cold towel rub (1213); cold enema (1405) with simultaneous fomentation (1328) to the back; hot enema (1406) followed by cold towel rub (1213) or cold mitten friction (1209).

5. **Coma or Collapse.**—Hot-blanket pack (1197); colocylster (1407) at 80°; alternate compress or sponging to spine (1342); cold mitten friction (1209); hot and cold cephalic compress (1358); in case of collapse, short hot immersion bath (1126) followed by dry pack (1192); hot enema followed by dry pack (1192).

6. **Albuminuria, Nephritis.**—See 1537.

7. **Broncho-Pneumonia.**—See 1573.

8. **Paralysis.**—Fomentation to spine (1328) with cold mitten friction (1209); short hot-blanket pack (1197) or electric-light bath (1250) followed by cold mitten friction (1209); hot and cold friction over the affected part; applications of galvanism and

sinusoidal current; gymnastics, massage, and appropriate exercise.

9. **Neuritis.**—Fomentation (**1328**) over the course of the affected nerve for 15 minutes every 2 to 4 hours; during the interval, the heating compress (**1344**), well protected. Coloclyster (**1407**) daily; water drinking (**1423**), two to four pints; aseptic diet (**1626**); rest of affected part.

10. **Croup.**—Steam inhalation; inhalation of vapor arising from slaking lime; fomentation to throat 15 minutes every 2 hours; cold or very cold compress, changed every 15 minutes during the interval; hot blanket pack (**1197**); keep skin warm. Surgical interference is often necessary.

11. **Threatened Suffocation.**—Put the patient in a bath (102° to 105°), and pour cold water over the chest and spine. Cold mitten friction.

LOBAR PNEUMONIA.

Etiological Indications. 1498

1. Exercise special care to prevent pulmonary congestion from exposure of the shoulders or chest to chill by evaporation. Provide the patient with abundance of pure warm air; have a supply of oxygen at hand for immediate use if required.

Pathological Indications.

2. **Maintain General Vital Resistance.**—Cold mitten friction (**1209**) or cold towel rub (**1213**) two to four times daily, after some appropriate heating procedure, as fomentation (**1328**) to chest or back, hot-blanket pack (**1197**), or sweating pack (**1191**).

3. **Combat Local Congestion of the Lungs and Invasion of the Specific Bacillus.**—Fomentation (**1328**) to the chest before and behind, for 15 minutes every 3 hours. During interval, apply cold compress (**1318**) at 60°, changing every 15 minutes, or as soon as warmed. Lengthen the period between fomentations, and change the compress less frequently as temperature is lowered, the pain less, and the stage of the disease more advanced. Several ice-bags may be used in place of the cold compress, but the bags should be removed at least every half hour, and the chest should be rubbed until red and warm to maintain surface circulation and skin reflexes. The skin must be kept warm.

4. **Elimination of Poisons.**—Sweating pack (**1191**) continued

for 2 to 4 hours followed by cold mitten friction (**1209**) carefully administered. The sweating bath may be preceded by the short hot bath. Copious water drinking (**1423**). Neutral enema twice daily (**1404**).

Clinical Indications.

5. **Cough.**— Fomentations (**1328**) every 3 hours; heating compress (**1344**), changing every 15 to 30 minutes during interval. Steam inhalation (**1419**) 15 minutes every hour; sipping half a glass of hot water (**1429**) when inclined to cough; careful protection of neck and shoulders from chilling by contact with wet bedclothing. Keep shoulders covered. Fig. (186.)

6. **Pain in Chest.**— Revulsive compress (**1341**) covering the whole chest before and behind.

7. **Exudate.**— Alternate compresses (**1340**) for 20 minutes three times a day, with continuous well-protected heating compress (**1344**) during intervals after convalescence; for unresolved exudate, alternate fan douche (**1061**) or alternate spray (**1055**).

8. **Constipation.**— Daily cold enema (**1405**) or coloclyster (**1407**).

9. **Diarrhea.**— Enema (**1404**) at 96° after each movement; cold abdominal compress (**1318**), renewing every half hour. Fomentation (**1328**) every 2–4 hours if pain or tenderness is present.

10. **Tympanites.**— Hot enema (**1406**) followed by small cool enema (**1405**); cold coloclyster (**1407**) with soap; cold abdominal compress (**1318**) changing hourly.

11. **Gastro-Duodenitis.**— Fomentation (**1328**) over stomach and bowels or hot trunk pack (**1197**) every 3 hours. During intervals, cold compress (**1318**) at 60°, changing every 30 minutes; neutral enema (**1404**) daily.

12. **Jaundice.**— Large hot coloclyster (**1407**) at 105°, followed by small cold enema (**1405**) twice daily. Fomentation (**1328**) over the liver and stomach every 2 hours. During the interval, heating compress (**1344**), changing every 30 minutes.

13. **Weak Heart, Feeble Pulse.**— Cold compress (**1314**) or ice-bag (**1314**) over the heart for 15 minutes every 2 hours. Cold mitten friction (**1209**) every 2 hours. Prolonged neutral bath (**1130**) with ice-bag over heart, cold pour to back of head and upper spine at the end of the bath.

14. **Cyanosis.**— Hot-blanket pack (1197) for 15 minutes, followed by cold mitten friction (1209). Avoid exposure of the body to chill by evaporation.

15. **Headache.**— Ice compress (1314) to head, or ice-cap (1323); hot pack to legs (1393) and hips (1389), or other derivative treatment; hot and cold cephalic compress (1358).

16. **Nose-Bleed.**— Ice-bag (1314) to back of neck; short hot fomentations (1328) to face. See 1496, 4.

17. **Delirium.**— Heating wet-sheet pack (1183); ice-cap (1323) to head; prolonged sweating pack (1197).

18. **Insomnia.**— Neutral wet-sheet pack (1182).

19. **Cerebral Congestion.**— Hip and leg pack (1189); ice head cap (1323).

20. **Fever.**— Prolonged neutral bath (1130); wet-sheet pack (1179), cooling enema, 1405. See 1485.

21. **Subnormal Temperature.** See 752, 1486.

22. **Pain in Abdomen and Back.**— Hot-blanket pack (1197) or large fomentations (1328) over affected parts, followed by heating compress (1344).

23. **Capillary Bronchitis.**— Hot-blanket pack (1197) followed by sweating wet-sheet pack (1187). Hot enemas (1406) followed by cold friction (1209) carefully given. Fomentation (1328) to the chest followed by heating compress (1344) or chest pack (1373), to remain in place an hour, or until thoroughly warmed. Repeat bath when temperature rises to 102°.

24. **Contraindications.**— Brand bath and cold immersions.

General Method.— Maintain warmth and activity of the skin, taking special care to avoid chilling of the shoulders, which should be especially protected by a wrapping closely applied. Combat pulmonary congestion by local applications made as above directed. Keep the temperature down by carefully managed hydriatic measures such as the heating pack (1183), the hot-blanket pack (1197), followed by cold mitten friction (1209), and like measures, rather than cold immersion baths and cooling packs, which aggravate pulmonary congestion by producing retrostasis. Promote vital resistance by frequently repeated partial cold rubbings (1209), and thus sustain the vital powers until opportunity has been afforded for the development of autitoxins and the suppression of the disease by the natural healing processes.

ACUTE ARTICULAR RHEUMATISM.

1499 ***Etiological Indications.***

1. Absolute rest in bed. Abstinence from all solid food for a few days, allowing only ripe fruits, fruit juices, well dextrinized cereals (**1630**), and malted foods (**1631**). Avoid meats, animal broths, beef tea or extracts, eggs, oysters, cheese, and all foods rich in proteids.

Pathological Indications.

2. **Combat Inflammatory Process in Joints.**—Secure active cutaneous circulation by hot-blanket pack (**1197**) and sweating wet-sheet pack (**1187**); hot fomentations (**1328**) to the joints, followed by heating compress (**1344**). Keep the patient sweating until acute pain ceases and temperature falls.

3. **Prevent Extension of the Disease to the Heart, Lungs, Pleura, and Meninges** by promoting activity of the skin and kidneys, and building up the general vital resistance by carefully administered cold applications. The hot-blanket pack (**1197**), hot enemas (**1406**), hot trunk pack (**1367**), following each hot application by cold mitten friction (**1209**) administered carefully to all portions of the body free from local inflammation.

Clinical Indications.

4. **Encourage Elimination.**—The prolonged sweating bath administered by means of the hot-blanket pack (**1197**) continued for several hours, is a most valuable measure. The patient should not be taken out of the pack suddenly, but gradually, cold mitten friction (**1209**) being applied to each part until good reaction occurs before uncovering another portion. After rubbing, the surface should be carefully protected by flannel blankets. Free water drinking; large enema twice a day (**1404**).

5. **Pains in Joints.**—Hot-blanket pack (**1197**) followed by dry wrapping; fomentation (**1328**) to joints, repeated every 2 hours; during the interval a well-protected heating compress (**1344**) applied as soon as the fomentation is removed. Smear joints with vaseline daily.

6. **Fever.**—Hot-blanket pack (**1197**) continued to sweating, followed by sweating wet-sheet pack (**1191**) prolonged for several

hours, is the best means of lowering the temperature. When the temperature is very high, the neutral bath (**1130**), 92°–95°, may be employed. Ice compress to head and neck. Cold mitten friction (**1209**) or cold towel rub (**1213**) may be administered after the sweating pack (**1191**) or the hot-blanket pack (**1197**) two to three times daily.

7. **Profuse Perspiration.**— Do not check during early stage; simply wipe the patient with a dry cloth. If the temperature is very high, 104° to 105°, the graduated bath (**1120**) may be administered; the temperature should not be lowered below 85°. As the temperature is lowered, the patient should be rubbed with sufficient vigor to prevent chill. The cool enema (**1405**) may also be used in connection with the fomentation (**1328**) to the back. Be careful not to check perspiration suddenly, nor at all until acute symptoms subside.

8. **In Convalescence** encourage blood making by graduated cold baths (**1625**), especially cold mitten friction.

9. **Hyperpyrexia** (temp. 104° to 106°).—*a.* Prevent by ice-cap (**1323**), cold mitten friction (**1209**) at 50° to 40°, or cold towel rub (**1213**) at 60° to 50°, two or three times a day, when temperature rises above 101.5° F. May precede cold application by very hot sponging (**1204**).

b. Combat when temperature rises above 101.5° by mitten friction (**1209**), temperature 60°, every two or three hours, continuing until temperature falls to 101°. Continue application to each part until reddened, so as to prevent retrostasis (**671**). Graduated baths (**1120**) (102° to 85°) may be resorted to in obstinate cases, also the cool enema (**1405**). In all cases apply ice-cap (**1323**) and ice-collar (**1316**) to antagonize cerebral congestion and coma.

10. **Endocarditis, Pericarditis.**—The hot fomentation (**1328**) (not *very* hot) should be applied over the heart for half a minute at intervals of 1 hour. This should be followed by the ice-bag (**1314**) or cold precordial compress (**1383**).

11. **Pleurisy and Pneumonia.**— See **1498, 1573, 1574.**

12. **Cerebral Rheumatism.**— Ice (**1314**) to head; prolonged neutral baths (**1130**), 92°; coloclysters (**1407**) at 80° three times a day; ice to head and neck; cooling pack; sweating pack, repeating two or three times daily.

13. **To Prevent Permanent Damage of Joints.**— Simple flex-

ions of the joints as soon as the fever declines; short applications of alternate compress or alternate douche two to three times daily, after convalescence begins, with a well-protected heating compress during the interval.

14. **Articular Affusions.**—Alternate compress (**1340**) or alternate douche (**1044**) three times a day, well-protected heating compress (**1344**) during interval; galvanism to joint; cataphoresis; static electricity; massage; bandaging.

15. **Nodosities.**—Scotch douche (**1037**) or fomentations (**1328**) three times a day, heating compress (**1344**) during interval until tenderness is removed, then alternate douche (**1044**) three times a day, followed by well-protected heating compress (**1344**); massage; galvanism.

16. **Arteritis and Phlebitis.**—Fomentation (**1328**) over affected part every 2 or 3 hours for 20 minutes; heating compress (**1344**) during interval, wrung very dry, and protected with mackintosh (**1344**).

17. **Neuralgia.**—Revulsive compress (**1341**) followed by dry cotton poultice; renew every hour or two.

18. **Neuritis.**—Complete rest of part; fomentation every 2 to 3 hours, followed by well-protected heating compress (**1344**).

19. **Tachycardia.**—Cold precordial compress (**1383**) for 15 minutes every hour; avoid hot food and drinks; ice-bag over heart (**620**) during hot applications to joints and other parts.

20. **Diarrhea.**—Neutral enema (**1404**), 95°, after each stool; cold abdominal compress (**1318**), 60°, during intervals, changed every hour.

21. **Gastralgia.**—Hot and cold gastric compress (**1362**), heat to epigastrium (**1332**), cold to spine (**1372**). Hot water drinking (**1429**); dry diet of well-dextrinized cereals (**1630**).

22. **Periostitis and Osteitis.**—Very hot fomentation (**1328**) for 15 minutes every 2 hours, heating compress (**1344**) during intervals, well wrung and well protected with flannel and mackintosh. If suppuration, early opening with knife.

23. **Urticaria.**—Sponging with very hot water (**1204**); hot saline or alkaline sponging (**1206**); prolonged neutral bath (**1130**).

24. **Contraindications.**—Cold immersion baths and cold douche.

General Method.—Aid the elimination of lactic acid by promoting cutaneous activity. This is also the best means of relieving the articular pains. The patient should be drenched with water through both the stomach (1423) and rectum (1404), to encourage profuse perspiration, and prevent undue increase in the specific gravity of the blood. Tonic and antipyretic measures must be used with great care, and so managed as to avoid retrostasis. Chilling the patient will increase the pain. The cold rubbings applied to maintain general vital resistance must be accompanied by hot applications to the joints, and if necessary, more extensive hot applications to the spine (1328) or legs (1393) to prevent chilling of the surface. Those hydriatic measures are most appropriate and efficient which aid heat elimination by dilating the surface vessels rather than by lowering the temperature of the skin.

CHRONIC RHEUMATISM. 1500

Etiological Indications.

1. A nourishing dietary excluding meats; avoid fruits and vegetables at same meal, all indigestible foods and dishes, tea, coffee, condiments, and excess of salt. Carefully graduated cold bathing daily (1625).

Pathological Indications.

2. **Increase General Vital Resistance.**—This is the most important indication in this disease, as in malarial infection, and in acute rheumatism and other infectious maladies. Short sweating procedures (1246, 1250) of any sort followed by short and graduated cold applications (1625) are the most important general measures.

3. **Swelling of Joints.**—Fomentation three times a day; during intervals, heating compress (1344) wrung dry and well protected by mackintosh; derivative massage.

4. **Pain.**—See 1499, 5; Scotch fan douche (1037).

5. **Stiffness of Joints.**—Fomentation three times a day, well-protected heating compress during intervals; alternate articular douche (1100); massage of joints and muscles (1461); massage douche (1066); prolonged neutral bath (1130).

6. **Cardiac Disease.**—See 1576.

7. **Dry Skin.**—Sweating pack (1191); electric-light bath (1250); oil rubbing (1232); cold mitten friction (1209); cold

towel rub (**1213**); wet-sheet rubbing (**1216**); vapor bath (**1246**); hot-air bath, especially electric-light bath (**1250**); Turkish bath (**1239**); sun bath (**1254**).

8. **Contraindications.**—Very cold baths, especially immersions. See **1010, 1103, 1174, 1201, 1209, 1213, 1216, 1217.**

See also Acute Rheumatism, **1499.**

TYPHUS FEVER.

1501 ***Pathological Indications.***

1. **General.**—See **1489,** 4, 5, 6.

2. **Prevent Visceral Congestion and Degeneration.**—Hot-blanket pack (**1197**) followed by sweating wet-sheet pack (**1187**) and prolonged neutral bath (**1130**), once or twice daily.

Clinical Indications.

3. **Fever.**—The graduated bath (**1120**), the prolonged tepid bath (**1123**), and the prolonged cooling pack (**1181**) are preferable to the Brand bath (**1150**), as tending less to produce visceral and cerebral congestion.

4. **Insomnia.**—The wet-sheet pack (**1179**) continued to the heating (**1183**) or sweating stage (**1187**). Repeat often as necessary and continue 2 hours or more if patient sleeps. Continuous cold to the head; ice-bag to neck and head.

5. **Delirium.**—Ice compress (**1314**) to head and neck; prolonged neutral bath (**1130**) or prolonged or repeated wet-sheet pack (**1179**).

6. **Cerebral Congestion.**—Fomentation (**1328**) to the upper spine; ice compress (**1314**) to the head and face; ice-collar (**1316**); ice-cap (**1323**); hot and cold cephalic compress (**1358**); wet-sheet pack (**1179**); hot-blanket pack (**1197**).

7. **Pain in Legs.**—Fomentation (**1328**) to the lower spine; hot hip (**1389**) and leg pack (**1393**) followed by wet-sheet pack (**1179**) or cold towel rub (**1213**).

8. **Persistent Vomiting.**—Ice-bag (**1314**) to the epigastrium; hot and cold gastric compress (**1362**); hot and cold trunk pack (**1367**); lavage (**1401**), if persistent.

9. **Complications.**—See **1507.**

General Method.—Combat cerebral congestion by carefully maintaining a warm and active skin. Cold immersion baths (**1114**) when applied must be of brief duration and the brain must be carefully protected by an ice-collar (1316) and ice-cap (1323) during the application. Less intense refrigerative measures are preferable because of the danger attending strong retrostasis in this disease. In other particulars the management of this disease is essentially the same as that of typhoid fever.

YELLOW FEVER.

Pathological Indications. 1502

1. **Maintain General Vital Resistance.**— Short hot applications followed by cold mitten friction (1209) or wet towel rub (1213) every 3 to 6 hours. Copious water drinking (1424); cool enema (1405) twice a day, more often if vomiting is persistent.

2. **Elimination of Poisons.**— Prolonged neutral bath (1130); water drinking (1424); enemas (1404). See 1473, 1474.

Clinical Indications.

3. **Chill.**— Dry pack (1192); hot water drinking (1429).

4. **Headache.**— Ice-cap (1323); hot and cold head compress (1358).

5. **Pain in Loins and Legs.**— Hot hip and leg pack (1197), trunk pack (1196). Fomentation over lower back (1328).

6. **Delirium.**— Ice-cap (1323), wet-sheet pack (1183) to heating stage.

7. **Cerebral Congestion.**— Ice-cap (1323), or ice-collar (1316); hot leg pack (1393); prolonged neutral bath (1130).

8. **Gastric Irritation.**— Fomentation (1328) over stomach every 2 hours; during interval heating compress (1344) at 60° renewed every 20 minutes; ice-bag (1314) to epigastrium; hot and cold gastric compress (1362) or hot and cold trunk pack,

9. **Vomiting.**— Ice pills; if necessary, withhold liquid foods. and administer food and water by enema (1404); gastric lavage. Ice-bag over sternum; ice to spine; fomentation over stomach.

10. **Constipation.**— Cold enema (1405) twice daily; soap enema.

11. **Albuminuria.**— Fomentation (1328) to the back every 2 hours for 15 minutes; during interval, heating compress (1344), well protected; hot-blanket pack (1197) for 30 minutes, followed by short cold friction (1209) and wrapping in dry blankets (1192); repeat every 4 hours. Ice-bag over ster-

num; continuous abdominal heating compress (1344), changing every 20 or 30 minutes. Copious enema twice daily (1405).

12. **Collapse.**—Hot-blanket pack (1197); hot enema (1406); cold mitten friction (1209); cold compress over heart (620); fomentation over heart (1328) for 30 seconds, cold compress (1314) 10 minutes; repeat.

13. **Jaundice.**—Prolonged neutral bath (1130); large hot enema (1404) twice daily; copious water drinking (1423); fomentation (1328) over liver every 3 to 6 hours for fifteen minutes, heating compress (1344) during the intervals.

14. **Convulsions.**—Short hot bath (1126) followed or accompanied by cold affusion (1103) to head and spine; alternate compress (1342) to spine; heating wet sheet pack (1183).

15. **Coma.**—Alternate spinal compress (1342) or sponging (1342); hot enema (1406); cold friction (1209); ice-cap (1323).

General Method.—Combat visceral congestion from the start by maintaining a warm and active skin. Copious enemas (1404) and water drinking (1423) will encourage elimination of the poison while the frequently repeated cold rubbings stimulate vital resistance. The hydriatic method bids fair to rob this disease of its terrors, as shown by the experience of Jackson and others more than a century ago and numerous observers in more recent years.

INFLUENZA, LA GRIPPE.

1503 ***Pathological Indications.***

1. **Increase General Vital Resistance and Aid Elimination of Poisons.**—Sweating baths followed by vigorous cold applications; hot-blanket pack (1197) or hot immersion bath (1126); hot leg bath (1299) with fomentations (1328) to chest or spine, followed by cold mitten friction (1209), cold towel rub (1213) or wet-sheet rub (1216); sweating pack (1191, 1197). Copious water drinking (1424); large enema (1404) once or twice daily.

Clinical Indications.

2. **Pain in Head, Back, and Legs.**—Very hot leg pack (1393) till general perspiration begins, followed by cold mitten friction (1209), or cold towel rub (1213), keeping limbs very warm.

3. **Fever.**— Sweating wet-sheet pack (1187) and neutral bath (1130); cold mitten friction (1209); cold towel rub (1213); copious water drinking (1424); cooling enema (1405).

4. **Bronchitis, Broncho-Pneumonia, Pleurisy.**— See 1570, 1571, 1572, 1573, 1574.

5. **Headache.**— Hot and cold head compress (1358), fomentation to face (1328) especially over eyes.

6. **Nausea.**— Ice-bag (1314) over stomach.

7. **Vomiting.**— Hot and cold trunk pack (1367); withhold liquids.

8. **Diarrhea.**— Neutral enema (1404) after each movement. Cold abdominal compress (1318), changing every 15 minutes.

9. **Colic.**— Hot enema (1406); hot fomentation (1328) over abdomen.

10. **Inflammation of Eye or Ear.**— Fomentation (1328) over affected part; derivative treatment to legs — hot leg bath (1299); hot foot bath (1297); prolonged leg pack (1393).

11. **Neuritis.**— See 1543.

12. **Typhoid Influenza.**— See Typhoid State (1507, 17).

13. **Rheumatoid Influenza.**— Hot-blanket pack (1197) 2 to 3 hours once or twice daily, followed by cold mitten friction (1209) carefully administered, and wrapping in dry flannels. Repeat pack twice a day. Fomentation (1328) over especially painful parts, several times daily, followed by heating compress (1344) during interval.

14. **Thoracic Influenza, Bronchitis.**— See 1570.

15. **Lobar, and Broncho-Pneumonia.**— See 1498, 1573.

16. **Catarrhal Jaundice.**— See 1534, A.

17. **Meningitis.**— See 1495.

18. **Nephritis.**— See 1537.

General Method.— Combat pulmonary and visceral congestion by maintaining warmth and activity of the whole cutaneous surface, giving special attention to the lower extremities so as to divert blood away from the cranial and pulmonary cavities. Sweating procedures (1197, 1233, 1250) may be employed with vigor and frequently repeated if followed by short cold rubbings (1209) administered in such a way as to avoid general chilling of the surface.

CHOLERA.

1504 ***Etiological Indications.***

1. **Prevent Further Infection.**—Boil drinking water, administering acid fruit juices to destroy cholera germs; avoid milk, meat juices, broths, which afford excellent nutrient media for the comma bacillus. Also avoid all solid food till convalescence is established.

Pathological Indications.

2. **Increase Vital Resistance.**—Hot full-bath (**1126**) or hot-blanket pack followed by cold mitten friction (**1209**) or cold towel rub (**1213**); hot-blanket pack (**1197**); short hot bath (**1126**) or hot enema (**1406**), followed by cold friction (**1209**) until surface is red.

3. **Combat Visceral Congestion.**—Hot-blanket pack (**1197**) followed by vigorous cold rubbing with mitt (**1209**) or towel (**1213**).

4. **Encourage Elimination.**—Prolonged neutral bath (95° to 98°) (**1130**); copious water drinking.

Clinical Indications.

5. **Vomiting.**—Lavage (**1401**); lavage with distilled water or boiled water containing 1 part pure hydrochloric acid to 4,000 parts of water (10 to 12 drops pure hydrochloric acid to the quart of water).

6. **Diarrhea.**—Large warm enema after each stool (**1406**), at first adding soap to the water. Cold compresses to the abdomen, changed every 20 minutes. Hot enemas, 108° to 110°, three to four pints. Hot enema, three to four pints, containing five to eight drams of tannic acid to the quart. Repeat every 2 hours.

7. **Cyanosis.**—Vigorous cold friction (**1209**); hot-blanket pack, followed by cold friction; dry pack with cold over heart; hot enema (110°), followed by cold friction.

8. **Scanty Urine.**—Hot enema (**1406**), frequently repeated; ice-bag (**1314**) over lower third of sternum. Hot-blanket pack (**1197**).

9. **Collapse.**—Alternate spinal sponging (**1206, 1342**) or compress (**1340**); cold friction (**1209**); hot enema (110°); alternate compress over heart.

10. **Cramps.**— Hot fomentations; short hot immersion bath (1126); rubbing of limbs.

11. **Heart Failure.**— Ice-bag or cold compress (1314) over heart for 15 minutes every 2 hours with general cold friction (1209).

12. **Contraindications.**— Prolonged hot baths; prolonged fomentations to abdomen.

General Method.— Relieve intense visceral congestion by maintaining warmth and activity of the skin; stimulate vital resistance by repeated cold rubbings (1209); while at the same time cleansing the stomach and bowels by frequent thorough washings, — gastric (1401) and rectal lavage (1410).

DENGUE, BREAKBONE FEVER.

Clinical Indications. 1505

1. **Chill.**— Dry pack (1192).

2. **Fever.**— Cooling pack (1189); hot-blanket pack (1197), followed by sweating wet-sheet pack (1187); prolonged neutral bath (1130); copious enema (1405) twice daily.

3. **Swollen Joints.**— Fomentation (1328) every 3 hours; during intervals, heating compress (1344), changing every hour.

4. **Cerebral Congestion.**— Ice-cap (1323); ice-collar (1316, 1327).

5. **During Remission.**— Sweating wet-sheet pack (1187) followed by cold mitten friction (1209) or towel rub daily (1213). Moist abdominal bandage (1351) at night. Copious water drinking (1423). Cold mitten friction (1209) twice daily.

6. **Convalescence.**— Graduated tonic treatment (1625); aseptic diet (1626); wet girdle (1347) at night.

General Method.— During the febrile period of the disease the method is essentially the same as that of other infectious fevers. Advantage should be taken of the intermission to build up the patient's resistance and fortify him against a return of the malady by means of cold friction (1209), towel rubs (1213), or wet-sheet rubs (1216) two or three times a day, and a simple, dry, highly nutritious, aseptic dietary (1626). The treatment should be continued for some weeks after the fever has disappeared, so as to prevent relapse.

PLAGUE.

1506 ***Pathological Indications.***

1. **Combat Visceral Congestion and Inflammation.**— Hot-blanket pack (**1197**) for one-half hour, followed by prolonged sweating wet-sheet pack (**1187**) 1 to 2 hours, repeating three times daily; copious water drinking (**1423**); large enema (**1404**) twice daily.

2. **Stimulate Resistance.**— Cold towel rub (**1213**) or mitten friction (**1209**) after each hot application, and at least as often as every 3 hours.

Clinical Indications.

3. **Pain in the Neck and Legs.**— Hot hip (**1389**) and leg pack (**1393**) or fomentation (**1328**) to the back every 3 or 4 hours, followed by heating compress (**1344**) to the back, changing hourly during the interval.

4. **Pain in the Head.**— Fomentation (**1328**) to the back of head for 5 minutes every 2 hours, followed by ice-cap or cold compress (**1314**); hot and cold head compress (**1358**).

5. **Gastric Hemorrhage.**— Hot trunk pack (**1197**) for 5 minutes, followed by ice-bag (**1314**) over the stomach; hot pack to hips (**1389**) and legs (**1393**), followed by continuous heating compress (**1344**) to each leg separately. Repeat every few hours if necessary.

6. **Intestinal Hemorrhage.**— Hot hip (**1389**) and leg pack (**1393**) for 10 minutes, followed by heating pack (**1344**) to each leg separately, ice-bag (**1314**) to abdomen. It is well to apply the ice-bag during hot applications.

7. **Renal Hemorrhage.**— The same as preceding, except that the ice-bag (**1314**) should be applied over the lower third of the sternum.

8. **Typhoid State.**— See (**1507**, 17).

9. **Collapse.**— Short hot immersion bath (**1126**) or hot-blanket pack (**1197**) for 15 minutes, followed by vigorous cold friction (**1209**) and warm wrapping of the body, repeated every 2 or 3 hours, if necessary.

10. **Cramps in Legs.**—Hot pack to legs (**1393**) followed by friction of the limbs with oil or vaseline.

11. **Buboes.**— Fomentation (1328) every 2 hours for 15 minutes; during interval, ice compress (1314) or heating compress (1344), whichever affords most relief. Lancing if suppuration occurs, then apply a cotton poultice over an antiseptic dressing with thorough drainage.

12. **After Reaction.**— Neutral bath for an hour to an hour and a half twice daily, followed by oil rubbing. Feed patient with fruit juice and well-dextrinized cereals (1630), grape juice, raspberry juice, buttermilk, kumyss.

General Method.— Maintain most intense activity of the skin by sweating baths (1197, 1233, 1250), followed by short cold rubbings (1209), thus relieving visceral congestion, and exciting vital resistance to combat the disease.

COMPLICATIONS COMMON TO ACUTE FEBRILE DISORDERS.

Digestive System. 1507

1. **Gastritis.**— Fomentation (1328) every 3 hours, followed by heating compress (1344) at 60°, to be changed every 30 minutes during interval.

2. **Entero-Colitis.**—Large hot enema (1406), 105°, followed by neutral enema (1404), 96°, after each movement. Fomentation (1328) to abdomen every 3 hours. Heating compress (1344) at 60° during intervals, changed every 30 minutes.

3. **Peritonitis.**— Hot soap enema (1406) 3 times daily; fomentation (1328) every 3 hours; heating compress (1344) at 60° during interval, changing every 30 minutes.

4. **Pericarditis, Endocarditis.**— Fomentation (1328) for 30 minutes every hour, followed by ice-bag (1314) or cold compress, (1318) to be removed for 5 minutes every 15 minutes. Hot hip (1389) and leg pack (1393) if extremities are cold. Cold mitten friction (1209) to maintain surface circulation.

5. **Phlebitis, Arteritis.**— Hot-blanket pack (1197) followed by cold mitten friction (1209), carefully avoiding the affected part; or hot pack (1197) to affected limb 15 minutes every 3 hours. The hot application should be followed by the heating compress (1344) which is changed after the next hot application, and retained during the interval.

6. **Laryngitis.**—Steam inhalation (**1419**); fomentation to throat (**1328**) every 3 hours with heating compress (**1344**) during interval, renewed every 15 minutes at first, later once an hour. Derivative applications to legs,—hot foot baths (**1297**), hot leg packs (**1393**), heating leg pack (**1183**). Repeat three to four times daily. Fomentation (**1328**) for 15 minutes every 3 hours, with well-protected heating compress (**1344**) between, changing once an hour. Derivative treatment to lower extremities. Steam inhalation (**1419**) 15 minutes every hour.

7. **Broncho-Pneumonia.**—Fomentation to chest (**1328**) every 2 hours, heating compress (**1344**) at 60° during the interval, changing every 30 minutes; hot-blanket pack (**1197**) for 15 minutes, followed by heating (**1183**) or sweating wet-sheet pack (**1187**), one to three applications each 24 hours.

8. **Pleurisy.**—Fomentation (**1328**) every 15 minutes until pain is relieved. Repeat every 3 hours; well-protected heating compress (**1344**) during interval. Tight bandage about chest if necessary to control pain.

9. **Nephritis, Albuminuria.**—Hot-blanket pack (**1197**) for 30 to 60 minutes two to three times in 24 hours. Follow by cold friction (**1209**). Protect the surface, and maintain vigorous surface circulation. Large enema (**1404**) 3 times a day; copious water drinking (**1424**); fomentation (**1328**) to lumbar region every 4 hours for 30 minutes, followed by heating compress (**1344**) during interval; ice-bag over lower sternum.

10. **Edema.**—The same treatment as above (9) with the addition of the cold precordial compress (**1383**) 15 minutes every 2 hours.

11. **Delirium.**—Ice-cap (**1323**); ice-collar (**1316**); heating wet-sheet pack (**1183**) continued 1 to 2 hours. Prolonged tepid or neutral bath (**1130**).

12. **Paralysis.**—Ice-cap (**1323**), ice to spine (**1372**); alternate with fomentation (**1328**) for 3 minutes every 15 minutes, repeating four times. Repeat every 4 hours.

13. **Convulsions.**—Ice-cap (**1323**); ice to spine (**1372**); hot hip (**1389**) and leg pack (**1393**). Hot immersion bath (**1126**) 105°, 5 to 8 minutes, with ice to head and neck (**1314**).

14. **Abscess.**—Fomentation (**1328**) for 15 minutes every 2 hours; heating compress (**1344**) at 60° during interval. Renew every 15 to 30 minutes.

15. **Visceral Inflammation.**—Large hot fomentation (1328) over inflamed part for 15 minutes every 2 hours. During the interval, heating compress (1344) at 60°, renewed every 15 minutes during the acute stage. Later, fomentation (1328) 3 times a day, with continuous heating compress (1344) during intervals.

16. **Threatened Gangrene.**—Alternate compresses (1340) every 3 hours, heating compress (1344) or dry heat during intervals.

17. **Typhoid State.**—Aseptic diet (1626); copious water; drinking (1423); neutral enema (1404) (95°) daily; prolonged neutral (1130) or tepid bath (1123); graduated bath (1120) Brand bath if no contraindications (1150, 1489, 65). See Typhoid Fever (1489, 5, 15, etc.).

PULMONARY TUBERCULOSIS.

Etiological Indications. 150

1. Destroy sputum; avoid swallowing sputum; live in the open air and sleep in cool, well-ventilated rooms.

Pathological Indications.

3. **Increase General Vital Resistance.**—Graduated cold baths (1625), twice daily; fattening dietary; systematic exercise; out-of-door life; cool, dry, elevated climate; very short electric-light bath (1250) daily, or three times a week.

Clinical Indications.

4. **Anemia.**—Cold bath twice daily; food rich in fat and blood-making material; easily digested foods rich in proteids, such as kumyss, buttermilk, purées of peas, etc., (1626, 1630, 1631.)

5. **Indigestion—Anorexia.**—Dry aseptic dietary (1626), kumyss, malted cereals (1631). Wet girdle (1347); ice-bag over the stomach half an hour before meals. See Gastric Catarrh (1520) and Hypopepsia (1521).

6. **Chill.**—Rest in bed, dry pack (1192), hot water drinking (1429).

7. **Cough.**—Fomentation (1328) to chest, followed by heating chest pack (1373); sipping hot water when inclined to cough.

8. **Pain.**—Revulsive compress (1341) 15 minutes two or three times daily; during intervals, well-protected heating compress (1379).

9. **Pulmonary Hemorrhage, Pulmonary Congestion.**— Very hot application to spine between shoulders. Ice to chest (**1314**), ice to hands (**1302**). Hot leg pack (**1393**). Keep the extremities warm. Elevate the chest and shoulders.

10. **Fever.**—Neutral pack (**1182**), 15 to 20 minutes. Free water drinking (**1423**). Rest in the horizontal position until the daily evening temperature becomes nearly normal.

11. **Night Sweats.**—Very hot sponging (**1204**) at bedtime.

12. **Hypopepsia.—Atonic Dyspepsia.**—Daily general cold applications (**1625**); ice-bag (**1314**) over stomach for half an hour before meals.

13. **Diarrhea.**—Enema (**1404**) at 95°, after each movement followed by cold abdominal compress (**1318**) at 60°, changing every half hour. Rest in bed till checked.

14. **Cough.**— See **1570**, 4-7.

15. **Laryngitis.**—See **1568**.

16. **Emaciation.**—See **1516**.

17. **Contraindications.**— Avoid general cold baths when hemorrhage is threatened, as immersion bath, affusion and cold sitz-bath, also Turkish and Russian baths.

General Method.— The great object to be kept in mind in the hydriatic treatment of this disease is to build up the patient's vital resistance by carefully graduated cold applications repeated two or three times daily. The intensity of the application should be steadily increased from day to day in order to secure good results. No patient is too feeble to receive hydriatic treatment of some sort, and by careful graduation persons of feeble physique but in whom the disease is not yet far advanced may be trained to receive very vigorous cold applications with excellent effects. In making the cold applications care must be taken to avoid chilling of the patient, the ill effects of which will be at once manifest by aggravation of the cough (**1625**).

TUBERCULOSIS OF LYMPH GLANDS, SCROFULA.

1509 ***Pathological Indications.***

1. **Increase General Vital Resistance.**— Graduated cold applications (**1625**); sun baths (**1254**); cold air baths; gymnastics; out-of-door life; aseptic diet rich in fats and proteids (**1626**); residence in elevated region.

Clinical Indications.

2. Revulsive (**1341**) or alternate compress (**1340**) over swollen glands twice a day. During intervals, flannel-covered heating compress (**1344**) renewed before becoming dry.

3. Suppurating glands must be treated surgically. Removal of the glands is sometimes necessary.

WHOOPING COUGH.

1. **Increase Vital Resistance.**—Cold mitten friction (**1209**) 1510
or cold wet-hand rub (**1213**) three times a day.

2. **To Relieve Cough.**—Chest and neck pack (**1373**) changing every four hours. Copious drinking of hot water (**1429**) especially just before coughing paroxysm. The patient should drink three to eight pints of water daily.

3. Neutral bath (**1130**) daily for a half-hour, followed by cold mitten friction (**1209**) to promote activity of the skin and kidneys.

4. The disease can not be greatly shortened, but the strength may be maintained, suffering mitigated, convalescence facilitated, and grave sequela prevented by the faithful employment of the above measures, which should be continued, not only during the active stage of the disease, but for several weeks after the beginning of convalescence.

LITHEMIA, URIC ACID DIATHESIS.

Etiological Indications. 1511

1. A spare aseptic diet (**1626**), especially avoiding beef tea, animal broths, and also tea, coffee, or cocoa. Use fruits freely. Kumyss or buttermilk is preferable to raw milk. In extreme cases, fruit diet for a few days (**1627**). Out-of-door life; abundant exercise; dry, cool climate; daily cold bathing.

Pathological Indications.

2. **Increase Oxidation of Proteid Wastes.**—Hot bath (**1126**), prolonged sufficiently to elevate body temperature 2° to 4°; sweating wet-sheet pack (**1191**); dry pack (**1192**); vapor bath (**1246**); hot-air (**1233**) or Turkish bath (**1239**). Electric-

light bath (**1250**), or hot full-bath (**1126**), followed by dry pack (**1192**); follow all hot baths by a short, cold application adapted to the patient's condition, cold mitten friction (**1209**), cold towel rub (**1213**), wet-sheet rub (**1216**), dripping sheet (**1217**), shallow bath (**1174**), cold rain douche (**1047**). Follow bath by prolonged moderate exercise, or massage and manual Swedish movements. Inhalation of oxygen; oxygen enema.

3. **Encourage Elimination of Tissue Wastes.**— In addition to above, water drinking (**1423**); free use of fruit juices and carbonated distilled water; wet girdle (**1347**) day and night; cool coloclyster (**1407**) daily, if bowels are sluggish.

4. **Increase Alkalinity of Blood.**— Exercise; cold baths; cold air bath (**1470**); sweating baths; fruit diet (**1627**).

Clinical Indications.

5. **Swollen and Painful Joints.**— Fomentation (**1328**) two to four times daily, heating compress (**1344**) during intervals, well-protected with mackintosh and cotton or flannel covering.

6. **Painful Joints, not Swollen.**— Revulsive compress (**1341**) three times a day, followed by deep massage of limb above the joint and light centrifugal friction (**1224**) of the joint; during intervals, dry pack or cotton poultice (**1388**) to the joint.

7. **Stiff and Enlarged Joints.**— Alternate jet or spray (**1044, 1055**) or the alternate compress (**1340**), followed by thorough massage of the joint with passive joint movements, applied twice daily, well-protected heating compress (**1344**) during intervals.

8. **Headache and Migraine.**— See **1562,** 6, 7, 8, 11, 12.

9. **Neurasthenia.**— See **1554.**

10. **Neuralgia.**— See **1545.**

11. **Insomnia.**— See **1564.**

12. **Muscular Pains.**— See **1513.**

13. **Gall Stones.**— See **1534** B.

14. **Renal Colic.**— See **1536.**

15. **Irritable Prostate.**— See **1594,** 2.

16. **Arterio-Sclerosis.**— See **1577,** 8.

17. **Bright's Disease.**— See **1538.**

18. **Contraindications.**— Prolonged cold baths.

General Method.— Diminish the production of uric acid by regulation of diet (**1626**); increase the destruction of uric acid by exercise, prolonged hot baths (1197, 1233, 1250), followed by short cold applications (1209, 1213); increase elimination of uric acid by copious water drinking (1423).

GOUT.

Etiological Indications. 1512

1. Avoid meats, tea, coffee, tobacco, sometimes even milk and eggs; take daily sufficient exercise in the open air to cause perspiration, followed by short cooling bath. Diet: fruits, dextrinized cereals, nuts, kumyss, buttermilk (1626-1631).

Pathological Indications.

2. **Encourage Tissue Change, Especially Oxidation of Proteid Wastes.**— Prolonged sweating baths — vapor (1246), Turkish (1239), electric-light (1250) or hot-air bath (1233), sweating wet-sheet pack (1187), dry pack (1192), hot-blanket pack (1197), followed by daily cold bath, carefully given, and nicely graduated (1625). Out-of-door life.

3. **Maintain Normal Alkalinity of the Blood.**— Tonic graduated cold applications (1625), free use of fruits; avoid flesh foods, tea, coffee, and alcohol.

See Lithemia (1511).

A. Acute Form.

Clinical Indications.

4. **Headache.**— Water drinking (1423); enema (1404); hot and cold cephalic compress (1358) with hot foot (1297) or leg bath (1393).

5. **Migraine.**— Lavage (1401); revulsive compress to seat of pain (1341); hot leg (1299) or foot bath (1297); enema (1404); hot enema (1406); fomentation over stomach (1328); fomentation over spine (1328); alternate spinal compress (1342).

6. **Constipation.**— Cold enema (1405).

7. **Hemorrhoids.**— If inflamed, hot fomentations (1328) to relieve pain, followed by cold compress (1314) to anal region and buttocks; cool enema.

8. **Pruritis Ani.**— Very hot anal douche (1087).

9. **Pain and Swelling of Joints.**— Elevate limb; cooling compress (1318); change soon as warm.

10. **Fever.**— Hot-blanket pack (1197) followed by prolonged neutral bath (1130).

11. **Scanty Urine.**—Water drinking (**1423**) (distilled carbonated water) (**1428**); enema (**1404**) twice daily. See **1537.**

12. **Retrocedent Gout.**—For coma or delirium, cold to head and neck (**1314**); large enema (**1404**); hot-blanket pack (**1197**); hot immersion (**1126**).

13. **Cardiac Complications, Syncope.**—Hot enema (**1406**); alternate compress to spine (**1342**).

14. **Gastro-Intestinal Disturbance by Retrocession.**—Fomentation (**1328**) over stomach; hot trunk pack (**1197**); hot immersion (**1126**) or hot-blanket pack (**1197**) with heating gastric compress (**1344**) during interval.

15. **Contraindications.**—Avoid cold baths; avoid immersion of affected parts in cold water, and general cold baths.

B. Chronic Form.

16. The general measures indicated above. See also **1511.**

17. **Increase circulation** in affected parts by hot fomentations (**1328**) followed by dry cotton pack (**1388**) or heating compress (**1344**); massage, at first derivative only; later, to joint itself.

18. **Constipation.**—Relaxing diet; wet girdle (**1347**); cold water drinking (**1423**); abdominal massage.

19. **Hepatic Congestion.**—Revulsive hepatic compress (**1341**) every 3 hours; heating compress (**1344**) during interval.

20. **Gravel.**—Copious water drinking (**1423**) and large enema (**1404**) daily. See Uric Acid Diathesis, **1511**.

21. **Melancholy.**—Vigorous sweating baths (**1191, 1250**) followed by short cold percussion douche to the spine (**1074**). See Melancholia (**1558**).

22. **Bronchitis.**—See Chronic Bronchitis, **1570**.

23. **Asthma.**—Scotch douche to legs (**1037**); large enema (**1404**); prolonged neutral bath (**1130**); fomentation (**1328**) to chest followed by the chest pack (**1373**).

24. **Epilepsy.**—See **1551.**

25. **Angina Pectoris.**—Fomentation (**1328**) over heart for 1 minute followed by cool compress (**1314**) for 10 minutes, repeat; hot foot bath (**1297**) or hot leg pack (**1393**); ice bag to spine (**1372**); rest in bed; keep extremities very warm.

General Method.—The general methods to be pursued in this disease are essentially the same as those applicable to the Uric Acid Diathesis, or Lithemia, **1511**.

ACUTE MUSCULAR RHEUMATISM.

Pathological Indications. 1513

1. See Acute Rheumatism, **1499**.

Clinical Indications.

2. The same as for acute articular rheumatism (**1499**) except that the local applications are made to the muscles instead of to the joints. Sweating baths (**1197, 1191**) especially the electric-light bath (**1250**) and the vapor bath (**1246**); long neutral baths (**1130**); fomentation (**1328**) over painful parts followed by the well protected heating compress (**1344**); water drinking (**1423**); aseptic diet (**1626**).

DIABETES.

Pathological Indications. 1514

1. **Increase Oxidation of Sugar.**—A large amount of moderate out-of-door exercise, especially respiratory exercise and daily cold baths.

2. **Increase Absorption of Oxygen.**—Graduated cold baths (**1625**); out-of-door exercise; breathing exercises; oxygen inhalation.

3. **Improve Intestinal Digestion.**—Cold percussion douche (**1035**) to spine; short cold fan douche (**1061**) to abdomen; wet girdle (**1347**) day and night; fomentation to abdomen twice daily; abdominal massage.

4. **Diabetic Diet.**—Eggs, buttermilk, kumyss, gluten biscuit, zwieback, fruits, except dates and figs, green peas, strawberries, spinach, greens, nuts and nut products of all sorts except chestnuts.

Clinical Indications.

5. **Sciatica.**—Hot leg pack (**1393**); Scotch douche (**1037**); rest in bed.

6. **Rheumatic Pains.**—Electric-light bath (**1250**) or sweating pack (**1191**) until patient perspires 5 to 8 minutes. Follow by a suitable cold application.

7. **Obesity.**—Vigorous exercise; monotonous diet; sweating baths (**1191, 1197**) three times a week; vigorous cold applications daily; dripping sheet rubs (**1217**); half bath (**1174**); cooling pack (**1189**); plunge bath (**1108**).

8. **Emaciation.**—Rest in bed; cold mitten friction (**1209**) or towel rubbing (**1213**); massage; diet rich in fats and proteids.

9. **Boils.**—Prolonged neutral baths (**1130**); tri-weekly soap shampoo.

10. **Pruritis.**—Prolonged neutral baths (**1130**) followed by cold mitten friction (**1209**) to sound parts of skin; neutral compress (**1339**).

11. **Somnolence.**—Copious water drinking (**1423**); hot enema (**1406**), repeated every 3 or 4 hours; prolonged neutral bath (**1130**) with cold affusion (**1103**), 60°, to head and spine at intervals of 15 minutes. Hot-blanket pack, 15 minutes (**1197**), followed by cold friction (**1209**) and dry pack (**1192**).

12. **Constipation.**—Enema (**1404**) at 70° daily; wet girdle (**1347**). See **1524.**

13. **Insomnia.**—Prolonged neutral bath (**1130**) at bedtime; neutral pack (**1182**), 30 to 40 minutes; neutral spray (**1057**) or broken douche (**1031**), 3 to 4 minutes at bedtime.

14. **Bronchitis.**—Chest pack (**1373**); steam inhalation (**1419**); Scotch douche (**1037**) to legs.

15. **Pulmonary Congestion.**—See **1572.**

16. **Edema of Legs.**—Rest in bed; cold precordial compress (**1383**), 15 to 30 minutes three times daily. Revulsive compress (**1341**) or Scotch douche (**1037**) to legs three times a day, ollowed during interval by heating compress (**1344**).

17. **Pneumonia.**—See **1498.**

18. **Cardiac Dilatation.**—Cold precordial compress (**1383**) or ice-bag (**1314**) over heart 15 minutes three times a day; effervescent bath (**1139**). Carefully graduated exercises by the Schott method.

19. **Threatened Gangrene.**—Alternate compress (**1340**) or pour (**1103**) to affected part and large adjacent area three times a day; protected heating compress (**1344**) during interval.

20. **Cirrhosis of Liver.**—Alternate hepatic compress (**1340**) or douche (**1044**) twice daily. During interval, well-protected heating compress (**1344**).

21. **Nephritis.**—See **1537.**

22. **Cystitis.**—See **1539.**

23. **Eczema.**—Alkaline bath (**1113, 1463**); or neutral bath (**1130**), 30 minutes twice daily; zinc ointment.

24. **Thirst.**—Frequent drinking of small quantities of cold water, as half a glass every hour. Sipping very hot water.

25. **Dry Skin.**—Vapor bath (1246) or prolonged neutral bath (1130), followed by oil rubbing daily (1232), or two or three times a week.

26. **Contraindications.**—If emaciated, avoid exercise and prolonged hot or cold baths.

General Method.—The general plan of treatment in this disease is essentially the same as that required in the treatment of obesity, which this disease closely resembles, but in cases of diabetes accompanied by emaciation, very cold procedures, especially cold immersions (1114), which are applicable to cases of obesity and cases of diabetes in which the patients are fleshy, must be carefully avoided, and the principal reliance must be placed upon short cold procedures which build up the patient's resistance while increasing oxidation of carbon to a moderate degree. Special attention must be given to improving the intestinal digestion, the faulty character of which is doubtless largely responsible for this disease.

OBESITY.

Pathological Indications. 1515

1. **Increase Oxidation of Hydrocarbons.**—Moderately prolonged cold baths, especially wet-sheet pack (1179); shallow bath (1174); cold rain douche (1047); dripping sheet (1217); shallow bath (1174); plunge bath (1108); exercise to the extent of fatigue several times daily. The cold bath may be advantageously preceded by the electric-light bath (1250), or some other form of sweating bath (1191, 1197) not too prolonged. Exercise should always be preceded by a cold bath of sufficient duration to lower the temperature a few tenths of a degree.

Clinical Indications.

2. **Cardiac Weakness.**—Cold precordial compress (1383) (except in fatty degeneration of heart) 15 to 30 minutes three times daily; graduated exercises, effervescing bath (1140).

3. **Bronchitis.**—See 1570.

4. **Albuminuria.**—See Nephritis 1537.

5. **Diabetes.**—See 1514.

6. **Rheumatic Pains.**—See 1499, 5.

7. **Contraindications.**—Avoid prolonged hot baths unless immediately followed by cold bath.

General Method.—Increase the consumption of carbon by prolonged cold baths (**1114**) and vigorous exercise while reducing the daily ration to the lowest point consistent with the maintenance of the patient's strength. The treatment must never be conducted in such a way as to diminish the patient's muscular or nervous energy. If the patient complains of feeling weak or debilitated, the vigor of the treatment must be diminished. There should be a steady gain in muscular strength accompanying the loss of flesh. The patient's strength should be determined at least weekly by the dynamometer so that his condition may be exactly known. Hot baths are especially debilitating.

EMACIATION.

1516 ***Pathological Indications.***

1. Rest in bed, fat- and blood-making diet (kumyss, buttermilk, eggs, dextrinized cereals [**1630**], malted or predigested cereals [**1631**]); graduated tonic treatment (**1625**). Fomentation (**1328**) over stomach twice daily followed by wet girdle (**1347**).

Clinical Indications.

2. **Persistent Vomiting.**—See **1519**, 3.

3. **Gastric Ulcer.**—Withhold food by mouth; rectal feeding; fomentation (**1328**) over stomach twice daily; well-protected heating compress (**1344**) during interval. Graduated hydriatic treatment. See **1625**.

4. **Chronic Gastritis.**—Rest in bed; abdominal fomentations (**1328**), 2 to 3 times daily; protected heating compress (**1344**) during interval. See **1520**.

5. **Intestinal Catarrh.**—Enema (**1404**) at 95° after each stool. During interval heating compress (**1344**) at 60°, changing every 30 minutes. See **1529**.

6. **Hypopepsia.**—Graduated tonic treatment (**1625**); ice-bag (**1314**) over stomach half an hour before each meal. See **1521**.

7. **Hyperpepsia.**—See **1522**.

8. **Diabetes.**—See **1514**.

9. **Insomnia.**—See **1564**.

10. **Tuberculosis.**—See **1508**.

11. **Chronic Malarial Infection.**—See **1490**.

12. **Chronic Bronchitis.**—See **1571**.

13. **Asthma.**— See 1571, 4.

14. **Drug Habits.**— See 1612.

15. **Pelvic Disease.**— See 1586–1592, 1596.

16. **Rachitis.**— See 1517.

17. **Scurvy, Purpura.**— See 1518.

18. **Contraindications.**— Avoid prolonged hot baths and cold immersion baths.

General Method.— The general plan of treatment must be such as to secure increased income of tissue-building material with a diminished outflow, hence the diet must be very simple, easily assimilable, and taken in as large a quantity as possible. Exercise must be diminished, or in grave cases suspended altogether. Moderate exercise may be allowed if necessary to maintain the appetite. Special attention must be given to increase of the appetite and improvement of digestion by suitable hydriatic applications. Cold applications must be very short and intense, so as to produce strong nervous impressions upon the nerve centers without to any considerable degree removing animal heat or increasing oxidation.

RACHITIS, RICKETS.

Pathological Indications. 1517

1. **Increase General Vital Resistance.**— Carefully graduated hydriatic treatment (1625) applied twice daily; aseptic dietary of substances rich in fats and proteids. Massage (1461); oil rubbing (1232); sun baths (1254); out-of-door life.

SCURVY, PURPURA.

Pathological Indications. 1518

1. **Increase General Vital Resistance.**— Neutral bath (1130) three times a week, 30 to 60 minutes; cold towel rub (1213) carefully administered twice daily; gentle massage. Aseptic dietary (1626); abundance of fruits, kumyss, buttermilk, dextrinized (1630) and malted foods (1631).

Clinical Indications.

2. **Local Pain.**— Alternate sponging (1204) or compress (1340); fomentation (1328), followed by heating compress (1344); rest in bed.

3. **Edema.**— Alternate compress (1340) or spray (1055); leg pack (1393); dry bandaging. Centripetal friction(1221).

ACUTE GASTRIC CATARRH.

1519 ***Etiological Indications.***

1. **Rest.**— Withhold food if necessary, administering food and water by enema for several days (**1404**).

Pathological Indications.

2. **Combat Local Inflammation.**— Fomentation (**1328**) for 15 minutes over stomach and bowels every 2 hours. During intervals, heating compress (**1344**) at 60°, changing every 30 minutes. Hot foot bath (**1297**); hot leg pack (**1393**).

Clinical Indications.

3. **Vomiting.**— Ice-bag (**1314**) to epigastrium; hot and cold gastric compress (**1362**); hot and cold trunk pack (**1367**); ice (**1372**) to spine opposite stomach; careful lavage (**1401**) if vomiting is persistent and rejected matters offensive.

4. **Pain.**— Revulsive compress (**1341**) 10 minutes every hour. Heating compress (**1344**) during interval.

5. **Fever.**— Hot-blanket pack (**1197**) 20 minutes, followed by cold half pack (**1196**); prolonged neutral bath (**1130**); cooling pack (**1189**), following fomentation (**1328**) over stomach.

6. **Contraindications.**— Cold immersion baths and general cold douche.

CHRONIC GASTRITIS.

1520 ***Etiological Indications.***

1. **Avoid causes,** as, mustard, pepper, vinegar, strong acids, even acid fruits; sugar, preserves, cheese, alcoholic beverages, tea and coffee, all indigestible and irritating substances, coarse vegetables, pickles, confectionery, and hasty eating.

2. **Physiological Rest.**— Avoid the use of fish, fowl, game, and all flesh foods, which excite the secretion of HCl and remain long in the stomach. Coarse vegetables, fried foods, fats, except in a natural emulsified condition, large meals, tea, coffee, wines, and all liquors are to be avoided.

Pathological Indications.

3. **Increase General Vital Resistance.**— Graduated cold baths (**1625**) twice daily.

4. **Combat Local Congestion.**— Gastric fomentation (**1328**)

three times daily, 15 min.; during intervals, heating compress (**1344**). Hot leg pack (**1393**) followed by heating compress (**1344**) to legs; Scotch douche (**1037**) to legs; hot leg bath (**1299**), followed by cold friction (**1209**) to legs. In acute exacerbations, withhold all food, rest in bed.

Clinical Indications.

5. **Mucus Vomiting in Morning.**— Omit the evening meal. Fomentation (**1328**) over stomach in evening followed by heating compress (**1344**) to be worn during the night; lavage (**1401**) at bedtime.

6. **Vomiting Soon after Eating.**— Hot and cold gastric compress (**1362**) or trunk pack (**1367**) half an hour before eating, to be retained 2 hours; dry food in small quantity; rest in bed after eating; ice-bag to spine after eating.

7. **Gaseous Eructations.**— Lavage (**1401**) once or twice a week; dry diet of predigested cereals (**1630**). Cold compress (**1314**); heating compress (**1344**) over stomach at 60°, changing every 4 hours. Massage for half an hour 2 hours after eating, if local irritation or tenderness does not contraindicate. Drink pint of hot water half an hour before eating. Avoid use of vegetables, or of vegetables and fruits at same meal.

8. **Abdominal Tympanitis.**— Abdominal heating compress (**1351**), 60°, changed every 4 hours; large soap enema (**1404**) or coloclyster (**1407**) two or three times a week, at 70°.

9. **Constipation.**— Graduated cold enema (**1409**) 70°, daily. Abdominal massage; wet girdle (**1347**); cold douche to abdomen (**1081**), fan (**1061**) or broken jet (**1010**), 20 seconds; cold rubbing sitz (**1309**).

10. **Hepatic Congestion.**— Fomentation (**1328**) over liver twice daily; during interval, continuous heating compress (**1344**).

11. **Emaciation.**— Rest in bed; mild tonic hydriatic treatment, carefully graduated (**1625**). Ice-bag (**1314**) over stomach half an hour before eating. See **1516**.

12. **Pain in Stomach.**— Revulsive compress (**1341**) over epigastrium; repeat several times daily if necessary. Avoid acid fruits, very hot foods, very cold foods, and concentrated sweets if they cause pain.

HYPOPEPSIA AND APEPSIA.

1521 ***Pathological Indications.***

1. **Increase General Vital Resistance.**—Graduated tonic hydriatic treatment (**1625**) twice daily; out-of-door life; cold-air bath (**733, 1470**); swimming.

2. **Increase Activity of Gastric Glands.**—Cold fan douche (**1061**) over stomach; cold percussion douche (**1035**) to dorsal spine; general cold douche (**1010**) or other cold procedure (**1625**); wet girdle (**1347**); external and internal galvanism of stomach. Drink a third of a glass of cold water half an hour before eating.

3. **Increase Motility.**—Cold gastric douche (**1094**) 3 hours after meals; small cold enema, retained, three to four hours after eating; abdominal massage; manual and mechanical Swedish movements; galvanization of cervical and abdominal sympathetic.

Clinical Indications.

4. **Indigestion, Biliousness.**—Hydrochloric acid being absent, flesh meats must be withheld. Aseptic diet (**1626**); avoid fried foods, rich gravies and animal fats, which lessen the secretion of HCl (Pawlow), cane sugar, and concentrated sweets. Hot applications over the stomach an hour after eating.

5. **Loss of Appetite.**—Ice-bag over stomach half an hour before each meal; hot and cold gastric lavage (page 886); cold mitten friction (**1209**) before breakfast; repeat before dinner if necessary; small cold enema (**1404**) or cold rectal irrigation (**1410**) before breakfast.

HYPERPEPSIA.

1522 ***Etiological Indications.***

1. Avoid irritating food substances, mustard, pepper, spices, condiments of all sorts, flesh foods of all sorts, excess of proteids, hot foods, mushes, farinaceous and sweet desserts, frequent meals.

Pathological Indications.

2. **Increase General Vital Resistance.**—Graduated tonic hydriatic treatment (**1625**) twice daily.

3. **Combat Irritation of Gastric Glands, or Hypersecretion.**—Revulsive compress (**1341**) twice daily, an hour before meals; continuous heating compress (**1351**) without mackintosh during

interval. Avoid cold douche over stomach and spine opposite, and prolonged cold baths. Hot douche (**1024**) or fomentation over stomach and spine opposite 3 to 4 times daily. Hot immersion bath (**1126**) at 105° for 15 minutes, or electric-light bath 10 minutes, half an hour before dinner. Follow by cold mitten friction (**1209**). Sip half a glass of hot water half hour before eating.

4. **Combat Toxemia.**— Sweating procedures; electric-light bath (**1250**); sweating pack (**1191**); vapor bath (**1246**); prolonged neutral bath (**1130**); follow hot baths by short cold application, as a wet-sheet rub (**1216**), cold towel rub (**1213**), cold shower (**1047**), douche with broken jet (**1010**). Water drinking (**1423**). Enema (**1404**) daily for a week or two, 70°, injecting a second portion to be retained.

5. **Flatulence of Stomach and Bowels.**— Cold abdominal compress (**1318**), changed every 4 hours; cold enema, following fomentation for 15 minutes twice a day.

6. **Painful Digestion.**— Hot fomentation (**1328**) an hour after eating for 15 minutes, followed by heating compress (**1344**) to be worn until next meal.

7. **Gastric Irritation with Vomiting After Eating.**— Hot and cold gastric compress (**1362**) or hot and cold trunk pack (**1367**) applied half an hour before eating and continued for 2 hours.

8. **Contraindications.**— Cold douche over stomach, cold shower, and prolonged cold baths of all sorts.

DILATATION OF THE STOMACH.

Etiological Indications. 1523

Aseptic diet (**1626**); avoid overeating, frequent eating, and gas-forming foods, also drinking large quantities at once. Give very simple dry dietary of well-dextrinized (**1630**) or predigested (**1631**) cereals or liquid diet,— kumyss, acid buttermilk, purées, or gruels prepared from predigested cereals, nut creams or emulsions.

Pathological Indications.

1. **Combat Gaseous Distension of Stomach.**— Lavage (**1401**) at regular intervals as required to prevent food accumuation. Cold gastric compress (**1314**) without impervious cover-

ing, changed every 4 hours; cold fan douche (**1061**) over stomach twice daily.

2. **Increase General Vital Resistance, Combat Autointoxication.**— Short sweating baths,— electric-light bath (**1250**); sweating wet-sheet pack (**1187**); hot immersion (**1126**) 4 to 6 minutes, at 105°; hot-blanket pack (**1197**); hot enema (**1405**). Follow each hot bath by a tonic application (**1625**).

Clinical Indications.

3. **Vomiting.**— Lavage (**1401**); withholding food; if persistent, feeding by nutrient enema; ice-bag (**1314**) over stomach and to spine opposite.

4. **Pyrosis.**— Hot water drinking (**1429**) before retiring at night; fomentation (**1328**) over stomach at bedtime, with wet girdle (**1347**) overnight; sipping half a glass of very hot water on rising in the morning. A few ounces of orange juice or other natural, unsweetened fruit juice a half-hour before eating.

5. **Enteroptosis.**— Massage with replacement of viscera, electricity to abdominal muscles; manual Swedish movements to strengthen abdominal muscles; cold fan douche (**1061**) to abdomen; abdominal supporter.

6. **Constipation.**— Graduated cold enema (**1409**); cold douche (**1010**) to abdomen; wet girdle (**1347**); regularity at stool. See **1524.**

6. **Pain.**— Fomentation over the abdomen (**1328**) followed by heating compress (**1344**), protected by flannel only.

Complications.

7. **Neurasthenia.**— See **1554.**

8. **Hysteria.**— See **1553.**

9. **Delirium.**— Hot-blanket pack (**1197**) followed by cold mitten friction (**1209**); heating wet-sheet pack (**1183**), succeeded by dry pack (**1192**); lavage (**1401**); coloclyster (**1407**).

10. **Coma.**— Lavage; coloclyster; hot and cold head compress (**1358**); hot and cold to spine (**1342**); hot-blanket pack (**1197**); hot enema (**1406**); ice-cap (**1323**); cold towel rub (**1213**) or cold mitten friction (**1209**).

11. **Cardiac Palpitation.**— Lavage (**1401**); ice-bag (**1314**) over heart 15 minutes every hour.

12. **Aortic Palpitation.**— Rest in horizontal position; ice-bag

(**1314**) over aorta; abdominal supporter when on feet; enema (**1404**) if colon is distended; gastric lavage (**1401**) if the stomach is foul.

13. **Anorexia.**— Graduated cold baths (**1625**); wet-sheet pack (**1179**) once or twice a week; short electric-light bath (**1250**) two to three times a week; sun bath (**1254**) daily; cold-air bath (**733, 1470**) daily; ice-bag over stomach half an hour before meals; cool sitz (**1305**); general and abdominal massage; manual Swedish movements; application of faradic or sinusoidal current to principal groups of muscles so as to cause contraction.

14. **Hiccough.**—Lavage (**1401**) when due to gastric irritation and stasis of food. Faradization, one electrode to spine, the other below ribs, right and left sides, of sufficient strength to contract the muscles strongly. Continue 5 to 15 minutes. Slowly sip half a pint of iced carbonated water; hold breath for half a minute; pressure with hands over the stomach, forcing the viscera up against the diaphragm. Hot and cold gastric compress (**1362**); ice-bag to back of neck; ice pills; ice-bag to epigastrium (**664**).

CONSTIPATION.

1. **Increase Peristaltic Activity.**— Drink half a pint to a 1524
pint of cold water before breakfast, preferably carbonated water. Increase bulk of food, with free use of fruit, especially apples, oranges, and figs. Granose is especially to be commended; also nut products, malted nuts, cereals, bran cakes, and figs. Small cold enema (**1404**); graduated enema (**1409**); fomentation (**1328**) over liver twice daily followed by heating compress (**1344**) during interval. Wet girdle (**1347**) at night. Abdominal massage. Cold fan douche (**1061**) to abdomen; cold percussion douche (**1035**) to spine. Cold plantar douche (**1083**) 1 to 3 minutes; cold rubbing sitz, 70° to 75° (**1309**), 5 to 20 minutes. Avoid complete emptying of colon, using small cold enema instead of a large quantity of warm water, except when necessary to relieve autointoxication, or remove hardened or impacted feces. If necessary, introduce into rectum, as high as possible, at night or before breakfast, to be retained till next stool, a small pledget of cotton saturated with raw linseed oil or with glycerin.

2. **Increase Activity of Intestinal Glands.**— Half a pint to a pint of water at bedtime, to be retained overnight; abdominal massage; wet girdle, without mackintosh (**1347**). Boracic acid powder before breakfast, introduction of absorbent cotton saturated with oil or glycerin at night or before breakfast.

3. **Remove Accumulated Fecal Matters.**—Large hot enema or coloclyster; neutral enema; warm soap enema; oil enema; glycerin enema (one part glycerin to four water) (**1404**). Repeat the application till bowel is thoroughly emptied, then inject a pint of water at 70° to 60° to tone the bowel.

4. **Dilatation of Colon.**— Graduated enema (**1409**); cold fan douche (**1061**) to abdomen and spine opposite; running cold foot bath (**1296**); cold rubbing sitz (**1309**); cold wet girdle, without mackintosh (**1347**), changing every 4 hours.

5. **Increase Strength of Abdominal Muscles.**— Cold fan douche (**1061**); cold plantar douche (**1083**); percussion abdominal douche (**1081**); cold abdominal compress (**1318**); renewed every 4 hours, without impervious covering; sinusoidal electricity; massage; special exercises, particularly head raising and legs raising while lying upon the back.

6. **Enteroptosis.**— Restore prolapsed bowels to position; strengthen abdominal muscles as indicated above; correct sitting position; abdominal supporter; replace viscera daily. See **1525.**

7. **Hemorrhoids.**—Long cold sitz bath (**1305**); cool anal douche (**1087**); cold anal compress (**1395**); small cold enema (**1405**); if inflamed, rest in bed, fomentations over the nates followed by cold compress (**1395**). Repeat fomentations every 3 hours. Surgery if necessary.

8. **Pain.**— If due to *fissure*, hot applications; sitting over steam. If due to *irritable rectum*, hot irrigation (**1410**). For *pain in the abdomen*, revulsive compress (**1341**); Scotch douche (**1037**); hot enema at 110°, followed by small cool enema (**1404**); revulsive sitz (**1311½**).

9. **Relieve Spasm of Sphincter Ani Muscle.**— Prolonged neutral (**1312**) or hot sitz bath (**1311**); warm rectal irrigation (**1410**); hot rectal irrigation (**1410**); fomentations (**1328**) over the nates. Dilatation sometimes required.

10. **Restore Sensibility of Rectum.**— Alternate irrigation of the rectum (**1410**); cold douche to lower spine and nates (**1076**).

Shallow cold sitz (1305); cold anal douche (1087); alternate anal douche (1046); sinusoidal electricity to rectum.

11. **Contraindications.**— Sweating baths sometimes induce constipation (1176), also abuse of the fomentation and the habitual use of the warm enema, which should be strictly avoided. If the enema is used daily, the temperature, at least at the conclusion, should be 65° to 75°, so that a tonic effect may be secured.

General Method.— Each case must be carefully studied with reference to the leading cause or causes which are operative in the individual case. Most important of these are,—a paretic or atonic condition of the intestine through disturbed or defective innervation; diminished intestinal secretion or an abnormal absorption of intestinal secretion resulting in unusually dry and solid fecal mass; dilatation of the colon, giving rise to accumulation; relaxation and weakness of the abdominal muscles with lowered intra-abdominal tension; hemorrhoids and other diseases of the rectum; prolapse of the colon and other abdominal viscera; loss of normal sensibility of the rectum; spasm of the anal sphincter.

ENTEROPTOSIS.

Etiological Indications. 1525

1. Correct sitting and standing positions; corrective gymnastics and manual Swedish movements; sinusoidal electricity to muscles of the trunk. Avoidance of waist constriction by belts, corsets, or heavy skirts. Cold fan douche (1061) to abdomen; cold plantar douche (1083).

Pathological Indications.

2. **Replace the Viscera.**— Replace viscera daily by abdominal massage, genu-pectoral position, inspiratory lifting, etc; abdominal supporter; combined support of abdomen and shoulders.

3. **Strengthen the Abdominal Muscles.**— Cold fan douche to abdomen (1061); cold plantar douche (1083; special exercises, particularly raising head, both legs, head and legs simultaneously or in alternation, inspiratory lifting; knee-chest position; electricity, applied so as to cause rhythmical contraction of abdominal muscles, preferably the slowly alternated sinusoidal current; swimming; Swedish gymnastics; abdominal massage.

Clinical Indications.

4. **Abdominal Tenderness and Discomfort.**— Fomentation (**1328**) twice daily; wet girdle (**1347**); abdominal supporter; hot enema followed by small cold enema (**1404**).

5. **Indigestion.**—Aseptic dietary (**1626**); massage to empty the stomach 2 hours after eating. Massage (**1461**) when required. See Hypopepsia and Dilatation of Stomach (**1521, 1523**).

6. **Pain between Shoulders.**—Fomentation (**1328**) to back; gastric heating compress (**1344**); abdominal supporter.

7. **Backache.**— Fomentation (**1328**); revulsive compress (**1341**); alternate sponging (**1206**) or compress (**1340**); heating spinal compress (**1355**); Scotch douche (**1037**); abdominal supporter.

8. **Neurasthenia.**— See **1554.**

9. **Headache.**— See **1554,** 11–15, **1562.**

10. **Hysteria.**— See **1553.**

11. **Nervous Asthma.**— Hot enema (**1406**); hot water drinking (a pint or more); fomentation to abdomen (**1328**); fomentation to back; wet girdle day and night (**1347**); hot and cold trunk pack daily (**1367**); abdominal supporter; galvanism to abdominal sympathetic; abdominal massage with replacement of viscera.

12. **Constipation.**—Graduated cold enema (**1409**). See **1524.**

General Method.—General tonic treatment to improve innervation; special massage to restore viscera to position; a properly adjusted abdominal supporter; special gymnastics for exercising the abdominal muscles; the daily application of electricity as a means of passive exercise of the muscles of the abdomen and loins; and the cultivation of an upright and forcible attitude in sitting and standing, the abdominal muscles being well drawn in, are the essential features of the rational method of dealing with this disorder.

GASTRIC ULCER.

1526 ***Etiological Indications.***

1. Rest in bed; rectal feeding for 2 weeks, repeating after a few days if necessary; bland aseptic liquid diet (**1626, 1628**); avoid solid food, condiments, flesh foods.

Pathological Indications.

2. Revulsive compress (**1341**) three times a day, heating compress (**1344**) during intervals; hot fomentation (**1328**) or hot douche to spine (**1074**).

Clinical Indications.

3. **Pain.**— Revulsive compress (**1341**); gastric fomentation (**1328**); heat to spine (**1335**); hot-blanket pack to hips and legs (**1393**).

4. **Vomiting.**— Ice pills; carbonated water; lavage (**1401**) if stomach is foul and no recent hemorrhage.

5. **Hemorrhage.**— Rest in bed; ice-bag over stomach; hot hip and leg pack (**1197**). Withhold foods and drink by stomach. administering water and food by enema.

NERVOUS DYSPEPSIA.

Pathological Indications. 1527

1. **Irritation of Solar Plexus and Abdominal Sympathetic.** — Fomentation (**1328**) twice a day; during interval, apply heating compress (**1344**), changing every 4 hours, except during sleep. Abdominal compress (**1351**) during the night; dry bandage (**1353**) during the day; abdominal supporter when enteroptosis exists.

Clinical Indications.

2. **General Weakness.**— Graduated cold baths (**1625**) twice daily; percussion douche to spine.

3. **Heartburn.**— Dry aseptic dietary (**1626**); gastric fomentation (**1328**) followed by heating compress (**1344**).

4. **Eructations and Regurgitations of Food.**— Fomentation (**1328**) over the stomach twice daily; continuous heating compress (**1344**) during the interval, without impervious covering, renewing every 4 hours.

5. **Spinal Irritation.**— Fomentation (**1328**) at night followed by heating spinal compress (**1355**) to be worn during the night; wet girdle (**1347**).

6. **Cold Extremities.**— Scotch douche (**1037**); running cold foot bath (**1296**); leg pack (**1393**); massage (**1461**).

7. **Headache.**— Hot and cold head compress (**1358**); alternate spinal sponging (**1342**), cool compress if congestion is present; massage to head and neck.

8. **Anorexia.**— Ice-bag over stomach half an hour before eating; cold spinal douche (**1074**); cold air bath (**733, 1470**); out-of-door life; small cold enema before breakfast, retained.

9. **Abdominal Weight and Tenderness.**— Abdominal supporter; hot fan douche (**1063**) to abdomen; hot foot bath (**1297**); revulsive sitz (**1308**); fomentation (**1328**) twice daily, followed by heating compress (**1344**).

10. **Excessive Peristalsis.**— Hot and cold abdominal compress (**1356**); abdominal fomentation twice daily, followed by wet girdle (**1347**) protected with mackintosh; abdominal supporter.

11. **Asthma** —Nervous or reflex asthma, is commonly associated with dilated or prolapsed stomach, and irritable lumbar sympathetic ganglia. The most important palliative measures are the hot and cold trunk pack (**1367**); fomentation (**1328**) over abdomen twice daily, followed by heating compress (**1344**) to be worn during intervals; hot enema (**1406**); hot immersion bath (**1126**); general tonic treatment (**1625**); Scotch douche to legs. See Enteroptosis (**1525**) and Dilatation of the Stomach (**1523**).

General Method.— The general method consists in improving the nerve tone, allaying general nervous irritability, lessening gastric irritation and improving the general nutrition by the appropriate measures as indicated above.

ACUTE GASTRO-INTESTINAL CATARRH IN CHILDREN,
1528 CHOLERA INFANTUM, SUMMER DIARRHEA

1. Withdraw all food; hot-blanket pack (**1197**) till skin is reddened; follow by cold mitten friction (**1209**) or cold wet-hand rubbing (**1213**). If temperature is high, heating wet-sheet pack (**1183**), repeated if necessary. Rest in bed.

2. **Persistent Vomiting.**— Gastric lavage (**1401**); ice-bag (**1314**) to stomach.

3. **Frequent Stools.**— Hot enema (**1406**), at 105° to 110° after every stool; fomentation (**1328**) to abdomen every 3 hours, followed by heating compress (**1344**), changing every 20 minutes.

4. **Pain in Abdomen.**— Revulsive abdominal compress (**1341**) for 15 to 20 minutes every hour or two.

5. **Collapse.**—Hot-blanket pack (1197) until warm, followed by prolonged neutral bath (1130) at 92° to 95°. Hot water drinking (1424); large warm (98°) enema (1406).

CHRONIC INTESTINAL CATARRH, CHRONIC DIARRHEA.

Pathological Indications. 1529

1. **To Lessen Congestion.**—Rest in bed. Enema (1404), 95°, after each stool, followed by half a pint of cold water. Fomentation (1328) to abdomen twice daily, 15 minutes; during interval, heating abdominal compress (1351) renewed every 2 hours. The heating compress should be covered with flannel only.

2. **To Discourage Bacterial Growth.**—Aseptic dietary, especially fruit juices, purées, dextrinized cereals, kumyss, beaten eggs. Cleanse colon by large hot enema daily, following by small enema (pint) of gallic or tannic acid solution (dram to pint).

3. **To Combat Weakness and Autointoxication.**—Short sweating baths, 3 to 8 minutes, and graduated cold baths (1625).

Clinical Indications.

4. **Pain in Abdomen with Tenderness.**—Fomentation (1328) to abdomen every 2 to 3 hours; hot enema (1406), 110°, after each stool; heating abdominal compress (1344) after each hot application, to be changed once an hour until the next hot application is made.

5. **Gas in Intestines.**—See 1520, 8.

6. **Gastric Symptoms.**—See 1520–1523.

7. **Neurasthenic Symptoms.**—See 1554.

8. **Mucous Stools.**—Large hot enema (1404) at 95° followed by small cold enema (1405); cold abdominal compress (1318) changed every hour. Revulsive sitz (1308) or compress to abdomen (1341); Scotch (1037) fan douche (1061) to abdomen.

9. **Frequent Stools.**—Abdominal compress as above; prolonged cool sitz (1309) at 75°, 15 minutes, followed by short hot affusion (1103) to spine, and wet-sheet rub (1216).

10. **Alternating Constipation and Diarrhea.**—Large warm (98°) soap enema (1406), or coloclyster (1407), once or twice a week; follow with small cold enema (1405); wet girdle (1347).

11. **Contraindications.**—Cold douche, protected heating compress, prolonged fomentations.

General Method.—Increase the general vital resistance and improve gastric conditions, regulating the diet so as to render the intestine an unfavorable habitat for the bacteria which constitute the chief cause of this disease; remove bacteria and masses of mucus and pseudomembrane by neutral enemas (**1404**), and follow by small enemas of gallic or tannic acid solution, which destroy the germs associated with this disease.

1530 ACUTE DYSENTERY, COLITIS.

1. Free water drinking (**1423**); an aseptic dietary; no animal broths or meat preparations (**1626**). Browned rice, kumyss, buttermilk, fresh ripe fruit, fruit juices, with well-dextrinized cereals (**1630**), are proper foods.

2. **To Combat Visceral Inflammation.**—Hot-blanket pack, (**1197**) with hot hip and leg pack (**1197**), followed by heating abdominal compress (**1344**), 60°, changed every 20 to 40 minutes; ice suppositories if the inflammation extends into the rectum. Cold sitz (**1305**), 75°, 15 to 30 minutes, with hot foot bath (**1297**). Cold irrigation of the rectum (**1410**). Rest in bed.

3. **To Relieve Pain.**—Very hot pelvic pack, with hot foot bath (**1297**); very hot enema (**1406**), 110°, followed by cold rectal irrigation (**1410**); repeat hourly if required.

1531 CHRONIC DYSENTERY, CHRONIC COLITIS.

Rest in bed; aseptic dietary (**1626**); graduated cold baths (**1625**) twice daily; cold rubbing sitz (**1309**); hot revulsive sitz bath (**1311**) 6 to 10 minutes daily, immediately preceded by a hot enema (**1406**).

If much pain is present, revulsive sitz (**1308, 1311**) once or twice a day. Moist abdominal bandage (**1347**).

1532 CHOLERA MORBUS.

1. Secure physiological rest of stomach and bowels by withholding food. Rest in bed.

2. **Vomiting.**—Ice-bag (**1314**) over stomach. Ice pills; ice compress to the throat. (**1314**). Fomentation (**1328**) to spine; ice-bag (**1314**) to spine; hot and cold trunk pack (**1367**); lavage (**1401**).

3. **Diarrhea.**—Hot enema (**1406**) after each stool; fomentation (**1328**) over abdomen every 2 hours, duration 20 minutes during interval, heating compress (**1344**) at 60°, renewed every 30 minutes. If the temperature is above 102°, prolonged neutral bath (**1130**) or hot-blanket pack (**1197**) followed by cold friction (**1209**) or cold towel rub (**1213**).

4. **Collapse.**—Hot-blanket pack (**1197**) 15 minutes, followed by cold mitten friction (**1209**).

5. **Cardiac Weakness.**—Ice-bag (**1314**) over heart.

APPENDICITIS. 1533

1. Withhold food. Rest in bed. Large hot enema (**1406**), repeated every 6 hours; fomentation (**1328**) 15 minutes every hour; during interval, heating compress (**1344**) at 60°, changed every 10 minutes. As inflammation is subdued, prolong interval between fomentations, and change cold compress less frequently. Fomentation at night followed by heating compress over affected region (**1344**) for several months, if necessary.

2. **Intestinal Obstruction.**—Large hot coloclyster (**1407**); hot bath (**1126**). If speedy relief is not obtained, surgical measures should be employed.

JAUNDICE. 1534

A. Catarrhal Form.

1. **General.**—Cold mitten friction (**1209**); cold towel rub (**1213**); rest in bed; aseptic diet (**1626**).

2. **Pain.**—Fomentation (**1328**) over stomach and liver for 15 minutes every 2 or 3 hours; during interval, heating compress (**1344**) at 60°, renewed every 30 minutes. Copious hot enema (**1406**), 110°, twice a day. After discharge of hot-water, an enema of one pint water at 70°. Hot trunk pack (**1197**); hot immmersion bath (**1126**) 104°, 10 min.; cold towel rub (**1213**), or wet sheet rub (**1216**).

3. **Fever.**—Sweating wet sheet pack (**1191**); vapor bath (**1246**); electric light bath (**1250**); copious water drinking (**1423**).

4. **Headache.**—Hot and cold head compress (**1358**); evaporating head compress (**1324**); cold cephalic compress (**1371**); hot sponging (**1204**) of back of neck.

5. **Itching.**—Neutral saline bath (**1464**); hot sponging (**1204**).

6. **Chill.**— Hot water drinking (**1429**); dry pack (**1192**).

7. **Gastric Catarrh.**— See Chronic Gastritis **1520.**

B. Biliary Colic — Gall-stone.

1. **General.**— Fruit diet (**1627**); water drinking (**1423**); liquid aseptic dietary (**1628**).

2. **Pain.**— Revulsive compress (**1341**) every two hours; continuous hot applications to hepatic region; hot coloclyster (**1407**), or enema (**1406**), every 2 hours; hot immersion bath (**1126**).

3. **Fever.**— Prolonged neutral bath (**1130**); hot-blanket pack (**1197**) followed by wet-sheet pack (**1216**); cold mitten friction (**1209**) or cold towel rub (**1213**).

4. **Nausea and Vomiting.**— Lavage (**1401**) if persistent. See **1519,** 3.

5. After acute attack, administer treatment for Gastro-intestinal Catarrh. See **1529.**

CIRRHOSIS OF THE LIVER.

1535 ***Etiological Indications.***

1. Avoid tea, coffee, tobacco, alcoholics, condiments. Aseptic dietary (**1626**).

Pathological Indications.

2. **Organic Changes in Liver.**— Alternate douche (**1044**), alternate compress (**1340**); Scotch douche (**1037**); flannel-covered heating compress (**1344**). Follow local application by genaral douche (**1010**,) or wet-sheet rub (**1216**).

Clinical Indications.

3. **Pain.**— Fomentation (**1328**); revulsive compress (**1341**) or douche (**1041**), with hot leg bath (**1299**) or pack (**1393**) followed by compress (**1344**), twice a day.

4. **Jaundice.**— Wet sheet pack (**1179**) followed by wet sheet rub (**1216**); electric-light bath (**1250**) followed by graduated shower (**1047**) or wet-sheet rub (**1216**).

5. **Dropsy.**— Scotch douche (**1037**) to legs and abdomen; trunk pack (**1349**); strong faradic application to abdomen.

6. **General Weakness.**— Carefully graduated tonic baths (**1625**); neutral bath (**1130**); neutral galvanic bath (**1451**); sun baths (**1254**); out-of-door life.

7. **Contraindications.**— Cold immersions and very cold general or prolonged cold douche.

RENAL COLIC.

1. **During Attack.**— Rest in bed; diet of fruit (**1627**), kumyss, or buttermilk; hot water drinking (**1423**); hot enema (**1406**), repeat every two hours; hot immersion bath (**1126**) cold to head and over the heart, if the bath is greatly prolonged; hot trunk pack (**1197**) renewed hourly; revulsive sitz (**1308**); cold precordial compress (**1383**) if heart is weak or much excited. 1536

2. **To Prevent Attacks.**— Combat lithemia. See **1511**.

3. **Vomiting.**— Ice pills; ice to throat.

4. **Urinary Suppression.**— Hot-blanket pack (**1197**) followed by dry sweating pack (**1192**).

ACUTE NEPHRITIS.

Pathological Indications. 1537

1. **Relieve Renal Congestion.**— Congest the skin by means of the hot trunk pack (**1197**), hot-blanket pack (**1197**), or hot immersion bath (**1126**) continued to perspiration, followed by friction, avoiding deep massage procedures. Rubbing until vigorous perspiration is induced. Maintain active cutaneous circulation; fomentation to loins for 30 minutes every 3 or 4 hours, heating lumbar compress (**1344**) during interval.

2. **Encourage Renal Activity.**— Ice-bag (**1314**) over lower third of sternum; hot enema (**1406**); hot water drinking (**1429**); prolonged neutral bath (**1130**).

3. **Encourage Elimination of Toxins.**— Hot (**1406**) or cold enema (**1405**) twice daily. Prolonged hot-blanket pack (**1197**); sweating wet-sheet pack (**1191**); electric-light bath (**1250**); vapor bath (**1246**); copious water drinking (**1423**).

Clinical Indications.

4. **Nausea.**— Hot and cold gastric compress (**1362**); ice-bag over the stomach (**1314**); sipping very hot water (**1429**).

5. **Diet.**— Fruit juice; fruit purées; buttermilk or kumyss.

6. **Cardiac Weakness.**— Ice-bag (**1314**) over heart for 15 minutes every 2 hours; cold mitten friction (**1209**); cold towel rub (**1213**) 2 or 3 times daily.

7. **Contraindications.**— Prolonged general cold applications, Brand bath, cold douche, cold affusion.

General Method.— Absolute rest in bed; maintaining a warm and active skin even to the extent of perspiration; an aseptic, liquid dietary (**1628**) to encourage free diuresis, copious water drinking.

CHRONIC NEPHRITIS, BRIGHT'S DISEASE.

1538 1. **General.**— Aseptic dietary (**1626**); especially avoid meats and condiments; buttermilk or kumyss diet or exclusive fruit diet (**1627**) during acute attack; tea, coffee, tobacco, and alcoholic liquors to be strictly avoided.

2. **Maintain activity of skin** by warm woolen clothing, dry friction (**1221**), applied daily; cold mitten friction (**1209**) followed by dry friction (**1221**); oil rubbing (**1232**). Carefully graduated cold applications (**1625**). Electric-light bath (**1250**) followed by cold towel rub (**1213**). Sweating bath (**1197**) twice a week at bedtime, followed by cold mitten friction (**1209**).

3. **Acute Exacerbation.**— Apply treatment recommended for acute Bright's disease (**1537**).

4. **Dropsy.**— Short electric-light bath (**1250**), followed by cold mitten friction (**1209**) or cold towel rub (**1213**), water drinking (**1423**), one to two pints twice daily; efferverscent bath (**1139**).

5. **Contraindications.**— Cold immersions, prolonged cold douche, frequently repeated, or prolonged hot baths.

General Method.— The essential features are a carefully regulated regimen adapted to the patient's condition, warm clothing, avoidance of chill, frequent neutral baths (**1130**), very gentle tonic measures, copious water drinking (**1423**), perfect digestion and bowel action, an aseptic dietary (**1626**), out-of-door life, avoidance of exposure to cold and excesses of every description especially sexual and dietetic excesses.

CYSTITIS AND IRRITABLE BLADDER.

1539 1. **Inflammation.**— Copious water drinking (**1423**), revulsive sitz (**1308**) twice a day; hot leg packs (**1393**) followed by dry heat to legs; neutral bath (**1130**) 20 to 40 minutes two or three times a week; prolonged neutral sitz (**1312**); cold friction; cold towel rub (**1213**); fomentation (**1328**) over bladder; bladder irrigation (**1411**); hot enema (**1406**); hot pelvic pack (**1390**); aseptic dietary (**1626**).

2. **Irritable bladder,** inflammation not present. Very hot sitz (**1311**) for five minutes, followed by neutral sitz (**1312**) for 10 to 20 minutes. Hot pelvic pack (**1390**); heating compress (**1344**) over perineum and genitals; revulsive sitz (**1308**); hot rectal irrigation (**1410**).

3. **Contraindications.**—Cold sitz, cold immersion, cold douche, cold foot bath.

INCONTINENCE OF URINE.

1. **To Increase Energy of Bladder.**—Cold plantar douche 1540
(**1083**) 1 to 2 minutes; cold running foot bath (**1296**); cold percussion douche (**1035**) to hips and legs, 60° to 65°; cold douche (**1076**) to lumbar region; cold fan douche (**1061**) at 65° over bladder. Cold rubbing sitz (**1309**). Irrigation with normal saline or boracic acid solution; begin at 100°, and lower temperature 1° daily to 80°.

2. **Relieve Vesical Irritation.**—Revulsive sitz (**1308**); hot pelvic pack (**1390**); prolonged neutral sitz (**1312**) following revulsive sitz (**1308**). Neutral douche to lower spine (**1103**); Scotch douche to feet and legs (**1037**); hot bladder irrigation, 100°–115°.

3. **Improve General Nerve Tone.**—Cold mitten friction (**1209**) or cold towel rub (**1213**); cold pelvic pack (**1390**); general cold douche (**1010**); shallow bath (**1174**); wet-sheet rub (**1216**).

NOCTURNAL INCONTINENCE IN CHILDREN.

1. **Improve General and Local Nerve Tone.**—Cold affusion 1541
(**1103**) at 75° at bedtime, followed by neutral pour (**1103**) to spine, 2 minutes, 96°. Sea-bathing (**1147**) and swimming. Avoid water drinking for 2 hours before retiring. Aseptic dietary (**1626**). Meats and salt especially to be avoided.

2. **Relieve Constipation** and flatulence when present by wet girdle (**1347**), graduated enema (**1409**); if necessary, carefully graduated cold baths (**1625**); cool enema (**1405**), and proper diet.

3. **Diminish Acidity of Urine,** by free use of fruit and water drinking in the forenoon.

PERITONITIS.

A. Acute Form.

1542 1. Rest in bed; fluid diet; fruit-juice without sugar; gruels of dextrinized or malted cereals (**1630**); withhold food 24 to 48 hours.

2. **Albumin in Urine.**—Hot-blanket pack (**1197**) and other sweating measures to maintain cutaneous activity, repeated every 2 to 4 hours.

3. **Fever.**—Hot-blanket pack (**1197**) followed by cold mitten friction (**1209**); prolonged neutral bath (**1130**); fomentation (**1328**) to abdomen with cooling wet-sheet pack (**1189**) at the same time.

4. Enema (**1404**) at 80°, repeating, to remove gas; add soap to water if necessary to secure movement. Fomentation (**1328**) every 2 hours for 15 to 20 minutes. During interval, heating compress (**1344**) at 60°, changing every 5 minutes while the body temperature is elevated, less frequently as temperature falls. Copious water drinking (**1423**); prolonged neutral bath (**1130**); cold precordial compress (**1383**) or ice-bag (**1314**) over heart for 15 minutes 2 or 3 times a day for cardiac weakness.

Prevent Obstruction.—Large enema (**1404**) three times a day from beginning, temperature 75°; soap and turpentine enema.

B. Chronic Form.

Aseptic dietary (**1626**), liquid diet (**1628**). Hot enema (**1406**) followed by fomentation (**1328**) to abdomen for 20 minutes, three times daily; well-protected heating compress (**1344**) during the interval. Copious water drinking (**1423**); graduated cold applications twice daily (**1625**). If temperature is elevated, neutral bath (**1130**) half an hour to an hour daily.

Contraindications.—Cold immersions, prolonged cold douche, cold affusion, cold wet-sheet rub, and cold sitz.

NEURITIS.

1543 ***Etiological Indications.***

1. Rest of affected parts until acute stage is over.

2. **Combat Toxemia.**—Sweating bath two or three times a week, preferably the electric-light bath (**1250**); follow sweating bath by a suitable cold application (**1625**).

Pathological Indications.

3. **Combat Inflammation.**—Local revulsive compress (**1341**) for 15 minutes every 2 to 4 hours, followed by heating compress (**1344**) during intervals; suitable derivative applications (**682**).

Clinical Indications.

4. **Pain.**—Scotch douche (**1037**); vapor douche (**1102**) followed by graduated fan douche (**1061**), gradually reduced from 100° to 80°; protect by dry cotton pack (**1388**) or heating compress (**1344**) covered with mackintosh.

5. **Paralysis.**—Alternate compress (**1340**); alternate douche (**1044**); percussion douche (**1035**) to spine and affected parts.

MULTIPLE NEURITIS.

Etiological Indications. **1544**

1. Rest in bed while the disease is rapidly progressive.

2. **Combat Toxemia.**—Prolonged neutral bath 1 to 2 hours, daily. Aseptic dietary (**1626**); avoidance of tea and coffee, tobacco and alcoholic liquors, and all excesses. Sweating, especially by electric-light bath (**1250**), 10 to 20 minutes, followed by cold mitten friction (**1209**).

3. **Combat Local Inflammations.**—Revulsive compresses, then heating compress or packing in dry cotton (**1388**); fomentations to spine, followed by heating compress. When affecting the lower extremities, hot foot or leg bath (**1299**); hot leg pack (**1393**); complete rest of the affected part.

4. **Improve the General Nutrition** by graduated cold baths (**1625**); massage; galvanic neutral bath (**1451**); out-of-door air with careful protection; sun baths (**1254**); aseptic diet (**1626**).

5. **Pain.**—See **1543**, 4.

6. **Paralysis.**—See **1543**, 5.

7. **Atrophy.**—Alternate douche (**1044**); galvanism or sinusoidal electrical current; massage; manual Swedish movements.

Contraindications.—During acute stage, carefully avoid cold applications unless very short and preceded by heat; avoid percutient applications so long as tenderness exists, that is, all forms of the douche. Avoid especially cold immersion baths, and very prolonged hot baths.

NEURALGIA.

1545 ***Pathological Indications.***

1. **Combat Toxemia when Present.**— Sweating bath followed by appropriate general cold bath (**1625**) three times a week; the electric-light bath (**1250**), vapor bath (**1246**), sweating wet-sheet pack (**1191**), are especially serviceable. Copious water drinking (**1423**); aseptic dietary (**1626**); dry friction (**1221**) of skin or oil rubbing daily after short sweating bath (**1250**), followed by tonic cold application (**1625**).

2. **Combat Anemia and General Weakness.**— Graduated cold applications (**1625**). Avoid increasing pain by preceding or accompanying the cold bath by a hot application to the affected part; cover or avoid the part during the cold application.

Clinical Indications.

3. **Pain.**—Fomentation (**1328**) or revulsive compress (**1341**) to the seat of pain. Scotch douche (**1037**) or alternate douche (**1044**); ice-bag (**1314**) sometimes more effective than heat. This is often the case when the parts are congested as shown by redness of the skin or throbbing sensation, and also when the nerves affected are extremely superficial.

4. **Reflex Neuralgias.**— Usually due to enteroptosis or hyperesthesia of the lumbar ganglia. Fomentation (**1328**) to abdomen twice daily; wet girdle (**1347**) during intervals; abdominal supporter. Avoid chilling after baths, and general prolonged cold applications, such as immersions, shallow and wet-sheet pack.

5. **Neuralgia of the Head.**— Employ derivative measures, as hot sitz bath (**1311**); hot leg bath (**1299**); hot pack to legs (**1393**); hot foot bath (**1297**); cold running foot bath (**1296**); heating wet-sheet pack (**1183**); fan douche to head (**1061**); hot and cold compress to head (**1358**); heat over the seat of pain. Fomentation (**1328**) to the abdomen twice daily, followed by heating compress (**1344**); very hot application to forearm of opposite side.

6. **Spinal Neuralgia and Lumbago.**— Fomentation (**1128**) to spine two or three times a day; during interval, heating compress (**1344**); hot and cold spinal pack (**1369**). Alternate compress (**1340**); Scotch douche (**1037**); hot trunk pack; hot half blanket pack; spinal fomentation with hot leg bath; rest.

7. **General Neuralgic Pain.**—Hot immersion bath (1126) 4 to 5 minutes followed by prolonged neutral bath (1130), 95°; hot-blanket pack (1197), electric-light bath (1250), vapor bath (1246) or sweating pack (1191) followed by dry pack (1192).

8. **Neuralgia due to Chronic Neuritis.**—Alternate compress (1340) or douche (1044); filiform douche (1064). In sciatica, Scotch douche, if persistent; nerve-stretching.

9. **Neuralgic Affections of Ovaries, Uterus, Rectum, Bladder, and Coccyx.**—Revulsive sitz (1308); hot pelvic pack (1390), followed by cold mitten friction (1209); hot enema (1406); hot vaginal irrigation (1413); hot and cold pelvic pack (1370, 1390); revulsive compresses over affected parts (1341).

10. **Gastralgia.**—Very hot fomentation (1328) over stomach and abdomen; hot trunk pack (1196); revulsive compress (1341) for 10 to 30 minutes over stomach, repeated every 2 hours, or as often as needed; hot leg pack (1393); hot water drinking (1429); hot enema (1406). Withhold food until pain is relieved. Aseptic diet (1626); if necessary, liquid diet for a few days (1628).

11. **Enteralgia.**—Abdominal fomentation (1328) 15 minutes every hour; hot enema (1406); heating compress (1344) applied at 60° during interval; graduated tonic treatment (1625).

12. **Erythro Melalgia—Red Neuralgia.**—Rest; elevation of the affected part. Cold compress (1318) changed every 20 to 30 minutes. Application of faradic current and the rapidly alternated sinusoidal current. Graduated tonic treatment (1625).

13. **Herpes Zoster.**—During eruption, dry cotton pack (1388); after, revulsive compress (1341) several times daily, heating compress (1344) during interval.

14. **Contraindications.**—Cold applications increase pain unless very carefully graduated, but are usually necessary for a permanent cure.

ACUTE MYELITIS

Pathological Indications. 1546

1. **Combat Inflammatory Process in Cord.**—Ice-bag (1314), continuously, changing for fomentations 5 min. every half-hour. Revulsive compress (1341) to the spine; fomentation (1328) for 20 minutes every 3 hours, during interval. Heating compress (1344) to spine, 60°, renewed every 15 minutes.

2. **After Acute Stage Has Subsided.**—Alternate compress (1340), or alternate douche (1044) to spine three times a day.

Clinical Indications.

3. **Pain and Paresthesia in Legs.**—Hot leg pack (1393); hot foot bath (1299); hot half-bath (1174); revulsive compress (1341) to spine several times daily, duration 15 to 60 minutes.

4. **Girdle Sensation.**—Hot trunk pack (1197) followed by cold friction (1209); wet girdle, well-protected (1347); fomentation to spine followed by heating spinal compress (1355).

5. **Neuralgic Spinal Pain.**—Fomentation (1328) or hot sponging (1204) of spine followed by heating compress (1344).

6. **Paraplegia.**—Alternate compress (1340) or fan douche (1061) to spine and legs; massage; galvanic, faradic, or sinusoidal electrical applications.

7. **Sensory Paralysis.**—Alternate spray (1044, 1055); alternate sponging (1204); alternate compress (1340); percussion douche (1035) twice daily. Static or faradic electricity.

8. **Muscular Spasm.**—Revulsive compress (1341) to spine. Fomentation (1328) over irritated muscular groups, followed by continuous heating compress (1344), repeating twice daily or as often as neccessary; heating spinal compress (1355).

9. **Hiccough.**—See 1523, 14.

10. **Gastric Crises.**—Hot and cold trunk pack (1367); revulsive gastric compress (1341); fomentation (1328) to spine; hot foot bath (1297); hot leg pack (1393); hot immersion (1126) or hot sitz (1311); galvanism to back of neck and epigastrium.

11. **Contraindications.**—Cold immersion and other general cold applications. Carefully avoid burning or blistering the patient with hot applications.

CHRONIC MYELITIS.

1547 ***Pathological Indications.***

1. Short sweating procedures, followed by graduated cold applications (1625) twice a day. Revulsive compress (1341) or fan douche (1061) to spine, temperature, 120°, 70°; prolonged neutral (92°) immersion baths (1130), 1 to 6 hours; heating compress to the spine (1355). Later stages, alternate douche or compresses to the spine (1342.)

Clinical Indications.

2. **Prickling Sensation in Legs.**—Scotch douche (**1037**), hot fomentations or affusion (96°) (**1328**) to spine and legs.

3. **During early stage** and exacerbations, neutral pour (**1103**) to spine, 96°, two to ten minutes, two or three times daily; absolute rest in bed; spinal fomentation every four hours, heating compress during intervals.

4. **Contraindications.**—Cold full bath, very cold douche, cold affusion, and all prolonged general cold applications. **1548**

SPINAL SCLEROSIS.

A. Lateral Sclerosis — Posterio-Lateral Sclerosis — Disseminated Sclerosis.

Pathological Indications.

1. **To Improve General Nutrition and Blood Movement.**—Graduated tonic baths (**1625**); massage carefully administered; manual Swedish movements; nutritious aseptic dietary (**1626**); sweating baths, especially the electric-light bath (**1250**) followed by cold mitten friction (**1209**), carefully administered; copious water drinking (**1423**).

2. **To Combat Local Morbid Processes.**—Fomentation (**1328**) to the back twice daily, followed by heating spinal compress (**1355**.) The heating compress may be applied at night and retained until morning. Hot-leg bath (**1299**) with fomentation to the spine; prolonged neutral bath (**1130**), 1 to 4 hours daily.

Clinical Indications.

3. **To Relieve Clonic Spasm and Nervous Irritability.**—Warm bath (96° to 100°); prolonged neutral affusion to the spine (93° to to 98°) heating spinal compress (**1355**) at night; neutral galvanic bath (92° to 98°) (**1451**), 10 minutes; galvanism of the dorsal spine and abdominal sympathetic with simultaneous spinal fomentation. Rest in bed when symptoms are progressing.

4. **For Muscular Weakness or Paralysis.**—Massage; manual Swedish movements; exercise of muscles by slowly alternated sinusoidal electrical current. Special gymnastics.

5. **Contraindications**—The cold douche and other general cold baths; prolonged hot baths; exercise to the extent of fatigue.

The patient should be kept in the open air as much as possible. Out-of-door gymnastics are especially useful.

B. **Amyotrophic Lateral Sclerosis.**

1. See (A) 1, above.

2. Prolonged neutral baths (**1130**), 1 to 3 hours daily; massage; manual Swedish movements.

3. **Contraindications.**—Avoid the use of electricity, the cold douche, prolonged hot baths, and general cold baths.

General Method.—Build up the general health by gentle tonic measures slowly increased in intensity (**1625**), suppressing the formation of toxic substances and promoting their elimination by a suitable dietary (**1626**), improvement of digestion and the employment of the other measures above indicated.

By the suppression of the active causes of the disease and the adoption of rational means for the improvement of general nutrition and especially of the nutrition of the cord, it is usually possible to arrest the disease, and not infrequently a considerable degree of improvement may be secured. Therapeutic measures must be most thoroughly and perseveringly employed. The progress of the disease may be delayed, even when it can not be altogether arrested.

LOCOMOTOR ATAXIA.

1549 1. **Improve General Nutrition.**—Careful cold mitten friction (**1209**) or cold towel rubbing (**1213**). Very carefully graduated cold baths (**1625**). Tonic pack (**1179**), protecting the spine by a dry towel, followed by cold friction (**1209**) and affusion (**1103**) or half-bath at 85° (**1174**).

2. **Combat Toxemia** by short sweating baths (**1191, 1246, 1250**), followed by appropriate graduated cold baths (**1625**). Prolonged neutral bath (**1130**), beginning at 96° and daily lowering the temperature to 90°; increase duration from 30 minutes to 2 or 3 hours daily. Copious water drinking (**1423**); coloclyster daily (**1407**).

3. **Improve Nutrition of Cord.**—Fomentation (**1328**) to the spine 110° to 120° twice daily, with heating compress (**1355**) during the interval. Thorough massage of the back; suspension, or spine-stretching by flexion of the trunk upon the thighs, or flexion of the thighs upon the trunk.

Clinical Indications.

4. **Ataxic Movements.**— Special exercises in small movements of each of the affected muscular groups.

5. **Lightning Pains.**— Prolonged warm fan douche to spine (**1103**), 95° to 100°, two or three times a day (pressure 2 to 5 lbs.).

6. **Gastric Crises.**— Very hot fomentation to the abdomen (**1328**) several times a day, followed by heating compress (**1344**) when lumbar ganglia are sensitive; continue for several weeks. Revulsive gastric compress (**1341**). See **1545,** 10.

7. **Local Pains.**— Revulsive compress (**1341**) and Scotch douche (**1037**) followed by heating compress (**1344**).

8. **Rectal Pain.**— Very hot anal douche (**1087**), 115° to 122°, with little pressure. Revulsive sitz (**1308**). Fomentation (**1328**) over buttocks. Hot rectal irrigation (**1410**).

9. **Paresis of Bladder.**— Daily irrigation (**1411**). Cold plantar douche (**1083**).

10. **Constipation.**— See **1524.**

11. **Trophic Changes — Charcot's Joints.**— Fomentation (**1328**) to the parts when painful, three times daily, with heating compress (**1344**) during the intervals. Apply mechanical support when necessary. Galvanism and the rapidly alternating sinusoidal electrical current.

12. **Contraindications.**— Cold immersions, cold applications to spine, general cold douche, very hot applications.

General Method.— Build up the patient's general health by gentle tonic measures, carefully avoiding such applications of cold water as are found to increase pain or aggravate other symptoms; combat the local morbid process in the spine by the measures above indicated, and restore the power of co-ordinated movement in the affected muscular groups by special gymnastic training.

CEREBRAL APOPLEXY.

1. **During Attack.**— Rest, head and shoulders raised; cold compress to head (**1371**); tepid enema (**1404**); warm extremities by hot-water bags or hot pack. Ice-collar (**1316**). 1550

1. **After Attack.**—Cold mitten friction (**1209**) twice daily; well-protected wet girdle (**1347**) night and day; carefully graduated cold baths (**1625**); prolonged neutral bath (**1130**); wet-sheet pack (**1179**). After a few weeks, electricity to affected muscles; man-

ual Swedish movements; carefully graduated exercises; massage; cold or alternate douche (**1044**) to affected muscles.

EPILEPSY.

1551 1. Abstemious, dry, aseptic dietary (**1626**), chiefly fruits and grains; vigorous out-of-door exercise to the extent of fatigue daily. Prolonged neutral bath (**1130**) daily; sweating process (**642, 1233–1255**) two or three times a week; graduated cold procedures (**1625**), avoiding prolonged and intense applications.

2. **When Attack Is Threatened.**—Coloclyster (**1407**) twice daily; copious water drinking (**1423**); neutral pack (**1182**); ice to head (**1314**); rest in bed. If aura in hand or foot precedes attack, the seizure may sometimes be averted by placing the part in cold water.

3. **After Attack.**—Rest; cold to head; cold mitten friction (**1209**) or cold towel rub (**1213**); half-bath (**1174**); Scotch douche (**1037**) to legs, and percussion douche (**1035**) to spine.

General Method.—Train the patient to a vigorous regimen, a simple abstemious dietary (**1626**), abundance of outdoor exercise, the daily employment of the prolonged neutral bath (**1130**); followed by short, moderately cold applications (**1625**); copious water drinking (**1423**); regulation of all the vital functions, avoidance of all sources of nervous irritation and exhaustion.

CHOREA.

1552 ***Etiological Indications.***

1. Combat anemia and improve general nutrition by graduated tonic applications (**1625**); copious water drinking (**1423**); large enema or coloclyster (**1407**). Fomentation to abdomen (**1328**) morning and night, heating compress during intervals. Secure mental quiet by isolation if necessary. The patient should be kept in the open air. Out-of-door life and rhythmical gymnastics are especially useful.

Clinical Indications.

2. **Insomnia.**—Prolonged neutral bath (**1130**) or douche (**1031**); wet girdle (**1347**).

3. **Agitation.**—Neutral spinal pour (**1103**); wet-sheet pack (**1179**).

4. **Constipation.**—See 1524.

5. **Indigestion.**—See 1520–1525.

6. **Irregular Movements.**—Neutral pour to spine (1103) daily; prolonged neutral bath (1130); special gymnastics.

7. **Endocarditis.**—Ice-bags over the heart (1314). See 1576.

General Method.—Improve the nerve tone by tonic measures and careful attention to nutrition. Train the patient to better mental and moral control, and combat the choreic movements by systematic gymnastic training.

HYSTERIA.

Pathological Indications. 1553

1. Tonic, reconstructive, and sedative measures. Graduated cold applications (1625) are of the first importance; must be carefully managed at first; application twice daily, short, intense. Prolonged neutral bath (1130) in cases due to autointoxication. Out-of-door life; generous aseptic diet (1626); suitable moral and mental surroundings.

Clinical Indications.

2. **Convulsions.**—Neutral bath (1130); neutral pack (1182); hot-blanket pack (1197); hot and cold spinal compress or sponging (1342); hot enema (1406); hot half-bath (1174) with tepid affusion (1103) to head and spine; heating spinal compress (1355).

3. **Coma.**—Alternate compress or sponging to spine (1342); cold mitten friction (1209); hot half bath (1177); cold, or hot and cold, compress to head (1358).

4. **Vomiting.**—Hot and cold gastric compress (1362); dry diet (1629); rectal feeding; gastric lavage (1401); ice to the epigastrium; (1314) ice pills.

5. **Anorexia.**—Ice-bag (1314) over stomach half an hour before meals; alternate compress (1340) to epigastrium, twice daily. Alternate lavage (1401); cold douche (1074) to spine and epigastrium (1079).

6. **Cough.**—Fomentation (1328) to spine; sipping hot water (1429); chest pack (1373). Cold compress to the throat (1381); gargling hot water (1400) several times daily.

7. **Muscular Paralysis.**—Alternate affusion or douche (1044, 1103); alternate compress (1340); cold affusion (1103);

cold douche (**1047**); massage douche (**1066**); massage; manual Swedish movements; electricity.

8. **Contractions.**—Fomentations to affected parts (**1328**) followed by heating compress (**1344**). Revulsive douche (**1041**).

9. **Trembling.**—Neutral affusion (**1103**) to spine, 92° to 96° 15 minutes.

10. **Incontinence of Urine.**—Percussion douche (**1035**) to spine; neutral sitz (**1312**) 15 to 30 minutes.

11. **Retention of Urine.**—Hot sitz (**1311**), 5 minutes, followed by cold plantar douche (**1083**). Cold perineal douche (**1084**); cold douche to the lumbar region (**1076**) and hypogastrium (**1079**); cold rubbing sitz (**1309**).

12. **Anesthesia or Paresthesia.**—Alternate douche (**1044**) or compress (**1340**); cold percussion douche (**1035**) to spine; cold rubbing of affected part with hand or friction mitt (**1209**) after a hot fomentation (**1328**) for 5 to 10 minutes.

13. **Hyperesthesia — Pain.**—Hot fan douche (**1061**); fomentation (**1328**) followed by heating compress (**1344**); revulsive compress (**1341**). Cold douche to the symmetrical part of the opposite side (**1022**).

14. **Loss of Muscular Sense.**—Alternate douche (**1044**); massage douche (**1066**); cold percussion douche (**1035**).

15. **Visceral Neuralgia.**—Very hot fomentation (**1328**) over the affected part 20 minutes twice daily, followed by heating compress (**1344**) during the interval; revulsive compress (**1341**); Scotch revulsive fan douche (**1041**).

16. **Motor Paralysis.**—Alternate douche (**1044**); massage douche (**1066**); cold percussion douche (**1035**).

17. **Hiccough.**—Hot trunk pack (**1196**); heating gastric compress (**1344**); sipping ice-cold carbonated water; lavage (**1401**).

18. **Syncope.**—Heat to neck (**1382**); short cold application to chest and face. Alternate compress to spine (**1342**); percussion of the chest with the hands dipped in cold water or with the end of a cold towel; vigorous centripetal friction (**1223**); rhythmical traction of the tongue.

19. **Spinal Irritation.** — Fomentation (**1328**) to the spine twice a day, followed by continuous heating compress (**1344**) during the intervals; Scotch fan douche (**1061, 1037**); fomentation (**1328**) followed by affusion (**1103**) for 5 minutes, 80° to 85°.

20. **Anal Spasm.**—Hot anal douche (**1087**) or hot, shallow sitz (**1311**) (102° to 106°). General applications of faradic, static, galvanic, or sinusoidal electrical currents are also useful in connection with massage, manual Swedish movements, and regulated gymnastics.

21. **Aphonia.**—Ice-bag to the throat (**1314**); with general cold douche (**1037**).

General Method.—Improve the patient's general health by vigorous tonic measures continued during many months or even years. Improve the general nutrition by a nutritious, simple, unstimulating dietary (**1626**). Combat special symptoms by the hydriatic measures indicated above, together with suitable mental and moral treatment.

NEURASTHENIA.

This is not a distinct pathological entity, but a group of symp- 1554
toms due to various etiological influences and connected with various morbid states.

Etiological Indications.

1. Rest-cure for those who have been overworked nervously and physically, and for those who need a rapid gain of fat and blood; muscular exercise and diversion for those who are mentally and nervously tired.

Pathological Indications.

2. **Combat Autointoxication.**—Aseptic diet (**1626**); fruit diet (**1627**); daily neutral baths (**1130**) (1-3 hours); sweating procedures (**642, 1233-1255**) of short duration (3-6 minutes) followed by suitable cold applications (**1625**); hot enema (**1406**) daily; copious water drinking (**1423**); out-of-door life.

3. **Combat Exhaustion.**—Rest for the overworked. Improve digestion in cases of starved dyspeptics by appropriate measures. Foods rich in fats and proteids are especially important. Tonic cold applications carefully graduated (**1625**); especially percussion douche to spine.

4. **Check Exhausting Discharges** by appropriate measures as Menorrhagia (**1588**), Leucorrhea (**1591**, 3), Spermatorrhea (**1596**).

5. **Relieve Reflex Irritation.**—If sexual, rectal, prostatic, or urethral irritation, employ revulsive sitz (**1311**), prolonged neu-

tral sitz (**1312**), rectal and urethral irrigation, hot foot bath (**1297**), hot pelvic pack (**1390**). For ovarian irritation, in addition to above, hot vaginal irrigation (**1413**), 15 to 20 min.

6. **Irritation of Solar Plexus and Sympathetic Ganglia.**— Fomentation (**1328**) over abdomen three times daily; during intervals, heating compress (**1344**); abdominal supporter.

Clinical Indications.

7. **Improve General Nerve Tone.**— Graduated cold applications (**1625**). The cold percussion douche (**1035**) to spine is the most efficient of all measures; general cold douche (**1010**); very hot douche (**1024**) (110° for 30 seconds), followed by graduated or cold douche (**1037**).

8. **Indigestion.**— See **1520–1525.**

9. **Constipation.**— See **1524.**

10. **Intestinal Catarrh.**—See **1529.**

11. **Headache.**— Hot and cold compress (**1358**); revulsive compress (**1341**); alternate spinal compress or sponging (**1342**); hot foot bath (**1297**); running foot bath (**1296**).

12. **Frontal Headache.**— Revulsive compress (**1341**) to forehead and eyes; hot and cold trunk pack (**1367**); derivative applications to feet and legs (**682**).

13. **Congestive Headache.**— Ice-bag (**1314**) to back of head and cold compress (**1314**) to face; ice-collar (**1316**); hot and cold cephalic compress (**1358**); hot foot bath (**1297**); hot leg pack (**1393**); heating compress to legs (**1344**); cold running foot bath (**1296**); alternate foot bath (**1298**); felt shoes.

14. **Occipital Headache.**— Hot compress (**1286**) or sponging (**1206**) to upper spine and occipital region. Revulsive compress (**1341**); hot and cold cephalic compress (**1358**).

15. **Nervous Headache.**— Fomentation (**1328**) to seat of pain, with simultaneous hot foot bath (**1297**); gastric lavage (**1401**). Daily cold enema (**1405**) to relieve constipation if present. Special attention to the diet; a dry aseptic (**1626**) diet is indicated, avoiding milk. See Migraine (**1555**).

16. **Sensation of Band around Head.**— Hot sponging (**1206**) or hot compress (**1286**); alternate sponging (**1206**) of neck and upper spine; massage to head.

17. **Sensation of Pressure at Vertex.**— Hot foot bath

(1297), cold compress (1314) to head; ice-collar (1316); sleep with head elevated; heat to feet and legs if cold.

18. **Pain in Eyes, Intolerance to Light or Use in Reading.**—Light fomentation over eyes and forehead (1264); protect eyes from bright light; facial massage and massage to eyes; an oculist should be consulted, as the temporary use of glasses to correct muscular insufficiency due to deficient innervation or some slight optical defect may be useful or necessary.

19. **Backache.**—Fomentation (1328) to abdomen; wet girdle (1347); abdominal supporter; alternate spinal sponging (1206) or compress (1340); Scotch douche (1037) to spine; revulsive sitz (1308).

20. **Neuralgia.**—See 1545.

21. **Insomnia.**—See 1564.

22. **Vertigo.**—Fomentation (1328) to stomach followed by wet girdle (1347). Gastric lavage (1401) when indicated. Bathing face or top of head with very hot water, or hot compress (1286) for 2 minutes, followed by cool compress (1318), 15 seconds; heat to back of neck in anemia of the brain (1262).

23. **Anorexia.**—Cold bag (1314) over stomach for half an hour before meals, with cold compress or water bag (1314) to epigastrium; cold mitten friction (1209) or cold towel rub (1213).

24. **Muscular Weakness, Especially in Legs.**—Cold percussion douche (1035) to spine; alternate douche (1044) to legs.

25. **Mental Depression.**—Sweating bath followed by short general cold douche (1010); neutral bath (1031) for 1 hour daily; neutral pack (1182); cold percussion spinal douche (1035); alternate spinal sponging (1342) or douche (1044).

26. **Fidgets.**—Fomentation (1328) to abdomen followed by wet girdle (1347); empty colon, if loaded, by enema (1404); abdominal supporter; revulsive sitz (1311); neutral pour to spine (1103).

27. **Dreams.**—Neutral bath (1031) for half an hour before going to bed; wet girdle (1347); evaporating head cap (1324); elevate head of bed; avoid eating after 4 P. M. except fruit.

28. **Flushings.**—Scotch fan douche (1061) to abdomen, especially the umbilical region; percussion douche (1035) to spine; alternate spinal douche (693, 1342); wet girdle (1347).

29. **Cold Extremities.**—Scotch douche (**1037**) to legs and feet, followed by standing shallow bath (**1174**); fomentation to abdomen (**1328**) twice daily, followed by heating compress (**1344**) during intervals; alternate foot bath (**1298**); massage to feet and legs; cold friction (**1209**).

30. **Perspiration when Sleeping.**—**1508**, 11.

General Method.—While not recognizable as a distinct malady, it is convenient from a practical standpoint to consider neurasthenia as a disease. The tonic effects of cold water are essential in the treatment of neurasthenic conditions. The management of cold applications in such a way as to secure the tonic effects desired without aggravating any of the patient's symptoms is a problem which taxes to the utmost the skill and experience of the hydriatic physician. Special attention must be given to the digestion, improvement of nutrition, regulation of the bowels and the relief of prominent and distressing symptoms by suitable palliative measures.

MIGRAINE.

1555 ***Etiological Indications.***

1. **Prevent Formation of Uric Acid.**—Avoid use of meats, also tea and coffee, etc.; aseptic dietary (**1625**); out-of-door life.

Pathological Indications.

2. **Eliminate Uric Acid.**—Hot baths, especially moderately prolonged sweating baths (**1191**) followed by short cold baths; electric-light bath (**1250**); wet-sheet pack (**1179**); vapor bath (**1246**); prolonged neutral bath (**1130**); water drinking (**1423**).

3. **Lower Arterial Tension.**—Hot immersion, 102°, 5 to 10 min. (**1126**); hot leg bath (**1299**); or pack (**1393**); hot enema, 100° to 204° (**1406**); rest in bed; exclusive of light.

Clinical Indications.

4. **Pain.**—Hot foot bath (**1297**); alternate spinal compress or sponging (**1342**); revulsive compress (**1341**) to seat of pain; local application of ice-bag (**1314**) in some cases: hot leg pack (**1393**); protect the eyes from light.

5. **Nausea and Vomiting.**—Lavage (**1401**); ice pills; ice (**1314**) to stomach and spine opposite.

6. **Constipation.**—Coloclyster (**1407**). See **1524**.

7. **Gastric Disorders.**— 1519-1527.

8. **To Prevent Attack.**— Lavage (1401); fruit diet (1627); large coloclyster (1407); water drinking (1423).

9. **To Relieve Hyperesthesia of Lumbar Ganglia.**— Abdominal fomentation (1328) twice daily; continuous heating compress (1344) during interval. Abdominal supporter.

General Method.— Every case is curable by sufficiently prolonged treatment, carefully managed. The general nervous system must be built up by measures essentially the same as those indicated for neurasthenia (1554, 3) and other conditions requiring tonic treatment. The causes must be removed, especially autointoxication and morbid reflex influences arising from dilatation of the stomach, enteroptosis, and indigestion.

INFANTILE CONVULSIONS.

Etiological Indications. 1556

1. Regulate diet, withholding meats and all indigestibles. Avoid cow's milk if curds are present in the stools. Daily cold bath, wet-hand rub (1201) or cold towel rub (1213).

Pathological Indications.

2. When due to autointoxication from intestinal irritation, large hot enema (1406). If undigested food is present in the stomach, lavage (1401). For immediate relief, hot-blanket pack (1197); warm bath (95° to 98°) (1123), 1 to 2 minutes. If not quickly relieved, remove from bath, and employ cold affusion (1103) to head and spine. Alternate hot and cold affusion if necessary. Apply wet girdle (1347), changing every 4 hours.

WRITER'S CRAMP.

1. **General.**—Scotch douche (1035, 1074) to spine and 1557
affected muscles twice daily. Neutral affusion (1103) to spine 10 minutes daily; neutral bath (1130), 1 hour at bedtime. Cold mitten friction (1209) twice daily following other treatment. Shallow bath 1 to 3 minutes (1174); prolonged neutral bath (1130); massage and passive exercises (1461).

2. **Paresis.**—Cold percussion douche to spine (1037, 1074) following warm rain douche (1047). Alternate douche (1044) to affected muscles. Gymnastics; passive exercises and massage of affected parts; sinusoidal or galvanic electricity.

MELANCHOLIA.

1558 ***Pathological Indications.***

1. **For Anemia and Malnutrition.**— Fomentation (**1328**) to abdomen followed by cold mitten friction (**1209**) twice daily; aseptic diet (**1626**); water drinking (**1423**); air bath (**1470**); electric-light bath (**1250**); sun baths (**1254**); rest in bed; massage; manual Swedish movements; galvanization of cervical and abdominal sympathetic.

2. **For Cerebral Anemia** (usually present).— Warm compress (98° to 100°) to back of neck 15 minutes three times daily.

3. **To Diminish Blood Pressure** (usually excessive).— Warm immersion bath (**1126**), 98° to 100°, 10 to 20 minutes, twice daily; heating wet-sheet pack (**1183**); heating trunk pack (**1196**), 30 minutes, twice daily; neutral douche (94°), pressure 10 to 20 pounds, duration 2 to 4 minutes.

4. **For Autointoxication.**— See **1559**, 4.

Clinical Indications.

5. **Insomnia.**— See **1564.**

6. **Anorexia.**— Lavage; feeding with tube; see **1401.**

7. **Constipation.**— Laxative diet, fruit, granose, malted cereals (**1631**); cool enema. See **1524.**

8. **Indigestion.**— See **1521, 1522.**

9. **Cold Extremities.**— See **1554**, 29; **1527**, 6.

10. **Dry Skin.**— See **1609.**

11. **Mental and Nervous Irritability.**— Neutral bath (94° to 96°, 30 minutes to 2 hours); heating wet-sheet pack (**1183**); wet girdle (**1347**); heating spinal compress (**1344, 1355**).

12. **Contraindications.**— Avoid cold immersions and all very cold general applications, which by raising blood pressure and exciting the irritable cerebral structures aggravate the condition.

General Method.— A patient suffering from melancholia requires essentially the same therapeutic measures as the neurasthenic with the special moral treatment and control indicated.

MANIA.

1559 ***Pathological Indications.***

1. **For Malnutrition.**— Graduated tonic baths (**1625**); generous aseptic diet. See **1558**, 1.

2. **To Increase Blood Pressure.**— Hot baths — electric-light (**1250**), hot immersion (**1126**), 100° to 102°, 8 to 15 minutes, hot leg (**1299**) or sitz bath (**1311**), 108° to 115°, 8 to 12 minutes, followed by shallow (**1174**) at 68° to 74°, affusion (**1103**) at 70° to 60°, or percussion douche at 60° to 50°, duration 20 to 40 seconds; ice-bag over heart for 15 minutes every 2 hours.

3. **To Diminish Cerebral Hyperemia.**— Short hot immersion (**1126**) or shower (**1047**) followed by douche (**1010**) at 70° to 60°, 20 to 40 seconds, light pressure; hot (106° to 115°) leg (**1299**) or sitz bath (**1311**); ice-collar (p. 779); cephalic compress (**1371**); wet girdle, well protected (**1347**); heating wet-sheet pack (**1183**).

4. **For Autointoxication.**— Aseptic diet (**1626**), if necessary, fruit (**1627**) or kumyss diet (**1628**); coloclyster (**1407**) daily for a few days; long neutral bath (**1130**), 30 to 60 minutes.

Clinical Indications.

5. **To Relieve or Prevent Exhaustion.**— Rest in bed; tonic treatment (**1625**) twice a day.

6. **For Fever.**— Local antiphlogistic measures (**698**) as may be indicated; neutral bath (**1130**); cooling pack (**1189**).

7. **For Insomnia.**— See **1564.**

8. **For Constipation.**— Cool enema (**1409**). See **1524.**

9. **Indigestion.**— See **1521, 1522.**

10. **Contraindications.**— Avoid very hot or prolonged cold baths; avoid cold to head when face is pale.

CONFUSIONAL, PUERPERAL; POST-FEBRILE, POST-OPERATIVE, TOXIC INSANITIES.

1. **Malnutrition.**— Rest; careful tonic treatment (**1625**). **1560**

2. **Autointoxication.**— Aseptic dietary (**1626**); fruit diet (**1627**) for 3 or 4 days; warm baths, electric-light (**1250**), sweating pack (**1191**) followed by short cold applications; wet-sheet rub (**1216**) or douche (**1010**); copious water drinking (**1423**); coloclyster daily (**1407**) for a week or two.

3. **Puerperal Lesions or Complications.**— Curettement, hot vaginal irrigation (**1413**); neutral (**1312**) or tonic sitz (**1309**).

4. **Fever.**— Absolute rest in bed; prolonged tepid bath (88° to 92°, 30 to 60 minutes); cooling enemas (**1405**); cold cephalic compress (**1371**); copious water drinking (**1423**).

5. **Alcoholism.**— Withdraw alcohol at once; withhold food for 3 days; nutritive enemas; copious water drinking (**1423**); neutral coloclyster (**1407**) daily for a week.

6. **Uremia.**— See Acute Nephritis, **1537**.

7. For other Clinical indications, see Simple Mania above.

8. **Contraindications.**—The same as those of Mania, when conditions coincide. Especially avoid all intensely exciting procedures.

General Method.— In most cases essentially the same as for Mania, giving special attention to the particular etiological element which may be a prominent factor in the case. In certain cases, the symptoms are those of Melancholia, and the treatment must be modified accordingly.

GENERAL PARESIS.

1561 ***Pathological Indications.***

1. **Malnutrition.**—Vigorous but graduated tonic measures (**1625**); rest in bed. See **1558**, 1, also Neurasthenia, **1554**.

2. **Cerebral Hyperemia.**—Continuous ice-cap (**1323**). See **1562**, 1.

3. **Disturbed Arterial Tension.**—If excessive, see **1558**, 3; if diminished, see **1559**, 2.

4. **Autointoxication.**—See **1559**, 4.

Clinical Indications.

5. **Insomnia.**—Ice-cap (**1323**); neutral bath (**1130**) or douche (**1031**); wet girdle (**1347**); wet-sheet pack (**1179**). See **1564**.

6. **Constipation.**—Cool enema (70°); wet girdle (**1347**); cold abdominal douche (**1081**); abdominal massage. See **1524**.

7. **Retention of Urine.**—Catheterization; irrigation of the bladder (**1411**); cool rubbing sitz (**1309**), 70° to 65°, 3 to 6 minutes; cold spray to feet (**1055**); cold plantar douche (**1083**); cold hypogastric douche (**1080**) (75° to 60°); running foot bath (**1296**).

HEADACHE.

1562 The following grouping of headaches is made for practical convenience alone, and is not offered as a scientific classification:—

1. **Hyperemic Headache.**— Rest, head and shoulders elevated; heat to feet and legs — foot bath (**1297**), leg bath (**1299**), leg pack (**1393**), Scotch douche (**1037**); cold to head and neck (**1314**), enema at 102° (**1406**); well protected wet girdle night and day (**1347**); wet sheet pack (**1179**); neutral spray, 2 to 4 minutes (**1057**), moderate pressure.

2. **Anemic Headache.**— Hot bag to back of neck; fomentation (**1328**) over painful part; rest in bed with head low; general treatment for anemia. See **1580.**

3. **High Pressure Headache.** — Abstemious aseptic diet; prolonged warm or neutral bath daily, with cool compress to head; hot leg (**1299**) and foot baths (**1297**); Scotch douche (**1037**) to legs; heating compress (**1344**) over heart.

4. **Dyspeptic Headache.**— Gastric lavage (**1401**) if stomach is foul; enema (**1405**) if constipated; dry, aseptic diet (**1626**) two meals a day, or fruit only at night.

See **1119** to **1523**. For palliation, hot and cold cephalic compress (**1358**); avoid sleeping soon after eating, though a short nap is sometimes beneficial.

5. **Headache Due to Enteroptosis.**— Abdominal supporter; wet girdle at night (**1347**); abdominal massage; cold abdominal douche (**1081**); sinusoidal current to muscles; galvanization of cervical and abdominal sympathetic; for palliation, alternate spinal sponging (**1342**) or compress (**1340**); hot and cold head compress (**1358**).

6. **Toxic Headache.**— Due to uric acid, oxalates, urea, and other wastes, or to decomposition products absorbed from the alimentary canal. Sweating baths (**1125, 1197, 1246, 1126**) followed by cold douche (**1010**), wet-sheet rub (**1216**), or shallow (**1174**); copious water drinking (**1423**); enema (**1405**) or coloclyster (**1407**) daily or tri-weekly; out-of-door life; air-bath (**1471**); aseptic diet.

7. **Periodical Headache, Nervous Headache, Bilious Headache, Migraine, Hermicrania.**— Dry, abstemious, aseptic diet (**1626**); out-of-door life; air-bath (**1470**); gastric lavage and large enema (**1401**) the day before attack is due (**1406**); tonic treatment (**1625**); wet girdle (**1347**); abdominal supporter if enteroptosis exists.

8. **Rheumatic Headache.**— Sweating bath, **1499**, 12, daily;

hot foot bath (**1297**) or leg pack (**1393**), fomentation to painful part for 10 to 15 minutes, followed by heating compress (**1344**). See Uric Acid Diathesis **1511**.

9. **Neurasthenic Headaches.**—See **1554**, 11–15.

10. **Clavus.**—Very hot foot bath (**1297**), with fomentation over painful point for 10 minutes, repeated every 2 hours; carefully graduated cool baths (**1625**). Heating compress at night; protect well from cold during the day.

11. **Renal Headache.**—Copious water drinking (**1423**); enema (**1405**); hot bath (**1126, 1250, 1246, 1197**); ice-bag over lower sternum, with hot and cold compress to head (**1358**). See Acute Nephritis (**1537**); and Chronic Nephritis (**1538**).

12. **Hepatic Headache.**—Aseptic diet (**1626**); fruit diet (**1627**); water-drinking (**1423**); graduated enema (**1409**); fomentation over liver twice daily, 15 min., heating compress during the intervals. Out-of-door exercise; air-bath (**1470**); breathing exercises; abdominal massage. For palliation, revulsive compress to head (**1341**); hot and cold head compress (**1358**), with derivative applications to legs (**1299, 1393, 1037, 1250**); graduated tonic treatment (**1625**).

13. **Organic Headaches** (tumors, inflammation, syphilis, abscess,, trauma, general paresis).—Very hot and frequently repeated derivative applications to legs, with short, often repeated revulsive compress to head, followed by cold or heating compress.

14. **Headache Due to Disease of Eye, Ear, Nose, and Teeth.**—Correct diseased condition by surgical or other means. Hot foot (**1297**), or leg (**1299**) bath, with revulsive compress (**1341**) over painful parts.

15. **Coldness, Numbness, Pressure, Band Sensation, Etc.**—Improve vasomotor tone by tonic measures (**1625**); massage of head and neck; revulsive compress (**1341**) to spine, head, and face; hot and cold head compress (**1358**); static breeze. See Neurasthenia **1554**.

Supra-orbital Headache.—Hot foot bath with revulsive compress above the eye-brow, but not covering the eye; avoid exposure to cold; rest eyes, protecting from light; general tonic treatment (**1625**). Hot foot (**1297**) or leg pack (**1393**).

16. **Temporal Headache.**—Fomentation (**1328**) over side of head, face and ear, for ten minutes, followed by warm dry com-

press, repeated every two hours, between attacks, tonic treatment (**1625**), local massage, galvanism, sinuosoidal current. Fat- and blood-making diet (**1626**). See Lithemia (**1511**).

17. **Mastoid or Post-Auricular Headache.**— Fomentation for 10 minutes to side of head followed by cotton poultice or well-covered heating compress. Otherwise the same as 16, above. See also 4 and 14.

18. **Cervico-Occipital Headache.**— Revulsive compress to back of head and neck. Otherwise the same as 16, above. See Neurasthenia **1554.**

19. **Uterine Headache** (Pain or pressure at vertex).— Revulsive sitz (p. 766, 770); abdominal supporter; wet girdle (**1347**); application of sinusoidal electricity to uterus; central galvanization; hot and cold head compress (**1358**); massage of head; static breeze to head. Correct any ovarian or uterine disease present. See neurasthenia **1554.**

20. **Fever Headache.**— Ice-cap or cold cephalic compress (**1371**); ice-collar (**1316**); ice-bag over heart (**1314**): cooling pack (**1189**); prolonged neutral bath.

THERMIC FEVER, HEAT STROKE, SUN STROKE, HEAT EXHAUSTION.

1. **Thermic Fever.**— Increase heat elimination. Pour from a **1563**
height water at 60° or less, while two persons rub the patient vigorously. Give special attention to the spine. Ice compress to the head and neck (**1318**). Continue until the temperature falls to 101°; cool enema (**1405**); cold water drinking (**1426**) when possible. Ice-bag to the head and neck (**1314**) during cold affusion (**1103**). As soon as the temperature falls to near the normal point, sweating wet-sheet pack (**1183, 1191**).

2. **After-Treatment** should consist of daily graduated cold applications (**1625**). The head should be thoroughly cooled before each application.

3. **Neurasthenia.**— See **1554.**

4. **Insomnia.**— See **1564.**

5. **Heat Exhaustion.**— Hot immersion bath (**1126**), 3 to 8 minutes; hot-blanket pack (**1197**); hot enema (**1406**) followed immediately by short cold mitten friction (**1209**), cold wet-sheet rub (**1216**), afterward wrapping in warm blankets.

6. **Threatened Cardiac Failure.**—Cold bag over heart (**1383**) for 15 minutes every hour; cold mitten friction (**1209**) every 2 hours; hot-blanket pack (**1197**) 10 minutes, followed by cold towel rub (**1213**). Hot enema (**1406**) followed by cold enema (**1405**); artificial respiration.

INSOMNIA.

1564 ***Pathological Indications.***

1. **To Relieve Cerebral Congestion.**—Neutral douche (**1031**) 3 to 5 minutes at bedtime; cold douche (**1010**); hot leg bath (**1299**); running foot bath (**1296**); heating wet sheet pack (**1183**) followed by rubbing wet sheet (**1216**); wet girdle warmly covered and protected with mackintosh (**1347**); heating leg pack (**1393**); dry heat to the feet and legs; hot leg pack (**1393**) followed by cold mitten friction (**1209**) to the legs; heating compress to legs, or leg pack at bedtime, to be prolonged during the night; wet-girdle and leg pack over night; Scotch douche (**1037**) to the legs at 102°, 2 minutes, 60° 15 seconds; neutral douche (**1031**), 3 to 5 minutes; evaporating head-cap (**1324**); downward stroking of head and neck; galvanization of the cervical sympathetic.

2. **Relieve Irritability of the Cerebral Cell.**—Prolonged neutral bath (**1130**) at bedtime; neutral-wet-sheet pack (**1182**). Enema (**1404**) if constipation or flatulence are present.

3. **Irritability of Solar Plexus or Lumbar Ganglia.**—Abdominal fomentation (**1328**) followed by abdominal heating compress (**1351**), changing every 6 hours. Avoid eating anything but fruits after 4 P. M. Copious water drinking (**1423**). Colo-clyster (**1407**), especially if the bowels are inactive, as constipation is a frequent cause of insomnia through producing irritation of the abdominal sympathetic.

4. **Excessive Cardiac Activity.**—Ice-bag over heart (**1383**). Galvanism to spine and cervical sympathetic.

5. **Fidgets, or Restlessness.**—Warm affusion to spine (**1103**), 95° to 98°. Tepid sponging (**1204**); rubbing of limbs; rubbing spine (**1221**); massage of head.

6. **General Irritability.**—Neutral wet-sheet pack (**1182**); neutral immersion bath (**1130**); neutral fan douche (**1031**) or shower (**1047**) 2 to 4 minutes.

General Method.—There may be said to be three forms of insomnia: Sleeplessness may be due to (*a*) congestion of the brain; (*b*) irritability of the cerebral cell, or to (*c*) a combination of these two conditions. Which of these conditions is present in any individual case must be carefully determined, and the treatment adjusted accordingly, as above indicated.

PRURITIS.

1. Neutral fan douche (1061), 95° to 100°, 10 to 15 minutes. 1565
Drying by gently patting over Turkish sheet or towel. Prolonged neutral bath (1130) 94° to 96°. If temperature sense is perverted, employ higher or lower temperature.

2. **Winter Pruritis of Lithemia.**—Very hot Scotch douche, (1037), 1 to 2 minutes, 115° to 122°, followed by cool douche 70° 30 seconds; prolonged neutral bath (1130), 92°.

3. **Pruritis of Genitals or Anus.**—Prolonged cold compress (1318) or ascending douche (1058, 1087) when no eruption is present; with eruption, very hot spray followed by evaporating compress and a suitable lotion or unguent. If the skin is thickened, very hot or alternate douche (1044) or revulsive douche (1041) to affected parts, with considerable pressure, three times a day.

NASAL CATARRH.

A. Acute Catarrh—Acute Coryza.

1. Sweating bath at bedtime (1216, 1126, 1191, 1250) 1566
followed by a short cold application,—wet-sheet rub (1216), cold towel rub (1213), cold douche (1010); hot foot bath (1297) with very hot compress to face (1286); steam inhalation (1419); water drinking (1423).

2. **To Prevent.**—Cold bath daily, or twice a day (1625); out-of-door life; avoid excessively warm clothing and warm living or sleeping rooms in winter. Wear linen next the skin summer and winter.

B. Chronic Catarrh.

Etiological Indications.

3. Avoid taking cold, and when an acute catarrh is contracted, cure as soon as possible. See Acute Catarrh 1566, 1, 2.

Pathological Indications.

4. **Increase Activity of the Skin and Tone of Cutaneous Vessels.**—Short sweating procedures, especially the electric-light bath (**1250**) and wet-sheet pack (**1179**) continued until the sweating stage, followed by short cold applications,—wet-sheet rub (**1216**), shallow (**1174**), or cold douche (**1010**); neutral bath at bedtime (**1130**), 20 to 30 minutes, 3 times a week; daily cold morning bath; cold towel rub (**1213**); cold shower (**1047**) or rubbing shallow (**1174**). All sweating baths ought, if possible, to be taken just before retiring at night. During cold weather, oil rubbing (**1232**) two or three times a week.

5. **Improve General Nutrition by Correcting Existing Digestive Disorders.**—See **1520, 1521, 1523.** Out-of-door exercise, especially sun-baths (**1254**) and swimming.

6. **Relieve Nasal Congestion.**—Alternate compresses to the face (**1340**); alternate sponging or compresses to the cervical spine (**1342**); running cold foot (**1296**) bath if extremities are cold; nasal secretions must be removed by antiseptic spray or vaporizer; hypertrophies, polypi, etc., require surgical interference.

General Method.—Build up the general health by tonic measures, employing tonic cold procedures (**1625**) of some sort at least twice daily. Avoid hot baths and too warm clothing and expose the body as much as possible to the open air. Use great care to avoid taking cold by undue exposures; but gradually train the body to the point of enduring exposure without injury. The intestinal disease, which is simply a local manifestation of a general condition of lowered vital resistance, must have the benefit of such local measures as are indicated above.

PHARYNGITIS—TONSILITIS.

A. Acute Form.

1567 1. Rest in bed, room of uniform temperature. Spare diet consisting chiefly of fruits (**1626, 1627**). Avoid meats of all sorts. Copious water drinking (**1423**), especially carbonated water.

2. Hot-blanket pack (**1197**); sweating wet-sheet pack (**1183**); vapor bath (**1246**); electric-light bath (**1250**); hot immersion bath (**1126**) followed by dry pack (**1192, 1191**) or other sweating procedure once daily, followed by cold mitten friction (**1209**), cold wet-sheet rub (**1216**), or cold douche (**1010**). Fomen-

tation (**1328**) to the throat three times a day; cold compress (**1381**) between, changed every 15 to 30 minutes. Enema (**1404**) if bowels are inactive. Hot gargle (**1400**) every few minutes if throat is very sensitive. Ice-bag to throat if inflammation is intense. Inhalation of antiseptic vapors; use of steam inhaler (**1419**), 10 to 14 minutes hourly, or almost continuously. If tonsil suppurates, it should be lanced.

B. Chronic Pharyngitis or Tonsilitis, Clergyman's Sore Throat.

1. Aseptic dietary (**1626**); out-of-door life; open air gymnastics; swimming.

2. Fomentation to throat at bedtime (**1328**), followed by throat pack (**1381**) during night; hot gargle (**1400**) three times a day.

3. Electric-light bath (**1250**); sweating pack (**1191**); vapor bath (**1246**), or other sweating bath, three times a week, followed by suitable cold application (**1625**). Daily cold bath on rising. Moist girdle (**1347**) to be worn during the night. If necessary remove tonsils and vegetations in throat or post-nasal region.

LARYNGITIS.

A. Acute Form.

See Acute Coryza (**1565**). Steam inhalation (**1419**), for **1568**
10 minutes hourly; heating compress to throat (**1382**) without mackintosh; avoid use of voice while very hoarse.

B. Chronic Form.

1. **Increase General Vital Resistance, and Invigorate the Skin.**—Graduated cold baths (**1625**); sweating bath (**1197, 1246, 1250**) or prolonged neutral bath (**1130**) at night, two or three times a week. Follow sweating procedure by any suitable cold application.

2. **To Relieve Local Congestion.**—Steam inhalation (**1419**) every 4 hours for 10 minutes; fomentation (**1328**) at night, followed by well-protected neck compress (**1382**) to be worn during the night.

3. **Cough.**—See **1569**, 4–7.

CROUP.

1569 ### A. Acute Catarrh of Larynx.

Hot bath with cold to head; hot water drinking (**1429**); cold mitten friction (**1209**) every 3 hours; inhalation of vapor arising from slacking lime; cold compress, 60°, over throat, changed every 10 to 20 minutes; hot-blanket pack every three or four hours, 15 minutes; keep feet, legs, and arms very warm. Surgical interference often necessary.

B. False Croup, Laryngismus Stridulus, Spasmodic Laryngitis.

Etiological Indications.

1. **Prevent attacks** by hardening the skin by daily cold bath (**1625**). Remove nasal obstruction, hypertrophies, or adenoid vegetations. Antiseptic inhalations.

2. **Prevent Chilling of Shoulders** during sleep, by warm sleeping jacket. Proper clothing.

Pathological Indications.

3. **Develop Resistance.** — Graduated tonic applications (**1625**); out-of-door life; careful regulation of clothing.

4. **Relieve Congestion** if spasm is severe by hot-blanket pack (**1197**) or hot immersion bath (**1126**). Repeat every three to six hours. Hot half-bath (**1174**) with cold affusion (**1103**) to head, back, and chest. Follow bath by ice-cold heating compress to neck (**1382**) to be changed every two to four hours. Fomentation to cervical and dorsal spine for 15 minutes each time the ice compress is changed.

5. **To relieve spasm,** compress the phrenic nerve by pressure just above the sternal intersection of the sterno-cleido-mastoid muscle; percuss chest with end of cold wet towel, or dash cold water over chest and back.

6. **Bronchitis.**— If present, chest pack (**1373**); repeat in four to six hours; cold mitten friction (**1209**) twice a day. Steam inhalation (**1419**) and copious water drinking (**1423**) when bronchial or laryngeal catarrh exists.

ACUTE BRONCHITIS.

Etiological Indications. 1570

1. **Increase Resistance.**—Graduated cold applications (1625) daily; out-of-door life; daily air bath (1470); avoid excessively warm clothing, and very warm sleeping or living rooms.

Pathological Indications.

2. **Eliminate Toxins.**—Moderately prolonged sweating procedures (1250, 1246, 1233, 1191) followed by cold applications.

3. **Relieve Visceral Congestion.**—Electric-light bath (10 to 20 minutes) (1250), sweating pack (1191), 1 to 2 hours, or vapor bath (1246) 6 to 15 minutes, followed by rubbing wet sheet (1216) or cold douche (1010); hot bath at bedtime (1126) for 6 to 10 minutes, followed by prolonged neutral bath (1130) 20 to 40 minutes. Apply daily or twice a day, hot hip (1389) and leg pack (1393), followed by cold towel rub (1213).

Clinical Indications.

4. **Cough.**—Chest pack (1373), to be changed every 6 hours. If temperature is elevated, change chest pack every 2 to 4 hours. Copious water drinking (1423), 2 to 3 pints daily.

5. **Irritable Cough, without Expectoration.**—Sipping very hot water; gargle hot water (1400); steam inhalations (1419); avoid mouth breathing; keep air of room warm (75° to 80°), and moist with steam; carefully avoid exposure of back of neck, chest, or shoulders to drafts, or chill by evaporation during treatment.

6. **Cough with Viscid Expectoration.**—Copious hot water drinking (1423); fluid diet (1628); fomentation to chest (1328, 1380) every two hours, followed by heating compress (1373).

7. **Painful Cough.**—Fomentation to chest (1328) every two hours; tight bandage about chest to restrain movement if necessary; revulsive compress (1341) for 15 minutes every two hours or often as needed, dry cotton chest pack (1388) between 1571
applications.

CHRONIC BRONCHITIS.

1. **Improve General Resistance.**—Graduated cold treatment (1625); aseptic dietary (1626); warm dry climate; outdoor life.

2. **Cough.**— Chest pack (**1373**) protected by impervious covering. Copious water drinking (**1423**), 3 to 6 pints daily, steam inhalation (**1419**). See **1570.**

3. **Ineffective Cough.**— Increase expulsive power by rubbing or percussion of the chest with the hand dipped in ice water, or slapping the chest with a cold, wet towel.

4. **Asthma.**—Cold fan douche to back of chest (**1061**), followed by heating chest pack (**1373**); revulsive compress to chest (**1341**); Scotch douche to legs (**1037**); hot foot (**1297**) or leg bath (**1299**); hot leg pack (**1393**); hot enema (**1404**); if sympathetic is irritable, wet-girdle (**1347, 1348, 1367**); chest pack (**1373**), well protected.

5. **Emphysema.** — Alternate compress or douche to spine (**1342**); cold mitten friction (**1209**); cold towel rub (**1213**); wet-sheet rub (**1216**); wet girdle covered with flannel only (**1347**); leg packs (**1393**); cold precordial compress (**1383**) 15 to 30 minutes three times a day.

General Method.—The general method is the same as that for intestinal catarrh. See **1529.**

PULMONARY CONGESTION.

1572 1. **Active Congestion.**—Fomentation to back (**1328**), cold compress to chest (**1318**) with hot leg pack (**1393**), followed by cold friction and dry heat (**1192**) to legs; short cold applications to hands and arms (**1209, 1213**), followed by hot packs to arms (**1328**); Scotch douche to legs (**1037**); hot leg bath (**1299**) with very cold compress to chest (**1314**) before and behind. Change compress as soon as warmed.

2. **Passive Congestion of Chest.**—Apply fomentation (**1328**) over chest for 10 minutes every hour; during interval, cold compress (**1314**), renewing every fifteen minutes, rubbing surface well at each change. Most often occurs in fevers (hypostatic congestion). Prevent by frequent change of patient's position. Apply same derivative measures as for active congestion (See above).

3. **Pulmonary Hemorrhage.**—Ice compress to chest (**1314**); remove, and rub the chest with dry warm flannel 1 to 2 minutes every 15 minutes; hot leg pack (**1393**), very hot sponging of the upper half of the spine. Place hands in ice-water 1 to 2 minutes; maintain skin circulation by dry rubbing (**1221**). Keep

patient very quiet. After hemorrhage ceases, graduated cold treatment (1625) to increase resistance and combat the disease to which the hemorrhage is due. See Pulmonary Tuberculosis 1508.

BRONCHO-PNEUMONIA.

For general measures See Lobar Pneumonia (1498). 1573

1. **Bronchial Irritation.**—Steam inhalation (1419), 15 minutes every hour; fomentation (1328) to chest every 2 hours for 15 minutes, followed by heating compress (1373); hot-blanket pack.

2. **Cyanosis.**—Short hot half-bath (1174); pour cold water over head, spine, and chest to induce cough, if cough is checked or inefficient while secretion is abundant. It is well to have the patient sit in a tub with a small amount of hot water (1174), while a cold affusion (1102) is administered followed by vigorous rubbing, and wrapping in dry blankets in bed.

3. **Heart Failure.**—Cold precordial compress (1383) 15 minutes every hour. Also see 1578, 1, 5.

4. **After Convalescence Begins.**—Chest pack (1373) night and day. Graduated cold applications (1625) to build up general resistance.

PLEURISY.

A. Acute Form.

1. **General.**—Improve general resistance by cold applications two or three times daily (1625, 1201, 1209, 1213); hot leg bath (1299) if extremities are cold. Water drinking (1423); aseptic dietary (1626). 1574

2. **Pain.**—Very hot fomentation (1328) for 10 minutes over affected side. Revulsive compress (1341); limit movement of lung by tight bandage to the chest. Repeat every 2 hours. During interval, apply either cold (1318) or heating compress (1344) as best suits the case.

After Convalescence.—Alternate chest douche (1044) or alternate compress (1340) if necessary to absorb exudate. Apply three times a day, continuous heating compress (1344, 1373), with mackintosh covering, during interval.

3. **Exudate.**—Alternate compress or spray three times a day; graduated general tonic applications (1625). Prolonged neutral bath (1130) half an hour to an hour daily.

B. Chronic Form.

1. Neutral bath (**1130**) at night three times a week, of 20 to 30 minutes' duration. Graduated cold (**1625**) daily. Fomentation (**1328**) to chest three times a day, or revulsive spray (**1041**), or compress (**1341**); well-protected heating compress (**1344**) during the interval.

2. Aseptic dietary (**1626**). Gymnastics to expan dchest after removal of fluid if necessary to overcome adhesions.

3. **Tubercular Pleurisy.**—Short revulsive compress (**1341**) (5 minutes) for relief of pain, three or four times a day, or often as necessary; flannel-covered heating compress (**1344**) during intervals; graduated tonic measures (**1625**).

NOCTURNAL ASTHMA.

1575 Neutral bath (**1130**) at bedtime; wet girdle (**1347**); copious water drinking (**1423**); enema before retiring (**1404**); graduated cold baths (**1625**); renal douche (**1098**). Cold coloclyster (**1407**) daily in cases of toxemia with dilated colon. Correct any existing gastric disturbance.

Sweating process when skin is inactive (**1250, 1246, 1197, 1191**) followed by cold bath of appropriate form (**1625**).

PERICARDITIS, ENDOCARDITIS.

1576 1. **To Combat Inflammation.**—Continuous ice-bag (**1383**) over heart, or precordial compress at 60°, changed every 15 minutes. Remove ice-bag every 15 minutes, rub chest with dry flannel until skin is red.

2. **To Energize Heart and Maintain General Vital Resistance.**—Cold mitten friction (**1209**); cold towel rub (**1213**) twice a day.

3. **Fever.**—Prolonged neutral bath (**1130**); neutral wet-sheet pack (**1182**).

4. **Pain.**—Fomentation (**1328**) for 1 to 3 minutes every half-hour; cold compress changed every 15 minutes during interval.

5. **Myocarditis.**—Employ all the means above recommended, except, avoid ice-bag over heart.

ORGANIC CARDIAC DISEASE, VALVULAR DISEASE OF THE HEART.

1. General tonic measures, carefully graduated (**1625**); moderate antiseptic dietary (**1626**), avoiding hot foods, tea and coffee, alcoholic drinks, condiments, flesh meats, and indigestibles. 1577

Pathological Indications.

2. **To Increase Energy of Heart.**—Ice-bag over heart (**1383**) for 15 minutes, gradually increased to 1 hour, twice a day. If limbs are swollen, rest in bed until swelling disappears. Effervescent bath (**1139**) one to three times weekly; massage; leg packs. Special gymnastics (Schott).

Clinical Indications.

3. **Dyspnea.**—Elevate the head and shoulders when patient is ying down; cold compress to chest (**1318**) and hot pack to legs (**1393**); change compress every 15 to 20 minutes; at each change, rub the surface of the chest with dry flannel until red.

4. **Pain.**—Very hot fomentation (**1328**) over seat of pain for 3 minutes; follow by heating compress (**1344**) at 60°, changing every 20 minutes; repeat every two or three hours; revulsive compress (**1341**); hot and cold gastric compress (**1356**).

5. **Insomnia.**—Elevation of head and shoulders or head of bed; wet girdle (**1347**); neutral bath (**1130**) for half an hour at bedtime, or neutral douche (**1031**) 3 to 4 minutes at bedtime.

6. **Headache.**—Prolonged neutral bath (**1130**); copious water drinking (**1423**); cool enema (**1404**); hot-blanket pack (**1197**) with ice-bag over the heart (**1383**); ice-cap (**1323, 1371**). If kidneys are diseased, apply fomentation over loins with ice-bag over heart and lower third of sternum.

7. **Dropsy.**—Rest in bed; hot blanket pack (**1197**) followed by sweating wet-sheet pack (**1191**) ending with cold friction (**1209**); leg packs (**1393**); electric-light bath (**1250**) or vapor bath (**1246**) for lower half of body; ice-bag over heart during hot baths; massage; effervescing bath (**1139**).

8. **To Energize the Heart and Encourage Peripheral Circulation.**—Wet sheet rub (**1216**); cold towel rub (**1213**); Scotch douche (**1037**) at 102°, lowering without sudden change to 80° during first applications. At each succeeding application, a temperature 1° lower until 65° or 60° is reached. Cold friction

(**1209**); fan douche (**1061**) over chest without pressure at 75°, duration 10 or 15 seconds.

9. **Cardiac Hypertrophy.**—Rest in bed; ice-bag over heart for 1 hour three to four times daily; prolonged neutral bath (**1130**), 92° to 94°, 20 to 60 minutes; neutral pack (**1182**) 20 to 40 minutes; graduated cold baths (**1625**); heating abdominal compress (**1351**); gentle massage; centrifugal friction (**1224**).

10. **Hepatic Congestion and Hypertrophy (Nutmeg Liver).**—Alternate compress (**1340**); alternate douche (**1044**) with slight pressure; heating compress (**1344**), covered with flannel only during the night; if pain is present, revulsive compress (**1341**); treatment for relief of portal congestion. See **1278, 1279**.

11. **Pulmonary Hemorrhage.**—See Pulmonary Congestion (**1572**, 2, 3).

12. **Cough.**—If acute, **1572**, 2; if chronic, chest pack, flannel covered (**1373**); warm covering of arms; heat to legs; intermittent precordial compress (**1383**).

13. **Palpitation.**—See **1578**, 3.

14. **Angina Pectoris.**—Ice-bag to dorsal spine (**1372**); hot leg pack (**1393**); short fomentation (30 secs.) over heart, followed by warm dry compress.

15. **Gastric Catarrh.**—See **1520**.

16. **Arterio-Sclerosis.**—Prolonged neutral bath (**1130**) three times a week at bedtime. Carefully graduated cold baths (**1625**). Aseptic dietary (**1626**); gentle massage; moderate exercise.

17. **Contraindications.**—Cold immersion baths, cold douche, Russian bath, very hot or prolonged warm baths. Avoid such exercises as produce swelling of feet, cough, dyspnea. Ice-bag over the heart, and the ice-cold precordial compress must be avoided in cases of fatty heart.

In general, cases of valvular disease of the heart require, during the *first stage*, carefully graduated cold baths with moderate exercise. During the *second stage*, rest in bed, ice-bag over the heart for 15 to 30 minutes two to three times daily; very carefully administered tonic treatment, such as cold mitten friction, cold towel rubbing, graduated into more vigorous measures (**1625**); skillful massage and carefully graduated exercises. In the *third stage* complete rest in bed, with the application of special measures for the relief of dropsy (**1582**), and the careful employment of the same measures necessary for the second stage. The general aim is to energize the heart and lessen its work by increasing the activity of the peripheral heart (1139).

FUNCTIONAL CARDIAC DISEASES.

1. **Shock, Collapse, Cyanosis.**— Hot fomentations (1328) or 1578
hot-blanket pack (1197) for 10 to 15 minutes, or hot immersion bath (1126) 3 to 6 minutes, followed by cold mitten friction (1209); cold towel rubbing (1213) or wet-sheet rubbing (1216), continued until surface is reddened, applying every 2 to 3 hours, or two to three times daily, as may be necessary; ice-bag over heart, or cold precordial compress (1383), 15 minutes, repeating every hour; alternate compress to spine (1342); hot enema (1406); keep patient warm by hot bags and flannel blankets; alternate compress (1340) over heart if necessary; heat to head if face is pale.

2. **Tachycardia.**—Rest in bed; ice-bag over heart (1383); gastric lavage (1401) if indicated; cold enema (1404) or coloclyster (1407) to relieve constipation; if abdominal ganglia are sensitive, abdominal fomentation (1328) followed by heating compress (1344) to be repeated every 6 hours; neutral bath (1130) for half an hour, 92° to 94°; gastric lavage if stomach is foul.

3. **Cardiac Palpitation.**—Rest in bed; cold precordial compress (1383); ice-bag to the cervical region (1314); cold frictions (1209); cold douche (1047) following hot foot bath (1297); wet-sheet rub (1216); shallow bath 78°, one-half minute (1174); gradually accustom patient to cold applications (1625); hot and cold gastric compress (1362), or trunk pack (1367); gastric lavage (1401); enema (1404).

4. **Aortic Palpitation.**— Usually due to toxins or other irritants of the abdominal sympathetic. Fomentation (1328) to abdominal region for 10 minutes followed by heating compress (1351) to be renewed every 4 to 6 hours; if enteroptosis is present, abdominal supporter; ice-bag over aorta. Relieve constipation if present by cool enema (1404), 75° to 65°. Gastric lavage if required. Wet girdle (1347) at night without impervious covering.

5. **Feeble Heart, without Fatty Degeneration.**— Cold precordial compress (1383) 15 minutes daily; increase 5 minutes each day until duration is 30 to 40 minutes. Percussion douche

to the spine (1035); vigorous cold friction (1209) to extremities. Avoid prolonged cold applications or prolonged chilling.

6. **Decrease Work Required of the Heart.**— Dilate surface vessels and increase their activity by cold mitten friction (1209), cold towel rub (1213), wet-sheet rub (1216), shallow bath, 72° to 75°, one-half minute (1174). If necessary, precede the short cold application by a short heating procedure as a fomentation to the spine (1328), vapor (1246), hot immersion (1126), or electric-light bath (1250) for 3 to 5 minutes, or hot sponging (1206).

7. **Remove Toxins.**— Lavage (1401); coloclyster (1407); water drinking (1423).

8. **Slow Pulse.**— Alternate sponging or compress to spine (1342); hot water drinking (1429); dry friction (1221); massage; carefully graduated cold baths (1625).

9. Avoid hot baths, or if a warm bath is necessary, make very short (102° to 104°), and follow with short, cold application.

CHLOROSIS.

1579 ***Etiological Indications.***

1. **Correct Enteroptosis.**— Abdominal Supporter; abdominal massage; corrective exercises; cold abdominal douche (1081); electricity.

Pathological Indications.

2. **Increase Vital Resistance.**— General graduated cold procedures (1625) twice daily.

3. **Combat Autoxintoication.**— Aseptic diet (1626); sweating bath to beginning perspiration, electric-light bath (1250) or sun bath (1254) followed by short cold application (1625).

Clinical Indications.

4. **Low Blood Count.**— See Anemia 1580, 1.

5. **Constipation.**— See 1524.

6. **Vaso-Motor Spasm.**— General Scotch douche (1037); alternate immersion (105° to 110°, 30 seconds, 80° to 70°, 15 seconds); simultaneous Scotch douche (1037).

7. **Visceral Anemias.**— Visceral douches (1088–1099), alternate (1044), Scotch (1037) short percussion (1035); alternate compress over part (1340), followed by well-protected heat-

ing compress (1344); Mackintosh-covered wet girdle at night; cool enema (75° to 68°), 1 to 3 pints, daily.

ANEMIA.

Etiological Indications.

1. **Increase Blood-Making Process.**— Graduated cold applications (1625). The electric-light bath (1250) is especially valuable as a means of heating before general cold applications (1637); aseptic dietary (1626), substances rich in proteids and fats; rest in bed, if patient is emaciated; out-of-door life; cold air baths (1470); sun baths (1254); sea bathing (1147); massage; manual Swedish movements; electricity; oxygen inhalation. static. 1580

Clinical Indications.

2. **Neuralgia.**—See 1545.
3. **Hyperpepsia.**— See 1522.
4. **Hypopepsia.**— See 1521.
5. **Chronic Gastro-Intestinal Catarrh.**— See 1519, 1529
6. **Loss of Appetite.**—See 1521, 5.
7. **Vomiting.**— See 1523, 3.
8. **Constipation.**— See 1524.
9. **Enteroptosis.**— See 1525.
10. **Gastric Dilatation.**— See 1523.
11. **Gastric Ulcer.**— See 1526.
12. **Fever.**— Prolonged neutral bath (1130) daily; fomentation to spine (1328) followed by wet-sheet pack (1179).
13. **Nervous Excitability.**— Neutral bath (1130); heating compress to spine (1344); neutral rain douche (1050).
14. **Dropsy.**— See 1582.
15. **Palpitation of Heart or Aorta.**— See 1578, 3, 4.
16. **Metrorrhagia or Menorrhagia.**— See 1588.
17. **Chronic Nephritis.**— See 1538.
18. **Malarial Cachexia.**— See 1490, 17.
19. **Vaso-Motor Spasm.**— See 1579, 6, 7.

General Method.— Cold water is the most valuable of all curative measures in anemia. Apply twice daily, graduating carefully (1625). Autointoxication arising from dilatation (1523) or prolapse (1525) of the stomach, or chronic constipation (1524), is often the principal cause to be combated (1473-1475).

PERNICIOUS ANEMIA.

1581 1. **Combat Autointoxication.**— Electric-light bath (**1250**) vapor bath (**1246**), or hot-blanket pack (**1197**), 5 minutes, followed by cold bath (**1625**) twice a week. Aseptic dietary (**1626**).

2. **Indigestion.** — See Hypopepsia (**1521**). Aseptic diet (**1626**).

3. **Promote General Nutrition and Blood Making.** —Graduated tonic baths daily (**1625**); ice-bag over the stomach half an hour before each meal. See Anemia **1580.**

4. **Cerebral Anemia.**— Rest in bed with foot of bed raised. Warm flannel about the neck to promote cerebral circulation. Warm compress to back of neck if patient is inclined to faint.

5. **General Method.**— The same as for simple anemia (**1580**).

GENERAL DROPSY, ANASARCA, OR MALEOLAR EDEMA.

1582 1. Rest in bed; ice-bag over heart 15 to 30 minutes three times a day; graduated cold treatment twice daily (**1625**); heating pack to legs (**1393**); water drinking (**1423**); sweating procedures when due to renal disease (**1250, 1191**); wet girdle (**1347**), changing every 2 hours.

2. **Palpitation.**—See **1578,** 3.

3. **Nervous Irritability.**— Prolonged neutral bath (**1130**) 30 to 60 minutes every other day; alternate spinal compress.

4. **Vomiting.**— Lavage (**1401**); ice-bag over stomach; hot and cold trunk pack (**1367**); ice-bag to lumbar region.

5. **Fever.**— Prolonged neutral bath (**1130**), daily or more often; cold mitten friction (**1209**); cold towel rub (**1213**).

EXOPHTHALMIC GOITER.

1583 ***Pathological Indications.***

1. **Enlarged Thyroid.**— Ice-bag over gland, continuously, removing for five minutes every half-hour; galvanization of cervical and abdominal sympathetic.

2. **Anemia.**— Carefully graduated cold wet hand rub (**1201**), mitten friction (**1209**), and towel rub (**1213**). See **1580.**

3. **Autointoxication.**— Aseptic diet (**1626**); coloclyster (80°) daily; neutral bath, 20 to 30 minutes daily (**1130**); water drinking (**1423**).

4. **Nervous Irritability and Exhaustion.**— Rest in bed; carefully graduated cold baths (**1625**).

Clinical Indications.

5. **General Feebleness.**— Graduated cold applications (**1625**).
6. **Emaciation.**— Rest; diet rich in fats and proteids (**1626**).
7. **Palpitation.**— See **1578**, 3, 4.
8. **Insomnia.**— See **1564**.
9. **Neuralgia.**— See **1545**.
10. **Diarrhea.**— See **1529**.
11. **Constipation.**— See **1524**.
12. **Gastric Irritability.**— Hot and cold gastric compress (**1356**); revulsive compress (**1341**). See Chronic Gastritis (**1520**), Hypopepsia (**1521**), Hyperpepsia (**1522**).
13. **Jaundice.**— See **1608**.
14. **Tremor.**— Short spinal fomentation (5 minutes) followed by heating compress (**1344**) for several hours daily.
15. **Contraindications.**— Very hot or cold general applications.

General Method.— This disease is probably an autointoxication. As the patients are generally very feeble, the measures employed must be at first very gentle, and must be very carefully graduated to avoid any aggravation of symptoms (**1625**).

MYXEDEMA.

Graduated cold baths (**1625**); massage; galvanism to abdominal sympathetic; electric-light bath (**1250**) or other sweating procedure (**1246, 1233, 1191**) followed by appropriate cold baths (**1213, 1216, 1010**). Ice-bag over heart during hot applications. Train patient to use of cold douche (**1010, 1017, 1625**) as soon as possible. Strong percussion douche (**1035**) to spine when it can be borne. 1584

General Method.—This condition is doubtless due to autointoxication and lack of some element supplied to the body by the thyroid gland. Hydrotherapy alone is beneficial in many cases, but hydriatic measures may be best employed in connection with the systematic use of the dried sheep's thyroid.

ARTHRITIS DEFORMANS, RHEUMATIC GOUT.

1. **General Restorative Measures.**—The diet must be specially nourishing and digestible, rich in fats and proteids (**1626**). See 1585

Emaciation (**1516**). A warm, rather dry, and uniform climtae is most desirable.

2. Carefully graduated cold applications (**1625**), preceded by very short hot applications; fomentation (**1328**) to spine or the electric-light bath (**1250**) 3 to 5 minutes, and the sun bath (**1254**), followed by cold mitten friction (**1209**) are especially suitable; massage; manual Swedish movements; oil rubbing (**1232**); wet girdle (**1347**).

Clinical Indications.

3. **Fever.**—Prolonged neutral bath (**1130**) at 92°; fomentation (**1328**) to spine followed by cold friction (**1209**) or towel rub (**1213**).

4. **Frequent Pulse.**—Cold precordial compress (**1383**) or ice-bag for 15 to 30 minutes three times a day.

5. **Pain in Joints.**—Revulsive compresses (**1341**) followed by cotton poultice (**1388**); local vapor bath (**1249**); local electric-light bath (**1250**).

6. **Neuralgia of Hands.**—Hot hand bath (**1302**) followed by cotton poultice (**1388**).

7. **Radiating Pains.**—Fomentation (**1328**) to spine three times a day, heating compress (**1344**) during interval, well protected with mackintosh; revulsive compress (**1341**) to spine; galvanic or sinusoidal electricity to trunk, arms, or legs, as indicated.

8. **Numbness and Tingling of Hands and Feet.**—Fomentation to spine, hot or alternate sponging of limbs (**1204**), repeated three times a day; faradic or sinusoidal electricity.

9. **Muscular Cramps.**—Fomentation (**1328**) or hot immersion of affected parts two or more times daily; during interval, well-protected heating compress (**1344**); hot sponging; firm bandaging. Protect patient from chill.

10. **Muscular Atrophy.**—Alternate douche (**1044**), compress (**1340**) or sponging; massage; massage-douche (**1066**); sinusoidal electrical current (**1446**) applied to affected muscles.

11. **Joint Deformities.**—For thickening of synovial membrane or accumulation of fluid in joints or bursæ, apply alternate douche (**1044**); alternate compress (**1340**); massage-douche (**1066**); Apply to joint dry flannel bandage or cotton poultice (**1388**).

12. **Contraindications.**—Cold douche to painful joints; long sweating processes and prolonged general hot applications.

General Method.—Improve the general health by general tonic measures, especially carefully graduated cold baths (**1625**), massage and general applications of electricity, combating local manifestations of the disease by local applications of massage and other palliative measures above recommended.

PELVIC PAIN.

1. Remove all known causes—tight bands, heavy skirts, tight shoes, cold extremities, sexual excess. **1586**

2. Rest in horizontal position, with proper general treatment for any existing general or local morbid condition, as anemia (**1580**), neurasthenia (**1554**), hysteria (**1553**), enteroptosis (**1525**), constipation (**1524**), or any discoverable pelvic disease. See **1590, 1591, 1592, 1619**.

3. If *neuralgic*, hot hip and leg pack (**1389, 1393**) or very hot revulsive sitz (pp. 766, 770) three times a day; hot bag over seat of pain, heat to feet and legs. Very hot vaginal irrigation (**1413**).

4. *If due to chronic congestion*, hot hip and leg pack (**1389, 1393**) every 2 to 4 hours, with abdominal heating compress (**1351**); and heating leg packs (**1393**) during interval.

5. *If due to inflammation or acute congestion*, hot hip and leg pack (**1389, 1393**) or hot and cold pelvic pack (**1370**) every 2 to 4 hours, followed by continuous heat to legs with cooling compress to lower abdomen, external genitals and inner surfaces of thighs. Vaginal irrigation (**1413**) at 105° for 15 minutes every 3 hours, apply ice-bag over seat of pain during hot vaginal irrigation and hot hip and leg pack.

DYSMENORRHEA.

1. Rest in bed during period. **1587**

2. **When Due to Ovarian Disease** (beginning before flow).—Hot hip and leg pack (**1389, 1393**); hot-blanket pack (**1197**); fomentation (**1328**) over hypogastrium; hot pelvic pack (**1390**); revulsive sitz (pp. 776, 770); hot rectal irrigation (**1410**) followed by hot foot bath (**1297**) if flow is checked; hot douche (99° to 102°); very hot immersion (105° to 110°) 5 to 8 minutes.

3. **When Due to Uterine Disease** (beginning with and accompanying flow).—Hot hip pack (**1389**) with hot foot bath

(**1297**) followed by cold compress to hypogastrium and inner surfaces of thighs for 30 to 40 seconds. For treatment between periods, see **1591**.

4. **When Due to Inflammatory Disease of Appendages.**— Hot enema (**1406**); hot fomentations (**1328**); hot pelvic pack (**1390**); hot-blanket pack (**1197**).

General Method.— In addition to the local measures for relief of pain which have been indicated above, it is in most cases necessary to combat some general disorder to which the local disease may be more or less directly related. See Anemia (**1580**), Neurasthenia (**1554**), Hysteria (**1553**). General tonic measures must be employed between the menstrual periods. In chronic ovarian congestion, apply the hypogastric compress (**1318**) during the night; administer daily the revulsive sitz (pp. 766, 770) or hot pelvic pack (**1390**), and the very hot vaginal irrigation (**1413**), 115° to 120°, 15 minutes. In cases of deficient development, as in infantile uterus or vasomotor spasm of the uterine vessels, employ the revulsive sitz, alternate genito-urinary douche (**1099**), tonic sitz (**1309**), pelvic and general massage, and local galvanic and sinusoidal electrical applications.

Applications of electricity and surgical measures are often required for permanent relief, but a surprisingly large number of cases are curable without surgery; hence hydriatic measures should be perseveringly tried before resorting to surgical procedures.

METRORRHAGIA AND MENORRHAGIA.

1588 1. Hot vaginal irrigation (**1413**); short hot hip pack (**1389**); hot foot bath (**1297**), followed by cold compress to hypogastrium (**1314**) and inner surfaces of thighs. In obstinate cases, cold vaginal irrigation (**1413**). Moderately prolonged, very cold, shallow sitz (50° to 65° for 5 to 15 minutes) (**1309**), accompanied by hot foot bath (**1297**) when other measures fail; hot douche (**1024**) to lower spine, hypogastrium, inner surfaces of thighs, twice daily during intervals.

2. **Contraindications.**— Prolonged hot sitz, hot douche, hot leg, foot, and sitz baths, and in some cases even fomentations and hot vaginal irrigation must be avoided. It is equally necessary to avoid short cold applications to the lower spine, abdomen, thighs and feet, as the reflex effects of such applications increase pelvic and uterine congestion.

General Method.—It is always highly important to inquire closely for all possible causes of the profuse flow. The cause may be simple anemia (**1580**) from defective nutrition, constipation (**1524**), sexual excess, enteroptosis (**1525**), uterine displacement (**1619**), ovarian or tubal disease (**1592**), uterine inflammation or congestion (**1591**). The most common cause is vegetations of the endometrium, which must be removed by surgical measures. The operation must be followed by treatment for chronic metritis (**1591**). In many instances, several of these conditions may be combined. Such general and local measures must be employed as have been suggested above and elsewhere, and it is rare that treatment is not very speedily followed by most gratifying results.

AMENORRHEA.

1. Tonic sitz (**1309**); cold pelvic pack (**1390**, 1); graduated tonic baths (**1625**) twice daily; short very cold douche to lower spine (**1076**), hypogastrium and inner surfaces of thighs; pelvic massage daily, and especially when period is due. 1589

2. **Suppressed Menstruation.**—Short cold douche to spine, thighs, and hypogastrium (**1099**) daily or twice a day; hot foot bath (**1297**) or hot-blanket pack (**1197**) during interval between the periods. Intrauterine applications of the faradic or sinusoidal electrical current; hot hip pack (**1389**); warm vaginal irrigation (**1413**), 95° to 100°.

3. **General Method.**—It is very necessary to treat the patient rather than her malady. Apply such measures as may be required for relief of anemia (**1580**), chlorosis (**1579**), indigestion (**1521–1523**) or any other disturbance of the nutritive functions.

PELVIC PERITONITIS, CELLULITIS.

Etiological Indications.

1. Surgical and puerperal asepsis; care to avoid exposures at menstrual periods; protection of feet and legs in damp and cold weather; proper clothing. 1590

Pathological Indications.

2. **Increase Resistance.**—Cold mitten friction (**1209**) or cold towel rub (**1213**) two to four times a day, protecting pelvic viscera by simultaneous hot foot or leg pack (**1393, 1394**) or by hot bag to sacrum and cold compress to hypogastrium.

3. **Combat Local Inflammation.**—Hot hip and leg pack (**1389, 1393**) 20 minutes every 2 hours; during intervals, cold compress (**1318**) at 60° to hypogastrium, pudenda and inner surfaces of thighs, with heat to feet and legs, or ice-bag over seat of pain, hot bags or fomentations to feet, hips and thighs; hot and cold pelvic compress (**1364**) with ice-bag over seat of pain; continue 20 to 40 minutes, and repeat when needed; hot vaginal irrigation (**1413**) (110° to 120°), one gallon, every 4 hours.

4. **Encourage Resolution.**—After acute stage has passed, apply alternate compress (**1340**) for 30 minutes three times a day; during interval, heating compresses (**1344**), changing every 2 hours, or as soon as well warmed; graduated tonic baths (**1625**); alternate vaginal irrigation (110°, 80° to 70°); later, pelvic massage.

Clinical Indications.

5. **Pain.**—Fomentation (**1328**) or revulsive compress (**1341**) every 2 to 4 hours, or oftener if necessary.

6. **Constipation.**—Large hot enemas (**1406**) twice a day during acute pain and inflammation; later, graduated cold enema (**1409**).

7. **Chill.**—Anticipate chill by wrapping patient in warm blankets with hot bags to trunk and limbs; hot water drinking (**1429**).

8. **Septic Fever.**—Add to local measures, if fever is high, hot-blanket pack (**1197**) 10 to 15 minutes, followed by sweating wet-sheet pack (**1183, 1191**) prolonged neutral bath (**1130**). If suppuration occurs, surgical interference is generally indicated.

9. **Anemia.**—See **1580**.

10. **Contraindications.**—Avoid cold immersions; partial cold applications, such as the cold-mitten friction and the cold-towel rub, must be used instead.

CHRONIC METRITIS AND PELVIC CONGESTION.

1591 1. Graduated cold applications (**1625**); hot vaginal irrigation (**1413**), 10 to 15 minutes, twice daily; hot-blanket pack to legs (**1393**) with cold pelvic pack (**1390**), continued to sweating stage, followed by cold friction (**1209, 1213**) or wet-sheet rub (**1216**).

Clinical Indications.

2. **Pain.**—Prolonged neutral sitz bath (**1312**) 95° to 97°, duration, 15 to 20 minutes.

3. **Leucorrhea.**—In addition to the above measures, antiseptic vaginal irrigation, bichloride 1 to 5,000, or permanganate 1 to 200. In certain cases, cool irrigation, 75° to 65°, produces better results than hot irrigation. Constipation (**1524**) and portal congestion (**1279**) must be relieved. Cervical catarrh and erosions often require the use of the curette.

4. **Acute Inflammation.**—If attacks of inflammation occur, rest in bed; hot hip or leg pack (**1389, 1393**); hot and cold pelvic compress (**1364**) or hot and cold pelvic pack (**1370**).

OVARITIS AND SALPINGITIS.

A. Acute Form.

1. Rest in bed; hot vaginal irrigation (**1413**) twice daily; hot 1592
pelvic pack (**1390**); hot leg pack (**1393**) or hot foot bath (**1297**) twice daily, followed by cold friction (**1209**). If suppuration of tubes occurs, operation is usually necessary. During the first few days, ice-bag over inflamed part, interrupted at intervals of 1 to 3 hours by fomentatation for 15 minutes or hot and cold pelvic compress (**1364**) for 30 minutes; heat to limbs.

2. **Contraindications.**—General cold applications, and cold applications to the feet.

B. Chronic Form.

1. Rest in bed with hips elevated; neutral bath (**1130**) 15 to 30 minutes three times a week; hot pelvic pack (**1390**) morning and night followed by general cold friction (**1209**) and heating compress (**1344**) over the hypogastrium to be retained until the next hot application. The heating compress should be well covered. If pain is intense, employ a hot hip and leg pack (**1389, 1393**) twice daily, with the heating compress during the interval. The circulation of the lower extremities may also be encouraged by a prolonged heating compress applied to each leg separately (**1393**) 2 or 3 hours once a day. Vigorous cold friction with towel or mitt should be applied to the legs on removal of the pack (**1209–1213**). Keep the feet and legs warm.

2. Hot vaginal irrigation twice daily (**1413**); hot rectal irriga-

tion (**1410**) once daily if exudate in pelvis is extensive; sinusoidal current with very rapid alternations; pelvic massage.

3. General tonic applications (**1625**); general massage; manual Swedish movements; sun baths (**1254**); out-of-door exposure with proper protection, carefully avoiding chill; fat and blood-building diet. See Emaciation (**1516**).

4. If suppuration is present, drainage. Removal of the diseased appendages is sometimes required, but in most cases this may be obviated by the proper application of hydriatic measures at the outset.

STERILITY IN WOMEN.

1593 When not due to organic diseases, may often be cured by a course of hydriatic treatment. A course of graduated cold applications (**1625**) is most efficient. The cold rubbing sitz (**1309**) is highly useful. Remove catarrhal conditions of uterus and vagina and subinvolution by means of hot vaginal irrigation (**1413**) followed by tonic sitz (**1309**).

PROSTATITIS.

1594 1. Revulsive sitz bath (p. 770); hot rectal irrigation (**1410**); irrigation of bladder (**1411**), if bladder does not empty itself. Neutral sitz (**1312**), 30 to 60 min. Cold mitten friction (**1209**).

2. **When painful,** revulsive sitz (pp. 770, 766). Fomentation or the Scotch douche to perineum (**1084**), with little pressure. Rectal irrigation (**1410**) in chronic cases. Hot enema (**1406**) when bowels are constipated.

3. **Chronic Enlargement with Induration.**—Good results often follow the use of the following measures: alternate rectal irrigation (**1410**); shallow cold rubbing sitz (**1309**) 4 to 8 min.; cold pelvic pack (**1390**) with hot leg pack (**1393**); massage of prostate; graduated tonic baths (**1625**); ice-bag to perineum, with hot hip and leg pack, 15 to 30 min.

4. **Contraindications.**—When pain is present, avoid general cold baths, cold sitz and foot baths, and chilling of feet. Absolute sexual continence is essential.

ACUTE ORCHITIS.

1595 Rest in bed. Elevation of scrotum upon a tense broad band of cloth placed about the thighs close to hips. Hot pelvic pack

(**1390**) or hot hip pack with cold compress over genitals (**1364**), every 3 hours. During intervals, cold compress at 60° over perineum, genitals, and hypogastrium, with heat to feet. Tepid enema (**1404**) twice daily; cold mitten friction (**1209**) or cold towel rub (**1213**) twice a day; prolonged neutral bath (**1130**) or neutral pack (**1182**) to control temperature if necessary.

SPERMATORRHEA.

1. Graduated cold applications (**1625**) to improve general con- **1596**
dition.

Clinical Indications.

2. **General Nervous Irritability.**—Prolonged neutral bath (**1130**) at night. See Neurasthenia (**1054**).

3. **Irritable Prostate, Irritable Urethra.**—Prolonged neutral sitz (**1312**), 30 to 60 minutes, at bedtime; Scotch douche to perineum (**1084**) with little pressure; tepid rectal irrigation (**1410**) at 80°.

4. **Relaxed Ejaculatory Ducts.**—Rubbing cold sitz (**1309**), cold or alternate irrigation of rectum (**1410**); cold douche to feet and legs (**1082**); cold percussion douche to lower spine (**1074**). Bowels must be kept regular by the cool enema (**1405**) if necessary, and proper diet. An aseptic dietary (**1626**) is essential. Condiments must be strictly avoided. Cooling sound (**1416**), 70°, for 5 minutes daily.

5. **Contraindications.**—When losses are frequent or parts irritable, avoid cold sitz baths and prolonged hot baths.

SEXUAL IMPOTENCE.

Graduated cold baths (**1625**); cold douche to spine (**1074**), **1597**
especially lower part; cold rubbing sitz (**1309**), beginning at 60°, lowering temperature 5° daily to 60°; duration of bath 3 to 8 minutes. Patient should be vigorously rubbed to prevent chilling. If urethral irritation is present, short (2 to 4 minutes) revulsive sitz (pp. 766, 770); cooling compress (**1395**), 5 minutes daily.

PRIAPISM.

Immersion bath (**1112**), 100° for 1 minute, 90° for 5 minutes; **1598**
gradually lower temperature to 75°, and continue for 5 minutes;

lower minimum temperatures 1° daily to 60°; hot douche to lower spine (**1074**) and thighs for 30 seconds; follow by general neutral douche (**1031**) 2 to 3 minutes with considerable pressure (20 to 30 lbs.); prolonged general neutral bath (**1130**) 30 to 40 minutes; Spinal affusion (**1103**) 5 minutes, 98°.

IRRITABLE RECTUM.

1599 ***Pathological Indications.***

1. **Increase Vital Resistance.**— Graduated tonic baths (**1625**).

2. **Combat Local Inflammation.**— Prolonged cool sitz (**1308**), 75° for 15 minutes; cooling compress (**1395**) to nates, anus, perineum, and genitals; cleanse rectum after each stool; render fecal matters soft and bowels regular, by diet and other measures. See **1524.** Rest in horizontal position; hot rectal irrigation (**1410**) daily or oftener; prolonged cold anal douche (**1087**) with little pressure.

Clinical Indications.

Pain.— Revulsive compress (**1341**); ice-bag to anus; fomentation (**1328**) to nates and perineum; hot hip pack (**1389**); hot foot bath (**1297**); hot hip and leg pack (**1389, 1393**); hot vaginal irrigation (**1413**).

Spasm.— Hot sitz (**1311**); sitting over hot water (p. 707).

Constipation.— See **1524.**

Pain in the Back.— Scotch douche to back (**1037**); hot sitz (**1311**); wet-girdle (**1347**).

HEMORRHOIDS.

1600 1. **Portal Congestion.**— Running cold foot bath (**1296**); hot foot (**1297**) or leg bath (**1299**); hot leg pack (**1393**); scotch douche to feet and legs (**1082**); wet girdle (**1347**). (See also **1278, 1279**).

2. **Constipation.**— See **1524.**

3. **Diarrhea.**— See **1528.**

4. **Irreducible Prolapse.**— Rest in bed; lying on the face; knee-chest position if required. Ice compress (**1314**); bathing parts with ice water; daily small cold enema after stool; relieve bowels while lying in horizontal position; avoid straining; abdominal supporter. In many cases, surgical measures are necessary.

5. **Inflamed Hemorrhoids.**—Rest in bed with feet and hips elevated; knee-chest position if necessary; ice-cold compress (1395) pressed firmly against anus; ice suppositories; very shallow ice-cold sitz.

6. **Pain.**—If due to inflammation, short hot fomentation (1328) followed by cold compress applied to the anus and nates (1395), with hot foot bath (1297) at the same time; repeat fomentation hourly or every two hours; prolonged tepid sitz (1304), temperature 85° to 80°; hot hip and leg pack (1389, 1393), followed by cold compress over nates, perineum, and lumbar region (1395).

SYPHILIS.

1. **First and Second Stages.**—Eliminative baths—vapor 1601
(1246), electric-light (1250), sweating pack (1191), followed by short cold tonic applications—wet-sheet rub (1216), graduated douche (1017), or cold towel rub (1209); outdoor life; regular habits, aseptic dietary (1626), especially careful avoidance of meats, tea and coffee, tobacco, alcoholic drinks, and all indigestible and unwholesome foods.

2. **Skin Eruptions.**—Prolonged neutral bath (1130).

3. **Syphilitic Cachexia.**—Electric-light baths (1250); sun baths (1254); water drinking (1423); wet girdle (1347); cold mitten friction (1209); cold towel rub (1213); rubbing wet-sheet (1216).

4. **Anemia Due to Long-Continued Use of Mercury or Iodide of Potash.**—Galvanic bath (1457) two or three times a week, and carefully graduated tonic baths (1626); water drinking (1423).

5. **Nocturnal Pains.**—Prolonged neutral douche (1031), 5 minutes at bedtime; fomentation to the spine; alternate compress to spine.

6. **Insomnia.**—Prolonged neutral bath (1130) at bedtime; wet girdle (1347) to be worn during the night; See 1564.

7. **Syphilitic Ulcers.**—General eliminative and tonic measures, sweating bath daily (1250, 1191) followed by short cold applications (1625); prolonged immersion of the affected parts (1107), or antiseptic dressing.

8. **Indolent Ulcers.**—Alternate spray to ulcer, with measures indicated above, twice daily for 10 minutes.

9. **To Induce Absorption of Gummata.**—A fruit dietary (1627) for 3 days, prolonged sweating bath (1191) daily, electric-light bath (1250), vapor bath (1246), or sweating wet-sheet pack followed by a vigorous cold application, as a cold douche or rubbing shallow (1174). Continue long as indicated.

10. **Contraindications.**—Avoid prolonged very cold baths, especially cold immersions. Such baths are especially harmful when mercury is being taken. Avoid prolonged hot baths in cachectic and anemic patients, also when patient's temperature is elevated.

General Method.—The important thing to be accomplished in the treatment of this malady is the reconstruction of the body by the regulation of the patient's habits, and by the employment of proper hydriatic measures. Hydrotherapy often affords an excellent means of determining the diagnosis in a doubtful case by bringing out the characteristic eruption.

INFLAMMATIONS OF THE EYE.

1602 1. **External Inflammations.**—Light fomentations (1328) for 15 minutes every 2 hours; frequently renewed cooling (1318) compress during interval.

2. **Inflammations of Eyeball.**—A fomentation (1328) covering the eye and extending to the forehead, for 15 to 20 minutes or until the skin is well reddened (1282). Repeat as often as necessary to relieve pain. Employ the frequently renewed (5 to 15 minutes, 60°) heating compress (1344, 1282) during the interval between hot applications.

SKIN DISORDERS.

1603 **Chilblains.**—Alternate foot bath (1298); Scotch douche to feet (1037); alternate douche (1044, 1082); hot foot bath (1297) followed by flowing foot bath (1296); foot pack (1394).

1604 **Burns.**—The evaporating compress (1324); the cool irrigating compress (1326); if very extensive, the prolonged or continuous neutral bath (1130).

1605 **Erythema.**—Cool evaporating compress (1324), or irrigating compress (1326); neutral compress (1339).

1606 **Pruritus.**—Prolonged neutral bath (1130); copious water drinking (1423); large enema (1404); daily aseptic dietary; (1625) effervescing bath (1139).

Eruptions.—*If dry*, not irritable, prolonged neutral bath (1130). *If scaly*, alkaline bath (1463). *If moist* and irritable, cool evaporating compress moistened with soda solution, 1 ounce to the gallon; emollient bath (1462). *If skin is thickened*, as in chronic eczema, hot or alternate spray or compress for 10 to 15 minutes three times a day. If skin is extensively damaged, as in pemphigus, confluent smallpox, bad burns, the continuous neutral immersion bath (1130) until the skin is healed. 1607

Jaundice.—Copious water drinking (1423); large enema (1404) twice daily; sweating bath for 15 minutes,—electric-light (1250), vapor (1246), hot immersion (1126), wet-sheet pack (1179), followed by prolonged neutral bath (1130). Administer sweating bath once daily, or even twice, if patient is not too weak. For general tonic effects apply cold mitten friction (1209) or cold towel rub (1213) twice daily. Alternate compress over the liver twice daily, with heating compress (1344) over the liver or flannel covered wet girdle (1347) during intervals. 1608

Dry Skin.—Short sweating bath, electric-light (1250), vapor (1246), hot air (1233), Turkish (1239), hot immersion (1126), hot-blanket pack (1197), dry pack (1192), sweating wet-sheet pack (1187, 1191), followed by a cold bath suited to the patient's general condition (1625), and massage (fulling and friction) (1461). 1609

Hyperidrosis.—Vapor bath (1246), sweating electric-light bath (1250), followed by Scotch douche to spine (1037, 1074) and general cold douche (1010). 1610

For sweating feet, Scotch douche (1037) to feet with extremes as great as possible; alternate foot bath (1298), heating compress to feet during night (1394) with cold friction of feet in the morning on rising.

Baldness.—General tonic measures (1625); shampoo of scalp with cold water three times a day; some antiseptic lotion to destroy the parasitic cause of the disease. 1611

DRUG HABITS.

A. Alcoholism.

1612 **General.**— 1. Aseptic dietary (**1626**), especially fruits. Meats and flesh foods must be strictly prohibited, also meat juices, broths, and all preparations of flesh. Fomentation (**1328**) over the stomach twice a day with wet girdle (**1347**) between applications; short sweating baths,— electric-light bath (**1250**), sweating pack (**1191**) followed by wet-sheet rub (**1216**). Graduated cold baths (**1625**) twice a day.

2. **Insomnia.**— Neutral bath at bed-ime, 94° to 96°, 20 to 60 min.; wet girdle at night. See Insomnia (**1564**).

3. **Vomiting.**— Ice pills, ice-bag over stomach, hot and cold gastric compress (**1362**). See **1519**, 3.

4. **Delirium Tremens.**— Rest in bed; hot immersion bath (**1126**) 5 minutes, hot-blanket pack (**1197**) followed by sweating wet-sheet pack (**1179, 1191**); neutral bath (**1130**) 1 to 2 hours or longer twice a day; ice-cap (**1314, 1371**); hot fomentations (**1328**) over stomach and abdomen, every 3 hours for 15 minutes; during interval, heating compress (**1344**) changing every 30 to 60 minutes. Copious water drinking (**1423**); large enema (**1404**) daily. Exclusive fruit diet (**1627**) for 2 or 3 days.

5. **Counteract Narcotic Effects of Alcohol.**— Cold shower; water drinking (**1423**) or enema (**1404**) followed by short cold douche to spine (**1074**) and lower sternum. Repeat every hour or two if necessary, until the toxic effects disappear. Gastric lavage (**1401**), followed by cold or alternate irrigation (**1401**).

6. **Nephritis.**— Usually present in acute alcoholism. See **1537.**

7. **Gastritis.**— See **1519.**

General Method.— The patient must be placed in a proper environment; isolation and confinement may be required. Suitable mental and moral influences must be brought to bear.

B. Opium, Cocaine, and Chloral Habits.

1. Rest in bed. Sweating baths,— electric-light bath (**1250**), vapor bath (**1246**) twice a day for 3 days before withdrawing the drug. Follow bath by vigorous cold applications. While withdrawing the drug, the leading symptoms may be successfully combated as follows: —

2. **Nervousness, Restlessness, "Indescribable Sensations."** — Prolonged neutral bath (**1130**) 92° to 94°, ten minutes; neutral douche (**1031**), 92°, 2 to 4 minutes.

3. **Cardiac Weakness.**— Cold precordial compress (**1383**) or ice-bag over heart (**1314**); alternate applications to spine (**1342**); cold mitten friction (**1209**); cold towel rub (**1213**), repeating treatment hourly if necessary.

4. **Vomiting.**— Hot and cold trunk pack (**1367**); ice-bag over stomach and spine; hot-leg pack (**1197**).

5. **Diarrhea.**— Hot enema (**1406**) after each movement; cold abdominal compress (**1284, 1314**) changed every 30 minutes.

6. **Local Pain.**— Revulsive compresses (**1341**); alternate or hot and cold compress (**1340, 1356**).

7. **Insomnia after Withdrawal.**— Wet-sheet pack (**1179**); prolonged neutral bath, 20 to 60 minutes (**1130**); prolonged neutral spray (**1031**) 3 to 5 minutes; heating leg pack (**1393**); wet girdle (**1347**); cold head cap (**1314, 1371**). See **1564**.

General Method.— Same as for alcoholism (**1612**). Withdraw gradually within two or three days.

C. Tobacco Habit.

Drop the drug at once. Put the patient to bed. Sweating procedures,— electric-light bath (**1250**), vapor bath (**1246**), sweating wet-sheet pack (**1179, 1191**), twice daily; follow with short cold application, as shallow bath (**1174**), wet-sheet rub (**1216**), or cold douche (**1010, 1023**). Alternate spinal compress (**1342**) three times a day; wet girdle (**1347**) day and night, renewing three times daily. Copious water drinking (**1423**); large coloclyster (**1407**) daily.

D. Tea and Coffee Habit.

1. Discontinue the use of the drug at once. If necessary, employ some harmless cereal substitute. Neutral bath (**1130**) at bedtime. Fomentation over abdomen (**1328**); alternate sponging of the spine (**1342**); cold mitten friction (**1209**) or cold towel rub (**1213**) before rising in the morning. Wet girdle (**1347**) night and day, changing morning, noon, and night; short sweating wet-sheet pack (**1191**) or vapor bath (**1246**) two or three times a week followed by a cold application (**1625**).

2. **Constipation.**— Graduated enema (**1409**). See **1524.**

3. **Diarrhea.**— Neutral enema (**1404**) after each movement; cold abdominal compress (**1318**) every half-hour.

4. **Nervous Headache.**— See **1554,** 15.

5. The diet should consist chiefly of fruits (**1627**) and liquid foods (**1628**) for a few days; the patient should be gradually accustomed to a dry dietary (**1629**).

APPLICATIONS OF HYDROTHERAPY IN SURGICAL CASES.

1613 **Contusions.**— Fomentation (**1328**) three times a day, 10 to 15 minutes, with protected heating compress (**1344**) during the interval; if heat and swelling are great, change the compress every 15 minutes; as swelling and heat diminish, renew less frequently.

1614 **Fractures.**— Apply a fomentation (**1328**) or a revulsive compress (**1341**) for 10 or 15 minutes before application of the permanent dressing. When possible, the revulsive compress should be applied two or three times daily. This will afford the patient much comfort in relief from pain, and will expedite the healing process. Apply massage to portion of the limb which is accessible. In cases of compound fractures which are inoperable, the continuous neutral bath may sometimes be employed with advantage.

1615 **Dislocations.**— If necessary, apply large fomentations (**1328**) over the joint, or a hot immersion bath (**1026**) to relax the muscles before reduction; after reduction, apply the revulsive compress (**1341**) three times daily with heating compress (**1344**) during intervals. Apply massage to the limb, carefully.

1616 **Sprains.**— Very hot foot bath (**1297**) or hot pour (**1103**) for 15 minutes three times a day; firm bandage and absolute rest during intervals. Derivative massage (**1225**) the second day, increasing the vigor of the application and approaching nearer to the joint daily. Gentle massage and flexion of joint after third day.

1617 **Pott's Disease.**— In the early stage, when fever is present, rest in bed with careful tonic hydriatic measures in addition to the proper surgical treatment. Cold wet-hand rubbing (**1201**), the cold mitten friction (**1209**), and the cold towel rub are especially valuable measures. Later, more vigorous measures may be employed (**1625**). See Pulmonary Tuberculosis (**1508**).

Scoliosis.— The treatment of this and all other forms of spinal curvature due to deficient muscular development or irregular muscular action, may be greatly facilitated by combining with corrective gymnastics, massage, and electricity, the tonic and energizing effects of hydrotherapy. Administer daily or twice daily, carefully graduated tonic measures (**1625**), and in addition apply to the back the cold jet (**1074**), cold percussion douche (**1035**), or alternate douche (**1044**). 1618

Uterine Displacements.— Retroversion, procidentia, and some other forms of uterine displacement require mechanical and surgical treatment in most cases, but hydrotherapy is almost essential for a radical cure. Administer daily vaginal irrigation (110° to 115° when pain is present, 80° to 70° when pain is not a prominent symptom); tonic sitz (**1209**); graduated tonic measures (**1625**). See also Enteroptosis (**1525**). 1619

Abdominal Surgery.— Hot vaginal irrigation (**1413**) daily, the hot or cool cleansing enema or coloclyster daily (**1407**), water drinking (**1423**), and general tonic hydriatic measures (**1625**) either alone or in combination with eliminative procedures, electric-light bath (**1250**), vapor bath (**1246**), hot-air bath (**1233**), sweating pack (**1191**), are of the highest value as means of preparing a patient to undergo the ordeal of an abdominal operation. In suitable cases, in which immediate operation is not imperative, these simple measures, combined with an aseptic dietary (**1626**), employed for one or two weeks, enormously increase the patient's prospects for a safe and quick recovery, and prevent many of the complications to which this class of patients are especially liable. Tonic hydriatic procedures are equally useful in hastening the progress of convalescence; and such measures as the cold wet-hand rub (**1201**) and the cold mitten friction (**1209**) are most valuable means of increasing vital resistance, energizing the heart and central nervous system, and combating shock and collapse immediately after operation and may be advantageously employed two or three times a day during the weeks following. 1620

A hot enema (**1406**), hot vaginal irrigation (**1413**), hot foot bath (**1297**), even a hot bag to the spine or the epigastrium, will often obviate the use of an opiate to relieve the suffering in a laparotomy case, a very important consideration as every abdominal surgeon will recognize.

Pelvic inflammation following operation should be combated by the measures elsewhere indicated. See **1590.**

The ice-bag renders invaluable service in combating threatened cardiac failure; Apply over the heart for 15 minutes every 2 hours when necessary, but not continuously. The ice-bag to the throat or over the stomach, or applied to the spine opposite, will often check vomiting. Persistent vomiting may be relieved in many cases by gastric lavage, whether following an abdominal operation or in any case after the use of an anesthetic.

1621 **Surgical Shock.**—Hot bags and blankets about the patient; hot enema (**1405**); alternate compress to spine (**1342**); fomentation to spine (**1328**) immediately followed by cold mitten friction (**1209**); ice-bag over heart (**620**) for 15 minutes every 2 or 3 hours; hot or alternate irrigation of stomach (**1401**).

1622 **Anesthesia.**—Cold compress (60° F.) or ice-bag over heart during operation. Change every 15 minutes, with rubbing of chest until red at each change. After ether, apply heating chest pack (**1374**) to be changed every 4 hours. In all cases when not contraindicated, as in rectal cases, for example, administer an enema at 96° to encourage renal activity. Control vomiting by ice-bag to throat, over stomach, or to the spine opposite. Lavage, if bilious or fecal vomiting occurs and is persistent.

1623 **Hemorrhage.**—Hydriatic procedures, both hot and cold, afford most admirable means of checking hemorrhage when properly used, as has been elsewhere indicated. See **697** and **1496,** 4.

1624 **Surgical Fever.**—The various antipyretic measures which have been elsewhere recommended (**711–745**) are of equal value in the treatment of febrile conditions due to surgical procedures, or to traumatism. The ice-bag (**1314**), the cooling compress, (**1318**) and the frequently renewed heating compress (**1344**) are of great service in combating local inflammation, which is a most common cause of febrile conditions in surgical cases. The cold mitten friction (**1209**), cold towel rub (**1213**), cool enema (**1405**), cold head compress (**1371**), and usually copious water drinking (**1423**), are measures of the greatest value in combating surgical fever and preventing septic infection by building up general vital resistance.

GRADUATED SCHEME FOR TONIC COLD APPLICATIONS.

1. **Wet-Hand Rubbing (1201).**—In extremely feeble patients apply to back only, then from day to day increase the area, adding chest, arms, and lower legs; then cover arms, chest, back, and entire legs; finally the entire surface. Begin the application with water at 65° or even 70°, and lower the temperature 1° or 2° daily to 40°, or even to 34°. 1625

2. **Cold Mitten Friction (1209).**—Begin with water at 60°, dipping once only. Lower the temperature 1° or 2° daily to 40°, then gradually increase the number of dips from one to four.

3. **Cold Towel Rub (1213).**—Begin at 65°; lower the temperature 1° or 2° daily to 40°. Wring towel at first very dry. Wring less from day to day, until a saturated towel is used.

4. **Wet-Sheet Rub (1216).**—At first wring the sheet very dry, in water at 65°. Lower temperature 1° daily to 55°; wring sheet less dry at each application till a saturated sheet is used. Increase the duration of application from ½ minute to 2 minutes.

5. **Dripping Sheet (1217).**—The same as preceding until rubbing is completed, then, the sheet being well warmed, a pail of water 5° lower than the water in which the sheet was wet is poured over the patient and the rubbing renewed. This may be repeated three or four times.

6. **Shallow Bath (1174).**—Begin at 75°; lower temperature 1° daily to 60°; duration at first ½ minute, gradually increasing to 3 minutes.

7. **Pail Douche (1103).**—Begin at 75°; lower the temperature 2° daily to 60°; at first two pails only, gradually increase to six.

8. **Cold Douche (1010).**—Temp. 70° to 60°. Precede by a warm shower. Lower the temperature 1° daily, increasing the pressure; the duration is also increased from 5 or 10 seconds to 15 or 20 seconds. Percussion douche (1035) to spine when possible.

ASEPTIC DIETARY.

Meats of all sorts, oysters, fowl, game, meat juices, beef tea, 1626
animal broths, and all meat preparations are carefully and rigidly excluded because of the presence of tissue wastes, uric acid, crea-

tin, creatinin, and other toxic substances, together with ptomains, the product of putrefactive change.

Coarse vegetables, as cabbage, celery, lettuce, roots of all sorts, string beans, spinach, and greens, must generally be avoided, for the reason that their indigestibility leads to their retention in the stomach and colon, and thus encourages fermentative processes. Cauliflower, tender asparagus roots, green peas, purées of peas, beans, and lentils, excluding the skins of these seeds, are allowable, if not the very best. Eggs in the form of egg-nog, prepared without wine or brandy, slightly boiled or poached eggs, and soft custards, prepared without sugar, are readily taken. In many cases of gastric dilatation, eggs must be avoided. Raw, fresh milk is admissible in a small proportion of cases only. In the majority of cases, milk is well tolerated only in the form of kumyss, kumyzoon, buttermilk, cottage cheese, peptonized milk, junket, or in combination with cereals, as in milk gruel or porridge, and in not a few cases nothing containing milk can be eaten without injury.

Ripe fruits of all sorts are of the highest value because of the germ-destroying acids which they contain. Fresh fruits are best, but cooked fruits are valuable. Cane sugar as sweetening is admissible only in small quantities. Some fruits, as prunes and figs, are most digestible in the form of purées. Olives should be taken only when thoroughly ripened, as indicated by a black or very brown color. Dried fruit must be very thoroughly cooked. Fresh fruits, with hard flesh, should be discarded, especially apples, pears, and cherries that are not thoroughly ripened. Fruit juices, especially grape juice, orange juice, and the juice of limes and lemons or raspberries, and blackberries, and jellies made without sugar, are wholesome. Preserves and pickled fruits are indigestible, and must be discarded.

Cereals have a high nutritive value, and are readily digestible when cooked at a sufficiently high temperature (300° to 320°), to thoroughly dextrinize the starch, as in zwieback, granose, granut, granola, browned rice, and crystal wheat. Mushes, farinaceous gruels, blancmange, boiled potatoes, mashed potatoes, puddings, farinaceous desserts, fermented breads, dumplings, ordinary crackers, biscuit, and most ordinary cereal preparations are difficult of digestion in the dilated or feeble stomach, and give rise to fermentation and other changes and encourage gastrointestinal catarrh.

Malt, malt honey (meltose), honey, if sterilized by heating in a double boiler at boiling point for half an hour, malted milk, malted nuts, and bromose, represent preparations which contain starch in the predigested form of maltose (in honey, levulose, and glucose).

Nuts are practically free from starch, consisting chiefly of fats and albuminous substances. They closely resemble meat in composition, but are more nourishing and palatable when properly prepared. They may be eaten fresh or crushed in the form of nut butter and various other combinations and preparations, such as nuttolene, protose, nut meals, bromose, and malted nuts. Ordinary fresh nut meats are very digestible if thoroughly chewed. Peanuts are more nearly allied to beans than to nuts, and must be cooked to render them digestible; roasting renders them very indigestible, unless very carefully managed.

Fruit Diet.—When rapid sterilization of the alimentary canal 1627
is required, fasting, or better still, an exclusive fruit dietary, is the best course. Fruits consist chiefly of water, with a small amount of thoroughly digested starch in the form of fruit sugar or levulose, and various acid flavors, and almost nothing requiring the action of the digestive fluids. It is important that the fruit should enter the stomach in the form of a smooth pulp. Fruit swallowed in masses is very difficult of digestion. Imperfectly ripened apples or pears, and grapes swallowed without separating the seeds are often a source of indigestion, being retained so long in the stomach that fermentation occurs. Fruit skins and seeds should always be rejected.

When the dietary consists wholly of fruit, food may be taken four times a day, and the patient may be allowed to take as much as he likes.

A modified fruit dietary is often sufficient. At dinner the patient takes fruits and grains, and perhaps a small amount of nuts or nut preparations, with fruits only for breakfast, and the same for supper, if a third meal is taken.

Intestinal asepsis may also be promoted by an exclusive dietary of acid buttermilk or kumyss. The patient should take three or four quarts of kumyss in four portions, say at 7 A. M., 11 A. M., 3 P. M., 7 P. M. Zwieback, or toasted granose flakes or biscuits, may be eaten at the 7 A. M. and 3 P. M. meals.

An exclusive diet of fruit or kumyss is usually not required for more than a short period, as two to six days. If greatly prolonged, the patient will be weakened.

An aseptic dietary is best for all, sick or well. It is especially demanded in typhoid and all other acute fevers, in the rheumatic or uric acid diathesis, in diabetes, obesity, and other nutritive disorders, in indigestion accompanied by a dilated stomach or a prolapsed stomach, in intestinal catarrh and all cases of bacterial infection of the stomach or intestines, in infectious jaundice, arteriosclerosis, hepatic cirrhosis, all forms of autointoxication, in Bright's disease of the kidneys, malarial cachexia, pulmonary tuberculosis, eczema, and other forms of skin disease, apoplexy, neurasthenia, anemia (Haig has shown that flesh-eating causes anemia in consequence of the uric acid present), especially in pernicious anemia, and acute infections and inflammatory disorders, visceral inflammations of every description,— acute and chronic,— epilepsy, insanity, hysteria, in diseases of children of all forms, in insomnia, before and after grave surgical operations, in the treatment of the alcohol, morphia, cocaine, and tobacco habits, and most acute and chronic disorders.

Indigestible substances and dishes of all sorts must be avoided. In this list must be included pickles, spiced pickles, green olives, preserved and brandied fruits, fried foods, rich pastry, cheese, griddle cakes, ices, ice-cream, tea, coffee, cocoa, beer, and alcoholics of every description. Condiments of every sort must also be interdicted, as mustard, pepper, peppersauce, ginger, cayenne, capsicum, horseradish, chillies, curries, and hot sauces of every sort.

1628 **Liquid Diet.**— Fruit juice, malted nuts, almond cream, gluten gruel, granola, softened zwieback, malted milk, buttermilk, kumyss, kumyzoon, kumyss-nog, protose broth, vegetable broth, fruit soup.

1629 **Dry Diet.**— Toasted granose flakes, toasted granose biscuit, zwieback, toasted whole-wheat wafers, toasted wheat sticks, blanched almonds, blanched filberts, steamed figs, bromose, malt honey, malted nuts, nuttolene, nuttose, granola, granut.

1630 **Dextrinized Cereals.**— Well-toasted bread, zwieback, browned or roasted rice, parched wheat or corn (gofio), granose, granola, granut, crystal wheat, toasted wheat flakes.

1631 **Malted or Predigested Foods.**— Syrupy extracts of malt, malt honey, malted milk, malted nuts, bromose, granut.

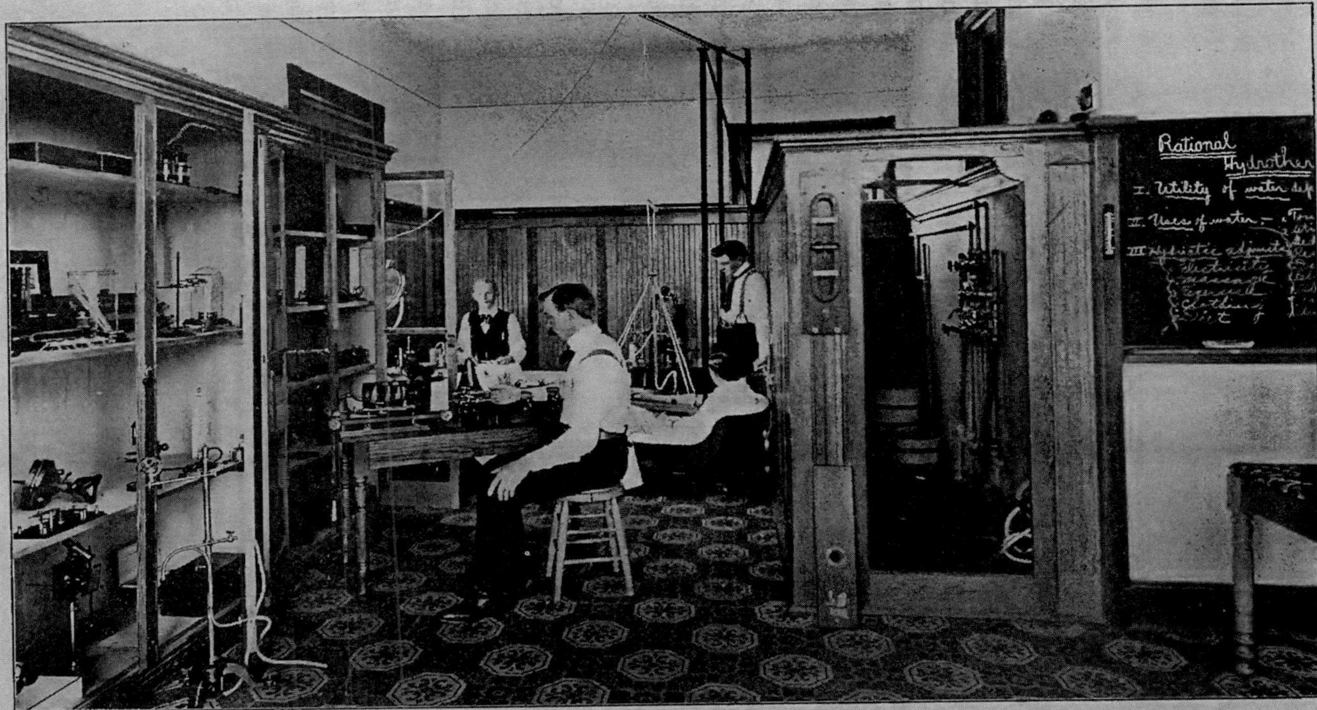

FIG. 248. A CORNER IN THE BATTLE CREEK SANITARIUM LABORATORY OF EXPERIMENTAL HYDROTHERAPY (p. 1107).

A BRIEF SUMMARY OF EXPERIMENTAL WORK DONE IN THE HYDRIATIC LABORATORY OF THE BATTLE CREEK SANITARIUM.

THE first experimental work done by the author in the study of scientific hydrotherapy was begun in the summer of 1875. During the twenty-six years which have since elapsed, experimental inquiries of various sorts have been carried on almost constantly, and particularly during the last ten or twelve years. Within the last year an attempt has been made to review the entire field of physiological experiments upon which the fundamental principles of hydrotherapy rest. In this work a large share of the experimental work which has been done by others has been repeated, and a considerable number of new experiments have been devised. In the following pages the author presents the results of a few of the many hundreds of experiments made in the laboratory under his supervision. Most of the work has been done under the author's direction by one of his able assistants, Dr. Elmer F. Otis, aided by trained nurses and medical students. The faithful work of Messrs. Wolfsen, Swartwout, Larson, Lemon, and Selmon, medical students, entitles them to mention among the many who have contributed excellent service in various capacities in prosecuting the extensive and laborious studies briefly presented in this summary, which have involved an amount of painstaking effort which can be appreciated only by those who have engaged in similar work.

The purpose of presenting the results of these laboratory studies is to place before the profession some of the tangible facts that constitute the data upon which the foundations of scientific hydrotherapy are laid, and which constitute this the most thoroughly rational of all branches of therapeutics.

EXPERIMENT I.—*Showing the increase of heat production resulting from vigorous exercise* (*page 81*).

(*a*) R. A. S., a young man aged 21, weight 140 lbs., rode twenty-two miles upon a bicycle in two hours over an ordinary country road. The rectal temperature on starting was 98.9°. At the close of the ride the rectal temperature was 103.3°; increase, 4.4°. The patient perspired very freely, showing increase of elimination; but notwithstanding, the increase in heat production was sufficient to cause an accumulation of heat amounting to 554.4 heat units (140×4.4×.9=554.4).

(*b*) F. W. W., aged 25, weight 160 lbs., Sept. 30, 1900, ran four miles in forty minutes. The rectal temperature on starting was 98.8°; at the end of the course, it was 102.2°; increase, 3.42°, indicating an increase in the rate of heat production sufficient to store in the body, notwithstanding increased heat elimination, heat amounting to 490 heat units (160×3.4×.9 = 489.6).

(*c*) L. H. W., a young man aged 30, weight 150 lbs., Oct. 4, 1900, swam for twenty-five minutes in water at 70°. The rectal temperature on entering the water was 99°; immediately on coming out of the water, it was found to be 100.2°; increase, 1.2°. In this case a considerable amount of heat was without doubt absorbed by the water, so that the actual increase in heat production is not shown by the increase in temperature; nevertheless the amount of heat accumulated was considerable, amounting to not less than 162 heat units (150×1.2 ×.9=162).

EXPERIMENT 2.—*Showing that heat production is increased by cold applications of brief duration (page 82).*

L. H. W., a young man aged 30, weight 166 lbs., received a percussion douche for thirty seconds, followed immediately by moderate exercise. The rectal temperature before the application was 99°; immediately afterward, 99.6°, an increase of .6°. The elevation of temperature was maintained for forty-five minutes. This observation has been repeated upon many subjects with similar results. The reaction following a short cold application results in increased heat elimination; notwithstanding, heat accumulation occurred in this case to the extent of 90 heat units (166×.6×.9=89.6). During the first moments following a short cold bath there is an elevation of temperature from diminished heat elimination.

EXPERIMENT 3.—*Showing the method of determining the rate of heat elimination by means of the bath-tub calorimeter (page 87).*

This method was first used by Liebermeister more than a score of years ago. It was independently devised and utilized by the author in 1892.

Four hundred pounds of water at a temperature of 68.4° was placed in an ordinary bath tub, the temperature of the room being 71.5°. Under these conditions the temperature of the water remained practically stationary. A young man, F. W. W., aged 25, weight 160 lbs., with a rectal temperature of 98.8°, was immersed in the water. At the end of fifteen minutes the temperature of the water was found to have risen 1.5°; the subject's temperature had also risen .2°. By simple calculation, it appears that the water had absorbed 600 heat units from the subject ($400 \times 1.5 = 600$), while his temperature had not only not fallen, but was actually slightly raised. The ordinary rate of heat production and elimination is about 7.2 heat units per minute. Under the conditions above named, the loss was 40 heat units per minute without lowering of the body temperature, showing an increase of heat production amounting to more than five and a half times the ordinary rate ($40 \div 7.2 = 5.55$).

EXPERIMENT 4.—(*Page 87.*)

The conditions being the same as in the preceding experiment, the subject, E. F. O., a young man aged 26, weight 105 lbs., temperature 98.4°, was immersed in the bath for five minutes. At the close of the experiment the body temperature was found to be 98.6°. The temperature of the water was raised .4°, amounting to 160 heat units, sufficient to reduce the temperature of the patient, if heat production had been suspended, 1.5° ($160 \div 105 = 1.5$). The normal rate of heat elimination for a patient weighing 105 lbs. would be about 30 heat units in five minutes. In the calorimeter, the amount eliminated was 160 heat units, or more than five times the normal amount.

EXPERIMENT 5.—(*Page 87.*)

(*a*) The subject, A. W. P., a young man aged 27 years, weight 165 lbs., was placed in the bath calorimeter with water at a temperature of 75.3°. At the end of five minutes it was found that the temperature of the water had risen to 76°, an increase of .7 of a degree, indicating that the body had given off 280 heat units.

The body temperature had also fallen from 98.4° to 98°, representing a loss of 59 heat units. Subtracting 59 from 280 we have 221 heat units, representing the amount of heat actually produced by the body during the five minutes. At the ordinary rate, the amount of heat produced during this period would be about 37.5 heat units. There was hence an increase in heat production amounting to 183.5 heat units, and heat production was excited to the extent of about five times the ordinary rate (221—37.5=183.5÷37.5=4.89).

(*b*) The young man was then given a hot shower bath for ten minutes, at which time the body temperature was found to be 99°. He was then placed in the calorimeter with the water at 76°. At the end of five minutes the temperature of the water was raised to 77.1°, while the patient's temperature had fallen to 98°, indicating a loss of 440 heat units.

(*c*) On removal from the bath, the patient was wrapped in blankets, and allowed to remain covered until warm, when he was returned to the calorimeter with the water at a temperature of 77.5°. At the end of five minutes the temperature of the water had risen .3°, showing a loss of heat communicated by the subject to the water amounting to 120 heat units.

(*d*) T. J., a young man aged 23, weight 160 lbs, in the second week of typhoid fever The mouth temperature was 104.4°; rectal 104.8°. The patient was immersed in the bath-tub calorimeter containing 400 pounds of water at 70.2°, with room temperature at 63°. He remained in the calorimeter five minutes, during which time surface friction was kept up constantly. At the end of the experiment, the patient's temperature by mouth was 101.2°, by rectum, 102°. The temperature of the water had risen to 72.1°. As previously noted, the temperature of the water was cooling by evaporation at the rate of .2° every five minutes.

From the above it appears that the water of the bath absorbed in five minutes 680 heat units (72.1—70.2—.2=1.7×400=680). Of this amount, 403.2 heat units is accounted for in the lowering of body temperature (104.8°—102° = 2.8°×160×.9* = 403.2). There was thus a temporary increase of heat production during the bath, amounting to 7.4 times the normal, while heat elimination

* The specific heat of the body is .9 that of water.

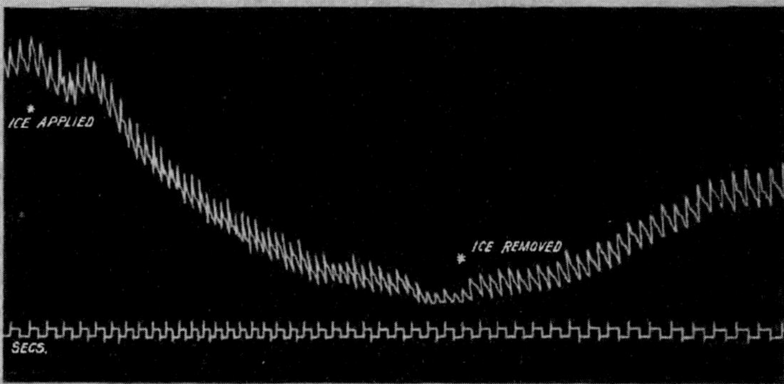

Fig. 249 (Exp. 16). Plethysmographic Tracing Showing Shrinkage of Blood-vessels in Hand Produced by Ice Applied to Opposite Hand (p. 1114).

Before. After.

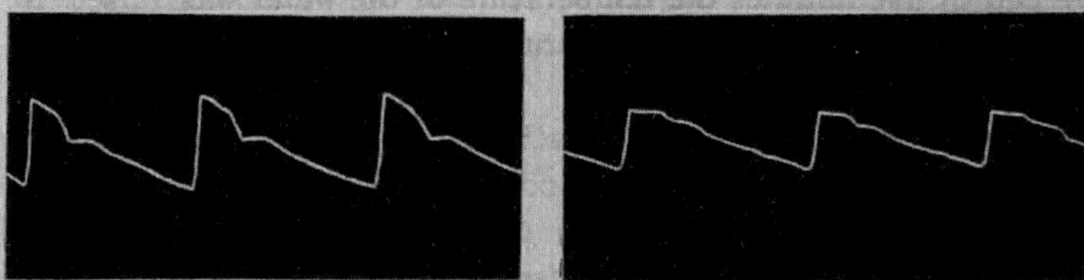

Fig. 250 (Exp. 17). Sphygmographic Tracing Showing Contraction of Vessels of Arm Produced by Applications of Ice to Axilla (p. 1114).

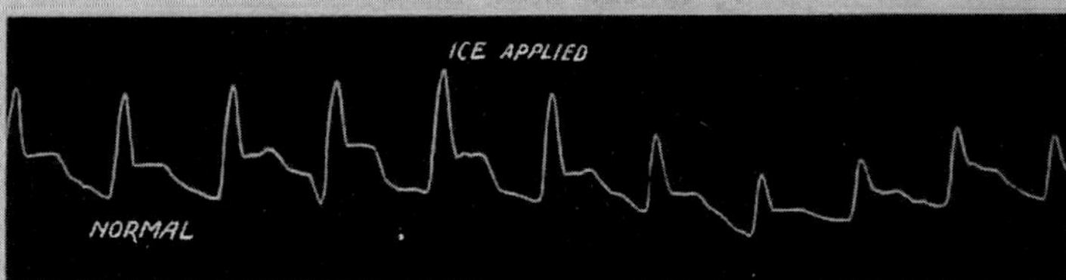

Fig. 251 (Exp. 18). Sphygmographic Tracing of Radial Pulse Showing Contraction of the vessels of the Forearm Resulting from Application of Ice to Bend of Elbow (p. 1114).

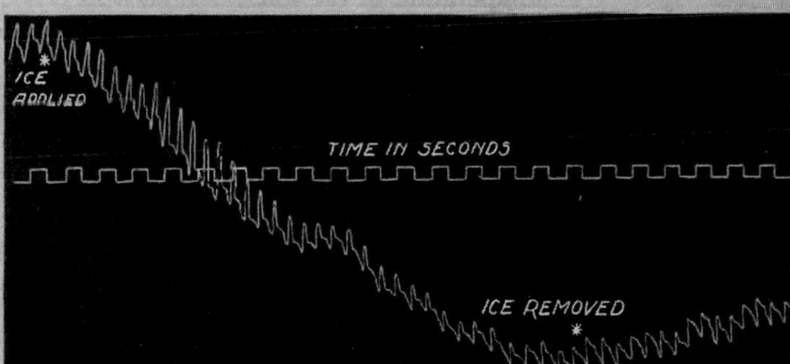

Fig. 252 (Exp. 19). Plethysmographic Tracing Showing Diminution in the Volume of the Forearm Resulting from Application of Ice to Elbow (p. 1114).

was increased to 18 times the normal rate. Heat elimination was thus increased in a febrile case nearly two and a half times as much as heat production. The heat elimination was increased 2.4 times as much as in a normal subject (Exp. 5 (*a*)), while heat production was increased only 25 per cent. This explains the great value of the cold rubbing bath as a means of reducing temperature in fever.

EXPERIMENT 6.— *Observations respecting the influence of various procedures upon heat elimination by means of d'Arsonval's calorimeter (Fig. 24, page 89).*

(*a*) The subject, L. H. W., a young man aged 30, weight 166 lbs., was placed in calorimeter such as is shown in Fig. 24, page 89, with his clothing removed, in a room at a temperature of 70°. The rate of air movement as shown by the anemometer, was 123 feet per minute.

(*b*) The same subject was placed in an electric-light bath for sufficient time to redden the skin, but not to produce perspiration, and then placed in the calorimeter. The rate of air movement was found to be 140 feet per minute.

(*c*) The same subject was given an electric-light bath to the extent of producing profuse perspiration. He was then placed in the calorimeter, and the rate of air movement was found to be 170 feet per minute, showing a very considerable increase in the rate of heat elimination due to elevation of the temperature of the skin.

(*d*) The same subject was given a cold percussion douche for two minutes (temperature of the water 60° F.). When placed in the calorimeter, the rate of air movement was found to be 70 feet per minute. In ten minutes, when reaction had taken place, the rate was found to be 110 feet per minute.

EXPERIMENT 7.—(*Page 89.*)

(*a*) The subject, R. A. S., a young man aged 21, weight 140 lbs., was placed in the calorimeter in a room at 86°. The rate of air movement, as shown by the anemometer, was found to be 70 feet per minute. After the administration of a cold wet-sheet rub, the rate of movement was found to be 97 feet per minute. Seven minutes later, when reaction had taken place, the rate of movement had increased to 110 feet per minute.

(*b*) After a very cold percussion douche (56°) the rate of movement was found to be reduced to 92 feet per minute.

(*c*) The same subject was placed in a wet-sheet pack, and removed at the beginning of the heating stage. When placed in the calorimeter, the rate of air movement was found to be 98 feet per minute.

(*d*) After a hot blanket pack and while perspiring freely, the same subject produced an air movement of 122 feet per minute.

(*e*) The subject was made to exercise moderately until general perspiration was induced. He was then placed in the calorimeter with the result of producing an air movement of 90 feet per minute. The difference between the results in this experiment and in (*c*) was doubtless due to the fact that in the latter the temperature of the skin was raised by the prevention of heat elimination, while in the former there was increase of heat elimination, with increase in heat production.

EXPERIMENT 8.—*Showing the effects of partial cold applications in lowering the surface temperature (page 104).*

The subject was a young man aged 26, weight 153 lbs. The temperature of the hand, as obtained in the palm with the hand closed, was 98.4°. The hand was immersed in water at 40° for one minute, then removed and lightly dried, when the temperature was found to be 90°. The temperature rose to 95° in five minutes, and to 97.8° in ten minutes. Only at the end of fifteen minutes was the initial temperature reached.

EXPERIMENT 9.—*Comparison of the reaction produced by percussion and friction with that of the heating compress (page 105).*

A heating compress was applied to the upper arm of a healthy young man for twenty minutes. The compress consisted of a linen cloth wrung as dry as possible out of ice-cold water, wrappe dabout the arm, and covered with several layers of flannel tightly applied. Immediately afterward, percussion and friction movements were begun upon the arm of the opposite side, and continued during the whole period of twenty minutes. At the end of this time, the pack was removed. On comparison, it was found that the degree of redness of the skin on the two arms was practically equal.

EXPERIMENT 10.—*Showing the influence of cold upon perspiration (page 105).*

The electric-light bath was applied to the leg of a young man for fifteen minutes until profuse perspiration of the limb was produced. Water at 60° was then dashed upon the leg, with the result that perspiratory activity was instantly suspended.

EXPERIMENT 11.—(*Page 106.*)

The subject, M. M. M., was a young man aged 35. By means of an asthesiometer the normal tactile sensibility of the subject was found to be such as to enable him to recognize the two points of the asthesiometer when separated 2 mm. After immersion for five minutes in water at 60°, it was necessary to separate the points 3.5 mm. to enable the subject to distinguish them. Five minutes' immersion at 40° increased the distance to 6 mm.

EXPERIMENT 12.—*Showing the effect of short cold applications upon cardiac activity (page 107).*

(*a*) The subject, R. R. H., was a young man aged 21 years, weight 115 lbs., pulse 74. Gently slapping the chest over the heart with the end of a towel wrung out of cold water, half a dozen times, raised the pulse rate to 86.

(*b*) In another subject with normal pulse (66), the cold percussion douche at 65° increased the pulse rate to 86.

EXPERIMENT 13.—*Showing the increase of arterial tension resulting from cold applications of short duration (page 107).*

The subject, R. A. S., a young man aged 21, weight 140 lbs., presented a normal pulse rate of 81, with a tension, as shown by Gærtner's tonometer (Figs. 239, 240, page 931), of 9.5 cm. of mercury. Upon the application of a douche at 55°, the pulse rate was immediately increased to 90, and the tension to 10 cm.

EXPERIMENT 14.—*Showing the effect of prolonged cold applications in slowing the heart (page 107).*

(*a*) The subject, a man aged 40, weight 140 lbs., pulse rate 76. was in water at 55° for ten minutes, when the pulse rate was found to be reduced to 50°. The tension was decidedly increased.

EXPERIMENT 15.—(*Page 107.*)

(*b*) The subject, E. F. O., a young man aged 26, weight 105 lbs., pulse 74, was placed in a shallow bath at 70° for three minutes. The pulse rate at the close of the bath was 60, with tension greatly increased. This observation was made by the author's colleague, Dr. W. H. Riley, in August, 1895.

EXPERIMENT 16.—*Showing that ice held in one hand produces a contraction of the blood-vessels of the opposite hand* (*page 108*).

The subject was a young man of 35 years, weight 172 lbs. One arm was placed in the glass cylinder of a plethysmograph. A piece of ice was placed in the opposite hand, with the result shown in the accompany inggraphic, which is a photo reproduction of the original (Fig. 249).

EXPERIMENT 17.—*Showing that the application of ice to the axilla causes contraction of the arteries of the arm* (*page 108*).

The subject was a young man aged 27, weight 165 lbs. The accompanying tracing was obtained by means of Dudgeon's sphygmograph (Fig. 4, page 60) immediately before and after the application of ice to the axilla (Fig. 250 *a* and *b*.)

EXPERIMENT 18.—*Showing the effect of the application of ice to the bend of the elbow in diminishing the weight of the up stroke in sphygmographic tracings obtained from the radial pulse* (*page 108*).

The subject was a young man aged 26, weight 105 lbs. By Marey's sphygmograph the accompanying graphic was obtained, showing the normal tracing and the effect produced by the application of ice to the bend of the elbow (Fig. 251).

EXPERIMENT 19.—*Showing by means of the phthysmograph the effect of the application of ice to the bend of the elbow in diminishing the capacity of the blood-vessels of the hand and forearm* (*Fig. 252, page 109*).

EXPERIMENT 20.—*Showing the effect upon the pulse rate of a prolonged cold immersion with friction.*

The subject, J. T. M., a vigorous young man of 32 years, weight 170 lbs., with normal pulse rate of 80, was placed in a cold immer-

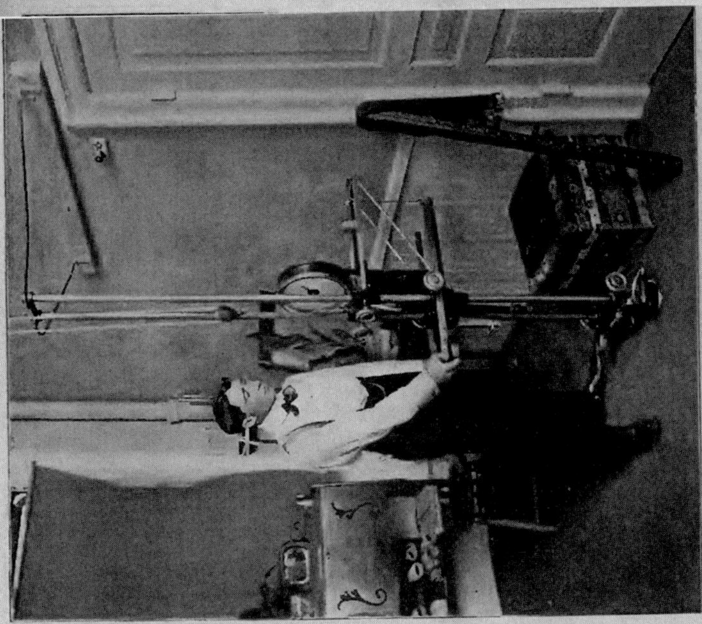

FIG. 253 (EXP. 44). UNIVERSAL DYNAMOMETER (p. 1122). (Kellogg)

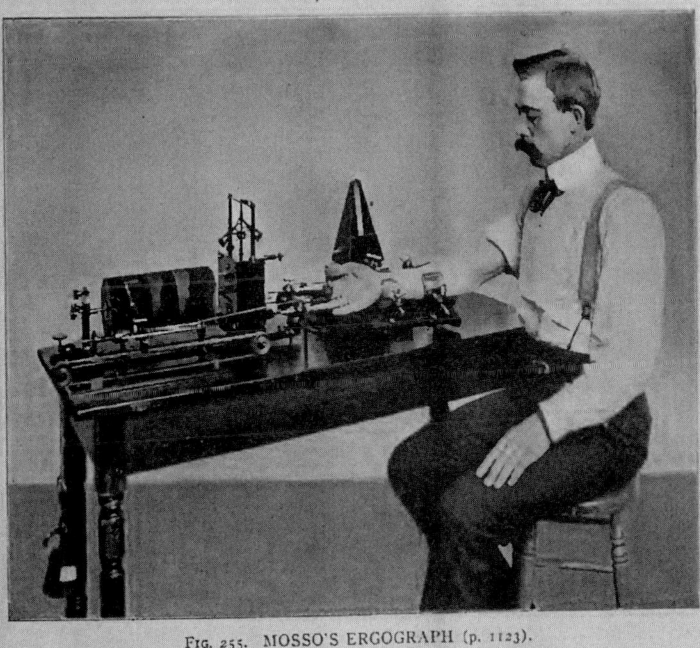

FIG. 255. MOSSO'S ERGOGRAPH (p. 1123).

sion bath at 45° for twenty minutes, friction being applied at the same time. At the end of the experiment the patient's pulse was 58.

EXPERIMENT 21.—*Showing the effect of cold beverages upon the pulse rate and tension (page 109).*

The subject, A. E. L., was a young man aged 26 years, weight 165 lbs., a normal pulse of 66, blood pressure 13.5 cm. as determined by Gærtner's tonometer. Five glassfuls of weak lemonade at 50° were swallowed quickly. Examination of the pulse, made almost immediately after, showed it to be slowed to 52, while the arterial tension, as indicated by the tonometer, was 14.5 cm.

EXPERIMENT 22.—*Showing the effect of the cold enema in lowering the body temperature (page 110).*

(*a*) For the purpose of determining the effect of a cold enema on the normal subject, water at 70° was passed in and out the colon continuously for forty-five minutes, the subject being a young man of 21 years, weight 140 lbs. The mouth temperature rose from 97.8° to 98° during the application. Forty-five minutes after the conclusion of the experiment, the rectal temperature was 94°, and at the end of one hour and a quarter 98.1°, still nearly 2° F. below the normal rectal temperature.

(*b*) The subject, M. G., a young man aged 22, suffering from typhoid fever, first week presented a temperature of 104.2°. Three large enemas were administered in rapid succession, the temperature being 66°, 62°, 62°. The result was a reduction of the body temperature within one hour to 99.2°. So marked a result as this is not always obtainable, but temperature reduction is decided whenever this measure is faithfully employed.

EXPERIMENT 23.—*Showing the effect of the application of the cold douche to the chest in increasing the depth of the respiratory movements (page 110).*

The accompanying tracing was made by the author's pneograph (see Figs. 25, 26, p. 110). The increased amplitude of the respiratory movements continued for fully one minute. When the cold application is general, the amplitude is still more decided, and continues or a longer time (see Fig. 26, p. 110).

EXPERIMENT 24.—*Showing the restorative effects of the cold douche* (*page 112*).

M. J. N., a man of 21 years, weight 136 lbs., rode, Aug. 26, 1900, 35 miles on a bicycle within two and a half hours, at the end of which time he was very much fatigued, not being accustomed to long riding. The muscular capacity of the subject, as shown by the author's dynamometer (Fig. 253), was 6,870 lbs. At the conclusion of the ride, the dynamometer showed reduction of nearly 1,000 foot pounds, or 5,955 lbs. A cold (55°) percussion douche was administered for thirty seconds, having been preceded by a hot shower for thirty seconds. A second test with the dynamometer was then made, and the total strength was found to be increased to 6,555 lbs., a gain of 600 lbs. The sensation of freshness and vigor experienced by the subject as the result of the cold douche was so marked that he expressed himself as being quite relieved from any sense of exhaustion.

EXPERIMENT 25.—*Showing diminution of the rate of transmission of impressions over a nerve trunk as the result of a cold application made along the course of the nerve* (*pages 110, 114*).

In the subject selected, the rate of time required for the patient to make a signal after an impression made upon the finger was .11 seconds. After the elbow of the same arm had been packed in ice for five minutes, the time required was .22 seconds.

EXPERIMENT 26.—*Showing the local increase in the blood count resulting from a cold application* (*pages 110, 121*).

To the subject, W. E. P., a medical student, a short, hot abdominal fomentation was applied, followed by a snow compress at 40° applied to the abdomen for twenty minutes. The blood count made before and after the application gave the following results: Before, 4,450,000 red blood cells, 4,900 white corpuscles; after, 4,950,000 red cells, and 10,100 white cells. The hemoglobin was 96 per cent before and 99 per cent after the application. Examination made fifteen minutes later showed the blood count to be practically the same as before the application.

EXPERIMENT 27.—*Showing the effect of the cold epigastric douche, or the ice-bag applied to the epigastrium, in increasing the amount of hydrochloric acid in the gastric secretion (page 122).*

The subject, L. H. W., was a vigorous young man aged 30, weight 166 lbs. A careful examination of the stomach fluid drawn at the end of an hour after an Ewald test meal, showed the total calculated acidity to be .150, free hydrochloric acid .126.

A second test meal was given after the application of a cold percussion douche to the epigastrium and the spine opposite at 55° for two minutes. The chemical examination showed the calculated acidity to be .286, and free hydrochloric acid .156. An increase in the calculated acidity of 90 per cent, and in the amount of free hydrochloric acid of 24 per cent.

EXPERIMENT 28.—*Showing the influence of thermic applications upon heat production and heat loss* (page 123).*

The subject, F. W. W., a young man aged 25, weight 160 lbs., was placed in a bath-tub calorimeter containing 400 pounds of water at a temperature of 68.4°. At the end of five minutes the temperature of the water was raised .7 of a degree, representing a heat loss by the subject amounting to 280 heat units. The body temperature during the application fell .8 of a degree, representing 115.2 heat units (160×.8×.9=115.2), leaving 164.8 heat units resulting from heat production during the time covered by the experiment.

EXPERIMENT 29.—*Showing the effect of a hot spray in lessening heat production (page 123).*

The subject, A. W. P., aged 27, weight 165 lbs., was placed in a bath-tub calorimeter at 77.5°, after taking a spray bath at 106°. At the end of five minutes, the temperature of the bath had risen .3°, showing the absorption of 120 heat units (400×.3=120). The rectal temperature showed a drop of .6 during the application, amounting to 99 heat units. Subtracting 99 from 120 leaves 21 heat units, representing the amount of heat actually produced during the five minutes. The normal amount of heat produced during this time should be, for a man weighing 165 pounds, at the rate of about 7.5 heat units per minute, or 37.5 heat units for the

*For the method of employing the bath-tub calorimeter, see page 87.

five minutes, from which it appears that there was a lowering of the heat production amounting to 16.5 heat units in five minutes, presumably as the result of the short hot spray, the natural effect of which is to diminish heat production by reflex influence upon the thermic centers.

EXPERIMENT 30.—(*Page 126.*)

(*a*) The subject, S. R. A., a young man aged 26, weighing 128 lbs., was first placed in a bath-tub calorimeter with water at a temperature of 82.4°. The temperature of the water was raised .18° in five minutes. The patient's temperature at the beginning of the bath was 98.6°, at the end 98.3°. From this data it appears that 400 pounds of water absorbed from the subject 72 heat units, o which amount 34.2 is accounted for by the fall of the body temperature, and 37.8 heat units were produced during the five minutes, an amount of heat practically the same as that normally produced within the time named.

(*b*) Later the same subject was placed in a bath at 77°, being rubbed during the entire period of five minutes, at the end of which time the temperature of the bath was found to be raised .54. The subject's temperature had in the meantime fallen .1 of a degree (from 98.8° to 98.7°). Of the heat absorbed by the water, 216 heat units, 11.5 heat units were accounted for by the fall of body temperature, leaving 204 heat units to be accounted for by increased heat production, about six times the amount that would have been developed if heat production had continued at the normal rate. The great increase of heat loss shown as the result of friction, in this case amounting to nearly 300 per cent, was without doubt due to the fact that there was very marked constriction of the surface vessels during the first immersion (Exp. 29), with goose-flesh appearance, whereby the heat elimination was interfered with to an unusual degree.

EXPERIMENT 31.—*Showing the effect of the application of the cold proximal compress to the arm* (*page 128*).

The subject, R. R. H., was made to immerse his elbow in a bath at 50°. The temperature of the hand at the beginning of the experiment was 90.5. After two minutes, the temperature of the hand was 87°. The temperature still remained below normal twenty minutes after removing the arm from the bath.

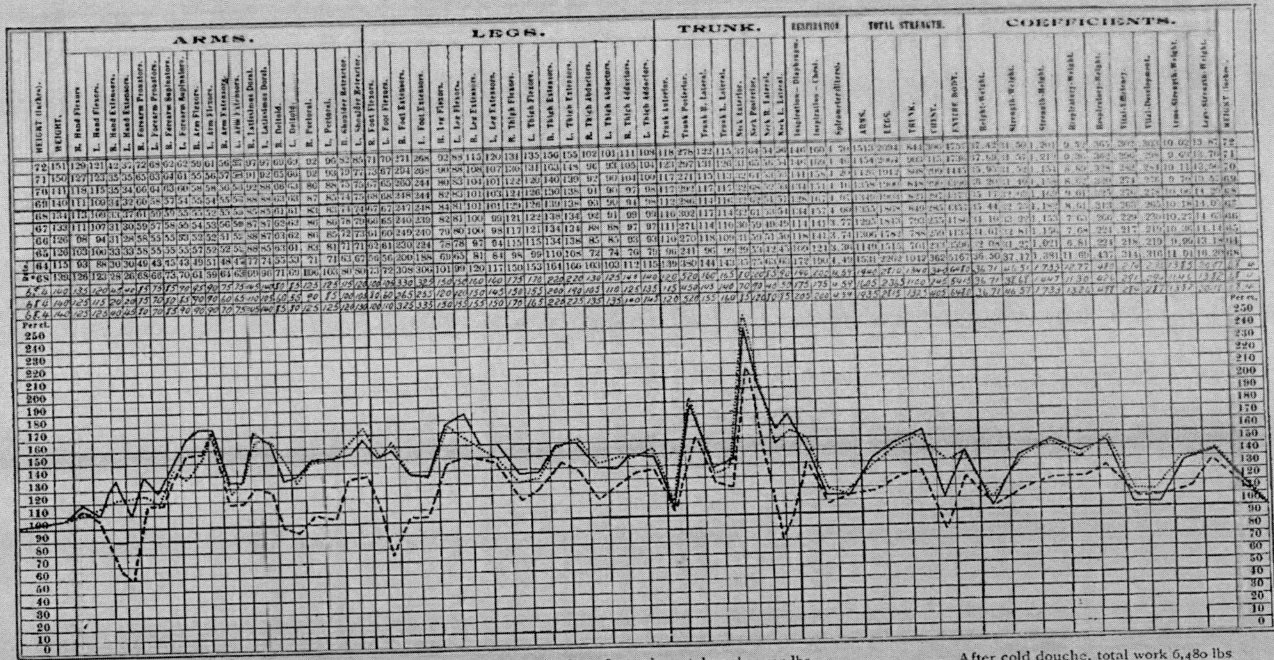

——— Normal, total work 6,480 lbs. - - - - - - - After bath 112° 12 min, total work 5,415 lbs. .... After cold douche, total work 6,480 lbs

FIG. 254. PHYSICAL CHART SHOWING THE EFFECT OF A GENERAL HOT BATH IN DIMINISHING MUSCULAR CAPACITY (p. 1123).

EXPERIMENT 32.—*Showing the effect of cold water in the stomach upon the temperature of the overlying skin (page 128).*

The subject, R. A. S., a healthy young man, was made to take seven glasses of water at 55°. The surface temperature at the epigastrium, taken before the water was swallowed, was found to be 97.6°; after, 95.1°, a loss of 2.5° (see Exps. 64, 65, and 73).

EXPERIMENT 33.—*Showing the influence upon the general temperature and the circulation of the ice-bag applied over the heart (page 128).*

The subject, A. C. S., having a normal pulse of 80, and a tonometer reading (Gærtner) of 10 cm. of mercury, with mouth temperature of 99°, was placed in a reclining position, and an ice-bag applied over the heart. After three minutes, the pulse was found to be 72 and the tonometer reading was raised to 12 cm. At the end of one hour, the mouth temperature was found to be 98.5°. The rectal temperature was lowered one degree (from 100° to 99°).

EXPERIMENT 34.—*Showing the effect of copious water-drinking and large cold enemas, in lowering the general temperature (page 128).*

(*a*) The subject, A. C. S., was a young man of 23 years, weight 137 lbs. His mouth temperature was 98°; rectum, 100°. Copious enemas at 70° were administered at intervals of twenty-five minutes for an hour and a half. The mouth temperature was then found to be 96.9°, and the rectal 95.2°.

(*b*) The subject, A. J. M., was made to drink seven glasses of weak lemonade at 59° F. The rectal temperature was reduced from 100° to 98.7°. The surface temperature at the epigastrium was reduced from 94° to 92°.

EXPERIMENT 35.—*Showing that friction accompanying partial cold immersion favors reaction (page 133).*

The subject placed his hand in water at 40°F. for one minute. Before immersion, the surface temperature of the hand taken in the palm with the hand closed, was 98.4°. After removing the hand and wiping it, the temperature was found to be 90°. In a room at 70° the normal temperature was regained at the end of fifteen minutes.

Repeating the same experiment under the same conditions, with the exception that the hand was rubbed vigorously during immersion in the water, the normal temperature was regained at the end of ten minutes.

EXPERIMENT 36.—*Showing that percussion accompanying a cold application favors reaction* (*page 134*).

(*a*) The subject, A. C. S., aged 23, weight 137 lbs., was immersed in a bath at 56° for 40 seconds, then gently dried and wrapped in a woolen blanket. The initial temperature of the surface was 97.6°. Immediately following the bath the surface temperature was found to be 94.1°. At the end of thirty minutes the temperature of the skin had become the same as before the immersion.

(*b*) To the same subject was administered a percussion douche at a temperature of 50°, pressure 35 lbs., duration 40 seconds. The initial temperature was 97.6°. After the douche, the skin temperature was found to be 94.6°. The initial temperature was recovered at the end of ten minutes.

(*c*) In an experiment with the same subject under like conditions, the ordinary jet douche with pressure of 35 lbs. was followed by complete reaction with return of normal surface temperature, in twelve minutes.

EXPERIMENT 37.—*Showing the advantage of friction in connection with general cold immersion in promoting reaction* (*page 134*).

(*a*) The subject, A. C. S., a young man aged 23, weight 137 lbs., was placed in an immersion bath at 56° for forty seconds. The initial surface temperature (abdomen) was 98.1°; immediately following the bath, 96.1°. The initial temperature was regained at the end of twenty-seven minutes.

(*b*) The same subject was immersed in a bath at 56° for 40 seconds with vigorous friction during the bath. The initial surface temperature was 97.6°. Immediately after the bath the surface temperature was 94.1°. The initial temperature was regained in eighteen minutes.

(*c*) A wet-sheet rub was administered to the same subject, the sheet being wrung from water at 40°. The initial temperature was 97.6°; immediately following the bath, 96.1°. The initial temperature was regained at the end of five minutes.

EXPERIMENT 38.—*Showing the influence of exercise upon reaction (page 134).*

(*a*) A cold bath at 55°, duration 20 minutes, with friction, was administered to J. T. M., a young man aged 32, weight 170 lbs. Full reaction, as indicated by a return of the surface temperature to the initial point, was complete only at the end of four hours, the patient in the meantime remaining quiet. The subject was cold and shivered considerably for some time after the bath.

(*b*) The same procedure, in the same subject, with identical conditions, but followed by moderately vigorous exercise, secured complete reaction in fifteen minutes.

EXPERIMENT 39.—(*Page 139.*)

The subject, H. R. P., placed his hand in water at 50° for one minute. The initial temperature taken with the closed palm was 97°. Immediately after the immersion it was found to be 90°. The normal temperature was regained in nine minutes.

EXPERIMENT 40.—*Showing the effect of heat and cold upon the surface circulation (page 143).*

(*a*) The subject, L. S., was a young woman aged 23, just convalescing from typhoid. The blood pressure, as determined for the middle finger of each hand by Gærtner's tonometer (Figs. 239, 240, page 931), indicated a pressure of 7 cm. mercury. The two hands were immersed, the right hand in ice-water, the left hand in hot water, for five minutes, at the end of which time the tension was found to be, for the right hand, 5.5 cm.; for the left, 9 cm., a difference of 3.5 cm.

(*b*) The same experiment made in healthy subjects showed a difference of about 1 cm. of mercury.

This experiment very clearly shows the influence of cold in contracting the surface vessels, and of heat in dilating the vessels and exciting the surface circulation.

EXPERIMENT 41.—*Showing the influence of heat upon the tactile sensibility (page 145).*

The subject, A. C. S., was a young man aged 23, weight 137 lbs. The two points of the asthesiometer were distinctly felt upon the back of the hand at a distance of 20 mm. After immersion in water at 117° for four and a half minutes, the two points were distinct only at 30 mm. Temperatures of 98° to 95° produced no effect.

EXPERIMENT 42.—*Showing the effect of general hot applications upon the blood pressure and pulse rate (page 147).*

The subject, R. R. H., was a young man aged 21, weight 115 lbs. Before the experiment, with the subject reclining, the pulse was 92, radial tension 9 cm., as determined by Gærtner's tonometer (Figs. 239, 240, page 931). The couch, the subject lying upon it, was pushed into an electric-light cabinet without any exertion on his part. Within a minute the radial pulse fell to 54, and the tonometer showed a rise of pressure in the peripheral vessels to 10 cm. At the end of five minutes, the subject was perspiring moderately. The pulse was then found to be 66, the tonometer reading 8 cm. At the end of 20 minutes the pulse was 92, the tonometer reading 7 cm. The subject was then withdrawn from the cabinet. The pulse rate immediately fell to 86, but some time elapsed before the blood pressure rose to normal.

EXPERIMENT 43.—*Showing the effect of heat and cold upon the volume of the tidal air of respiration (page 149).*

(*a*) The subject, R. A. S., was a young man aged 21, weight 140 lbs. The normal amount of tidal air was determined to be 43 cubic inches. The patient was placed in an immersion bath at 108°. At the end of twelve minutes, the amount of tidal air was found to be 27 cubic inches. Ten minutes after the bath, the tidal air was 33 cubic inches; 30 minutes after, 37 cubic inches. This experiment shows a loss in the volume of the respired air amounting to 37.5 per cent.

(*b*) A wet-sheet rub at a temperature of 40° was administered toa young man, O. R. C., aged 25, weight 142 lbs. The initial volume of tidal air was 28 cubic inches. The volume of tidal air immediately after the treatment was 35 cubic inches, an increase of nearly 26 per cent.

(*c*) The subject, F. J. W., was a young man aged 25, weight 127 lbs. The initial volume of tidal air was 33 cubic inches. Cold mitten friction was administered at 45° for two minutes. Immediately after the application the tidal air was found to be 51 cubic inches, an increase of 55 per cent.

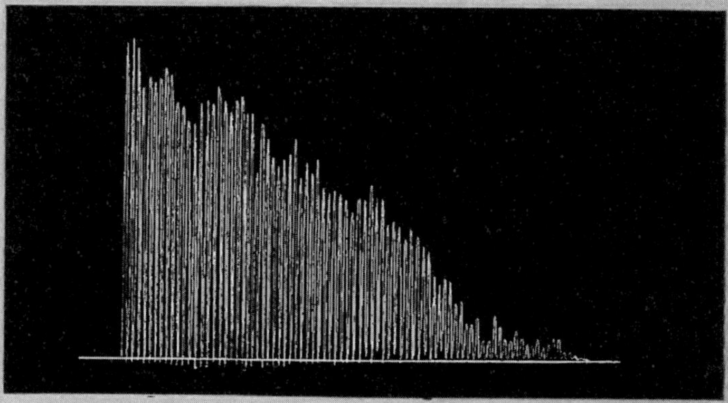

Fig. 256 (Exp. 45). Ergogram Obtained by Means of Mosso's Ergograph, Showing Normal Fatigue Curve of a Young Man, R. A. S. Total work, 4.994 kgm. (p. 1123).

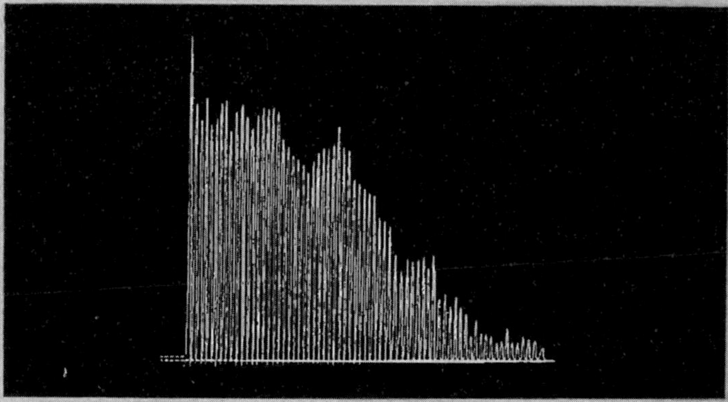

Fig. 257 (Exp. 45). Ergogram Showing Fatigue Curve of R. A. S. after a Spray at 113° for Fifteen Minutes. Total work, 4.432 kgm. (p. 1123).

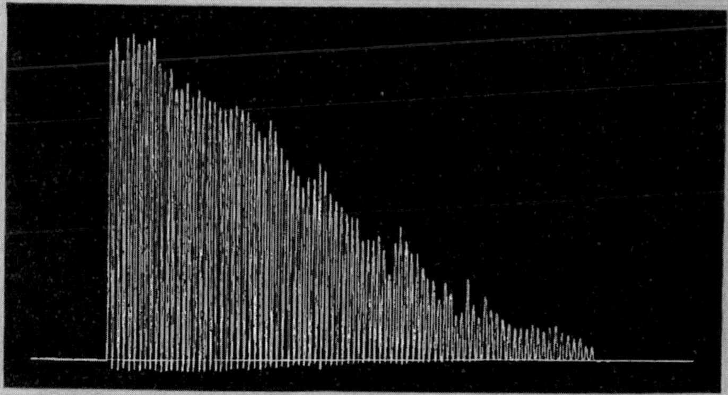

Fig. 258 (Exp. 45). Ergogram Showing Fatigue Curve of R. A. S. after a Cold Spray Following a Hot Bath. Total work, 6.094 kgm. (p. 1124).

(*d*) E. F. O., a young man aged 25, weight 105 lbs., was given a wet-sheet pack for one hour. The sheet was wrung as dry as possible, from water at 45°. The amount of tidal air before the application of the wet sheet was 27 cubic inches. Two minutes after the sheet was applied, the amount was 36 cubic inches, an increase of 33⅓ per cent; fifteen minutes later, 33 cubic inches. The amplitude of respiratory movement gradually lessened, until at the end of an hour, when the experiment terminated, the amount of tidal air was 28 cubic inches. The experiment thus showed an increase in the amount of air received into the lungs during the entire period, amounting to an average of 18.5 per cent. The subject was lightly covered to prevent excessive heat accumulation, thus maintaining the pack in the neutral stage.

EXPERIMENT 44.—*Showing the depressing effects of the general hot bath by its influence upon muscular capacity (page 150).*

The subject, W. P. L., was a young man of 21 years, weight 140 lbs. His total muscular strength, as shown by the Universal Dynamometer (see Fig. 253), was 6,480 lbs. (Fig. 254). The full immersion bath was administered at 112°, duration twelve minutes. At the conclusion of the bath, the strength was tested again, and found to be 5,415 pounds, a loss of 1,065 pounds, or more than 16 per cent. The subject felt very much weakened and depressed by the experiment, from which he was quickly recovered, however, by the application of a spray douche at 50° for thirty seconds. His strength was again tested, and found to be 6,480 pounds, or exactly the same as at the beginning of the experiment. This experiment also illustrates the marvelous properties of cold water as a restorative agent.

EXPERIMENT 45.—*Showing the effects upon muscular capacity of a cold bath following a hot immersion bath (page 151).*

(*a*) The subject, R. A. S., was a young man aged 21, weight 140 lbs. The strength of the flexor muscle of the middle finger of the right hand was determined by means of Mosso's ergograph (Fig. 255), and is shown in the accompanying graphic (Fig. 256). The total work was 5.290 kgm. A hot spray was administered at 113° for fifteen minutes. Another ergogram was obtained (Fig. 257), and the amount of work done was found to be 5.235 kgm., showing a loss of .562 kgm., or 11 per cent. A cold spray was then administered at 60°, duration ten minutes, and the ergogram shown in Fig. 258 was obtained. The amount of work recorded was 6.094 kgm., an immediate increase of more than 16 per cent, and an increase of 15 per cent over the total work recorded at the beginning of the experiment.

(*b*) In a similar experiment with the same subject, in which the Universal Dynamometer was used as a means of determining the effects of the applications, the hot bath produced a loss of 915 pounds, or 13 per cent of the total strength, while the cold bath produced a gain of 1,267 pounds, or 18 per cent, the subject having a total muscular capacity at the end of the experiment 5 per cent greater than at the beginning.

EXPERIMENT 46.—*Showing the effects upon the body temperature of a general application of heat (page 158).*

(*a*) The subject, A. C. S., was a young man aged 23, weight 137 lbs. A Russian bath was administered at 115°, duration twenty-five minutes. The initial body temperature was, mouth, 98.6°; rectal, 99.9°. At the conclusion of the bath, the mouth temperature was 102.4° and the rectal temperature 102°, an increase of 258.9 heat units (137×2.1×.9=258.9).

(*b*) An electric-light bath was administered (1891) to a young man aged 22, weight 145 lbs. The subject's temperature was normal at the beginning of the experiment, and was raised by the bath in five and one-half minutes 1.6° F. (mouth). The surface temperature was elevated during the same period 2.3° F.

EXPERIMENT 47.—*Showing the effects of the hot immersion bath on the body temperature (page 158).*

The subject, W. E. P., was a young man aged 35, weight 120 lbs. He was placed in a full bath at 104° for thirty minutes. The initial body temperature was, mouth, 98.7°; rectal, 99.6°. At the end of the experiment, the mouth temperature was found to be 102.3°; and the rectal temperature, 102.8°, an increase of 3.2°, representing 345.6 heat units (120×3.2×.9=345.6). The amount of heat normally produced in thirty minutes would be 216 heat units (7.2×30=216). This leaves 129.7 heat units to be accounted for by absorption or increased heat production. Some

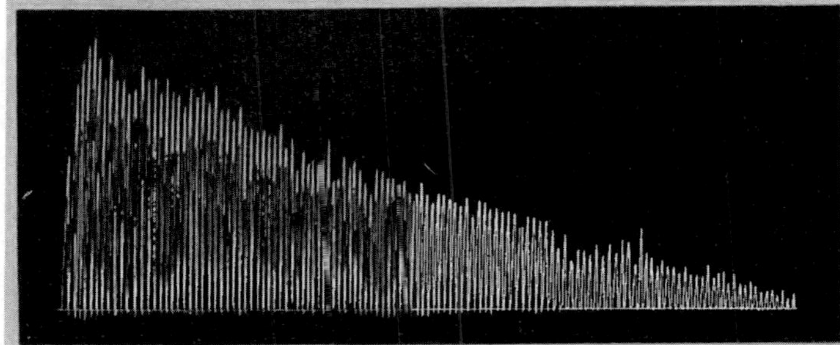

Fig. 259 (Exp. 50). Norma Fatigue Curve of A. E. L. Total work, 5.395 kgm. (p. 1125).

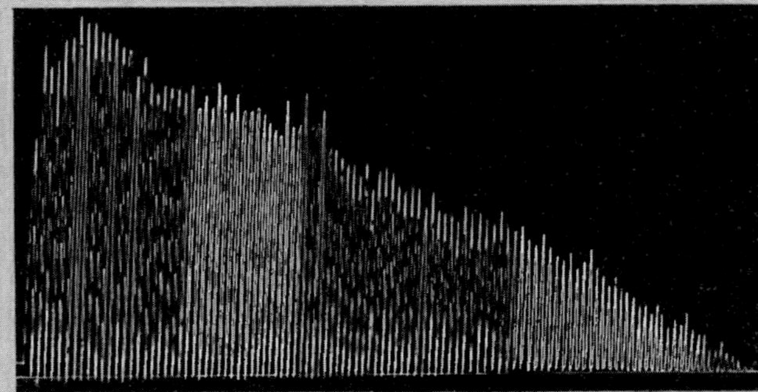

Fig. 260 (Exp. 50). Ergogram Showing Fatigue Curve of A. E. L. after Application to Forearm of a Douche at 60° for One Minute. Total work, 6.925 kgm. (p. 1125).

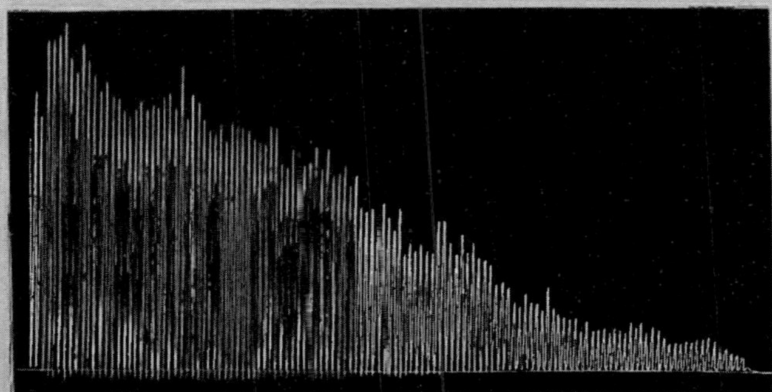

Fig. 269 (Exp. 56*b*). Normal Fatigue Curve of a Young Man, the Subject of the Experiment. Total work, 8.033 kgm. (p. 1128).

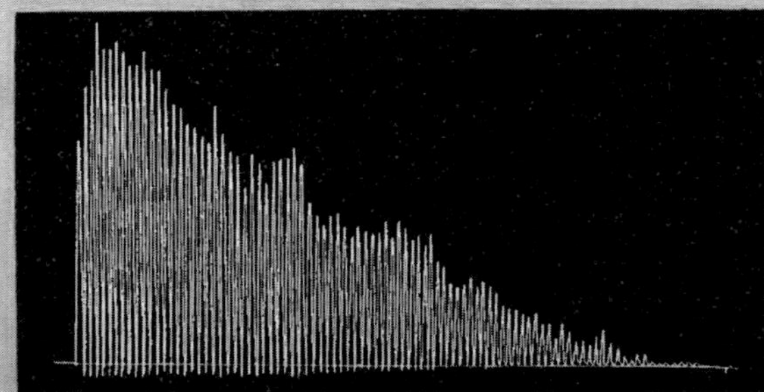

Fig. 270 (Exp. 56*b*). Fatigue Curve Obtained from the Same Subject after an Immersion Bath at 104° for Twenty Minutes. Total work, 4.459 kgm. (p. 1127).

heat was doubtless absorbed by the body during the bath, but it seems reasonable to believe that the great accumulation of heat was due to diminished heat elimination with increased heat production, rather than to the mere absorption of heat.

All general applications which interfere with heat elimination at the ordinary rate, produce similar results.

EXPERIMENT 48.—*Showing the effect on body temperature of a bath at the temperature of the body* (*page 159*).

The subject, W. E. P., was a man aged 35, weight 120 lbs. The body temperature determined just before the experiment was, mouth, 98.5°; rectal, 101.2°. The subject was placed in an immersion bath at 100° for one hour. The mouth temperature was then found to be 101.9°; the rectal, 101.8°.

EXPERIMENT 49.—*Showing the effect of dry friction upon the surface temperature* (*page 166*).

Friction with the dry shampoo brush was administered for thirty minutes to a subject, W. E. P., aged 35, weight 120 lbs. The surface temperature, taken at different parts of the body before and after the experiment, showed a gain of from 1.5° to 4°, an average of 2.7°.

EXPERIMENT 50.—*Showing the effects of a partial cold application in increasing muscular capacity* (*page 300*).

The subject, A. E. L., was a young man aged 26 years, weight 151 lbs. His normal ergogram is shown in Fig. 259. The total work recorded was 5.395 kgm. After the application to the forearm for one minute, of a douche at 60°, the ergogram shown in Fig. 260 was obtained, and the total work recorded was 6.925 kgm., an increase of 30 per cent.

EXPERIMENT 51.—*Showing the effect of friction in connection with the cold bath in increasing heat elimination* (*page 304*).

The subject, E. F. O., a young man aged 26, weight 105 lbs., was placed in a bath-tub calorimeter containing 400 pounds of water at 70°. Without friction the temperature of the water rose at the rate of .72° F. in five minutes. When friction was applied, the temperature of the water rose at the rate of 1.08° F. every five minutes. By calculation it appears that the rate of heat elimination was, without friction, 57.6 heat units per minute; with friction, 86.4 heat units, an increase of 50 per cent.

EXPERIMENT 52.—*Showing the effects of the cold enema upont he body temperature in a normal, healthy person* (*page 318*).

The subject, L. H. W., was a young man aged 30, weight 166 lbs. The initial temperature was, mouth 99°; rectal, 99.7°. The temperature of the water administered was 70° F., the amount, 8 pints. This quantity was introduced in three portions within 57 minutes, each succeeding portion being introduced immediately after the discharge of the preceding. At the end of the experiment, the mouth temperature was found to be 98.4°, a decrease of .6°; the rectal temperature was 94°. The axillary temperature at the beginning of the experiment was 97.2°; at the end, 97.6°. The rise in axillary temperature which usually occurs in connection with the cold enema is due to the contraction of the mesenteric vessels, producing a movement of blood toward the surface, especially of the upper portion of the body.

EXPERIMENT 53.—*Showing the effects of percussion in increasing the intensity of the reaction from cold.*

(*a*) The subject, W. P. L., was a young man aged 21, weight 140 lbs. The initial surface temperature obtained by placing a surface thermometer at a point near the umbilicus was 97.6°. A percussion douche was administered at 55°, duration forty seconds. Immediately after the application, the surface temperature, determined at the same point, was 94.6°. The initial temperature was reached at the end of fourteen minutes. (See also experiment 36.)

(*b*) The subject, A. G. F., was a young man aged 23, weight 132 lbs. The cold compress and the percussion douche were simultaneously given at 65° for five seconds, to opposite and corresponding parts. After the cold compress, the time required for reaction was forty seconds, whereas after the percussion douche with pressure at 30 lbs., the circulatory reaction appeared in five seconds.

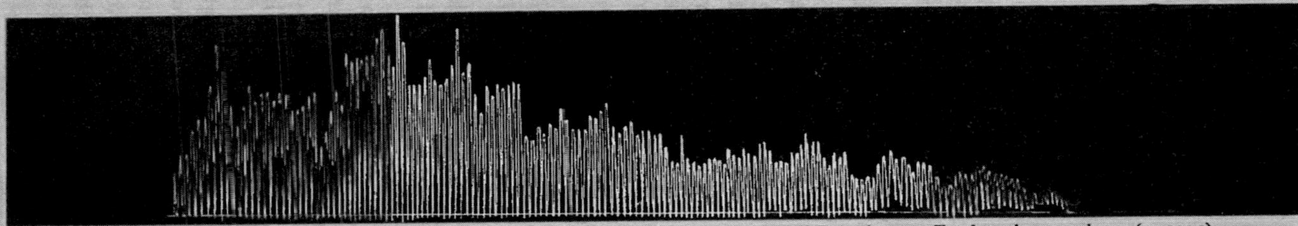

Fig. 261 (Exp. 54). Normal Fatigue Curve of a Young Man Who Was the Subject of Experiment. Total work, 1.312 kgm. (p. 1127).

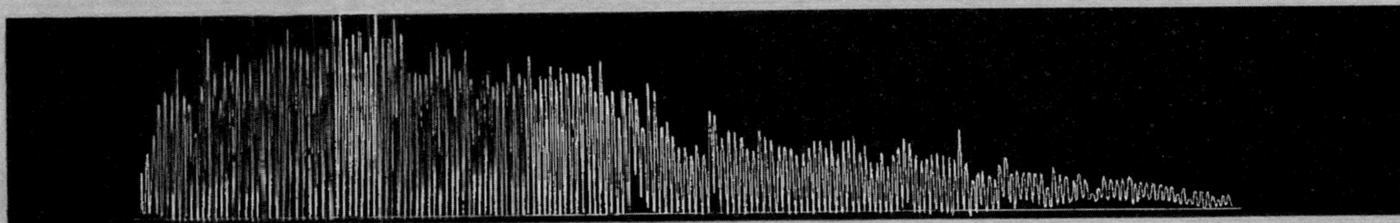

Fig. 262 (Exp. 54). Fatigue Curve Obtained from the Same Subject as the Preceding after a Douche at 55° for Fifteen Seconds. Total work, 1.527 kgm. (p. 1127).

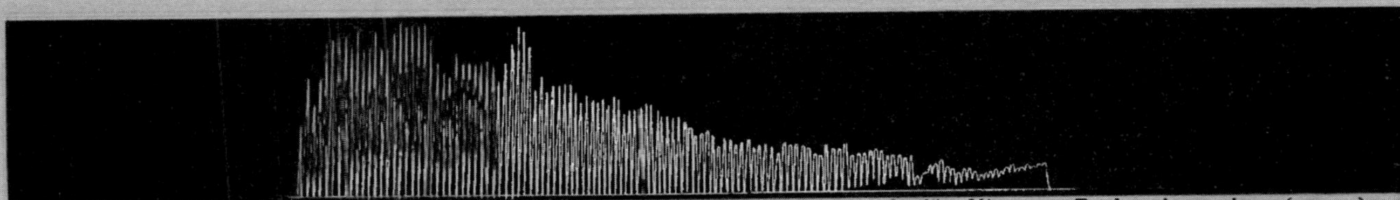

Fig. 263 (Exp. 54). Fatigue Curve Obtained from the Same Subject after a Douche at 115° for Five Minutes. Total work, .927 kgm. (p. 1127).

EXPERIMENT 54.—*Showing the effect of cold applications upon the muscular response to electrical currents (page 438).*

The amount of work done before and after the application was measured by Mosso's ergograph (see Fig. 255, page 1123), in which a spring resistance was substituted for the weights (this modification was suggested by Dr. E. Otis). The results obtained are shown in Figs. 261, 262, and 263. Fig. 261 shows the normal curve. The amount of work done was 1.312 kgm. After a douche at 55° for fifteen seconds, as shown in Fig. 262, the work done was 1.527 kgm. After a douche at 115°, duration five minutes, the ergogram shown in Fig. 263 was obtained, and the amount of work registered was .927 kgm. The capacity for muscular work was thus increased 16.4 per cent by the cold douche to the arm, and diminished 29.3 per cent by the hot douche. The increased amount of work done was due to the more energetic contraction of the muscles.

The observation was constantly made that the resistance of the skin is increased to a marked degree after a cold application; that is, after the application of cold to the parts while the current is passing there is immediate decrease in the reading of the milliampèremeter, while an application of heat produces the opposite effect, without any change in the adjustment of the rheostat.

EXPERIMENT 55.—*Showing the effect of the general cold douche on the capacity for muscular work (page 438).*

The subject, A. E. L., was a young man aged 26, weight 151 lbs. His normal fatigue curve is shown in Fig. 264. After the administration of a general douche at 60° for three minutes, a second ergogram was obtained, shown in Fig. 265. The amount of work registered before the douche was 8.282 kgm.; after the douche the total work was 11.966 kgm. an increase of 44 per cent.

EXPERIMENT 56.—*Showing the effects of heat and cold on the capacity for muscular work (page 438).*

(*a*) The subject, A. E. L., a young man aged 26, weight 151 lbs., gave the normal fatigue curve shown in Fig. 266; total work, 6.371 kgm. A general douche at 56° for fifteen seconds was then administered, and another ergogram obtained, shown in

Fig. 267. The amount of work registered was 8.448 kgm., an increase of 32 per cent. A general hot douche (temperature 112°, duration fifteen min.) was then administered, and another ergogram obtained, shown in Fig. 268. The total amount of work done was 4.155 kgm., a decrease of 33 per cent.

(*b*) On another occasion, a hot immersion bath was given the same patient at 104° for twenty minutes with the following result: Normal fatigue curve, shown in Fig. 269; amount of work registered, 8.033 kgm. After the bath, the fatigue curve shown in Fig. 270 was obtained, showing a notable depression. The amount of work registered was 4.459 kgm., a decrease of 44 per cent.

EXPERIMENT 57.—*Showing the effects of very hot applications in producing an initial slowing of the pulse with subsequent increase* (*page 448*).

In the subject, A. C. S., a young man aged 23, weight 137 lbs., the normal radial pulse rate was found to be 70. The arterial tension, as indicated by Gærtner's tonometer (see Figs. 239, 240, page 931), was 9 cm. The subject was placed in an immersion bath at 102°. The pulse immediately fell to 61. At the end of fifteen minutes, the pulse rate was 87, and the tonometer registered 6 cm., showing a marked fall in blood pressure.

By comparison with Experiment 40, it will be noted that local hot applications produce a rise in blood pressure, as indicated by the tonometer, while general hot applications produce a fall, as shown above. Thirty minutes after the bath, the pulse rate was 60 and the tonometer reading 8 cm.

EXPERIMENT 58.—*Showing the effects of the cold and the neutral immersion bath on capacity for muscular work* (*page 529*).

(*a*) The subject, A. E. L., was a young man aged 26, weight 151 lbs. The normal fatigue curve obtained is shown in Fig. 271. The total amount of work done was 5.817 kgm. After a general douche at 55° for fifteen seconds, the fatigue curve shown in Fig. 272 was obtained, and the amount of work registered was 8.642 kgm., an increase of 48.5 per cent.

(*b*) A neutral immersion bath administered to the same subject produced practically no effect on the capacity for muscular work, as shown in the normal fatigue curve presented in Fig. 273. Total work, 5.789 kgm.

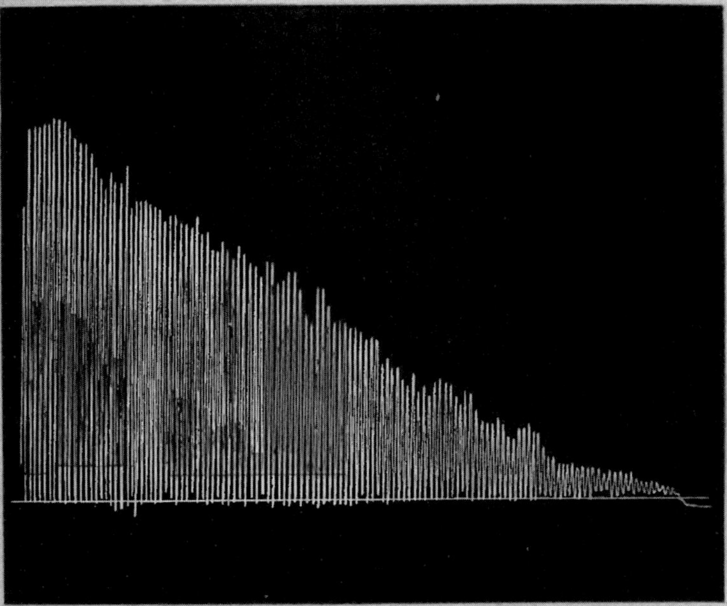

Fig. 264 (Exp. 55). Normal Fatigue Curve of A. E. L. Total work, 8.282 kgm. (p. 1127).

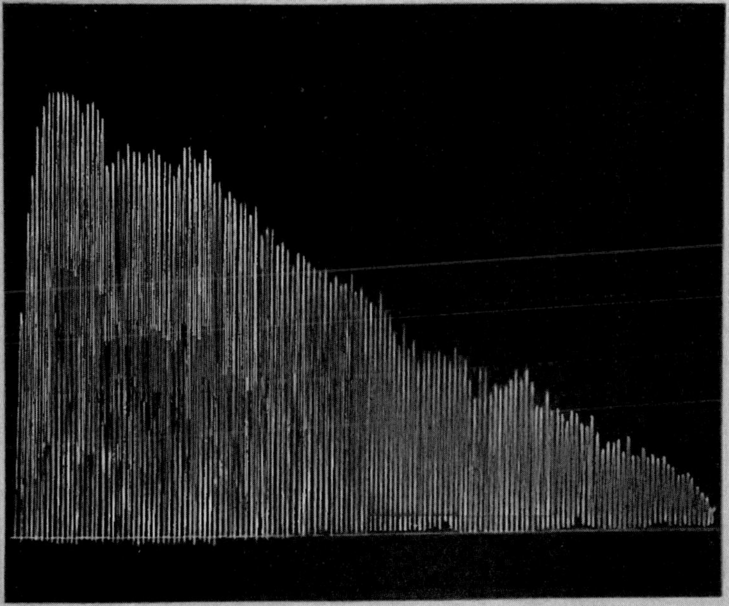

Fig. 265 (Exp. 55). Fatigue Curve of A. E. L. after a General Douche at 60° for Three Minutes. Total work, 11.966 kgm. (p. 1127).

EXPERIMENT 59.—*Showing the effects of the cold shallow bath on capacity for muscular work* (*page 597*).

The subject, W. P. L., was a young man aged 21, weight 140 lbs. A shallow bath was administered at 65° for two minutes, with the result of increasing the capacity for muscular work 32 per cent, as shown in the fatigue curves presented in Figs. 274 and 275.

EXPERIMENT 60.—*Showing the effects of a tonic application of the wet-sheet pack upon muscular work* (*page 615*).

The subject, W. P. L., aged 21, weight 140 lbs., gave the normal fatigue curve shown in Fig. 276. The wet-sheet pack was applied at 60° for twenty minutes, after which the fatigue curve shown in Fig. 277 was obtained. The amount of work registered was increased from 4.791 kgm. to 5.456 kgm., or a gain of 14 per cent.

EXPERIMENT 61.—*Showing the effects of oiling the skin upon heat elimination by conduction* (*page 685*).

The subject, E. F. O., was a young man aged 26, weight 105 lbs. When placed in a d'Arsonval calorimeter (see Fig. 24, page 89) in a room at a temperature of 82° F., the movement of air was at the rate of 100 feet per minute. The subject was then removed from the calorimeter and smeared with vaseline. Upon returning to the calorimeter, the rate was 55 feet per minute, a decrease of 45 per cent.

Numerous observations made with the bath-tub calorimeter agreed with the above results.

EXPERIMENT 62.—*Showing the effects of Russian, electric-light, and Turkish baths upon the body temperature* (*page 704*).

(*a*) The subject, A. C. S., a young man aged 23 years, weight 137 lbs., was given a Russian bath at 115° for twenty-five minutes. At the beginning of the bath, the pulse rate was 56; rectal temperature, 99.9°. At the conclusion of the bath, the pulse rate was 130; rectal temperature, 102°, an increase of 258.9 heat units ($137 \times 2.1 \times .9 = 258.9$). The normal amount of heat produced in twenty-five minutes is about 180 heat units, leaving 78.9 heat units to be accounted for either by increased heat production or absorption. Other observations indicate the probability of an increase in heat production.

(*b*) The subject, V. P., aged 26 years, weight 130 lbs., was placed in an electric-light bath for twenty-three minutes. At the beginning of the bath the pulse rate was 82; rectal temperature, 99.9°. At the end of the bath, the pulse rate was 134; rectal temperature, 101.4°; mouth temperature, 102°, an increase of 175.5 heat units ($130 \times 1.5 \times .9 = 175.5$). The amount of heat normally produced during the time covered by the experiment is about 165.6 (23×7.2), almost exactly the amount represented by the elevation of temperature. As heat elimination, either by radiation or evaporation, is not interfered with during this bath, the increase was probably the result, in part, at least, of augmented heat production.

(*c*) P. H., a young man aged 25 years, weight 150 lbs., was given a Turkish bath for one hour at 146° to 158°. At the beginning of the bath, the pulse was 49; rectal temperature, 98.9°. At the end of the experiment, the pulse rate was 59; rectal temperature, 100.6°, and respiration increased from 13 to 19 per minute. The elevation in temperature represented an accumulation of 229.5 heat units. In many subjects more marked effects are produced.

EXPERIMENT 63.—*Showing the influence of the cold proximal compress upon the temperature of distal parts* (*page 760*).

The subject, A. C. S., was a young man aged 23, weight 137 lbs.; initial temperature, axilla, 99.8°; palmar surface, hand closed, 98.1°. The elbow was immersed in water at 42° for thirty minutes, at the end of which time the axillary temperature was 100.8°, and the hand temperature, 96.1°.

EXPERIMENT 64.—(*Page 774.*)

The surface temperature of the cheek was determined to be 97.3°. Ice was then placed in the mouth, and held in contact with the mucous surface of the cheek for fifteen minutes. The temperature of the cutaneous surface was reduced to 89.6°.

EXPERIMENT 65.—(*Page 774.*)

The temperature of the inner surface of the cheek was taken, and found to be 98.6°. By the application of ice to the outer surface of the cheek for fifteen minutes, the temperature of the inner surface was reduced to 90° F.

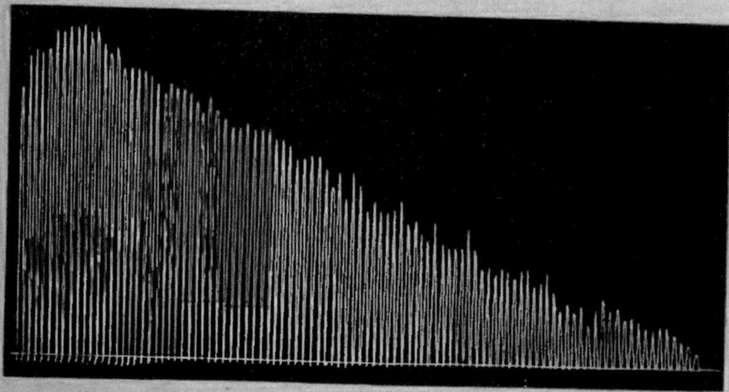

Fig. 266 (Exp. 56*a*). Normal Fatigue Curve of A. E. L. Total work, 6.371 kgm. (p. 1128).

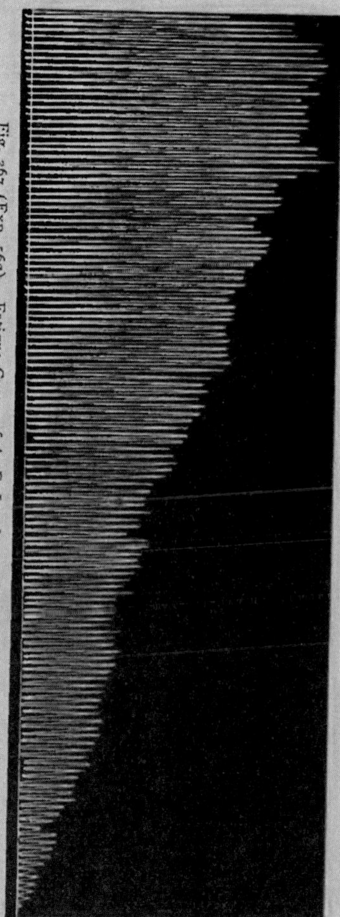

Fig. 267 (Exp. 56*a*). Fatigue Curve of A. E. L. after a General Douche at 56° for Fifteen Seconds. Total work, 8.448 kgm. (p. 1128).

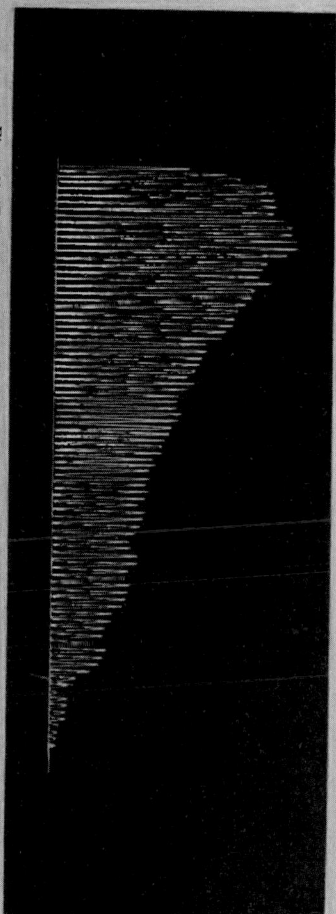

Fig. 268 (Exp. 56*a*). Fatigue Curve of A. E. L. after a General Douche at 112° for Fifteen Minutes. Total work, 4.155 kgm. (p. 1128).

EXPERIMENT 66.—(*Page 774.*)

The subject, F. G. L., was a young man aged 21, weight 135 lbs. The rectal temperature was taken and found to be 99.8°. An ice compress was applied to the abdomen and sacrum. At the end of thirty minutes, the rectal temperature had fallen to 98.6°, clearly showing the value of these applications in rectal and pelvic inflammations. It should be borne in mind that the reduction in internal temperature resulting from a cold application to the cutaneous surface is not due to the abstraction of heat from, or direct cooling of, the internal part, but is brought about indirectly through the reflex contraction of the blood-vessels of the part, and the lessened tissue activity resulting from diminished blood supply.

EXPERIMENT 67.—(*Page 774.*)

In a subject whose initial rectal temperature was 99.8°, an ice compress to the abdomen and sacrum, combined with the hot foot bath, reduced the rectal temperature in one hour and ten minutes to 97.4°.

EXPERIMENT 68.—(*Page 791.*)

(*a*) An ice compress was applied to the knee of a young man, W. P. L. The initial temperature of the foot was 94°. At the end of thirty minutes the temperature was reduced to 91.5°.

(*b*) An ice compress applied about the thigh for forty-five minutes reduced the temperature of the foot from 94° to 91°.

(*c*) An ice bag applied to the axilla for thirty minutes reduced the temperature of the hand from 97° to 96°.

(*d*) An ice collar applied to the neck produced the following results: The initial pulse of the subject, V. P., was 77; the temperature, taken in the external auditory meatus, 98°; mouth temperature, 97.8°; rectal, 99°. At the end of fifty minutes the pulse was reduced to 56; the temperature of the external auditory meatus was 93°; mouth temperature, 93.7°; rectal, 98.4°. The pulse was reduced 21 beats; the temperature of the external auditory canal, 5°; the mouth, 4.1°; and the rectal temperature, .6°.

EXPERIMENT 69.—*Showing the rate of heating of the abdominal compress protected with flannel only* (*page 826*).

Three experiments were made on a subject, a young man, A. E. L., aged 26, weight 151 lbs. The procedure consisted of the application of an ordinary heating abdominal compress, using a linen cloth for the moist layer, covering with flannel, employing different thicknesses in the different experiments. The temperature of the water used was 59° F., the room temperature 77° F. The temperature was taken at the end of the first and second minutes, then every two minutes afterward until the maximum temperature was reached. The results were as follows:—

(*a*) Employing one layer of flannel to cover the wet compress, the temperature at the end of the first minute was found to be 81.5°; the maximum temperature, 86.5°, was reached at the end of eight minutes.

(*b*) With two layers of flannel, the temperature was found at the end of the first minute as in the preceding experiment, 81.5°. The maximum temperature of 89.3° was reached at the end of ten minutes.

(*c*) The moist bandage was covered with four thicknesses of flannel. Temperature at the end of one minute was 82.5°; the maximum temperature of 91.8° was reached at the end of ten minutes.

EXPERIMENT 70.—*Showing the rate of heating of the heating abdominal compress, when protected with mackintosh or other impervious material* (*page 826*).

These experiments were made with the same subject as the preceding and the conditions were the same:—

(*a*) With one thickness of flannel, the maximum temperature 91.4° was reached at the end of fifteen minutes.

(*b*) With two thicknesses of flannel, the maximum temperature of 92.1° was reached at the end of twenty minutes.

(*c*) With four thicknesses of flannel, the maximum temperature of 93.6° was reached at the end of twenty minutes.

(*d*) With eight thicknesses of flannel, the maximum temperature of 94.7° was reached at the end of twenty minutes.

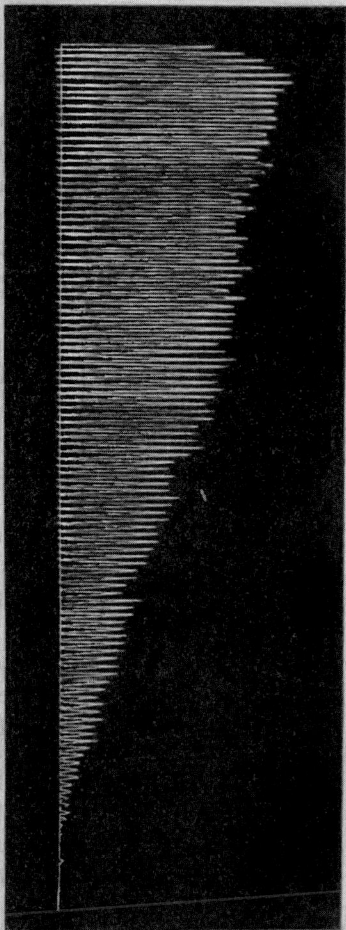

Fig. 271 (Exp. 58). Normal Fatigue Curve of A. E. L. Total work, 4.791 kgm. (p. 1128).

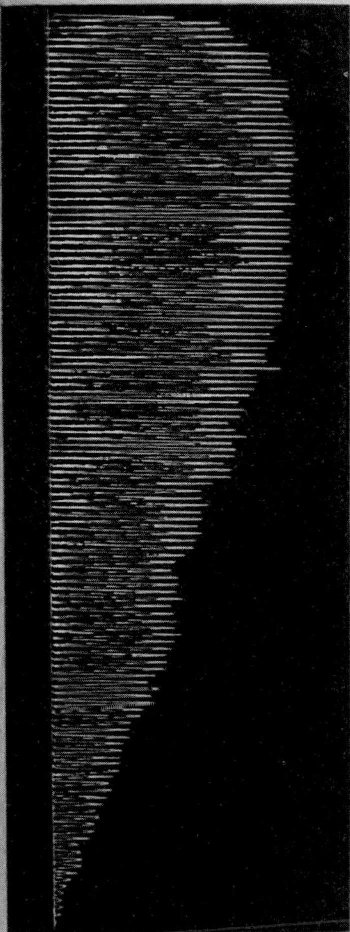

Fig. 272 (Exp. 58). Fatigue Curve of A. E. L. after General Horizontal Jet at 55° for Fifteen Seconds. Total work, 8.642 kgm. (p. 1128).

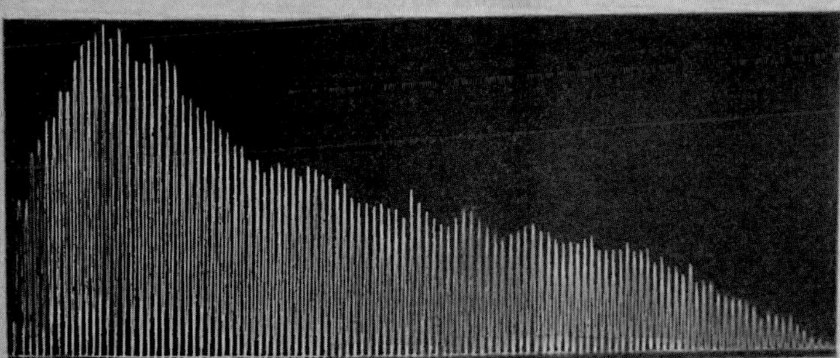

Fig. 273. (Exp. 58). Fatigue Curve of A. E. L. after Neutral Immersion Bath. Total work, 5.789 kgm. (p. 1128).

EXPERIMENT 71.—*Showing the effect of the chest compress upon the volume of tidal air (page 862).*

The subject, J. C. B., was a young man aged 27, weight 132 lbs. The normal amount of tidal air was 507 c.c. The application of the chest compress, wrung from ice-water, produced an immediate increase in the depth of the respiratory movements and the volume of the tidal air rose at once to 751 c.c., an increase of 48 per cent. At the end of twenty minutes, when the experiment terminated, the amount of tidal air was 604 c.c., 20 per cent more than at the beginning. The average increase for the whole twenty minutes was 170 c.c., or 33 per cent.

EXPERIMENT 72.—*Showing the effects of the cold precordial compress upon the rate and force of the heart beat (page 868).*

(*a*) The subject was a young man aged 35, weight 122 lbs. A sphygmographic tracing obtained before the application of the compress, is shown in Fig. 207 (*a*), page 868; pulse rate, 72. A cold application, consisting of an ice-poultice one foot square, was applied over the heart and left chest. The effect was an immediate increase of the pulse rate to 76 for two minutes. The pulse was then slowed, becoming at the end of three minutes 72. A second sphygmographic tracing was then taken, shown in Fig. 207 (*b*), page 868. Comparison of the two tracings shows clearly the increased tension resulting from the application.

(*b*) The subject was a patient, Mr. W., suffering from severe collapse following a prolonged and complicated abdominal operation for the removal of impacted gallstones. Before the application of the compress, the patient's pulse was so weak that it could not be felt at the wrist. When counted by means of the stethoscope placed over the heart, it was found to be 120. An ice-bag was applied over the heart with the result that the pulse could be counted at the wrist, the rate was slowed to 87, and the tension, which was zero as indicated by Gærtner's tonometer, rose to 5 cm.

(*c*) The subject, R. M. B., was a young man aged 23, weight 130 lbs.; pulse, 80; tonometer reading, 13. After the application of cold to the precordial region, there was an immediate increase in tension to 17. In two minutes the tension fell to 16, and the pulse to 70. At the end of twenty-five minutes, the pulse was 64, and the tonometer reading 15.

EXPERIMENT 73.—*Showing the effect of cold-water drinking upon the axillary temperature and the surface temperature as determined at the epigastrium* (*page 928*).

The subject, A. G. M., was a young man aged 26, weight, 153 lbs.; axillary temperature, 97.7°; mouth, 98.7°; rectal, 99.2°; surface temperature at the epigastrium, 97°. The patient drank in rapid succession seven glasses of lemonade at 58°. A fall in the axillary temperature was noted in five minutes. At the end of twenty minutes, the axillary temperature was 96.1°; mouth, 98°; rectal, 98°; surface temperature at the epigastrium, 92°.

The great fall in surface temperature at the epigastrium, after drinking ice-water, may be utilized as a means of locating the stomach and determining its size and contour. The interesting fact that a very marked depression in the surface temperature of the skin overlying the stomach takes place as the result of drinking a quantity of ice-water, was first noted by Dr. F. J. Otis (1898), while a medical student, engaged in carrying out experimental researches under the direction of the author.

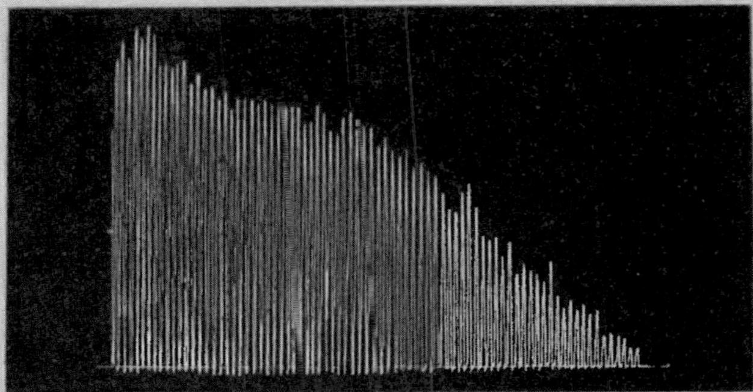

Fig. 274 (Exp. 59). Normal Fatigue Curve of W. P. L. Total work, 5.761 kgm. (p. 1129).

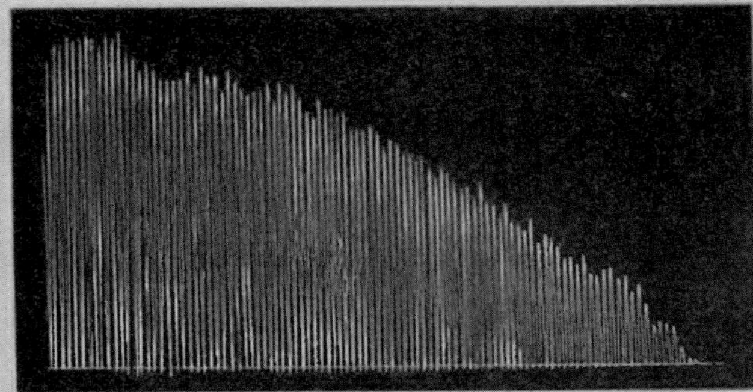

Fig. 275 (Exp. 59). Ergogram of W. P. L. after Shallow Bath at 65° for Two Minutes. Total work, 7.589 kgm. (p. 1129).

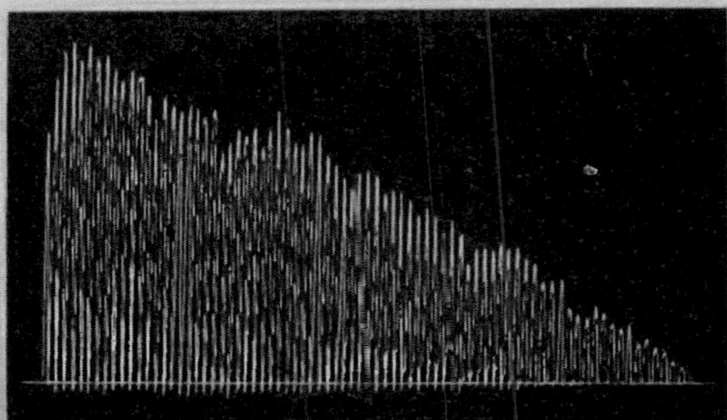

Fig. 276 (Exp. 60). Normal Fatigue Curve of W. P. L. Total work, 5.761 kgm. (p. 1129).

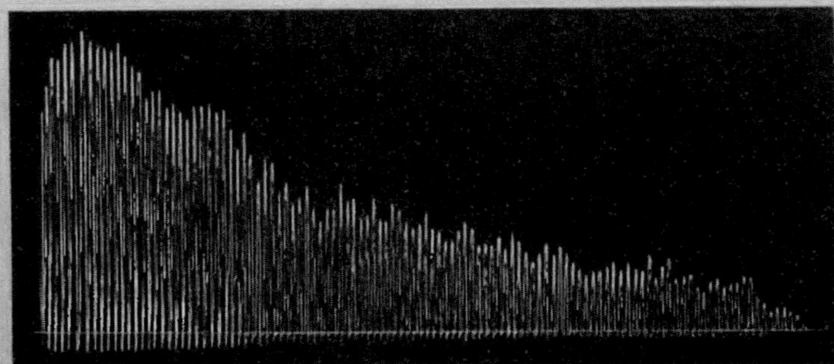

Fig. 277 (Exp. 60) Fatigue Curve of W. P. L. after a Wet-Sheet Pack at 60° for Twenty Minutes. Total work, 5.495 kgm. (p. 1129).

BIBLIOGRAPHY.

WITH very few exceptions all the following authorities have been consulted in the preparation of this work, and a considerable number are referred to in foot-notes in the preceding pages. This list, however, is not presented as by any means complete. The bibliography of hydrotherapy has within the last few years grown to enormous proportions. It is believed, however, that the major part of what is worth reading upon this subject may be found in the works named below. The authorities indicated by numeral reference marks are referred to in Parts I and II.

1. Landois & Sterling. Text-book of Human Physiology, 1891, page 174.
2. Landois & Sterling. Text-book of Human Physiology, 1891, page 113.
3. Waller, Augustus. Human Physiology, 1891, page 59.
4. Landois & Sterling. Text-book of Human Physiology, 1891, page 228.
5. Landois & Sterling. Human Physiology, 1891, pages 780–783.
6. Landois & Sterling. Human Physiology, 1891, page 230.
7. Waller, Augustus. Human Physiology, pages 280–281.
8. Schüller. Archiv für Klinische medicin, 1874.
9. Landois & Sterling. Human Physiology, 1891, page 427.
10. Naumann. Zur Lehre von dem Reflex, 1872.
11. Gillebert-Dhercourt. Annales de la Société d'hydrologie médicale, 1870.
12. Franck, François. Travaux dur laboratoire du professeur Marey. Tome 1.
13. Vinaj & Maggiori. Blätter für Klin. Hydrother., 1893.
14. Centralblatt für innere Medicin, 1893, page 1017.
15. Archiv für experimentelle Pathologie und Pharmakologie.
16. Thayer, W. S. Johns Hopkins Hospital Bulletin, 1893.
17. Strasser, A., and Buxbaum, B. Fortschritte der Hydrotherapie, 1897.
18. Landois & Sterling. Human Physiology, 1891, page 548.
19. Fleury, Louis. Traité Thérapeutique et clinique d'hydrothérapie, page 144.
20. Fleury, page 160.

21. Bottey, Fernand. Traité théorique et pratique d'hydrothérapie médicale, 1895.
22. Oliver. London Lancet, 1896.
23. Beni-Barde. L'Hydrothérapie dans les maladies chronique et les maladies nerveuses, 1894.
24. Maggiori & Vinaj. Blätter für Klinische Hydrotherapie 1892, Vol. II, No. 15; Vol. III, No. 7, also page 67.
25. Hénocque, Albert. Annales de la Société de Biologie, 1887.
26. Pflüger's Archiv, 1871. Jahrg IV, pages 57-90.
27. Beni-Barde. Les douches locales en hydrothérapie, Congrès d'hydrologie, 1889.
28. Bottey, Fernand. Traité théorique et pratique d'hydrthérapie médicale, 1895, page 117.
29. Bottey, Fernand. Annales de la Société d'hydrologie médicale, 1886, page 60.
30. Draper. New York Medical Journal, 1888.
31. Leyden. Archiv für Anat. u. Phys., 1867–68.

Baginsky. Lehrbuch der Kinder Krankheiten, 1896, page 292.

Barra, M. P. L'usage de la glace de la neige et du froid, Aggrégé au collège de Lyon.

Barthélemy, T. Etude sur de Dermographisme, Paris.

Baruch, Simon.

The Treatment of Typhoid Fever, Medical Record, Vol. 37, No. 12, pages 318, 355.

Causes and Treatment of the Summer Diarrhea of Infants, Medical News, 1890.

The Status of Water in Modern Medicine, 1890.

A Plea for the Practical Utilization of Hydrotherapy, Gaillard's Medical Journal, New York, 1890, Vol. 1, pages 24–54.

Hydrotherapy in Europe, Medical Record, Oct. 11, 1890.

Hydrotherapy and Mineral Springs (Hare's American System of Practical Therapeutics), Phila., 1891. Vol. 1, page 453.

A Plea for the More Methodical Management of Chronic Diseases, Dietetic Gazette, January, February, March, 1892.

The Uses of Water in Modern Medicine, Geo. G. Davis, Detroit, 1892.

Conditions Indicating Change of Air and Baths in the Summer Diarrhea of Children, Medical News, June 18, 1892.

Practical Data on the Application of Water in Some Intractable Diseases, Medical Record, Vol. 43, page 5, 1893.

Discussion on Therapeutic Reflections, Medical Record, Nov. 4. 1893, pages 597, 598, and Vol. 44, No. 19, page 580.
Diagnostic Bath in Typhoid Fever, N. Y. Med. Jour., Sept. 2, 1893.
A Plea for Physiological Remedies, Therapeutic Gazette, 1893.
Logic vs. Sentiment in Therapeutics, Medical Record, Dec. 23, 1893.
Rationale of Hydrotherapy, Medical Record, Oct. 27, 1894.
Water the Ancient and Ready Remedy, Editorial, Medical Record, March, 1894.
Methods of Fostering the Interests of Medical Science, Presidential Address before the South Carolina Med. Assn., 1894.
Non-Medicinal Remedies in Anemia, N. Y. Med. Jour., May 15, 1895.
Kneipp's Water Cure in the Light of Medical History, New York Medical Journal, 1895, pages 522–525.
Das Wasser in der Aertztlichen Praxis, Trans. by Dr. Friedrich Grosse, Stuttgart, 1895.
The Clinical Aspect of Dyspepsia, Transactions South Carolina Medical Association, 1895.
Importance of Precision in the Technique of Hydrotherapy, Medical News, Feb. 22, 1896, Discussion Medical and Surgical Reporter, page 686, 1896.
Tubbing in Typhoid Fever, Discussion, Medical Record, Nov. 7, 1896, page 692.
Riverside Association Hydriatric Department, Medical News, May 2, 1896, page 500.
Hydrotherapy in Typhoid Fever, Medical News, April 25, 1896, Vol. 68, No. 6.
The Management of Pneumonia Patients, Medical News, Jan. 2, 1897, and American Med. & Surg. Bulletin, Dec. 19. 1896.
Recent Advances in Hydrotherapy (Hare's System of Practical Therapeutics), Phila., 1897, Vol. 4, pages 17–36.
Cold Compresses in Pneumonia, Medical News, January, 1897.
Ueber die Wichtigkeit der Praecision in der hydriatischen Technik, Fortsch. der Hydrotherapie, Festschrift, Wilhelm Winternitz, Wien und Leipzig, 1897, pages 96–118.
Fehlgriffe in der Hydrotherapie, New York Medical Monatschr., 1897, Vol. 9, pages 129–143.
Lecture on the Practical Application of Hydrotherapy, Philadelphia International Clinics, 1897.
Faulty Hydrotherapy, Jour. of the Amer. Med. Assn., May 13, 1897.

Discussion of Typhoid Bathing at the County Medical Society, Medical Times, February 1897, page 56.

Pneumonia, Editorial, Medical Record, Jan. 9, 1897, page 14.

Some Desperate Cases of Typhoid Fever Treated with and without Baths, Medical Record, Oct. 1, 1898.

The Principles and Practice of Hydrotherapy, Wm. Wood and Co., 1898.

Die praktische Anwendung der Wasserheilkunde, Monatschr. f. prakt. Wasserheilkunde, München, 1898, Vol. V., pages 145–155.

Hydriatische Technik und wissenschaftliche Hydrotherapie, Blätter f. klin. Hydrother., Wien., 1898, Vol. VIII, page 211.

The Present Status of Hydrotherapy, Editorial, Medical News, Vol. 75, No. 28, 1899.

Modern Management of Pneumonia, New York Medical Times, February, 1899, page 49.

Hydrotherapy (Hare's System of Practical Therapeutics), Vol. 1, 1900.

Principles and Practice of Hydrotherapy, London, 1900, Bailliere, Tindall & Co.

The Treatment of Pneumonia, New York Medical Journal, Vol. 69, No. 1, page 16.

Practical Data on Continental Health Resorts, Medical News, Vol. 71, No. 2, page 53.

Hydrotherapy in Pneumonia of Children, Medical News, Vol. 73, No. 21, page 652.

Discussion on Practical Data on the Application of Water in Some Intractable Diseases, New York Medical Times, Vol. 23, No. 12, page 380.

The Clinical Aspect of Dyspepsia, Medical Record, Vol. 48, No. 14, page 469.

Baum, S. On the Effects of Cold Wet Friction, Wien. Med. Presse, 1893. XXXIV, 1921, 1967.

Bell, John. Treatise on Baths. Ed. 2, Phila., 1859.

Beni-Barde, Joseph-Marie-Alfred.

Manuel Médical d'Hydrothérapie, 1883.

Les Douches Locales en Hydrothérapie. Congrès d'Hydrologie, 1889.

L'Hydrothérapie, dans les maladies chroniques et les maladies neurveuses, 1894.

Bernard, Cl. Études Physiologiques sur quelques Poisons Américains, Paris, 1864.

Leçons sur la chaleur animale, Paris, 1876.

Bernard, P. Ann. de la Société d'Hydrol., Paris, 1894.
Blätter der Hydrotherapie, Bände I.—IX.
Bottey, F. Ann. de la Société d'Hydrol. Med., 1886.
Traité Théorique et Pratique d'Hydrothérapie Médicale, 1895.
Bouchard, Ch. Leçons sur les Auto-Intoxications, Paris, 1887.
Traité de Médecine, 1899-1901.
Bougarel. Ann. de la Société d'Hydrol. Med., Paris.
Brown-Sequard. Archives de Physiologie, Vol. III, pages 497–502.
Brunner. Berliner Klinische Wochenschrift, 1891, page 505.
Cameron, Charles. The Baths of the Romans, London, 1772.
Centralblatt für Innere Medicin, 1893, page 1017.
Couette. Étude Expérimentale sur l'Action Thermique de l'Eau Froide en Applications Hydrothérapeutiques.
Currie, James. Medical Reports, 4th ed.
Currie and Fordyce. On Fever, Medical Reports, 1797.
Dauchez. Bull. Gen. de Therap., 1884, page 153.
Descantes. Revue d'Hydrologie, Paris, 1896, page 51.
Dickinson, W. H. Recherches sur l'effet produit sur la circulation par l'application prolongée de l'eau froide à la surface du corps de l'homme, Jour. de la physiol. de l'homme, Paris, 1858, Vol. I, pages 72–89. Also Abstr. transl., Proc. Roy., Med. and Chir. Soc. Lond., 1806–1807, Vol. I, pages 77–80.
Draper, W. H. On Hydrotherapy, External and Internal. Trans. New England Academy of Medicine, 1892, 1893. Vol. IX, page 145.
Dujardin-Beaumetz, Georges. On Cold Baths in Nervous Diseases, Especially Douches, Immersions, Affusions, Wet Sheet Rub. Trans. latin. Boston M. & S. G. Vol. CVIII, pages 169–172.
L'Hygiène Thérapeutique, Paris, 1888.
Duval. Heating Compress, Ann. de Cher. et d'Orthod., 1896. Vol. IX, pages 73, 76.
Duval, E. Traité Pratique et Clinique d'Hydrothérapie, Paris, 1888.
Edes, Peter. Use of Water, an Abridgement of the second edition of a work written by Dr. Currie on The Use of Water in Diseases of the Human Frame, Aug. 12, 1799.
Fleming. Physiology of the Turkish Bath. Glasgow.
Flint, Austin. On the Researches of Currie and Recent Views Relating to the Remedial Use of Water, Louisville Practitioner. Vol. XI, 1875, pages 1-29.
Franck, Francois. Travaux sur Laboratoire du Professeur Marey. Tome 1.
Fleury, Louis. Traité Thérapeutique et Clinique d'Hydrothérapie, Paris, 4th ed., page 144, 1875.

Frey. Experimentelle Studien über die Wirkung der heissen Luft und Dampfbäder, Archiv. für Psychiatrie, Berlin, 1880. Vol. XI, pages 266-270.

Gillebert-Dhercourt. Ann. de la Société d'Hydrol. Med., 1870.

Gilles de la Tourette. Progrès Médical, 1890, page 101.

Glatz. L'Hydrothérapie Tonique et Revulsive. Cong. Period, internal, d. sc. med. Compt. rend. Geneve, 1878, page 524.

Graham, Thos. J. The Cold Water System, London, 1843.

Graham, Robert Hay. Graefenberg, London, 1844.

Hayem, Georges. Physical and Natural Therapeutics, 1895.

Hebra. On the Continuous Bath. Wien. Med. Woch., 1877, also 1865, pages 893, 920, 940.

Hippocrates. Aphorisms on Affusions, Sect. 5, pages 20, 23, 42, 46. The Genuine Works of, Trans. from the Greek by Francis Adams.

Hénocque, Albert. Comtes Rend. des Séances et Mémoires de la Société de Biologie. Tome IV, 1887, page 678.

Joffroy. Thèse d'Aggregation, Paris, 1878, page 176.

Kellogg, J. H. Early Observation in the Disease now known as Friedrich's Ataxia, Modern Medicine and Bacteriological Review, December, 1898. Reprint of paper published in the Archives of Electrology and Neurology, 1875.

The Uses of Water in Health and Disease, 1876.

Report of Thirty-five Successive Cases of Typhoid Fever Treated by Hydrotherapy, with no Death. Read before the Calhoun Co. (Mich.) Medical Association, 1877.

Bouchard's Bath in Typhoid Fever, The Bacteriological World and Modern Medicine, November, 1891.

The Effect of Warm Baths upon Assimilation, Bact. World and Modern Medicine, 1892.

Reaction in Cold Bathing, Bact. World and Modern Medicine, 1892.

Sanitarium Methods, Bact. World and Modern Medicine, 1892.

The Non-Surgical Treatment of Ovarian Diseases, Modern Medicine and Bact. World, 1893.

Rational Therapeutics of Typhoid Fever, Modern Medicine and Bacteriological World, September, 1893.

Hydrotherapy, Modern Medicine and Bact. World, Aug. 1893.

Substitutes for Alcohol, etc. Medical Temperance Quarterly, July, 1893.

The Incandescent Electric-Light or Radiant-Heat Bath. Read before the American Electro-Therapeutic Association at the Fourth Annual Meeting, New York City, Sept. 25-27, 1894.

Hydrotherapy in Acute Pulmonary Disease, Modern Medicine and Bacteriological Review, 1894.
Hot Water in Infantile Maladies, Modern Medicine and Bact. Review, March, 1894.
The Prolonged Hot Bath in Chronic Joint Disease, Modern Medicine and Bact. Review, March, 1894.
Hydropathic Treatment of Fever, Modern Medicine and Bact. Review, March, 1894.
The Warm Bath, Modern Medicine and Bact. Review, Jan., 1894.
Charlatanry in Hydrotherapy, Modern Medicine and Bact. Review, October, 1895.
Migraine, Its Cause and Radical Cure, Modern Medicine Pub. Co., 1895.
Diabetes, Modern Medicine, September, 1895.
The Ice Compress in Pneumonia, Modern Medicine and Bact. Review, March, 1896.
The Cure of Incurables. Transactions of the Michigan State Medical Society, 1896.
The Cure of Chronic Invalids by Regimen and Training. Transactions of the Pan-American Medical Congress, Mexico City, 1896. Modern Medicine, Nov. and Dec., 1897; Jan., 1898.
The Rational Treatment of Catarrhal Affections of the Nose and Upper Air Passages, Modern Medicine and Bact. Review, September, 1896.
Anwendung von Wärme nach einer neuen Methode. Fortschritte der Hydrotherapie, Festschrift zum vierzigjährigen Doctorjubiläum des Prof. Dr. W. Winternitz. Wien, 1897.
Thermic Applications by a New Method, Modern Medicine and Bact. Review, April, 1897.
A New and Successful Method of Treatment of the Opium Habit and Other Forms of Drug Addiction. Read at the 27th Annual Meeting of the American Association for the Study and Cure of Inebriety, Boston, Mass., Dec. 7, 1897. Modern Medicine, June, 1898.
The Therapeutic Effects of Water, Modern Medicine and Bact. Review, 1898.
Hydrotherapy in Typhoid Fever Fifty Years Ago, Modern Medicine and Bact. Review, April, 1898.
The Hydriatic Treatment of Tuberculosis. Read before the American Climatological Association, Washington, D. C., Medical News, Nov. 10, 1900.
Klar. Wiener Klinische Wochenschrift, 1895, page 180.
Krull. Berliner Klinische Wochenschrift, 1877.

Kuhn. Monograph, Paris, 1854.

Kuhner. Int. Klin. Rundschau, Wien., 1894.

Landois and Sterlin. Text-book of Human Physiology, 1891, pages 113, 174, 228, 230, 427, 548, 780–783.

Langenbeck. Deutsche Klinik, 1855. No. 39, pages 409-419.

Large, E. Recherches Physiologiques sur les Bains de Vapeur Sèche. (Hamman, Bains, Tures.)

Lasèque. Arch. Gen. de Med., 1874, page 132.

Lemarchand. Annales de la Société d'Hydrologie, Med., Paris, Compt. rend. 1892-93. Vol. XXXVIII, pages 247-275.

Lepine and Flavard. On Effects of Cold Bath on Urea and Acid Phosphate Elimination. l'Union Médicale, 1880, page 722.

Leyden. On Water Retention in Fever a Cause of Diminished Heat Elimination, Arch. of Anat. and Phys., 1867-68.

Liebermeister. On Heat Elimination in Malarial Fever, Deutsch. Arch., 1868. Vol. V, page 217.

Maggiori and Vinaj. Blätter für Klinische Medicin, 1892. Vol. II, No. 15; Vol. III, No. 7, page 67.

Mays. Transactions of the Philadelphia County Medical Society, 1895, page 302.

Naumann, Präger, Viet. 1867.

Zur Lehre von dem Reflex, 1872.

Osler, William. Johns Hopkins Hospital Reports, page 321.

Oliver. London Lancet, 1896.

Paessler. Kongresz für Innere Medicin, Wiesbaden, 1896, pages 256-266.

Paulson, David. Morphinism, Modern Medicine and Bact. Review, December, 1898.

Treatment of the Morphine and Allied Habits, Modern Medicine and Bact. Review, August, 1898.

Porter. On the Physiological Action of the Cold Bath, Journal of the Post-Graduate Medical College, New York, 1897. Vol. XXII, pages 113-125.

Pflüger's Archiv. 1871. Jahrg. Vol. IV, pages 57-90.

Rand, Howard F. Sexual Neurasthenia, Modern Medicine and Bact. Review, December, 1898.

Rendu. Journal de Médecine et de Chirurgie Pratiques, 1893, page 209.

Revue d'Hygiéne Thérapeutique, June, 1893, page 164.

Richardson, B. W. The Application of Cold Water to the Cervical Region for Reduction of Pyrexia, Medical Times and Gazette, London, 1874, pages 1, 312.

Riess, Arch. für Klin. Auflage, 1889–90.

Riley, W. H. The Physiological Action and Some Therapeutic Uses of the Cold Bath, Modern Medicine and Bact. Review, September, 1895.

The Non-Medical Treatment of Insomnia, Modern Medicine and Bact. Review, December, 1896.

The Apoplectic Pulse, and Its Treatment by the Cool Shower Bath, Modern Medicine and Bact. Review, Feb. 1, 1898.

Robinson, Byron. The Vaginal Douche, Modern Medicine and Bact. Review, June, 1896.

Roe, J. T. On Use of Water in Typhoid, Pneumonia, Malarial Fever, and Appendicitis, Trans. Luzerne Co., Pennsylvania Medical Society, 1896.

Romberg. Berliner Klinische Wochenschrift, 1895.

Russel, A. Remarks on the Use of Cold Water in the Congestive and Collapsed Forms of Fever, Transl. by J. M., Lexington, Ky. 1833.

Schott, Theodore. Blätter Klinische Wochenschrift, 1880, pages 4, 7–9, 17, 35, 372.

The Treatment of Cardiac Neuroses, Medical Record, March 11, 1899, page 345.

Schroth, Johann. Die Heilmethode des Naturarztes, 1846.

Schüller. Archiv. für Klinische Medicin, Leipzig. Vol. XIV, 1874, pages 103, 429, 566.

Scoutetten, H. Rapport sur l'Hydrothérapie, Paris, 1844.

Shovosky. On the Physiological effects of the Foot Bath, Lyon Médicale, 1883, page 541.

Smith, J. The Curiosities of Common Water, Fourth Edition.

Smith, T. On the Effects of Cold Water Given Internally, or Applied Externally in Four Cases of Abdominal Inflammation, Edinburgh Medical and Surgical Journal, 1813, Vol. IX, pages 287–299.

Stewart, Chas. E. Chronic Constipation a Symptom Resulting from a Disordered State of the Sympathetic Nervous System, Its Causes and Cure, Journal of the American Medical Association, May 26, 1900.

Hydriatic Measures in the Treatment of Diarrhea, Report of a Case, Modern Medicine, April, 1901.

The Hydriatic Treatment of Typhoid Fever, Report of a Case, Modern Medicine, March, 1901.

The Hydriatic Treatment of Pleurisy with Effusion, Report of a Case, Modern Medicine, July, 1900.

Storoscheff, H. On the Physiological Effects of the Cold Clyster, Blätter für Klinische Hydrotherapie, August, 1893.

Strasser, Alvis, and Buxbaum, B. Fortschritte der Hydrotherapie-Festschrift zum Vierzigjärhigen Doctorjubiläum des Prof. Dr. W. Winternitz, 1897.

Thayer, W. S. Johns Hopkins Hospital Bulletin, Baltimore, 1893. Vol. IV, pages 37-40.

Thermes. Ann. de la Société d'Hydrol., Paris, 1879-80.

Tokada, S. Treatment of Disease by Cold Baths in Japan Seven Hundred Years Ago, Tokei Iyi Shinshi, Tokio, Feb. 5, 1881.

Verrier, E. Précis d'Hydrothérapie Scientifique, 1895.

Vigoroux, R. Neurasthénie et Arthritisme, 1893, page 308.

Vinaj and Maggiori. Blätter für Klin. Med., 1893.

Von Generesch. Progrès Médical, 1893, page 162.

Waller, Augustus D. Human Physiology, 1891, pages 59, 280, 281.

Washington, B. H. On Use of Hot-Blanket Pack in Dysmenorrhœa, Nashville Journal of Medicine and Surgery, 1877. Vol. XIX, pages 3, 15, 157.

Wertheimer, M. Académie des Sciences, 1893, page 44.

Winternitz, Wilhelm. Zur Rationellen Begründung einiger hydrotherapeutischer Proceduren, Jahrb. d. k. k. Gesellsch. d. Aerzte in Wien, 1865.

Das methodische Wassertrinken, Zeitschr. f. prakt. Heilkunde, 1865-67.

Ueber rationelle Anwendung von kalten Umschlägen, Sitzungsber. d. k. k. Gesellsch. d. Aertze in Wien, 1866.

Erfahrungen über die hydrotherapeutische Behandlung von chirurgischen Erkrankungen, Zeitschr. f. prakt. Heilkunde, 1867.

Die hydrotherapeutische Behandlung der Diarrhoe im Kindesalter, auf Grundlage physiologischer Wasserwirkungen und klinischer Erfahrungen, Jahrb. f. Kinderhk., 1868.

Ueber Revulsion und Ableitung, Wiener med. Wochenschr., 1868, und Jahrb. f. Balneol., 1869.

Zur Hydrotherapie des Typhus. Ein Beitrag zur Fieberlehre. Wiener med. Presse, 1869.

Kritische und experimentelle Beiträge zur Lehre von dem Einflusse der Wärmeentziehung auf die Wärmeproduction. Jahrb. d. k. k. Gesellsch. d. Aertze in Wein, 1871.

Ueber die Principien der Wirkungsweise thermischer Einflüsse auf den Organismus. Arch. f. Balneol. u. Hydrol., 1871.

Die Kühlkappe, ein Apparat zu Kopfumschlägen. Demonstration im Wiener med. Doctoren-Collegium, 1871.

Die hydriatische Methodik in fieberhaften Krankheiten. Wiener med. Presse, 1871. Abgerdruckt im Jahrb. f. Balneol.

Choleraschutz und Cholera-Behandlung. Allg. Wiener med Ztg., 1872. Blätter f. Klin. Hydrother., 1892, Heft 7.

Hydrotherapie bei Erkrankungen der Respirationsorgane. Poliklinischer Vortrag. Pester med.-chir. Presse, 1873.

Die feuchten Einpackungen als antipyretische Procedur. Jahrb. f. Balneol. u. Hydrol., 1875.

Der Psychrophor, die Kühlsonde. Ein Mittel zur Heilung von Spermatorrhoe, Pollutionen, Impotenz und chronischer Gonorrhoe. Berliner klin. Wochenschr., 1877.

Die Hydrotherapie bei dem Geburtsact. Wiener med. Presse, 1877.

Die Hydrotherapie auf physiologischer und klinischer Grundlage. Vorträge für Aerzte und Studirende. I. Band: Thermische Einflüsse auf Innervation und Circulation. Wien, 1877.

On the Use of Cold Compresses and Friction, Practitioner, London, 1878.

On the Action of the Thermal Application to the Skin upon the Circulation in the Brain and Other Organs, Practitioner, 1878.

Die Aufgaben der Hydrotherapie bei der Lungenphthise. Wiener Klinik, 1881.

Die Hydrotherapie. Ziemssen's Handbuch der allgemeinen Therapie, II. Band, 3. Theil. Leipzig, 1881.

Ein Fall von Hysteroepilepsie bei einen Manne. Wiener med. Blätter, 1885.

Influence de la chaleur et du froid sur la tonicité de vaisseau et de tissus, Compt. rend. du premier Congr. internat. d'Hydrol. et Climatol. de Biarritz, 1886.

Zur Pathogenese der Infectionskrankheiten. Klinische Studien aus der hydriatischen Abtheilung der allgemeinen Poliklinik. Heft I, 1887.

Die Physiologischen Grundlagen der Hydrotherapie. Wiener med. Presse, 1887.

Zur Pathologie und Hydrotherapie der Lungenphthise. Klinische Studien aus der hydriatischen Abtheilung der allgemeinen Poliklinik, 1887, Heft 2.

Zur Behandlung der croupösen Pneumonie. Offene Briefe an Herrn Prof. Oskar Fränzel in Berlin. Internat. klin. Rundschau, 1887.

Zur Pathologie und Hydrotherapie des Fiebers. Klinische Studien aus der hydriatischen Abtheilung der allgemeinen Poliklinik in Wien. Herausgegeben von Professor Winternitz. Hert 3, 1888.

Influence de l'eau froide ou chaude et de l'action mécanique sur la circulation, Compt. rend. de la deuxième session du Congr. internat. d'Hydrol., Paris, 1889.

Die Wasserheilanstalt in Kaltenleutgeben. 2. Auflage, nebst einer Statistik der 25jährigen Krankenaufnahme. Braumüller, 1890.

Infectionskrankheiten und Hydrotherapie. Blätter f. klin. Hydrother., 1891, Heft 1.

A New Hydropathic Treatment for Dyspepsia. Bacteriological World and Modern Medicine, December, 1891.

Ueber Neuralgien und ihre hydriatische Behandlung. Blätter f. klin. Hydrother., 1892, Heft 1.

Die erste Klinik für Hydrotherapie. Blätter f. klin. Hydrother., 1892, Heft 2.

Diarrhoe, Brechdurchfall, Cholera und Wassercur. Blätter f. klin. Hydrother., 1892, Heft 10.

Ueber Leukocytose nach Kälteeinwirkungen. Centralbl. f. d. med. Wissensch. und Blätter f. klin. Hydrother., 1893.

Hydrotherapie und chronischer Gelenksrheumatismus. Blätter f. klin. Hydrother., 1893, Heft 1.

New investigations concerning Changes in the Blood Resulting from Applications of Heat and Cold, Trans. in Modern Medicine and Bacteriological Review, December, 1893.

Zur physikalischen und diätetischen Therapie der Magenkrankheiten. Blätter f. klin. Hydrother., 1894, Heft 2, 3 u. 6.

Die Hydrotherapie der Lungenphthise. Vortrag, gehalten in der Balneologischen Gesellschaft in Berlin. Deutsche med. Wochenschr., 1896.

Kurzer Abriss der Hydrotherapie. Börner's Reichs-Medicinal-Kalendar, 1. Theil, 1897.

Hydrotherapy in Fevers, Trans. in Modern Medicine and Bacteriological Review, May, 1897.

Angina diphtheritica und ihre hydrotherapeutische Behandlung.

Artikel "Hydrotherapie" in Eulenburg's Real-Encyclopädie der med. Wissensch. 1. und 2. Auflage.

Winternitz, Wilhelm, and Pospischil. Neue Untersuchungen über den respiratorischen Gaswechsel unter thermischen und mechanischen Einflüssen. Blätter f. klin. Hydrother., 1893, Heft 1-5.

Winternitz, Wilhelm, and Strasser, Alois. Hydrotherapie, Berlin, 1898.

Wratsch. Lyon Médicale, 1883, page 541.

INDEX.